TEXTBOOK OF THE
PRINCIPLES AND PRACTICE
OF NURSING

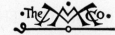

THE MACMILLAN COMPANY
NEW YORK · CHICAGO
DALLAS · ATLANTA · SAN FRANCISCO
LONDON · MANILA
IN CANADA
BRETT-MACMILLAN LTD.
GALT, ONTARIO

Textbook of the Principles and Practice of Nursing

FIFTH EDITION

BERTHA HARMER, R.N., A.M.

Late Director of the School for Graduate Nurses,
McGill University, Montreal, Canada

REVISED BY

VIRGINIA HENDERSON, R.N., A.M.

Research Associate, Yale University School of Nursing, New
Haven, Connecticut. Formerly Associate Professor of Nursing
Education, Teachers College, Columbia University, New York
City. Formerly Instructor in the Norfolk Protestant Hospital,
Norfolk, Virginia, and the Strong Memorial Hospital,
Rochester, New York

NEW YORK   *The Macmillan Company*   1960

Library of Congress catalog card number: 55-12634

PREFACE TO THE FIFTH EDITION

This text is intended as a guide to instructors and students of nursing, and as a general reference for nurses practicing in hospital or clinic, office or home. I am persuaded that the best way to meet the needs of student and graduate alike is first to present the scientific principles that underlie practice and then to suggest the methods that embody these principles, rather than merely to recommend any one method of a particular institution or agency. Where I have found conflicts in experimental evidence and expert opinion, they are reported; in such cases the recommended method may represent, in certain respects, my own weighing of evidence or opinion. Actually no claim is made for any procedure that it is the best possible practice. I have emphasized the tentative nature of the scientist's conclusions, hoping that the nurse reader will be stimulated to continue to think of herself as a student and of her practice as subject to modification with every major advance in the biological and social sciences.

While virtually the entire text has been rewritten, the organization remains essentially unchanged. Part I, "The Place of Nursing in Health Service," is a definition of nursing as I interpret it, and a discussion of the preparation of the nurse and of her place in current health programs. Part II, "Fundamentals of Nursing Care," while stressing underlying principles, shows in detail how to help a person meet his fundamental health needs. Part III, "The Role of Nursing in Health Evaluation and Diagnostic Techniques," describes the nurse's role in assessing the patient's nursing needs and his physical and emotional status, and in assisting him with the diagnostic measures prescribed by the physician. Part IV, "The Role of Nursing in Therapeutic Measures," deals with the nurse's role in giving, or assisting patients with, prescribed therapy. Finally, in Part V, "Common Problems in Nursing Practice," are discussed selected problems that the nurse commonly encounters, such as the following: How to care for a person with a local or systemic infection; how to nurse the patient who is about to undergo surgery or who is recovering from it; and how to nurse the unconscious or the dying. Those chapters in Part V of the fourth edition that described nursing care in specific diseases have been omitted. Although in some cases they were used to illustrate a disease category or a larger problem, their inclusion may have suggested to the reader a broader scope for the book than in fact it had. Students and practitioners in each clinical service will prefer, I believe, to consult specialized texts for help in meeting the particular needs of the person with diabetes, for instance, or heart disease, or scarlet fever, or the one undergoing a brain operation or a thyroidectomy.

An early chapter is devoted to planning nursing care around the requirements of the individual. The importance of understanding what the patient's illness means to him and his family is stressed. This clearly demands of the nurse, as well as of other medical workers, considerable knowledge of the cultural and social settings in which their patients live.

Throughout the text I have proceeded on the premise that nursing is a service to both well and sick; and that all branches of medicine have their preventive and therapeutic aspects. I have tried also to indicate the concepts that mind and body are inseparable, that structure and function affect each other, and that physical and emotional health are interdependent. For this reason I abandoned an earlier intention to include a section on the "psychiatric aspects of general nursing." Instead, I have tried to point out that every aspect of nursing has an emotional, or psychological, component. This is an inescapable conclusion if one believes that every thought or emotion has its physical expression even though the manifestation is often too minute or fleeting for measurement. I believe that, if this concept were applied, it would convert all general nursing into a preventive psychiatric service which might materially reduce the incidence of fully developed mental disorder.

Rehabilitation as an aspect of nursing is another pervasive idea that refused to be confined to any part of the text, although one chapter is devoted to a summarization of the subject. If the aim of *all* medical care is to help *every* patient to increase his emotional and physical independence, rehabilitation is a psychosocial and physical process which should begin as soon as anyone comes under treatment for disease or disability. Unless medical workers look upon rehabilitation as applicable to every person in all stages of illness (except the final one), the patient may develop in an early stage unnecessary helplessness that must be painfully relinquished when later the medical staff and his family and friends expect him to be self-reliant. This does not mean that the value of sympathy with the unavoidable, and sometimes healing, dependence of the sick and injured should be ignored.

All material of a strictly referable nature, such as lists of abbreviations and tables of measurement, have been placed in the Appendix. For the convenience of the reader who may be familiar with the metric but not the apothecaries' system, or vice versa, equivalents have been given throughout the text.

Since women predominate in the occupation of nursing and men in that of medicine, the nurse is referred to as "she" and the doctor as "he." I hope this will offend neither the man nurse nor the woman physician.

I wish I could mention each person who has helped me revise this text. It is impossible, however, to gauge all I have learned from the graduate nurses with whom I, as a teacher, have been associated, nor has it been practicable to list under "References" all the written works of others that I have consulted in preparing the manuscript.

To those who have revised certain chapters, or parts of them, I am deeply grateful: to Dr. John Hampden Hobart for preparing Chapter 19; to Miss Margaret Gibson for her work on Chapter 24; to Miss Virginia Dericks for revising Chapter 39; and, particularly, to Miss Barbara Russell, not only for revising Chapters 27,

42, and parts of others, but for her competence and understanding as the pub-lisher's editor. To Mr. W. Holt Seale and The Macmillan Company, who have been embarrassed by the delays in publication, I wish to express my appreciation of their continued support and patience.

The major burden of typing and initial editing of the manuscript was borne by my sister, Miss Lucy R. Henderson, and Mrs. Joseph E. Johnson contributed, with the same generosity, these invaluable services; to both of them I am particularly indebted. Mrs. Richard Landon, Miss Bessie Carroll, and Mr. Wilbur Baily also assisted in typing; Mrs. Jan van Tijn aided with the typing and some of the library research; Miss Marion D. Cleveland, Miss Cecile Covell, and Dr. David V. Habif read and criticized various chapters.

The total number of illustrations has been increased, and the majority are new. The Clay-Adams Company of New York City has made for this text, or supplied from their stock of purchasable medical Kodachromes (Medichromes), illustra-tions, many of them photographs. I thank Mr. Edgar Nebel, of this firm, for his expert photography and also the administration of the Columbia-Presbyterian Medi-cal Center, who put their facilities at my disposal when the photographs were taken. I acknowledge the kindness of the American Hospital Supply Corporation and Becton, Dickinson and Company in lending many of the items of improved equip-ment shown in some of these photographs.

For the original figure drawings in this volume, I am indebted to Miss Lalah Durham and Mr. Scaisbrooke L. Abbot; for some of the diagrams to Mr. Harry Guillaume; and for the architectural scheme in Chapter 7 to Mr. Jesse L. Orrick.

To the authors and publishers who have allowed me to quote or to use illustra-tions from their works, I extend my thanks, as well as to the manufacturers who have provided illustrations of their equipment.

The economics of textbook publishing imposes limits to size and scope. Regret-ting that this is so, I nevertheless take full responsibility for the text. Likewise, I am responsible for any errors it may contain.

V. H.

May, 1955

CONTENTS

PART V. COMMON PROBLEMS IN NURSING PRACTICE

APPENDIXES

TEXTBOOK OF THE
PRINCIPLES AND PRACTICE
OF NURSING

PART I. THE PLACE OF NURSING IN HEALTH SERVICE

CHAPTER 1. THE PRACTICE OF NURSING AND PREPARATION OF THE NURSE

1. **DEFINITION OF NURSING AND THE FUNCTION OF THE NURSE**
2. **NURSING AND WHAT IT OFFERS AS AN OCCUPATION**
3. **PREPARATION OF THE NURSE FOR GENERAL NURSING**
4. **PREPARATION OF THE NURSE FOR SPECIALIZATION**

1. DEFINITION OF NURSING AND THE FUNCTION OF THE NURSE

What is nursing and what is the function of the nurse? These are questions every person who chooses nursing as a vocation should try to answer. While they may be answered in terms of what each person in his experience has seen and heard, definitive answers are not easily found. The American Nurses' Association[1] is searching for a satisfactory definition of nursing; many analyses that have been made of the function of the nurse have failed to give the final answer. J. C. Meakins[2] entitles a thoughtful article written in 1948 "Nursing Must Be Defined."

Most definitions of nursing are so general and/or inclusive that while they suggest an extensive and vital role for the nurse they apply equally to other types of medical service. In 1937 the American Nurses' Association defined (professional) nursing as:

A blend of intellectual attainment, attitudes and mental skills based upon the principles of scientific medicine acquired by means of a prescribed course in a school of nursing affiliated with a hospital, recognized by the state and practiced in conjunction with curative and preventive medicine by an individual licensed to do so by the state.*

Substitute "physical therapy" and "school for physical therapy" and the statement is almost as valid. Other definitions, such as that in the 1937 *Curriculum Guide for Schools of Nursing*,[3] tell us that nursing is, in effect, helping the person to keep well, or regain his health if he is ill. This fails to differentiate nursing from other

* "Professional Nursing Defined" (editorial), *Am. J. Nursing,* **37:**518, (May) 1937.

1

vocations such as medicine, occupational therapy, or physical therapy that have this same over-all purpose. Annie W. Goodrich indicates the depth and breadth of the service of nursing in the following definition:

Nursing is that expression of social activities that seeks under qualified instruction and direction to interpret through action the findings of the medical and social sciences in relation to bodily ills, their care, cure and prevention, including all factors, personal and environmental, that bear upon the achievement of the desired objective, a healthy citizenry.*

Again most workers in the general field of medicine and health would accept this as a statement of the nature of their service, although some groups might want to remove, modify, or interpret the phrase "through qualified instruction and direction" if applied to them.

A national committee made up of nurses from many parts of the United States worked intensively for two weeks in 1947 to produce a statement on "the probable nature of nursing" in the latter half of this century. The following is the kernel of their thought as given by Esther Lucile Brown in her report *Nursing for the Future:*

. . . the professional nurse will be one who recognizes and understands the fundamental [health] needs of a person, sick or well, and who knows how these needs can best be met. She will possess a body of scientific nursing knowledge which is based upon and keeps pace with general scientific advancement, and she will be able to apply this knowledge in meeting the nursing needs of a person and a community. She must possess that kind of discriminative judgment which will enable her to recognize those activities which fall within the area of professional nursing and those activities which have been identified with the fields of other professional or nonprofessional groups.†

The phrases "health needs," "nursing needs," and "how these needs can best be met" still must be explained if the statement is to help the reader who is trying to differentiate between the practice of nursing and the other medical arts.

William Osler commented at the turn of the last century on the varied and enlarging functions of the nurse. He wrote:

. . . . Nursing as an art to be cultivated, as a profession to be followed, is modern: nursing as a practice originated in the dim past, when some mother among the cave-dwellers cooled the forehead of her sick child with water from the brook, or first yielded to the prompting to leave a well-covered bone and a handful of meal by the side of a wounded man left in the hurried flight before an enemy.‡

As the needs of humanity change, with different times and conditions, out of the same impulse to serve, nursing has developed broader interests and functions.

* Goodrich, Annie W.: *A Definition of Nursing* (privately printed), 1946; also "Report of the Biennial," *Am. J. Nursing,* **46:**741, (Nov.) 1946.

† Brown, Esther Lucile: *Nursing for the Future.* Russell Sage Foundation, New York, 1948, p. 73.

‡ Osler, Sir William: *Aequanimitas and Other Addresses.* Blakiston Co., Philadelphia, 1925, p. 163.

We find in the dictionary that "nursing" has a wide range of meanings, which, however, fall into the following three groups according to the basic ideas expressed. Nursing means (1) to "nourish," "to cherish," "to protect," "to support"; it means "to sustain," "to conserve energy," "to keep in good health," and "to avoid injury"; (2) it means "to train," "to cultivate," "to educate," and "to supply with whatever promotes growth, development, or progress"; (3) "to give curative care and treatment to the sick and infirm." Hugh Cabot,[4] talking to a graduating class of nursing students in 1934, spoke of the overlapping between medicine and nursing and the trend toward the assumption by the nurse of more and more medical activities. He suggested that custom alters the definition of nursing and that definitions designed for one age won't fit another.

A glance at history helps explain the elusive boundaries between the various fields of medical and health practice. It is startling to realize that up to fifty years ago, or thereabouts, the only attendants who gave direct personal service to the patient were the doctor and the nurse. With the expansion of scientific knowledge, hygienic, diagnostic, and therapeutic procedures multiplied. Equipment was elaborated and specialization developed rapidly, particularly within medicine; specialization within nursing is here, but it came more slowly. Possibly because the general practitioners in medicine, and more particularly in nursing, were so inadequately prepared to carry the varied functions involved in the total care of the patient, many of their early functions have been taken from them and developed by other groups outside the vocations of medicine and nursing. At any rate where we once had a team composed of the patient, the doctor, and the nurse we now have in addition medical social workers, nutritionists, physical therapists, occupational and play therapists, clinical psychologists, rehabilitation and vocation officers, health educators, medical clerks, laboratory technicians, and others. All of these workers have functions that doctors and nurses once had, however inexpertly and inadequately they fulfilled them. With so many new vocations it is naturally difficult to determine the best contribution each worker can make to the total program of health service and medical care. It is especially difficult because in many parts of the country, and in some situations everywhere, the doctor and the nurse still find themselves working alone; they must assume in such cases the functions of the social worker, the physical therapist, the clinical psychologist, and so on.

Even when a community is economically able to provide experts in every field it is not always practical or desirable to send a dozen different kinds of specialists into a home, or to a patient's bedside in the hospital. Granted that much of this division of labor improves medical care, sooner or later the optimum in specialization will be reached. Even now it might be profitable to prepare fewer kinds of workers more thoroughly so that they can assume a larger share of responsibility for the total care of the individual. In order to meet the person's health needs it is necessary to know him and his family, and this can only be accomplished by being with them and studying them. At the present time it is not unusual for a hospital patient to have as many as 25 different persons contributing directly to this medical and nursing care within a 24-hour period. No one person is with them long enough to know their individual problems.*

In any age, under any provision for medical care, each type of worker on the medical team should be recognized as having a peculiar or *unique* function, no matter how many functions he has in common with others. Certainly the members of each vocational group should be more competent in performing some activities than are the workers in any other vocation. This brings us to the question: What *is* *nursing* that is not also medicine, physical therapy, social work, etc.?; and what is *the unique function of the nurse?* The writer assumes responsibility for the following analysis but cannot take full credit for it since association with hundreds of nurses, and others interested in nursing, has contributed inestimably to clarification of these concepts—right or wrong. They are presented in the hope that they may help others, whether they agree or disagree, to develop a working concept of the place of nursing in our society.

Nursing is primarily assisting the individual (sick or well) in the performance of those activities contributing to health, or its recovery (or to a peaceful death) that he would perform unaided if he had the necessary strength, will, or knowledge. It is likewise the unique contribution of nursing to help the individual to be independent of such assistance as soon as possible. Nursing has a part in other activities that contribute toward the accomplishment of what Goodrich refers to as "a healthy citizenry," just as medicine, whose unique function is diagnosis and therapy, may be engaged cooperatively in all activities concerned with health in its fullest meaning. From the preceding definition of nursing the definition of the *unique* function of the nurse follows: *To assist the individual, sick or well, in the performance of those activities contributing to health or its recovery (or to a peaceful death) that he would perform unaided if he had the necessary strength, will, or knowledge. It is likewise her function to help the individual gain independence as rapidly as possible.* This aspect of her work, this part of her function, she initiates and controls; of this she is master. In addition (or as part of this defined function if it is broadly interpreted) she helps the patient to carry out the therapeutic plan as initiated by the physician. She also, as a member of a co-operative medical team, assists its other members, as they in turn assist her, to plan and carry out the total program of care. No one of the team should make such heavy demands on another member that he or she is unable to perform his or her special, or unique, function. Nor should any member of the medical team be diverted by nonmedical activities such as cleaning, clerking, and filing, as long as his or her unique task must be neglected. All members of the team should consider the person (patient) served as the central figure, and should realize that

---

* Visiting a large dairy, the writer was interested to find that the management had recently switched from a functionalized assignment of work to a case (cow) assignment system. Each employee (previously assigned "functions") is now responsible for the total care of 15 or 16 cows. He cleans, feeds, and (hand) milks his cows. As one of the men explained, "Now we know the cows, they know us, they are healthier, and we like it better." If cows flourish with understanding, individualized attention, how much more important must it be to the human organism!

primarily they are all *"assisting"* him. If the patient does not understand, accept, and participate in the program of care, the effort of the medical team is largely wasted. The sooner the person can care for himself, even carry out his own treatments, the better off he is.

This concept of the nurse as a substitute for what the patient lacks to make him "complete," "whole," or "independent," be the lack physical strength, will, or knowledge, may seem limited to some who read this. The more one thinks about it, however, the more complex the nurse's function as so defined is seen to be. Think how rarely one sees independence, completeness, or wholeness of mind and body! To what extent good health is a matter of heredity, to what extent it is acquired, is controversial but it is generally admitted that intelligence and education, by and large, tend to parallel health status. If then each man finds "good health" a difficult goal to reach, how much more difficult is it for the nurse to help him reach it! She must, in a sense, get "inside the skin" of each of her patients, in order to know what help he needs from her. She is temporarily the consciousness of the unconscious, the love of life for the suicidal, the leg of the amputee, the eyes of the newly blind, a means of locomotion for the newborn, knowledge and confidence for the young mother, a "mouthpiece" for those too weak to speak, and so on.

It is this necessity for estimating the individual's need for hourly care, encouragement, and training that makes nursing a service of the highest order. Many of the activities involved are simple until their adjustment to the particular demands of the patient makes them complex. In health, for example, breathing is effortless; the nurse who places a patient in position for proper chest expansion following a rib resection, or who operates a respirator, performs a complex function. Eating is effortless with appetite; when that is lacking it becomes a problem for the nurse. To brush the teeth seems easy to most persons (actually few know enough about mouth hygiene); to thoroughly clean the mouth of an unconscious patient is so difficult and dangerous that few skilled nurses accomplish it effectively and safely.

Perhaps enough has been said to indicate that the primary responsibility of the nurse is that of helping the patient with his daily pattern of living, or with those activities that he ordinarily performs without assistance: breathing, eating, eliminating, resting, sleeping and moving, cleaning the body and keeping it warm and properly clothed. She also helps to provide for those activities that make life more than a vegetative process: namely, social intercourse, learning, occupations that are recreational and those that are productive in some way. In other words she helps him to maintain or create a health regimen that, were he strong, knowing, and filled with the love of life, he would carry out unaided. It is this intimate, demanding, and yet inexpressibly rewarding service that the nurse is best prepared to render.

In addition to this primary function she helps the patient to carry out such treatments, prescribed by the physician, as he cannot perform unaided.

Albert Schweitzer, who left successful musical and theological careers to be a medical missionary, says he wanted to be able:

. . . to work without having to talk. For years I have been giving myself out in words and it was with joy that I had followed the calling of theological teacher and preacher. But this new form of activity [the practice of medicine] I couldn't represent to myself as being talking about the religion of love but only as an actual putting it into practice.*

He quotes Goethe's *Faust,* "In the beginning was the Deed." Nursing is a service primarily of deeds. These deeds can be reduced to mechanical, or even crude, acts; if performed by the intelligent, sensitive, educated, and skillful nurse they constitute a fine art.

Esther A. Werminghaus in her biographical sketch of Annie W. Goodrich says:

Gradually a new symbol is emerging. . . . Miss Goodrich has referred to her as "the complete nurse." A few schools can produce a good many complete nurses, but it is Miss Goodrich's unfaltering contention that all nurses must be complete nurses before we can expect to realize the great social potentialities of professional nursing.†

2. NURSING AND WHAT IT OFFERS AS AN OCCUPATION

Men and women choose vocations for different reasons; they may seek spiritual or material rewards, but usually they are compelled by ideals as well as the necessity for earning a living. Nursing as defined in this text offers immediate and powerful satisfaction to the humanitarian who wants to give a direct service to his or her fellow man. It is interesting that Gandhi and Walt Whitman both sought this type of satisfaction through nursing, as have thousands of the finest men and women in almost all periods of history. Undoubtedly many practicing nurses, in all ages, have gone into this vocation with the highest motives.

The leaders of modern nursing, by and large, believe that if nursing is to attract able men and women in sufficient numbers it must offer not only the satisfaction of a vital service to mankind, but it must be a vocation that is highly valued by society, and society must be willing to pay as much for the service of the nurse as it is for the services in rival fields into which potential nurses may be drawn if nursing cannot offer comparable rewards. Most students of human behavior think it is possible for people to serve others most sympathetically and effectively when they are themselves happy and secure in the esteem of their associates.

There are differences of opinion as to whether all nursing should have professional status; that is, whether all nurses should be educated in professional schools and should enjoy the privileges and assume the obligations of a profession.

The following are Abraham Flexner's criteria by which he measured the professional status of vocations:

1. They involve essentially intellectual operations accompanied by large undivided responsibility.

* Schweitzer, Albert: *Out of My Life and Thought* (translated by C. T. Campion). Henry Holt & Co., Inc., New York, 1933, p. 114.
    † Werminghaus, Esther A.: *Annie W. Goodrich; Her Journey to Yale.* The Macmillan Company, New York, 1950, p. 7.

2. They are learned in nature and their members are constantly resorting to the laboratory and seminar for a fresh supply of facts.

3. They are not merely academic and theoretical, however, but are definitely practical in the aims.

4. They possess a technique capable of communication through a highly specialized educational discipline.

5. They are self-organized, with activities, duties and responsibilities which completely engage their participants and develop group consciousness.

6. They are likely to be more responsible to public interest than are unorganized and isolated individuals, and they tend to become increasingly concerned with the achievements of social ends.*

Using these criteria some nurses, and some critics of nursing, say that only the administration and teaching of nursing represent a professional service; others say that to this list should be added nursing service to the individual patient where there is a high component of teaching, such as is found in so-called public health nursing, and also the nursing care in a clinical specialty for which the nurse has had special preparation. Another point of view is that nursing, as defined in this chapter, is essentially complex, depending for its full expression on a profound knowledge of the nature of man and at least some familiarity with a large body of medical science. This is comparable to the position educators take that all teaching, even the teaching of children in nursery school, is a service of a professional nature and demands professional preparation. The point is made that all teachers should have a deep understanding of children and should be able to apply this in attempting to meet the varying needs of individual children. Such a hypothesis leads us to assume that the preparation for nursing will, like the preparation for all the vocations that demand an understanding of the total personality, move into the colleges and universities. There is unquestionably a trend in this direction. There were 64 schools of nursing in this country offering a degree in 1935[5] as compared with 215 in 1954.[6]

While studies proceed, committees meet, and discussion runs high on whether nurses should be divided into classes, in what type of schools they should be educated, and what should be the nature of the course, there is unmistakable evidence that an increasing number of nurses can be said to meet the measurable standards set up by Flexner.

The term "professional nurse" is generally applied to the graduate of a recognized nursing school (usually a three-year course) who has met the requirements for "a registered nurse" in a state in which she is licensed to practice. All such schools in this country now require the candidate to be at least a high-school graduate, or the equivalent. It has been proposed that the term "professional nurse" be reserved in the future for graduates of nursing schools affiliated with colleges and universities that can claim to meet the standards of other professional schools. It is more likely that with the upgrading of nursing schools, as with the upgrading

---

* Flexner, Abraham: "Is Social Work a Profession?" *Proceedings of the National Conference of Charities and Corrections,* Chicago, Ill., 1915, p. 578.

of medical schools, no attempt will be made to take away from graduates of schools known in their day as professional a title in common usage.

As nursing takes its place beside the more established professions, and as the colleges assume responsibility for the education of nurses, it is possible that the titles bachelor, master, and doctor of nursing will be used to designate, as in other professions, the thoroughness of the nurse's preparation for her work.

There were 300,533 registered "professional" nurses reported to be practicing nursing in this country in 1949. Two thirds as many more (almost 200,000) were registered but inactive. It is reported that in 1950 there were 297,310 persons giving some sort of nursing service in hospitals under the titles "practical nurse," "attendant," "nurse's aide" (volunteer and paid), "orderly," and "ward maid." Their preparation varies from a two-year planned program to none at all. In addition to the so-called "professional" and so-called "auxiliary" nursing personnel whose numbers *can* be counted there are women (and men) all over the country whose numbers *cannot* be estimated who are giving nursing care in homes where no trained workers of any sort are available. It is recognized that the need for nurses far exceeds the supply. As long as this condition exists nursing care must be given to the helpless, sick, and disabled by the best person available to that family in each situation, regardless of how much knowledge or skill he or she has.

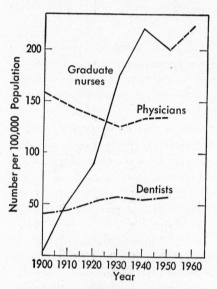

Figure 1. Number of physicians, dentists, and graduate nurses per 100,000 population, 1900-1950. (National League for Nursing, Department of Hospital Nursing: *News Letter,* **2:**1, [Dec.] 1952. Source: adapted from US Public Health Service data.)

The US Women's Bureau, with the help of the national nursing organizations, estimated in 1949 that if we were to maintain current standards, we would need 477,700 professional nurses in 1955, as compared with the 1949 supply of 300,533 active nurses. If, however, the standards of nursing care in the psychiatric hospitals were raised to those in nonpsychiatric hospitals, and if medical care (including nursing) were available to all economic classes, the need for nurses would, right now, approach 1,000,000.[7] (The number of trained teachers in the United States, reported by Karl Bigelow in 1944, was 1,093,000. About 85 per cent were college graduates.)[8]

There is little doubt that all the men and women who can be recruited into nursing will find full employment for many years to come, or until our preventive health program yields richer dividends.

More nurses (44,185) entered nursing schools in 1950 than in any previous peacetime year. The number admitted in 1953 was 43,327. This represents a drop of 2.1 per cent over the peak year. The number of men admitted in 1953 (332) dropped 35 per cent over the 1950 peak of 508.[9] The number of schools that will accept men students jumped from 68 in 1941 to 181 in 1951.[10] While women seem to have pre-empted the field of nursing in this age, there is no reason to believe that this situation will or should persist. There have been periods of history, during the Crusades, for example, when men nurses were numerous. If improvement of employment practices, of working conditions, and of nursing schools continues, more men as well as women will inevitably be drawn to nursing.

In an effort to make the present nurse power go as far as possible, many attempts have been made to differentiate between nursing services that require a greater or less degree of nursing judgment and skill, with an assignment of different grades of services to better and less well-prepared persons. One method of doing this is to assign the "professional nurse" to the patients whose care is thought to present the more difficult problems, while those whose care is believed to be less complex are assigned to the "practical nurse," the "attendant," the "nurse's aide," or some other member of the auxiliary nursing group.

A second plan for spreading the "professional nurse" power is to have the "professional nurse" supervise the care of all patients, and/or carry out the more complex procedures involved in this program of care. Other categories of nursing personnel work with the "professional nurse" to give each patient total nursing care, each nurse performing her relatively more complex or less complex part. In other words, each patient has a "team" of nurses assigned to him and all contribute to the planning and execution of his care. Some persons insist that under any plan the nursing care of *all* patients should be supervised by the "professional nurse" when it is given by the nonprofessional worker.

A third, and most widely accepted, method of conserving professional nurse power is to limit her activities to *nursing care,* while assigning to others the numerous non-nursing functions that the graduate or professional nurse has had for so many years. For example, ordering supplies, cleaning and sterilizing equipment, and serving food. Many agencies are eliminating from the functions of the graduate nurse staff everything that is not a service to the person (mind and body) of the patient. Administering and teaching and keeping the records of this practical service (or nursing care) are included as an integral part of the nursing function.

The position is taken in this text that all "nursing care" as just indicated is essentially complex because it involves constant adaptation of procedures to the needs of the individual. Care of the chronically ill may be as difficult as, or more difficult than, that of the acutely ill; preventive nursing is as complex as curative; patients of all ages and with all diagnoses present their peculiar problems to the nurse. The term "nurse" as used hereafter (unless otherwise indicated) will refer to a man or woman with a minimum general education represented by graduation from high school, having been prepared for nursing in a recognized basic program of from two and a half to three years. It is hoped, however, that the text will be useful to all nurses everywhere, no matter what their preparation, who are attempting to "get inside the patient's skin" and supplement his strength, will, or knowledge according to his needs.

Many analyses have been made of the activities that constitute modern nursing. The one by Ethel Johns and Blanche Pfefferkorn[11] is the most general, but nursing functions have changed greatly since this study was made. Studies of clinical services like orthopedics and tuberculosis give a more complete list within that specialty. Nell Beeby[12] attempted to show some of the more intangible aspects of the nurse's work by listing the problems, or "situations," the nurse meets in obstetrics. The latter study indicates clearly the variety and complexity of the nurse's work. Other analyses have attempted to differentiate between those activities that require more and those that require less knowledge and judgment; those that require more and less skill. Such lists serve as a basis for differentiating between the functions of the better and less well-prepared nurse. The weakness of this last classification lies in the assumption that the patient's condition or needs are static. If they are assumed to be changing and unpredictable, we see that each time the nurse assists the patient with any aspect of his health, or therapeutic program, she may have an opportunity to teach or encourage him to acquire increasing independence—in other words to rehabilitate him. This requires a great deal of judgment, and the personality of the nurse is in itself a therapeutic factor. What the nurse says, which cannot be prescribed, the hopefulness of her attitude, may have as great an influence on the patient's recovery as what she actually does for him.

If the practice of medicine and the practice of nursing are fine arts, as some believe, the kind of a person the doctor or the nurse is becomes a matter of great importance. Lin Yutang expresses this same idea, with reference to the fine arts, in an article comparing painting and drawing in the East and the West.

Here we are faced with the central problem of art, the problem of personality in art. The achievement of a special atmosphere is like achieving a special outlook in philosophy or a special style in writing. The atmosphere, the outlook, the style must come from the personality and must be a natural outgrowth from it. It is not something that can be imposed from the outside by any trickery in technique. Hence, in training an artist, the Chinese always insist on the cultivation of a high moral personality. The final test of a great art is, according to the Chinese, does it show a high personality? The technique may be flawless and yet the personality may be lacking.*

In like manner the technique of the nurse may be flawless, but her performance lacking in character. Practiced sympathetically, nursing, like all the medical arts, makes heavy demands if sympathy is correctly interpreted as "the willingness to suffer with another." Florence R. Weiner[13] thinks the interest (or love) shown the patient by the nurse is the most essential element of her service. She believes, however, that it is only when the nurse is made to feel her own worth (or is herself beloved) that she can express this warmth in her work.

In an effort to arrive at a sound basis on which to build a curriculum, the National League of Nursing Education[14] attempted to list the qualities the nurse

---

* Yutang, Lin: "East to West in Art," *Magazine of Art,* **31**:70, (Feb.) 1938.

should have, as well as what she should do. It is generally agreed that personality cannot be reduced to a formula, and that it would be a mistake to try to make all nurses behave in the same way; nevertheless, there seems to be some reason to believe that successful nurses have certain characteristics in common, and that these characteristics can be cultivated without making nurses too much alike.

3. PREPARATION OF THE NURSE FOR GENERAL NURSING

All professional registered nurses in this country must complete a basic course of study that measures up to standards set by a state agency. (Members of the agency are usually recommended for office by a professional body but appointed by the governor of the state.)* The length of the basic nursing course varies from two and a half to three years; at the end of this period the student receives a diploma. If the nursing school is affiliated with a college or university, the student may receive a bachelor's or a master's degree in nursing, according to the academic program of study that has preceded or accompanied the professional course. Quite naturally this type of preparation for nursing takes longer than the diploma program. Of the 1141 schools that offered the basic nursing course in 1954, there were 215 schools with some sort of collegiate affiliation, having basic programs leading to a degree. During 1953, 29,308 students were graduated from schools of nursing offering the basic course.[15]

The main divisions of the basic nursing course are: (1) the biological and physical sciences, (2) the social sciences, (3) the medical sciences, and (4) the nursing arts.

The biological and physical sciences are a necessary part of the nurse's preparation because she must have some understanding of body functions, she must know what is normal activity in order to recognize subnormal or pathological activity. The more thorough the nurse's knowledge of physiology, the more intelligent is she likely to be in promoting her own health and that of others. A study of chemistry and physics is essential to even a superficial understanding of physiology, pathology, and therapeutics. It is impossible to explain the processes of digestion without going into the chemical changes that take place in the alimentary tract, and it is equally impossible to understand the mechanical aspects of respiration and the therapeutic use of oxygen without some knowledge of the physical principles governing the behavior of gases. The rules of hygiene may be memorized and blindly adhered to, but this rarely results in the most successful practice and is never an adequate preparation for the health teacher. The nurse must know why certain food elements are essential in the diet and the most available and economical sources of these foods, if she hopes to give her patients real help in food selection. She must have an accurate knowledge of the characteristics of the organisms that cause disease if she expects to develop practices, or to guide others in developing practices, that protect the individual from communicable disease.

* National nursing organizations have set up an accrediting agency that approves schools of nursing on a national basis.

The social sciences have to do with the study of individual and group behavior, social relationships, and social welfare. This part of the nursing program usually includes courses in psychology, the dynamics of human behavior, sociology, special social problems related to the work of the nurse, and the history of nursing.

A study of psychology gives the nurse a more thorough understanding of herself and by so doing enables her to look at her personal problems more objectively. It also helps her to assess her personality as a therapeutic agent. Medical workers, to an almost greater extent than any other professional group, must learn to deal dispassionately and yet sympathetically with human beings. Instead of being irritated or offended by signs of anger or distrust in the behavior of a sick person, they must try to understand what causes them. Although tolerance and sympathy are desirable attributes in anyone they are essential qualities in the nurse. She is more likely to be tolerant and sympathetic with those whose behavior is different from her own if she knows something about personality structure and mental mechanisms. She will discover that the way so-called normal persons react to embarrassment, fear, and frustration differs greatly and that normal reactions may be seriously altered by illness. The nurse's feeling toward the patient must be as free as possible from blame or censure. It is much easier for her to acquire this attitude if she has learned to place the emphasis on motives underlying behavior rather than on manners. A study of psychology should help her to do this and to meet more adequately the emotional needs of the individual.

A study reported briefly by the National League of Nursing Education in *A Curriculum Guide for Schools of Nursing,* referred to on page 1, shows that a nurse who is able to adjust well to nursing situations is said to be resourceful, considerate of others, able to cooperate, cultivated, and possessed of a sense of social and professional responsibility. Some of these characteristics have their origin in good feeling, in kind and generous impulses that the novice in nursing may possess to as great a degree as the veteran; but this unfortunately is not enough. Misguided kindness may in some cases do as much harm as a malicious act. If the nurse hopes to be resourceful and to show intelligent consideration for all sorts of people, regardless of their race, religion, or nationality, she must have some knowledge of personality development and of the beliefs and customs of different groups.

Many persons have been brought up in the midst of a fairly homogeneous society. They have had no intimate acquaintances whose customs are very different from their own, and this tends to give them an exaggerated sense of the importance of behaving as the members of their group behave. Even a superficial knowledge of sociology teaches us that there are many patterns of group behavior, and that it is characteristic of each group to think its set of customs, habits, and manners the best. The "good life" may be the goal of all, but each culture may be approaching it along a different path.

The nurse who has no knowledge of religious beliefs in relation to dietary customs may, in serving a meal that is acceptable to those of her race and creed, be asking a person from another race and religion to eat food that is prohibited by the laws of his faith. Without some knowledge of racial and national customs, the nurse who is attempting to teach a foreign-born mother the care of her new baby is often dealing with an unseen handicap. The mother, fearing that she will be ridiculed or criticized by the nurse, may not say that the nurse's suggestions run counter to long-established customs of her people.

If the nurse is to develop a sense of social and professional responsibility, and to act intelligently in response to it, she must understand existing social conditions. She should have a clear concept of what she can do as an individual, and as a member of the nursing profession, to further health conservation. A study of the history of nursing shows her the part that has been played by nurses in the past, and this may strengthen her interest, direct her efforts, and stimulate her imagination.

A study of community resources, living conditions, social legislation, and mortality and morbidity rates is essential in the preparation of any medical worker if she is to act effectively in promoting the health of people in her community. For many reasons the nurse should be familiar with public health regulations. She should be able to select and help her patients to purchase food and drugs that have a guarantee of quality; she should know how to report a nuisance or a public danger; and she should know the regulations affecting the care of patients with such conditions as tuberculosis and venereal disease. These are only a few examples of the kinds of social information the nurse should have.

The medical sciences include what is known about the cause, the signs and symptoms, the occurrence, prevention, treatment, and probable outcome of disease. This covers a vast field of knowledge, so complex that many areas of specialization exist within it. The nurse cannot be expected to go deeply into the study of medical science; on the other hand, it is impossible for her to give a high quality of nursing care unless she can intelligently observe and report signs of disease, or deviations from normal; unless she knows the effect the physician hopes to get from prescribed treatment and unless she has some idea of the length of time the patient is likely to be ill. In order to cooperate effectively in the physician's therapeutic plan for the patient the nurse must have a body of knowledge that falls within the realm of medicine.

The first course in medical science deals with general principles, or concepts; the remaining courses are concerned with the various branches of medical practice —medicine, surgery, obstetrics, pediatrics, and psychiatry. Before studying any particular disease condition, such as pneumonia, diabetes, cancer, clubfoot, cataract, or dementia precox, it is very desirable to know some general principles of medical science, such as the principle that diseases of similar origin are likely to be manifested by similar signs and symptoms. For example, diseases caused by microorganisms usually produce a rise in body temperature, an increased pulse rate, an increase in white blood cells, a sensation of heaviness or fatigue, and local signs of inflammation if the organisms are successfully attacking a part of the body where the reaction of the tissues can be observed.

Having acquired this picture of the typical reaction of the body to an invading microorganism, the study of the prevention, treatment, and nursing care of specific bacterial diseases, such as tuberculosis, is greatly simplified.

In like manner the introductory medical science course deals with general methods of diagnosis and with the principles of therapy in types of disease, such as infection, nutritional deficiency, or degenerative change.

Early in her basic preparation the nurse should learn something about the incidence of disease, especially in that part of the country in which she expects to work. The conquest of disease is a romantic thrilling story. Nurses have an important part to play in medical research; their observations, and records of their observations, are essential in the study of both normal and abnormal states; nurses make and assist in making tests that lead to improved methods of diagnosis and treatment; and in other ways too numerous to mention they help to build up bodies of data leading to so-called "medical discoveries."

In the *nursing arts* courses the student learns to apply her knowledge of the sciences and develops skill in many nursing activities. She acquires the ability to "size up," or analyze, a nursing situation in order to determine a patient's nursing needs, to make a plan for his nursing care, and to cooperate with the other workers in the hospital and the community who are concerned with the patient's total care and welfare.

In the first part of the student's preparation, she is introduced to the fundamentals of nursing. These include assisting the patient with all body functions— eating, eliminating, breathing, regulating body temperature, protecting the body with clothing, sleeping, resting, moving and exercising. She also helps the person to provide for companionship, recreation, and occupation. As she helps the patient she also encourages him to acquire and assists him in acquiring independence. In the introductory nursing course the student learns to do these things for the less seriously ill, and she participates to only a limited extent in the therapeutic and diagnostic program prescribed by the physician. Little emphasis is placed at first on the patient's diagnosis and the pathology involved, although the student is encouraged to learn as much as she can about the social and medical history of each person to whom she is assigned.

A good deal of difference of opinion exists as to what constitutes the most desirable order, or sequence, of clinical experiences for the student of nursing. It is usual to have her first learn to give the "fundamentals of nursing care" to mildly ill or convalescent adult patients who are undergoing treatment in the medical and surgical divisions of the hospital. She is assigned to patients whose care presents no very difficult medical or social problems and at least a portion of which can be safely and satisfactorily undertaken by the less experienced person. In any case, the responsibility for planning and executing the total nursing plan for the patient is in the hands of an older nurse. The young student assists the older nurse, works under her direction, and gradually assumes more and more functions as her professional judgment matures and she learns new skills. The patients assigned to her care are selected in such a way as to give her opportunity to work with nursing problems of increasing complexity.

The medical and surgical services offer a wide range of experience for the student nurse. She studies and takes care of patients with diseases produced by microorganisms and foreign proteins, with nutritional disorders, new growths, injuries such as fractures, and functional disorders. While assigned to these services, she goes to the operating room and the dietary and physical therapy departments, all of which have special contributions to make to her preparation. She may have a block of experience in these departments or she may go to them with her patients as they are sent there for treatment.

From the adult medical and surgical divisions of the hospital, the student goes to either the maternity or children's division. In these services she is confronted with new problems, and she learns new skills and the adaptation of fundamental nursing care to the particular needs of the mother and infant. Since reproduction is a physiological function and the newborn period one in which the individual requires care because he is helpless rather than because he is sick, obstetrical nursing is chiefly a matter of health guidance for the mother, assistance to the mother during and immediately following delivery, and hygienic care of the infant. Therapy in many diseases or conditions is simply a matter of aiding nature; in obstetrics it is especially so, and therefore the care of mothers and infants gives the student nurse a particularly good opportunity to see a medical and nursing program that is largely health teaching and hygienic care. This service may be said to belong in the field of preventive, rather than curative, medicine. Some educators believe that students of nursing might profitably be assigned to this service first.

In pediatric nursing it is as important to learn to take care of well children as to take care of those who are sick. Pediatrists and nurses, particularly those whose work takes them outside the hospital, are giving as much time to the prevention as to the treatment of disease in infancy and childhood. The nurse should be prepared to recognize normal physical and mental behavior in adults in order to promote her own health and that of adult patients; but it is, if anything, more important that she be able to distinguish normal and abnormal growth and development in children because abnormalities can be cured most readily if they are treated in childhood. Psychiatrists echo the poet who said, "The child is father to the man." Since adult behavior is largely determined by experiences in infancy, childhood, and youth, it is hard to nurse adults intelligently without an understanding of behavior characteristics in all ages. Many adults never progress beyond childish patterns, and sick adults may regress to earlier stages of mental and emotional development. It is possible that experience in the care of infants and children might be placed earlier in the curriculum. At present it usually follows medical and surgical nursing and often obstetrics.

The essentials in child care are the same as those in the care of adults, but there are many adaptations of adult nursing procedures to be learned because of the differences in understanding sensitivity, size, functions, and interests. If the nurse is to be successful in taking care of children she must learn to work with and through the parents; she must know how to interest, divert, entertain, comfort, and teach the child in a wholesome constructive manner. These are very special abilities that can only be acquired through study and experience in working with children. There is much to be said in favor of combining the obstetrical and pediatric nursing courses since they are so largely interdependent.

In the latter part of her basic preparation, the student nurse has an opportunity in many schools to assist in the care of patients with mental disorders. Experience in psychiatric nursing is usually placed in the third year of the course because it is thought to be one of the most difficult phases of nursing. Some educators are of the opinion, however, that it should come earlier so that the student will be better prepared to recognize, interpret, and deal intelligently with abnormalities in the behavior of patients in every clinical service. Illness is always accompanied by some deviations from "normal" mental behavior. Anyone associated with sick people knows how common it is to see them extremely depressed, irritable, or critical; unnaturally reserved, suspicious, anxious, or hysterical. Whether these symptoms are manifested in a patient with pneumonia or dementia precox the nurse must learn to understand their cause and to deal with them as she would with physical symptoms such as loss of appetite, motor weakness, retention of urine, or constipation.

The student should be helped to realize that her experience in "mental nursing" begins with her first and ends with her last contact with the sick. Mind and body are so closely related that when one is sick the other also is sick, and for this reason therapy should be as carefully adapted to the mood as to the physical condition of the patient. The care of persons with acute and serious psychiatric disorders may be reserved for the senior student, but she should be prepared to undertake this by having consciously dealt with similar but milder conditions in the medical, surgical, pediatric, and obstetrical services.

In psychiatry great emphasis is placed on the special therapies such as occupational therapy, physical therapy, and various forms of psychotherapy. Since there are usually experts in these fields associated with a psychiatric department the student has a particularly good opportunity, in caring for the mentally ill, to learn how to administer therapeutic baths and packs, to use games, handicrafts, and other forms of recreation as therapeutic agents; she should acquire judgment as to when and how to use such psychic agents as encouragement and persuasion in giving nursing care. Actually all of these special therapies should be available to every sick person and should be used by medical workers according to the needs of the individual regardless of his diagnosis.

In all these nursing arts courses the student is expected to take every opportunity that offers itself to study the preventive aspects of nursing, to learn the cause of the patient's disorder, to follow him after he leaves the hospital, and to learn as much as possible about the home care of the sick. Hospital workers, including student nurses, may easily acquire the habit of thinking that most illnesses are treated within the walls of institutions. While there has been a phenomenal increase in hospital admissions in recent years, a great deal of illness is treated in homes. Of the 334,733 nurses recorded as "active" in 1951, 52 per cent were working in hospitals and schools of nursing, the remainder (almost half the total) were nursing in homes, schools, industries, health clinics, and doctors' offices.[16]

In discussing what each clinical service has to offer as a basis for more effective nursing care of all patients a change in the organization of our present curriculum suggests itself. It may be that in the future the nursing program will be organized around nursing problems, and those fundamental to all services will be given early, with the more specific problems serving as a basis for the latter part of the program. For examples of the more general, or fundamental, problems: the adaptation of nursing care to the age of the patient, meeting the special demands of the common emotional disturbances, the care of the person with a fever, the care of the un- conscious and of the dying patient. These are problems the nurse faces in every clinical service. Problems that are more specific include: nursing care of the burned patient, of a person with amputation of a leg or arm, nursing during delivery or during the prenatal or post-partum period, and nursing care of the premature infant. A few schools are experimenting with different sequences of clinical experience and with different types of organization of the clinical content within the blocks of clinical experience.

The basic course is designed to prepare nurses for general nursing in homes or institutions. Preparation for specialized forms of nursing requires postgraduate study and experience.

4. PREPARATION OF THE NURSE FOR SPECIALIZATION

The basic nursing preparation is not designed to make the graduate nurse a specialist in any of the clinical fields. In order to qualify as an expert practitioner, teacher, or administrator, in any branch of nursing, experience and study beyond that offered in the undergraduate program are needed. Postgraduate courses are given in colleges and universities, and also in schools under hospital or private ownership and control. Many colleges and universities offer programs of study for the graduate nurse that lead to a bachelor's, master's, or doctor's degree. Some other types of institutions offer opportunities for study and experience.

In 1953 there were 114 universities and colleges offering programs for graduate nurses leading to a degree. There were 11,877 professional, or graduate, nurses enrolled in these programs.[17]

Some of the specialties within the field of nursing are the following: (1) spe- cialization for practice in any one of the clinical fields, such as obstetrics or psychiatry; (2) administration of a nursing school, or of a nursing service, in hospitals and clinics and other health agencies, private or public; (3) teaching in schools of nursing, in hospitals, clinics, and other community health agencies.

There are also closely allied fields, such as hospital administration, midwifery, physical therapy, and social service, for which nurses may fit themselves through additional preparation.

SUMMARY

Nursing is an important and useful occupation that has attracted an increasing number of women and men into its ranks until there are now more than 500,000 registered "professional" nurses in the United States and territories. Of the 334,733 who were active in 1951 approximately 52 per cent were in hospitals and schools of nursing, 13 per cent in public health and industrial nursing, 21 per cent in private duty, 9 per cent in offices, and the remaining 5 per cent is unclassified. The vast majority of nurses are women although this occupation is drawing an increasing number of men. Almost one out of every 122 entrants to "professional" schools of nursing in 1954 were men. In addition to the "professional" nursing personnel there were 347,369 paid auxiliary workers in hospitals in 1953 and many unclassified and unlisted persons giving nursing care in homes. While there are more nurses today than there have been before, the demand far exceeds the supply in every field. In 1950 a ratio of one active registered nurse to 401 people existed, but it is generally conceded that this is not a sufficient number to meet the health needs of the country.[18, 19]

The work of the nurse is an integral part of the national and local programs that are planned to help human beings maintain a high standard of health. The boundaries of the fields of medicine, nursing, social service, and other specialties are not very well defined, and the work of the different groups often overlaps. While the aim of all these workers may be to help the patient to attain or maintain a high standard of health, or to be relieved of unnecessary discomfort when a return to health is not possible, each should function as an authority within a given area. The nurse is especially qualified to help the patient to perform those health functions that he would perform unaided if he had the strength, will, and/or knowledge. While she is doing this, she helps him to acquire or regain his independence as soon as possible. The physician directs the program of therapy, and in some cases the nurse may serve as his agent. As his agent and in emergencies, she administers treatment that belongs in the field of medicine rather than nursing. A high quality of service to the patient necessitates the close cooperation of those attending him.

The term nursing may be used to cover a wide range of human activities. In this country, the title "nurse" most often refers to the graduate "professional nurse" who is eligible for registration or certification because she has completed a course of study of approximately three years in an accredited school of nursing. Nurses who can qualify as applicants and who pass state-board examinations for registration on graduation make up the professional nursing group. There is a movement on foot to place all such schools under college or university auspices. In 1950 about 86 per cent of these schools were still under the control of hospitals.

The basic or undergraduate nursing course is from two and a half to three years in length. There were, in 1953, 1148 such schools under university, college, hospital, or private control. These schools graduated 29,308 students in 1953. The largest number (40,744) ever to graduate in a peacetime year was in 1947.[20] The basic nursing program of study is made up of courses in (1) the physical and biological sciences, (2) the social services, (3) the medical sciences, and (4) the nursing arts. Students in these schools should if possible have experience in caring for well children, for mothers and infants, for men, women, and children who have medical and surgical conditions, and those who are mentally ill. The basic course is designed to prepare nurses for general practice. Postgraduate experience and study are available for those members of the profession who desire to qualify as experts in the clinical branches of nursing and those who expect to teach or administer a school or nursing service.

The work of professional nurses is vital and varied in its character; because of its variety and impelling interest, it appeals to many different natures. A study of successful nurses seems to show that there are a number of common characteristics among them, but this does not mean that the successful nurse is "a type." There is the science of nursing, but equally important is the art of nursing. In its highest form, nursing calls for the same qualities that are found in most persons who work successfully in other professional fields—sensitiveness to people and their moods, insight into human nature, an ability to distinguish what is true from what is false, the capacity for sustained effort, and the mastery of the techniques involved.

REFERENCES

1. "Research and the A.N.A. Program for Studies of Nursing Functions" (editorial), *Am. J. Nursing,* **50:**767, (Dec.) 1950.
2. Meakins, J. C.: "Nursing Must Be Defined," *Am. J. Nursing,* **48:**622, (Oct.) 1948.
3. National League of Nursing Education, Committee on Curriculum: *A Curriculum Guide for Schools of Nursing.* The League, New York, 1937, p. 20.
4. Cabot, Hugh: "What Is the Future of Nursing?" *Trained Nurse and Hosp. Rev.,* **92:**229, (Mar.) 1934.
5. Petry, Lucile: "Basic Professional Curricula in Nursing Leading to Degrees," *Am. J. Nursing,* **37:**287, (Mar.) 1937.
6. American Nurses' Association: *Facts about Nursing, 1954.* The Association, New York, 1954, p. 68.
7. American Nurses' Association: *Facts about Nursing, 1951.* The Association, New York, 1951, pp. 13, 93 (1949 ed., p. 11).
8. Bigelow, Karl: *Teachers for Our Times.* American Council on Education, Washington, D.C., 1944, p. 12.
9. American Nurses' Association: *Facts about Nursing, 1954.* The Association, New York, 1954, pp. 60, 61.
10. American Nurses' Association: *Facts about Nursing, 1951.* The Association, New York, 1951, pp. 39, 41, 44, 53.
11. Johns, Ethel, and Pfefferkorn, Blanche: *An Activity Analysis of Nursing.* Committee on the Grading of Nursing Schools, National League of Nursing Education, New York, 1934.
12. Beeby, Nell: "Where and What Shall We Teach?" *Am. J. Nursing,* **37:**64, (Jan.) 1937.
13. Weiner, Florence R.: "Professional Consequences of the Nurse's Occupational Status," *Am. J. Nursing,* **51:**614, (Oct.) 1951.
14. National League of Nursing Education, Committee on Curriculum: *op. cit.,* p. 593.
15. American Nurses' Association: *Facts about Nursing, 1954.* The Association, New York, 1954, pp. 54, 58, 68.
16. American Nurses' Association: *Facts about Nursing, 1954.* The Association, New York, 1954, p. 11.
17. American Nurses' Association: *Facts about Nursing, 1954.* The Association, New York, 1954, p. 73.

18. American Nurses' Association: *Facts about Nursing, 1954.* The Association, New York, 1954, pp. 8, 11, 61, 130, 131.
19. United States Department of Commerce, Bureau of the Census: *Statistical Abstract of the United States, 1950.* US Government Printing Office, Washington, D.C., 1950, p. 11.
20. American Nurses' Association: *Facts about Nursing, 1953.* The Association, New York, 1953, pp. 54, 65,

Additional Suggested Reading

Barbour, George B.: "The Genuine Article. Don't Palm Off a Counterfeit Self on Your Patient," *Am. J. Nursing,* **50:**342, (June) 1950.

Bayne-Jones, Stanhope: "The Role of the Nurse in Medical Progress," *Am. J. Nursing,* **50:**601, (Oct.) 1950.

Bennett, Bertina A.: "Development of Modern Nursing," *Nursing Mirror & Midwives J.,* **91:**97, (May) 1950.

Brown, Esther Lucile: *Nursing as a Profession,* 2nd ed. Russell Sage Foundation, New York, 1940.

————: *Nursing for the Future.* Russell Sage Foundation, New York, 1948.

Chayer, Mary E.: *Nursing in Modern Society.* G. P. Putnam's Sons, New York, 1947.

Conner, Mary C.: "Accreditation—Stimulant or Narcotic?" *Am. J. Nursing,* **47:**484, (July) 1947.

Curran, Jean A., and Bunge, Helen L.: *Better Nursing. A Study of Nursing Care and Education in Washington.* University of Washington Press, Seattle, 1951.

Gelinas, Agnes: *Nursing and Nursing Education.* Commonwealth Fund, New York, 1946.

Goodrich, Annie W.: *The Social and Ethical Significance of Nursing.* The Macmillan Company, New York, 1932.

Langford, William S., et al.: "The Professional Person: A Mental Hygiene Resource," *Ment. Hyg.,* **32:**262, (Apr.) 1950.

Mayo, Leonard W.: "Organizing the Community for Nursing Service," *Am. J. Nursing,* **48:**649, (Oct.) 1948.

Nahm, Helen: "A Follow-Up Study on Satisfaction with Nursing," *J. Appl. Psychol.,* **34:**343, (Oct.) 1950.

National League of Nursing Education: *Essentials of a Good School of Nursing,* 2nd ed. The League, New York, 1942.

————: *Problems of Collegiate Schools of Nursing.* The League, New York, 1945.

————: *State-Approved Schools of Nursing,* 15th ed. The League, New York, 1950.

Scheele, Leonard A.: "Looking Ahead with the Nursing Profession," *Am. J. Nursing,* **50:**631, (Oct.) 1950.

Stewart, Isabel M.: *The Education of Nurses.* The Macmillan Company, New York, 1943.

Williams, Dorothy R.: *Administration of Schools of Nursing.* The Macmillan Company, New York, 1950.

World Health Organization, Expert Committee on Nursing: *Report of the First Session,* Series No. 24. The Organization, New York, 1950.

CHAPTER 2. HEALTH PROGRAMS AND NURSING RELATIONSHIPS

1. VALUE OF HEALTH AND HUMAN LIFE
2. CONDITIONS AFFECTING COMMUNITY HEALTH
3. OUTSTANDING ACCOMPLISHMENTS IN CONTROL OF DISEASE AND PROMOTION OF HEALTH
4. IMPORTANCE OF ORGANIZATION IN HEALTH WORK
5. INTERNATIONAL, NATIONAL, STATE, AND LOCAL HEALTH AGENCIES
6. SOCIAL AGENCIES IN THE COMMUNITY INDIRECTLY CONCERNED WITH HEALTH PROMOTION
7. PLACE OF THE HOSPITAL IN THE COMMUNITY HEALTH PROGRAM
8. WHAT THE NURSE AND OTHER HEALTH WORKERS SHOULD KNOW ABOUT THE COMMUNITY

1. VALUE OF HEALTH AND HUMAN LIFE

Human life, or capital, exceeds in economic value all other material resources of a nation. Louis I. Dublin and Alfred J. Lotka[1] say it defies measurement. A healthy population, in its broadest sense, is the best measure of a people's prosperity. Its value in terms of human happiness is immeasurable. In the preamble of the charter to the World Health Organization, health is defined as "the state of complete physical, mental and social well-being and not merely the absence of disease or infirmity."*

There is a growing realization that this natural wealth is the *quality of health* rather than life itself, that margin of mental and physical vigor that allows a person to work most effectively and to reach his highest potential level of satisfaction in life. Peoples of different cultures attach importance to health in varying degrees. In spite of our growing knowledge of, and interest in, health, we apparently do not yet consider it of primary importance. A series of national conferences, beginning with the National Conservation Commission in 1909, have made "Reports to the President," calling attention to the tangible and intangible waste that results from our failure to apply what is known about health conservation.

* World Health Organization: "Charter," *J.A.M.A.*, **131**:1431, (Aug.) 1946.

A study has recently been completed on personal consumption expenditures, by type of products, in the United States, 1952. According to this report, the "civilian money income"—$218,130 millions—was spent as follows:

Table 1. Personal Consumption Expenditures, by Type of Product, United States, 1952
(in millions of dollars)

PRODUCT	PERSONAL CONSUMPTION EXPENDITURES		PER CENT OF TOTAL
All products		218,130	100.0
Food, alcoholic beverages, and tobacco		77,750	35.6
Food	63,725		29.2
Alcoholic beverages	8,870		4.1
Tobacco	5,155		2.3
Household operation		27,601	12.6
Clothing, accessories, jewelry		25,199	11.5
Housing		24,014	11.0
Transportation		22,509	10.3
Recreation		11,716	5.4
Medical care and death expenses		10,852	5.0
Personal business		9,961	4.6
Personal care		2,515	1.2
Private education and research		2,199	1.0
Religious and welfare activities		2,148	1.0
Foreign travel and remittances (net)		1,666	0.8

Source: US Department of Commerce, Office of Business Economics: *Survey of Current Business,* National Income Number, Vol. 33, No. 7, July, 1953, Table 30, pp. 22-23.

Obviously, if we, and other peoples of the world, spent more on education and medical care and less on nonessential commodities and destructive agents such as tobacco, cosmetics, liquor, and the tools of warfare, a level of health could be reached that we can now only barely imagine.

The Report of the Committee on Costs of Medical Care in 1933 and the Report of the Health Survey by the United States Public Health Service in 1935–1936 showed that expenditures for medical care varied greatly, expenditures by families with higher incomes being ten times more than those of the poorer families, even though the latter had greater need for them. It was believed then that a $35 to $40 per capita expenditure for health (including dental care) would provide adequate medical care.[2] This figure would be doubled with the present dollar value. In 1949 it was estimated that the average private expenditure for medical care was $54 per capita. In 1947 families with an income of less than $1000 spent $28, and those with incomes of $5000 and over spent $288.

The total expenditure for civilian medical and health services in 1949 was over $10 billion. (Of this amount about $8 billion is personal expenditure and $2 billion public expenditure.) This amounts to a per capita expenditure of $70 for civilians. In addition, very large sums were spent by the military establishments, the Veterans Administration, and some other federal agencies on medical care and research.[3, 4]

Even these figures give no correct impression of the cost of illness. Josephine Roche concluded that whenever $1 billion is spent on medical care by families whose incomes are less than $2500 a year, more than half this amount is lost to them in wages.[5]

It is often said that we in the United States have the best medical care in the world, and it is clear that larger and larger sums are spent on health in this country. With the rising cost of medical care it is hard to use this as an index of improvement in the national health program, and sometimes the gains in the program seem to be offset by unfavorable environmental conditions or destructive forces. Of the World War II draftees 45 per cent were rejected in contrast to 30 per cent in World War I.[6]

Nevertheless, most authorities would probably agree that the average man of this generation is increasingly aware of the importance of health. He knows more about the way he functions and about the prevention and cure of disease. He is willing to spend each year larger and larger sums to "buy" health. The life span increases steadily, and the key has been found to control of disease caused by micro-organisms, even though degenerative diseases are on the increase and admissions to mental hospitals mount rapidly.

In summary, it seems that modern man recognizes the value of human life (economists give a specific figure for the value of an infant, an adult, and a middle-aged man), but he has not learned to control those forces that are inimical to health, particularly mental health; and even in this country the people have not yet spent enough money and effort, or distributed them well enough, to take full advantage of the enormous store of knowledge that medical scientists have accumulated. Further discussion of the subject is beyond the scope of this text. This chapter indicates some outstanding health achievements and problems, and some plans for the future; it outlines the organization, or the machinery, for health promotion and it points out the particular place of the nurse in this program.

2. CONDITIONS AFFECTING COMMUNITY HEALTH

Many factors contribute toward establishing a high standard of health within a community. In this country there are areas in which the death and sickness rates are extremely low, and others in which the rates are appallingly high, as compared with the total death and sickness rates for the country as a whole. It is possible here to suggest only some of the outstanding causes.

An economic status that provides an adequate diet, shelter, medical service, and other minimal health essentials is almost certainly the most important contributory factor in producing a high standard of health in any geographical area. In a health survey made by the United States Public Health Service, a higher sickness rate was reported among the 1,000,000 underprivileged families studied than existed among those with incomes of $3000 or more. The death rate from all causes was found to be more than twice as high for the unskilled worker as for the professional. In families with an annual income of $500 the annual infant death rate was 168 in 1000 live births; in families having an annual income of $3000 or more, the annual death rate was 30 in 1000 live births. The incidence of "chronic diseases" was about twice as high for the families with a low economic status as in well-to-do families.[7] Comprehensive health programs, therefore, include plans for adequate nutrition, recreation, and housing.

Education is another important factor the effect of which is difficult to isolate and measure, since the economic status tends to rise with the educational level and the more intelligent persons tend to secure the best education. There can be little doubt that a knowledge of the essentials of health and familiarity with community resources are a protection for the individual. As the level of general education rises in a community, the morbidity and mortality rates may be expected to fall. Education will only be effective, however, if it stimulates *interest* in health. As long as people value wealth, power, or pleasure more than mental and physical health, knowledge alone will not protect them.

The provision of medical services and health facilities is a third factor on which the health status depends. Roche attributed, in large part, the high sickness and death rates among the unemployed and families on relief to the inadequate medical care that they received. Only a small proportion of patients with disabling illnesses received full-time nursing care. While 10 per cent of the families with incomes of $3000 or more had adequate nursing care, less than 5 per cent of families with incomes smaller than this had full-time nursing care. It is often pointed out that persons with higher incomes need less medical care and receive more, while underprivileged families have greater need for medical service and receive less. This, of course, is an argument for an extension of tax-supported medical service not only for the sake of the so-called underprivileged, but for the sake of the population as a whole, which benefits from improved conditions.

In 1900 there was one physician to every 578 persons. The ratio declined until 1920 when there was one to every 730 persons. In 1949 there was one physician to every 741 persons, but if only those in active practice were considered, there was one physician to every 982 persons in the population of the United States.[8] During the period from 1900 to 1920 the standards of medical education were raised, and the profession as a whole was more concerned with quality than with quantity. Some medical leaders maintain that there is today an adequate supply of doctors in this country, but few deny that many areas are badly in need of doctors. Bernhard J. Stern shows that for the country as a whole there were in 1938 46 physicians per 100,000 in the poorest counties with per capita annual incomes of less than $100, whereas there were 171 per 100,000 in counties with an average per capita income of $600 or more. Medical workers under a fee-for-service system find it difficult to earn what they consider an adequate living in rural areas; they also gravitate to areas where modern hospital facilities are available and they concentrate most attention on the acutely ill, giving relatively less attention to the care of the chronically ill (including mental illness) and very little attention to preventive medicine. Where doctors are scarce, nursing and all other types of medical service are also likely to be inadequate. (The need for more nurses was discussed in Chapter 1.)

Dublin and Lotka[9] have shown that the morbidity rates among the Metropolitan Life Insurance policyholders were lower than for the population as a whole. They believe that this is largely the result of the health-education program of the company as well as the home nursing, which was furnished to policyholders until 1952. Demonstrations have been made of the way in which sickness and death rates may be lowered in metropolitan and rural areas through a program of health education and the increase of organized medical service. These demonstrations have been financed by private endowments, such as the Commonwealth Fund and the Milbank Memorial Fund.

Many students of sociology have called attention to the close relationship between poverty, sickness, vice, and crime. Howard W. Green[10] shows in a series of maps of Cleveland that in the city districts where the housing rates are lowest the tuberculosis rate is appallingly high, juvenile delinquency most marked, and the houses of prostitution most numerous.

Some doubt may exist as to what is cause and what is effect; but, whether sickness results from poverty or poverty from sickness, it is plain to see that the total social picture has to be taken into consideration if health conditions are to be materially improved.

3. OUTSTANDING ACCOMPLISHMENTS IN CONTROL OF DISEASE AND PROMOTION OF HEALTH

While we cannot be smug over the health accomplishments of this era there is no doubt that our means of controlling disease and improving health are immeasurably greater in this age than at any other period of history. *Medical practice is emerging from an art that was based on a meager body of knowledge and vague theories of "fluxes" and "humors" into a science growing out of present knowledge of cell physiology.* The microscope and modern laboratory methods in chemistry and physics have revolutionized the study of physiology and consequently the practice of medicine. Claude Bernard's[11] pronouncement that in effect health consists in keeping the lymph constant around the cell is so simple that many persons hear it and assume that they have always known it. He pointed out that all vital mechanisms of the body, varied as they are, have but one object: to preserve the constant conditions of life in the internal environment. Actually it is a most profound observation, and in it medicine and nursing have a sure guide. Disease is a state in which one or more components or conditions of the cell fluids are out of equilibrium: temperature, water, salts, nutrients, gases, or hormones. The constancy of the fluid around the cell may also be disturbed by foreign substances, bacteria, their toxins, other poisons or mechanical obstacles that prevent free circulation of this fluid. Some persons believe that so-called "mental disease" is as much a disturbance of this internal environment as is so-called physical disease. Emotions can produce a disequilibrium in hormones, nutrients, salts, gases, and water just as completely as can toxic substances that are swallowed, or growths that interfere mechanically with the circulation.

The realization that health consists in this equilibrium of the fluid surrounding body cells does not endow us with the ability to maintain it, and disease will not be conquered until the answers are found to the problems involved and until man is able and willing to maintain an emotional balance, to eat a complete diet, to avoid living and nonliving toxic agents and mechanically injurious agents. Science has provided us with the best tools man has devised, but we have not yet learned to use them except in specific and limited areas. Our greatest failure is in the realm of the spirit, the mind, or the emotions. The increase of mental illness indicates that with all the new methods at our disposal for the maintenance of nutritional equilibrium, for the removal of obstructions to the circulation of body fluids, for the destruction of invading organisms, we have not learned much about the control of injurious psychic forces. Hope lies in the fact that so many people recognize this great need. All doctors, nurses, and others who work in education, the ministry, and medicine are urged to have some psychological and psychiatric training; and the medical and theological schools in this country cannot ac-commodate all the well-prepared applicants who intend to work for spiritual, mental, or emotional harmony through medicine and the ministry.

Alexis Carrell, comparing modern man's gain in physical development with his disproportionate gain in stamina and moral force, says:

It is certain, nevertheless, that health is improving. Not only has mortality decreased but each individual is handsomer, larger, and stronger. Today, children are much taller than their parents. An abundance of good food and physical exercises have augmented the size of the body and its muscular strength. . . . However, the longevity of the men proficient in all kinds of sports is not greater than that of their ancestors. It may be even less . . . we know that the products of modern education need much sleep, good food, and regular habits. Their nervous system is delicate. They do not endure the mode of existence in the larger cities, the confinement in offices, the worries of business, and even the every-day difficulties and sufferings of life. They easily break down. Perhaps the triumphs of hygiene, medicine, and modern education are not so advantageous as we are led to believe.*

In spite of Carrell's doubts the medical world takes great pride in the fact that the average life span was 68 years in 1950 in the United States in contrast to 49.2 years in 1900. It is true that the gain is largely due to improved maternal and child health and that the life expectancy at 40 is not so much greater than it was 50 years ago. It is also clear that the gain is much greater among white people than among the nonwhite.

In 1948 the life expectancy of nonwhite males was 58.1 years as compared with 65.5 for white males, and 62.5 years for nonwhite females as compared with 71 years for white females. These racial differences in longevity are, how-ever, lessening in this country. The average length of life is influenced by the daily

---

* Carrell, Alexis: *Man the Unknown.* Harper & Brothers, New York, 1935, p. 19.

per capita consumption of food. Countries that have a consistent food shortage have the lowest life expectancy, and the countries with a high life expectancy have a more nearly adequate national diet. The Scandinavian countries, Australia, and New Zealand are the only ones whose average length of life exceeds that in the United States.[12]

Table 2.   The Ten Leading Causes of Death in the United States 1900 and 1948*

RANK	CAUSE OF DEATH	DEATH RATE PER 100,000 POPULATION	PER CENT OF DEATHS FROM ALL CAUSES
	1948		
	All Causes	989	100.0
1	Diseases of heart	323	32.7
2	Cancer	135	13.7
3	Cerebral hemorrhage	90	9.1
4	Accidents	67	6.8
5	Nephritis	53	5.4
6	Pneumonia and influenza	39	3.9
7	Tuberculosis	30	3.0
8	Premature birth	27	2.7
9	Diabetes mellitus	26	2.6
10	Arteriosclerosis	19	1.9
	First ten causes	809	81.8
	1900		
	All Causes	1719	100.0
1	Pneumonia and influenza	202	11.8
2	Tuberculosis	194	11.3
3	Diarrhea and enteritis	143	8.3
4	Diseases of heart	137	8.0
5	Cerebral hemorrhage	107	6.2
6	Nephritis	89	5.2
7	Accidents	72	4.2
8	Cancer	64	3.7
9	Diphtheria	40	2.3
10	Meningitis	34	2.0
	First ten causes	1082	63.0

* Dublin, Louis I.: *The Facts of Life from Birth to Death*. The Macmillan Company, New York, 1951, p. 105.

Most authorities attribute the saving of maternal and child life to the *control of infections*—the most conspicuously successful accomplishment of medical science.

Diseases caused by microorganisms usually produce *acute* illness. Fifty years ago such diseases were responsible for more than two thirds of the deaths in our registration area. Today the situation is reversed, and four fifths of the deaths that occur yearly are caused by diseases ordinarily classed as *chronic*. (See Table 2.) Students of public health believe that these diseases are not necessarily increasing, however. They call attention to the fact that more persons are now living to middle age, when tumorous growths and degenerative processes are most likely to manifest themselves.

It has been demonstrated that when the cause and the mode of transmission are known and a protective serum, or specific drug, is available, a communicable disease can be practically wiped out. Yellow fever, malaria, typhoid fever, and diphtheria are examples of such diseases. Their occurrence in any numbers is considered a disgrace in a well-organized community. Almost any communicable condition, regardless of what is known about the causative organism, can now be controlled by isolation of infected persons so that epidemics of all sorts are becoming less and less common. In spite of well-developed methods of control, however, we are far from having reached the goal in the prevention of communicable diseases. Although the tuberculosis rate has been falling in this country since 1900, when it was the second cause of death, *it still ranks seventh in the 1948 list;* diarrhea and enteritis had dropped from the third to a rank below ten. However, among the families studied in the Health Survey in 1935–1936 these intestinal infections were the eighth most frequent cause of death.[13, 14]

The means of arresting and preventing the spread of syphilis are so well established that the Scandinavian countries had practically eliminated the disease before World War II. While incidence figures are always estimates from discovered cases it is believed that the incidence of syphilis in Sweden was 7 cases in every 100,000 of the population whereas the rate varied in different parts of the United States from 1800 to 20,000 in every 100,000. Thomas Parran, as Surgeon General of the United States Public Health Service, promoted a campaign that reduced the incidence of syphilis until World War II reversed the trend, as all wars have done. Now the incidence is again declining. Wilson G. Smillie,[15] applying the ratio, found in an intensive survey of Birmingham, Alabama, in 1946, that the rate for this country might have been at that time 3 per cent with infections among nonwhites outnumbering those among whites 15 to 1. E. Gurney Clark says that an official of the US Public Health Service estimates that in 1949 2 per cent of the population, if tested, would be found to have positive serologic tests for syphilis. The US Public Health Service reported 45.3 cases of detected syphilis for every 1000 men in the selective service examinations. A higher rate is found, generally speaking, in families with low incomes.[16, 17]

Rapid and effective methods of treating syphilis as well as other infections with the modern "miracle drugs" (sulfa drugs and antibiotics) have made startling gains in their control. A new era in therapy has opened up, and it is not possible to estimate the changes that sulfa, the antibiotics, and comparable agents will make in the control of disease. (See Table 16 in Chapter 41.)

Modern obstetrics makes childbirth far less hazardous today than it was fifty or even twenty-five years ago, but the maternal death rate shows that clean and skillful medical and nursing care is not available to a large proportion of the population. Smillie believes that two thirds of the maternal deaths in this country could be prevented.

To illustrate what good medical and nursing supervision can accomplish in reducing the maternal death rate, Carolyn C. Van Blarcom[18] cites the work of the Frontier Nursing Service established in consultation with the State Department of Health in Kentucky in 1925. The midwifery and nursing service reports that, in its first 1000 deliveries in the mountainous regions of Kentucky, there were no deaths from puerperal causes and the stillbirth and neonatal death rate was reduced to one third the current rate for this country.

Great strides have been made in reducing the infant death rate here and abroad. Much of this gain has been due to eliminating from the public market grossly contaminated milk. Improved feeding methods and the discovery of the significance of vitamins in the diet have saved infants and children from nutritional diseases, such as scurvy and rickets.

The development in the field of nutrition should certainly receive honorable mention in even the briefest review of medical progress. Not only have dietary cures been discovered for true nutritional diseases, such as scurvy, beriberi, and pellagra, but, in almost every branch of medicine and surgery, therapy has been improved by more scientific methods of feeding. Experiments with animals and studies made with regional and national diets have helped to establish nutritional needs for various ages and for conditions such as pregnancy. Experts in this field are putting forth the startling theory that certain traits of personality can be weakened and intensified by diet. Ruth F. Harrell[19] has demonstrated that the learning accomplishment of children in manual and mental skills could be increased approximately 15 per cent by the addition of vitamins to what was thought to be an adequate diet. Recent studies indicate that dental caries can be controlled by improved dietary habits.

The diet in the United States as a whole is often said to be more adequate and varied than that of any other nation. Students from other countries come here to study feeding methods in hospitals and schools. In spite of this fact, there are large areas of the country in which the diet of the average family is deficient in certain essentials. When economic conditions limit food selection, few families know enough to provide the necessary food elements. There is a great deal to be done through health education along these lines and further discoveries to be made through research. The chemistry of nutrition is so new that its students consider they have barely scratched the surface in discovering its secrets.

The development of aseptic surgery and modern anesthesia has entirely altered the outlook for those who must undergo operations. A hundred years ago surgeons expected wounds to become infected, whereas today an infected wound is considered a serious accident. The use of the new chemotherapeutic agents and antibiotics has still further reduced the incidence and duration of surgical infections. Prior to the middle of the last century operations were performed without the aid of an anesthetic proper. In some cases the patient would be made drunk with alcohol or drugged with opium or mandrake. Surgery performed under these conditions could not fail to produce a severe nervous shock. Anesthesia has been made progressively more effective, less dangerous, and less unpleasant from the patient's standpoint. Surgical treatment has been improved in so many ways that the hazards are enormously reduced and the person returned to normal living much sooner.

Scientific organic therapy is a comparatively recent addition to medical science. The control of diabetes with insulin, hypothyroidism with thyroid extracts, pernicious anemia with preparations of liver, and the effective treatment of other conditions with the secretions of the pituitary, adrenal, and thymus glands are among the great blessings modern medicine has brought to mankind. The idea of treating disease with secretions of the body and organs of animals is not new. Medical historians call attention to the ancient practice of compounding remedies from the spinal cords or brains of animals and from the urine and blood of human beings. Today, organic therapy is based on the findings in blood chemistry, x-ray photographs, and other accurate means of detecting deviations from normal in the size and function of glands; it has become a rational procedure. Unfortunately, the discoveries in this field are no more universally applied than they are in other fields of modern therapy. Diabetes, which can be satisfactorily controlled by diet and insulin, ranked as the *ninth commonest cause* of death, as reported by Dublin.

The discovery of cortisone and ACTH has an unpredictable significance in the control of diseases, such as arthritis, that have not responded markedly to any previously known remedies. As effective agents are discovered for the control of diabetes, pernicious anemia, Addison's disease, and many other conditions that were fatal fifty years ago, the association of the terms "incurable" and "chronic" is less and less justified.

When we turn to *mental illness* there seem to be few brilliant achievements to point out. For the most part the causes are a matter of conjecture and the treatment one of helping the person to gain insight, or to be re-educated, to rid himself of his fears, and to build up his physical resistance. Psychoanalysis, shock therapy, and surgical interruption of nerve pathways are more or less recent additions to psychiatric therapy. They have improved, but not revolutionized, the treatment of the mentally ill. It is possible that as more is learned about the functions of glands and about human nutrition a physiological approach to psychiatry will be developed to produce more startling results.

Hospitals for the mentally ill are absurdly understaffed. Psychiatry and psychiatric nursing make excessive demands upon the imagination and the patience of the worker. They require to a greater extent than any other branch of medicine a thorough understanding of human nature. The cure is often slow and difficult. For these or other reasons this specialty has failed to attract an adequate number of physicians and well-prepared nurses. Few persons realize that about one half of the hospital beds in this country are occupied by the mentally ill.[20, 21] Because of the social opprobrium attached to mental disease, there is a tendency on the part of patients and their families to keep "a nervous breakdown" a secret, and so it is again surprising to most of us to learn how many individuals have been patients, at one time or another, in mental hospitals. While psychoanalysis has achieved a certain popularity, often caricatured in current literature, there is need for more general knowledge of the early symptoms of mental disease, for a recognition of the value of early treatment, and for a more hopeful outlook and open manner of dealing with psychiatric conditions. Mental disease is often called our most serious public health problem. James M. Mather[22] gives it this emphasis in a summary of outstanding health service needs. He reports that in Canada in 1950 there were 49,163 mentally ill whose care cost $30,000,000. This is five times the budget of the World Health Organization. In point of numbers affected and acuteness of suffering there is no problem facing humanity comparable to the control of mental disease. Dublin says:

Currently about one in every 20 persons spends part of his life in an institution for mental patients. . . . More than half of the hospital beds in the country are occupied by mental patients. . . . There is no evidence that mental illness is more prevalent in any given age group today than fifty or a hundred years ago, but it is true that a greater proportion of the total population is now hospitalized for mental disease. While some authorities might question the statement many of them believe that the high incidence of mental illness is an indictment of our culture. It is a problem that must be attacked at its roots by all groups in our society.*

This summary of the progress that has been made in raising health standards touches upon only a few of the outstanding achievements. The suggested health problems facing medical workers and the public at large are only a sampling of the total list, but in all these, as in nearly every aspect of therapy and health education, nurses have taken an active part. In the control of communicable disease, it is the nurse who most constantly applies the principles of microbiology in preventing the transfer of disease-producing organisms from one individual to another. In hospitals, in private practice, and as the representative of official health agencies, she teaches persons with communicable conditions to care for themselves in such a way that they will not be a menace to others. She administers protective and curative agents prescribed by the physician, and makes and records observations, which are an essential part of the study of all disease.

In the maternity program the nurse has been especially conspicuous. In clinics and in homes she works with the physician in teaching and supervising prenatal hygiene. She provides the obstetrician with aseptic conditions under which to work in the delivery room. She, more than anybody else, protects the newborn infant from harmful elements in his environment. She protects the mother after delivery from those microorganisms that 50 or 60 years ago in many large hospitals attacked and killed one out of every two women who were delivered. The fall in the maternal death rate is probably due as much to the nurse's constant attention to asepsis as to the increased skill of the obstetrician.

Nurses have helped to reduce the infant death rate by teaching mothers home nursing, by giving instruction and supervision in the preparation of feeding, by working with the physician in the care of sick infants, and by participating in research of various kinds.

* Dublin, Louis I.: *The Facts of Life from Birth to Death.* The Macmillan Company, New York, 1951, pp. 313-14.

Progress in nutrition has been the result of the combined efforts of nutritionists, chemists, physiologists, physicians, nurses, and social workers. A nurse does not ordinarily prepare or supervise the preparation of food in institutions. All women, and particularly nurses, should have some knowledge of this art, however. The nurse is often responsible for food selection within the range allowed by the prescribed diet; she gives assistance and instruction to the patient or his family about food selection and budgeting funds available for food. She helps to plan for the spacing of feedings and helps the patient to eat when he needs such assistance. In this, as in all fields of medical research, she participates by her constant observation of the patient and by recording these observations.

Aseptic surgery is usually the result of the work of the surgeon, the nurse, and the technicians who prepare surgical supplies. The success of modern anesthesia is likewise due in large part to more effective preoperative nursing care and to the intelligent observation of the patient by the nurse as he is recovering.

The improvement in the care of the mentally ill lies partly in the wholesome hygienic regimen made possible very largely by nurses. The nurse helps these sick people, who have often lost interest in their personal appearance, to keep themselves clean and neat; she helps to rouse them from their indifference to take a walk or play a game; she encourages them to eat and often feeds them when they would not get sufficient nourishment if left to themselves; and she induces sleep and rest with the use of baths, massage, and hot drinks. A more imaginative, individualized type of nursing service is gradually replacing the routine care that has been given. Where the well-prepared nurse is available, the psychiatrist can share with her the responsibility for the psychotherapeutic program. It is only in places where good nursing is available that such harmful practices as restraint, confinement, and widespread use of drugs to quiet violent persons can be so reduced that they are ordered for the benefit of the patient rather than protection of personnel.

The emphasis here is on nursing because this text is for nurses, and the purpose of this discussion is to impress students and members of this profession with the relationship of nurses to the total health program. It is so essential, however, that each group appreciate the need for understanding and cooperation with other groups that the total program is discussed in some detail.

4. IMPORTANCE OF ORGANIZATION IN HEALTH WORK

Health promotion and medical care of the sick have been a decentralized, divided, and chiefly local responsibility until comparatively recent years. Bureaus concerned with health have been scattered through many departments of the federal government in contrast to the centralized Ministry of Health commonly found in most national governments. State health departments have set up regulations and established standards but have left the county or city health department free to provide service to the individual without much interference as to kind and quantity. In general the services of the public health, or tax-supported, agencies have been educational or of a nature to protect the citizenry from dangers in the environment. This has been interpreted to include hospitalization of persons with communicable disease (including tuberculosis) and mental illness. It has also grown to include all kinds of medical care for the wards of the government: Indians, military personnel, and veterans. Gradually the general medical care of the indigent has come to be included in the list of tax-supported services. In contrast to these tax-supported "public health services" there are the medical care and health promotion of the major part of the population that have been, and still are, a private or voluntary service. It is furnished by individual practitioners and by private or voluntary health agencies. Selskar M. Gunn and Phillip S. Platt,[23] in a monograph on the subject, say that there are at least 20,000 voluntary health agencies exclusive of hospitals, most of them concerned with the control of a particular disease and working, more or less, independently.

To sum up, the task of maintaining a healthy people is divided among many agencies. The first big division of the task is between public and private agencies. The functions of the two groups are not always clear cut, but even when they are there is so much overlapping and so inadequate a system of getting the individual to the proper agency, or practitioner, that his need often goes unanswered.

The responsibility of the state for providing an education for everyone has been accepted by the people of this country, and every state has the machinery for providing it. Federal aid for education is advocated by some as a nationwide means of improving the quality of education; it is feared by others who believe that federal aid will mean interference with the right of the state to control its educational system. There is considerable evidence that this country is moving toward the same concept of public responsibility for the health of the individual that we have assumed for his education. The same belief is held by some that federal aid is necessary in order to provide adequate health services in certain areas; the same fear exists that it will bring with it federal control. Whether or not it is universally acceptable, the federal government is playing an increasingly important role in health promotion.

A brief listing of events since the turn of the century shows that we are moving toward (1) concentration of health functions in one federal department or agency; (2) extending the functions of federal, state, and local tax-supported health agencies; (3) interpreting the function of the tax-supported agency as that of promoting the health of the individual by all types of service rather than that of protecting the well person from the sick; (4) districting the nation into workable health units; (5) coordinating the work of all health agencies, public and private, by national, state, district, and even more local health councils; and (6) distributing the cost of medical care by a system of insurance.

It is not practicable to do more than list the following events in this text. Nurses will find it profitable to study them through the writings of such authorities as Michael Davis, Joseph W. Mountain, Smillie, Stern, and Dublin.

1909   Report to President Theodore Roosevelt by the National Conservation Commission on National Vitality: Its Waste and Conservation.

1921   Formation of the National Health Council with the objective of coordinating the activities of the member agencies, official (public) and voluntary (private).

1930   White House Conference on Child Health and Protection, called by President Hoover.

1933   Publication of *Costs of Medical Care*—a study made by Ira S. Falk et al. under the auspices of the American Medical Association and other national health agencies that showed adequate medical care was not universally available, nor was it economically possible for a large proportion of the population. This gave impetus to the development of sickness insurance.

1935   Report to President Franklin D. Roosevelt by the Committee on Economic Security, including recommendations on health and welfare, that served as a basis for the Social Security Act adopted by Congress in this same year. The bill provided for assistance for the aged, the unemployed, the blind, the crippled, and grants-in-aid to improve maternal and child care. It also extended public health services and provided for increase in trained health personnel.

1935–36 "The Health Survey"—a study made by the United States Public Health Service: A house-to-house canvass of almost three million people in 19 states. On the basis of the data collected the conclusion was reached that the incidence of illness was higher in low-income groups and that where the need was greatest the care was least adequate.

1938   The National Health Conference, held as an Interdepartmental Committee to coordinate health and welfare activities.

1939   Senate Bill 1620—a bill incorporating the recommendations of the National Health Conference and presented to Congress by Senator Wagner. The bill proposed a national health and welfare program that in effect would have made the protection of the individual's health and welfare a public responsibility. The expense of the program was to be met by national compulsory health insurance. While this bill, like its successors, has never passed the houses of Congress, President Truman's administration promoted comparable legislation.

1940   A *recommendation* of the American Public Health Association approving in principle the assumption of the curative function by local health units. This action endorsed the concept that the public health program should not separate preventive and curative medicine, but should develop in the community a unified and complete health service that would help the individual to develop his maximum potential vitality.

1940–50 Expansion of voluntary sickness insurance with the present estimate that about 50 per cent of the population is insured in some way against illness and accidents. Most insurance plans provide for hospitalization and medical emergencies or acute illness; they are not an effective protection in chronic illness and are not within the reach of the lowest income group. Some states and local communities are setting up insurance plans to meet more completely the needs of the people.

1946   The Hospital Construction Bill (Hill-Burton Bill S. 191)—a bill passed by Congress appropriating $75,000,000 annually, for a period of five years to increase hospital facilities.

1946–48 Creation of a World Health Organization by the United Nations, with formal establishment in 1948. The United States became a member in 1948. Seventy-five nations belonged to the organization in 1950.

1937–50 Bills passed providing federal funds to be used by state agencies, and in some cases national programs for research, education, or medical care in tuberculosis, cancer, maternal and mental health, venereal and heart disease.

1949 The Housing Act passed by Congress, establishing a long-range federal program for slum clearance, urban development, and low-rent housing.

1950 Meeting in Washington of the National Conference on the Aging, proposed by President Truman and sponsored by the Federal Security Agency.

1948 Conclusions reached by the National Health Assembly (reported in *America's Health: a Report to the Nation,* Harper & Brothers, New York, 1949):

   (a) more public health facilities, doctors, and nurses are needed, particularly in rural areas;

   (b) localities with low-capital incomes and substandard facilities should receive supplementary funds from federal and state governments to assist them to obtain adequate health resources;

   (c) research and medical education should be aided by government funds;

   (d) the insurance principle, as a method of spreading sickness costs in a predictable fashion, should be extended;

   (e) health insurance should be supplemented by use of tax resources to provide for low-income groups and other persons for whom special public responsibility is acknowledged;

   (f) high standards of service should be encouraged through greater coordination of services of physicians, hospitals, and other health agencies.

1953 Establishment of the Department of Health, Education, and Welfare which coordinates the activities of many federal health agencies in one department.

Obviously, what has been accomplished so far would not have been possible without the *organized* efforts of medical and nonmedical workers. The fall in the nation's death rate from diphtheria is an example of the cooperation of parents, school boards, public health officials, hospital authorities, nurses, and physicians who have instituted state and local programs for diagnosis, isolation, and preventive and curative therapy. Toxin-antitoxin is produced and distributed by state and local health departments, and examination of material from the throat made in their laboratories. School boards require that each child be tested for susceptibility with the Schick test, and that all those who are shown to be susceptible be given toxin-antitoxin. Hospitals isolate and care for persons who, failing to receive preventive treatment, contract the disease. Physicians and nurses employed by official and nonofficial health agencies give home care and instruction and supervise the isolation of patients who are not taken to the hospital. Physicians report every case of diphtheria coming under their observation to the local health department, and report deaths, so that special precautions may be taken in the burial of bodies infected with diphtheria and vital statistics may be compiled.

In like manner the control of tuberculosis, syphilis, dysentery, and all those conditions for which the means of prevention or control are known, depends upon, or will depend upon, the extent to which the resources for combating them are organized and the degree to which cooperation exists among the various groups of health workers.

In spite of the opposition in some quarters to so-called socialized medicine, the functions of official health organizations—that is, tax-supported agencies—are constantly enlarging and the volume of work increasing. A system of disease control that leaves everything to private enterprise has never adequately protected the health of either the privileged or underprivileged. Private or voluntary institutions and individual workers are learning to value cooperation with public agencies more highly.

Communities are organizing health councils whose functions are to collect and apportion funds for the support of the agencies represented to study the needs of the community, the facilities, and the activities of the various agencies. Such a study serves as a basis for planning more adequate and less wasteful health service. In many places there is unnecessary duplication of effort in some directions and uncared-for needs in others. The most satisfactory type of community health organization is one in which there is some central control and direction, so that all agencies, public and private, are working together.[24]

Any nurse who hopes to take an intelligent part in the community health program should know and be able to use the existing machinery for health promotion. She should be able to promote the establishment of, and work in, community health councils. It is part of her professional obligation to be informed about the health needs of the community and to further legislation which she believes will help supply these needs.

5. INTERNATIONAL, NATIONAL, STATE, AND LOCAL HEALTH AGENCIES

There are many books on public health that give a full account of the origin, control, aims, and functions of the more important health agencies. Such detailed information goes beyond the scope of this text. The following is nothing more than a birds'-eye view of the subject, and may be supplemented by some of the texts listed at the end of the chapter.

Classifications of health agencies are based on (1) control, (2) scope or area served by the agency, (3) function, or type of service rendered, and (4) the class of persons served. Control depends upon the source from which the organization receives its support; and, since this is such an important factor in determining both scope and function, agencies are usually classified according to whether they are (1) public or official, that is, supported by tax funds, or (2) voluntary or private, which means that they are supported by private funds.

It would not be practical here to give the long list of categories of agencies according to the nature of their service as used in directories of social agencies. A classification of this kind includes headings such as: family welfare work, hospital social work, maternal and child welfare, rehabilitation and placement of the handicapped, convalescent care, and occupational therapy.

The system of classification that places agencies under the class or group of persons they serve includes headings such as: infants, the aged, the foreign-born, and mental defectives.

Both these types of classification are lengthy and difficult and will not be discussed in this text. The following classification gives types of agencies according to the area they serve, and their control:

Classification of Health and Welfare Agencies According to Scope and Control

A. INTERNATIONAL
   1. *Public or Official Agencies:* Those supported by public funds from the national governments represented. *Example*—World Health Organization.
   2. *Private or Voluntary:* Those supported by private funds* from sources such as membership fees and endowments, and engaged in activities that are international in their scope. *Example*—International Council of Nurses.

B. NATIONAL
   1. *Public or Official Agencies:* Those administered by appointees of the federal government and supported by funds from federal taxes, and engaged in activities that are national in their scope. *Example*—Public Health Service. (Reorganization Plan I of 1939 transferred the Public Health Service from the Department of the Treasury to the Federal Security Agency; by Reorganization Plan I of 1953 and the act approved April 1, 1953 [Pub. Law 13, 83rd Cong.; 67 Stat. 18], the Federal Security Agency became the Department of Health, Education, and Welfare.)
   2. *Private or Voluntary:* Those supported by private funds from sources such as membership fees and endowments, and engaged in activities that are national in their scope. *Example*—American Medical Association.

C. STATE
   1. *Public or Official:* Those administered by appointees of the state government represented, supported by funds from the state treasury, and engaged in activities that are state-wide in their scope. *Example*—New York State Department of Health.
   2. *Private or Voluntary:* Those supported by private funds from sources such as membership fees and endowments, and engaged in activities that are state-wide in their scope. *Example*—Virginia Conference of Social Work.

D. LOCAL (COUNTY, TOWNSHIP, MUNICIPAL)
   1. *Public or Official:* Those administered by appointees of county, township, or municipal governments, and engaged in activities affecting one of these local areas. *Example*—Cattaraugus County Health Department, New York State.
   2. *Private or Voluntary:* Those supported by private funds from sources such as gifts, endowments, membership or patients' fees, and engaged in activities affecting a county, town or city, or a section of one of these. *Example*—Visiting Nurse Service of New York City.

Public or Official Health Agencies. In the preceding classification of official health agencies it was stated that they may be international, national, state, county, or municipal organizations.

* Public funds are in some cases allocated to private organizations when they perform some service that is recognized as a public responsibility. A good example of this is the payment of public funds to a private hospital that undertakes the care of public charges (indigents) in the community.

Ernest L. Stebbins,[25] in Kenneth F. Maxcy's text, *Rosenau's Preventive Medicine and Hygiene,* dates the beginning of international health organization from the efforts of the Egyptian Quarantine Board in 1831 to control the spread of plague in Europe by cooperative measures of the nations affected. In 1851 the first formal International Health Council was held in Paris; this Health Council finally succeeded in establishing an International Office of Public Health in Paris in 1909. A few years earlier the International Sanitary Conference of American Republics established the International Sanitary Bureau which became the Pan-American Sanitary Bureau in 1924. These two international organizations, one with headquarters in Paris, the other in Washington, were absorbed by the Health Section of the League of Nations and became regional offices of this body in 1923.* The work of this agency and the health work of the United Nations Relief and Rehabilitation Administration (1943) were taken over by the World Health Organization, established in 1948 as a specialized agency of the United Nations.

The stated purposes of the World Health Organization are:

1. To assist governments upon request in strengthening health services.
2. To promote improved standards of teaching and training in health, medical, and related professions.
3. To provide information, counsel, and assistance in the field of health.
4. To promote, in cooperation with other specialized agencies where necessary, the improvement of nutrition, housing, sanitation, recreation, economic or working conditions, and other aspects of environmental hygiene.
5. To promote cooperation among scientific and professional groups which contribute to the advancement of health.
6. To promote maternal and child health and welfare; to foster the ability to live harmoniously in a changing total environment.
7. To foster activities in the field of mental health, especially those affecting the harmony of human relations.
8. To promote and conduct research in the field of health.
9. To study and report, in cooperation with other specialized agencies where necessary, administrative and social technics affecting public and medical care from preventive and curative points of view, including hospital services and social security.

There were, in 1950, 75 member states. The official budget for 1950 was $7,500,-000, made by the World Health Assembly with the hope that member nations would contribute at least this much or more. Willard L. Thorp[26] comments on the inadequacy of this sum for the "huge tasks" of the agency. Because the organization is new, relatively undeveloped, and very limited by the budget, it has concentrated its efforts on a few health problems in what might be called "trouble spots." Priority has been given to malaria, tuberculosis, venereal disease, and yaws; to child and maternal health and nutritional programs and to the improvement of environmental conditions in places where they are thought to be responsible for a

* The regional offices of the World Health Organization in 1950 were in New Delhi, India (for South East Asia), in Alexandria, Egypt (for the Eastern Mediterranean), the Pan-American Sanitary Bureau in Washington, D.C. (for the Americas), and the Geneva, Switzerland, head office (serving temporarily as regional office for Europe, Africa, and the Western Pacific).

"significant proportion of deaths." It is generally agreed that such programs can succeed only where there are funds and technical assistance provided. Lowell L. Reed[27] urges upon all medical workers a point of view and a habit of work that makes them assume responsibility for world health. Thorp says "world-wide health improvement has become a major concern of American Foreign Policy. . . . Progress depends upon health, food production, and education."*

National, or federal, health work in the United States is carried on in a number of federal agencies under cabinet ministers, administrators, or commissioners (see Fig. 2). In most countries there is a Ministry of Health just as there is a Ministry of the Treasury, of Agriculture, and of Commerce, from which all health work emanates. The National Health Board established in the latter part of the last century, as a part of the plan to control a yellow fever epidemic, was an abortive attempt to centralize federal health work. It was not possible to accomplish much in the way of reorganization since the office was discontinued in 1882. Transference of important health bureaus from other departments to the Federal Security Agency and recently to the Department of Health, Education, and Welfare represents successful efforts in the past decade to centralize the federal health work.[28, 29]

The work of United States Public Health Service, formerly in the Federal Security Agency and now in the Department of Health, Education, and Welfare, is the most extensive and varied of any health agency. Since World War II the Veterans Administration's health service has also assumed great importance because the number of veterans served is so large and because the quality of its service, including that of rehabilitation, is so outstanding.

According to the United States Government *Organization Manual 1953–54,* the major functions of the United States Public Health Service are:

(1) to conduct and support research and training in the medical and related sciences, and in public health methods and administration; (2) to provide medical and hospital services to persons authorized to receive care from the Service, to aid in the development of the Nation's hospital and related facilities, and to prevent the introduction of communicable diseases into the United States and its possessions; and (3) to assist the States and other governments in the application of new knowledge to the prevention and control of disease, the maintenance of a healthful environment, and the development of community health services.†

This is obviously a very extensive program. That of the Children's Bureau, in the Social Security Administration under the Department of Health, Education, and Welfare, is another federal service that has a far-reaching effect. Its functions are to (1) develop standards of child care, (2) conduct research and report on conditions that affect the welfare of children, and (3) working through state programs to promote maternal and child health, services to crippled children, and all child welfare activities.

* Thorp, Willard L.: "New International Programs in Public Health," *Am. J. Pub. Health,* **40**:1479, (Dec.) 1950.
† P. 314.

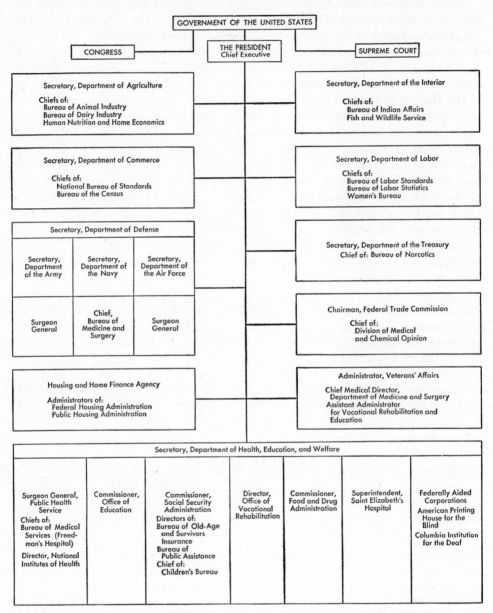

Figure 2. Administrative plan of the chief federal agencies concerned with health and related programs, 1953-1954. (Based on data from *United States Government Organization Manual 1953-54*. Federal Register Division, National Archives and Record Service, General Services Administration, Washington, D.C., revised as of July 1, 1953.)

(Note: The federal government transferred in July, 1955, responsibility for the health of Indians from the Bureau of Indian Affairs, in the Department of the Interior, to the US Public Health Service, in the Department of Health, Education, and Welfare.)

Health education and health promotion are also furthered by the Office of Education, transferred in 1939 to the Federal Security Agency.* Health among the Indians, wards of the federal government, is promoted through the Bureau of Indian Affairs, which remains in the Department of the Interior.

Nurses serve as administrators, consultants, and workers in all these agencies mentioned, and the value of their contribution is more fully recognized each year.

The Bureau of the Census in the Department of Commerce collects, compiles, and analyzes statistics on population births, the causes and incidence of death, employment, income, and other data. Such figures are essential in estimating the health needs in a community, in determining whether climatic factors affect the incidence of a disease, in establishing the relationship between economic conditions and the death rate, and many other problems in the realm of medical science.

The work of the National Bureau of Standards in the Department of Commerce has had a marked effect upon health. This bureau, either alone or in cooperation with the Food and Drug Administration in the Department of Health, Education, and Welfare, or some other branch of the government, sets up standards for drugs, foods, and for all sorts of articles used in hospitals, clinics, and the home care of the sick. "U.S.P." on a drug container means that the preparation is made according to the formula in the *United States Pharmacopoeia*. When a manufacturer advertises rubber tubing as "made according to the US government specifications," it is a recommendation of quality. The establishment of universally recognized standards has protected the public from injurious or ineffective products.

Through the Departments of Agriculture and Commerce, plant and animal diseases that affect man's health indirectly are studied and controlled, and the public is protected from contaminated fish and dairy products. The Bureau of Human Nutrition and Home Economics in the Department of Agriculture carries on a program of instruction that helps to raise health standards in the home.

A study of the functions of the federal health services shows that they are so set up as to allow the states freedom in planning and conducting their programs. The federal government gives actual medical care to certain of its personnel including the armed services, under certain conditions to ex-service men, and to Indians living as wards of the government; it operates to prevent the spread of communicable disease from abroad and between states; and it tests, publishes reports of, and controls the manufacture of biological products affected by interstate commerce. The remainder of its program consists of allocating—usually matched— funds for building, educating personnel, conducting research, public education, and furnishing technical assistance and consultation service to state health officials.

As has been noted, the federal government, working through state governments and agencies, is taking a more and more active part in the national health program.

A *state health department* serves the people in that state largely by assisting the local health organizations. When a local organization (for example, a county health department) is not prepared to deal with the health problems in the com-

* By Reorganization Plan 1 of 1953, the Federal Security Agency became the Department of Health, Education, and Welfare.

munity, the state department may send workers to assist the local health officers or it may take charge of the program. The authority of the state is supreme, although the state may delegate considerable authority to a large health department in a city such as Chicago.

Harry Mustard calls attention to the difference between the powers of local control assigned to the federal and state governments. He says:

The federal government may assist and advise the state on its internal health affairs, but not supersede it, as the authority of each is distinct. The local government, however, has only the authority which the state delegates to it. Though the state may assume control in health matters, it seldom does. To do so would be somewhat comparable to the situation where the state militia supersedes the local sheriff or police, under martial law.*

A comparison of a state and a local health organization shows that they have approximately the same divisions or sections; for example, there is the Division of Public Health Nursing in the state and there is likewise the Division of Public Health Nursing in the local health organization. The same is true of Divisions of Mental Hygiene, Communicable Disease, Tuberculosis, Vital Statistics, and other aspects of health work. The administrative plans of all the 48 state health departments are not identical; however, most of them are similar to the one that is shown diagramatically in Figure 3.

The official local health organization may be a county, a township, or a city health department. Its functions vary with the community and the funds available for health work. The efficiency of the organization and the type of men and women appointed as officers and staff also affect the quantity and quality of health service given by this agency. Smillie lists the following as fundamental functions of a local health organization:

It is a basic principle that the direct responsibility for health protection rests upon the official health department of the local self-governing unit—be it village, township, county, or municipality. . . . Local health departments function on the social theory that the community is responsible for protection of its members against the special hazards of community life.†

He outlines the following administrative divisions, or bureaus, and their activities about as follows: (1) *Communicable disease control* includes providing public health laboratories, enforcing isolation and quarantine regulations, and instructing patients and their families; (2) *vital statistics* is concerned primarily with collecting data on births and deaths, but this division may also collect, analyze, and report data on the incidence of disease and other matters related to the health of the community; (3) *environmental sanitation* concerns itself with "the condition" and "arrangement of houses in relation to one another and to adjacent buildings," the

---

* Mustard, Harry S.: *An Introduction to Public Health,* 3rd ed. The Macmillian Company, New York, 1953, pp. 51–52.

† Smillie, Wilson G.: *Preventive Medicine and Public Health,* 2nd ed. The Macmillan Company, New York, 1952, pp. 509–10.

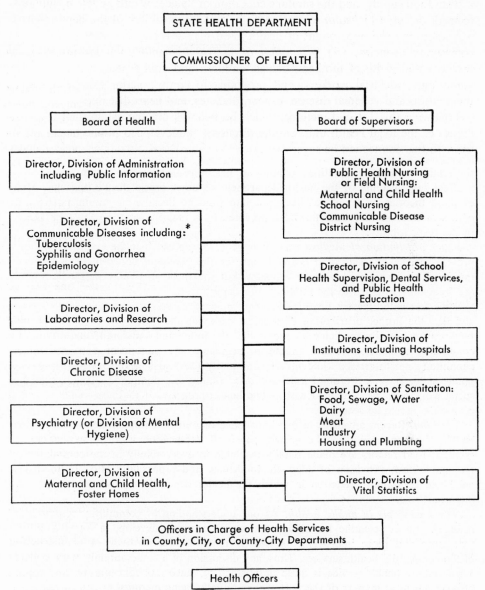

STATE HEALTH DEPARTMENT

COMMISSIONER OF HEALTH

Board of Health

Board of Supervisors

Director, Division of Administration including Public Information

Director, Division of Public Health Nursing or Field Nursing:
Maternal and Child Health
School Nursing
Communicable Disease
District Nursing

Director, Division of Communicable Diseases including:*
Tuberculosis
Syphilis and Gonorrhea
Epidemiology

Director, Division of School Health Supervision, Dental Services, and Public Health Education

Director, Division of Laboratories and Research

Director, Division of Institutions including Hospitals

Director, Division of Chronic Disease

Director, Division of Sanitation:
Food, Sewage, Water
Dairy
Meat
Industry
Housing and Plumbing

Director, Division of Psychiatry (or Division of Mental Hygiene)

Director, Division of Maternal and Child Health, Foster Homes

Director, Division of Vital Statistics

Officers in Charge of Health Services in County, City, or County-City Departments

Health Officers

* This and other divisions may provide health and morbidity data although the emphasis is still on preventive health in public services.

Figure 3. Administrative plan of a county, city, or county-city health department. (State organizational pattern is similar.)

disposal of excreta and waste, the provision of clean or unpolluted water and air, a clean food supply, and the sanitary condition of "places where people congregate" to work or eat; (4) *health education* "is a joint responsibility of the department of education and the department of health" and may involve cooperation with many community agencies; (5) *promotion of individual health* includes programs to promote the health of mothers, babies, children and young people of school age, adults and industrial workers; and programs to control major diseases, such as tuberculosis and venereal disease, cancer, diabetes, and heart disease.

Following this list of functions, which he believes are the established responsibilities of the local health unit, Smillie discusses "undeveloped public health activities." In this connection he says:

Certain community functions relating to health promotion are, in theory at least, a direct responsibility of the health department or other official health agencies. Many of these theories have not yet been put into practice because of administrative difficulties or because they have not been accepted by a majority of the people as a direct public responsibility.

Better distribution of medical care. It is generally agreed that the community should provide medical, nursing, and hospital care for the poor and unfortunate of the community. This is a public welfare function, but the medical aspects of public welfare are frequently assigned to the public health department.

Some farsighted leaders have insisted that medical care is an essential health service, and that the proper distribution of medical care, together with provision of adequate facilities for curative medicine, at a cost that the individual and family can afford, is a community responsibility, and should be regulated and administered by the official community health service. Students of community life also believe that social and economic status have a profound influence upon family and community health, and thus social work must be combined with public health programs if the best results in health promotion are to be secured.

Nutrition. Recent advances in our knowledge of nutrition show conclusively that the health of a community can be greatly improved if provision is made so that all the essential food factors are made readily available to every family in the community, at reasonable cost. Provision of adequate foodstuffs, and proper utilization of food, is a combined community function in which the health department plays an auxiliary but important role.

Newer concepts in public health. As our understanding of community responsibility changes, and as scientific knowledge and social concepts develop, it seems axiomatic that more and more improvements will be made in the methods of administration of the community health services. Thus, any discussion of a static administrative unit for a community health service is quite unsatisfactory, since our concepts of the function of government in matters of this sort are continually being modified.*

Programs of local health units are very unequal in their extent and in the quality of service given. This inadequacy and inequality led to a nationwide study, a report of which was made in 1945 by Haven Emerson and Martha Luginbuhl[30] and published by the Commonwealth Fund. The report indicates that although more than half of the counties in the United States have an organized health service on a full-

* Smillie, Wilson G.: *op. cit.,* pp. 512–13.

time basis over 40,000,000 persons lack good local public health service. While the value of the county unit is recognized, its development has lagged because many counties are sparsely settled and for this, or other reasons, are very poor. In some cases legal difficulties have stood in the way of county organization. The recommendation in this report is that health districts be constituted on the basis of population, per capita wealth, and other factors—not on county lines.

The American Public Health Association backs the recommendation of Emerson's committee that a local health unit serve an area with a population of not less than 50,000 persons. The staff should include at least one full-time medical officer, sanitary engineer, and sanitarian, ten public health nurses, three clerks, and part-time clinicians. The program should provide for the essential services of (1) vital statistics, (2) community sanitation, (3) control of communicable disease and preventable diseases, (4) laboratory services, (5) maternal and child health services, and (6) public health education. Leonard Scheele,[31] writing in the *Social Work Year Book,* says it is estimated that not more than 4 per cent of the population is served by health units staffed according to these minimum standards. As improved health units are organized, district health councils are formed to study and provide for the health needs of the district. All health agencies, including hospitals, are considered in the planning. There is a trend toward coordinating under one administration all public agencies, hospitals, clinics, and bureaus giving educational, preventive, and curative services.

Recent federal and state appropriations have considerably extended most health services. Many writers in the field of public health call attention to the rapid extension of the work of tax-supported health agencies. They seem to be gradually taking over a great deal of what was done by voluntary agencies. Nursing care of the sick in their homes is one of the few functions that is still almost entirely in the hands of private visiting nurse organizations. Unless there is a marked change in public opinion with relation to the government's responsibility for the protection of people's health, there is every reason to suppose that there will continue to be an increase in "socialized medicine" or the health service given by official agencies, and that it may be extended to include nursing in homes.

Private or Voluntary Health Agencies. Gunn and Platt say the growth of private or voluntary health agencies in this century is phenomenal. Excepting the American Red Cross and the tuberculosis societies there was in 1900 scarcely a local health agency, whereas, including the Red Cross, 20,000 is a conservative estimate for 1945. The difficulties growing out of such rapid expansion were recognized early. In 1913 a committee was formed to study functions and relationships. This led to the development of a permanent joint organization, the National Health Council. Official agencies worked in this council in an advisory capacity. Primarily, the council is a coordinating body for voluntary health agencies. Gunn and Platt, studying the problem of coordination for the National Health Council, have recommended a thorough reorganization of the council on a national level, and the establishment of *one* unified and central voluntary health agency in each community.

The tendency of interested persons to form a health agency for the control of one disease, or *cause,* has resulted in a duplication of effort in fund raising, administration, and actual service to the public. The recommended reorganization is in line with the recent emphasis on the treatment of a person, and complete health service to a family, in contrast to the treatment of a disease. Some health and welfare agencies are very successful in providing a total centralized health, recreational, and welfare service to families. A good example of this is the former service at Peckham, England. The work of this community center is described as *The Peckham Experiment*[32, 33] by those who developed it, and the reports deserve careful study. This philosophy has had a marked influence in many countries; the positive achievements set an example, and the weaknesses that resulted in its closing serve as a warning.

Voluntary health agencies are more properly designed to perform the services not supplied by official agencies. Until recently they have offered the major share of the person-to-person health service in this country. It is not so easy to say this now with the extension of service in recent years by official agencies. Dean A. Clark reports in the *Social Work Year Book* for 1949 that 78 per cent of all hospital beds of all types are owned and operated by federal, state, and local governments. The federal government has assumed the responsibility for the care of veterans, the armed services, the Indians, certain other government employees, and seamen. State governments provide care for the mentally ill and the tuberculous, and give many special services, such as rehabilitation.

Gunn and Platt define a voluntary health agency as:

An organization that is administered by an autonomous Board which holds meetings, collects funds for its support chiefly from private sources, and expends money, whether with or without paid workers, in conducting a program directed primarily to furthering the public health by providing health services or health education, or by advancing research or legislation related to health, or by a combination of these activities.*

It is clear that public and private health agencies are giving the same kind of service. The scope of each is a controversial question which cannot be discussed here in any detail.

Voluntary agencies are classified according to the area served, as international, national, state, and local, and may be grouped in various way according to their chief function as child welfare agencies, convalescent homes, psychiatric clinics, etc.

Many national voluntary agencies join forces to form an *international* agency. The governing body is often made up of the national presidents. The International Council of Nurses is an example.

All professional groups of health workers have *national* organizations. Examples of these are: the American Nurses' Association, the American Medical Association, and the National Dietetic Association. There are other national agencies whose membership includes various types of workers who unite to carry forward a special

* Gunn, Selskar M., and Platt, Phillip S.: *Voluntary Health Agencies*. Ronald Press, New York, 1945, pp. 15–16.

aspect of the national health program. Examples of such agencies are the American Heart Association, the National Tuberculosis Association, the National Committee for Mental Hygiene, the National Association for the Prevention of Blindness, and the American Society for the Control of Cancer.

Such agencies as have been mentioned vary greatly in their functions. Some are service organizations; others raise funds with which they aid either official or non-official agencies to administer a health service; many of them put all their efforts into health education and research. All together, they play an important part in the total health program.

Since it is difficult to administer any sort of service on a national scale, it will be seen that most of the private national health organizations operate through *state organizations*. In some cases the work started within the state and spread throughout the country, and in other instances the original organization was a national one and from its membership the state chapters, committees, or associations were formed. All professional health workers have state organizations. Membership dues for the state organization ordinarily include the fee that gives the individual membership in the national organization. National organizations tend to form state units, and state units are again broken up into *local units*. In nursing, for example, the American Nurses' Association has state branches, and state associations have district branches; these district organizations may cover an area of from one to ten or more counties. The American Medical Association has the same type of organization. The association for the control of tuberculosis has state and local chapters as well as a national organization.

Besides the local health agencies that are a part of a parent organization, there are many independent local agencies. Some of the more important of these are hospitals, clinics, visiting nurse associations, convalescent homes, and research laboratories.

All communities need a coordinating council of social agencies. The systematic exchange of data on families served by health and welfare agencies is important. Effective methods of referring families to agencies is also essential. Community health councils are rapidly increasing in number and usefulness.

6. SOCIAL AGENCIES IN THE COMMUNITY INDIRECTLY CONCERNED WITH HEALTH PROMOTION

It is difficult to distinguish between the organizations that are designed primarily to promote health and those that indirectly affect the health of the people in a community. The following definition of *public health* given in the *Social Work Year Book,* suggests a wide range of activities and the necessity for many types of organizations.

The term *public health* comprehends the sum of all of those measures designed to postpone mortality and to promote the health and physical well-being of the population concerned. The state of the public health is everywhere and always influenced by a multitude of factors. Hardly any great change whether economic, social, or technological fails to have direct and often recognizable influence on the health of large numbers of people. It is the task of public health to promote the beneficial and minimize the harmful effects of our changing environment. A broad conception of the general principles of health work includes the whole field of curative as well as preventive medicine. Provision for furnishing each individual in the community with the best attainable hygienic supervision and medical care, under economic conditions which will make their utilization easy of attainment, is necessary.*

Accepting such a definition and the implication that health means a normal mental and physical state, it is easy to see that almost all of our social institutions have some effect upon health. For instance, a vocational placement service may help the handicapped to establish his maximum potential mental health just as truly as a physical therapy service helps him regain the use of his muscles. Schools for the deaf, the dumb, and the blind are of more use to such persons than hospitals; juvenile and family relation courts are close kin to the mental hygiene clinics; and nursery schools provide expert guidance for young children and help prevent physical defects and abnormal behavior. All of these agencies and many others play such an important part in the total health program of the community that nurses cannot afford not to know about them or to ignore their own responsibility for cooperation with such agencies.

The American Association of Social Workers publishes the *Social Work Year Book* which lists and gives the functions of the most important national agencies and many state agencies. It also summarizes trends in health administration and legislation. This national directory is a useful tool. Every health worker should have for reference also a directory of the social agencies in his or her community. Agencies are usually grouped according to function and the functions listed alphabetically, so that if a physician or a nurse wants to send a patient to a convalescent home it is a simple matter to find a suitable one. All those concerned with nursing should learn to help others make the most effective use of the facilities at their disposal.

7. PLACE OF THE HOSPITAL IN THE COMMUNITY HEALTH PROGRAM

The concept of the function of the hospital is changing so rapidly, and hospitals vary so much in character, that it is hard to describe the position of the average present-day hospital in the community and harder still to say what it will be in ten years. Most people in this country think of a hospital as concerned primarily with the care of the sick; they are also accustomed to think of it as a practice field in which to learn the medical arts. The functions of research, preventive medicine, health education, and total rehabilitation of the chronically sick and handicapped are not so generally expected by the public, or assumed by the hospital. The typical voluntary hospital of the past, and even of the present, is

* Kurtz, Russell H. (ed.): *Social Work Year Book 1937: A Description of Organized Activities in Social Work and in Related Fields.* Russell Sage Foundation, New York, 1937, p. 365.

more or less autonomous, and if it is not supported by a community fund it may be practically independent of all other community agencies except the regional health department with which it must cooperate in such things as reporting births and deaths, and communicable disease.

This latter type of institution is passing and in its place there will be hospitals that are an interlocking part of a regional plan for providing a total medical and health program. Such regional planning often crosses state boundaries. Located at the hub, a "medical center" will offer all kinds of medical care and health

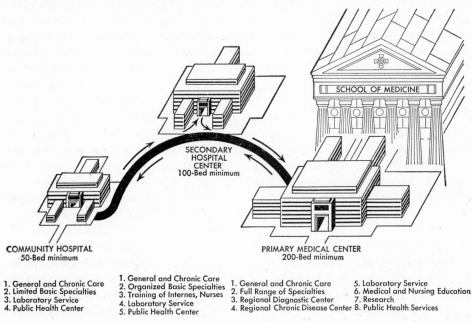

SCHOOL OF MEDICINE

SECONDARY
HOSPITAL
CENTER
100-Bed minimum

COMMUNITY HOSPITAL
50-Bed minimum

PRIMARY MEDICAL CENTER
200-Bed minimum

	1. General and Chronic Care		
1. General and Chronic Care	2. Organized Basic Specialties	1. General and Chronic Care	5. Laboratory Service
2. Limited Basic Specialties	3. Training of Internes, Nurses	2. Full Range of Specialties	6. Medical and Nursing Education
3. Laboratory Service	4. Laboratory Service	3. Regional Diagnostic Center	7. Research
4. Public Health Center	5. Public Health Center	4. Regional Chronic Disease Center	8. Public Health Services

Figure 4. Relationship of regional hospitals. Flow of patients and services, coordinated hospital plan, New York State. (From New York State Joint Hospital Survey and Planning Commission, Albany, New York, 1949, p. 12.)

service: medical care with its various special therapies, dental care, health education of the public and medical education for personnel, services of the public health department, and rehabilitation including vocational placement. Patients will receive care in the hospital and clinic, but from this center many kinds of workers will be sent to extend into his home the care the person needs. It is recognized that smaller regional hospitals should surround this medical center, giving such care as they are prepared to give with the help that can be gotten from the larger institution. Likewise, these smaller regional or "district hospitals" will be surrounded by emergency, often rural, units that can give a very limited service but that, nevertheless, can be valuable because, since they will be articulated with the district hospitals and the medical center, they can transfer and refer patients promptly to those institutions prepared to give them the help they need.[34, 35]

Many experiments with the closer incorporation of the hospital in a total scheme for health promotion are in progress. In Rochester, New York; Columbus, Georgia; in Barry County, Michigan; to mention a few places, steps have been taken in this direction. Montefiore and Bellevue Hospitals in New York City have made considerable contributions to the home care program, and the Institute of Physical Medicine and Rehabilitation in the latter hospital is a notable effort to extend the services of the civil hospital beyond the traditional limits.[36, 37, 38] The idea for a new pattern has been prevalent for a long time, but the old mold is hard to break. About twenty years ago the Committee on the Costs of Medical Care[39] recommended a unified type of health service to the community, emanating from a medical center. The Study Committee of the Joint Hospital Survey for New York made a similar recommendation for this metropolitan area in 1937. In that year John Ellis, writing on the place of the hospital in the community, said:

Few will disagree with the thesis that the hospital will increasingly be the central and strategic factor in medical care and medical education. Not many will deny that the hospital of the future is bound to be an important center of consultation service. . . .

In their external affairs, the hospitals must lose their intense individualism and become part of a broad social welfare program. They must realize that they are only one element in the community resources for the care of the sick. They must be integrated with other similar health services.

It is probable that the future will see the expansion of hospital councils, composed of trustees of voluntary institutions, public health officials, and public officers who are responsible for the support of indigents in need of hospitalization.*

One effect of this unification of medical service, of particular interest to nurses, is the wiping out of the line between what is now called public health nursing and institutional nursing. Visiting nurse organizations, both public and private, even at the present time have offices in hospitals, most often in the outpatient department. As medical centers develop out-service staffs—that is, physicians, nurses, and other workers who visit patients in their homes—it will be necessary to prepare institutional nurses for home nursing or to bring about a more thorough amalgamation of the various nursing groups in the community. This seems altogether desirable, since institutional workers will in this way become more conscious of the public's need for health teaching and the adjustment of social problems, and the public health worker will, through contact with a hospital, tend to keep in closer touch with the field of medical science.

As tax-supported hospital service extends its scope, the relationship with voluntary hospital service requires clarification and adjustment. It is part of the over-all question of how much medical care the American people want provided for them by government and how much they want left to private initiative. When this question is answered a little more definitely, a more satisfactory system of cooperation between public and private agencies can be developed.

* Ellis, W. John: "How Shall the Hospital Develop to Meet the Demand of the Future?" *Hospitals,* **11**:49, (Oct.) 1937.

8. WHAT THE NURSE AND OTHER HEALTH WORKERS SHOULD KNOW ABOUT THE COMMUNITY

Many useful types of service are given by persons who work from day to day without much thought of anything except what lies immediately before them. Some nurses, who are good technicians, work in this way, doing little to stimulate their imaginations or to broaden their concepts of nursing. Not seeing the larger problems, however, they may waste their energies worrying over trifles, and, like Chicken Little, run around crying that the skies are falling; or, if they are of a carefree disposition, they may be unconcerned when serious issues are at stake that will affect not only themselves but the profession as a whole and the public at large. Needless to say, those nurses, doctors, dentists, or medical social workers who recognize and live up to the responsibilities of their professions have the widest influence and probably derive the greatest satisfaction from their work. With the close cooperation between welfare groups that exists today and the promise of still greater unification of medical services, it does not seem possible for members of any of these professions to work with maximal effectiveness without knowing a good deal about the community.

In order to be a well-informed medical and health worker, it is desirable to have some knowledge along the following lines: (1) the nationalities, races, and religions represented by the people of the community and the characteristic ways of living among these different groups; (2) the general level of intelligence, the interest of people in, and their knowledge of, laws governing healthful living; (3) the economic status of persons living in different districts of the community; (4) the social agencies and the health facilities available to the people; (5) the local health government and its relationship to the state and national government; and (6) the machinery for the passage of health legislation and the ways in which the individual in the community may make his influence felt when questions affecting the health and welfare of the community are up for discussion before bodies of lawmakers. Nurses should welcome opportunities to keep up, through the daily newspapers, with what is going on locally; to observe the work of other health agencies; to take part in discussions of current health problems, and to work in coordinating committees and agencies.

SUMMARY

In estimating the resources of a nation, human life and the health of the people are said to exceed all other economic resources. While a growing health consciousness is apparent here and in many other countries, our knowledge of how to prevent and control disease far exceeds its application. The average life span has been increased 20 years since 1870 and the incidence of many diseases materially reduced, but conditions, for which the means of prevention and cure are well known, still rank high among the common causes of death. In order to raise health standards, the main problems seem to be the establishment of an economic status that provides people with the necessities of life, general education that will stimulate a desire for and knowledge of health, and the provision of adequate medical service and facilities. Intensive health-supervision programs, sponsored by philanthropic foundations, have demonstrated the effectiveness of such measures. An important factor in such health demonstrations has been the improvement and extension of community nursing services. The part that nursing care plays in raising health standards is recognized and has added not only to the dignity but to the interest of the nurse's work.

The necessity of cooperation among health workers was never greater or more generally emphasized than it is today. Realization that rapid modes of travel make it possible to spread infection from one continent to another in a few hours suggests the importance of an international program for the control of communicable disease, developing under the World Health Organization. Each country has its national plan of health work. States, counties, cities, and townships also have their health programs, and there is a definite relationship between the national, state, and local agencies. Where health work is carried on by governmental agencies and is supported by public funds (taxes and governmental forms of insurance), it is called *public health,* or *"socialized medicine"* if the service is of a medical nature. About one half the amount spent on medical care in this country comes from public funds. There are thousands of private, national, state, and local health agencies. These agencies are supported by gifts, membership fees, and patients' fees. There is a growing tendency to place the general direction of all the health work of a given locality in the hands of a community health council. Forward-looking groups and individuals are recommending that health districts be formed on the basis of population and resources of the area in place of the present county and municipal health units. The new health district would be served by a medical center and outlying coordinated district and rural hospitals. Hospitals would give not only hospital care (or in-service) to the people in their district but also all types of medical care in homes through an out-service department.

There are few, if any, public or private agencies giving medical care that do not consider the nurse an essential member of their staffs. She has taken an active part in health and morbidity programs and in medical research. It is significant that the period of time in which professional nursing has existed is also the period in which greatest advances have been made in medical science.

Because the health of an individual is so dependent upon food, shelter, clothing, and suitable occupation, the work of welfare agencies is difficult to classify into those that relate to health and those that do not. All types of welfare agencies are recognizing their interdependence and the importance of a more unified family health service. Medical workers are being urged to study the people, the conditions, and the health facilities within their communities in order that they may give the best possible service to the persons in their care. In almost every community better planning, closer coordination, and simplification of health services are needed.

REFERENCES

1. Dublin, Louis I., and Lotka, Alfred J.: *The Money Value of Man,* rev. ed. Ronald Press, New York, 1946, p. 5.
2. Stern, Bernhard J.: *American Medical Practice in the Perspectives of a Century.* Commonwealth Fund, New York, 1945, p. 108.
3. Hodges, Margaret B. (ed.): *Social Work Year Book 1951: A Description of Organized Activities in Social Work and in Related Fields.* American Association of Social Workers, New York, 1951, p. 304.
4. Dublin, Louis I.: *The Facts of Life from Birth to Death.* The Macmillan Company, New York, 1951, pp. 86-87.
5. Roche, Josephine: "Medical Care as a Public Health Function," *Am. J. Public Health,* **27:**1221, (Dec.) 1937.
6. Perrot, George St. J.: *Findings of Selective Service Examinations; New Steps in Public Health.* Milbank Memorial Fund, Annual Report, New York, 1945, p. 22.
7. Dublin, Louis I.: *op. cit.,* p. 84.
8. Stern, Bernhard J.: *op. cit.,* pp. 103-39.
9. Dublin, Louis I., and Lotka, Alfred J.: *Twenty-Five Years of Health Progress; A Study of the Mortality-Experience Among the Industrial Policy Holders of the Metropolitan Life Insurance Company.* Metropolitan Life Insurance Co., New York, 1937, p. 345.
10. Green, Howard W.: *Population Characteristics by Census Tracts.* Cleveland Plain Dealer Co., Cleveland, 1931.
11. Bernard, Claude: *Introduction to the Study of Experimental Medicine* (translated by Henry C. Greene). The Macmillan Company, New York, 1927.
12. Dublin, Louis I.: *op. cit.,* pp. 396-99.
13. US Social Security Administration, Bureau of Research and Statistics: *Medical Care and Costs in Relation to Family Income; A Statistical Source Book,* 2nd ed. US Government Printing Office, Washington, D.C., 1947, p. 54.
14. Roche, Josephine: *op. cit.*
15. Smillie, Wilson G.: *Public Health Administration in the United States,* 3rd ed. The Macmillan Company, New York, 147, pp. 103-9.
16. US Public Health Service: *Venereal Disease Fact Sheet, No. 6.* US Government Printing Office, Washington, D.C., 1949.
17. Clark, E. Gurney: "Is Venereal Disease No Longer a Problem?" *Am. J. Syph.,* **34:**401, (Sept.) 1950.
18. Van Blarcom, Carolyn C.: *Obstetrical Nursing,* 3rd ed. The Macmillan Company, New York, 1933, p. 461.
19. Harrell, Ruth F.; *Effect of Added Thiamine on Learning* (Contributions to Education No. 877). Teachers College, New York, 943, pp. 55-56.
20. Rennie, Thomas A. C., and Woodward, Luther E.: *Mental Health in Modern Society.* Commonwealth Fund, New York, 1948, p. 154.
21. US Bureau of the Census: *Hospitals: Statistics and Directory Section,* Part 2. US Government Printing Office, Washington, D.C., 1949, p. 16.
22. Mather, James M.: "Trends in Community Health Services," *Canad. J. Pub. Health,* **41:**381, (Sept.) 1950.
23. Gunn, Selskar M., and Platt, Phillip S.: *Voluntary Health Agencies.* Ronald Press, New York, 1945, p. 3.
24. Colcord, Joanna C.: *Your Community: Its Provision for Health Education, Safety and Welfare.* Russell Sage Foundation, New York, 1947.
25. Maxcy, Kenneth F. (ed.): *Rosenau's Preventive Medicine and Hygiene,* 7th ed. Appleton-Century-Crofts, Inc., New York, 1951, p. 1436.

26. Thorp, Willard L.: "New International Programs in Public Health," *Am. J. Pub. Health,* **40:**1479, (Dec.) 1950.
27. Reed, Lowell L.: "Local Responsibility for World Health," *Am. J. Pub. Health,* **40:**1363, (Nov.) 1950.
28. Mountin, Joseph W.: *Guide to Health Organization in the United States.* Public Health Service in the Federal Security Agency, Washington, D.C., 1946.
29. United States Government, Federal Register Division: *Organization Manual 1953-54.* National Archives and Record Service, General Services Administration, Washington, D.C., 1953.
30. Emerson, Haven, and Luginbuhl, Martha: *Local Health Units for the Nation.* Commonwealth Fund, New York, 1945, pp. 2, 12, 14, 329-33.
31. Hodges, Margaret B. (ed.): *Social Work Year Book 1949: A Description of Organized Activities in Social Work and in Related Fields.* Russell Sage Foundation, New York, 1949, p. 383.
32. Pearse, Innes, and Crocker, Lucy H.: *The Peckham Experiment: A Study of the Living Structure of Society.* Yale University Press, New Haven, 1944.
33. Chance, M. R. A.: "Where from Peckham," *Lancet,* **1:**726, (Apr.) 1950.
34. Mountin, Joseph W., et al.: *Health Service Areas: Requirements for General Hospitals and Health Centers.* US Public Health Service, Washington, D.C., 1945.
35. Ryder, Brooks: "Regionalization of Medical Services in New England," *Am. J. Pub. Health,* **40:**602, (May) 1950.
36. Slee, Vergil N., Director, Barry County Health Center, Hastings, Michigan: Personal communication to the writer.
37. Hilbert, Hortense: "Extending Hospital Care to the Home," *Pub. Health Nursing,* **41:**378, (July) 1949.
38. McGibony, J. R., and Block, Louis: "Better Patient Care Through Coordination," *Pub. Health Rep.,* **64:**1499, (Nov.) 1949.
39. Falk, Isidore S., et al.: *The Costs of Medical Care: A Summary of Investigations on the Economic Aspects of the Prevention and Care of Illness.* University of Chicago Press, Chicago, 1933, p. 426.

Additional Suggested Reading

Doull, James A., and Kramer, Morton: "The First World Health Assembly," *Pub. Health Rep.,* **63:**1379, (Oct.) 1948.
Emerson, Haven (ed.): *Administrative Medicine.* Thomas Nelson & Sons, New York, 1951.
Ewing, Oscar R.: *The Nation's Health: A Ten Year Program: Report to the President.* US Federal Security Agency, Washington, D.C., 1948.
"Incidence of Disease" (editorial), *Pub. Health Rep.,* **65:**548, (Apr.) 1950.
Kogel, Marcus D., and Kruger, Alexander W.: "New York City's Long-range Program for Extending Hospital Care into the Home," *Hospitals,* **24:**35, (Feb.) 1950.
Lawson, Mabel G.: "Nurses and the British National Health Service," *Am. J. Nursing,* **51:**31, (Jan.) 1951.
Mountin, Joseph W.: "Organizing for the Newer Public Health Programs," *Pub. Health Nursing,* **42:**562, (Oct.) 1950.
Mustard, Harry S.: *Government in Public Health.* Commonwealth Fund, New York, 1945.
————: *An Introduction to Public Health,* 3rd ed. The Macmillan Company, New York, 1953.
National Health Council: *The National Health Council and Its Member Organizations.* The Council, New York, 1948.
Rabson, S. M.: "Sudden and Unexpected Natural Death: V. Census of Death Classified by Sex and Age," *A.M.A. Arch. Int. Med.,* **86:**361, (Sept.) 1950.

"Reported Mortality Rates per 100,000 Population Continental United States 1933-48" (editorial), *J. Ven. Dis. Inform.*, **32**:81, (Mar.) 1951.

Richardson, Henry B.: *Patients Have Families.* Commonwealth Fund, New York, 1945.

Scheele, Leonard A.: "Cooperation Between Health and Welfare Agencies: A Health Officer's View," *Pub. Health Rep.*, **66**:163, (Feb.) 1951.

Sinai, Nathan, et al.: *Health Insurance in the United States.* Commonwealth Fund, New York, 1946.

Smillie, Wilson G.: *Preventive Medicine and Public Health,* 2nd ed. The Macmillan Company, New York, 1952.

Springett, V. H.: "A Comparative Study of Tuberculosis Mortality Rates," *J. Hyg.*, **48**:361, (Sept.) 1950.

US Social Administration, Bureau of Research and Statistics: *Medical Care and Costs in Relation to Family Income.* US Government Printing Office, Washington, D.C., 1947.

US Social Security Board, Bureau of Research and Statistics: *Medical Care Insurance: A Social Insurance Program for Personal Health Services* (79th Congress, 2nd Session, Senate Committee, Print No. 5). US Government Printing Office, Washington, D.C., 1946.

Whitby, Lionel: "Can Disease Be Prevented?" *Brit. M. J.*, **4691**:1272, (Dec.) 1950.

World Health Organization: "Charter," *J.A.M.A.*, **131**:1431, (Aug.) 1946.

————: *What It Is, What It Does, How It Works,* 4th ed. The Organization, Geneva, Switzerland, 1950.

CHAPTER 3. THE HOSPITAL

1. FUNCTIONS OF THE HOSPITAL

The Care of the Sick. The words *hospice, hotel,* and *hospital* all come from the same root, *hospes,* which means host. Hospitals were originally guesthouses for the shelter of the homeless and for the entertainment of travelers. In modern times, however, the chief function of the hospital has been the care and treatment of the sick. An increasing percentage of the sick go to hospitals as family living quarters decrease in size, as medical treatment grows more complex, and as hospital insurance brings the cost of hospitalization within the reach of many who couldn't otherwise afford it.

It was suggested in Chapter 2 that the hospital of the future would extend this care of the sick within its walls to the medical supervision and nursing care of the sick within the health district served by the hospital. Many hospitals have outpatient departments, or clinics, for the care of the ambulatory sick. Some maternity hospitals have had a well-organized delivery and post-partum "out-service" for many years. Generally speaking a home care program for the sick extending from the institution is a new development in hospital practice. This plan has so much promise that it was discussed at some length on page 49, as part of the general health program.

Health Supervision and Prevention of Disease. The preventive aspects of medical work have been given so much emphasis in all phases of medical practice that it would be strange indeed if hospital services had not been broadened in some places to include health supervision and preventive therapy. In their outpatient departments some hospitals are giving routine health examinations, supervision of women during pregnancy and the post-partum period, supervision of infants and well children, and other services to persons in normal conditions. Hospitals prevent the spread of disease by isolating patients with communicable conditions and help to raise the standard of health in the community by health teaching.

The hospital staff reduces the recurrence of disease by helping the patient to change those aspects of his way of life that led to illness. It is well recognized that unhappy personal relationships, uncongenial employment, lack of employment, or insecurity of any kind undermines health and induces disease. The patient's condition may improve temporarily while he is in the hospital, removed from his social problems, but if these problems remain unsolved when he goes home the condition that necessitated hospital care is likely to recur. One or more medical social workers are commonly assigned to each clinical service; their function is to help patients in the adjustment of financial difficulties, employment problems, securing suitable living conditions, and so on. Vocational guidance experts, psychologists, rehabilitation officers, nurses, physicians, and other workers in many hospitals contribute toward a rehabilitation program that prevents the recurrence of crippling conditions.

As the modern hospital extends its medical service to the sick in their homes, it seems reasonable to assume that it will provide for a more extensive health supervision within its health district. To what extent the organized care of the sick and public health service will, or should be, combined is discussed by Haven Emerson in Bachmeyer and Hartman's *The Hospital in Modern Society*.[1] Some communities are experimenting in a thorough amalgamation of health and morbidity services. The Commission on Hospital Care in the United States has said:

> The individual hospital is only one unit of a large, complex, and interrelated health program which should cover the entire community in which it operates. . . . Hospitals as a group alone and in association with organizations of physicians, nurses, and public health workers, have responsibility for developing a well-rounded, closely integrated service which meets all the health needs of all of the people.*

In Barry County, Michigan, the county hospital and the county health unit are under one roof, have one medical director, and have a unified record system. Hospitals in many cities that provide home care services keep the patients receiving this care on their roster, furnish patients with drugs and necessary equipment from the hospital, and have a unified record system. As the medical workers from the hospital find themselves serving patients in their homes, it is inevitable that they will see the patient's problem as related to the total family welfare and that their service will grow more and more into a family health service, combining preventive and morbidity aspects. Titles such as the "Responsibility of the Hospital in Realizing a Community Health Program"[2] are common in medical literature. In his monograph *Patients Have Families* Henry B. Richardson,[3] analyzing the effectiveness of the medical service given a family in a large metropolitan hospital, traces a large part of the illness in the mother and daughters to an uncorrected physical condition of the father. His conclusion that patients must be treated as members

* Commission on Hospital Care: *Hospital Care in the United States*. Commonwealth Fund, New York, and Harvard University Press, Cambridge, Mass., 1947, p. 610.

of the family (the social unit) goes unchallenged by most medical workers nowadays.

The Education of Medical Workers. Physicians, nurses, dietitians, social workers, physical therapists, hospital administrators, and others are taught within the hospital much of what they must learn in order to practice their professions. Without hospitals or their equivalents, it would be impossible to give an adequate preparation for almost any type of modern medical service.

Medical Research. With their laboratory facilities, trained personnel, numbers of patients, and accumulation of records, hospitals offer medical workers opportunities for investigation that are not available elsewhere. This research is thought to be such an important factor in the successful practice of medicine and in the advancement of medical science that all physicians seek, and are urged to make, some connection with a hospital.

It has been pointed out that there is a trend toward the establishment of a close association between the small rural hospitals and research centers and between all hospitals and other community health organizations in order that their personnel may have access to adequate research, diagnostic, and therapeutic facilities. The free flow of patients and workers to and from these research centers and district hospitals should foster all kinds of medical research.

2. CLASSIFICATION AND NUMBER OF HOSPITALS

Ways in Which Hospitals May Be Classified. Hospitals may be grouped according to (1) the *type of service* they offer the community and (2) their *ownership* or *control*. They are graded according to the *quality of service they give,* as measured by such hospital standards as those set by the American College of Surgeons.

Classification of Hospitals, According to Clinical Service Offered. Hospitals that treat many different kinds of conditions are called *general;* those that limit their services to one class of patients, or to persons who have the same kind of disease or condition, are *special* hospitals. The special hospitals include among others the following: maternity; children's; convalescent; chronic; eye, ear, nose, and throat; tuberculosis; orthopedic; skin and cancer; neurological; and mental hospitals.

In 6340 registered hospitals in this country in 1950 there were 1,456,912 beds. Of the total number of registered hospitals in the United States in 1948, 4589 were general hospitals. The largest group of special hospitals, 586, were for mental and nervous disorders. There were 438 hospitals for the care of the tuberculous. All other special hospitals totaled 722. A better comparison, however, is to say that roughly 50 per cent of the beds were in neuropsychiatric hospitals, 38 per cent in general hospitals, and 12 per cent in tuberculosis hospitals.[4]

The majority of our hospitals are small. About 70 per cent of the general hospitals have less than 100 beds. Too many of them are understaffed and poorly equipped. G. D. Crain, Jr.,[5] believes that there may be as many as 8000 hospitals in this country, which, if true, would mean that approximately 1500 are not registered. The upgrading of small hospitals through affiliations with larger hospitals and other agencies is discussed in this chapter.

Table 3. Number and Types of Hospital Beds in the United States, 1950*

TYPE OF HOSPITAL	HOSPITALS	BEDS	BASSINETS	ADMISSIONS	AVERAGE CENSUS
Total	100.0	100.0	100.0	100.0	100.0
Federal	5.5	12.8	2.7	6.6	11.7
Governmental, nonfederal	24.2	58.4	15.9	18.8	63.2
Private, nonprofit	49.3	25.3	71.5	66.1	22.4
Proprietary	21.0	3.5	9.9	8.5	2.7

* Dublin, Louis I.: *The Facts of Life from Birth to Death.* The Macmillan Company, New York, 1951, p. 90.

Classification According to Control.   Hospitals fall into two main classes, according to control and ownership; these are *governmental* and *nongovernmental*. Governmental hospitals are those owned by the federal government, that is, the hospitals of the Army, the Navy, the United States Public Health Service, the Bureau of Indian Affairs, and the Veterans Administration, and those owned by the state, city, and county governments. Governmental hospitals are sometimes called *public hospitals*. They may offer one or many types of clinical service.

Nongovernmental hospitals (70 per cent of the total in 1950) are owned by churches, fraternal orders, individuals or groups of individuals in partnership, by corporations, and by industries such as railroads. Nonprofit-making hospitals comprise about 80 per cent of the total number. If hospitals depend upon their earnings for support and are organized to make a profit on their services, they are designated as *proprietary* hospitals. About one fifth of the hospitals in this country in 1950 fell into this class; however, these hospitals are usually small, and out of the total hospital beds in this country only 3.5 per cent were in proprietary hospitals. The occupancy of governmental hospitals is relatively higher than that of nongovernmental institutions. There were over a million beds (71.2 per cent of the total) in governmental hospitals as against an approximate one-half million beds (28.8 per cent of the total) in nongovernmental hospitals. The average census in government hospitals was 74.9 as compared with 25.1 in nongovernmental hospitals.[6]

Supply of Hospital Care in Relation to Need.   The real need for hospital care, based on the demands of a definition of health such as that given on page 21, has not been met. On the basis of state surveys the US Public Health Service[6] estimated in 1949 that an additional 900,000 beds were needed. They set 12 beds per 1000 of the population as a possible goal. The Hospital Survey and Construction

Act passed in 1946 made federal funds available to states for hospital construction. This has increased and improved the distribution of facilities. The 1950 Census shows 6430 registered hospitals and 1,456,912 beds amounting to 9.6 beds per 1000 population, including the armed forces. An analysis of these figures shows that in some parts of the country the supply of hospital beds is more than double that in other parts. It is also clear that certain clinical specialties and age groups are provided for more adequately than others. For example, more beds are needed for the mentally ill, for those with communicable disease, particularly tuberculosis, and for the aged. Students of this subject urge that general hospitals include communicable disease and psychiatric units in their building plans since so many persons admitted to general hospitals for other conditions fall, after diagnosis, into one of these two categories, and that the special needs of elderly patients should be considered.[7, 8, 9]

Standardization of Hospitals. Medical groups have recommendations for hospital construction, organization, and practice that serve as standards by which the quality of hospital service can be measured. Hospital administrators, physicians, nurses, dietitians, and other medical workers hope by establishing standards to improve hospital service, but they are interested also in having some means of determining what institutions offer adequate educational opportunities for students in their respective fields. The national associations representing these professions have, therefore, either singly or in groups, set up standards of hospital construction and practice. The responsibility of the various agencies concerned was under analysis by a joint committee in 1952.

The American College of Surgeons at present surveys and grades hospitals having more than 25 beds, and the list of these hospitals is published annually, the institutions being classed as *fully approved, provisionally approved,* or *not approved.* The Council on Medical Education and Hospitals of the American Medical Association also surveys and grades hospitals, listing those that are suitable and those that are unsuitable for medical education.[10, 11]

An attempt has been made through a number of studies to set minimal standards of hospital nursing care although nursing has not been represented on major standardizing bodies. The most tangible result is the recommendation for minimum hours of nursing care per patient, these hours varying with the type of service. In the *Hospital Nursing Service Manual,*[12] for example, it is recommended that provision be made for an average of 3 to 3½ hours of nursing care for adult medical patients in each 24 hours, 2½ to 3 hours for obstetrical cases (mothers), and 4½ hours for sick children from 2 to 5 years, and so on. Standards such as these, based on current rather than ideal practice, are often misleading.

There is always danger in using standards arbitrarily and in applying standardization to human behavior, which cannot be standardized, but there is little doubt that the standardization movement has improved hospital practice. While much has been accomplished in this direction, there are many technical aspects of hospital work, such as the process of sterilization, preparation of supplies, and the design of equipment, that could and should be standardized.

3. POSITION OF THE PATIENT IN THE HOSPITAL

Responsible adults go to and leave the hospital of their own free will. Exceptions to this are the psychiatric patient who is committed to an institution and the person who is under legal custody. Children and temporarily irrational patients are brought to hospitals by parents or guardians. If such patients leave the institution when the results of this step are injurious or disastrous, the institution may be sued for negligence. In case a patient demands his discharge from the hospital against the advice of the physician and refuses to sign a statement to this effect, the physician should tell him in the presence of several persons what the results may be. For the protection of the medical staff and the hospital, the patient's record should contain the physician's witnessed statement of the circumstances and what was said. Patients with communicable diseases are subject to public health regulations, and may not be free to leave the hospital except under conditions that will give full protection to others.

Treatment cannot in most cases be legally forced upon a rational adult patient nor can parents be made to agree, in most instances, to have their child treated in any manner of which they disapprove. When the patient or his guardian shows marked lack of confidence in the prescribed treatment, however, the physician usually prefers to give up the case. For the protection of the surgeon and the hospital, the patient or his guardian always signs a statement of consent to any operation that is to be performed. It is only in an emergency in which life is endangered that a surgeon assumes responsibility for operating without this written permission.[13]

The position of the patient in the hospital is that of a paying guest. Even when he is unable to pay his own fees, the public or the community finances his stay in the hospital, and the hospital staff itself is not "giving" its services.

Hospitals are organized to serve the public—they depend upon patients for their existence, and their personnel should try to make these institutions what the thoughtful members of the community want them to be. The average person going to a hospital probably expects, primarily, adequate medical attention from the various professional groups concerned with his care; in addition to this, he expects the same provision for his physical comfort and protection he would find in a good hotel. In some cases this may be as much as the individual desires or needs, but in many instances, it is not. Sick persons are often thrown off their balance—they are dependent, sensitive, frightened, and emotional, so that they want and need the kindness, consideration, and support they would get from their family and friends if they were at home. This element in hospital care, which is neither technical competence nor efficient institutional management, is what makes the patient's position in the institution a difficult one to define. The recognition of this element by the hospital staff or their failure to recognize it accounts in a large measure for the popularity of some hospitals and the unpopularity of others.

4. COST OF HOSPITAL CARE

The American Hospital Association in 1949 estimated that the hospitals in this country represented an investment of more than 6½ billion dollars. The capital investment is provided almost entirely by the general public, either through taxation or voluntary contributions. Government hospitals provide care for over 95 per cent of the neuropsychiatric patients and the majority of tuberculous patients; the federal government provides medical care for Army and Navy personnel, veterans, and Indians.

The average cost per patient day rose from $3.25 in 1930 to $13.09 in 1948. Louis I. Dublin[14] gives the figure $14.06 for 1948 and says that the average income per patient per day in general hospitals was $11.74. Nathaniel W. Faxon[15] discussing the cost of hospital care in *The Hospital in Contemporary Life* notes, however, that the per capita income has risen in direct proportion to the cost of hospitalization. (He thinks that we could meet the increased cost if we did not spend an excessive amount of the national income on liquor, tobacco, cosmetics, and other nonessentials. See p. 22.) Obviously the cost varies with the quality of the accommodations, the service given to the patient, the part of the country in which the institution is located, current salaries, the price of commodities, and other factors. It should be borne in mind also that these figures are based on the kind of care that was given at that time, which may or may not have been of such quality as to be of optimal benefit to the patient.

After all possible sources of waste are eliminated within the hospital, there is obliged to be an increase in the cost of care as standards of care are raised. Good hospital care depends not alone upon the ability of the personnel to provide it. The public must decide how much it will pay for hospital care, or, in other words, what quality of care it desires. The hospital administration must make every effort to help in the solution of this problem by expending the funds that are available on those aspects of care that will contribute most to the patient's total and ultimate welfare.

5. LOCATION AND PHYSICAL PLAN OF THE HOSPITAL

Location.   A hospital should be accessible to the people of the area that it serves. When it is possible, a site should be selected that has the advantages of quiet, beautiful surroundings, and freedom from smoke, dust, and odors. An elevated site is often chosen because it affords the possibility of better light, ventilation, drainage, and a spacious outlook. Mental hospitals, convalescent homes, and tuberculosis sanatoria are usually built in the suburbs or the country in order to make it economically possible to provide ample grounds. When a person has an acute illness and recovers rapidly, progress is not so much affected by the surroundings; on the other hand, beauty and harmony in the environment may be a most important therapeutic agent in the treatment of a mental or physical disorder that runs a long and tedious course.

While Blue Cross patients in 1950 had an average hospital stay of 7.5 days (an increase over war years), there are mounting numbers of patients with degenerative diseases who average 122 days of disability or illness, orthopedic impairments with 306 days disability, and neuropsychiatric patients with 190 days disability.[16]

Plan and Structure of Buildings. Hospitals are often beautiful in outline and in detail. Old and new they represent some of the most interesting buildings in the world. *Styles in hospital architecture* have changed with the demands of present-day life, the new methods of steel construction in building, and our modern concept of beauty.

During the first quarter of the century, a period of great hospital expansion, hospitals were often built on the pavilion plan. This is a series of buildings connected by corridors. A pavilion is usually devoted to a special clinical service or class of patient. This pattern was thought to be ideal because an outside exposure was made possible for every room, and, since each pavilion was operated more or less independently, the plan combined the merits of the large and small institution.

Lately, there has been a marked change in the architectural trend. Ours is sometimes spoken of as the "vertical age of architecture," and so we see hospitals climbing into the skies along with other public buildings. New types of steel structure have made skyscrapers possible, and they have the advantages, even in a congested district, of sunlight, a view from the windows, and some relief from the noise of traffic.

Another reason for a compact style of architecture is that it is believed to be more efficient to centralize many hospital services. Patients can be admitted and discharged through one department, operations performed in one suite of operating rooms, physical therapy concentrated as much as possible in a centrally located department, diets prepared in one main kitchen, equipment sterilized in one place, and supplies issued from one storeroom. The rambling pavilion type of hospital presents a more difficult problem in the transportation of patients and supplies to and from these central departments than does the vertical plan in which elevator service provides a rapid means of transportation.

In general, new buildings show the simplicity of outline and the integrity of design characteristic of modern architecture. The expert hospital designer, however, takes into account the architecture of the locality and adapts this style in such a way as to make the hospital building fit into the community and at the same time fulfill its functions.

The general scheme, decoration, and furnishing of the building are affected by the amount of money available. In highly endowed institutions handsome accommodations may be found for patients and staff. Where hospital grounds are limited, as in metropolitan areas, roof gardens are seen as substitutes. Buildings are often constructed so that practically every patient has access to a porch or balcony. Sitting rooms furnished with recreational facilities are provided on each corridor for patients and their visitors. Patients' rooms frequently have adjoining baths, suites are available for persons who wish to have a member of their family stay with them, and dining room accommodations for convalescent patients and their visitors are provided. In hospitals for convalescents and those not acutely ill we find many types of recreation rooms, and it is not unusual in children's hospitals to see nursery schools and classrooms for older children.

With the present emphasis on early ambulation and the maintenance of as normal living as possible during any illness there will be a more marked change in hospital

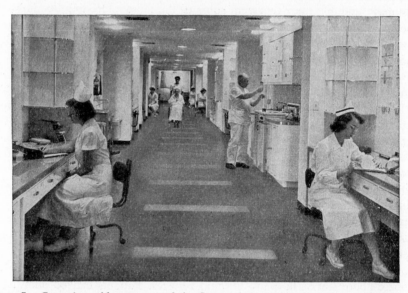

Figure 5. Central corridor on one of the floors of the Kaiser Foundation Medical Center is restricted to physicians, nurses, and other hospital personnel and is exclusively a work corridor. Visitors are routed through other corridors, thereby eliminating hospital traffic congestion.

Decentralized nurses' stations (*left and right foreground*) permit faster and more personal care and cut nurses' walking to one seventh that of the conventional floor plans. Nurses work in one unit only, and since at least one graduate nurse is part of the staff for each unit, the traditional "head nurse" is unnecessary.

Each clinical unit has eight beds, and each two-bed room is provided with complete bathroom facilities. Rooms open onto this corridor used by hospital personnel and onto an outer corridor used by patients and visitors. (Courtesy of Kaiser Foundation Medical Center, Los Angeles, Calif.)

construction. Hospitals will look more like hotels, clubs, or dwellings, and there will be more rooms in which patients can congregate for meals and recreation. As patients are encouraged to move about the hospital and to acquire or maintain their independence, the following conditions and facilities should be provided: (1) Sufficient space between beds or other furnishings to make it possible for patients in wheelchairs or on crutches to move about freely; (2) doorways, even those to bathroom cubicles and telephone booths, large enough to admit a wheelchair; (3) ramps as substitutes for steps; (4) railings along corridors, as well as beside toilets and bathtubs; (5) greatly increased bathroom facilities with tubs so arranged that those helping a patient with a bath can stand on either side of the tub; (6) tubs provided with seats so that weak and elderly patients can sit during a bath and a surgical patient with an abdominal dressing can take a tub bath and keep the dressing dry; (7) improved facilities for washing the hair and cleaning the mouth and for all aspects of the toilet; (8) conference rooms where groups of patients may assemble for the discussion of common health problems; (9) rooms equipped so that patients can learn to launder clothing, use a stove and a refrigerator, get across a street or mount a bus with whatever handicap illness or accident may have brought them; and (10) recreational facilities such as game rooms, libraries, radios, television, movies, pianos, studios and shops for arts and crafts and even for learning certain trades. Pedestal tables in libraries, shops, recreational, dining, and other communal rooms will make it possible for patients in wheelchairs to work, eat, and enjoy recreation with others.

If general hospitals are designed to meet present-day needs more completely, they will include special divisions for the care of patients with communicable and psychiatric conditions. All hospitals should have some rooms so well insulated that noisy, excited patients will not disturb others; provision should also be made for protection of irrational, suicidal, and homicidal patients.

In new hospitals and in an increasing number of existing hospitals, *patient-nurse intercommunication systems* are being installed. This system provides a two-way voice communication between the patient and the nurse; at the same time the customary signal light over the door of the patient's room and a corresponding light in the nurse's floor station flash on. Such an intercommunication system is reassuring to the patient because he knows his call is receiving immediate attention; it also means that time is saved for the nursing staff since a trip to the patient's unit to find out what he wants or needs is unnecessary. Intercommunication systems are made so that the patient can turn off the mechanism in order to ensure privacy during visiting hours and when he so desires.

With the recognized shortage of nurses and other more highly prepared workers a greater effort will be made to provide centralized workrooms, as in hotels, where equipment may be cared for and dispensed by personnel employed for this purpose. Utility rooms for individual services will be constructed to make better use of laborsaving machinery and to encourage the use of non-nursing personnel for all cleaning, sorting and dispensing of linen, clothing, toilet articles, and medical supplies.

The most carefully planned institutions provide ample and convenient working space for the personnel and at the same time arrange workrooms so that they cannot be seen by patients and visitors; likewise business offices are detached from the main lobby of the hospital. Space is allocated for hostesses, information clerks, and messengers at entrances to the hospital and the clinical divisions, not only to provide attention and direction for patients and visitors but also to prevent the interruption of work by medical and nursing personnel. In the clinical divisions, offices are provided for the medical and nursing staffs. A separate room should be set aside for the purpose of reporting and recording. Service, treatment, and storage rooms as well as elevators are centrally located on each division, but are made as inconspicuous as possible and treated in various ways to muffle noise. (Stairways and elevator shafts are often enclosed for the control of noise and fire.) Sitting rooms and dressing rooms for the nursing staff on the clinical divisions are not unusual. Clinical classrooms and conference rooms on each service facilitate the instruction of patients and any groups of students there may be in the hospital. Throughout the building, corners and edges are rounded, and crevices of all kinds are avoided to make cleaning and general upkeep as easy as possible.

The *protection of patients and personnel* is safeguarded in modern hospitals as it never has been in the past. Buildings are constructed almost entirely of fireproof materials. Metal doors that seal off one section of a building are used to localize fires if they occur. Extinguishing devices that surround the fire with a noninflammable gas, or sprinkling systems, are installed in some institutions. Automatic alarms and other features in hospital buildings lessen the danger of fire. Mechanical devices, such as furnaces, boilers, elevators, and sterilizers, are installed in duplicate so that hospital operations will not be delayed during periods when repairs are made. Skeleton lighting systems operated on batteries are provided in some cases, so that, if catastrophes occur that put the community power plant out of working order, this independent unit is available. Hospital windows are designed so that they will not open far enough to allow any one to fall through them, elevators will not move while the doors are open, and in many other ways hospital buildings have been improved to protect those who use them.

Concealed methods of *lighting* enhance the appearance, comfort, and efficiency of modern hospitals. Good natural lighting and ventilation with large, low, and well-spaced windows are noticeable in most new structures. *Modern heating systems* are automatically controlled, with the units often concealed in floors and ceilings. As air conditioning becomes more general our common methods of heating and ventilating undergo marked changes. At the present time some institutions are air-conditioned throughout, and many hospitals have installed this system in special departments, such as operating suites, and in clinical services for the treatment of allergies.

Interior decoration of hospitals has undergone a marked change. In the beginning of what we consider the modern public health movement, sanitation was the keynote. William Ernest Henley in this verse expressed a common impression of the hospital:

> My confidence all gone,
> The gray-haired soldier-poster waves me on,
> And on I crawl and still my spirits fail—
> These corridors and stairs of stone and iron,
> Cold, naked, clean—half work-house and half jail.*

Early in the century the typical hospital was bare and usually white; tiles and painted iron furniture were everywhere. Carbolic acid and formaldehyde odors were

* Henley, William Ernest: *In Hospital*. Thomas B. Mosher, Portland, Maine, 1908, pp. 3, 5.

so pervasive that everything and everyone in the hospital smelled of them. Henley said, "The atmosphere suggests the trail of a ghostly druggist." Outside the institution staff members were often told on introduction: "You must be a doctor," or "You must be a nurse." In an effort to make the hospital "sanitary," curtains, rugs, pictures, and unnecessary objects were removed from the patient's rooms and even from the entrance halls, dining rooms, and corridors. The average hospital was a very austere place. Lately there has been a reaction against the forbidding appearance of such institutions. *Color* is used freely in walls, floor coverings, and draperies; windows are treated more or less as they are in homes. Many hospitals have so far departed from the "sanitary tradition" as to have pictures on the walls of patients' rooms. (It is interesting to note in this connection that Florence Nightingale suggested changing the pictures in rooms for the sick as a means of diversion for the patients.) Hospitals for the well-to-do and a few private psychiatric hospitals look like fine inns or hotels.

Floors may be made of plastic, cork, wood, tiling, terrazzo, or marble. These materials are often used in several colors to make a pattern. To lessen fatigue and muffle the sound of footsteps on the harder floors, areas on which people stand or walk constantly are covered with a resilient material, such as linoleum or cork.

Walls are usually painted with washable paint. Pastel shades are most often used in patients' rooms. Stronger colors are found in reception and dining rooms. The walls of lobbies, libraries, auditoriums, and other public rooms may be paneled or made of marble. Walls are insulated to make room temperature more equable and to reduce heating costs. Walls built of two layers of porous blocks with a heavy paper between insulate and reduce noise. Ceilings are often covered with sound-absorbing materials to cut down the *noise* made within a room. Silent mercury light switches and improved plumbing have still further controlled the noise in hospitals.

The costliest hospitals are not necessarily the most pleasing to look at or the most convenient. Efficiency is achieved through wise planning and organization; beauty, by good proportions, harmonious color combinations, and suitable furnishings. All that is essential to the recovery of the patient, as a matter of fact, may be provided in very simple surroundings. There is a good deal of danger that medical workers who learn to take care of patients, and some patients who recover in luxurious hospitals, may be poorly prepared to deal with the problem of sickness in the average home. In hospital planning, as in all phases of health work, essentials should be stressed and provided before attention is given or money spent on nonessentials. Nurses and all other major groups of the hospital staff should be represented on planning committees.

6. ORGANIZATION OF THE HOSPITAL

A Typical Plan of Organization. With hospitals under the ownership and control of governments, churches, universities, industries, and individuals, it is not surprising to find differences in hospital organization. There are, however, certain

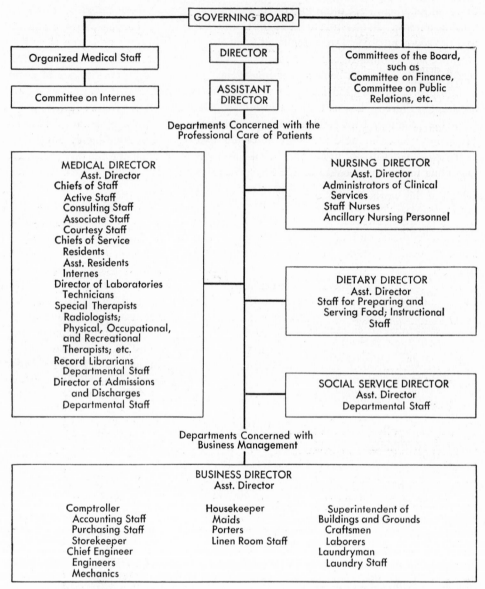

Figure 6. Organization of a hospital. (*Note:* It is the opinion of the writer that rehabilitation is a joint responsibility of all clinical services, and, therefore, no special department is shown.) (After MacEachern, M. T.: *Hospital Organization and Management*, rev. ed. Physicians Record Co., Chicago, 1940.)

features of organization common to many hospitals, and Figure 6 represents the organization plan of a typical hospital.

In almost every hospital there is a body that may be known as the board of governors, trustees, or directors. The American Hospital Association defines the duties of this board as follows:

To determine the policies of the institution with relation to community needs.

To see that professional standards are maintained in the care of the sick.

To coordinate the professional interests of the hospital with administrative, financial, and community needs.

To direct the administrative personnel of the hospital in order to carry out the above policies.

To provide adequate financing both as to securing a sufficient income and as to enforcing businesslike control of expenditure.*

Much of this work may be accomplished through committees, and this central board may delegate authority to its committees, to the medical staff, and to the chief executive officer. This officer, who is given the title of superintendent in some hospitals, or director in others, administers the policies of the board of directors and is responsible to them for the successful management of the institution. Obviously, it is impossible for one person to be an authority in all the various departments of the hospitals; therefore, each special aspect of the work is under a director of that division, and the director of the hospital delegates to these persons the authority that enables them to operate their departments effectively. Malcolm T. MacEachern[17] gives two main divisions of hospital work: the first is concerned with "business management," and the other with the "professional care of patients." The auditing, purchasing, issuing of supplies, engineering, housekeeping, laundry, and supervision of buildings and grounds comes under business administration. Each of these departments is in charge of a supervisor who may be responsible to the business director, or in smaller institutions to the director of the hospital. The medical, nursing, dietary, and social service departments are jointly concerned with the professional care of patients. Each department has a director, and under each departmental director are varying numbers of assistants and supervisors who are in charge of smaller divisions of work within the department.

The Relationship of the Hospital to Professional Schools. Students of medicine, nursing, physical therapy, occupational therapy, social service, or hospital administration may all be found in hospitals. There are many hospitals, however, in which there are no students of any kind. If there are students the organization of the hospital and the organization of the schools it controls, or with which it is affiliated, should be separate and distinct and the relationship of the two organizations clearly defined.

The director of any one of these professional schools may be a person who holds no hospital appointment. In many cases, however, the director is at the head of one of the departments of the hospital. For example, the director of the nursing

* American Hospital Association and American College of Hospital Administrators: *Code of Hospital Ethics*. American Hospital Association, Chicago, 1941, p. 3.

school may also be the director of the nursing service. In this case she has two distinct functions. As director, or dean of the school, she is responsible to the governing board of the school; as the director of the nursing service she is responsible to the director of the hospital. The director of the school has various administrative and teaching assistants, or instructors. Some of these instructors also may be members of the hospital staff. When such persons hold joint appointments they are responsible to the director of the nursing service for the performance of their hospital duties and to the director of the school for the performance of their educational function.

Students may pay a fee to the hospital for its use as a practice field; the benefits to the institution may be thought to cancel the benefits to the individual; or the hospital may pay the student for his or her services during the learning period. If the student is a paid member of the hospital personnel, the institution must assume responsibility for the student's work and may demand a reasonably high standard of performance and conformity to hospital regulations. Because of the serious nature of hospital work, there is in all cases a distinct understanding between the hospital and school authorities to the effect that students' activities are to be confined to those that they can perform without danger to others, that students use methods acceptable to the institution, and that they work under the supervision of the hospital staff when adequate supervision is not provided by the school.

SUMMARY

The modern hospital is an institution that is still chiefly concerned with the care of the sick, but a great deal of health service is given in hospitals, and representative professional groups are recommending that hospitals serve as centers in which most, or all, preventive and curative medical services of the community are coordinated. Under this coordinated plan the health center's staff would supply or supervise medical care in the hospital and in the homes of the area it serves. Experience outside the hospital makes doctors, nurses, and other hospital personnel more effective; on the other hand, access to hospital facilities and a knowledge of newer methods of treatments as developed in the hospital add competence to the private practitioner and the visiting nurse. The continuity of medical and nursing care for the patient that is possible under this coordinated program has unlimited promise.

Hospitals are classified according to the type of service they give and their control. About two thirds of all the hospitals in this country are general hospitals —that is, they admit patients with many different kinds of conditions. Of the special hospitals, the largest group is the one in which patients with mental diseases are treated. There are more beds in institutions for the care of persons with mental diseases than there are in the general hospitals.

Hospitals may be owned and administered by the federal, state, or local government, in which case they are called *governmental or public* hospitals; or they may be owned by individuals or groups of individuals, in which case they are called *nongovernmental or private* hospitals. Professional organizations have set standards for hospital construction and operation. The practice of surveying hospitals, grading them by these standards and publishing the results, is a large factor in the improvement of hospitals.

The patient in the hospital is ordinarily there of his own free will. He may accept or reject the proposed medical treatment, and leave at any time. If the individual is not responsible for his actions, a member of his family or a friend serves as his guardian, and holds the hospital staff accountable for the patient's protection. Persons committed to mental hospitals, prisoners of the law undergoing medical treatment, and persons with communicable diseases are free to leave the institution only under certain conditions.

The majority of hospitals are nonprofit-making. Hospital care is expensive, and since sickness often reduces the person's earning capacity, more than 37 million persons were enrolled in 1950 in the Blue Cross, or voluntary hospital insurance plan, which enabled them to distribute the expense of hospitalization over the entire year. The cost of hospital care for the indigent patient is met by the community, or by individuals or societies in the community. Hospital facilities in this country are unevenly distributed, certain communities, economic classes, and disease groups being more adequately provided for than others.

There is a marked improvement in hospital architecture, both without and within. The hospital of the present day is likely to be built as a compact unit in order to make its operation economical. It is constructed in such a way that it is well ventilated, well lighted, uniformly heated, and in some cases air-conditioned. The stark whiteness and drab coloring of past years are giving way to a much more varied and interesting use of color. Colorfast dyes, improved methods of cleaning fabrics, and changing conceptions of sanitation and bacteriology—all make it possible to furnish sitting rooms and bedrooms in hospitals as they are furnished in homes. Modern hospitals are not only more convenient and more attractive in appearance but also are safer than those built in former times. The hazards of fire, mechanical injury, and infection are reduced by improved design and construction.

Hospital organization varies considerably in different institutions, but there are some features that are almost universal. An understanding on the part of the staff of the principles of hospital administration and of the specific organization plan of the institution stimulates cooperation and efficiency in hospital operation. The governing board, the executive officers, the staff workers, and students should know what their functions are and for what, and to whom, they are held responsible. A hospital has atmosphere, or personality, that does not lend itself to analysis. It is almost impossible to enumerate the factors that contribute toward either a pleasant or an unpleasant atmosphere, but mutual understanding and respect. the recognition of common standards of work, and a common goal are certainly some important elements. Medical care has become so complex that the highest quality of medical service is achieved only through coordinating the efforts of many persons.

REFERENCES

1. Bachmeyer, Arthur C., and Hartman, Gerhard (eds.): *The Hospital in Modern Society.* Commonwealth Fund, New York, 1943, p. 747.
2. Groulx, Adélard: "Responsibility of the Hospital in Realizing a Community Health Program," *Canad. Hosp.,* **27:**30, (Aug.) 1950.
3. Richardson, Henry B.: *Patients Have Families.* Commonwealth Fund, New York, 1945.
4. US Bureau of the Census: *Hospitals: Statistics and Directory Section—June, Part 2.* US Government Printing Office, Washington, D.C., 1949.
5. Crain, G. D., Jr.: "We Need Official U.S. Census of Hospitals," *Hosp. Management,* **70:**39, (Nov.) 1950.
6. US Public Health Service: *The Nation's Needs for Hospitals and Health Centers.* US Government Printing Office, Washington, D.C., 1949, p. 33.
7. McDougall, J. B.: "Role and Responsibility of the General Hospital in the Diagnosis and Treatment of Tuberculosis," *Bull. World Health Organ.,* **3:**325, 1950.
8. Kline, Carl L.: "Should the General Hospital Provide Psychiatric Services?" *Wisconsin M. J.,* **49:**901, (Oct.) 1950.
9. Sternberg, M. R.: "The General Hospital in Community Planning for the Aged," *Geriatrics,* **5:**231, (July-Aug.) 1950.
10. American College of Surgeons: *Manual of Hospital Standardization.* The College, Chicago, 1946.
11. Allen, Arthur W.: "The Hospital Standardization Program of the American College of Surgeons," *Bull. Am. Coll. Surgeons,* **36:**22, (Jan.) 1951.
12. American Hospital Association and National League of Nursing Education: *Hospital Nursing Service Manual.* National League of Nursing Education, New York, 1950, p. 30.
13. Hayt, Emanuel, and Hayt, Lillian R.: *Legal Guide for American Hospitals.* Hospital Textbook Co., New York, 1940, pp. 235, 268, 272, 369.
14. Dublin, Louis I.: *The Facts of Life from Birth to Death.* The Macmillan Company, New York, 1951, p. 88.
15. Faxon, Nathaniel W. (ed.): *The Hospital in Contemporary Life.* Harvard University Press, Cambridge, Mass., 1949, p. 264.
16. Dublin, Louis I.: *op. cit.,* pp. 85, 89.
17. MacEachern, Malcolm T.: *Hospital Organization and Management,* 2nd ed. Physicians Record Co., Chicago, 1946, p. 74.

Additional Suggested Reading

"American College of Surgeons Continues Hospital Standardization Program" (editorial), *Hosp. Management,* **70:**33, (Nov.) 1950.
Arestad, F. H., and McGovern, Mary A.: "Hospital Service in the United States, 30th Annual Presentation of Hospital Data by the Council on Medical Education and Hospitals of the American Medical Association," *J.A.M.A.,* **146:**109, (May) 1951.
Bryan, Helen M., and Peterson, Muriel: "Two-Way Communication System," *Am. J. Nursing,* **50:**639, (Oct.) 1950.
Cherkasky, Martin: "The Montefiore Home Care Program," *Am. J. Pub. Health,* **39:**163, 1949.
Corwin, E. H. L.: *The American Hospital.* Commonwealth Fund, New York, 1946.
Ginzberg, Eli: *New York (State) Hospital Study: A Pattern for Hospital Care: Final Report.* Columbia University Press, New York, 1949.
Hayt, Emanuel: "Hospitals Should Insure Their Patients," *Hospitals,* **25:**46, (Jan.) 1951.
"Hospitals in the New World" (editorial), *M. Press,* **224:**627, (Dec.) 1950.

Johnson, Roy: "Decorating the Hospital Properly—the Backdoor to Morale," *Hosp. Management,* **69:**138, (May) 1950.

McGibony, J. R., and Block, Louis: "Better Patient Care Through Coordination," *Pub. Health Rep.,* **64:**1499, (Nov.) 1949.

Neergaard, Charles F.: "Hospital Construction," *Canad. Hosp.,* **27:**38, (Jan.) 1950.

Northrup, M. W., et al., " 'Race Track' Plan Cuts Down the Distance from Nurses' Stations to Patients' Rooms," *Mod. Hosp.,* **75:**59 (Oct.) 1950.

"Opinions on General Hospital Bed Occupancy" (editorial), *Hospitals,* **24:**24, (May) 1950.

Pfefferkorn, Blanche, and Rovetta, Charles A.: *Administrative Cost Analysis for Nursing Service and Nursing Education.* American Hospital Association, Chicago, and National League of Nursing Education, New York, 1940.

Southmayd, Henry John, and Smith, Geddes: *Small Community Hospitals.* Commonwealth Fund, New York, 1944.

US Public Health Service: *The Hospital Act and Your Community.* US Government Printing Office, Washington, D.C., 1947.

————: *The Nation's Needs for Hospitals and Health Centers.* US Government Printing Office, Washington, D.C., 1949.

Willard, W. R.: "Relationship of the Health Department and the Hospital with Special Reference to a Regional Hospital Council for Connecticut," *Connecticut State M. J.,* **14:**1089, (Dec.) 1950.

Zintek, A. R.: "Treatment of Communicable Diseases in General Hospitals," *Wisconsin M. J.,* **49:**936, (Oct.) 1950.

PART II. FUNDAMENTALS OF NURSING CARE

CHAPTER 4. THE PLAN OF CARE
FOR THE PATIENT

1. MEANING OF THE PLAN OF CARE
2. THE ROLE OF THOSE WHO PARTICIPATE IN MAKING AND CARRYING OUT THE PLAN OF CARE
3. IMPORTANCE OF A UNIFIED PLAN OF CARE
4. PLACING THE RESPONSIBILITY FOR STUDYING THE PATIENT AND PLANNING HIS NURSING CARE
5. WHAT THE NURSE SHOULD KNOW ABOUT THE PATIENT IN ORDER TO PLAN NURSING CARE
6. SUGGESTED FORMS FOR CASE STUDIES
7. SOURCES FROM WHICH THE NURSE SECURES INFORMATION ABOUT THE PATIENT
8. PLAN OF NURSING CARE AND SUGGESTED FORMS FOR WRITTEN PLANS
9. MEASURING THE SUCCESS OF THE PLAN OF NURSING CARE AND ITS EXECUTION

1. MEANING OF THE PLAN OF CARE

Everybody has some sort of design for living, and the concept of a health plan as part of this design is not confined to the medical world. Each person as he grows up deliberately or unconsciously develops a life pattern that is an adaptation of his native culture to his particular needs and desires. Different as these individual patterns often seem, the underlying needs, or urges, are similar. All human beings want security (food, clothing, and shelter) and desire love and approval; we also crave variety, adventure, achievement, including learning, and, in varying degree, we search for the ultimate good, the ethical force that man sees in his God, or his religion.

Some medical workers in every age have seen the difficulty, or even impossibility, of separating from the total life pattern those activities affecting health. We realize now that the extent to which and the way in which man satisfies these basic cravings are a measure of health. Medical care that ignores any of man's fundamental needs is unconsciously fighting nature, an unconquerable force, an incomparable ally. The plan of patient care should therefore be made with the recognition that the person under treatment is constantly longing for security, approval, love, adventure, accomplishment, learning or diversion, and a renewal of his faith in God or a universal ethical principle. Medical workers cannot provide patients with all this, but they can help them create an environment and set up a plan that makes possible the satisfaction of these cravings. The sick are suffering not so much from a disease as from its threat to their economic security, to their relationships with others, and to those activities that bring variety, entertainment, or pleasure into their lives. Sickness may also threaten the patient's faith in the ultimate "goodness" of life; he cannot believe in a God that lets such terrible things happen to him, or he may fear that he has lost favor in the sight of God, considering his illness a punishment for real or imagined sins.

Medical workers study the patient's history; they try to gather the salient facts about his occupation, his position in the family and community, and his emotional ties. Usually a more specific study is made of the habits that, for him, constitute daily care.

These habitual ways of dressing, bathing, eating, eliminating, exercising, resting, sleeping, as well as working and playing, tend to get so fixed and so essential to physical comfort and peace of mind that interruptions of the day's routine cause vague, or even acute, discomfort. Few children are so inflexible, but many adults are disgruntled if deprived of their morning coffee or daily bath. They are "off schedule" and lack the unconsciousness of the body which is part of a sense of well-being. Most readers will recognize this reference to their daily program; many persons have in addition weekly, monthly, or yearly plans that include rest periods and visits to doctors and dentists for health appraisals. The kind of regimen developed depends upon a person's intelligence, knowledge, his economic resources, and the value he puts on health. Ideally, each person would develop such a way of living as to enable him to realize his optimum usefulness and happiness; actually, this rarely happens. The "average man" has no such standard and is content with his health program as long as he can work, play, and sleep with relative freedom from anxiety, discomfort, fatigue, or pain. He loses confidence in his plan only when signs of disease are marked or persistent. At such times he is likely to ask for medical advice, and he then becomes a "patient." As a "patient" or "trainee" he expects the medical workers to help him modify his way of living so that health will be restored, or, if a cure is impossible, suffering relieved. Few persons, however, are willing or able to scrap their established regimen for an entirely new one. Wise doctors and nurses will therefore learn as much as they can about the individual's habits so that, in helping him to make a new plan, they can build on the foundation of his established pattern. *This modification of the patient's manner of living and the provision for making such a modification possible is the meaning of the plan of care as discussed in this text.*

The plan is intended to promote better health, to develop independence, to bring about the cure of disease when possible, and if incurable to reduce suffering to a minimum, and finally to make death easier.

Some plans of care may be carried out by the patient himself under direction of the physician. More often they require the cooperation of others, as, for example, the family, the nurse, the nutritionist, the physical therapist, the occupational therapist, the social worker, the minister, the vocational adviser, the psychologist, or others. Obviously, it is important that all those who carry out the plan have a common understanding of the goal of therapy.

When independence, or rehabilitation, is recognized as the primary and ultimate aim, as the writer believes it should be in most cases, the plan provides for the patient's optimum participation throughout the illness. This requires so much encouragement and guidance by the medical team that too often they, like the busy or impatient mother, find it quicker and easier to act for the person than to encourage or teach him, and so he develops dependency.

Some medical workers look upon rehabilitation as "the third phase of treatment," considering it a process to be carried out for selected patients in a special service, or rehabilitation center. Others believe that it is inherent in good medical care, that it should be practiced by every medical worker in every situation, and that every patient should be rehabilitated to the extent demanded by his condition.

This means that throughout the time the patient, or trainee, is under treatment, consideration is given to the part he should play in every therapeutic and hygienic activity. He should never be a passive recipient of care when he would ultimately benefit by participating in, or even assuming responsibility for, the activity.

When rehabilitation is looked upon as a separate program to be carried out by experts after ordinary medical personnel have done what they could for the patient, it too often happens that the work of these experts is doubled or tripled and the patient has to be brought to independence by slow stages of unlearning a dependence he need never have developed. Every patient could be so nursed and so treated by the physician and special therapists that he would be able on discharge to carry out all of these daily activities that give us what we call independence, or as many as are consistent with an irreversible disability, if he has one.

Figure 98 is a list of daily activities that embody our concept of independence. Anyone who can do all of these things unaided is "rehabilitated." It is apparent that the independence of a patient undergoing an appendectomy is threatened for only a few hours or days, whereas that of the person who is blinded or paralyzed in all extremities is permanently curtailed. In between these two extremes lie all those with moderate to severe handicaps of short or long duration. The activities listed in Figure 98 could be kept in mind or the form actually used in the care of all patients. This form was developed by Mary E. Brown and George G. Deaver at the Institute for the Crippled and Disabled in New York City; similar lists are now used in rehabilitation centers all over the world. The forms have brought this invaluable concept into clear focus and wide usage. It is difficult to conceive of a more practical guide for medical workers, but its application requires acceptance, understanding, and teamwork.[1]

A plan of care that brings an individual through a long illness into productive employment and useful living involves a wide variety of skills and the cooperation of many persons. It is costly, and few receive this comprehensive medical care. The physical facilities are not always available, but more often failure is the result of an inadequate number of well-prepared medical workers who know how to work toward the objective of independence for every patient.

While conscientious and trained medical workers never use haphazard methods, it would be misleading to imply that written plans of patient care and stated goals for therapy and rehabilitation can be found in the average health agency. *It is hard to imagine anything requiring more insight, knowledge, skill, and cooperative effort on the part of the sick person, his family, and medical workers than making a plan of care as interpreted here.*

Whenever a group of persons undertake a joint enterprise, each should have an understanding of his function. Before any further details about planning patient care are given, an attempt is made to differentiate between the parts played by those involved.

2. THE ROLE OF THOSE WHO PARTICIPATE IN MAKING AND CARRYING OUT THE PLAN OF CARE

The Patient and His Family. If the individual is rational, his understanding, interest, and cooperation are of the greatest importance both in planning and carrying out the program of care. While he is in an institution it may be possible to force a regimen upon him, but even in the hospital his cooperation is essential to successful therapy; ultimately, the health of the individual will depend upon his initiative and ability to care for himself. The plan of care, therefore, should be made with the assistance, the suggestion, and certainly the approval or acceptance of the patient. He is, after all, more concerned than anyone else with his condition and future welfare.

In order to make him realize the importance of a suggested regimen, it may be necessary to give him considerable guidance. A blind faith in the wisdom of his medical advisers may be sufficiently powerful to induce a patient to follow the plan made for him; but most individuals prefer to have something to say about what he will do or have done for him, when it shall be done, and who shall do it. If the patient does not agree to the conditions that his medical advisers believe to be *essential* to effective therapy, they may refuse to treat him. This they seldom do and then not until every effort has been made to help the patient understand the reasons for the proposed treatment. More and more it is believed that plans for medical care should be made in consultation with the relatives (or friends) involved.

In his text, *Patients Have Families,* Henry B. Richardson[2] has shown the waste of effort in treating a patient without consideration of the family situation. The failure of medical education along these lines has led to the practice of having medical students follow a hospital patient for a year or more after his discharge.

One such experiment is described in *Medical Care of the Discharged Hospital Patient*[3] by Frode Jensen and his associates. Wendell Muncie makes observations in psychiatry that might be applied to general practice.* In Chapter 2 attention was called to *The Peckham Experiment,* the account of a center where families (never individuals) registered and received health and sickness services. Margaret L. Shetland,[4] in her study of their work, describes a family health service provided by the Community Service Society of New York. Examples of ways in which the patient and his family participate in the plan of care are given later in this chapter and throughout this text.

The Physician. All diagnostic and therapeutic procedures are prescribed by the physician. Certain of these he carries out himself with the patient, his family, the nurse, or special therapists, but many are left entirely to others. Those who perform therapeutic procedures prescribed by the physician might be called, in legal terms, the doctor's agents. This, however, is an oversimplification of a rather complex problem. If other workers act as agents of the physician, he might be responsible for supervising and training them, but actually this is not the case. In practice, the physician prescribes physical and occupational therapy carried out by independent professional workers, and many of the therapeutic procedures he prescribes are so consistently performed by nurses that the doctor considers them nursing procedures. The strict differentiation between medicine and nursing was made in Chapter 1.

While most patients' plans for personal cleanliness, feeding, elimination, rest, sleep, exercise, diversion, and occupation are left to the professional nurse, in certain conditions, William R. Houston has pointed out in his *Art of Treatment,*[5] the regulation of this nursing care is of great concern to the physician, because it is the chief therapeutic agent. In tuberculosis, for example, the physician may prescribe the number of baths, the amount of rest and exercise, the spacing of meals, and the nature of any diversion and occupation permitted the patient. In this disease the patient's recovery depends partly upon the nice adjustment of his hygienic regimen. Ordinarily, however, the doctor leaves only the most general prescription for "bed rest" or "general diet" and expects the nurse to arrange feedings, periods of sleep, rest, and diversion around his plan of therapy. He may indicate the time at which treatments are to be given and diagnostic tests made; he always indicates their frequency; often he leaves their timing to others. When the physician has no other professional workers associated with him in the care of the patient, he will necessarily have many more problems and carry greater responsibility in making and executing the total plan of care than when he is working in a modern hospital situation.

Medicine is so highly specialized that most medical programs are the result of collaboration among a number of doctors. One physician or one surgeon is usually in charge, and others act as consultants, unless doctors practice as a group and arrange to share the responsibility for all patients. With the growing belief that

* For example, see Muncie, Wendell: "The Therapeutic Situation As It Concerns the Family with Special Reference to the Other Marital Partner," *Am. J. Psychotherapy,* **4:**595, (Oct.) 1950.

mind and body are inseparable and that disease affects both aspects—the psyche and the soma—the psychiatrist's help is more often sought. It is increasingly difficult to say one person is physically and another mentally ill. In some cases physical symptoms may be more noticeable and more measurable, and in others the personality changes may stand out, but both are present in some degree. The plan of therapy is then often the product of pooled medical judgment.

The Psychologist and Other Social Scientists. In assessing the psychic component of illness and the potential abilities of patients, psychologists and sociologists are valuable members of the therapeutic team. As residents or consultants, clinical psychologists are employed in most psychiatric services and in rehabilitation centers. Their help is sought increasingly where psychometric tests are indicated, and where interviewing and counseling are needed. Many long-term plans of care include provision for the psychologist's participation through one or more of these channels.

The cause of illness is increasingly sought in conflicts that arise in the social setting. Harry E. Moore suggests that psychosomatic conditions may have several bases, which he believes include the physiological, emotional, and social. When an illness cannot be explained satisfactorily after considering the first two, often knowledge of the patient's social background will be an important factor in understanding the present illness. "Bereavement, domestic difficulties, love affairs, thwarted ambitions, along with social class and group membership, are factors in diagnosis into which we have just begun to delve."*

The Nurse. The function of the nurse has been discussed in Chapter 1 and is suggested in the preceding paragraph dealing with the physician's role. Her major function is providing for, or helping the patient to provide for, his hygienic needs. By this is meant eating, eliminating, sleeping, resting, exercising, controlling body temperature by clothing and regulation of environment, communicating with others, and such activities as bring variety, refreshment, and accomplishment (including learning) into the day. The patient may need the nurse's help in making or executing the plan, or in both. It is the nurse's ultimate aim to make him independent of her as soon as possible. This hygienic regimen is arranged with reference to the diagnostic, therapeutic, and relief-giving measures prescribed by the physician. Obviously all medical workers should cooperate so that the timing, or spacing, of the activities involved provide a plan of optimum benefit to the patient.

A secondary, but nonetheless important, function of the nurse, is working with the patient, the physician, special therapists, and other members of the medical team in planning and giving the patient the assistance he needs with the diagnostic, therapeutic, and rehabilitation measures, prescribed or planned by them. If the patient is young, very ill, or comatose, he may be a passive participant. In this cooperative effort all workers should constantly keep the patient's welfare in the forefront and pay less attention than in the past to protocol. Since the functions of the doctor, the nurse, the dietitian, the social worker, the vocational guidance expert, and the special therapists are determined by custom and by the availability

* Moore, Harry E.: "Social Factors in Health," *Dis. Nerv. System,* **11:**244, (Aug.) 1950.

of their services, what each does will differ from time to time and place to place. While the nurse's activities should include only those that she is prepared to carry out safely and effectively, it is obvious that she will assume the heaviest responsibility for interpreting the physician's plan of therapy in the home, or in hospitals where there are no medical internes. Likewise, the physician's and the nurse's functions are enlarged when there are no social workers or special therapists in the picture. Houston, in discussing "resources of nursing" with respect to relief of pain, advocates giving the nurse an opportunity to exercise her clinical judgment more freely than custom permitted at the time he wrote. He says: "Another defect in hospital management of patients arises from the failure to do small things for the patient's comfort, because the doctor's orders refer only to the broad lines of treatment and cannot provide for every contingency."*

The writer believes that nurses should attach prime importance to effective performance of their major function and, having safeguarded this, should then participate in the total plan of care according to the special demands of the situation and their preparation for competent performance of additional functions.

If the nurse consistently encourages the patient's optimum participation in his hygienic and therapeutic program, she must spend a large part of her time encouraging, guiding, or teaching.[6] Her ingenuity, understanding, and skill are taxed to the utmost as she helps the paralyzed, incontinent patient to acquire control over the bladder or rectum; the spastic child to feed himself; or the blind diabetic to give himself insulin. Much of her teaching is unconscious and is an inseparable part of everyday practice so that she doesn't consider it teaching. Plans of nursing care are most complete and most effective guides, however, when a conscious effort is made to arrange a definite time each day for helping patients with specific procedures: for example, teaching a preoperative patient the exercises he will use postoperatively, how he will turn in bed and lift himself on the bedpan; or, as another example, planning spaced practice in manipulating crutches so that a person is adept in their use before leaving the hospital.[6]

Nursing, like medicine, is developing its specialties, and many plans of nursing care should be, for example, the cooperative effort of a medical and a psychiatric nurse, a surgical and a pediatric nurse. Collaboration between the nursing departments within a hospital or health agency with a pooling of nursing judgment is improving the quality of nursing care in many places.

Without presuming to enumerate or assess the schools of psychiatric thought, it can safely be said that most workers now accept the premise that emotional stability depends upon constructive or happy personal relationships. The fundamental need to feel useful, to be loved and approved of, exists among the sick to as great an extent as among the well. Too often the patient is sick because these basic needs have not been met. How difficult it will be then for him to get well in the average hospital environment where he may feel not only useless but a burden, where young doctors, nurses, and other personnel control his activities, and where he

* Houston, William R.: *The Art of Treatment.* The Macmillan Company, New York, 1936, p. 110.

may find only the most impersonal professional interest. Often in psychiatry there is a deliberate plan to cast the nurse in the role of the mother or the sister with the intention that she can therefore give the patient the interest and thoughtful sympathetic care this relative might supply. Other workers may play the role of a father or an older brother. In pediatric services doctors are prescribing for infants "ten minutes of T.L.C." (tender, loving care) at stated intervals during the day. Too often in general medical and surgical services no attempt is made to analyze and meet the emotional or psychic needs of the patient. It is partly the nurse's responsibility to provide for this in the plan of care if she accepts the thesis that all nursing has its psychiatric aspects.

Nutritionists.   The physician prescribes the patient's diet; but if an expert in this field is available, he relies on her to estimate quantities, to plan appetizing combinations of food, to get variety and balance in the diet, and to supervise its preparation. The nutritionist is often expected to guide patients in purchasing, planning, and preparing foods; she cooperates with the physician, the nurse, and the patient in arranging suitable hours for feedings and in selecting foods. She may play an important role in the rehabilitation of some patients.

Social Worker, Vocational Guidance Expert, and Rehabilitation Officer.   It was remarked earlier that the threat to economic security made by illness may involve far more suffering than the pain connected with the disease. Worry over finances, disrupted family relationships, or unemployment not only delays recovery but may be the underlying cause of organic pathology. While the physician and nurse should have a sufficient knowledge of the community resources to enable them to advise the patient and his family, their burden will be lightened if specialists in social work and vocational guidance are participating in the patient's care. They give patients expert assistance in financial problems, in job placement, in finding and being admitted to health and welfare agencies, in securing housekeeping and other services demanded by sickness, and in other health problems too numerous to list.

The Chaplain.   If we accept the thesis that each man has a faith he lives by, it follows that he finds comfort in the presence and counsel of a representative of this faith, especially in the stress of birth, illness, and death. A man's faith or "religion" may be so unorthodox, so individual, that it is difficult to find "a representative" of his school of thought, but even such a person often recognizes that he is strengthened or calmed by the spirituality of another, although their faiths are dissimilar. With the growing realization that emotional stress has its counterpart in physical stress, comes the acceptance of the minister, the priest, or the rabbi as a member of the therapeutic team.[7, 8]

Otis Rice, discussing "the religious needs of the patient" in Mildred L. Montag and Margaret Filson's text, lists as "religious and emotional problems" the intangibles of illness—strangeness, loneliness, anxiety, fear, questioning, guilt, hostility, and grief. He thinks the nurse, who is so constantly with the patient, should be prepared to recognize signs of these "intangibles" and relieve them according to her resources. Many who write on the social-psychological aspects of illness say that the relationship between the nurse and patient is itself therapy—constructive therapy where the nurse is a whole, or complete, individual with some self-knowledge and understanding of her effect on others; destructive when she is herself unbalanced, incomplete, and unaware of the qualities that elicit from the patient fear, distrust, anger, resentment, ridicule, disdain, indifference, or any other emotion that interferes with a therapeutic, sympathetic relationship.* Given a sympathetic relationship between the patient and the nursing staff, much of the strangeness, loneliness, anxiety, fear, and other "intangibles of illness" can be minimized, but it is obvious that many of these reactions are too deep to be uprooted easily. And so we find that if, for example, the obstetrician thinks a Roman Catholic woman's physical condition indicates interruption of a pregnancy, the priest must be brought in to discuss this problem with the family and the medical workers; or if a therapeutic diet is in conflict with the dietary laws of the orthodox Jew or Hindu, the rabbi's or swami's counsel may be necessary in resolving the conflict. Such specific cases, however, in no way suggest the variety of situations in which the religious leader, whatever his title, can help in the psychological aspects of patient care. This is so generally accepted that present-day literature abounds in articles and books attempting to resolve the conflict between the cleric and the psychiatrist, to deny the existence of a conflict, or to define the realms in which each functions. As many writers point out, the priest and the physician were once the same man, and are today in some cultures.[7, 8, 9]

In this country there is a growing tendency to appoint full-time or part-time chaplains to the staffs of health agencies and to provide a place for religious services —often a room used by many denominations. The most elementary symbols of the faith, such as military chaplains wear, may give comfort to patients. Special training, sometimes an interneship, is available to hospital and military chaplains that prepares them to work more effectively with the sick, their families, and medical personnel. These trainees may even elect to serve as medical orderlies or technicians for a limited period so that they may understand the problems of illness more thoroughly and, themselves, feel more at home in its presence. Those who have had this experience are likely to be especially helpful in planning and carrying out a program of care.

Ministers, priests, or rabbis who are a part of the regular staff, who move naturally and easily among the sick, give most comfort. To the person who has had no previous hospital experience the representative of his church at his bedside is a most familiar figure, a link with his life outside and often with his most highly charged emotional experiences. While in some cases the patient may consider

---

* The concept of wholeness or saneness and self-knowledge is ancient. The philosophy that ruled Greece in the days of her greatness is based on it. In more recent times Johannes Brahms, with no psychological training in the modern sense, wished he could find more "complete persons" in Hamburg. Florence R. Weiner decries present-day conditions that make it difficult for the nurse to realize her potential development ("Professional Consequences of the Nurse's Occupational Status," *Am. J. Nursing*, **51**:614, [Oct.] 1951), and along these lines George B. Babour's article is suggestive: "The Genuine Article; Don't Palm Off a Counterfeit Self on Your Patient" (*Am. J. Nursing*, **50**:342, [June] 1950).

the chaplain's visit an ominous sign, this is not so likely to be true if he sees him visiting other patients, obviously recovering or in good condition. To the patient who is convinced that he is dying, no one is more welcome. Henry K. Beecher has written on the relationship of the physician to the chaplain and that of the chaplain to the patient. He has said that "knowledge of imminent death, when correctly imparted, does good . . . that anguished hope gives way to tranquillity. . . ."* Seriously ill persons are restless and uneasy until a chaplain or a religious representative has visited and talked with them. Such spiritual assistance gives the patient comfort and surcease at this critical stage of his illness.

Rice says: "The nurse is usually the key person in relating the clergyman to her patient."† Only with the knowledge and approval of the physician does the nurse arrange the initial visit of the chaplain to her patient, or a conference with the family and medical personnel on the plan of care, but she may call to the chaplain's attention signs indicating the patient's need for his presence; in certain situations she fails in her service to the patient when she does not do so. If, for example, a Roman Catholic patient is in danger of dying or is going to have an operation, the priest should be notified at once.‡

Health services should have a written guide to help medical personnel work more effectively with religious representatives. It could give directions for reaching them; it could list the rituals of the various denominations, indicating what the clergyman might like provided when he comes to the health agency to perform the rite, and it might describe the significance of the ritual and suggest the conditions under which it is performed by the clergy or a lay person. For example, the Roman Catholic priest administers Baptism, Confession, Communion, and Extreme Unction to the sick, but if the nurse fears that the newborn infant may die before he can be baptized in the faith of his parents, she also may baptize him by sprinkling water on his forehead and saying, "I baptize thee in the name of the Father, and of the Son, and of the Holy Ghost." It is well for nurses to know that orthodox Jewish male infants are circumcised by the Rabbi on the eighth day after birth, and that this is both a religious and social ceremony. When the mother and infant are in the hospital, the plan of care should make provision for this ceremony.

It is impossible to discuss thoroughly in a text of this sort so complex a subject as the religious needs of the patient and the functions of the chaplain in the care

* Beecher, Henry K.: *Resuscitation and Anesthesia for Wounded Men; The Management of Traumatic Shock.* Charles C Thomas, Publisher, Springfield, Ill., 1949, pp. 11, 12.

† Montag, Mildred M., and Filson, Margaret: *Nursing Arts,* 2nd ed. W. B. Saunders Co., Philadelphia, 1953, p. 360.

‡ It may be helpful to nurses to learn the following forms of spoken addresses for the ordained clergy: "Mister" for most Protestant ministers who are not bishops. "Pastor" is used for some Lutheran, and "Father" for some Episcopal ministers; "Doctor" is preferred by some Protestant clergymen who hold such a degree. Roman Catholic priests are addressed as "Father" unless they hold other titles, and the Jewish clergyman is addressed as "Rabbi." Rice suggests that when the nurse is in doubt she should say "Doctor," never "Reverend," which is only proper in written address. Some other titles are "Swami" for a Hindu priest and "Muezzin" for a Mohammedan. (Montag, Mildred M., and Filson, Margaret: *op cit.,* p. 360.

of the sick. While special aspects are discussed in other chapters, it is hoped that
what is said here emphasizes the importance of the clergy as a member of the therapeutic team and the obligation of medical personnel to make possible the observation of those religious practices that are significant to each patient.

Special Therapists.   Medical care encompasses such a wide range of skills
that experts have been developed to take over certain elements from the doctor
and nurse. So, in a fully staffed medical center, there are physical, occupational,
recreational, and special therapists as well as numerous technicians. The special
therapists mentioned have professional standards of selection and preparation.
Without their participation the plan and execution of patient care are often incomplete, for no other workers are so highly trained in their specialties. The technician
is a key worker in many situations. The man who makes a wearable leg for an
amputee or an artificial eye for a patient who has just lost a natural one holds
an important place on the rehabilitation team. As specialties multiply, however, the
task of coordination and cooperation enlarges, and the service to the patient grows
less personal. Morton A. Seidenfeld,[10] discussing the psychological aspects of
medical care, makes a plea for helping the patient to understand his illness and
for orienting medical personnel to a patient-centered program where his psychological needs are recognized and met as carefully as his physical; but he doubts that
you can orient a "platoon" of workers to a patient's emotional problems. When the
disadvantages of segmented care are recognized as outweighing its advantages, the
pendulum will swing, and we will begin to prepare fewer types of workers more
thoroughly, each of whom will give a wider variety of services.

3. IMPORTANCE OF A UNIFIED PLAN OF CARE

Economy of Planning.   In medical and health services each person's case
should be looked upon as a problem. The question is: How may this man, woman,
or child be helped to regain or maintain his health so as to be a happy and useful
citizen? Or, if this is impossible, how may he be made as comfortable as possible
for the rest of his life? Since no two persons are alike, this problem is always an
individual one. Although the hospital routine provides patients with the necessities
of life, and often with comforts, it is not always consistent with the main therapeutic
aims; likewise, in home nursing the desired ends probably cannot be reached by
fitting the patient into the regimen of the household. In each case, time, effort,
and money expended on treatment are conserved if the patient and the persons in
attendance upon him have made out, and are attempting to follow, a definite plan
based on the needs of the patient and the circumstances of his situation.

Coordination and Cooperation in Planning.   When several workers are responsible for planning and giving care to a patient, it goes without saying that
some means must be devised to coordinate their efforts and direct them toward a
common goal. The obvious means are providing for discussion of the work, or for
a written plan to which everyone refers, or for both.

In some organizations a regular time is set aside for discussing the care and

PLAN OF NURSING CARE

Name _De Santa, Mrs Angela_   Division _A Medical_   History Number _629781_

Hour	Date 4-23-39 23	24	25	26	27	28	29	Treatments and Nursing Care	Notes to Assist in Giving Care
A.M. 7:00	+ + +							Offer bedpan, measure and record output / Bathe face and hands / Clean mouth, urge to drink water	Observe aseptic precautions as in respiratory infections / Prevent exertion by patient / Use menthol flavored mouthwash. Use toothbrush.
7:30	−							Pineapple juice, Coffee with 40 cc of 20% cream and gruel with cream	Don't force feeding if patient is nauseated. Substitute other liquids allowed in diet if preferred. Report inability to take fluids (Indication for infusion)
8:00	+ + +							Take temp, pulse and resp. (rectal temperature) / Offer bedpan; if patient does not defecate / Give cleansing enema (1% sod. bicarb. sol.)	Note especially character of respiration / Give enema slowly, under low pressure. Good results obtained with 500 to 600 c.c.
8:30	+ +							Pump breasts / Give bath	Use extra blanket and hot water bottle at feet during bath; avoid unnecessary exposure. Work quickly, prevent unnecessary exertion by patient
9:00	+ 9a. 1115							Apply flaxseed poultice to right chest / Codeine sulphate /03 Gm. (H) if in pain	Cover anterior and posterior chest wall excluding breast. Fix poultice in place with binder
9:30	+ +							Remove poultice. Leave dry binder over breasts / Offer bedpan / Change position	Cover nipples with gauze dressings. Do not apply binder tightly enough to limit respirations
10:00	+							Lemonade with Cerelose or ginger ale with 20% Cream, or substitute	
10:30								Rest period	
11:00								"	
11:30	+ +							Take temp., pulse and respiration / Clean mouth, urge to drink water	
12:00	−							Broth with egg or 40 cc. of 20% cream and gelatin with Cerelose, or substitute	
P.M. 12:30	+ 9a. 1215							Offer bedpan / Sponge and rub back, straighten bed / Codeine sulphate /03 Gm. if in pain	Remove binder for back-care. Leave properly adjusted / See that water in bottle at feet is hot
1:00								Rest period	
1:30								"	
2:00	+ +							Visitors / Flaxseed poultice	Visitors for short periods. Limited to immediate family. Discourage patient talking. Mrs De Santa especially wants to see husband and sister Mary.
2:30	+ + + +							Remove poultice. / Change position / Clean mouth	
3:00	+							Malted milk with 40 cc. of 20% cream, or substitute / Rest period	
3:30								Rest period	
4:00								"	
4:30	+ + −							Take temp. pulse and resp. / Offer bedpan / Codeine sulphate /03 Gm. (H.) if in pain	
5:00	+ +							Clean mouth / Broth or gruel with 40cc of 20% cream, or substitute	
5:30	+							Pump breasts if necessary	
6:00	+ +							Poultice to right chest / Urge to drink water	See that water in bottle at feet is hot.
6:30	+ + +							Remove poultice / Offer bedpan / Bathe face hands and back. Rub back	Leave binder applied to breasts.

+ Indicates that item of care or treatment is carried out.

− Indicates that item of care or treatment is omitted purposely. The explanation of the omission is given in the nurse's notes on patient's condition. In recording the administration of medications, the nurse's initials and the time of administration are given.

Figure 7. Form filled in to show plan of nursing care from 7 A.M. to 7 P.M. By checking the items of care in the columns to the left as they are given, the form combines a plan and a record of nursing care. (See Chapter 11, Fig. 55, for form for nurse's notes used in conjunction with this plan of care.)

85

Hour	Date						Treatments and Nursing Care	Notes to Assist in Giving Care
P.M. 7:00	+						Visitors	Limit to short visits from immediate family
7:30								
8:00	+ + +						Take temp. pulse and resp. Clean mouth Apply poultice to right chest	
8:30	+ + +						Remove poultice Offer bedpan Rub back . Leave in most comfortable position	See that water in bottle at feet is hot
9:00	+ + EW 9:20						Straighten bedding and arrange unit to induce sleep Hot broth or substitute Codeine sulphate /03 Gm Codeine prin	Night light does not seem to disturb patient and facilitates care
9:30								
10:00								
10:30								
11:00								If not sleeping report at late medical rounds
11:30								
12:00	+ + +						Take temp. pulse and resp. if awake Urge to drink water Offer bedpan	See that water in bottle at feet is hot and that patient is warm
A.M. 12:30	+ + Mc. 1:45						Apply poultice if in pain Change position Codeine sulphate /03 Gm (H) if in pain	
1:00								
1:30								
2:00								
2:30								
3:00								
3:30								
4:00	− −						Take temp. pulse and resp. if awake Urge to drink water Offer bedpan	See that water in bottle at feet is hot
4:30	− −						Apply poultice if in pain Change position Codeine sulphate /03 Gm. (H.) if in pain	
5:00								
5:30								
6:00								
6:30								

Figure 8. Plan of care from 7 P.M. to 7 A.M. (Reverse side of form shown in Fig. 7.)

progress of patients. These meetings, called *case conferences,* may be attended by doctors, nurses, dietitians, social workers, and others concerned with the patient's care. Formal meetings are not always possible or desirable, and the workers may depend upon their daily association in caring for the patient for opportunity to develop a coordinated scheme.

Some form of written plan is to be found in almost every case, however. For example, it is the custom for physicians to put all orders for medical treatment in writing; physicians and nurses keep written records of what they observe in the patient's behavior or condition. Less frequently, there is a written record of what either the physician or the nurse plans to do for the patient in the future. Figures 7 and 8 show a form for a written plan of nursing care that outlines what the nurse plans to do for the patient hour by hour. What she hopes to accomplish with nursing care over the time the patient is expected to be in the hospital, and the plan of home care that she makes in cooperation with the patient, the family, and the social worker before the patient leaves the hospital would be stated or implied in plans made subsequently.

The therapeutic plan for a patient with lung abscess today would differ from this one set up in 1939. Since this case history serves the purpose of this chapter, it has not been replaced by one of a later date. The brief note on modern treatment of lung abscess will be of interest to the reader.

Jim S. Jewett and George E. Dimond, reviewing the literature on lung abscess and reporting their observation of 28 cases in the last 2 years, say:

"Within the past decade, the medical regimen for lung abscess has included postural drainage, bronchoscopic aspiration and irrigation, artificial pneumothorax, intravenous injections of arsphenamine and guaiacol, rectal instillations of ether in oil, and the oral administration of potassium iodide and sulfonamides. The data reported by Rosenblatt (1940) indicate the hazards and ineffectiveness of such treatment. Of 72 patients with putrid lung abscess treated medically only 9 per cent were improved or cured, and 91 per cent unimproved or dead."* Other studies of more than 4000 cases showed a mortality of 34.4 per cent with medical treatment persisting through 1948. These results led to the surgical removal of the abscess and surrounding area in some instances. Many physicians and surgeons favor this treatment today. Jewett and Dimond, however, report a "radiographic cure" of 10 out of a series of 12 persons with the administration of intramuscular penicillin and aerosolized, or inspired, penicillin. Antibiotics are the agents of choice in current therapy, but authorities cited believe that a follow-up program is necessary for assurance that persons so treated are really cured.

Figure 9 shows a form which may be used in conjunction with the nursing plan to emphasize important points in the treatment and care of the patient. Written plans such as these enable a second nurse in attendance to take up the care of the patient where the first nurse left off, and provide a means of communication between the nurses and other medical workers contributing to the total program of care.

A nurse must know a good deal about the person and the way he lives to plan nursing care. She must make a preliminary study in order to institute a regimen

* Jewett, Jim S., and Dimond, George E.: "Medical Management of Acute Lung Abscess Report in 12 Cases," *Dis. Chest,* **18:**478, (Nov.) 1950.

suited to the patient's needs, and must continue to study the patient and the situation in order to modify the plan as conditions change. This power of analysis varies greatly according to the native intelligence, the sensitiveness, and experience of the nurse. The ability to collect significant information and to observe accurately is useful to everyone, but it is particularly essential in the practice of the medical arts.

Patient De Santo, Mrs Angela

Date	Doctors Orders	Emphasis in Nursing Care
4-23-39	Diet - Pneumonia fluids Measure intake and output Sod. bicarb. enema (1%) o.d., s.os. Pump breasts p.r.n. Codeine sulphate /o3 Gm. q.4h. p.r.n. Flaxseed poultice to right chest q.4h p.r.n. White blood count and differential o.d.	Force fluids but avoid producing nausea. Report low fluid intake as indication for infusion. Relieve pain by change of posture with support and measures prescribed by doctor. Limit exertion - Limit visiting. Try to relieve apprehension.

Figure 9. Card which may be used to give a summary of doctor's orders and points to be emphasized in nursing care. (Not a permanent part of the patient's record as is the form shown in Figs. 7 and 8.)

4. PLACING THE RESPONSIBILITY FOR STUDYING THE PATIENT AND PLANNING HIS NURSING CARE

It is a principle of good medical care that each patient is under the care of a particular physician. Other doctors work through the physician in charge of the case, who presumably knows more about the individual than anyone else. A physician does not consider himself qualified to treat a person until he has made an examination and secured a medical history. His plan of therapy is based on these findings.

Some nurses believe that a similar principle applies to nursing. It is becoming more and more general to assign a patient to one nurse who makes it her business to study the patient's particular nursing needs. The nurse is as dependent upon a thorough knowledge of the patient in planning nursing care as the physician is in mapping out a plan of therapy. The nurse to whom the patient is assigned becomes responsible for his nursing care. Other nurses who relieve her when she goes off duty or who work with her follow the nursing plan she makes. In some situations the patients are assigned to a "team" of nurses. In this case the team leader assumes responsibility for the plan of care. If a patient is assigned to a student nurse, the student may study the individual and arrange a program for him, but a graduate nurse must take the ultimate responsibility.

5. WHAT THE NURSE SHOULD KNOW ABOUT THE PATIENT IN ORDER TO PLAN NURSING CARE

Factors That Affect Nursing Care. The nurse should have such knowledge as shows her what kind of nursing care the patient needs. She must know the *sex* and *age* of the patient; she should know his *race, nationality,* and *religion* in order to understand his language difficulties and the way he thinks and feels about many things. A Roman Catholic, for instance, should not be served meat on Friday; an orthodox Jew will not want to eat meat unless the animal was killed under conditions prescribed by his faith. Many aspects of treatment, such as circumcision, have a religious significance for certain peoples. The nurse must understand and show respect for religious and racial customs if she hopes to give the highest type of service.*

Since the nurse must constantly seek to gain the cooperation of the patient through explanation of what is being done for him, or what he must do for himself, she should try to make a fairly accurate estimate of his *native intelligence* and his *previous experience,* particularly with respect to health practices. A technical explanation of a procedure may frighten rather than reassure one patient, whereas it may interest and please a more informed person who has had many illnesses. Such terms as *enema, lumbar puncture,* and *catheterization* may mean absolutely nothing to one individual and yet be familiar terms to another.

If nursing care is to conform to the general outlines of treatment, the nurse must know the *physician's diagnosis* and his *plan of therapy.* It is important to know not only the diagnosis but also the *severity of the condition.* A person with a mild heart condition may be able to take his own bath, assume almost any position in bed with comfort, exercise moderately, and talk to friends for several hours without being tired by the exertion. One with an acute or severe cardiac disease, however, should often be spared the slightest effort; he may be comfortable only when he is supported in a sitting posture, and absolute quiet may be essential to his recovery.

The *mental state* of the individual may have as much influence on nursing care as the physical condition. The hyperactive, exuberant, optimistic, talkative person often needs long periods of rest and some limit set to his activity, while the hypoactive, discouraged, depressed patient needs encouragement to do many things and to spend more time with others.

Since the plan of care is directed toward prevention of future illness, as well as toward the cure of the present one, the nurse should know the *direct* and *indirect causes* of the condition for which the patient is treated. It is essential that she know

---

* Joseph Gaer's *How the Great Religions Began* (Dodd, Mead and Co., New York, 1951) is a helpful introduction to the study of comparative religion.

his *occupation and economic status,* his resources, and his dependence upon others, including his *need for guidance in health procedures.* She should, of course, know what workers are participating in his care and the responsibilities of each; and she should be familiar with the community facilities in order that she may help patients and their families to use them.

6. SUGGESTED FORMS FOR CASE STUDIES

Collecting all such information about the patient is known as *a case study.* William Osler and great doctors in all ages have stressed the present practice of teaching medicine through the study of individual cases. It seems self-evident that the nurse cannot make an effective plan for care of the patient without preparing a case study. When the particular needs of a patient are not analyzed, the inevitable result for him is a routine pattern of care. The study need not necessarily take written form. If the nurse is to discuss the case in a conference, however, she may find it valuable to make notes on the salient facts and the way in which they affect nursing care; or, if she is preparing a study of the patient to be published or read by others, she may give this information in a narrative form. The following are samples of a longer narrative type and a shorter working analysis, both of which are used as a basis for planning nursing care.

CASE REPORT OF A YOUNG WOMAN WITH A LUNG ABSCESS
(Longer Type of Case Study)

Angela De Santo is a young married woman 23 years of age. She was born in this country of Italian parentage. Her father is a day laborer, and his family lives in a crowded Italian section of ———— (a large city). Mrs. De Santo is the eldest of seven children. She was taken from school at the age of 14 to help support the family by working in a dress factory, where she was employed until December, 1938.

About a year ago Angela (Romano) married Michael De Santo, a young man her own age, employed as a presser in a cleaning agency. The couple took a three-room basement apartment in a house near her parents, for which they pay a monthly rent of $35. According to the report from the social service department, it is in poor repair and badly ventilated.

Mrs. De Santo was earning $30 to $40 weekly when she gave up her job; Mr. De Santo has a smaller and more uncertain weekly wage, usually around $20 to $25. They thought themselves well off until Mrs. De Santo's pregnancy. She particularly resented this because of the expense involved and because it meant that she would have to give up work at the factory. The pregnancy was normal, and she was employed up to the last three months. When the baby came, Mrs. De Santo said she was surprised to find that her resentment had vanished and that she was glad she had not had an abortion, which she had at one time considered. The baby was born in the hospital, and the expenses were met on an easy-payment plan. Mrs. De Santo had a difficult labor, which lasted 2 days. The baby was delivered by forceps, without injury to the mother or child, so far as was known at the time. Young Michael, now 2 months old, is with his grandparents, the Romanos.

Both Mr. and Mrs. De Santo are bright and attractive looking. Neither one has more than a grade-school education, but they are teachable, ambitious, and eager to have a nice home, both for their own sake and for the sake of their child.

Mrs. De Santo noticed signs of her present illness on April 10, about ten days after her return from the maternity hospital. When the visiting nurse came for one of her regular post-partum calls, Mrs. De Santo said that she had a cold, was coughing, and felt chilly most of the time. The nurse took Mrs. De Santo's temperature, said she had some fever, and that she should stay in bed and call a doctor. This same nurse came to see the patient daily after this and urged that the baby be sent to his grandmother. The parents were unwilling to part with him, and since there was no one to care for him except herself while her husband was at work, Mrs. De Santo was obliged to get in and out of bed. Her condition grew steadily worse, and the third day, after the doctor was called, he sent her to the hospital. By this time Mrs. De Santo was thoroughly frightened by a pain under the right shoulder blade, which she described as terrible, making her unwilling to speak or move.

Dr. Livingston, who examined Mrs. De Santo 6 weeks ago, on admission to the women's medical division of the hospital, made the following notes on her condition.

"The patient is suffering with intense pain in the right chest on breathing and coughing, with sudden onset the day of admission; milder generalized pain extends throughout the chest. Breathing, which occurs at the rate of 30 times a minute, is shallow and difficult. Breath sounds are diminished throughout chest, no rales heard or change in quality of breath and voice sounds. Coughing, which occurs every few minutes, produces small amounts of blood-tinged sputum, and the patient says she has a very unpleasant taste in her mouth. The throat is not inflamed. Milk exudes from the nipples on slight pressure, and the breasts are moderately filled. There is no tenderness in the slightly distended abdomen. The pulse rate is 148 per minute, and the quality is full and bounding. There is pallor rather than cyanosis, and the skin is hot and dry to the touch. The patient's temperature is 41° C (105.8° F), and there is a constant sensation of chilliness. The pupils are mildly dilated and react to light.

"Mrs. De Santo appears to be an acutely ill woman who is anxious about her condition. (She says she is afraid she has tuberculosis.) Her manner is pleasant and cooperative, but she was excited and apprehensive during the physical examination."

After this examination the tentative diagnosis was *lobar pneumonia of the right lung.* Drs. Parks and Simon saw Mrs. De Santo on the day of her admission, and they thought her symptoms more indicative of a *lung abscess.* In an effort to arrive at a satisfactory diagnosis and a more accurate index of her condition, the following tests were made: Blood was cultured to see whether any microorganisms were present; it was tested for specific substances which indicate the existence of infections from types of pneumococci. A routine Wassermann test for syphilis also was made. White blood cell counts were made to see whether there was a total increase and, if so, among which kinds of white cells; the red blood cells and hemoglobin content were estimated to determine whether or not the patient was anemic. The sputum was cultured, and the types of microorganisms studied in the hope of identifying those causing the disease. The second day after admission an x-ray picture of the chest was made to see whether the affected area could be defined. The fluid output, as compared with the intake, was measured throughout the patient's illness in order to check the status of the organs of elimination, especially the kidneys.

Findings from these tests, made over a period of 4 to 5 days, supported the diagnosis of a lung abscess. Dr. Hanson, who made a series of x-ray pictures at varying intervals throughout, expressed his opinion that a necrotic area (dead tissue) had formed in the lung following the blocking of the blood supply to that area by a clot in a blood vessel. This might have occurred following childbirth. Dr. Hanson suggested that the abscess, or necrotic area, ruptured into the pleural sac surrounding the lung, causing acute pain characteristic of pleurisy. Identification of a causative organism was never satisfactorily accomplished, the sputum showing no predominant strain. Fever and the white cell count of 18,000 to 20,000 per milliliter of blood (about twice the normal number) were indications of infection. A red blood cell count of 3,880,000 (the normal is from 4,500,-000 to 5,000,000) and a hemoglobin of 75 per cent showed a mild anemia. A blood pressure of 120/75 was considered normal, and the elimination by the kidneys satisfactory.

During the first 2 weeks, Mrs. De Santo's temperature ranged between 38° and 40.6° C (100.4° and 105° F), gradually subsiding until at the present time there is no elevation. Severe pain in the right chest continued for 2 weeks, gradually diminishing and finally disappearing altogether. There was little discharge accompanying the cough at first, but about the tenth day of her illness the patient began to cough up large quantities of very foul, purulent sputum.

Since there was doubt about the diagnosis at the time of admission, the treatment prescribed by Dr. Livingston was conservative and in the main designed to support vital processes and relieve pain and discomfort.* After the existence of a lung abscess was established and pus appeared in the sputum, the patient was placed in a position to favor drainage (the head lowered) twice a day. Codeine sulfate was prescribed immediately for relief of pain and to control the cough, and phenobarbital to induce sleep and rest. Icecaps and poultices were applied to the chest during the first few days but were soon discontinued. A creosote mixture, administered by inhalation with a wire and gauze mask, was ordered to combat the foul odor of the sputum and with the hope that it would have a mild disinfecting action on the respiratory tract. Mrs. De Santo objected to this treatment so strenuously that it was discontinued. A daily cleansing enema, or colonic irrigation, was ordered if needed during the first 2 weeks; after this the bowel movements were regulated with mineral oil. During the acute stage of her illness, a high-caloric fluid diet, similar to that used for pneumonia patients, was prescribed, and solid food added after the first week until Mrs. De Santo was having a high-caloric, high-vitamin, anticonstipating diet. Ferrous sulfate was prescribed for the anemia.

The care of Mrs. De Santo presented an interesting and complex nursing problem. The patient had had no other hospital experience except her recent one as a maternity patient, and was apprehensive about every treatment. Although she made an effort to follow the suggestions of the physicians and nurses, the acute pain induced by any movement made her unwilling to move. She cried almost constantly the first few days, when awake, and not under the influence of codeine. Another source of distress of a different nature was the separation from her child and her anxiety over what would happen to her baby and her husband if she did not get well. Other difficulties in the first stages of her illness were the nausea and vomiting that often prevented effective oral

* Antibiotics were not available for treatment of lung infections in 1939.

feeding, the disagreeable taste in the mouth, the odor of the sputum that was sickening not only to her but to nearby patients, the breasts filled with milk, the distended abdomen, the tendency to constipation, the periods of excessive sweating, and the sensation of chilliness.

A tentative schedule of nursing care was planned for Mrs. De Santo for the first 2 days. Frequent visits of physicians and technicians and changes in therapy as the nature of her condition became better established made it difficult to carry out any schedule. The plan was constantly modified to meet the needs of the case. Figure 8 shows the nursing care as planned and carried out, with only minor changes, on the third day. Nursing care followed substantially this same program for the first week with new medical "orders" incorporated, and discontinued treatment indicated.

On admission to Ward A, Mrs. De Santo was assigned to Miss Capelli (a graduate staff nurse) and the writer (a senior student nurse). Together we worked out the plan of care for the duration of the patient's illness. Since Miss Capelli was on duty from 3 to 11 P.M. and I from 7 A.M. to 3 P.M., we were able to give the major share of care, the night staff assuming responsibility for Mrs. De Santo from 11 P.M. to 7 A.M.

After examination of the patient, it was thought wise to put her in the small ward where she could have quiet, where she would be visible from the nurse's station, and where her serious condition would disturb as few patients as possible.

The acute need at first seemed to be the relief of pain. Strapping the chest and giving codeine (0.09 gm [1.5 gr]) by hypodermic gave partial relief. Ice bags were fastened to a pillow in order to keep the weight of the bags off the chest and then placed against the chest wall. Discomfort resulted, and when this was reported to Dr. Livingston the treatment was discontinued. Flaxseed poultices were prescribed the next day, and their warmth seemed to make Mrs. De Santo feel more comfortable. Care was taken to see that the poultice was not more than 46° C (114.8° F) when applied and that it was held in place with a loose binder, so that body movements were not unduly restricted. The poultice covered the major part of the right chest, back, front, and sides but did not extend over the breasts. A hot-water bottle was placed at the feet; extra blankets and a flannelette gown were used to overcome the sensation of chilliness. During the first few days the clothing had to be changed frequently, as periods of profuse sweating occurred; cleansing baths were given daily. As long as the sensation of chilliness persisted, very warm water was used for baths and little exposure of the body allowed, the bath being given between blankets, with a hot-water bottle at the feet. At no time was the temperature sufficiently elevated to warrant reducing measures.

Mrs. De Santo's cough throughout the first month of her illness was very distressing. It interfered with rest and sleep and, being violent and spasmodic, caused so much movement of the irritated pleura that the pain was at times excruciating. Codeine was used in an attempt to control it. Cough mixtures with a syrupy base were distasteful during the period of nausea but were used later with some success.

Nausea persisted intermittently for the first week, as a result of giving codeine so frequently, but this was thought necessary for the relief of pain. Nourishing foods were taken during this period only after coaxing and were sometimes vomited immediately. Glucose solution, 5 per cent, was administered intravenously once daily if the fluid intake fell below 1500 cc in 24 hours.* A variety of drinks were tried in an effort to find something that would not be distasteful. Ginger ale was tolerated and even when

---

* Fluid balance was less well understood in 1939. Other dietary elements would be given with the glucose today.

mixed with cream; the latter made a very nourishing drink. To help relieve nausea, noise was reduced to a minimum, and disagreeable odors combated by ventilation and general cleanliness. The scent of an alcoholic solution of camphor was pleasant to the patient. It was sprinkled on a paper handkerchief.

As recovery progressed, Mrs. De Santo developed not only a good appetite but an ambition to eat heartily so that she could get well. During her stay in the hospital, Miss Warner, a dietitian, gave the patient some guidance in the selection of a diet to correct constipation and the anemia. In order to spare her every possible exertion, a colonic irrigation with a constant in and out flow (rather than an enema) was given on the days when the patient was sickest. The importance of establishing normal evacuations with regularity, diet, and exercise was emphasized to Mrs. De Santo, and before her discharge from the hospital she made great progress. She tried to use the bedpan each morning after breakfast, and if this was unsuccessful, in order to encourage habit formation, an enema was given then rather than later in the day.

Engorgement of the breasts of this post-partum mother was prevented by the use of the breast pump twice a day for 3 days, then once a day for 4 days; at the end of this time there seemed to be no further necessity for the treatment. A soft binder with dressings over the nipples was kept on the patient to prevent soiling the gown. A tight binder could not be used to discourage the secretion of milk since this might have tended to limit respiratory movements in the unaffected side of the chest. The acute pain in the right chest made the patient instinctively reduce to a minimum all movement in this area. Mrs. De Santo was so much more comfortable lying on the right side that it was difficult to persuade her to change her position as often as desirable. When it was necessary to turn on her back to use the bedpan, she was urged to stay in that position for a little while. In all positions she was supported with pillows to relieve muscle strain.

During the second week when the diagnosis of lung abscess was established and there was evidence of pus in the sputum, postural drainage was used twice a day, at 10 A.M. and 8 P.M. The foot of the bed was elevated 45 cm (18 in.) for 15 minutes; two pillows were placed under the abdomen and the head turned on the side. While in this position, Mrs. De Santo was urged to cough in order to drain purulent material from the abscessed area. She found this position unpleasant, but after she thoroughly understood its purpose, she was very cooperative and succeeded in bringing up a good deal of discharge. The foul odor of the sputum was offensive and its appearance repellent. Covered paper cartons, half filled with moistened sawdust, weighed before and after use, determined the number of grams collected. A fresh container was supplied twice a day or oftener. The sputum amounted to as much as 200 gm in 24 hours during the third week of illness. A menthol mouthwash was used after each period of postural drainage, and the teeth were brushed thoroughly two or three times a day.

The physical aspects of care were by no means the most difficult problem in nursing Mrs. De Santo. At the time of her admission, she was in a highly excited and frightened state. Her remarks, and conferences with her husband and sister, showed that she was afraid she had tuberculosis; she knew this would necessitate separation from her husband and child and would cost more than they could afford. Unfamiliarity with hospitals made her apprehensive about all treatments. During the first two weeks of her illness, when she was in pain, she did not show undue concern about her baby; later, however, she tended to worry for fear he was being fed irregularly and "spoiled."

While strenuous efforts were made to effect a physical cure an equally earnest attempt was made to get at the basis of Mrs. De Santo's anxieties, to help her dispel imaginary troubles, and to work out a solution for those that were real.

It was possible for the physicians to convince Mrs. De Santo that she did not have tuberculosis. She was told that she had an acute infection of the lung of a type that could be cured with care. In answer to her questions she was advised that she should stay in the hospital about a month, but that the doctor, the nurses, and the social workers would work out a plan with her family for the payment of the hospital fees, the care of her child, and whatever physical help she needed during convalescence. Reassurance came gradually through these combined efforts. As her condition improved, she was given more definite information about the plan of payment to the hospital and the convalescent home to which she would be discharged. Since her illness has not left her with any disability, rehabilitation is uncomplicated.

It was obvious from the time of admission that Mrs. De Santo needed something else to think about besides the possible eventualities of her illness. During its acute stage entertainment or occupation was contraindicated by need for rest. In order to give her something to look forward to, however, special visiting privileges were allowed her husband and her sister. As her physical condition improved, books and magazines were furnished by the library, her bed was wheeled to the sun porch where she could listen to the radio, and later she was encouraged and helped by her nurses to knit a baby's sweater. In the past week she has been crocheting doilies, the pattern and materials for which were furnished by Mrs. Bemis, an occupational therapist.

Mr. and Mrs. De Santo were advised to move to a suburban district where they could get an apartment with more sunlight and where they would have easier access to the outdoors. With the assistance of the social service department, this was accomplished. The charge for hospitalization was reduced to a minimum, and the payment adjusted so that it was not an unreasonable burden.

Mrs. De Santo will be discharged day after tomorrow, having spent 7 weeks in the hospital. She will go to the ———— Convalescent Home (a Catholic institution), and arrangements have been made to have the baby there with her. Physician, dietitian, and nurses have helped Mrs. De Santo to make out a daily plan of home care for herself and the baby. This plan includes a specific time for sleep, rest, exercise, for housework, and for care of the baby. The anemic condition present on her admission to the hospital has improved sufficiently to make further medication unnecessary; however, she is urged to select her diet with especial care to see that each day it includes cooked cereal, a quart of milk, an orange or a tomato, a potato, dark bread, and an egg, with beef liver at least once a week, and a variety of vegetables.

Such a case history gives a vivid picture of what can be done for patients when the various medical specialists in a modern hospital work together in their interest.

CASE STUDY
(In Brief)

An analysis of factors influencing nursing care made the second day after admission of patient as a basis for planning nursing care.

Patient: De Santo, Mrs. Angela, age, 23 years; nationality, USA; parentage, Italian. Service: Medical Div. A. Date of admission: 4/21/39. Discharge:

FACTORS INFLUENCING NURSING CARE	WHAT THEY SUGGEST IN TERMS OF NURSING CARE
1. *Diagnosis* (tentative): lobar pneumonia? lung abscess? empyema?	1. *General nature of nursing care suggested by the diagnosis:* Care given any acute respiratory disease with precautions to prevent the spread of infection by discharge from the nose and throat. If presence of abscess is established, special posture will be used to favor drainage.
2. *Social history and health record:*	2. *Care must be modified by patient's past experience, social and economic status:*
a. Family history: Grew up in an apartment in a crowded section of ——— with 6 sisters and brothers; father a laborer. Parents affectionate, active, emotional. The patient worked in a factory from age of 14 until a few months before baby was born. No record of mental disease, tuberculosis, or syphilis in the family.	a. Limited economic resources suggest that patient may worry about cost of hospital care. Social service worker has been notified; has interviewed husband. Limited social and educational background makes an explanation of hospital customs and all treatment in simple terms especially important. Put patient in ward with other Italians if possible.
b. Marriage: One year to Michael De Santo, 24 years of age, presser in a cleaning establishment. Mrs. De Santo earned $30 to $40 weekly at piece work, husband $20 to $25. They have an apartment for which they pay $35 a month. Wife resented pregnancy because it cut down income; wanted abortion. Is glad now she didn't have it; devoted to baby. Child is now with grandparents. Husband attentive and considerate on visits.	b. Try to learn whether patient is worried about care given child by grandparents. If she is, suggest ways to the family of reassuring her. Encourage her to talk about the baby to comfort her for the enforced separation from her family. Later, in cooperation with social service department, investigate home to see whether conditions are suitable for convalescence and whether satisfactory arrangements can be made for care of child.
c. Health history: Diseases of childhood, no serious illnesses; happy nature; weight has remained constant as adult (118 lb) except during preg-	c. Since Mrs. De Santo is not accustomed to illness and to hospitals, especial care may be needed to prevent or relieve fear and anxiety. She

CASE STUDY (*Continued*)

FACTORS INFLUENCING NURSING CARE	WHAT THEY SUGGEST IN TERMS OF NURSING CARE
nancy. Birth of child only hospital experience. "Eats everything"; drinks wine, no hard liquor; does not smoke; good appetite; tendency to constipation. Takes very little exercise. Appears well nourished, normal physical development.	should be helped to overcome constipation through an understanding of the importance of regularity in evacuation, proper diet, and exercise. Measures used during illness should be designed to help establish a regular time for defecation.

3. *History of present illness:*
Symptoms of cold with cough, chilliness, fever, and weakness 5 days after return from maternity hospital. Visiting nurse, on post-partum follow-up visit, urged patient to go to bed and call doctor; this she did after second day. Patient unwilling to leave baby to care of grandmother, but was frightened by severe pain under right shoulder blade that attacked her suddenly 3 days ago, and agreed to come to hospital. On admission, said she was afraid she had tuberculosis.

3. *History of present illness may influence nursing care and preventive measures to be taken later:*
History of illness shows that Mrs. De Santo is very much attached to her child, and this may be used to influence her later to cooperate with medical advisers, so that she can make a rapid recovery. The fact that patient is known to the local visiting nurse association means that there is one source from which information about her living conditions may be sought and that nursing supervision during convalescence is very likely available through this agency. Reassurance about the nature of her illness should be given by the physicians if she continues to be anxious.

4. *Present signs and symptoms:*

   a. Intense pain in right chest increased by deep respirations.

4. *Nursing care designed largely to relieve symptoms of illness:*

   a. Patient will be most comfortable lying on right side since that will splint the affected lung and allow freedom of movement on unaffected side. Change to dorsal recumbent position every 4 hours to stimulate circulation and relieve muscle strain. Support with pillows. Discourage talking; provide paper handkerchiefs and paper sputum cup for discharge from cough.

   b. Violent episodes of coughing, with small amounts of blood-tinged sputum. Shallow breathing with par-

   b. In counting respiration, place hand lightly beside left chest wall and count movements.

CASE STUDY (*Continued*)

FACTORS INFLUENCING NURSING CARE	WHAT THEY SUGGEST IN TERMS OF NURSING CARE
ticularly limited excursion in right chest. Respirations around 30 per minute.	
c. Temperature ranging between 38.9°–39.4° C (102°–103° F) (dropped from 40.6° C [105° F] on admission).	c. and d. Hot-water bottle at feet will be comforting. Covering should be light and warm. As temperature fluctuates, there is likely to be excessive perspiration, and care must be taken to provide dry clothing as need arises. Important to get patient to drink large quantities of water, and high-caloric diet if temperature elevation continues. Make record of intake and output of fluids.
d. Skin pale, hot, dry; complains of sensation of chilliness much of the time.	
e. Pulse ranging between 120–130 per minute (dropped from 142 on admission). Systolic arterial pressure of 120, diastolic pressure 80.	e. To lessen tax on heart, limit motor activity and emotional excitement if possible, although the increase in the pulse rate and the blood pressure recordings indicate a fairly satisfactory reaction of the circulatory system to the toxemia.
f. Intermittent nausea, no appetite; abdomen slightly distended.	f. Do not force foods that are distasteful but keep a record of oral intake so that it may be supplemented intravenously if indicated. (Ginger ale is acceptable at present.) Record vomiting when it occurs, so that physician may determine need for infusion. Use cold compresses on forehead; hot-water bottle on abdomen; menthol mouthwash after vomiting. Prevent unnecessary noise at bedside and avoid making the patient talk. Reduce odors to a minimum.
g. Milk exuding from nipples; breasts slightly distended.	g. Breasts emptied with pump twice daily or oftener if indicated. Use loose soft binder to keep milk from soiling gown.
h. Rational but anxious. Tries to be cheerful but cries often when left alone. Looks acutely ill. Voice weak, uncertain.	h. Give as constant nursing care and supervision as possible. Very careful explanation of all treatments. An assured, quiet, and cheerful manner

CASE STUDY (*Continued*)

FACTORS INFLUENCING NURSING CARE	WHAT THEY SUGGEST IN TERMS OF NURSING CARE
	on the part of the nurse may help to give Mrs. De Santo more confidence in her chances for recovery. Conversation with her family may help to explain the cause or causes of her extreme anxiety.
5. *Laboratory findings:* a. Blood Hemoglobin 75 per cent. Red blood cells 3,880,000 per cubic centimeter. White blood cells 18,300 with marked increase in polymorphonuclear cells. b. Urine No sugar, albumin, casts, or other abnormal constituents. c. X-ray report (not yet received).	5. *Laboratory findings, like diagnosis, important leads in nursing care:* a. Encourage patient to eat foods in prescribed diet that are high in iron content.
6. *Treatment prescribed by physician:* Date: 4-21-39. a. Diet—pneumonia fluids.* b. Right side strapped. c. Ice bag to right chest. d. Pump breasts as need is indicated. e. Codeine sulfate 0.03 gm (0.5 gr) every 4 hours if necessary to relieve pain. f. Measure intake fluids and output of urine. Date: 4-22-39. g. Discontinue ice bag to chest.	6. *Nursing care built around prescribed medical treatment:* a. Feedings scheduled about 8-10-12-3-5-8. Try out different fluids to discover which the patient likes and tolerates when nauseated. b. Observe skin for irritation from adhesive. c. Bandage ice bags to rubber-covered pillow and allow patient to lie against them. e. Try to relieve pain by posture and physical agents as prescribed before giving codeine, which is possibly causing nausea. Administer codeine before rest periods in the day and at night in order to get maximum benefit from the drug. Group treatments so that there will be periods in the day when patient need not be disturbed.

* Present-day treatment would include a more complete diet. If not tolerated orally it would be given parenterally.

CASE STUDY (*Continued*)

FACTORS INFLUENCING NURSING CARE	WHAT THEY SUGGEST IN TERMS OF NURSING CARE
h. Apply flaxseed poultice every 4 hours to right chest.	h. Poultice should extend over posterior and side of right chest wall (not over breasts). Hold in place with chest binder with shoulder straps, so that patient's movements are not restricted. Binder should not be tight enough to restrict respiration.
i. Cleansing enema every day if necessary.	i. Offer bedpan after breakfast, and if patient is unable to have a defecation, give enema at this time to help her to establish the habit of regular defecation. Enema should also be given before bedding is changed to avoid soiling fresh linen. Give enema with patient on right side in a comfortable position with legs drawn up. If effort seems to exhaust patient, report to physician who may prefer to have a colonic irrigation given.
j. Culture of sputum. k. Differential blood count.	j. In collecting sputum, see that specimen is raised from the bronchi by coughing.

7. SOURCES FROM WHICH THE NURSE SECURES INFORMATION ABOUT THE PATIENT

Patient's Record.   When a physician takes over the treatment of a person, he asks him or his family a series of questions and records the answers on a medical history form; he then examines the patient and records his findings; from time to time he makes notes on the patient's progress. The social worker gets social data either by asking questions or writing to the patient's home or place of employment, or by visits to his family, friends, school, or working situation. The attending physician and the admitting officer in the hospital also may obtain information on his social and economic status. Technicians who make diagnostic tests for the physician send reports to him that are incorporated in the patient's record. All these data are accessible to the nurse, but if they do not give the information required for effective nursing care, she may talk with the physician, the social worker, the dietitian, or other medical associates.

Patient, Family, and Friends.   If the nurse is an informed and keen observer, she will find the patient himself the best source of information. She is with a sick person more than is any other medical attendant, and by studying him she can make an estimate of his physical and mental condition. In some cases the patient is unnatural during the physician's visit and so misleads him; or should a disease be characterized by periodic attacks of pain or convulsive seizures, the physician may not be present when these occur and is obliged to depend upon the nurse's observations. She is more likely than anyone else to see the patient with his family and his friends, and this gives her an opportunity to form some idea of his relationships.

The psychiatric nurse's understanding and care of mentally ill patients are very important. It may be said that the nurse plays a parental role in the real and fantasy life of such patients. During the prescribed treatment, the nurse serves as an intermediary between the patient and the doctor. This is true not only for the psychiatric nurse but for the nurse in general.

Some patients, when talking with the doctor, may feel they are taking too much of his time. If this happens, then the patient will not feel free to tell the doctor about his fears as well as other facts he thinks are unimportant. Because the nurse is with the patient for longer periods of time, the patient will frequently tell such items to the nurse. The nurse does not seem so forbidding to him, and he appreciates her friendliness and interest.

All nurses, including the student nurse, have opportunity for making observations on which therapy is based as well as contributing to the prescribed treatment.

Leo Alexander has been giving a lecture annually to students at the Boston City Hospital for a number of years. During the lecture on the role of the nurse in dealing with chronic progressive neurologic disease, he always asks this question: " 'How many of you have been asked by patients—especially during night duty —what their chances are, whether they will live or die, remain crippled or well?' " He continues his comments with: "Invariably, all hands go up. This experience has impressed me with the need for teaching nurses the proper attitudes toward diagnosis and prognosis so that they will adequately interpret them, as well as help to motivate the patients properly toward therapy."*

The nurse may ask the patient or members of his family certain questions, and in fact must do so on many occasions in order to modify nursing care according to the individual's needs and preferences; however, she must avoid unnecessary and annoying questions. Throughout her association with him she should try to keep the patient from thinking that she is idly curious. What should and should not be said to patients is a subject about which it is impossible to make hard and fast rules. In the last analysis, the judgment of the nurse will have to guide her. In this case she will do well to remember that most individuals respond to a genuine professional interest in their condition by volunteering information that they think will be helpful to the physician and the nurse; they are not likely to resent questions if they are told why the questions are asked, and if the reasons seem to them to be good ones.

It is a tradition of the profession that physicians and nurses hold in confidence information volunteered by the patient as well as what they may have discovered while attending him. In most states the courts cannot force the doctor, the priest, or the nurse to divulge this information. Anything they learn about the patient is

* Alexander, Leo: *Treatment of Mental Disorder*. W. B. Saunders Co., Philadelphia, 1953. pp. 417–18.

to be used solely as a means of giving better service. Medical workers who consistently observe this principle are the ones in whom the patients are most likely to confide. A nurse who criticizes, ridicules, or betrays the confidence of one patient to another will thereby make her listener fear that he will be the subject of her conversation with someone else.

Professional Records Dealing with the Same Condition.   The third main source of information the nurse may use is the indirect help she gets from studying records of patients who have had similar conditions, or by studying textbook descriptions. In this way she may learn symptoms the patient is likely to have, their significance, the cause of the condition, if known, and the usual treatment. If she is caring for well persons she should know the physiological range in development or function and how normal development or function is maintained.

There is, of course, danger in trying to fit the care of the patient into the textbook picture. Patients vary in their reaction to disease; the determination of the patient to get well may hasten his recovery or a loss of interest in life retard it. A Spartan spirit or an inability to express himself may mask symptoms of disease and make diagnosis difficult. In many cases patients' conditions are incorrectly diagnosed. For these and other reasons, the nurse must constantly remember that she is caring for an individual and not a disease, and she must adjust her care to his changing condition and needs.

The nature of a case study has been given in detail, and the way in which this influences the plan of nursing care; the latter has been discussed in general terms. All this is in preparation for the following analysis of what goes into a nursing plan, and suggestions as to the forms that may be used for written plans. Both content and form are illustrated by giving a plan of care for Angela De Santo, the patient whose history has just been studied.

8. PLAN OF NURSING CARE AND SUGGESTED FORMS
FOR WRITTEN PLANS

Aspects of Care to Be Provided For in the Plan.   The activities shown in the plan of nursing care might be grouped in the following manner:

1. Activities that are concerned with hygienic care
   a. The methods by which the environment is regulated
   b. The ways in which personal care is provided
      (1) Cleanliness of skin, mouth, nose, hair, and nails
      (2) Elimination
      (3) Body mechanics: posture—lying, sitting, and standing; changing from one posture or position to another; and exercise
      (4) Rest and sleep
      (5) Variety, diversions, occupations, companionship
      (6) Nutrition
2. Nursing measures used for the relief of pain and discomfort
3. Activities prescribed by the physician for their therapeutic and relief-giving effects.

The plan of nursing care shows the sequence of these activities. It should indicate also which activities the nurse performs for the patient, which he can perform with her help, and which he can perform unaided. It is obvious that as the patient's condition and needs change, the activities and their sequence should be changed, which means that the plan is in a constant state of revision. Obviously the plan of care that the hospital staff is assisting the patient to carry out while he is in the institution must be modified when he goes home. The schedule of care must always be made with reference to the available facilities; otherwise it will be looked upon as impractical, and there will be a tendency to disregard it altogether.

While the patient is acutely ill in the home or hospital, there is an hour-by-hour schedule of activities, the larger part of which is carried out by the nurse. When the patient is not acutely ill, or if he is recovering from an illness, the plan may be a less detailed long-term program; it may show daily, weekly, or monthly activities that the patient carries out for himself. Suggestions of the physician and the nurse may relate to exercise, dietary schedules, rest periods, or any other aspects of care.

It is possible to carry out a schedule of care without a written plan, but the advantages of a written plan are obvious, especially when a number of persons are responsible for its operation and some way must be devised to ensure continuity of service to the patient. There are many forms that may be used. Each hospital and clinic and physicians in private practice design forms to suit their particular purposes. Those on pages 85, 86, and 88 are suggested as useful types.

Forms for Written Plans of Nursing Care.   The form used for the hourly plan of care should provide space to list the various items of care; it should also provide space for notations on the patient's preferences, special precautions to be taken in giving a treatment, and other items that will help the nurses give more effective care. It is possible to combine with the plan a system of recording what is done for the patient by introducing a space opposite the activity for a check mark to indicate that the particular item of care has been given. If such a device is used, the accompanying notes on the nurse's observation of the patient may be reduced to brief summaries at stated intervals in a 24-hour period. She usually makes observations on physical and mental symptoms, her estimate of his general condition, records of elimination, and any other significant signs.

The scheme of care may be revised by replacing the old plan with a new one or by drawing lines through canceled items and adding new items in appropriate spaces. Patient and the nurse may become slaves to the plan unless flexibility is emphasized and revisions facilitated. The plan is made to serve them, and when it works any other way, it is either a poor one or is misused.

9. MEASURING THE SUCCESS OF THE PLAN OF NURSING CARE AND ITS EXECUTION

Maintenance of Health in Preventive Nursing.   In any nursing program for a healthy individual, there is no better indication of successful care than his vigor and freedom from disease. A nurse is always cooperating with others in health programs, so that it is difficult to determine what measure of "credit" is due her. In this country where nurses are the largest single medical group and consequently give the most service to the patient, in point of time, they can assume that the success of a community project is some indication that they are working effectively. Nurses, working with doctors in schools, expect to see, as a result of their combined efforts, a reduction in the occurrence of colds, local infections, digestive troubles, headaches, poor posture, and other minor ills and defects. Successful nursing in schools, then, would be evidenced by the practice of good hygiene by the students.

Districts in which hospitals and community nursing services are well organized should show not only lower morbidity and mortality rates, but also general improvement in health practices. While the results of preventive nursing are more convincingly demonstrated by statistics on a large group of persons, *it is nevertheless what the nurse accomplishes with the individual that is measured.*

Patient's Recovery and Return to Health.   In the case of a sick person, the success of the program of care is strikingly demonstrated by his recovery. Nurses are often heard to express their preference for taking care of a critically ill patient. His recovery gives them satisfaction and leaves them with a sense of achievement. There is more drama in nursing those who are acutely ill than those who are chronically ill or mildly ill. The changes during an acute illness are more obvious. While the patient is struggling against the forces of disease, the skilled nurse thinks for him, anticipates his needs, and supplies his wants, thereby making the individual very *dependent* upon her. Nurses and doctors sometimes give the patient and his family the impression that they take more interest in getting the patient over the critical stage of illness than in helping him to become *independent* during convalescence and in giving him the guidance that prevents a recurrence. Nurses or doctors who make the patient rely upon them unduly may be as mistaken as the mother who discourages self-reliance in her child. Nursing sick persons is not completely successful unless the patient is helped to maintain and acquire optimum independence throughout all stages of his illness. Normal habits of living should be re-established as rapidly as the condition of the patient permits rehabilitation.

Relief of Pain and Discomfort.   The control of pain and discomfort is the joint responsibility of the patient's medical attendants, but of this group the nurse probably carries the largest share. The doctor prescribes narcotics and with surgery and other forms of therapy may remove the cause of pain, but the main purpose of many nursing activities is to make the patient comfortable. Well-planned nursing care, skillfully executed, makes the patient actually *look* comfortable; for example, he appears relaxed and in an easy position; the bedclothes, pillows, and his clothing are so arranged that there is no pull or strain on any part of the body; his skin, hair, and nails look well cared for. There is order in the room; it is free from glare; there are no disagreeable odors; and the temperature is within the range of comfort. Whenever she gives a treatment, the capable nurse avoids causing unnecessary pain or discomfort. If the daily nursing care makes the patient uncomfortable, there is usually something wrong with its plan or the way it is carried out unless the patient has "intractable" or uncontrollable pain. When the patient's disease is self-limited and there is hope of recovery, a plan of care that effects a cure is the main consideration. On the other hand, when the person has an incurable and painful disease, the chief aim of the doctor and nurse may be simply to make him comfortable. In such a case the estimate of the success of the nursing plan is measured almost entirely by the relief given the patient.

Confidence of the Patient, His Family, and Friends. A sign of successful nursing is the establishment of mutual confidence and respect between the nurse and the patient, his family, and his friends. In community health work, cooperation with the family is stressed because the nurse must frequently depend upon members of the patient's household for assistance; but in the hospital the family and friends are likely to be given less consideration because the need for their cooperation, while it exists, is less evident. The patient's peace of mind, and consequently his physical condition, is affected by the feeling of confidence his family shows in his medical attendants. The respect and liking of the patient and members of his household are an important indicator of successful nursing, and without it almost any plan, no matter how technically correct, is likely to fail.

Cooperation with Other Medical Workers. It has been pointed out repeatedly that the most successful medical service is given when all those associated with the care of the patient are working together to accomplish a common purpose. A nursing plan that furthers this ideal and stimulates pleasant working relationships between the doctor, the nurse, the dietitian, the social worker, and special therapists has accomplished a good deal. The satisfaction of her associates in the care she gives her patients is one of the signal marks of successful nursing. While professional loyalties should never take precedence over the welfare of the patient, in the writer's opinion, mutual respect and confidence between medical workers are an essential element of the highest type of service for the patient. Plans for nursing care should be made with consideration for those concerned with giving the care as well as for the patient. In hospitals the welfare of one patient must not be sacrificed for that of another. This means that the hours of service available to patients and the available supplies must be distributed with consideration for the demands of each individual. Nurses who take unfair means of benefiting their patients at the expense of others are likely to lose the support of the persons with whom they work. An intelligent patient senses the attitude of those around him and is favorably affected by the harmony that exists. The nurse who works well with others not only gets greatest personal satisfaction but also gives better patient care than one who doesn't.

Increased Nursing Ability. With the care of each patient the nurse should feel that she has added something to her store of knowledge and has increased her professional skill. If she does not have this satisfaction of having worked out a problem successfully, it is very likely there was something wrong with the care she gave the patient, and she should try to find out in what respect she failed. Nothing could be more helpful to nurses than collecting and studying clinical nursing plans used for their patients. With each plan, notes should be kept on the condition of the patient, the reasons for, and the degree of success or failure of, the nursing measures employed.

SUMMARY

The plan of care for the patient includes an hour-by-hour and a long-term program designed with reference to the patient's particular needs and the conditions under which he lives. In some cases the latter type is all that is needed. The program or plan is made by the physician in collaboration with the patient and his family, the nurse, the dietitian, the social worker, special therapists, and other medical workers associated with him in care of the patient; in some cases the minister may play a significant role. The person for whom the plan is made, if he is not too sick and has reached the age of reason, participates in making and executing the plan, since his cooperation is essential to its success. It is important that all concerned with the patient's program of care should know the central therapeutic aim. It is equally important that there should be a schedule of care for the patient, known to all those who are responsible for its execution, in order to prevent omissions and overlapping.

Cooperation among workers and consistency in treatment and care are fostered by case conferences and by the use of written plans of care kept with the patient's record. Written plans of care seem to provide the surest means of making the schedule known to all concerned. Planning treatment and care on an individual basis means that those who plan it must acquire a certain amount of information about the patient in order that they may analyze his needs. Such data make up the *case studies* in medicine, nursing, and social work. All professional workers in attendance upon the patient share the responsibility of making this study; therefore, a record system that makes the findings of each available to all should be used. Every category of medical worker should have a clear understanding of their functions in relation to planning and executing the care of the patient. If they are not defined, there is likely to be overlapping and omissions.

The effectiveness of the plan of care and of the way in which it is carried out is demonstrated in various ways. The nurse may measure her success in preventive nursing by what she thinks she has contributed toward keeping the individual well. In nursing those who are sick, the recovery and rehabilitation of the individual in the shortest possible time is what the nurse, in cooperation with other medical workers, hopes to accomplish. In nursing those who have an incurable and painful disease, her success is judged largely by her ability to relieve the patient's discomfort. Success in nursing is evidenced by a spirit of friendliness and cooperation between the nurse and the patient, his family and his friends, and between the nurse and other medical workers. Any manifestations of effective nursing in the behavior of others and her own consciousness of having solved problems in a situation that comes within her province give the nurse increased professional confidence. It is difficult to imagine anything that offers more satisfaction than a well-conceived and skillfully executed plan of nursing care.

REFERENCES

1. Brown, Mary E.: "Daily Activity Inventory and Progress Record for Those with Atypical Movement," *J. Occup. Therap.,* **4:**195, (Oct.-Nov.) 1950; **4:**261, (Nov.-Dec.) 1951; and **5:**23, (Jan.-Feb.) 1951.
2. Richardson, Henry B.: *Patients Have Families.* Commonwealth Fund, New York, 1945.
3. Jensen, Frode, et al.: *Medical Care of the Discharged Hospital Patient.* Commonwealth Fund, New York, 1944.
4. Shetland, Margaret L.: *Family Health Service: A Study of the Department of Educational Nursing of the Community Service Society.* Institute of Welfare Research, in cooperation with the Department, New York, 1943.
5. Houston, William R.: *The Art of Treatment.* The Macmillan Company, New York, 1936, p. 85.
6. Priest, Prudence I.: "Teaching Patients to Take Care of Themselves," *Am. J. Nursing,* **52:**1493, (Dec.) 1952.
7. Leavy, Stanley A.: "Psychiatry in Its Relation with Religion," *Connecticut State M. J.,* **14:**1015, (Nov.) 1950.
8. Hiltner, Seward: *Religion and Health.* The Macmillan Company, New York, 1943.
9. Leslie, Robert C.: "Religion and the Mentally Ill," *Am. J. Nursing,* **51:**255, (Apr.) 1951.
10. Seidenfeld, Morton A.: *Psychological Aspects of Medical Care.* Charles C Thomas, Publisher, Springfield, Ill., 1949, p. 17.

Additional Suggested Reading

Atkins, Elizabeth S.: "When Patients Go Home," *Am. J. Nursing,* **43:**987, (Nov.) 1943.

Buell, Bradley, et al.: *Community Planning for Human Services.* Columbia University Press, New York, 1952.

Cabot, Richard C., and Dicks, Russell L.: *The Art of Ministering to the Sick.* The Macmillan Company, New York, 1936.

Cobb, Stanley: *Emotions and Clinical Medicine.* W. W. Norton & Co., New York, 1950.

Field, Minna: *Patients Are People.* Columbia University Press, New York, 1953.

Garrett, James F. (ed.): *Psychological Aspects of Physical Disability.* US Office of Vocational Rehabilitation, Washington, D.C., 1952.

Gilbert, Ruth: *The Public Health Nurse and Her Patient,* 2nd ed. Commonwealth Fund, New York, 1951.

Hinsie, Leland E.: *The Person in the Body.* W. W. Norton & Co., New York, 1945.

Jones, Maxwell, et al.: *The Therapeutic Community.* Basic Books, Inc., New York, 1953.

Linton, Ralph: *Cultural Background of Personality.* Appleton-Century-Crofts, Inc., New York, 1945.

Langford, William S., et al.: "The Professional Person: A Mental Hygiene Resource," *Ment. Hyg.,* **32:**262, (Apr.) 1950.

Maves, Paul B.: "The Church in Community Planning for the Aged." *Geriatrics,* **5:**339, (Nov.-Dec.) 1950.

May, Rollo: *The Meaning of Anxiety.* Ronald Press Co., New York, 1950.

Montag, Mildred M., and Filson, Margaret: *Nursing Arts,* 2nd ed. W. B. Saunders Co., Philadelphia, 1953.

Pearse, Innes, H., and Crocker, L. H.: *The Peckham Experiment.* Yale University Press, New Haven, 1945.

Peplau, Hildegarde: *Interpersonal Relations in Nursing.* G. P. Putnam's Sons, New York, 1952.

Romano, John: "Emotional Components of Illness," *Connecticut State M. J.,* **7:**22, (Jan.) 1943.

Scheele, Leonard A.: "Cooperation between Health and Welfare Agencies: A Health Officer's View," *Pub. Health Rep.,* **66:**163, (Feb.) 1951.

Simmons, Leo W., and Wolff, Harold G.: *Social Science in Medicine.* Russell Sage Foundation, New York, 1954.

CHAPTER 5. ORGANIZATION AND CARE
OF THE ENVIRONMENT

1. HEALTH ESSENTIALS IN THE ENVIRONMENT

Homes and hospitals may be of very simple construction and yet provide every essential for health. Briefly, these essentials are: (1) access of light during the day and adequate artificial lighting when there is insufficient daylight; (2) provision of an atmospheric temperature and humidity that promotes normal body function; (3) sufficient air movement to evaporate sweat and favor vascular changes within the skin; (4) atmospheric or gas pressures within man's tolerance; (5) provision for disposal of excreta and waste; (6) removal of appreciable quantities of dust, injurious chemicals, and pathogenic bacteria from the air; and (7) reasonable cleanliness of all surfaces and furnishings that the individual is likely to handle. Order, freedom from disagreeable odors and noise, harmony of color and design in the immediate surroundings, and the opportunity for privacy affect the mental state and indirectly the physical welfare. Individuals vary, however, according to temperament and training in their desire for quiet, beauty, and privacy, whereas the conditions listed above are truly essential to well-being. It goes without saying that a healthful environment provides facilities for all the physiological functions, such as eating, sleeping, and evacuation; that the dwelling is reasonably free from fire hazards, faulty construction, and insect and animal pests.

Henry E. Sigerist in his contribution to *When Doctors Are Patients** expresses his feelings about hospital atmosphere:

And so with three incurable diseases I have been very fortunate and I only wish that things may continue as they are for a few more years, so that I may complete my work. And I also wish that I may be granted to end my life at home and not in the hospital. I have a horror of the hospital, that blend of penitentiary and third-class hotel. Of course, we need hospitals and we must be grateful that there are so many excellent ones. Many examinations and treatments are impossible or at least very difficult outside of a hospital. But it is a dreary place, nevertheless, with its sterile-looking rooms, bare walls, high beds, and the necessary but rigid routine that makes it so difficult to rest in a hospital. The rooms are obviously made not to live in but to be treated in; and even the flowers that friends so kindly send us rarely succeed in brightening the room, because they are no organic part of it and rather give it the appearance of a funeral parlor. How much nicer it is to be sick at home where we have our books, where the cat takes the place of a hot-water bottle, and where we may count on a decent cup of tea to the very end!

Those accustomed to living surrounded by every convenience and comfort lose sight of the fact that these things are not essential to health or happiness. The nurse who finds the organization of the patient's surroundings one of her functions must not be discouraged if only the necessities can be provided, for the patient who has proper medical treatment and nursing care usually recovers as rapidly in simple surroundings as in luxurious ones.

2. MODIFICATION OF THE ENVIRONMENT IN SICKNESS

A Comparison of Environmental Needs in Health and Sickness.   Almost everything that contributes to a wholesome environment of persons in health may at one time or another require modification during sickness; for example, atmospheric temperatures normally desirable are too low for the burned patient; higher humidities than those ordinarily found indoors may be indicated for the person with bronchitis; atmospheres filtered free of pollens, or foreign proteins, are prescribed for the asthmatic patient; air containing a much higher concentration of oxygen than is found in nature is used in the treatment of many conditions characterized by lowered blood oxygen; airtight chambers with regulated atmospheric pressures are used to recompress and slowly decompress the patient with caisson disease, "the bends," or "diver's palsy"; and darkened rooms are used for patients with diseases in which there is photophobia, or hypersensitivity to light. It is possible to mention only a few examples of ways in which medicine uses special conditions within the patients' surroundings to treat disease. As more is learned about environmental medicine, hospital construction will be more highly specialized. Some present-day hospitals have controlled atmospheres throughout; many have special rooms with environmental modifications such as those just suggested.

* Edited by Max Pinner and Benjamin F. Miller; W. W. Norton & Co., New York, 1952, p. 17.

Function of the Nurse in Relation to the Patient's Environment. Radical changes in the patient's surroundings when used as therapy are prescribed by the physician; ordinarily he leaves to others provision of a wholesome and pleasant environment. Nurses should work closely with medical and hospital administrative personnel on environmental questions. The nurse, acting alone, cannot see that the persons under her care have adequate light, pure air, and other health essentials; she can, however, and often does take part in planning hospitals, schools, clinics, and other domiciles; in home nursing she may help the family to select the room for an infant or an invalid. In every situation the nurse who knows physiological and psychological reactions to temperature and humidity, light and color, gas pressures, odors, noise, and chemical impurities can organize and make the best use of the facilities available. Sanitation, architecture, and housekeeping, per se, are not nursing, but the nurse must know something about all these, and if the welfare of the patient demands it, she may be obliged to function in any of these fields. During epidemics of contagious diseases, she must teach and practice methods of sanitation, such as decontaminating drinking water and disinfecting excreta; and when her patient is very ill, the nurse may clean the room or prepare the food if she believes she can perform these services in such a way that the patient will be most benefited. In home nursing, the professional nurse may find it necessary to clean, wash, and cook, until a suitable person can be found to take over these tasks. Although housekeeping is not what the nurse is most highly qualified to do, and is misdirection of the energy that should go into nursing the patient, it is nevertheless a false idea of dignity to think that anything she is contributing to the total welfare of the patient is "unprofessional" or degrading. Sickness upsets a home, and if the nurse can help restore peace and order, she is giving a high type of service. When sickness disrupts the management of the house, a housekeeper should be employed to supply the domestic service that has sometimes, in the past, been confused with nursing care.

Ventilation, lighting, fire control, and similar topics are treated briefly in this chapter. For more details the reader is referred to texts and articles listed at the end of the chapter.

3. NATURAL AND ARTIFICIAL LIGHTING

Sources. Every gas, liquid, or solid object at temperatures above zero gives off radiant energy as a result of changes within the atom. The sun, called the natural source of radiant energy, gives off radiations continuously. Radiations are thought of as a stream of particles (photons), each carrying a quantum of energy. "The quantity of energy in each quantum is related to the frequency (per second) of the radiation and thus to the wave length—the higher the energy value of the quantum, the shorter the wave length."* Physicists classify electromagnetic radiations into seven groups according to wave lengths. A glance at Figure 149 giving

* Maxcy, Kenneth F. (ed.): *Rosenau's Preventive Medicine and Hygiene,* 7th ed. Appleton-Century-Crofts, Inc., New York, 1951, p. 966.

some names to these rays, familiar now to many persons, shows the short radiations to be those we fear, or know to be powerful—that is, the ones with a high-energy value. Radiations lying in the visible spectrum we recognize as those we see in a rainbow or a prism. As the sun's radiations ("sunlight") pass through the atmosphere to the earth's surface, many of the rays are scattered or absorbed. The ozone in the upper atmosphere absorbs the shorter ultraviolet rays; the water vapor, some of the infrared rays. Smoke, dust, gas, and water vapor scatter the rays, especially those with shorter wave lengths. Radiant energy has four different effects on the body: (1) the heating effect produced by infrared radiation; (2) the effect of the visual spectrum on the retina of the eye—which we call vision; (3) the effect of ultraviolet radiation; and (4) the ionizing effects of gamma rays and x-rays. All of these effects are dealt with to some extent in this text. The effect of the rays in the visible spectrum is involved in lighting, or illumination. The extent to which ultraviolet radiation has been confused with other effects of sunlight is discussed briefly.

Natural Light. While we can live without sight, it is hard to conceive a healthful life, in fact life at all, without sunlight. Physiologically and psychologically it is so important to us that buildings should be designed to admit adequate natural light to every room. There should be windows on at least two sides of the room whenever possible. Northern exposures are desirable in southern countries, and windows that face the south in northern latitudes. A well-lighted room has a window area equal to at least one fifth of the floor space, and to admit maximum light windows should reach nearly to the ceiling. A room is poorly lighted if it is very much brighter in one part than another. Windows, however, should be so placed that it is not necessary to face the light when working. Provision should be made for controlling glare. Contrasts in brightness are uncomfortable. Most eyes can tolerate outdoor sunlight because it is of uniform brightness. Visual acuity is cut down as one passes from a brightly lighted area to a darker one; therefore, passages and storage spaces should have ample illumination to prevent accidents. Rooms with pale walls and white ceilings are most easily lighted; dark, dull walls absorb much of the sunlight. Shining surfaces, however, contribute to glare, and flat finish for paint is recommended. Light or bright colors may be used to indicate danger areas or to call attention to an object or barrier that might be overlooked.[1]

Ordinary window glass absorbs the antirachitic ultraviolet radiation; for this reason it has been suggested that homes, hospitals, and schools be furnished with special window glass that permits the passage of ultraviolet rays. While this may be indicated in some treatment centers, Janet H. Clark[2] has pointed out that persons sitting for 20 hours in a room with such special glass outside the area of direct sunlight would get about as much ultraviolet radiation as they would receive from two-minutes' exposure to sunlight outdoors at noon.

The therapeutic effect of light has been greatly publicized in recent years. Mothers have been taught the value of sunlight in preventing rickets, and the vogue for sun-tanned complexions in adult circles needs no emphasis. The average person who goes in for this usually thinks it enhances the appearance, but he also believes that he is building up resistance to disease. Kenneth F. Maxcy says that no studies to date have shown that this practice increases resistance to respiratory or other infections. Some skin diseases do respond favorably to ultraviolet radiation, either with sunlight or lamps; on the other hand, excessive exposure to sunlight, as with sailors or farmers, particularly in southern latitudes, seems to predispose to skin cancer.[3] The use of ultraviolet lamps in homes without medical supervision is dangerous.

The public, unduly certain of the beneficial effects of prolonged exposure of the skin to intense sunlight, is equally convinced that the eyes must be shielded from the sun's rays. Again experts urge a more moderate course. Exposure of the eyes to snow or to radiation from the sand on beach or desert may be intensely irritating and, if of long duration, harmful to some eyes. Nature seems to have provided normal men with adequate protection against all ordinary exposures to visible light, and, in general, disuse weakens adaptive faculties. The National Bureau of Standards[4] has set up specifications for a variety of glasses that filter out ultraviolet, infrared, or excessive visible radiation to be worn in vocations that subject workers to these hazards.

Ward patients who are hypersensitive to light should use dark glasses or eyeshades so that normal lighting can be provided the other occupants. This is likewise the best way to treat photophobia in measles because sunlight helps to control the bacterial content of the air.

Artificial Lighting.   Just as the sun gives off radiations, enabling us to see as its rays fall on the earth, so likewise will solids and gases, when sufficiently hot, give off radiations in the visible spectrum. Carbon and tungsten filaments are commonly used in light bulbs, and mercury vapor in neon lights. Light in rooms is still measured, however, in terms of the amount of light given by an internationally standardized candle. A photometer is used to assess the amount of light.

Sidney A. Fox[5] says that a good norm for the average eye in daily occupations is about 12 foot candles of light. This is the amount of light given by a 40-watt electric bulb with a good reflector at a distance of 2 ft. If the work is closer to the source of light, the foot candles are almost doubled and, conversely, if the light bulb is moved to a greater distance from the work, it will give less light. A 100-watt bulb 10 ft away gives only 1 foot candle of light. The quality of the light is very much affected by the reflector. It is also affected by the contrasts and colors of objects on which it falls. Much less light is needed to read a page of black print on very white paper than to read the same print on gray paper. A person sewing on black cloth needs far more light than is needed for either white or gray. Dust on light bulbs and in the atmosphere cuts down illumination.[6] The nurse must bear in mind, too, that as persons grow older, they require more light. The middle-aged man or woman requires ten times as much light for clear vision as the young child. Persons with defective vision need more light, generally speaking, than those who see well, and, according to Fox, the light blue eye requires less light than the dark. Medical workers should be ever alert to special needs of patients and personnel.

Most rooms, particularly workrooms, should be uniformly and well lighted. An even distribution of light is best achieved by directing rays on a light (white) ceiling, from which they fall on all aspects of the room. When the occupants are using the eyes for close work, as in a library, a marked contrast between the light on the desks or tables and the surrounding area is undesirable. The constant adjustment to light and dark areas fatigues the muscles of accommodation. Reception and drawing rooms, where people do not need visual acuity, may be less uniformly lighted. Bedrooms in hospitals and homes should have adjustable lighting, but bright ceilings are of course contraindicated. Movable standard lamps or extendable lamps that can be attached to beds, other pieces of furniture, and the wall are convenient types for patients' rooms. Light should be adjustable in strength, and for night use a very dim light below the level of the patient's eyes should be provided. It is highly important that the rational bed patient have within his reach a light that he can control. The lamp should be behind and to the left of a right-handed person and to the right of the left-handed.

Psychological Aspects of Light in Illness.   Everyone is susceptible to the cheering effect of sunlight, and, while sickness occasionally makes an individual hypersensitive to light, it is a common mistake to darken "the sickroom."

Alfred W. Worcester,[7] a physician of long experience, commented on the tendency of the dying to turn toward light as vision waned. Nurses should help patients and their families to recognize the value of light and should use their influence in providing well-lighted dwellings for the sick and well. In hospitals, beds should be placed with reference to windows in such a way that the occupant does not face the light when lying on his back but is able by turning to see the outdoors. Since the patient's condition determines the positions he can assume, it may be desirable in hospital rooms to have signal and electric-light connections on two walls, so that several arrangements of the furniture can be made. It should be possible to regulate light with Venetian blinds or window shades. In rare cases it is necessary to shut out light almost entirely, although in most cases the eyes rather than the windows should be shielded.

The sick person's day is usually planned so that there are periods morning and afternoon when the room is kept light, not only for the beneficial effect of light but in order to facilitate medical and nursing care and to make it possible for the patient to read, to see his friends, or to be occupied in some way. There should likewise be rest hours, especially after meals, when the shades are drawn and the patient is encouraged to relax or sleep. Changes such as this in the environment help to give some variety to the day and to make the time pass more quickly. Good lighting, both natural and artificial, is important wherever human beings live because of its effect on mind and spirit as well as body.

4. REGULATION OF ATMOSPHERIC CONDITIONS

Conditions Affecting Health.   Temperature, air movement, humidity, radiation, atmospheric pressure, and the relative purity of air affect comfort and health.

Physicians attach less importance than they once did to sleeping outdoors, and experiments have exploded the theory that there is an injurious concentration of exhaled carbon dioxide in crowded rooms, but a relationship does exist between health and atmospheric conditions even though all its aspects are not understood. When the outdoor air is clean, the temperature neither too hot nor too cool for human comfort in relation to the prevailing humidity, and the atmospheric pressure within tolerable limits, dwellings can be adequately ventilated with doors, windows, and chimneys. This is called natural ventilation. An enclosed space is said to be *air-conditioned* when the contained air is circulated, impurities removed, and the temperature and humidity regulated. We are just entering a period when engineering and medicine have combined to provide man with the greatest atmospheric comfort he has ever known.

Temperature and Relative Humidity.   Tolerance of heat and cold depends upon the amount of moisture in the air; for this reason the two are considered together. Clarence A. Mills[8] in *Climate Makes the Man* develops the thesis that since even the food in cold and tropical climates differs chemically, man, played on by this and other climatic influences, has a set of characteristics typical of the cold, temperate, and tropical zones. One characteristic of the Northerner, who, according to Mills, has better food, is his abundant energy or drive. Arteriosclerosis and other degenerative diseases are thought by Mills to be associated with this temperament. He believes the peoples of cold climates wear themselves out. The less well-fed but easygoing Southerner, Mills thinks less susceptible to degenerative disease but an easy prey for the bacteria and protozoa surrounding him in such profusion. Marston Bates, in a study of the tropics, *Where Winter Never Comes*, questions most of our preconceived notions about hot countries. He points out that the "profusion of nature" in the tropics is reflected in the variety of indigenous diseases, mostly infectious. He also points out that "modern medicine" is a product of Western civilization and that it has consequently been most successful in nontropical areas.

In other words, disease conditions in the tropics are in part dependent on the cultural environment rather than the climatic environment. Diseases that we now think of as primarily tropical were once much more widely spread. Malaria, for instance, was common a hundred years ago in places like Denmark, Sweden, England, Connecticut, and Michigan. Bubonic plague was one of the diseases that swept across medieval Europe with disastrous effect. Yellow fever . . . was [once] the cause of a great epidemic in Philadelphia.*

He goes on to say that ". . . with the methods presently available, there is no technical reason why the tropics should not be just as healthy as any other part of the earth's surface." Bates thinks that many of the ills suffered by the non-native in tropical climates result from bringing into a hot climate habits of living unsuited to it. There is, on the other hand, a general acceptance of the theory that the white man is more susceptible than his dark-skinned brother to the excessive

* Bates, Marston: *Where Winter Never Comes*. Charles Scribner's Sons, New York, 1952, pp. 136, 153.

ultraviolet irradiation near the equator. Harold F. Blum[9] concludes that the higher incidence of cancer of the skin and lips in the southern part of the United States than is found in the northern part can be attributed to the difference in ultra-violet irradiation in these regions. Certainly, white races living in tropical countries develop more skin pigment, which is evidently nature's protecton. Anna M. Baetjer, discussing "Environmental Medicine" in the text, *Rosenau's Preventive Medicine and Hygiene,* implies that, given time for acclimatization, man can adapt himself to a wide range of temperature. She thinks there is at present little evidence to prove that environmental temperature and humidity in nature affect the quality of health.

Man is a warm-blooded animal whose temperature remains nearly constant regardless of the environmental temperature. He can lose or conserve heat, within limits, by physiological changes. When these limits are exceeded, hot or cold environments can be fatal. Heat is lost by man through the excreta and expired air but chiefly from the surface of the body by (1) radiation, (2) conduction-convection, and (3) evaporation of perspiration. In a hot environment the heart beats more rapidly, and the blood vessels dilate to bring more blood to the surface of the body where it can be cooled; sweating is increased so that heat can be lost from the body through its vaporization. Heat loss is further reduced by voluntarily seeking a cooler environment, by removing clothing that surrounds the body with insulating jackets of still air, and by cutting down muscular activity or the metabolic rate. Man can increase and conserve body heat by (1) increasing the metabolic rate with shivering, (2) reducing the circulating fluids in the skin by contracting the blood vessels and slowing the heartbeat, and (3) by decreasing the activity of sweat glands. Exposed to a cold environment, man seeks warmth, hunches himself to reduce the body surface, puts on more clothing, and increases metabolism with voluntary muscular exercise.

Tolerance for high environmental temperatures has been studied rather extensively with young men; less is known about the tolerance of older and younger persons. The Committee on Atmospheric Comfort of the American Public Health Association has summarized these data:

Young, healthy persons, working under the conditions defined in Table 1 [see footnote below] are capable of maintaining heat balance after having been acclimatized, with a pulse rate of less than 125 beats per minute and a rectal temperature of less than 101° [F] provided that the external work performed is not so high as to raise the metabolic rate above 240 Cal/hr. This is considered to be a practical rate of work capable of being sustained over a working day without much difficulty to physically fit persons.*

The ability of man to adjust to high temperature depends largely upon his condition. The following factors lower his tolerance:

Heavy physical work, lack of acclimatization, extensive dehydration, improper clothing, old age, lack of physical fitness, excessive adipose tissue, and a low rate of

* "Thermal Standards in Industry." Report of the Committee on Atmospheric Comfort (Constantin P. Yaglou, Chairman). *Fifteenth Yearbook, 1949-1950, Am. J. Pub. Health,* Pt. II, **40**:131, (May) 1950.

body surface area per unit of metabolic tissue. . . . [The last factor explains the suffering of babies in very hot weather.] Man can tolerate air temperatures as high as 150° F for short periods, whereas, for long periods under some conditions, he cannot tolerate even 85° F.*

Baetjer in Maxcy's text goes on to say when thermal strain raises the pulse rate to 140 beats per minute when sitting or 180 beats per minute when exercising, the person is on the borderline of collapse. When sweating for any length of time exceeds 1800 cc per hour, an individual at rest cannot sustain loss of so much fluid; when exercising, loss of 3900 cc is fatal. The loss of so much water or sodium chloride, which is in concentrations of 0.06 to 0.6 per cent in sweat, is dangerous. When the person makes a conscious effort to replace the fluids and salts lost, sweating is less dangerous. Working in high temperatures where 5 to 8 qt of sweat are lost per day, a person should take at least 15 gm (225 gr) of sodium chloride. A day's diet supplies two thirds of this amount; in addition, 5 gm (75 gr) should be supplied by drinking 5000 cc (5 qt) of 0.1 per cent sodium chloride solution or by taking the 5 gm (75 gr) of sodium chloride in tablets spaced throughout the day.[10] Clothing of light color should be worn because it reflects infrared rays. Fabrics should also be light in weight, dry quickly, and hold little air in its meshes.[11] Wet garments should be exchanged for dry before the wearer goes into a cool temperature. During excessive heat, hospital workers should be given frequent rest periods. Patients who can leave their beds periodically should be encouraged to sit in chairs, which allows more air movement around the body surface. Cold baths reduce body temperature to a slight degree, as do cold drinks. Atmospheric heat can be reduced by fans, coils of cold water, the use of heat-absorbing glass in windows, shades made of aluminum or painted with aluminum paint to absorb heat, and many other mechanical devices. Exposure to excessive heat may result in heat exhaustion, heat cramps, and heat stroke. These conditions are discussed in Chapter 43, under "Emergencies."

The physiological response to cold does not seem to give man great *tolerance for cold environmental temperatures.* Constantin P. Yaglou et al.[12] estimate that the inactive human body can endure less than 6 hours of exposure to air at +10° F; about 4 hours at −10° F; 1½ hours at −40° F; and 25 minutes at −70° F. Much shorter periods of exposure to cold water at these temperatures are tolerated. Age, amount of fatty tissue, physical fitness, physical exercise, and clothing—all affect adjustment to cold. Ordinarily, human beings prevent a drop of more than a few degrees of body temperature by muscular exercise and the use of protective clothing. If the body temperature falls to 27° C (80.6° F), the pulse rate and blood pressure drop; and numbness, weakness, and coma set in. Under these circumstances man is unable to do any of the things that would raise his temperature, and death occurs when the heart is no longer able to circulate the thickened (viscous) blood.[13] Recent experience with crymotherapy (the therapeutic application of cold) has demonstrated that under certain circumstances man can survive body temperatures between 27° and 31° C (80.6° and 87.8° F) for a week or more, but

* Maxcy, Kenneth F. (ed.): *op. cit.,* p. 944.

in such cases he is closely watched, and his temperature is raised if he shows signs of circulatory failure.

When it is not possible to provide patients with comfortably warm surroundings, they should be given several layers of clothing or bedding that holds air in its fibers and they should be encouraged to exercise. Warm socks and mittens are particularly helpful because skin temperature is always lowest in the extremities. Tight clothing should be avoided because it interferes with circulation. An outer windproof layer of clothing should be used when there is strong air movement.

Treatment of conditions caused by excessive cold, such as frostbite, are discussed in Chapter 43, under "Emergencies." It must be clear from the foregoing discussion that the *comfort zone* in environmental temperatures and humidity is relative since man can acclimatize himself very satisfactorily to high temperatures and, to a less extent, to low. In the United States, where fuel is more or less plentiful, buildings are kept uncomfortably warm in winter for most Europeans. C.-E. A. Winslow[14] says that the commonest error in the ventilation of living rooms and workrooms is the slight but injurious overheating. Figure 10 shows the comfort zones arrived at by the American Society of Heating and Ventilating Engineers. The relationship of temperature toleration to humidity and air movement is indicated.

Thermal Standards for Heated Buildings.   There is no point on the temperature scale that is the ideal indoor temperature for everyone. Individuals differ in their reactions to atmospheric conditions, and each person has periods of increased and decreased sensitivity to heat and cold. The ideal indoor temperature may be defined as one that does not make the person sitting in the room feel chilly, but is at the same time not warm enough to enervate or cause perceptible perspiration. Baetjer, in Maxcy's text, recommends a dry-bulb temperature of $20°$ to $22°$ C ($68°$ to $71.6°$ F) for men in sedentary occupations and as high as $24°$ C ($75.2°$ F) for women because they are more lightly clad. Higher temperatures may be indicated for the newborn, for the aged, or for the sick when a warm environment is used as a therapeutic agent. When an otherwise normal individual is supersensitive to cold, it is better to provide him with warm clothing than to raise the temperature of the room above $21.1°$ C ($70°$ F) so that the average person may enjoy his society. Room temperatures must be lower when the inhabitants are physically active. Baetjer thinks the temperature should not be allowed to fall below $16°$ C ($60.8°$ F) because chilling of the body is likely to occur as soon as activity ceases.

Steam and hot water are the two heating agents most commonly found in hospitals. In order to heat with steam, it is necessary for the water in the furnace room to be at boiling temperature; therefore, the radiators or pipes used in walls or floors are filled with steam and are uniformly hot. When hot-water systems are used, water of any temperature can be delivered to the radiators throughout the system; therefore, regulation of temperature is more easily accomplished. If there are large radiating surfaces in a room (open fires, stoves, furnaces, and heated walls), the inmates can tolerate a lower temperature than when the room is sur-

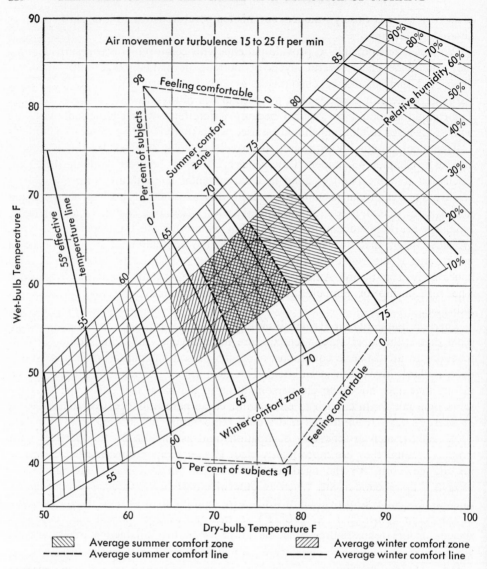

Figure 10. "Comfort or Effective Temperature Chart for Air Velocities of 15 to 25 FPM (Still Air)." (Copyright, American Society of Heating and Ventilating Engineers. From *A.S.H.V.E. Transactions,* Vol. 38, 1932.)

rounded by cold walls. Heated floors result in warm air around the feet and slightly cooler air around the head; this is desirable.

During summer heat and in tropical climates, it may be difficult and undesirable to lower the room temperature to 20° C (68° F). Mills,[15] in a discussion on methods of cooling room air, suggests that the difference between indoor and outdoor air should not exceed 8.3° C (15° F) because chilling is likely to occur if there is a more marked difference. Baetjer says physiologists believe that 7° to 9° C or 15° to 20° F between outdoor heat and air-conditioned (cooled) rooms is too great a difference. Some authorities recommend 24° C (75.2° F) as the lowest temperature for air-conditioned rooms in summer weather.

Rooms are cooled by introducing cold air through pipes or by cooling the room air with a refrigerating unit in the room itself. The principle underlying the heating and cooling of room air is virtually the same. In air-conditioned rooms windows and doors must be kept closed to exclude outside air.

In summary, there is general agreement that, when possible, indoor temperatures should range between 17.8° C (64° F) and 21.7° C (71° F). Lower temperatures are tolerated when the body is covered, as at night during sleep. An overheated environment is unwholesome because it enervates the individual, stimulates sweating, with consequent water loss, and produces an abnormal sensitivity to cold. Slight variations in temperature produced by air currents are desirable. Temperature toleration is affected by the moisture present and the amount of air movement in the atmosphere.

Because water is a better conductor of heat and cold than air, a person suffers from extremes of temperature more intensely as the amount of moisture in the atmosphere increases. A high content of moisture in the air intensifies the sensations of heat and cold, not only on account of the physical principle that water is a good conductor but also because evaporation of sweat from the skin is retarded. Very dry air, on the other hand, speeds up evaporation of sweat, a process that uses body heat; so this may also produce the sensation of chilliness under some conditions. Artificially heated homes are often excessively dry. A. P. Kratz[16] reported in 1931 that the estimated average relative humidity was about 20 per cent. Some authorities recommend pans of water on radiators or stoves when no special mechanism for humidification is included in the heating system. Others think such a device ineffective. Relatively inexpensive and effective humidifiers are now generally available.

Instruments—psychrometers and hygrometers—indicate the proportion of moisture in the air. When a given quantity at a given temperature contains as much water vapor as it can hold, without precipitation as rain or snow, the humidity is said to be 100 per cent; if it contains half this amount of water vapor, the humidity is said to be 50 per cent, and so on. The reading of a hygrometer, calibrated in terms of per cent, should therefore be taken to mean the relative amount of moisture in the air and not the actual water content.

Baetjer, in Maxcy's text, says that relative humidity plays only a small role in comfort except at very low and very high temperatures. The normal skin temperature exceeds the air temperature except in very hot weather; therefore, vaporization of sweat is, according to this authority, relatively constant in relative humidities of 15 to 75 per cent. The body compensates by increasing sweat production. When, however, this limit of compensation is reached and the entire body is covered with sweat, the relative humidity is the controlling factor in heat loss and high humidities cause great discomfort.

In certain disease conditions, such as bronchitis, it may be desirable to increase the relative humidity until a barometric reading of 80 per cent or more is reached. On the other hand, asthmatic patients are more comfortable when the inspired air has a relative humidity as low as 10 or 20 per cent.

Although outdoor humidity cannot be controlled by man, the water content of indoor air can be very accurately regulated. The relationship of humidity to health is not as well established as its relationship to comfort. When temperature and humidity are properly regulated, room air feels soft and warm.

Air Movement and Variability.   Warm air per unit of volume weighs less than cold and therefore tends to rise. Air currents of different temperatures have a refreshing effect on the body. They bring about circulatory changes and lower the skin temperature by increasing evaporation of sweat and also by carrying the air heated by the body away from it. High indoor and outdoor temperatures can be tolerated if there is sufficient air movement. On the contrary, discomfort from low temperatures is increased when there is marked air movement because rapid evaporation of sweat, with its accompanying heat loss, chills the body. Since outdoor air usually has the virtue of variability, it is much more refreshing than indoor air.

When natural ventilation by means of windows, doors, and fireplaces is not possible, air movement and variability can be secured by forcing cool air into the room through pipes and providing an outlet at a higher level for the lighter warmed air. With air conditioning it is now possible to approximate indoors the desirable features of outdoor air. Ordinary electric fans also may be used to set room air in motion, but must be used with caution because they are likely to make too strong air currents. Air movement of from 1 to 2 ft per second is considered desirable.

Regardless of what method of ventilation is used, care must be taken to avoid drafts, for their cooling effect is usually too marked to be wholesome. There is some evidence that chilling caused by a sudden drop in outdoor temperatures predisposes the person to acute respiratory infections; the danger of "drafts" is more controversial.[17] However, people fear them and are made uncomfortable by them. With a system of natural ventilation, deflectors should be placed in windows, screens used to protect the patient from air currents, and bedding and clothing provided according to atmospheric conditions. The resourceful nurse can usually find some way to keep rooms well ventilated, no matter how prejudiced the patient is against fresh air.

Air Pressure.   When man invades the ocean's depths or the stratosphere or even climbs very high mountains, atmospheric pressure must be considered in relation to health.

At sea level the atmosphere exerts a pressure of 14.7 lb per square inch on any object, including the body. This pressure decreases progressively with the altitude. At sea level the atmosphere supports a column of mercury 760 mm in height; at 50,000 feet above sea level, only 87 mm. (This mercury instrument is called a barometer, and atmospheric pressure is often called barometric pressure.)

Atmospheric pressure of 14.7 lb per square inch is spoken of as 1 atm (atmosphere); the pressure under water at 300 ft below sea level is equal to 10 atm or 147 lb per square inch. Because the atmosphere and the ocean exert an equal pressure over all parts of the living organism, the body is not destroyed by this enormous force. On the other hand, all animals are sensitive to marked changes in the pressures of gases (particularly oxygen) in air and water. The proportion of gases in the air is constant at all altitudes (nitrogen 79 per cent, oxygen 20.96 per cent, carbon dioxide 0.04 per cent, and traces of other gases), but at high altitudes, where the air pressure is low, the number of molecules of each gas in a given quantity of air is actually smaller and therefore the "partial pressure" of each gas is low. Under the circumstances the inhaled air is relatively poorer in oxygen, nitrogen, and carbon dioxide. At low altitudes the air in any given volume contains more molecules of each gas than that same amount of air at sea level. Since the concentration of oxygen and nitrogen in the blood is directly related to their partial pressures in the inhaled air, reactions to high and low altitudes are the result of lowered or raised concentrations of these gases in the tissues. It is for this reason that 18,000 is set as the highest altitude at which man can live and 300 feet as the lowest ocean depth at which man can work for even brief periods.[18] Man's body economy with relation to exchange of gases is apparently geared to the partial gas pressures near the earth's surface. Rachel L. Carson[19] says that marine animals who live near the surface of the ocean cannot sustain life in the ocean depths and that deep sea fish are thought to be destroyed when upheavals of the sea bring them to the surface. When human beings travel great distances into the air or the depths of the sea, they must surround themselves with airtight chambers in which gas pressures can be regulated or oxygen fed to them, just as in some diseases affecting the amount of oxygen available to the victim, he must be provided with an environment in which the contained gases are regulated to the patient's needs. (See Chapter 27.)

J. Bancroft, his associates,[20] and others have demonstrated that many discomforts and dangers to human beings in changing altitudes are overcome by gradual ascents or descents. Given time, the body can accommodate itself. Sudden ascents produce the *toxic symptoms of low gas pressures*. These are as follows: changes in pulse and respiratory rates and in blood pressure; headache; nausea and vomiting; fatigue; psychological symptoms of depression, or euphoria, or loss of memory; and, if the ascent is great enough, loss of voluntary muscle control, impairment of the special senses, coma, and death. Harry G. Armstrong[21] says that oxygen should be used at night when flying at 5000 ft or above because night vision is impaired; oxygen should always be used above 10,000 ft. Oxygen should be available to persons with symptoms of *anoxia* (oxygen deficiency) at any height, and unless the atmospheric pressure in the cabin of the airplane is maintained near that of sea level, persons with the following conditions should not fly: angina pectoris and coronary occlusion, if of recent occurrence; decompensated valvular heart disease; shock; severe anemia and asthma; pneumothorax; severe or complicated hypertension; pneumonia and severe bronchitis; and possibly gastric ulcers.[22] Effects of high altitude differ with the person's ability to adjust to it, the rapidity of ascent, and the duration. When a person exposed to high altitudes for a long time descends rapidly to sea level, when a miner goes down an air shaft, or when a deep-sea diver descends into the ocean, he may suffer on his return to sea level the *toxic effect of high gas pressure,* or of compression. If he dives deep enough or stays long enough he may be narcotized by the high concentration of nitrogen in his tissues or may have convulsions from an excess of oxygen, the physiological explanation of which is not entirely clear.[23] At 10 atm, or 300 ft below sea level, carbon dioxide is equivalent to 0.4 per cent at sea level, and, since man can tolerate up to 3 per cent with no serious effect, it is doubtful whether this gas is a trouble factor in high gas pressures. The symptoms experienced by man as he is *decompressed* occur from 2 to 12 hours after ascending from a low altitude and are believed to be caused by bubbles of nitrogen that in the higher altitude can no longer be held in solution in the blood. This condition is popularly called "the bends" because pain in the arms, legs, and abdomen makes the victim double up. He is fatigued and *dyspneic* ("the chokes"), nauseated and vomiting, and in severe cases there may be shock or paralysis. Death can and does result if the person is not again compressed and then decompressed gradually. Industries that expose workers to this hazard of low altitudes are replacing nitrogen with helium in the atmosphere (see Chapter 27) and are using great care to bring them gradually into higher altitudes. Nurses working in such industries and nurses in air transport services should make a more detailed study of the effect of gas pressures.

Purity of Air. Absolutely pure air is rarely if ever found; over the ocean and on mountain summits it is most free of contaminants. Air is, however, not considered "polluted" unless the concentration of foreign matter is high enough to harm plant or animal life. Impurities affecting human beings occur in the form of gases, vapors, and as fine, solid, or liquid particles that stay suspended in air (aerosols). Bacteria may be present on or in the solid or liquid particles. Baetjer, writing in Maxcy's text, still further defines the form of chemical contaminants in industry as liquids, gases, vapors, dusts, fumes, smoke, mists or fogs, and "smog, a popular term . . . to describe a combination of smoke and fog in the outdoor atmosphere. . . . Smogs are characterized by the general murkiness they impart to the atmosphere."* While most people have been aware that coal and stone dusts have resulted in occupational diseases among miners and stone cutters, there has been a tendency in recent years, even in medical circles, to discount the dangers of air pollution with inanimate matter. Convincing evidence is still lacking in many quarters, but recent publicized deaths in several areas, directly attributable to a combination of weather conditions and industrial air pollution, have aroused health officials and even average citizens.[24, 25] There is a wave of effort directed toward smoke control in cities and the making of more stringent regulations for the treatment of industrial contaminants. Some of the more important contaminants are the following: sulfur, fluorine, and chlorine compounds;

* Maxcy, Kenneth F. (ed.): *op. cit.,* p. 1037.

carbon monoxide and carbon dioxide; ozone; ammonia; formaldehyde; chlorinated aldehydes, ketones, and nitrites; acrolein; organic peroxide; soot, tar, and other organic mixtures and compounds.

Natural contaminants, such as pollens, are a menace to susceptible individuals. Microorganisms suspended in the air are a definite hazard in crowded areas. The increase in bacteria in relation to room occupancy has been demonstrated; air transmission of respiratory infections, especially those caused by viruses, is widely accepted. Maxcy says, "With the extreme use of radioactive chemicals and/or equipment the public may be exposed to atomic radiations through contamination of the air and water by radioactive waste products."* Hospital personnel are particularly exposed in the handling of radium, radioactive isotopes, and x-ray and fluoroscopic equipment.

In spite of this listing of dangers from air contaminants, chemically polluted air should not be considered an established cause of disease except in the case of such occupational diseases as silicosis, anthracosis, siderosis, and asbestosis, caused respectively by the inhalation of dusts of stone, coal, iron, and by fibrous forms of minerals called asbestos. Industrial workers undoubtedly need better protection from polluted air than they have at present. The general public should be more adequately protected from air contaminants that *may* affect general well-being by creating disagreeable odors, acting as a barrier to the sun, and possibly predisposing human beings to infections. Air with a high bacterial content is a definite hazard. In Chapter 7 there is a detailed discussion of the control of air contamination by bacteria. Crowded living quarters are unhealthful because the bacterial content of the air is high; they are uncomfortable because human bodies increase the temperature, block air currents, and, in some cases, give rise to unpleasant odors. It is known that exhaled carbon dioxide, even in the most crowded conditions, never reaches a concentration that could affect health or comfort.

In rural districts where the outdoor air is clean and crowded conditions rare, the provision of pure air presents little difficulty. In cities the air introduced into hospitals and other public buildings may be so full of injurious substances and unpleasant odors that it is desirable to wash the air by passing it through a vapor chamber or to kill bacteria with light rays or chemicals.

In discussing "the recommended indoor air supply" Baetjer says that the removal of odors, tobacco smoke, and "possibly infective agents" influences the requirement for introduction of outdoor air from the standpoint of health and comfort. The amount of outdoor air that can be tolerated with comfort depends also upon the number of persons in the room, the temperature of the outside air, the humidity, the temperature of the walls, the provisions for heating, and other conditions influencing atmospheric temperature and air movement. Health regulations for cubic feet of air space per person are set up with relation to the rate at which outdoor air is supplied to the room; the more outdoor air available to the inhabitant, the smaller air space he needs; the less outdoor air, the larger the

* Maxcy. Kenneth F. (ed.): *op. cit*, p. 901

space provided should be. The American Society of Heating and Ventilating Engineers suggests the following:

**Table 4. Minimum Air Requirements to Remove Body Odors
under Laboratory Conditions***

Heating season with or without recirculation. Air not conditioned.

TYPE OF OCCUPANTS	AIR SPACE PER PERSON CUBIC FEET	OUTDOOR AIR SUPPLY MINUTES PER PERSON CUBIC FEET
Sedentary adults of average socioeconomic level	100 200 300 500	25 16 12 7
Laborers	200	23
Grade-school children of lower socioeconomic status	200	38
Children attending private grade schools	100	22

* Adapted from American Society of Heating and Ventilating Engineers: *Heating, Ventilating, Air-Conditioning Guide.*   Published by the Society, New York, Vol. 29, p. 119, 1951.

To protect patients in wards and individuals living in open dormitories from diseases spread by droplet infection, it is recommended that beds be at least 8 ft apart from center to center. In the control of any communicable disease, more adequate protection in the way of cubicles or private rooms is advocated. Although the zone of greatest danger is the area immediately surrounding the infected individual, dust particles in the air may carry infectious material for appreciable distances. The desirability of submitting air, which may carry contamination, to the purifying action of sunlight or ultraviolet rays or chemical disinfectant aerosols is discussed in Chapter 7.

Suggested Procedure for Ventilation

1. Place a thermometer in an unprotected part of the room and, unless the occupant's condition indicates the need for a higher or lower temperature, try to keep it between 20° C (68° F) and 22.2° C (72° F) during the day. If the patient is sleeping well at night and can be kept covered and warm, temperatures as low as 4.4° C (40° F) are tolerated.

2. Keep a chart of the indoor temperature to encourage checking at regular intervals.

3. When the temperature is too high or too low in an air-conditioned building, adjust the regulator or notify the engineer; in rooms with natural ventilation, open the windows and doors as indicated. If the outdoor air is hot, place an electric fan so that it will blow over a pan of ice or a wet sheet. When the temperature is too low in rooms ventilated with doors and windows, it is obvious that these should be closed until the room is warm.

4. If a hygrometer is available, place one in an unprotected part of the room for determining the relative humidity. When the relative humidity falls below 35 or the air feels dry, place a pan of water on a stove or radiator. Wet cloths and growing plants also increase the moisture in the air. Dryness in room air may be more adequately corrected by making an outlet from steam pipes or by using a motor-driven humidifier that gives off water vapor day and night. Marked dampness is not likely to be a problem except in basement rooms and in certain climates. Airtight stoves, or almost any type of heating unit, will reduce the amount of moisture in the air. If it is necessary for sick persons to be in such rooms, especial pains must be taken to supply them with warm dry clothing.

5. To obtain air movement with natural ventilation, see that there are two openings to the outside air at different levels. This can be accomplished by raising the window from the bottom and lowering it from the top. The cold air enters through the lower opening and the hot air, being lighter, rises and passes out through the upper. Use deflectors in the windows or screens to protect sick persons from drafts. In case the patient is hypersensitive to air currents, ventilate his room through an adjoining room, or wrap him up periodically during the day as if he were going outdoors, and open the windows wide. In summer heat, use a fan, but do not allow it to blow directly on a person who must be still.

6. Keep room air clean by using wire or canvas filters for open windows in smoky cities. Reduce dust particles by proper methods of cleaning and allaying dust (discussed in Chapter 7). Protect the sick and well from contact with the exhaled air and vapor of others by allowing adequate space between beds, by covering nose and mouth in coughing and sneezing, by a purification system, such as ultraviolet radiation, and by specific isolation measures for those who are known to have communicable diseases.

5. WATER SUPPLY AND DISPOSAL OF WASTE

Water Supply.   There is great difference in the relative purity of water in both urban and rural communities. Purity is measured largely by the extent to which water is free from organisms that show pollution by excreta from human beings or animals. Sources of city water, if they are small lakes and reservoirs, are usually protected from pollution by restriction of habitation around their borders. In many cases where the water comes from large lakes or rivers, it is impossible to prevent habitation, and consequently a high bacterial count. In such cases the water is made relatively pure by physical processes, or natural means of purification, such as aeration, exposure to sunlight, sedimentation, oxidation, and storage in lakes with controlled animal and vegetable life. When these measures are unavailable or inadequate if used alone, water is treated with a chemical, such as chlorine.

Water in urban districts in this country is clean and should always be safe for drinking purposes in a community where there is efficient health service, although this does not necessarily mean that the water is sterile. It is not possible to deliver it to homes in this condition. Methods of testing water are in process of development, and standards are changing, but the standard most commonly accepted is that of the United States Public Health Service. The advisory committee on official water standards states that not more than 10 per cent of the 10-cc portions of water tested per month should show the presence of bacteria belonging to the coli group.[26]

When epidemics of intestinal diseases, such as typhoid fever and dysentery, occur either in town or country, health authorities may advocate decontamination of water used for drinking, dishwashing, and cleansing the face and hands. When in doubt about the purity of water, the nurse should decontaminate it without waiting for directions. Anyone who is anxious about water in a well or cistern may take a sample to the local health authorities for analysis.

Since heat destroys intestinal organisms, which are the menace in drinking water, water boiled for 5 minutes at sea level or longer at higher altitudes is safe for drinking purposes according to Edward W. Moore writing in Maxcy's text. Boiled water tastes flat. To reincorporate the air lost in the boiling process, pour the water from one vessel to another until its normal character is restored. Ralph E. Tarbett[27] says water can be made fit for drinking in emergencies by using chlorine in amounts to give 3 parts of available chlorine to a million parts of water. High-test chlorine preparations (H.T.H., or perchloron) or chlorine disinfectants, such as "Chlorox" or "Purex," sold at grocery stores as bleaching agents may be used. Keep a weak solution of chlorine on hand that is made by adding 6 level tbsp (3 oz or 96 cc) of chlorinated lime or 1½ oz of H.T.H., or perchloron, to 1 pt of water. Let this stand a few minutes and pour off the clear liquid. To make water fit for drinking add 3 drops of this liquid to 1 gal (4000 cc) of water.

Most people in this country are aware of the dangers of contaminated water, and the tin dipper is slowly disappearing, even from the back woods. Moore says, however, that we have replaced a common drinking cup with fountains that offer the same danger. The American Water Works Association says: "(1) Mouth-guards are a necessity; (2) the intermittent vertical jet fountain is unqualifiedly condemned; (3) continuous vertical jet fountains are open to suspicion; and (4) a slanting jet protected with a mouthguard is perfectly safe."* Moore urges the handling of ice with the same care as is used with food. Colon bacilli have been found in crushed ice, supposedly put there by handlers. Typhoid fever epidemics have been traced to ice yielding as many as 50,000 bacteria to the cubic centimeter that had survived for months embedded in the ice.

With the increased use of radioactive substances there is always danger of polluted drinking water. The US Atomic Energy Commission[28] has set up regulations to control the danger, although the problem has not been solved. Radioactive

---

* "Progress Report of the Committee on Sanitary Drinking Fountains" (editorial), J. Am. Water Works A., 5:110. (June) 1918.

liquids, if held for a time, are said to change into nonradioactive forms; contaminated water, if stored for a few days, should lose its radioactivity.

Most city waters are treated to control the growth of algae in reservoirs and to reduce the corrosive property of water and often to soften it—a process that may unfortunately remove fluorine. It is also treated with some form of carbon to control tastes and odors. Considering the difference in water according to the soil through which it flows and the number and variety of processes through which is passes before reaching the urban consumer, there is small wonder that water differs so much from one city to another.

So far, water has been considered in relation to purity; the *quality* of water in health promotion is also important. As far back as man's history goes, the virtue of water from special springs, rivers, and streams has been recognized. Through the centuries, spas and hospitals grew up around these "life-giving waters." Modern medicine takes a more skeptical view, but the relationship of goiter and dental caries to the chemical content of water in different regions of the United States has demonstrated the fact that the quality of natural waters can markedly influence health—at least in some aspects.

The addition of sodium fluoride or the less toxic sodium fluosilicate to public water for control of dental caries is discussed in Chapter 12. While simple goiter is endemic to regions where the iodine content of the water is low, and dental caries related to a lack of fluorine, there is a possibility that natural waters may have a higher content of some other minerals than is desirable. Cases have been reported recently in which babies have shown blood changes (methemoglobinemia) attributed to excess nitrates in well water.[29] Some writers suggest that through continued study of regional water a key may be found to other nutritional, or metabolic, diseases.

Disposal of Urine, Feces, and Vomitus. Sanitary disposal of excreta is of primary importance, for upon this depends the purity of drinking water, the cleanliness of vegetables eaten raw, and the safety with which children and adults can work and play in the soil. A large part of the inhabited earth is polluted with excreta because so many persons are ignorant of, or indifferent to, its danger. Some authorities believe that artificial fertilizers destroy the land and that they should be replaced by the natural fertilization of plant and animal life.[30, 31] The people of some overpopulated areas are dependent upon human excreta ("night soil") for fertilizer, and, when it is used untreated, it pollutes the land. Under such conditions the practice of storing the excreta for two to six weeks would reduce the serious danger that exists when fresh urine and feces are used. There are many sections of the United States where human dejecta are deposited on the ground and where outdoor toilets, or privies, are badly constructed and improperly tended. Rural homes and sometimes towns, and even cities, that have water-carried sewage fail to reduce the quantity of feces in circulation to the possible minimum, because the sewerage systems are badly designed or operated.

Some of the major diseases spread by the ingestion of excreta are caused by (1) bacilli—the *salmonellae*, causing typhoid, paratyphoid, and related focal infections, and the *shigellae* causing dysenteries; (2) the vibrio of cholera; (3) protozoa—chief of which is the *Endamoeba histolytica*, causing amebic dysentery; and (4) the worms or helminths—*Ancylostoma duodenale* and *Necator americanus* (hookworms), *Ascaris lumbricoides* (roundworm), *Trichuris trichiura* (whipworm), and *Strongyloides stercoralis* and *Enterobius vermicularis* (pinworm or seat worm). The extent to which these microorganisms and worms can be found in the intestinal tracts of the populace is an index of its sanitary practice. It has been supposed that hot weather favored the growth of these organisms and for this reason diseases caused by them were more prevalent in the tropical zone. It is now recognized that the *shigellae*, for example, live longer in cold waters than in warm and that the *salmonellae* survive freezing temperatures. Gilbert F. Otto, writing in Maxcy's text, says that amebae are widespread in cold temperatures and warm climates; he quotes an estimate that one fourth of the world's population is infected with hookworm and says that the pinworm is the most widely distributed of all worms infecting man. Stools from 5000 residents of New York City yielded only two positive *shigellae* cultures; comparable current surveys in Georgia, Texas, New Mexico, and California have showed as many as 20 per cent of the sample populations infected with these dysenteric bacilli.

Safe disposal of excreta means preventing its contact with human beings, insects, animals, foods eaten raw, such as shellfish or lettuce, and with water until all disease-producing quality has been destroyed by chemical action or by the forces of nature. The latter includes storage, drying, fermentation, filtration, sedimentation, the action of light and oxidation, and dilution. Modern sewerage is a system of pipes and underground drains that carry sewage from plumbing fixtures to a body of water or to a system of drains that supply irrigation to arid lands. Disposal of excreta for irrigation is rare in the United States. Excreta deposited in streams, lakes, or the ocean is soon converted into harmless and even useful food for animal and plant life. Communities not favored with bodies of water providing a natural means of purifying excreta treat sewage in a sewage-disposal plant to make it relatively harmless. Milton J. Rosenau,[32] writing in 1935, estimated that about four fifths of the population of the United States provided with sewerage systems empty untreated sewage into bodies of water. The *sanitary code* of each city or township should include regulations that enable the medical worker to know whether excreta from patients with enteric diseases should be disinfected before it is emptied in toilets or hoppers. Some cities attempt to keep nearby waterways clean for bathing and for protection of shellfish. In view of the widespread distribution of disease-producing organisms in the intestinal tracts of well persons, sporadic efforts to treat feces, urine, and vomitus from sick persons seem relatively useless. In rural communities or at camp sites excreta is deposited in trenches or pits. The deeper the pit the less danger there is of infecting flies, roaches, and animals; the more danger there may be, however, of contaminating the water supply. Covering fresh excreta with lime (calcium oxide) or with straw that is oiled and burned helps to reduce the hazard of disease. Trenches at camp sites should be filled with earth or sand as they are used. Persons in charge of temporary habitations, such as camps, and all householders should make a thorough study of sewage disposal. Nurses serving communities without modern sanitation may find that their first step is, through cooperation with other health workers, provision of toilets as well as education of the community in sanitary practices. Proper disposal of excreta, however, without control of vermin, infected animals, and particularly without the habitual washing of hands contaminated with excreta will not eliminate infectious conditions of the intestinal tract.

The sewerage system in most modern cities in the United States provides for the safe disposal of excreta by water carriage. Maxcy, discussing control of typhoid fever, says, "Disposal of untreated urine and feces by water-carried sewage is a safe practice in some areas if legally permissible."*

When excreta must be disinfected before disposal in the available sewerage system, Maxcy recommends the following agents: (1) lime water, 1:8; (2) cresol, 1:100; (3) carbolic acid, 1:20; (4) formaldehyde, 1:10. In all cases the fecal mass should be broken up with a stick, which is kept in a disinfectant solution or burned. The disinfectant should equal the volume of excreta and the mixture should be left in a covered vessel for 2 hours or more before it is emptied in the toilet. In the writer's opinion the odorless compounds, such as *diphenyl* should be used when phenols are selected. Lime, or calcium oxide, has the advantages of being nearly odorless and cheap. The bedpan must be disinfected by chemicals or heat. It is obvious that the disinfection of excreta *in the bedpan* is objectionable. When this method is adopted, the bathroom or workroom is filled with offensive odors, and the pan cannot be used again until sufficient time has elapsed for destruction of bacteria in the excreta.

Care of Sinks, Toilets, and Hoppers.   Nothing should be emptied into waste pipes that will not break up into small particles. It stands to reason that the larger the drainage pipe the less likely it is to clog; however, even very large openings will be obstructed if hair, matches, cotton fibers, and grease are emptied into them in appreciable quantities. Any indications that fixtures are out of order should be immediately reported.

Hoppers and toilets should have flushing rims. Toilet seats should be open in front and kept scrupulously clean. Paper covers for toilet seats in public places offer protection, and light rays are used to disinfect the surface. Long-handled mops or brushes should be available for washing the bowls of hoppers and toilets; these are usually kept in a disinfectant solution. Odorless chemicals should be selected for this purpose. Bathrooms and workrooms that are well ventilated and clean should be free from odors. Chemicals that mask rather than remove odors are nearly always offensive.

Disposal of Discharges from the Nose and Throat.   Even healthy individuals should be careful to protect others from their nasal and oral discharges. Paper handkerchiefs deposited in waste receptacles and burned are most desirable. Bathrooms should be provided with special basins over which the teeth may be cleaned. When washbasins are used for this purpose, they are unfit for washing the face,

* Maxcy, Kenneth F. (ed.): *op. cit.,* p. 204.

but if the basins must serve both purposes, care should be taken to use the water only as it flows from the taps. Discharges from mouth and nose may be deposited in toilets to avoid contaminating basins.

If patients have diseases that can be transmitted by oral and nasal discharges, contaminated paper handkerchiefs should be deposited immediately in a paper bag and then the bag and its contents burned. Water used in cleansing the mouth may be emptied into hoppers and toilets. In case the patient is coughing and expectorating, a sputum cup of some kind must be provided. A tightly covered paper carton is probably the best type because it can be burned with the contents. Sawdust in the cup absorbs the water in the sputum and helps to mask any disagreeable odor that may be present. To estimate the quantity of sputum, the container may be weighed when it is given to the patient and again before it is discarded; the difference in weight is the amount of sputum.

Disposal of Soiled Dressings and Similar Refuse. In some hospitals, dressings are reclaimed—that is, washed, sterilized, and used again for one purpose or another. If this practice is followed, dressings are collected in special mesh bags that can be placed directly in a washing machine or sterilizer. Such bags allow the water and detergent to come in contact with the contents and yet keep small pieces of gauze inside. When dressings are to be destroyed, they should be placed in waxed-paper bags or wrapped in several thicknesses of newspaper and placed directly in a refuse can. Waste cans with tops that can be operated by a pedal should be used whenever possible. The receptacle should be lined with a waterproof paper bag. This also reduces the danger of touching the contents when removed and taken to the incinerator. Contaminated refuse should always be destroyed by burning, and handling reduced to a minimum. Chutes leading to trash bins or incinerators are installed in many buildings. Such chutes can be constructed so that they may be flushed with water as often as necessary to keep them clean. Most modern plumbing includes waste disposal for almost any material.

Disposal of Garbage. Liquid food waste from well persons is emptied into sinks that are then considered contaminated until properly cleaned. If the plumbing does not provide appropriate mechanisms, solid waste is best collected in paper-lined, covered cans, or buckets, the lids of which can be operated with a pedal. Garbage pails or cans should be washed daily after emptying. Whenever possible, kitchens in homes and institutions should be provided with garbage disposal units.

In taking care of patients with communicable diseases, especially those of intestinal origin, such as typhoid fever and dysentery, all food waste from the tray must be disinfected or destroyed. Liquid waste is deposited in a covered container and disinfected with a chemical (described under disposal of excreta) or boiled for 10 minutes before emptying into a sink or hopper. Solid waste should be collected in paper bags and burned. Paper cartons are convenient if available; newspapers, if used in sufficient quantity, are satisfactory.

There is no aspect of cleaning, either in homes or institutions, that is of more importance than the efficient disposal of waste. If this is properly done, one of the greatest sources of disagreeable odors is eliminated, and repellent objects are immediately removed from sight. Because it is such a special problem, it has been discussed separately, but the housekeeping functions that the nurse must in some cases assume or direct make it necessary for her to know other fundamental principles of cleaning and sanitation.

6. PRINCIPLES AND METHODS OF CLEANING

Psychological Effect of Cleanliness and Order. There are many standards of cleanliness even in an economically favored country like the United States. What one person considers necessary in this respect may seem fastidious to his neighbor on the right and careless to his neighbor on the left. Generally speaking, however, most people respond favorably to symmetry and clarity of design in the arrangement of a room and cleanliness of walls, floors, and furnishings. Houses have personality and affect us in much the same way as human personalities. A disorderly room creates a sense of confusion, and suggests that the owner has an untidy way of living; on the other hand, a room that has a set scheme and is meticulously kept suggests a tenant who overemphasizes the importance of order and makes those who live with him uncomfortable. There is a nice feeling about a room that is free from dirt and dust, has balance, color, and harmony but at the same time has a look of being lived in. Austerity may be suitable in public buildings, but is to be avoided in dwellings. The danger of disease transmission and the necessity for economical methods of cleaning call for simplicity in hospital rooms, but efforts are now made to overcome an impression of severity by the use of warm colors and informal furnishings.

If the outlook of a person in good health is affected by his environment, that outlook is even more likely to be influenced during sickness. Those who are habitually orderly and clean are likely to be most sensitive to their surroundings, but even persons who seem unable to keep themselves and their belongings in order when well are very critical of disorder in the hospital. Teaching the value of cleanliness and order may be one of the nurse's most important services.

Dirt as a Carrier of Disease. A definite relationship exists between uncleanliness and certain types of disease since microorganisms found in the air are carried in dust particles. As has been pointed out, the number of bacteria at street level is many times greater than the number found 20 or 30 feet above. Bacterial counts in classrooms increase during periods when the pupils walk about. Flies, lice, bedbugs, and animal pests flourish in unclean houses and may be carriers of disease.

Dust itself is irritating to the exposed mucous membrane, and handling dusty, dirty objects may irritate the skin. The greater the number of persons living in a given area, the more danger there is from transmission of air-borne disease; for this reason and because very virulent strains of bacteria are likely to be found in hospitals, cleanliness is especially important.

In years past an infection known as *hospital sore throat* was a commonplace. When a patient contracts an infection in a modern hospital, it casts suspicion on all those who contribute to his care and the control of his environment. Order and cleanliness in hospitals, as in hotels, result from good institutional management. Most hospitals employ experts in this field; it is only when they do not that nurses must direct the housekeeping staff or take a more active part in ordering the environment. The nurse is rarely an expert in institutional management, and it is a waste of her special preparation for nursing to divert her energies to housekeeping; nevertheless, for the sake of the patient, she must be prepared to act in this role as she must often act for the physician, the nutritionist, or the social worker when they are unavailable. Because cleaning, laundering, and the care of furnishings are specialties, only the most fundamental principles can be set down in a text of this kind. More detailed information can be found in textbooks devoted to household arts and institutional management.

Methods of cleaning may be dangerous or safe, economical or wasteful, and the process may be unobtrusive or it may disturb everyone in sight or hearing. When ill, a person is likely to be supersensitive to odors, noise, and confusion, and in certain diseases the presence of dust in the atmosphere may be particularly harmful. Cleaning methods should be as silent as possible; odorless cleaning agents should be selected; and workers should be trained to operate unobtrusively.

The use of dampened or specially treated dustcloths or mops reduces dust and the danger of transmission of air-borne disease. Moist or oiled sawdust is sometimes sprinkled on floors before rooms are swept. Brushes and mops must be washed frequently. Dirty equipment cannot be expected to clean. A vacuum cleaner is most satisfactory since it draws all the dust directly into the vacuum chamber instead of scattering it about the room. Cleaners combining a rotating brush with suction are the most efficient. Control of dust is discussed in more detail on page 203.

Most *organic substances* are soluble in water and therefore not difficult to remove with ordinary cleansing agents. Fatty substances must be removed with fat solvents or emulsifying agents, such as gasoline, alkalies, soaps, and other detergents. Some organic substances combine chemically with fabrics, metals, and other materials and in so doing stain the surface. In such cases it may be possible to remove the stain, for example, from a metal surface with an abrasive, or it may be necessary to treat the fabric with a chemical. An oxidizing agent is commonly used to remove stains. Sunlight is sometimes effective as a bleach and is often employed to hasten chemical action. These examples are given to show that the nature of the "dirt" largely determines the choice of cleaning method. Dirt has been defined as "matter out of place."

Inorganic dirt is rarely as dangerous as organic because it does not encourage growth of bacteria. The total problem of cleaning, however, is largely one of getting rid of dust, mud, and mineral particles in city air. Metals combine with gases in the environment to form oxides and other compounds that coat surfaces; these must be removed for appearance and often for preservation of the coated articles.

Principles of cleaning are the same in all cases. Dirt or stain is removed mechanically by brushes or mops, by suction with a vacuum cleaner, or by an abrasive of some kind; if necessary, a solvent or detergent is used or a chemical that combines with the stain to make a different substance removable with a solvent. Cleaning agents are acid, alkaline, or neutral. It is important to know this property in selecting a detergent or a solvent and to consider its action on the article to be cleaned.[33] It is also important to select the most economical of the available agents. Large sums are wasted in hospitals through the use of expensive substances like "green soap" and ether for cleaning purposes.

7. ESTHETIC FACTORS IN THE ENVIRONMENT

Appeal to the Senses. A person's surroundings are attractive to him if they appeal to his senses; that is, if he enjoys looking at them; if he touches them with pleasure; if the atmosphere is fragrant or free from disagreeable odors, and free from noise. Close kin to these is the innate desire for privacy during certain aspects of the toilet, whenever treatments require exposure of the body, or when the individual feels that his illness necessitates behavior of any kind that would put him at a social disadvantage. There seems to be a universal desire to be alone at certain times, and a definite irritation when this privacy is invaded, especially without warning.

Beauty and Order in the Surroundings. Whether we are conscious of it or not, the *design* or arrangement of a room contributes to its harmony. Balance or symmetry is a cardinal principle, and furniture can often be rearranged so that large or dark pieces are placed on opposite walls or on either side of a door, window, or mantelpiece. Balance is sometimes achieved through the use of contrasting colors in curtains, screens, and furniture.

Through skillful use of *color* almost any room can be made attractive. With advances in industrial chemistry, colorfast dyes of every hue have been brought within the reach of all, but an appreciation of colors and the art of combining them are not universal. Certain principles may be learned that may help the average person with no special talent along these lines. For example, experts say that there should be a symmetrical use of dark, medium, and light tones in a room. Most persons respond favorably to rooms in which the dark tones are kept on or near the floor. Plain, light-colored walls make rooms look larger. The amount of sunlight and kind of artificial light available affect the selection of colors. Brightly lighted rooms, especially those with extensive window space, may be painted rich, even dark, colors; and paper or paint with a good deal of white should be used to reflect the light when this is meager. Warm colors, such as yellow and pink, are usually advocated for northern exposures; cool greens, blues, and grays are more suitable for sunny rooms.

Color preferences vary with race, age, and, to some extent, with sex, although there are strong individual likes and dislikes. Black is associated with death and mourning; but red is also worn as a symbol of bereavement by some peoples. A study of the tastes of children shows that they are partial to blue and red; young children seem to like vivid colors. Women are likely to surround themselves with pastel shades of the warm side of the spectrum; whereas men consider pastels effeminate, select deeper tones, and prefer the cooler colors. Blue is a general favorite and a first choice with men, and soft shades of red also are popular with men and women. White is considered glaring and is distasteful to most persons. When used by decorators, it is faintly tinged with cream or gray and combined with vivid colors for contrast.

Illness may or may not affect reaction to color; some authorities, however, think that color can be used as a therapeutic agent. Yellow, for example, is said to be exciting or stimulating and may be used for the depressed patient; lavender, gray, and gray blues are quieting and therefore indicated in rooms where sedative treatments are given; pink and rose are cheering, and because disease is likely to be depressing, free use should be made of such shades. It seems to be generally agreed that walls and floors should be colored rather than drab, but that soft shades should be used. Raymond P. Sloan[34] recommends colored ceilings, particularly for bed patients. His text has a helpful section on mixing paints. Vivid colors should be used in small objects for contrast. Flowers and pictures, if well chosen and properly placed, give charm to a room. Pictures may be changed for variety.

The care and arrangement of flowers is an item of no small magnitude in hospitals. In some countries, such as certain South American states, flowers are so closely associated with death that they are not sent to the sick. Here the well-to-do err on the other side, and so completely fill the sickroom with bouquets that the appearance of the room is marred, because there is seldom space enough for more than one arrangement of flowers on any piece of furniture. The container should be so placed that the entire outline of the bouquet can be seen. Containers should be chosen with care. The vase or bowl should not be higher and rarely greater in diameter than one third the length of the flower stems. Glass containers are suitable for roses and other flowers whose stems do not discolor the water. Vases of soft blues or greens, white or black, do not detract from the coloring of the bouquet. Experts in flower arrangement advocate putting the pale flowers of a mixed bouquet at the outer edge and making a vivid spot near the center or rim of the bowl with some of the highly colored flowers. Stems of individual blossoms should be of different lengths; otherwise, the effect is too regular, and all the color is centered in one plane. Unless each flower is put into the container separately and tangling of stems prevented, it is difficult to make a pleasing design.

To keep flowers fresh as long as possible, the stems should be cut on a slant under water; if this is not done, air gets into the openings of the stem and blocks the entrance of water. Removing the leaves from the length of stem that is to be covered by water helps to preserve the flowers and to prevent foul odors from decomposition of the foliage. Inhibiting the growth of bacteria prolongs the life of cut flowers. Preservatives act on this principle.[35]

Modern hospitals provide special rooms for the care of flowers so that other workrooms will not be cluttered with vases and the debris occasioned by flower arrangement. Nonprofessional workers who have some talent along these lines should arrange flowers. Volunteer workers often give this service. It is no longer thought that cut flowers in patients' rooms absorb oxygen. There is no necessity for removing them from the room at night except to get them out of a temperature that tends to wilt them. Flowers, such as lilies, which have a heavy fragrance, are often distasteful or even nauseating to the sick at any time, but may be especially noticeable at night. Patients attach great importance to the attention given their flowers. To them flowers are a symbol of the affection of their family or friends, and if the nurse takes no interest in them, it may denote to the patient indifference to his pleasure.

So far very little has been said about anything but the immediate surroundings of the patient. Nothing is more refreshing to the spirit of persons who are housed for any length of time than a lovely *outlook* from their windows. This the nurse cannot manufacture, but the furniture can be so arranged that the inmates will have the best possible view. Sometimes when a sick person must lie in one position and has little variety of scene, he will enjoy having a mirror placed so that he can see any moving objects that may be reflected. With suitable equipment most sick persons can and should be moved from one room to another or into the outdoors for variety of scene. It is rarely necessary to keep even a very ill person confined in one room.

Esthetic considerations should include freedom from unpleasant sights. Vessels of excreta, soiled dressings, and used linen should be covered and disposed of immediately. Trays of instruments and utensils that suggest painful treatments should be covered except when in use. Special passageways and service elevators are used in hospitals for the transportation of waste or any objects which would be repellent to patients and visitors.

Patients who are very ill, who are vomiting, or who for any reason present a painful appearance to other patients should be put in private rooms or screened if they must be cared for in multiple-bed units.

Concepts of beauty vary greatly with the individual, but pleasing proportions, balance, symmetry, order, harmonious coloring, and variety deserve universal consideration. It is particularly important that persons who are confused in mind and dispirited by illness should be surrounded by order and, if possible, by beauty.

Esthetic Sensations of Touch.   Metals, wooden surfaces, and fabrics may be attractive to look at and yet be unpleasant to touch. The choice of clothing and household equipment is influenced by this consideration, and very properly so. Sufferers from certain types of diseases, particularly those affecting the nerves of the skin, such as herpes or shingles, are particularly susceptible to irritation from rough fabrics and heavy clothing.

In health and sickness there is a tendency to like smooth surfaces, unless they are greasy, and to enjoy touching soft fabrics. Frank A. Geldard[36] reviews studies showing that textures regular in design are preferred if there are raised fibers in the textiles. Materials with curly fibers that have a nap hold air in their meshes and have a grateful warmth in winter but are unpleasant in hot weather. Few like the feeling of blankets or woolen material next to the skin except in severe climates and even then the sensation may be disagreeable. Warmth without weight is generally desired in blankets and bedclothes. The lightest covering may cause so much discomfort that it is necessary to support it on a framework or cradle (for further suggestions, see Chapter 15).

Freedom from Strong and Disagreeable Odors in the Surroundings.   Some odors, such as the fetid and the acrid, are so universally objectionable that there is no question as to whether they should be eliminated from the environment. Fetid odors in hospitals have their origin in body excretions, discharges from wounds, and necrotic areas. Sweat has an acrid odor, and so does formalin and other chemicals commonly used where there is sickness. Odors that are ordinarily pleasant may on occasion be objectionable. Nausea turns any one against favorite perfumes; unhappy associations can make the smell of a fruit or flower a disagreeble experience. The use of odors as a means of giving pleasure, or the opposite, is a highly subjective matter, differing with individuals and their moods. The safest practice is to keep the atmosphere as odorless as possible in public places, and particularly in hospitals. Medical workers should never use perfume and should avoid foods, such as onions, that make the breath malodorous. Many patients suffer from the smell of tobacco on the breath and hands of doctors and nurses. There is little evidence that oral chlorophyll and dentrifices reduce breath odors.[37] Soaps, detergents, and skin disinfectants as nearly odorless as possible should be selected.

Extravagant claims are made for chemical atmospheric deodorants, but physical measures are more effective. Dewey Palmer[38] lists the following as deodorizing processes in current use: dilution, sanitation, antisepsis, chemical neutralization of the odoriferous substance, oxidation, the use of other odors to mask the offensive odor, olfactory narcosis, electrostatic precipitation (filtration), and adsorption.* Dilution by air movement is very desirable when it is practical; the control of putrefaction with oxidizing, sanitizing, and disinfecting processes is effective, but the use of masking odors should be discouraged, as should olfactory narcosis. Electrostatic precipitation and the use of adsorbents, such as chlorophyll and activated carbon, are helpful. Motor-driven devices that suck air through a chamber containing an adsorbent are widely used with some measure of success. Any motor-driven air-conditioning system that constantly changes fresh air for stale is effective. Palmer says that cleanliness, or sanitation, which, of course, means removing the source, is the most satisfactory way to control odor. He recommends ultraviolet lights in storerooms to reduce bacterial growth, alkalis to neutralize acids, and the use of adsorbents when it is not possible to remove the material that is polluting the air. An absorbent, an oxidizing agent, or a bacteriostatic agent in impregnated dressings is sometimes used over wounds. Foul discharges, such as those in urinary drainage bottles, may be covered with toluol or some heavy oily liquid that prevents the escape of gases and hence controls the odor. When the source of a disagreeable odor cannot immediately be removed, an aromatic substance, such

* There is a widespread and persistent effort to produce an effective deodorant. Up-to-date and reliable data on commercial products are available from the National Bureau of Standards, Department of Commerce, Washington, D.C. Information on this subject at any time is soon misleading.

as ammonia or camphor, may be sprinkled about as a temporary measure; these chemicals are rarely distasteful to the ill and are usually considered refreshing. Winslow cites experimental evidence that disagreeable odors impair the appetite. The extent to which a hospital controls odors is to many persons an index of the quality of its total maintenance.

The Effect and Control of Noise. Baetjer, in Maxcy's text, defines noise as "discordant sound resulting from non-periodic vibrations of air." The characteristics of noise are pitch, quality, and intensity; or the number of double vibrations per second that strike the ear, the form of the sound waves, the amplitude of the vibrations set up in the vibrating body, and the nearness of the person to the vibrating objects. Sound intensity is most often mentioned in terms of the sensation produced by sound on the human ear. The *bel* or *decibel* (1/10 of a bel) is the name given this unit and is a measurement made with reference to the minimum audible sound. A low whisper 3 ft away has a noise intensity of 20 decibels; a jet engine, an intensity as high as 140 decibels.

Noise has been reported to affect man physically and psychologically. Intense noise may cause unsteady gait, nausea, headache, and weakness, and, if continued, irritability and apprehension. Intensities of 120 to 150 decibels sometimes cause temporary loss of hearing and may, if prolonged, cause permanent deafness. Sudden loud noises produce the physical changes typical of fear, such as increased arterial and intercranial pressure and decreased activity of the digestive system. It has been recommended that industrial noise not exceed 85 decibels.[39] It is obvious that control of noise is important physiologically, esthetically, and economically. Some investigations cited by Ralph M. Barnes[40] have shown that the output of work is not reduced by a moderate amount of noise, but that an increased effort is required to overcome the distracting effect.

A person sick at home should be placed, if possible, in the quietest room in the house while he is acutely ill, and it is perfectly proper for the nurse to suggest door silencers and other reasonable devices to reduce noise. Dead silence with no sign of activity may be frightening or depressing to a sick person and is particularly bad for patients who need diversion. Quiet, like every other therapeutic measure, must be used with discretion and with consideration for the individual's needs.

Hospital designers and hospital staffs are making efforts to reduce sounds of operation to a minimum. Walls and especially ceilings of workrooms and corridors are covered with materials (matted excelsior, shredded asbestos, or steel wool) that deaden sound. Hard, polished surfaces reflect and intensify noise; soft, porous materials absorb it. Double walls and doors that encase a chamber of air act as a barrier to sound waves. Rubber and similar materials for floors and working surfaces effectively muffle noise. Workrooms in clinical divisions should be segregated and, like elevators, separated from patients' rooms by corridors. Lights should replace bells, buzzers, or voices in call and alarm systems.

All portable equipment should be furnished with rubber-tired wheels or casters, and all parts kept tight to prevent rattling. Rubber bumpers on beds, wheelchairs, and carts of all kinds reduce noise and protect walls and door jambs. Racks for bedpans and similar objects may be coated with rubber; edges of hoppers, buckets, and such articles may be protected with rubber. Tops for pitchers and cans are available in rubber, and mats of similar composition are used on floor, table, sink, or shelves to deaden workroom noises.

Medical personnel are taught the importance of cultivating quiet, pleasing speech. Whispering is irritating to both sick and well. It is particularly undesirable around the apprehensive, who may fear it means that their condition is unfavorable. Both whispering and tiptoeing are objectionable because to most persons they suggest an anxious, fearful mood. Nurses, doctors, and visitors should avoid talking with one another within the patient's hearing, if he is not interested or if he is too sick to make the effort to attend to what is said. The positive use of sound or music as a therapeutic agent is discussed in Chapter 16.

Provision for Privacy. A part of the discomfort of hospital experiences for the average person is the necessity for exposing the body during physical examinations and treatments and for assistance during such physical acts as defecation, voiding, or vomiting. Added to this, in the case of the ward patient, is the necessity for staying in the room with strangers. Modesty is said by psychologists to be an acquired trait, which means that individuals differ markedly with respect to what embarrasses them. Although some patients give the impression that they have no modesty, hospital methods should be designed to protect the feelings of the most sensitive persons. Ward units should be provided with curtains that may be drawn around the bed when desirable; or screens used if curtains are not provided. In private rooms a screen may be placed between the patient and the open door. Revolving signs on doors that notify visitors when the patient is not to be disturbed give the patient a feeling of security and privacy. The practice of knocking, or otherwise announcing one's presence, is so generally observed that it seems almost unnecessary to say that the entire hospital staff is expected to follow this custom. Patients should be given as much privacy as possible; some are so sensitive that they dislike dressing, getting in and out of bed, or trying their strength by walking under observation. A nurse will often be surprised to find these acts performed during her absence, and may wonder why the patient did not wait for her to help him.

Providing an environment that does not offend the senses of the patient is not an easy matter but a task for imaginative, resourceful workers. There are numerous and varied possibilities for running counter to the prejudices and preferences of patients, and it is only by setting a high standard of institutional management that difficulties can be avoided.

8. SAFEGUARDING THE PATIENT FROM DANGERS IN THE ENVIRONMENT

Common Dangers in Health and Sickness. Possibilities of mechanical injury, electrical shocks, burns, poisoning, and infection are ever present in our surroundings. In 1949, accidents held fourth place as a cause of death in the United States.[41]

While 31,500 deaths were due to motor vehicles, 30,900 deaths were caused by home accidents, and about the same number by industrial and public accidents combined. The normal adult can, if he tries, substantially reduce the chance of having an accident or meeting accidental death; sickness, however, often distorts judgment and weakens, and in some cases destroys, the will to live. Some sick persons must be protected from accidental injury, as must children or the unconscious, but a more aggressive type of guardianship is necessary for the patient who has suicidal compulsions. Because plans of self-destruction are usually hidden by the patient and because such a sick person may seem normal mentally, large hospitals take definite steps, not considered necessary in homes, schools, or hotels, to prevent suicide.

Preventing Mechanical Injury. In order to keep patients from accidentally falling or intentionally throwing themselves from a window, the sashes should be made in such a way that they cannot be opened wide enough to admit a human form. For this same reason, porches are protected with glass, a heavy wire mesh, or metal framework. All elevators and similar mechanisms are equipped with safety devices. Handles, levers, and switches that operate physical therapy equipment are placed behind locked doors or controlled by keys kept by members of the staff.

Irrational persons may need restraint.* In such cases there is always the possibility that patients will injure themselves in fighting against the restraining device, and since the desire to be free is inherent, restraint of any sort is psychologically traumatic. Every effort should be made to use the least obvious and uncomfortable devices, and to give close supervision. There are so many measures that have to be followed in caring for and guarding a suicidal patient that it is difficult to cover the subject here. Sharp instruments, glass that may be broken, cords, belts, and all toxic drugs are kept under lock and key when it is suspected that some patients have suicidal intentions. Psychiatric services are so much more aware of this problem and so much better prepared to protect the patient that suicides are less likely to occur there than in other parts of the hospital. Many patients who are not classified as psychotic contemplate self-destruction. Louis I. Dublin,[42] who has made an extensive study of the subject, reports that suicides among men are three times more numerous than among women, and ill-health is the motive most frequently given by men. This suggests the importance of safeguarding all sick persons as much as it is possible to do so in an unobjectionable way.

Albert B. Siewers and Eugene Davidoff[43] compared attempted suicide in psychopathic and general hospital patients. Studying the records of 55,983 patients admitted to general hospitals and 1600 admissions to psychopathic hospitals they reported the following: one out of every 370 patients in the general hospital attempted suicide, while one out of 11 patients in the psychopathic hospital had "suicidal intent." They found that psychoneuroses predominated in the general hospital group, whereas in the mental hospital group functional psychoses were more prevalent. In addition they reported that the number of patients with organic

* Some states require hospitals to show written doctor's orders for all restraints or "protective devices."

illness comprised less than one third of all the cases in the two groups studied. In the mental hospital group, lesions of the central nervous system occurred more frequently, and in the general hospital patients, somatic disease. They found apparent motives elicited from the patients in both groups largely similar.

Smooth, even floors, fixed floor coverings, and well-lighted rooms help prevent accidents. Personnel and visitors must be warned when floors are wet, and movable objects kept out of passageways. Falls are not limited to those on their feet; it is not uncommon for children and sick people to tumble out of bed. In hospitals, beds are put on casters so that they may be easily moved, but this in itself constitutes a danger. Patients must be warned that in turning on their side and reaching for something from the bedside table there is a risk of falling; this is particularly true when inner-spring mattresses are used. It is very desirable to have a brake on at least one wheel or caster of any bed or similar piece of equipment.

Preventing Shocks and Burns from Electrical Fixtures.   Wiring for electricity should be done by trained persons in accordance with the regulations set by governmental authorities. For example, flexible electric-light cords, from wall or floor socket to fixture, should not exceed the prescribed length (8 ft in New York City), and all wires should be well insulated. As soon as the insulation has worn off metal wires that carry the current, the cord must be replaced. Cords should not be run under rugs or along door sills. In such positions the insulation is likely to be worn off and a spark created, which may cause fire as well as damage to the electric fixture. The National Board of Fire Underwriters tests electrical devices put on the market by manufacturers and either approves or condemns them. It is unwise to use equipment condemned by this board. All electrical appliances should be provided with signal lights that indicate that the current is flowing. It is highly desirable to have electrical wiring installed so that the circuit is automatically broken when overloaded.

Water is a good conductor of electricity, and it is not uncommon for persons to be shocked by touching an electric push button or switch with wet hands. Water must not be allowed to come in contact with electric pads or other appliances, because of the danger of short circuits. Each time that such devices are used at the bedside, they should be thoroughly insulated to reduce the danger of burning the patient or setting fire to the bedding.

Fire Prevention.   Modern buildings are often fireproof, the most effective means of fire control; but most houses in this country are inflammable. Some type of fire extinguishing system is always desirable, for even in metal, stone, and cement structures the furnishings are usually made of wood and combustible fabrics. Regardless of their construction, all hospitals are provided with some sort of fire extinguishers. In workrooms where appearance is not so important, sprinkling devices may be installed in the ceiling.

Fire doors that cut off burning rooms or portions of a corridor greatly reduce fire hazard; both sprinkling systems and doors may operate automatically by the action of high temperatures caused by fire occurring near them. As mentioned in Chapter 3, elevator shafts and stairways should be enclosed and made of fireproof materials. A water supply should be available in any part of the building for the use of the fire hose. Attempts to extinguish fire with water, however, are not only ineffective in some cases but destructive to equipment and injurious to patients; other measures also must be provided. All extinguishers operate on the same principle—the exclusion of oxygen from burning objects. Many devices contain chemicals, such as a soda solution and sulfuric acid, which, when combined, form carbon dioxide gas. When this gas surrounds the fire, it excludes oxygen as effectively as a water bath. The chemicals are usually mixed by inverting the container. Another type of extinguisher sprays the burning objects with a soap solution. Soapsuds spread rapidly over surfaces and in so doing exclude oxygen. Wool blankets or rugs thrown on a fire also exclude oxygen and extinguish flames. Some fire extinguishers contain substances that form phosgene, a poisonous gas, if used to extinguish fires occurring in oxygen tents; a fire of this nature can usually be extinguished with heavy blankets. When water and chemicals are not available in sufficient quantities for fire control, sand and other soils may be used to smother the flames.

Fire prevention, rather than fire control, should always be stressed. Most fires are a result of carelessness. Samuel J. Pope,[44] chief of the Boston Fire Department, estimates that about 90 per cent of fires are caused by smoking. In buildings where smoking is allowed, noninflammable receptacles for cigarette butts should be placed in corridors, and there should be an ample and obvious supply of ash receivers in every room.

Papers and rugs may reach the kindling point if allowed to collect in closets, attics, or any place where the temperature is likely to be high. Oil on paper or fabrics lowers the kindling point and thus increases the danger. Waste should be collected in metal containers; oiled mops and dustcloths and the clothing of workers in institutions should be stored in ventilated fireproof lockers.

So much publicity has been given to fires traceable to x-ray films that hospitals are now using the noninflammable acetate films instead of the combustible nitrous type. Old nitrous films that must be preserved as records should be stored in a separate fireproof room.

Accidents have occurred in operating rooms when a highly inflammable anesthetizing gas, such as nitrous oxide, has come in contact with cauteries or electric sparks. In an effort to prevent such accidents workers are required to wear only cotton clothing. Special shoes are worn, and furnishings are grounded to reduce static electricity. Pope calls attention to the importance of providing operating rooms, oxygen chambers, and storage rooms with vaporproof light globes that will prevent any gases from coming in contact with charged lighting filaments.

The entire hospital staff should be familiar with measures of fire prevention and control, but one individual should be responsible for the program. Each worker should know the procedure to follow in case of fire: how to turn in an alarm, use fire extinguishers, remove a patient to a place of safety, and to protect the nose and throat from smoke in leaving a burning building. Some hospital engineering staffs are so well prepared to deal with a fire that all medical workers are requested to turn in an alarm immediately, then to remain on the services to which they are assigned and to maintain the usual order while the fire is extinguished by those most expert in this task.

Protection from Poisons.   National and state legislative bodies have passed laws and formulated public health regulations to protect the public from the unwitting use of poisons. Druggists are not permitted to sell highly toxic and potent drugs without a prescription from a physician; labels must show the ingredients of patent medicines; and pharmacists are required to label highly toxic drugs as poison. The use of injurious chemicals as food preservatives or the employment of toxic sprays is regulated very carefully. Like all other medical workers, the nurse should keep herself informed about health legislation of this type and give her support to measures that provide thorough public protection.

In home nursing the risk of keeping poisonous drugs, cosmetics, or cleaning materials within the reach of children should be emphasized. When equally effective but harmless chemicals are available, they should replace dangerous ones. Some protection is given by keeping poisonous drugs in distinctive, well-labeled bottles stored in locked cabinets. In hospitals, drugs of a highly poisonous nature are always kept under lock and key. Some toxic antiseptic solutions, however, are usually found on open shelves in workrooms. Because it is difficult to recognize suicidal intentions, the use of *all* toxic chemicals should be reduced to a minimum and made as inaccessible to patients as possible.

Poisonous gases in the environment are not very likely to menace health or life. With modern methods of plumbing, sewer gas is no longer feared. Illuminating gas causes death by asphyxiation, and if ignited, a fire, when it escapes from fixtures in appreciable quantities. Because this gas has a strong and characteristic odor, its presence is usually detected before any harm is done. The important point to remember is not to light a match or make a spark in the room until the gas outlet is closed and the gas dissipated by opening windows to the outside air.

The practice of fumigating rooms in the control of communicable diseases has been superseded by the use of aerosols, ultraviolet rays, soap and water, and airing, letting in sunlight when possible. In cases where outmoded poisonous gases are used to exterminate vermin, mice, and rats, the greatest care must be exercised to protect human beings.

Extermination and Control of Vermin and Animal Pests.   Geographical location determines to some extent the varieties of insects and animals, but free travel increases the possibility that certain types of pests will become universally prevalent. In North America the common domestic pests are flies, mosquitoes, moths, bedbugs, pediculi, fleas, ticks, cockroaches, and rats and mice. There are poisonous spiders and other insects that have not been enumerated, but at the present time these are not commonly found inside dwellings.

The effectiveness of sanitary measures in the community largely defines the problems that the individual has to meet. Public health regulations have more influence upon the control of insect and animal pests than the efforts of private citizens; for example, mosquitoes must be exterminated by striking at their breeding places in swamps and stagnant water; rats are controlled in seaports by vigorous efforts to keep docks and storage houses free from foods; and the enterprise of many citizens may be useless in exterminating flies if there is no way of forcing livery stables and dairies to prevent their breeding in manure. Effective campaigns, however, combine the efforts of public agents with those of private householders.

The *dangers involved* vary with the nature of the insect or animal and the conditions in the environment.

The chief danger from pests is the spread of communicable disease. Insects may spread disease mechanically by contaminating food. Biting and sucking insects introduce microorganisms through their mouth parts or by defecating infectious feces on the puncture wound as they feed on their human host. Some diseases, for example, malaria, require an intermediate insect host, the mosquito, for the development of the invading microorganism.

Most insects that are a menace to human beings can and do live on animals. Lice, ticks, bedbugs, and fleas can all adapt themselves to human or animal hosts although each species has its favorite victim. The fact that fleas travel from house to house on infected rats to spread the plague among people made the control of the disease impossible until this fact was understood. To protect the population from insect-borne disease it is essential to know something of the habits and characteristics of the insect in relation to man, animals, and the environment. Domestic and wild animals may spread disease mechanically by harboring insects, and by their bite. When communicable disease transmitted by insects is endemic (ever present) in a community, the natives, particularly the underprivileged, are likely to develop an immunity. In poor, crowded, industrial districts, where infestation with lice is the rule, many persons develop an immunity to typhus fever. This fact makes such people far less fearful of the insect disease carriers than are newcomers. In many cases it requires a good deal of effort on the part of the visiting nurse to persuade a mother that it is important to get rid of the lice on her child's head. The writer often found this to be the case, and once nursed a mother who had never known freedom from these pests. This mother was entirely indifferent to the hundreds of bedbugs crawling over her bed and her infant's crib, even in broad daylight, although they are nocturnal in their habits and must have been an overwhelming army after dark. The mother showed little evidence of irritation from the bite of the bugs, but the infant was so covered with inflamed and infected bites that the condition might have been confused with impetigo. Even when insects do not transmit disease, they interfere with sleep. Unquestionably, all human parasites lower the health status and to a greater or lesser extent menace man.

Most institutions have contracts with exterminating companies that guarantee pest control by continuous service. While this is usually the most satisfactory way of handling the problem in hospitals, all medical workers—and, indeed, everyone —should have some knowledge of principles and methods involved. Conditions found in homes by nurses, such as the one mentioned above, may be reported to the local bureau of sanitation, but in some situations such expert service is not readily available, and the nurse might be able to give the family adequate help if she herself were well informed or knew where to get necessary information. Certain problems, such as the delousing of persons and the control of bedbugs, mosquitoes, and flies, are ever present in hospitals and schools and must be dealt with by the health service staff, either alone or in cooperation with exterminating experts. Nurses should have a thorough knowledge of insecticides and repellents used for these pests.

High standards of sanitation are particularly important where there is illness. The sick person is especially susceptible to infection, often irritable, and capricious in appetite. One small crawling object on his breakfast tray may turn him against all the food that is offered him, and the presence of one bedbug may disturb his sleep for many nights, even after the condition has been corrected.

Methods of pest control aim at (1) destruction by poison of the pests themselves, (2) making breeding impossible, (3) the protection of persons (and animals) from the pest, and (4) making the host repellent to the pest. The elimination of the disease spread by the pest is, of course, part of the total program.

Insecticides, Repellents, and Poisons.   In the last decade many new and effective insecticides and repellents have been developed. Most insecticides, repellents, and animal poisons are toxic to man. The particular advantage claimed for the new preparations is their low toxicity for human beings. Many authors suggest, however, that this cannot be proved until they have been used for years; nor can the effect on plant and animal life be fully estimated. Asa C. Chandler's[45] *Introduction to Parasitology* refers to a large body of the research in this field. Much of the material in the following pages is based on Chandler's text. This, or a similar work, should be consulted by the student who wants a detailed discussion.

The most reliable chemical for killing insects and animals in the past was hydrocyanic gas, which, together with sulfur dioxide gas, not nearly so effective, was widely used. The former is highly dangerous to man and pets, the latter less so, but sulfur is injurious to many household furnishings. Methyl bromide, arsenic, sodium fluoride, and nicotine sulfate are mentioned as other lethal agents that have been replaced by newer insecticides far less toxic to vertebrates. *Pyrethrum* and the oil-soluble pyrethrin were in use before World War II and are very effective— highly poisonous to insects, and only mildly toxic to man. They are made from a species of chrysanthemum. *Rotenone,* also extracted from plants, is in the same category.

Insecticides and repellents used in spraying devices often contain these chemicals. Pyrethrum is volatile, "knocks down," or acts immediately on flies, for example, and will kill them if used in sufficient quantities. If a slow-acting nonvolatile agent is added to such a substance, the effect is more lasting; therefore, many new insecticides contain pyrethrum and the more recent synthetic arrivals, such as *DDT* (dichlorodiphenyl trichloroethane), *clordane* (empirical formula, $C_{10}H_6Cl_8$), or benzene hexachloride (666), which act in from one-half to several hours. Lloyd E. Rozeboom, writing in Maxcy's text, says, "A mixture of 6 parts dimethyl phthalate and 2 parts each of Indalone and Rutgers 612 is known as 6-2-2 and is effective [as a repellent] against a greater number of arthropods than is any one of the ingredients."* This repellent rubbed on the skin will protect the user for several hours.

All of these agents act as contact poisons and do not depend for their effectiveness on being eaten by the insect as does Paris green (arsenic) sprayed on plants. Rotenone inhibits oxidation in tissues and is slow acting. It is used on crawling or burrowing insects and may take 48 hours to kill them.

The reader gets the impression that Chandler and Rozeboom in Maxcy's text give an almost unqualified approval of the use of DDT in limiting the number of certain insects that spread disease. In fact, they say that it is relatively harmless to man. Baetjer in her section of Maxcy's text that deals with environmental medicine discusses their great toxicity for man. She includes an excellent summary table of symptoms and treatment (taken from Lehman).† Morton S. Biskind decries its widespread and uncontrolled use. He says: 'Beyond question, no other substance known to man has ever before developed so rapidly and spread indiscriminately over so large a portion of the earth in so short a time." He states that it is "cumulatively stored in the body fat and is extremely toxic for many different species of animals"; and says the American Medical Association has warned, "The time to establish controls, voluntary or otherwise, is now, before possible tragic consequences occur."‡ Exponents of "organic gardening" believe that killing insects and using artificial fertilizers will destroy the balance of nature.[46] Responsible persons should be alert to developments that will help them to select and employ measures of control wisely.

Insecticides, repellents, and poisons for animal pests are used as fumigants (gases) or in the form of sprays, dusts, or pastes. They may be added to foods that attract the insect or animal, but in such cases great care must be taken to see that human beings (especially children) and animal pets do not eat the poisoned food.

Insecticides depending for their effectiveness upon contact with the pest should contain a chemical that will enable the lethal element to penetrate the insect's protective (waxy) coat. Sesame oil is an example of a substance used for this purpose. When insecticides are prepared as sprays, they are often carried in a volatile liquid, such as kerosene oil, which evaporates, leaving no trace of itself, but deposits fine particles of the lethal agent on surfaces in the environment and on the pests themselves.

The following topics are not given in order of importance, nor is the writer competent to make a choice.

Flies are probably the most common of the insect pests. Excreta from animals or people is the medium in which flies breed most prolifically. They lay eggs in any putrefying or fermenting organic matter; hence, garbage and also many foods

---

* Maxcy, Kenneth F. (ed.): *op. cit.,* p. 451.

† Lehman, A. J.: "The Toxicology of the Newer Agricultural Chemicals," *Bull. A. Food and Drug Officials,* **12**:82, 1948.

‡ Biskind, Morton S.: "Statement on Clinical Intoxication from DDT and Other New Insecticides," *J. Insur. Med.,* **6**:5, (Mar., Apr., May) 1951.

become breeding places if left exposed. The eradication of flies depends almost entirely upon the elimination of their breeding places. Excreta and manure from stables should be covered with straw and oil and burned; or, if used for fertilizer, they should be treated with chemicals to destroy the fly larvae. The action of sun, rain, and soil discourages the breeding of flies. Chemicals, sprinkled on the floors of barns, markets, and similar places, discourage fly breeding. Some cities have so successfully controlled this pest that screening houses is no longer necessary. When flies are prevalent, screening is important. Doors may be covered with wire netting carrying an electric charge strong enough to kill insects, but harmless to people. This method is used in some dairies where the use of DDT is contraindicated. When screening is not possible, patients with communicable disease should have their beds covered with a canopy of netting. Traps and swatters should give way to more effective methods of control.

Aerosol bombs, small thick-walled containers of volatile liquids containing insecticides under pressure, provide a convenient means of ridding a room of flies and mosquitoes. Chandler indicates that the mixture Freon (the volatile carrier, 8 per cent sesame oil, the activator, and the insecticides—DDT 5 per cent and pyrethrum 0.4 per cent) is relatively harmless to human beings. By releasing the pressure on the liquid the room may be sprayed quickly and occupied immediately, if necessary, but it is a wise precaution to leave the room unoccupied for a period of an hour after spraying. A similar mixture may be used, of course, in an ordinary hand spray. To make a room lethal or repellent to insects over a period of months, a heavy or "residual spraying" is necessary. Gaylord W. Anderson and Margaret G. Arnstein[47] say that 1 gal of a 5 per cent solution of DDT will cover 1000 sq ft of surface (0.2 gm per square foot).

Diseases most often spread by flies are those contracted by eating contaminated food. Examples of those known to fall in this group are the intestinal diseases, such as typhoid, dysentery, and cholera. Flies may contaminate food and drinking vessels with microorganisms that cause sore throat and may deposit anthrax, tetanus, or gas gangrene organisms in a wound. Unprotected ulcers may be infected with larvae deposited by flies.

In the United States "flies," unless otherwise indicated, refer to the domestic insect that, as a rule, does not bite and that spreads disease mechanically. It is believed, however, that the deer fly, horsefly, or biting fly, so often encountered outdoors, transmits tularemia from infected animals to man or other animals. In tropical countries, where the disease yaws is prevalent, flies are believed to be carriers; kala-azar is spread by sand flies, and African sleeping sickness by the tsetse fly.

Human beings or animals are made repellent to flies when sprayed or rubbed with indalone (n-butyl mesityl oxide oxalate), Rutgers 612, or dimethylphalate (2 ethyl 1, 3 hexanediol indol). These repellents were developed during and since World War II.

Mosquitoes, carriers of widespread and often fatal diseases, are said now to be, of all insects, the greatest threat to man. Hundreds of varieties have been described, but those of special interest to health workers are the *anopheles,* carrier of malaria, and the *Aedes aegypti,* which spreads epidemic yellow fever. The genus *haemogogus* is thought to be a factor in the transfer of jungle yellow fever, endemic in parts of South America and Africa. There is reason to believe that the endemic form of the disease transferred to new territory and "fresh meat" assumes the characteristics of the epidemic form.

The knowledge that mosquitoes breed in still water is the key to their control. Draining swamps and stagnant pools or making them unfit for breeding purposes by covering the surface with an insecticide, such as pyrethrin or DDT, are methods used. Spraying of poison dust may be effective on swamps, but an insecticide is added to an oil when it is spread on the surface of ponds. If water is used for ice or drinking purposes, it can be stocked with fish that eat the mosquito larvae.

Human beings are protected from adult mosquitoes, as they are from flies, by screens and netting over beds; by spraying rooms, porches, and doors with insecticides; and by applying repellents to the skin and clothing. Of the repellents mentioned, Rutgers 612 is said to be the most effective.

Mosquitoes spread malaria, yellow fever, dengue, jungle typhus, filariasis, and possibly other blood-borne diseases. The salivary glands of the mosquito are infected by biting a patient sick with the disease, and in biting the second individual the insect's saliva, laden with disease organisms, is introduced into his victim. It would seem to be possible for mosquitoes to spread disease as flies do—by carrying bacteria on their legs and bodies, but the habits of the former are very different from those of flies and they are not thought to be a menace in this respect.

Fleas have played a dramatic role in history. Parasites on rats and human beings, both subject to bubonic plague, fleas have laid waste vast cities as they plied between rodents and men, sick and well. Hans Zinnser, among others, tells the story in *Rats, Lice, and History.*[48]

More than 200 varieties of fleas are believed to exist. The *Pulex irritans* is said by some authorities to be primarily a human parasite. Plague is spread by the rat flea (*Xenopsylla cheopis*). Most species seem to prefer a particular animal host, but they can also adapt themselves to human beings. When a house is infested with fleas, it usually indicates the presence of rats or flea-ridden domestic pets.

The bite of an uninfected flea is not dangerous except that when scratching it a person may introduce microorganisms under the skin. The process of feeding, with many insects, stimulates defecation so that as the animal sucks the blood of his host, his excrement is deposited on the skin. When this excrement contains organisms pathologic to man, the insect bite is a serious threat. Infected insects, such as fleas or lice, produce disease when the host crushes them against the skin, if the skin is not intact. Even when fleas do not spread disease, they disturb sleep, rest, and waking comfort. They are always a direct or indirect cause of ill health.

The elimination of rats is essential in control of fleas. DDT powder 5 to 10 per cent in pyrophyllite or talc dusted on the coats of pet dogs and cats will make them fleaproof. Human beings may use this same powder on their own clothing, with or without pyrethrum. Dimethylphthalate is said to be particularly helpful in destroying fleas. Naphthalene flakes on the floor of a closed room were advocated by Rosenau before the newer preparations became available. In Maxcy's revision of Rosenau's text, Rozeboom says that benzene hexachloride is even more effective than DDT but that it must be used in concentrations of 1 to 2 gm per square meter of surface. Hydrocyanic gas is of course highly effective, but because it is so dangerous to man it is not recommended.

Ticks rank next to mosquitoes in spreading disease among men and are the greatest menace to animals of all the insects. Like all others, they may take many forms as they adapt themselves to different hosts and environments. Many species live outdoors on tame and wild animals, but some live in houses, as bedbugs do. The species sometimes found in houses is a bat tick. Ticks when not engorged resemble bedbugs in shape (see Plate I). Their bodies are leathery and very elastic and about the size of an adult bedbug. When full they may be half an inch long and look more like a light gray-brown bean than an insect. The *ornithodorous* and *dermacentor* species are important in North America.

When ticks are found attached to human beings or animals it is best to cover the insects' heads with an oil, lard, petroleum jelly, or a hydrocarbon, such as kerosene. If the ticks are found in the ear, a bland oil may be dropped in the ear. If the tick is torn from its attachment, the sucking portion is often left in the skin and infection results. The tick loses its hold when oil deprives it of oxygen. It is a wise precaution to apply a skin antiseptic to the bite.

Tick control involves dipping infested animals and spraying pastures with insecticides, using alternate fields to allow ticks to die out. An emulsion of benzene hexachloride is said by Chandler to be recommended by the Naval Research Institute. It is suggested that phenylcyclohexanol be used as an activator. Chandler finds that an emulsion of DDT 2.5 per cent applied once a month adequately protects dogs.

Ticks transmit Rocky Mountain spotted fever and tularemia to human beings, although the latter is often contracted from handling infected rabbits. Since bodies of ticks may contain infectious material, they should never be crushed but burned or dropped into kerosene oil.

Many people associate *bedbugs* with uncleanliness for the reason that this animal parasite is generally found in badly kept homes, hotels, and hospitals. Bedbugs usually infest a house by living and breeding in the cracks and crevices of beds, from which they emerge at night to feed on the blood of the occupants. They may hibernate in a house for as long as a year. They are very skillful in finding their prey. Young bedbugs are so small and light in color that they are difficult to see; a full-grown bedbug is more elongated and when it is not swollen with blood resembles a tick (see Plate I). The body is wingless, of a dark reddish-brown color, and appears to be smooth and hard, but under the microscope it is seen to be covered with fine hairs at the junction of each segment; the shape and size depend upon whether or not the body is distended with blood. There is a nauseating odor about these insects that may account in part for the extreme

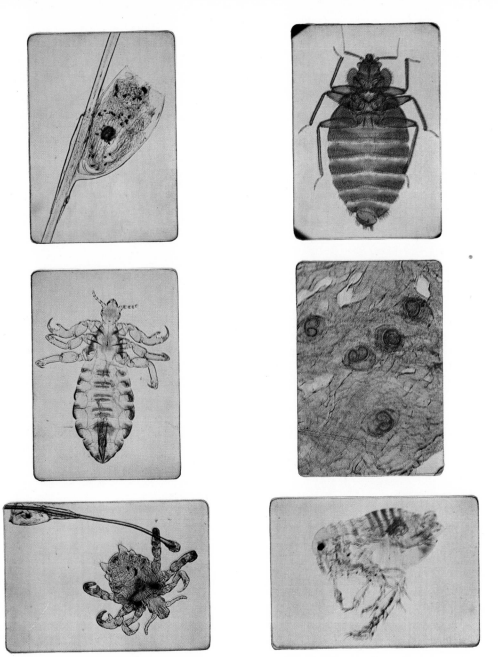

Plate I. Parasitic agents in diseases of man. (*Left, top to bottom*) Lice: hair shaft with nit (X 32); *Pediculus humanus* var. *capitis,* male (X 11.2); *Phthirius pubis,* female (X 14.4). (*Right, top to bottom*) *Cimex lectularius* (bedbug) (X 12.8); trichinosis: crushed specimen of muscle, calcified larvae (X 19.2); *Pulex irritans* (human flea) (X 19.2). (Courtesy of Henry E. Meleney, M.D.; Harry Most, M.D.; and Donald U. Moore, Ph.D.; and Clay-Adams Co., New York City.)

repulsion that is felt for them. According to Chandler, the bedbug is rarely found on animals, but a similar bug—a poultry pest—does attack man. The chief human parasites are the *Cimex lectularius* and the *C. hemipterus.* Pigeons and bats nesting in roofs may bring another type of bedbug into the house, but the typical bedbug is not carried by the bat.

In order to prevent infestation by bedbugs, buildings should be made as nearly insectproof as possible. The substitution of metals, concrete, and glass for wood construction helps to discourage these vermin. Constant vigilance is necessary in hospitals, however, to prevent patients and their visitors from bringing bedbugs into the buildings on their clothes or other belongings. The bugs cling to the clothing even while they are feeding on their host. The admitting division should be especially careful when storing patients' possessions.

Bedbugs hide during the day and come out at night; they generally inflict multiple bites, raising three or four small hard white elevations in a row. The sleeper is usually restless and anxious. If these signs occur a search should be made in the cracks of the bed and in the tufts of the mattress. It is sometimes difficult to find these insects. Poisonous gases, such as hydrocyanic gas, are very effective but very dangerous. The safer insecticides have replaced them. Good results can be obtained by spraying beds, mattresses, walls, and floors with DDT, chlordane, or benzene hexachloride. One and one-half ounces of a 10 per cent DDT dust sprayed on each bed is said to kill all bugs in 24 hours. This repels bugs for a period of three to six months.

If constantly exposed to bedbugs, human beings seem to develop an immunity to the irritation caused by their bite. A fresh victim may be very sick from the bites of a small army of bugs, and most people suffer from irritability and lassitude due to the interference with sleep. The itching is intense; the bite not actually painful, but burning. While it is possible for any infected biting insect to transfer blood-borne diseases, bedbugs have never been proved to be disease carriers. Chandler says that a few questionable claims are made that they are responsible for spreading infectious jaundice and undulant fever.

Lice, of which there are hundreds of varieties, are parasites of human beings, animals, fowls, birds, and plants. Three types belonging to two genera infest human beings: (1) *pediculus,* from which come the human head louse, *P. humanus var. capitus,* and the body louse, *P. humanus var. corporis* or *vestimenti,* and (2) *phthirius,* from which comes the crab louse, *P. pubis.* The latter lives in those parts of the body covered with short hairs: the pubes, the axillae, the eyebrows, and the eyelashes. The entire body of a very hairy man may be infested although the majority of infested persons harbor a relatively small number. In a study of school children by Kenneth Mellanby[49] it was found that a large proportion of infested heads might show as few as 1 to 10 lice. Cold and heat, removing the clothing, bathing, and brushing the hair all reduce the numbers.

While head lice and crab lice tend to stay on the host hidden by hairs, body lice cling to the clothing, and if a "lousy" person undresses, not one may be seen on the skin. Chandler says they cling to the clothing by their hind legs while they suck the blood of their host and lay their eggs on the clothing. The head and pubic lice lay eggs on the hairs, gluing them to the hairs with a waxy coating. The eggs hatch in 8 to 10 days, if they are not destroyed by excessive drying or moisture. The louse lives about 40 days if the temperature does not fall below 4.4° C (40° F) or rise above 52° C (125.6° F).

It is obvious that failure to bathe or change the clothing makes infestation by lice possible. Experiments with rats have shown that a diet low in vitamin B predisposes the rat to infestation, just as a sickly plant is more susceptible to attack by insects. Armies, ships' crews, prison inmates, all have suffered from lice for the reasons just indicated.

The presence of body lice is indicated by scratches on the skin and hemorrhagic specks on the body and by the person's habit of scratching. Occasionally they may be seen on the bedding. Clusters of nits (eggs), that look like oval particles of dandruff clinging to the hair, are usually found near the ears. Bites, or a pustular eruption, are seen near the hair line behind the ears. The louse is very small, grayish white, and hard to see; the crab louse has reddish legs. The fresh victim is highly sensitive to the bite and shows what is thought to be an allergic reaction. The veteran acquires an immunity, and often an indifference. With his resistance to the irritating chemical excretions of the louse, man also develops immunity to the diseases transmitted by the louse. In sections of the population where lice and typhus, for example, are present, such diseases tend to be endemic, low-grade infections in the native population that change to an epidemic and virulent form when the causative organism has new hosts unprotected by long exposure to the disease. Epidemics occur when "lousy" and "non-lousy" groups are thrown together, as in ships and army quarters.

Lice share with other bloodsuckers the transfer of typhus fever, trench fever, and relapsing fever. The first two are spread by the introduction of the feces of the infected louse into the puncture he makes as he sucks blood, while relapsing fever is thought not to be transferred through the bite but from body fluids of the louse, inoculating the host as he crushes the body of the louse against his skin. Crushing lice between the teeth, as is seen in some countries, may spread intestinal diseases. Rats, mice, and other animals may act as intermediary hosts and contribute to typhus epidemics as they have to those of plague.

It is obvious that a high standard of personal cleanliness tends to prevent infestation. The most fastidious person may pick up head lice from cloak rooms, trying on hats, or from chairs in public conveyances. Crab lice may be transferred from toilet seats and promiscuous sexual intercourse. Fortunately for the human race, whose numbers in certain countries have from time to time been decimated by typhus, new chemicals have made it possible to destroy these parasites quickly and easily. DDT kills the adult louse and nymph, and while it does not destroy the egg, its effect on the hair or clothing remains lethal to the louse until the eggs hatch into the nymph. In an extensive study in Scotland, Gaines W. Eddy[50] found more than 25 insecticides in common use, kerosene most often with olive oil or vinegar. None was entirely effective as used. Ten days after treating 1000 persons with DDT, no live lice were found.

Head lice are treated by shaking 10 per cent DDT powder in pyrophylite on the head from a perforated can. A teaspoonful is about enough for one person. The hair is not washed for about ten days in order to kill the nymphs as the eggs hatch. Body lice are treated by impregnating the clothing with DDT powder. In epidemics the entire population may be dusted by putting the nozzle of the spray pump up the trouser legs, sleeves, down the neck, and around the waist, using about 4 oz of powder per person. In hospitals, infested clothing may be treated with DDT powder or subjected to live steam, boiling water, or a hot iron. Crab lice are destroyed by applying 10 per cent DDT powder in 20 parts of cold cream, followed by a bath. A repetition of the treatment a few days later to take care of any nits that may have escaped is a safe procedure. Usually one application is sufficient.

The *cockroach* family has numerous branches that differ markedly in size and shape. The largest variety looks like a winged beetle and is 2 in. in length; the smallest type is less than an eighth that size. They are especially prevalent in crowded apartment houses, schools, stores, and similar places where they find food and moisture. Cockroaches are so dependent on water that they remain near plumbing fixtures and inhabit damp cellars. Any food or cellulose product left uncovered attracts and fosters cockroaches; some species even eat fabrics. Absolute cleanliness and the use of tightly covered containers for foods are the most effective measures in keeping them out of houses. Paper should not be used on kitchen and pantry shelves; leaking pipes should be repaired immediately. It is not difficult to poison cockroaches and to discourage them completely. Exterminating companies use mixtures containing chlordane (probably the most effective substance) and benzene hexachloride. DDT is not effective. If it is used at all, a heavy spraying of the emulsion is best. Poisonous gases are effective in destroying cockroaches, but, as Chandler says, they are as out of date as the horse and buggy except in killing rodents. Cockroaches may spread disease by contaminating food and utensils.

Moths are a serious menace to owners of woolen fabrics and furs. The flying moth lays eggs that hatch into the destructive larvae or worms. These insects flourish in warm, dark places and are more abundant in the spring. They are more likely to eat soiled than clean fabrics; they avoid strong odors and are killed by fumes of different chemicals.

To prevent loss from moths, keep materials they will eat clean, well aired, and, if possible, stored in light closets. After the winter season is over, furs, woolen clothes, and household goods should be cleaned and put away with flakes of camphor or paradichlorobenzene or stored in tar bags. Moth-repellant cakes, placed in a perforated container and hung in a closet, afford adequate protection. Packing clean clothes in tightly closed boxes or cedar chests to which the moths cannot gain access is effective. Cold storage, available only in large institutions and stores, is satisfactory protection.

Of all household pests, *rats and mice* are the most prevalent. They live in almost every climate and feed on a great variety of foods. Because they gain access to ships by ropes and gangplanks, they have in some cases carried disease from one continent to another. Certain laws require shipowners to use methods to prevent rats and mice from entering and leaving vessels. These animals are dangerous not only because they carry disease but also because they may bite human beings, especially infants, and gnaw matches, thereby causing fires.

To control these pests, all buildings should be ratproof; food should be inaccessible to them. Rats and mice may be trapped or poisoned. Mice are frightened and killed by cats and dogs; ferrets kill both rats and mice. Chemical poisoning is an effective means of destroying rodents. Because rats and mice cannot vomit, while human beings and most animals can, certain poisons toxic to all have been used in the past without danger. New chemicals have been recently developed that are highly toxic to rodents and comparatively nontoxic to man and other animals. The room in which poison is placed, however, should be closed if there are children or household pets about. Anderson and Arnstein recommend alphanaphthylthiourea, known as ANTU. In epidemics, "rat runs" are dusted with DDT to kill fleas and lice on the rats.

Like all living things, rats and mice may be destroyed by poisonous gases. This quick and complete method of exterminating pests is, however, rarely employed because of its difficulties and dangers. Of the gases formerly used hydrocyanic is the only one thought to be effective. Some health departments still advocate fumigation, but no recent texts have been found recommending it.

Parasitic worms constitute a distinct hazard in man's environment, the species depending upon the geographical area. Hookworm is a threat in warm countries where people go barefooted and unprotected from human excreta containing the worms. Obviously, methods of control depend upon proper sanitary facilities and wearing shoes. Roundworms, pinworms, tapeworms, and trichinella are taken in through the mouth. Their control is effected by cleanliness of everything that goes into the mouth, including food, and by good nutrition. Since it is difficult to make sure that meats do not contain disease-producing agents, thorough cooking of all meats, particularly pork that harbors trichinella, is important.

It is not possible to discuss all the live dangers in the environment, such as snakes and wild animals. Chapters 6 and 7 have been devoted to protection from pathogenic microorganisms. This material is placed early in the text since all nursing requires the practice of asepsis.

9. SELECTING AND MAKING BEDS

Importance of a Comfortable Bed.   As comfort, rest, and sleep are all important in maintaining health and in promoting recovery from disease, special attention, both in homes and hospitals, should be given to providing healthful beds and bedding. Skill in making a bed so as to ensure comfort is one of the first accomplishments of the housekeeper. Non-nursing personnel make empty beds in many hospitals, but the nurse should be skillful in making all sorts since in many situations she will prefer to prepare her patient's bed, or she may have to teach bedmaking to others.

Selection of Beds and Bedding.   A bed suitable for care of the sick, whether in the home or hospital, differs in certain important respects from that for the well. The sick person not only rests and sleeps but may have his meals, recreation, occupation, and exercise in it, and here all the bodily functions must be attended to. It should be adapted also to the needs of those who care for the sick so that their time and energy may be conserved.

The standard hospital bed is single, 6 ft and 6 in. long, 3 ft wide, and 26 in. from the floor. A lower bed is desirable for ambulatory patients. One that can be raised and lowered from the floor is ideal. It is simple in design; light; easily moved; easy to handle, clean, and disinfect; and is strong and durable. Hard-rubber casters or hard-rubber tires make it possible to move the bed without jarring the patient. The springs are usually woven wire, but box springs are also used. Adjustable beds, such as the Gatch bed, are now common. Motorized beds whose springs move slowly and constantly like a seesaw are used in circulatory disorders. Beds longer than standard and those with head- and footboards that can be lowered to mattress level should be available for special cases.

There is considerable economy in having the bed furnished with rubber bumpers that keep it clear of walls, door frames, and furniture; this also reduces irritation to the patient when the bed strikes an object. Paints used on babies' beds should always be free of lead, as babies frequently bite the frame with the resulting danger of lead poisoning.

The *bed in the home* is usually much lower and broader, and the linen and blankets are often shorter and narrower in proportion, all of which will require special adjustments when caring for the sick in the home. For instance, blocks may be used to raise the bed to the height that makes lifting and turning the person easier, and linen may be tied to the mattress to make it tight, smooth, and secure, or permanently mitered corners may be made. A piece of cloth sewed to the end of a short blanket at the foot makes tucking possible.

Mattresses for the hospital are generally made of stout, blue-and-white linen ticking (cotton ticking is not so cool or durable), stuffed with horsehair, felt, silk floss, cotton, or kapok. Horsehair mattresses are firm, cool, light, and, because they are nonabsorbent, easy to clean. Curled hair is the best type. Both cotton and kapok mattresses are hard and likely to be lumpy. Mattresses should be even, smooth, and firm to give a sense of support. Inner-spring mattresses are widely used in hospitals. They are the most acceptable type to many patients, and maintain their shape and resiliency over a long period. Many authorities in body mechanics condemn the use of inner-spring mattresses for sick or well, maintaining that they allow the body to sag and thereby encourage poor posture.

Sponge-rubber mattresses are proving very satisfactory in some situations. They have air cushions on the under surface, being constructed somewhat like a waffle, and are especially valuable for patients who must remain in bed over a long period. Sponge-rubber mattresses are inflammable and when burning give off a noxious gas. Unless properly protected with a fireproof cover they are a hazard. Compartmentalized air mattresses attached to a motor that progressively empties

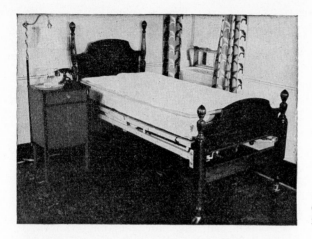

Figure 11A. Making the unoccupied bed. The mattress is covered with a plastic, waterproof, insectproof cover.

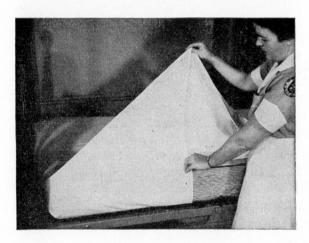

Figure 11B. To maintain the mitered corner the worker is holding the sheet against the mattress with the left hand as she drops the edge to be tucked with the right.

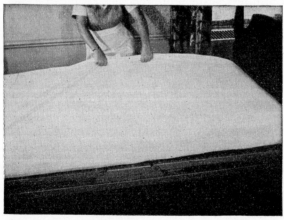

Figure 11C. Pulling the bottom sheet taut. This tautness is maintained because the worker tucks the sheet far under the mattress. (The edge of the sheet should almost reach the middle of the mattress.)

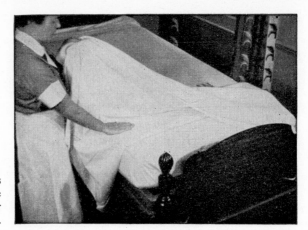

Figure 11D. The next step is making the horizontal pleat. Note that the pleat is made in the upper sheet and blanket simultaneously.

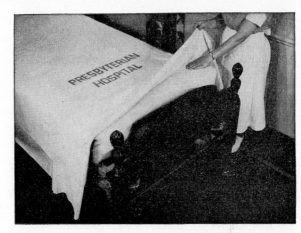

Figure 11E. Bring the pleat to the edge of the mattress.

Figure 11F. The finished bed. Note that the spread comes to the head of the bed and that the corners at the foot are square rather than mitered.

(Figs. 11 A-F, courtesy of Columbia-Presbyterian Medical Center, New York City, and Clay-Adams Co., New York City.)

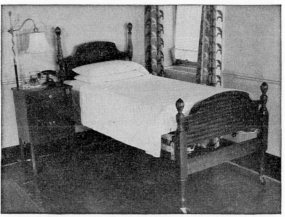

155

and fills with air the rubber compartments are available. They are called "alternating pressure" mattresses (see Fig. 148). All mattresses should be protected with washable covers or made with waterproof surfaces.

There are usually *two pillows* for each bed—one hard pillow stuffed with hair and one soft pillow stuffed with feathers (2½ to 3 lb). Foam- or sponge-rubber pillows are also very satisfactory. The hard pillow is used under the feather or rubber pillow for support to the head and shoulders and sometimes without the soft pillow for coolness. It is used for various other purposes, such as to support a limb or to hold it in a fixed position. Smaller pillows also are used for special support or comfort. For patients allergic to feathers, kapok or rubber pillows should be available. A very light rubberized silk or plastic cover with zipper fastening may be used successfully to protect the allergic patient.

A *rubber or plastic* sheet is used to protect the lower sheet and mattress. It must be without thin places or wrinkles. Because rubber prevents access of air to the skin, it delays evaporation and makes the patient feel hot and moist. In some hospitals quilted cotton pads instead of rubber draw sheets are used to protect the mattress unless the patient is incontinent. In homes, pads made of six thicknesses of newspapers inside a removable and washable cotton cover give satisfactory protection to the bed. Mattresses made with waterproof surfaces need less protection.

The *linen* consists of two large sheets, a draw sheet, a spread, and two pillow cases. The large sheets should be strong enough to stand pulling tightly and large enough to tuck in well under the mattress all around (72 by 108 in. is a good size). "The contour sheet" is a desirable substitute for the ordinary undersheet, for it stays tight indefinitely and saves the worker's time. The *draw sheet,* which may be made of single or double cotton, must be wide enough and stout enough to pull tightly and tuck well under the mattress. It is called a draw sheet because it is easily withdrawn, and formerly was made wide enough to be partly withdrawn in order to give the patient a cool place on which to lie. The *spread* should be light and easily laundered; dimity washes and wears well. *Pillow slips* should fit the pillows but not so tightly that they distort the shape.

Blankets should be light and warm. They are lighter in proportion to the warmth, depending upon the amount of wool present. A blanket with 60 to 80 per cent wool is generally used because a blanket with a cotton warp is durable and shrinks less in washing. The usual weight is from 4½ to 7 lb per pair.

The Art of Bedmaking.   The chief *objectives* in making a bed are comfort for the occupant and economy of materials, time, and energy. Finished appearance is also important.

The *method* of achieving these ends varies in hospitals and homes, but the following principles apply in all situations. To economize time and effort, everything necessary for bedmaking should be on hand before beginning. To ensure comfort the under sheet must be tight and smooth. "The contour sheet" with manufactured mitered corners eliminates the problem of getting a lastingly smooth lower sheet. If the ordinary kind of sheet is used, it should be placed perfectly straight on the bed; otherwise it will be impossible to make it tight.

The top of the mattress should be covered for protection and the linen tucked far enough under the mattress to keep it fixed, tight, and smooth. It is tucked in on one side and tightened as it is tucked in on the opposite side. Each article of bedclothing is placed on the bed and tightened separately. In the hospital a waterproof sheet extending from the shoulders to below the knees is used for protection of the mattress; but if the patient is continent and there is no gross discharge from the body, a quilted pad may be substituted. The protector must be smooth and well tucked in. In tightening the bedding, it is important to avoid altering the shape of the mattress, which should remain flat and even, with the corners firm and square.

The upper clothing should be tucked in neatly for warmth and security, but not too tight for comfort. Sufficient room must be allowed for turning the feet; they must not be forced into a cramped position by tight upper bedding. This makes the feet uncomfortable, numb, and chilly. If the patient is in bed long enough, tight upper bedding may cause a deformity called *foot drop*. To keep the covers loose, any one of several measures may be used: (1) Make a pleat in the sheet and blanket across the foot of the bed (see Fig. 11D); (2) make a longitudinal box pleat down the middle of the bed; (3) while tucking in the upper bedding, have the patient flex his knees; or (4) place a small mattress, board, or cradle (see also Chapter 15) at the foot of the bed. The upper sheet (wrong side up) should be tucked in well at the bottom, but left free at the top with enough to turn over the spread and blanket to protect both. Blankets, tucked in at the foot, should reach far enough to protect the shoulders. The spread covers the whole of the bed; it is usually left to fall free over the sides but is tucked in at the foot with square or envelope corners for security and appearance. The pillows should be snugly tucked into the corners of the case and should be flat and smooth.

When *stripping an empty bed to remake it,* put beside the bed one or two chairs in position to receive the bedclothes as they are removed. Pillows are taken off first, then the clothing loosened all around and removed one article at a time, each article being folded in quarters and spread over the chairs to air. Caution is used to prevent them from touching the floor. Care should be taken not to throw into the soiled linen container objects such as dentures, jewelry, instruments, and equipment such as a hot-water bag; all of which may be left in the bed through error. They may be lost or injured, and they damage laundry machinery. To avoid unevenness from constant pressure in one place, the mattress should be turned daily from head to foot when the patient can be removed from the bed.* An innerspring mattress need not be turned so often. It must not be bent, but swung around from head to foot and then flopped over from side to side.

The bed just described is adequate for those who sleep indoors in temperate climates. Special protection, however, must be provided in severe weather and climates.

---

* To some this is very important. A strong-minded acquaintance, up for the first time after a major abdominal operation, asked the person making her bed in the hospital to turn the mattress. Her request was refused. She replied, "Step aside," and turned the mattress herself.

Open-air Bed.   In the treatment of tuberculosis, it has been customary to require patients to sleep on open-air porches. This practice is becoming less common, but because sleeping in the open air is occasionally prescribed or necessary, it is essential that the nurse know how to dress the patient and make a bed in such a way that he is adequately protected. This protected type of bed is sometimes spoken of as a *Klondike bed,* because the severity of the winter in the Klondike region and the inadequately heated cabins that are used by campers make it necessary to provide extra warmth and insulating measures for sleepers.

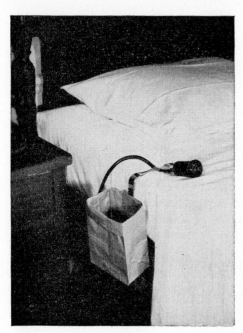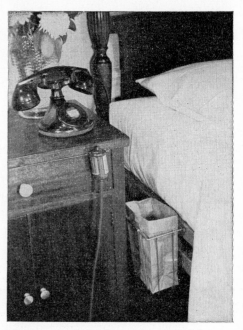

Figure 12. (*Left*) Shows a device that holds a bell cord and push button in place and provides attachment for a paper bag. (*Right*) Shows two separate devices for these two purposes. (Courtesy of Columbia-Presbyterian Medical Center, New York City, and Clay-Adams Co., New York City.)

Certain principles should be kept in mind when making a bed that is to be used in low environmental temperatures. One is insulation against drafts and moisture, another is provision of warm covering and heating devices, a third is the choice of fabrics that feel warm, and a fourth is the use of warm but lightweight covering and some means of keeping the weight of the covers off the patient, particularly off the feet.

Obviously, the amount of covering or protection varies with the climate and the patient's condition; therefore, this pattern must be modified to fit the situation. Place a winterweight blanket on the bedsprings in such a way that there is a sufficient amount left at the head of the bed to be drawn up over and to cover the head board. A second blanket is put over the lower half of the springs so that it can be brought up over the foot of the mattress. Place two more blankets of the same weight on the springs, leaving enough on each side to come over the mattress and cover it. The selvage of these blankets should be placed at the upper edge of the springs. Before placing the mattress on the springs, cover the area under the mattress with a piece of rubber sheeting or oilcloth. If this is not available, five or six thicknesses of newspapers provide good insulation. The bed is now made like any ordinary bed except that cotton blankets replace sheets. Use a footboard, a bolster, or large sandbags to keep the weight of the bed-clothes off the patient's feet. A cradle is not suitable because the large air pocket that it makes is too difficult to heat.

Before the patient gets into bed, a hot-water bottle or a heating pad is used to warm the bed and is left at his feet. Bags of heated sand are available in the country and are an effective means of providing warmth. If it is possible to roll the bed on to a porch it is desirable to make the bed in a warm room and have the patient get into it there. For baths, meals, and treatment, the patient is brought indoors.

As soon as the patient is in bed, tuck the top bedding in snugly but not so tightly that his movements are restricted. The blanket at the foot of the bed is then brought up like an envelope over the bottom of the mattress. Next bring the excess blanket hanging from each side of the springs over the pillows, folding the corners so that the blankets come under the chin and lap over the midline of the bed. The first blanket, which has been pinned in place over the head of the bed, is used to make a triangular-shaped windbreak on either side of the head of the bed. A sleeping bag is a good substitute for this bed.

The patient should wear outing-flannel night clothes, preferably pajamas. Sleeping socks, mittens, and a warm jacket with a hood (sometimes called a *parka*) are usually necessary. Occasionally a shoulder blanket that can be brought over the face is a necessity in very cold climates.

Patients who are on porches need especially careful supervision. They must be provided with a means of signaling attendants, and since there is always a good deal of danger that they may become chilled, there should be no possibility that their call will go unanswered for any appreciable time.

Care of Beds and Bedding. *Equipment* for beds (mattresses, pillows, blankets, linen) and its repair and renewal are among the heaviest items of expense in the hospital. Rigid economy and scrupulous care are essential in its use. The need for clean linen depends upon the amount of time the patient spends in bed. If he is up during the day, it is obvious that he does not need as frequent change of bed linen as he does when he is in bed day and night, and eats his meals in bed. Other considerations are unavoidable odors due, for example, to drainage from wounds and the incontinence of the patient. Hospitals should provide for the specific needs of each patient rather than make changing bed linen routine. Squares of rubber and soft paper should be used freely to prevent soiling sheets and blankets while treatments are given or when the patient uses the bedpan.

Special precautions should be taken in the care of blankets. Stains should be sponged off at once or the blankets sent to the laundry to have the stain removed. Cotton blankets should be used during treatments or when likely to be soiled. The supply, use, and provision for cleaning or washing blankets varies in different hospitals. Some hospitals have established modern laundries equipped with special machinery that makes it possible to wash blankets as frequently as desirable without shrinking or spoiling their appearance or making them harsh or uneven. Some modern laundries now clean blankets by steam, a method that is said not to shrink but to keep them soft and fluffy. In other hospitals not so equipped, blankets are sent to the cleaners to be dry-cleaned, or, if badly soiled, to the laundry.

After the discharge of a patient, in addition to the daily dusting of the bed and care of bedding, a more thorough cleaning is given than is possible when the patient is in bed. (Concurrent and terminal disinfection in homes and hospitals is discussed in Chapter 7.) All furniture and equipment should be examined to see whether it is in need of repair. Special attention should be given the mattress to see that there are no bedbugs in the tufts. Waterproof sheets and pillow cases should be scrubbed with warm water and soap, dried, and aired. When not in use, they should be rolled on or suspended over wooden rollers. Folding is likely to crack rubber or plastic. (Making the bed with a patient in it is discussed in Chapter 12, and changing and turning the mattress for a bed patient, in Chapter 15.)

REFERENCES

1. Maxcy, Kenneth F. (ed.): *Rosenau's Preventive Medicine and Hygiene,* 7th ed. Appleton-Century-Crofts, Inc., New York, 1951, p. 975.
2. Clark, Janet H.: "Ultraviolet Radiation in Relation to Health," *Nutrition Abstr. & Rev.,* 3:13, (July) 1933.
3. Maxcy, Kenneth F. (ed.): *op. cit.,* p. 981.
4. Stair, R.: *Spectral-Transmissive Properties and Use of Eye-Protective Glasses,* National Bureau of Standards, Circular No. 471. US Government Printing Office, Washington, D.C., 1948.
5. Fox, Sidney A.: *Your Eyes.* Alfred A. Knopf, New York, 1944, p. 94.
6. Weston, H. C.: *The Relation between Illumination and Visual Efficiency. The Effect of Brightness Contrast,* Medical Research Council, Industrial Health Resources Board, Report No. 87. H. M. Stationary Office, London, 1945, pp. 18, 29, 33.
7. Worcester, Alfred W.: *Care of the Aged, the Dying and the Dead.* Charles C Thomas, Publisher, Springfield, Ill., 1935, p. 19.
8. Mills, Clarence A.: *Climate Makes the Man.* Harper & Brothers, New York, 1942, pp. 9-67.
9. Blum, Harold F.: "The Physiological Effect of Sunlight on Man," *Physiol. Rev.,* 25:483, (July) 1945.
10. Maxcy, Kenneth F. (ed.): *op. cit.,* p. 946.
11. Newburgh, Louis H. (ed.): *Physiology of Heat Regulation and the Science of Clothing.* W. B. Saunders Co., Philadelphia, 1949, pp. 337, 339.
12. "Thermal Standards in Industry." Report of the Committee on Atmospheric Comfort (Constantin P. Yaglou, Chairman). *Fifteenth Yearbook, 1949-1950, Am. J. Pub. Health,* Pt. II, 40:131, (May) 1950.
13. Newburgh, Louis H. (ed.): *op. cit.,* pp. 264, 268.
14. Winslow, C.-E. A.: "Recent Advances in Our Knowledge of the Problems of Air-Conditioning," *Am. J. Pub. Health,* 27:767, (Aug.) 1937.

15. Mills, Clarence A.: "Artificial Climate—A New Service to Hospital Patients," *Mod. Hosp.,* **42:**57, (Oct.) 1934.
16. Kratz, A. P.: *Humidification of Residences,* Bulletin 230. Engineering Experiment Station, University of Illinois, Urbana, (July) 1931.
17. Maxcy, Kenneth F. (ed.): *op. cit.,* p. 954.
18. Maxcy, Kenneth F. (ed.): *op. cit.,* p. 996.
19. Carson, Rachel L.: *The Sea Around Us.* Oxford University Press, New York, 1951, p. 46.
20. Bancroft, J., et al.: "Observations upon the Effect of High Altitude on the Physiological Processes of the Human Body Carried Out in the Peruvian Andes, Chiefly at Cerro de Pasco," *Philos. Tr. Roy. Soc., London, s. B,* **211:**351, (Jan.) 1923.
21. Armstrong, Harry G.: *Principles and Practice of Aviation Medicine,* 2nd ed. Williams & Wilkins Co., Baltimore, 1943, p. 198.
22. Maxcy, Kenneth F. (ed.): *op. cit.,* p. 1000.
23. Bean, John W.: "Effects of Oxygen at Increased Pressures," *Physiol. Rev.,* **25:**1, (Jan.) 1945.
24. Stern, Arthur C., and Greenburg, Leonard: "Air Pollution: The Status Today," *Am. J. Pub. Health,* **41:**27, (Jan.) 1951.
25. Shrenk, H. H., et al.: *Air Pollution in Donora, Pa.: Epidemiology of the Unusual Smog Episode of October 1948,* Pub. Health Bull. No. 306. US Government Printing Office, Washington, D.C., 1949.
26. "Public Health Service Drinking Water Standards 1946," *Pub. Health Rep.,* **61:**371, (Mar.) 1946.
27. Tarbett, Ralph E.: "Emergency Sanitation Procedures," *Am. J. Nursing,* **42:**865, (Aug.) 1942.
28. US Atomic Energy Commission: *Control of Radiation Hazards in the Atomic Energy Program,* Eighth Semiannual Report, Pt. I. US Government Printing Office, Washington, D.C., 1950.
29. Comly, Hunter H.: "Cyanosis in Infants Caused by Nitrates in Well Water," *J.A.M.A.,* **129:**112, (Sept.) 1945.
30. De Castro, Josué: *The Geography of Hunger.* Little Brown & Co., Boston, 1952, p. 290.
31. Howard, Albert: *An Agricultural Testament.* Oxford University Press, New York, 1940.
32. Rosenau, Milton J.: *Preventive Medicine and Hygiene,* 6th ed. D. Appleton-Century Co., Inc., New York, 1935, p. 1131.
33. Wilton, Catherine J.: "Detergents," *Am. J. Nursing,* **50:**410, (Aug.) 1950.
34. Sloan, Raymond P.: *Hospital Color and Decoration.* Physicians Record Co., Chicago, 1944, pp. 77, 107.
35. Rockwell, Frederick F., and Grayson, E. C.: *Flower Arrangement in Color.* William H. Wise & Co., New York, 1940.
36. Geldard, Frank A.: "Somesthesis and the Chemical Senses," *Ann. Rev. Psychol.,* **1:**71, 1950.
37. Combes, Frank C., et al.: "Chlorophyll in Topical Therapy," *New York State J. Med.,* **52:**1025, (Apr.) 1952.
38. Palmer, Dewey: *The Problem of Odors in Institutions.* Hospital Bureau of Standards and Supplies, New York, 1947.
39. Sterner, James H., and Guild, Stacey R.: "Noise in Industry," *A.M.A. Arch. Ind. Hyg.,* **3:**232, (Mar.) 1951.
40. Barnes, Ralph M.: *Motion and Time Study.* John Wiley & Sons, Inc., New York, 1937, p. 105.
41. National Safety Council: *Accident Facts.* The Council, Chicago, 1950.
42. Dublin, Louis I.: *The Facts of Life from Birth to Death.* The Macmillan Company, New York, 1952, p. 262.
43. Siewers, Albert B., and Davidoff, Eugene: "Attempted Suicide; A Comparative Study of Psychopathic and General Hospital Patients," *Psychiatric Quart.,* **17:**520, (July) 1943.
44. Pope, Samuel J.: "Fire Hazards in Hospitals," *Hospitals,* **11:**91, (May) 1937.

45. Chandler, Asa C.: *Introduction to Parasitology with Special Reference to the Parasites of Man*, 8th ed. John Wiley & Sons, Inc., New York, 1950.
46. De Castro, Josué: *op. cit.*, p. 281.
47. Anderson, Gaylord W., and Arnstein, Margaret G.: *Communicable Disease Control*, 3rd ed. The Macmillan Company, New York, 1953, p. 440.
48. Zinnser, Hans: *Rats, Lice and History, Being a Study in Biography . . . with the Life History of Typhus Fever*. Little Brown & Co., Boston, 1935.
49. Mellanby, Kenneth: "Natural Population of the Head-Louse (*Pediculus Humanus Capitis: anoplura*) on Infested Children in England," *Parasitology*, **34**:180, (July) 1942.
50. Eddy, Gaines W.: "The Treatment of Head Lice with MYL and DDT Louse Powders and NBIN Emulsion," *Am. J. Hygiene*, **47**:29, (Jan.) 1948.

Additional Suggested Reading

American Public Health Association: *Basic Principles of Healthful Housing*, 2nd ed. The Association, New York, 1950.

Bendixen, T. W., et al.: *Studies on Household Sewage Disposal Systems*, Second in Series of Research Reports on Individual Sewage Disposal Systems, with lists of references, Pt. 2. US Public Health Service, US Government Printing Office, Washington, D.C., 1952.

Eadie, W. Robert: *Animal Control in Field, Farm, and Forest*. The Macmillan Company, New York, 1954.

Ehlers, Victor M., and Steel, Ernest W.: *Municipal and Rural Sanitation*, 4th ed. McGraw-Hill Book Co., New York, 1950.

Herms, William B.: *Medical Entomology*, 4th ed. The Macmillan Company, New York, 1950.

Klem, Margaret C., et al.: *Industrial Health and Medical Programs*, Statements, Tables, and Charts. US Public Health Service, US Government Printing Office, Washington, D.C., 1950.

MacEachern, Malcolm T.: *Hospital Organization and Management*, 2nd ed. Physicians Record Co., Chicago, 1946.

O'Hara, Dwight: *Airborne Infection, Some Observations on Its Decline*. Harvard University Press, Cambridge, 1943.

Sedgwick, William T.: *Principles of Sanitary Science and Public Health*, rewritten and enlarged by Samuel C. Prescott and Murray P. Horwood. The Macmillan Company, New York, 1935.

Simmons, James S., et al.: *Global Epidemiology*. J. B. Lippincott Co., Philadelphia, Vol. 1, 1944; Vol. 2, 1951.

Smillie, Wilson G.: *Preventive Medicine and Public Health*, 2nd ed. The Macmillan Company, New York, 1952.

Stone, Joseph E.: *Hospital Organization and Management*, 4th ed. Faber & Faber, Ltd., London, 1952.

US Public Health Service: *Water Pollution in the United States, Report No. 1 on Polluted Condition of Our Waters and What Is Needed to Restore Their Quality*. US Government Printing Office, Washington, D.C., 1951.

CHAPTER 6. ADMISSION AND DISCHARGE
OF THE PATIENT

1. **ADMISSION PROCEDURE WITH SPECIAL REFERENCE TO THE HOSPITAL PATIENT**
2. **DISCHARGE WITH SPECIAL REFERENCE TO THE HOSPITAL PATIENT**

1. ADMISSION PROCEDURE WITH SPECIAL REFERENCE TO THE HOSPITAL PATIENT

Receiving the Patient. Since first impressions are likely to be vivid and not easily erased, it is especially important that the patient, and those who are with him, receive the most courteous attention, and the patient himself the most effective medical service at the time of admission to an institution or during the initial home visit of a nurse or doctor. A hypercritical attitude toward medical groups, fear or prejudice against hospitals, or the morbid sensitiveness which often accompanies illness may turn a short delay, a moment of inattention, or a careless remark into a real grievance.

If the visiting nurse fails to make a favorable impression on her first visit to the patient, she may find it difficult to gain access to the home the next time she calls; institutional nurses and the hospital admitting staff, however, are less likely to discover their failures. The patient usually waits until he leaves the hospital to criticize it. He is, after all, at the mercy of the hospital personnel and fears that criticism may invite their disfavor. Unexpressed resentment, however, often makes the patient uncooperative, taciturn, or irritable. Since the patient bases his estimate of an institution on the sum total of his impressions while there, every contact he has with members of the staff, no matter what their positions, may indirectly affect his reaction to the care he receives.

The reception of the patient is now recognized to be of so much importance that in admitting services hospitals are employing hostesses and clerks who are especially qualified by virtue of their general poise and courteous manner to meet strangers and make them feel at ease. The hostess or clerk may ask the patient or his family for certain social data and escort or direct him to the proper department. The physician in charge of the patient's care is immediately notified

163

of his arrival, and the patient is soon turned over to medical workers. The manner in which the nurse and the physician receive and treat the patient is, after all, the most important aspect of his reception and admission to the hospital.

In a well-known psychiatric hospital in this country the director of the nursing service spends from one-half to one hour, or more, with each newly admitted patient. With her wide experience and mature judgment she should be able to help establish in the person a feeling of confidence. Her very title, if the person knows it, would tend to increase his sense of importance, which in illness is often at a low ebb.

Leo W. Simmons, a social anthropologist, directed a series of studies in 1951–1952 on the interpersonal relationship of patients, their relatives and friends, doctors, nurses, and auxiliary personnel. All those concerned should give thoughtful attention to his reports. The following excerpts from an article by him should help the nurse to understand the reaction of the average person on admission to the hospital. They also emphasize the healing power assigned by the writer to good relationships among the persons listed above.

In our American traditions, a man's home is still his fortress, if not his castle, and even though he becomes a "patient" there, he still retains a proprietary sense of his rights and privileges, and he can insist on being treated on his own terms. . . .

In contrast the sick man's personal prerogatives undergo very important changes when he is moved out of *his* home and *his* bed and into *our* hospital and into *one of our* beds. Whereas at home he retained his work-a-day apparel and accoutrements which provided a sense of competence and self-sufficiency, in the hospital all this equipage and the associated symbols of power are stripped from him and locked away out of his sight and reach—or even sent back home.

Moreover, at home physical surroundings were familiar and afforded a sense of security, while hospital surroundings are very different, strange and disquieting to say the least. The contrast between the physical environment of the home and of the hospital may be regarded even by the physician as sufficiently upsetting to justify some prescribed sedation, just to numb the patient's sensitivity to the disturbing ward activity, especially at night. Added to this is the general impression which a patient can easily acquire that something very serious is about to take place to call for such an important move.

The social environment changes even more radically. Members of the hospital staff begin to rule this man's life, and, not infrequently, they appear to hold his life, if not his death, in their hands. The resident physician can become nearly all powerful, and a little head nurse is the boss of the place in all but major matters. . . .

. . . . The social characteristics of the hospital (or its culture) tend to stimulate a considerable amount of dread and apprehension in the patient. To an ill-prepared and apprehensive person, some of the needed treatments can seem to be not far short of unfriendly intent and sometimes even torture. However well-meaning the staff, and however justifiable the treatment, if a patient worries about explanations which are never given or fails to understand them if they are, if he is full of misgivings and emotional sets against the procedure, and if he feels that he has been tricked or coerced into something more severe than was necessary, then stressful interpersonal relationships have already complicated the situation, and they may affect the course of treatment.

. . . . Sometimes it is easy to conclude that "headaches" and "heartaches" in our modern hospitals now surpass the physical pains, thanks perhaps to the almost miraculous "pain-killers." This accounts substantially, in my mind, for the increasing importance of the cultivation of improved interpersonal relationships in the very highly controlled hospital environment. . . .

There is in the sick man a *person* as well as a body. There are powers of personality within him for healing and for health, and also for sickness and death. Associated with him are other persons equally endowed with such powers. We know that the relationship of these persons to one another and to the patient are laden with both constructive and destructive possibilities. Every physician and nurse knows the difference it can make in a sick person to feel rejected and without interest in the fight for life on the one hand, or warmly wanted and stimulated to live on the other. . . .

In our attempts to explore the therapeutic possibilities of the interpersonal relationships in the treatment of disease, we have deliberately chosen to concentrate on certain of the key characters: the patient, his fellow patients, the physician, the staff nurse, the auxiliary help, the relatives and friends. . . .

. . . . Traditionally the nurse has been a servant at the bedside, not really a co-worker in the patient's care and therapy. But when the patient is treated seriously as a person instead of as a case, and therapy is boldly extended to utilize the resources of the personality, then the modern nurse is, both by training in our better schools of nursing and by the fact that she can spend so much more time with the patient, at some real advantage over the hurried and harried intern in her understanding of the patient as a person. . . .

Perhaps the most important [element] of all [in the hospital system] is the human resources latent in the nurse. . . .*

Simmons has been quoted at length in order to emphasize the therapeutic value he places on a sympathetic relationship between the patient and the nurse. There is no time at which this is more easily established, or more needed, than during the admission procedure. The interest in the patient must be genuine if it is to be effective. Francis Weld Peabody in a now famous lecture to medical students says this, which applies equally to nurses:

The good physician knows his patients through and through, and his knowledge is bought dearly. Time, sympathy, and understanding must be lavishly dispensed, but the reward is to be found in that personal bond which forms the greatest satisfaction of the practice of medicine. One of the essential qualities of the clinician is interest in humanity, for the secret of the care of the patient is in caring for the patient.†

The patient should be made to feel that the service in the agency is gladly given. The average patient is comforted and reassured by the confidence, ease, and

---

* Simmons, Leo W.: "The Manipulation of Human Resources in Nursing Care," *Am. J. Nursing*, **51**:452, (July) 1951.

† Peabody, Francis Weld: *The Care of the Patient*. Harvard University Press, Cambridge, Mass.. 1928. p. 48.

system with which medical workers carry out admission procedures. The majority of patients respond to the interest that is shown in their particular needs and problems. It should be apparent from the first contact with the patient that his care is planned on an individual basis.

Courteous attention should always be given to the family or friends of the sick person. Any failure in this respect reacts unfavorably on the patient as well as on those with him. Introductions should be made as in a home, and waiting children given toys, or adults something to read. Relatives or friends who bring the patient to the hospital usually like to go with him to the clinical service. They often want to meet and talk to the physician and nurse who will be in charge of the patient's program of care. If they wait in order to learn what is discovered in the initial examination of the patient, they should be made as comfortable as the facilities of the institution allow. Their cooperation in the care of the patient should be enlisted, and hospital regulations, such as visiting hours, should be explained to them, as well as the patient. This early meeting of the medical staff and the family or friends may serve to establish a relationship that is badly needed if the care planned for the patient throughout his illness is to take the family situation into account. When agencies such as that described in *The Peckham Experiment*[1] undertake to help individuals with health problems, a family health conference is considered an essential starting point.

Individualized Admissions.   An unfortunate term used in hospitals is *the admission routine,* which has an equally unfortunate counterpart in practice; that is, it happens too often that there is a stereotyped way of greeting people followed by a series of procedures to which everyone is required to submit, regardless of temperament and physical needs. It is true that there are certain administrative and diagnostic procedures that should be carried out in every case, but there are many ways in which the reception and initial treatment of patients should differ.

Nurses will find that consistent efforts to put themselves in the position of the patients they admit will almost inevitably make their reception of the individual more suitable and acceptable. With experience and genuine interest comes an ability to recognize signs of fear, excitement, embarrassment, pain, depression, and loneliness. Patients may have any or all of these sensations on entering a hospital, and the reception of each person should be designed to substitute a constructive attitude for a destructive one or to preserve a tranquil state of mind if one exists. Robert P. Knight[2] has pointed out that fear and embarrassment are expressed by deceptive attitudes of indifference, or even gaiety, so that the successful nurse must learn to be a real student of human nature. G. Canby Robinson,[3] and others since, has shown that more than half the persons treated in medical services of hospitals have conditions whose origins are emotional disturbance. This means that every nurse must be, in a sense, a psychiatric nurse, and every physician something of a psychiatrist.

It is the ideal of many hospitals to treat all who are admitted with *equal* consideration, regardless of nationality, race, creed, color, or economic status, but these factors of racial or personal differences also call for *special* consideration in their treatment. For example, the day laborer who is losing his job or means of livelihood because he is facing an indefinite period of hospitalization may have a sense of impending doom, and therefore should receive a different type of psychological treatment from the wealthy man with a similar disease condition whose economic status is not threatened. From the standpoint of the physical care of the patient, it is likewise obvious that the fastidious person who has prepared himself for admission to the hospital by making a careful toilet should not be subjected to the same procedures for cleaning the skin, hair, mouth, and nails that are necessary when a dirty, untidy person is admitted. Hospital regulations that deprive any patient, even temporarily, of his personal possessions, regardless of the patient's desire to have them or of his ability to take care of them, are open to criticism. Storage space to which the patient has free access should be provided on every clinical service.

Standardization of equipment and method result, as a rule, in a saving of time and money, and for this reason poorly financed and inadequately staffed hospitals are likely to give least consideration to the individual. When standardization is forced on an institution by economic necessity, an attempt should be made to explain to the patient that regulations objectionable to him have been set up for the good of the majority.

General Plan of Admission Procedure. In the plan for the admission of the patient, provision must be made for (1) transporting the patient to the proper clinical division; (2) getting preliminary medical and social data, and making arrangements for the payment of hospital fees; (3) safeguarding or properly disposing of the patient's belongings; (4) providing suitable clothing for the patient in some cases; (5) preparing the patient for the medical examination; (6) instituting preliminary diagnostic procedures; and (7) explaining hospital procedure and medical treatment. These aspects of admission are discussed in the following pages.

Transporting and Guiding the Patient to the Proper Department. Patients in health, and those who are not very ill, walk into the hospital and are escorted to the admitting department, if there is one, or directly to the clinical division by a hostess, a porter, or a nurse from the clinical service. Wheelchairs should be available for those who are too sick, weak, or lame to walk. Patients brought to the hospital in ambulances usually enter by a special door and are taken to the admitting department or clinical service on a stretcher and put to bed immediately. Stretchers also should be ready for very ill patients who are brought to the hospital in private conveyances.

In some hospitals all patients enter through the clinics of the outpatient department or an admitting office stationed within this department. Here it is determined where the patient should be treated, and the medical admission procedure is begun.

Getting Preliminary Social and Medical Data. The administrative department of the hospital is responsible for recording certain data essential for identification and payment of hospital fees. An admission officer from this department gets from the patient or his family the patient's name and address, his telephone number, the name and address of the nearest relative, friend, or guardian, the patient's employment, business address, and in certain cases the name of the employer. In some institutions prepayment of hospital fees is required; in others, a statement as to how the patient plans to meet the cost, including the use of hospital insurance. Patients obviously too ill to answer questions should be admitted immediately and the necessary data supplied by family or friends at the first opportunity. These preliminary data may be recorded in the admission department of a hospital, or in the clinical service where the admission procedure is completed. A member of the business administration staff may come to the clinical division to get the information from the patient, but other kinds of personnel, including nurses, may be asked to act for him or her. Medical social workers frequently take part in the patient's admission in order that problems requiring their help may have immediate attention.

In order to assign the patient to the proper service and to give immediate care suited to his condition, it is necessary to know the diagnosis, or suspected diagnosis, the duration of his illness, his particular handicaps, the name of the physician who sent him to the hospital and/or the staff physician to whom he is assigned. The patient's temperature, pulse, and respiratory rates are determined as soon as possible after he enters the hospital, because they are considered an important index of his condition and affect the procedure to be followed in preparing him for the medical examination and in giving emergency treatment. Before, during, and after the medical examination a detailed social and medical history of the patient's family and of the patient himself and an account of his present illness are taken by physicians and medical students, the latter often called *medical clerks*. The patient may be asked to write a part of this record. (For details of the medical history and examination, see Chapters 4 and 18.)

Safeguarding the Patient's Personal Belongings. In undressing the patient it should be remembered that his clothing, however old, dirty, or shabby, is probably the best that he has, for he no doubt dressed as well as he could when he came to the hospital, unless he was too sick to care. If his clothes are shabby, he will perhaps be very sensitive about them; but no word or look should indicate that the nurse is conscious of their condition. The worse the condition of the clothing the less likely it is that the patient can afford to have it carelessly handled. Lost articles must be replaced by the hospital. Negligence in handling patients' belongings brings criticism upon the institution and makes the personnel and other patients liable to suspicion. Hospitals are sometimes sued for loss of dentures, jewelry, and other possessions of value to the owner.

In private rooms, closets and chests of drawers are provided for clothing and other belongings, and thus their care presents comparatively little difficulty. If the patient is assigned to a service where no adequate provision is made for care of clothing, it is advisable to have relatives or friends return to his home immediately any clothes he will not use in the hospital, and especially any valuables, such as papers, jewelry, or money. If this is done the person assuming the responsibility

should sign a list of the articles he receives. A complete itemized list of everything belonging to the patient to be retained in the hospital must be made in
duplicate. This list should be checked with the patient, if he is not too sick, and he
should verify and sign it. The valuable articles should be tied up in a separate
package with one copy of the list and the patient's name, the unit number, the
date, and the nurse's signature recorded on it; then the package should be given
at once to the head nurse, who will transfer it to the safe kept for that purpose.
The duplicate list is given to the patient or kept by the head nurse.[4, 5]

Whether the patient is in a ward or in a private room, he should be discouraged from keeping money, jewelry, or valuable papers with him. When he is
not very ill and wishes to keep his watch, fountain pen, some money, rings, or
other effects, he does so at his own risk. If, later on, the patient's condition changes
and he cannot be held responsible, the nurse must list the articles and send them
to the office for safekeeping. The person in charge of valuables is usually bonded
to protect the institution. In ward services, where everything belonging to the
patient is stored in a bedside cabinet, it is not practical for a patient to keep many of
his personal belongings. Those that he will usually want or need are his dressing
gown, bedroom slippers, occasionally his own night clothes, his toilet articles,
writing materials, a few books, a watch, and in some cases a photograph, a piece of
jewelry, or an object that he cherishes and likes near him for sentimental reasons.

Increasingly, hospitals are providing lockers in wards near the bed of each
patient or providing a room for each person. It is unfortunate that so many hospitals
have, in the past, made such inadequate provision for patients' belongings.

Before the clothing is put away, it is examined for lice (pediculi) and bedbugs,
especially in the seams. If lice are found on clothing the condition is reported to
the doctor, who prescribes a delousing procedure. "Standing orders" for this exist
in most health agencies. (Delousing methods are discussed in Chapter 5.) In some
cases when clothing is infested, or *very* dirty, it is advisable to burn it. This must
first be explained to the patient or his relatives if he is very sick. The social
service will, if necessary, supply substitute garments.

Care of clothing varies in different hospitals. In some institutions a special
room is provided for the storage and protection of the clothing of "ward patients."
If necessary, the clothing is cleaned and pressed. All outer garments such as
coats and dresses are covered and hung. Scrupulous care of the clothing while
in the hospital plays an important part in the program of health education and rehabilitation of the individual. It is said that "the way to keep a man out of the
mud is to blacken his shoes." The clothing of a patient with an infectious disease
is put in special bags and containers, plainly marked, listed, and decontaminated,
before it is stored.

Restrictive regulations for care of personal belongings must be carefully explained because patients often resent the fact that so many of their possessions are
taken from them. Some of them feel like prisoners when their outer garments are
not available. If the individual understands that he can have his clothes at any

time he needs them and that the storage of his belongings is made necessary by a lack of storage space in ward services, he is not so likely to be resentful.

Providing the Hospital Patient with Suitable Clothing. Institutions must supply clothing for patients when articles brought by them are inadequate in supply, uncomfortable or inconvenient in cut, torn, soiled, or otherwise unsuitable for use in the hospital. Many patients are unable to provide themselves with private laundry service, and the administrative difficulty of getting clothing returned from the hospital laundry to patient-owners makes it impossible for the institution to provide this service for everyone. In some hospitals private patients wear their own clothing, and a laundry service is provided; or the family or friends see that fresh gowns or pajamas are available as required. In ward services, patients usually wear only clothing provided and laundered by the hospital.

In most hospitals the newly admitted patient is automatically undressed and put to bed in a nightgown. While this is often convenient for the examining physician, the practice is open to criticism unless the reason is explained and unless the person is encouraged to get up and dress if there is no longer any necessity for him to stay in bed. The value of maintaining as normal a regimen as possible during sickness is generally accepted as is the danger of continuous bed rest. For its physiological effect daytime activity should be encouraged; for its emotional value normal clothing and good grooming should be stimulated. Recovery is most rapidly promoted in hospitals that provide the patient with an opportunity to lead as vigorous and regular a life as his condition permits.[6, 7]

The clothing needed by the patient depends upon his age, his condition, the nature of his treatment, and the climate. The choice of clothing is particularly affected by his status, whether bedfast or ambulatory. Hospitals may supply nightgowns, pajamas, dressing gowns, shoulder wraps, leggings, caps, underclothes, dresses, coats, trousers, slippers, shoes, and even outdoor wraps. The economic resources of institutions vary; therefore the quantity and quality of the clothing supplied to patients must also vary.

Clothes have a more marked relationship to mental and physical health than most persons realize. Louis H. Newburgh[8] and Marston Bates[9] discuss the disastrous effects of forcing on a people, in the name of morals, customs of dress unsuited to their climate and mores. There are certain clothing needs, typical of each culture, that a health agency should attempt to supply, if the patient, or client, lacks them. In this country each hospital bed patient should have an adequate supply of clean, comfortable sleeping garments, and a shoulder wrap of some kind. He should be provided with a dressing gown or wrapper, socks or stockings, and slippers. Ambulatory patients who have their meals in dining rooms and mix with other patients should have underclothes and proper outer garments and shoes. Those who go outdoors need wraps suited to the weather. Bed patients who are given fresh-air treatment in cold climates must have special outing-flannel gowns or pajamas, woolen jackets, mittens, sleeping socks, and caps. For pelvic examinations and operative procedures, patients are dressed in special garments, and in some cases leggings are used.

While institutional clothing can perhaps never have the charm of that bought

especially for the individual, there is a noticeable trend toward the choice of becoming and cheerful garments. Colorfast dyes make it possible to use colors in all
types of garments. State hospitals that formerly provided uniforms for ambulatory
patients are now providing dresses of many colors, patterns, and styles. The choice of
a dress, a gown, or a jacket provides diversion for all persons, young and old. Interest
in the appearance is almost universal in healthy normal individuals.

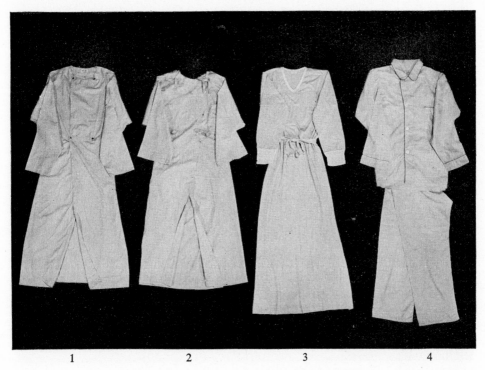

| 1 | 2 | 3 | 4 |

Figure 13. Gowns and pajamas: (*1*) a soft, gingham gown with lapping front suitable
for a man or woman; (*2*) the same gown fastened with tapes instead of snaps and made so
that it can be worn open in the front or back; (*3*) a jersey gown that is soft, absorbent, and
easily laundered; and (*4*) pajamas, preferred by most men and a few women, and desirable
for all patients who are sleeping on porches.

Nurses in homes and hospitals often have opportunities to select clothing for
the sick or to make recommendations for its selection. The following are some
suggestions in relation to specific articles.

Nightgowns should be loose in cut, allowing the patient to move without
restriction. A full-length opening simplifies nursing care. A back opening facilitates
the use of the bedpan; a front opening is convenient for pelvic dressings, examinations, and, in the care of obstetrical patients, for nursing infants. Figure 13 shows
a gown with a wide lap, tucks at the shoulders, and a special neck line that makes
the gown equally comfortable with the opening in the back or in the front.

Gowns should be made of a soft, absorbent, durable material. It is economically desirable that the material be one that does not require ironing. In Figure 13 a jersey or balbriggan gown is shown. Seersucker also is a satisfactory material for gowns if a good soft quality is selected. Knitted fabrics and Canton flannel are most comfortable when the patient perspires a great deal. A material that does not show the figure underneath is convenient because it makes it possible to appear modestly dressed without a second garment.

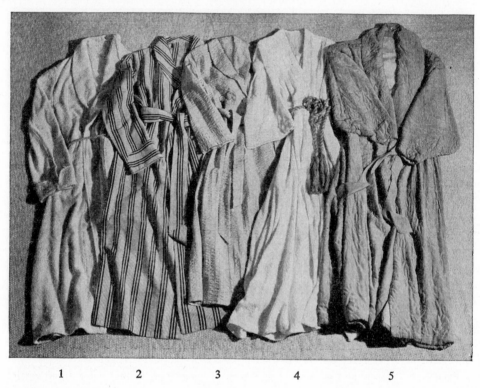

| 1 | 2 | 3 | 4 | 5 |

Figure 14.   Dressing gowns or wrappers: (*1*) a man's robe made of toweling; (*2*) a man's robe made of seersucker; (*3*) a woman's seersucker robe; and (*4*) a woman's robe made of toweling. All of these garments are inexpensive and launder satisfactorily. (*5*) A silk-and-wool quilted robe that is very warm and light.

It has been traditional to make hospital gowns short, or knee length, for the convenience of the nurse, or the surgeon, in caring for the patient. Since the majority of persons wear sleeping garments to the ankles, they are more likely to prefer this length when they are in a hospital. Long gowns are always preferred by patients who must get in and out of bed and who dislike the exposure likely to occur with short gowns. Certain operative procedures, dressings, and examinations may call for knee-length garments, but there seems to be *no good reason for the general use of short hospital gowns*. If the same gown is worn in the winter and summer, it is probably desirable to have it made with long, loose sleeves that can be rolled above the elbow in hot weather. The sleeve should be loose enough to allow for differences in the size of arms and to permit venipunctures and other procedures requiring exposure of the arm.

White sleeping clothes are generally acceptable, but many individuals enjoy wearing becoming pastel shades. Hospital gowns might well be available in white, blue, and pink. This is not uncommon in children's departments at the present time.

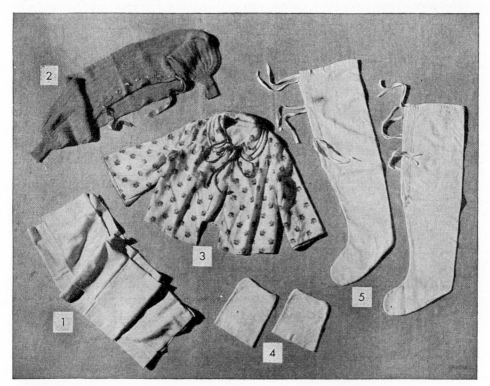

Figure 15.   Jackets, leggings, and caps: (*1*) a strip of flannelet serves the same purpose as the jackets (*2* and *3*) although they are more attractive looking; (*4*) knitted caps in two sizes; and (*5*) flannelet leggings often used to protect patients during operations.

Pajamas should be available for men patients who prefer them and who are not too sick to be exhausted by the effort required to put them on and take them off. Women patients on sleeping porches may also be more comfortable in pajamas.

Dressing gowns or wrappers should be available in different weights for hot and cold weather. Since cotton is less likely than wool, rayon, or nylon to change its texture in laundering, it is the preferred material. Terry cloth (bath toweling) is a satisfactory fabric for winter dressing gowns since it holds air in its meshes and is therefore warm; it does not require ironing, and has a pleasant, soft texture. In cold climates heavy outing flannel also is used for dressing gowns. Quilted robes are very warm, but are practical only for private use, since they should be dry-cleaned rather than washed. For summer weather, dressing gowns made of seersucker are comfortable, and, as they do not require ironing, are especially practical.

Like sleeping garments, dressing gowns, which must fit many shapes, should be loose in cut. They should have an ample lap in front and should come in several sizes. A variety of colors adds to the patients' pleasure in wearing them.

Shoulder wraps have been called *nightingales,* after Florence Nightingale, who advocated them. It seems obvious that a person who is temporarily living in bed

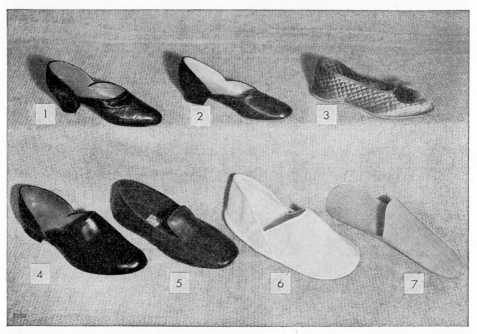

Figure 16.   Slippers suited to the needs of the sick: (*1, 2, 4,* and *5*) for ambulatory patients; (*3*) comfortable for a patient sitting in a chair; (*6*) a washable canvas slipper which the hospital may provide; and (*7*) a paper slipper, which can be worn only once and is suitable for use in examination rooms.

needs more protection for the arms while he or she is eating or reading than is afforded by the sleeves of gowns or pajamas. Many hospitals provide strips of outing flannel or small blankets to put over the shoulders. Many patients provide themselves with bed jackets, which need not be discussed here except to say that they should be soft, loosely cut, and easily washed or cleaned.

Caps must be adjustable, or made so that they will fit heads of varying sizes and shapes. They must be designed so that they do not cut or bind at the edge and so that they can be brought well down over the head and held in position. Stockinette is a soft elastic fabric woven in tubes of different sizes. Caps made of this material are comfortable, adjustable, inexpensive, and if made with a chin strap or a draw string at the edge are easily kept in place. A cap of this material is shown in Figure 15. Unless the patient is desperately ill, his or her morale will be raised by camouflaging caps used for therapeutic purposes. For women artificial bangs may be attached to silk kerchiefs or other suitable headgear. For men berets and skull caps of velvet, silk, or wool are appropriate.

Slippers should provide support and protection if worn by ambulatory patients. The quilted silk slipper shown in Figure 16 is suitable for the patient who gets up in a chair but does not walk about very much. Leather slippers are more practical for ambulatory patients. Silk and leather slippers are so expensive that few institutions can provide them, and in many cases the patient is unable to purchase slippers. The canvas slipper lined with Canton flannel illustrated in Figure 16 is an appropriate type for the hospital to provide. It costs very little, launders well, and is relatively durable. The crepe-paper slipper, shown next to the canvas slipper, is useful in examining rooms and departments where it is desirable to give protection for a short time only; these slippers are worn by only one person and are discarded after use.

In the admission of a patient one of the nurse's duties is to see that he is comfortably clothed, adequately protected from chilling, and conveniently dressed for the physician's examination. Before clothing the patient, however, a cleansing bath and special care of the nails may be indicated. In order to determine the need for this, certain tactful questions may be asked and certain observations can always be made as the nurse helps the patient to undress.

Observing the Patient. Without making it obvious that she is doing so, the nurse should note the general appearance of vigor, lassitude, or prostration in the patient. She should also note his color and his expression—all of which indicate whether he is in comparative health, mildly, or acutely, ill. The nurse should limit the exertion of the patient according to his condition. In helping him to undress, she should be able to get some idea as to whether he has good habits of cleanliness. Scratches and skin lesions on the body may indicate the presence of body lice. Any itching of the pubic region suggests the presence of pubic lice. Burns, rashes, bedsores, or any lesions present should be reported. Abnormality of movement or a paralysis of any part of the body should be called to the attention of the physician. (See Chapter 9 for full discussion of observing the patient.)

All medical workers who admit the patient, but particularly the nurse, who is with him most, should be alert to notice handicaps or limitations. A sensitive person notices signs of deafness, blindness, or dumbness and tries to protect the patient from psychic and physical trauma; the same is true in motor disabilities or in disturbances of equilibrium. The nurse should be familiar with the literature on the handicapped. In every case she should try through imagination to supply the particular needs of each person. For example, the deaf will appreciate distinct rather than overloud speech and care on the part of others to announce their presence; or a written list of the members of the staff. The blind need a thorough introduction to the environment with attention to the regular placement of everything they use; they also need complete verbal explanations and descriptions and the opportunity to feel as many objects as possible. The blind are peculiarly responsive to sounds and will judge their attendant's liking or sympathy by the tone of voice; they will likewise suffer from noise or meaningless sounds. Persons with serious speech difficulties should be provided with paper and pencil or a "magic" slate so that they can write their wants and with cards on which are printed routine needs such as "drinking water" or "more covering." Those with motor disabilities may need canes, wheelchairs, crutches, handles suspended over the bed, guide ropes, special utensils for eating or writing, and other aids.

Above all their physical needs, the handicapped want the understanding type of treatment that minimizes their disabilities. A blind practicing physician, writing under a pseudonym in *When Doctors Are Patients,* speaks for all those who have handicaps when he says:

Despite my best efforts to attain a serenity of spirit, I am still given to outbursts of irritability and to moods of depression, during which those I love are most likely to suffer. I own too that I have not been able entirely to overcome my aversion to those people whose efforts at patronizing kindness conceal but poorly the blend of smug pity and repugnance which lies beneath. Greatly to be cherished is the friend who keeps his pity buried deep and whose kindness does not cloy, but is kept faintly acid with the tang of humor and wit. The indulgence of a sense of humor is of great therapeutic value to those among the sightless so fortunately endowed; Thurber and *The New Yorker* are excellent substitutes for an appointment with the psychiatrist.*

All patients on admission, but particularly the handicapped, should be supplied as soon as possible with occupations suited to their conditions and interests. Observations by the nurse guide her and others in the provision of such materials as the patient wants and needs.

The nurse's observation of the patient should enable her to determine whether he needs immediate medical attention and what preparation should be made for the medical examination. Admission baths and shampoos are not given unless there is some reason to believe that they are indicated, either as preparation for the physical examination or for the patient's comfort.

The Admission Toilet.   If the patient is to have a bath on admission and his condition permits it, a tub bath is given. This is particularly desirable if portions of the body are noticeably dirty or if the treatment the patient is to receive will make it impossible for him to get into a tub for some time. Bed baths should be given to any patients who are very weak or ill.

Among patients admitted to the hospital, many will have established desirable habits of cleanliness and will be uncomfortable if these habits are disrupted. A few will object to the bath and particularly to the first bath on admission. Some object because they think it unnecessary and are rather insulted at the suggestion; others think too many baths bad for them, or fear they will catch cold. Some patients do not object to the bath, but from modesty or reserve dislike being bathed. A

* Pinner, Max, and Miller, Benjamin F. (eds.): *When Doctors Are Patients.* W. W. Norton & Co., New York, 1952, p. 55.

nurse should be tactful in overcoming objections, and must be tolerant of prejudices. The patient will soon learn to appreciate the beneficial effects of the bath. The admission toilet does not differ in any respect from the daily attention to personal cleanliness, except that in cases of neglect the cleansing process must be more thorough.

Brushing and combing the hair offer the nurse an opportunity to examine the scalp and the hair itself for pediculi and nits (eggs). If pediculi are present, treat-ment is prescribed by the physician and instituted immediately. (For a discussion of this topic and illustration of lice see Chapter 5.)

Immediate Preparation for the Medical Examination. Before a medical ex-amination is given, the rational patient should have a suitable explanation of the procedure unless he is familiar with it. An effort should be made to relieve, insofar as it is possible, the fear that so often accompanies the examination. The procedure commonly followed by the physician and nurse is described in Chapter 18.

2. DISCHARGE WITH SPECIAL REFERENCE TO THE HOSPITAL PATIENT

A serious illness in all its aspects usually makes a lasting impression. Discharge from the hospital should never come unexpectedly to the patient or to any of those attending him. The aim of the medical team, the patient, and his family, throughout his illness, is to make the patient independent; and from the first everyone looks forward to the day when he can leave the hospital. The position taken in this text, that rehabilitation is part of all complete medical care, is the position taken also by C. M. Gardner.[10] In some cases the person is discharged from one health agency to another better suited to his needs or his economic resources. In all cases the best results are gotten when those concerned agree upon the date and are ready for the discharge. In some institutions the doctor, nurse, and social worker meet weekly, or more often, to discuss plans for the discharge of patients or for continuing care. Ideally the patient and family concerned and representatives of all major departments contributing to his program of therapy should participate in such conferences. It is obvious that plans should be made far enough in advance to enable the staff of an-other agency, the family, and the patient himself to arrange things so that his needs will be met. In some cases he leaves the hospital cured and rehabilitated, ready to take up his former way of life; very often he faces a period of convalescence or training for a more limited existence. Hospitals differ greatly in the responsibility they assume for continuity of care. When the patient needs help from a second agency the professional personnel of the first agency can promote the patient's welfare by communication with the personnel of the second. This is usually ac-complished through "referral forms" (see Figs. 17 A and B). On the form the physician can make a note on treatment, the nurse, on nursing care, the social worker, on social problems, the physical therapist, on such treatment as he has been giving, the nutritionist, on nutritional problems, and so on. In special cases it is desir-able that workers in the second agency visit the patient while he is in the hospital so that they will know something about his problems when he arrives, and so that the patient will not feel entirely strange when he gets there. This exchange of information can be accomplished by letters, or telephone communication, or interagency conferences. In any event systematic use should be made of written referral forms similar to those shown in Figures 17 A and B.[11, 12, 13]

Some institutions are providing for continuity of care in homes by sending members of the hospital staff to see patients discharged from the hospital. Patients in some

---

REQUEST FOR PUBLIC HEALTH AND VISITING NURSE SERVICE

●

Washtenaw County Health Department and Affiliated Agencies

●

(Address)	(Office)	(Phone)
720 E. Catherine	Ann Arbor	2-5581
1761 Stamford Rd.	Willow Run	2892
26 S. Prospect St.	Ypsilanti	1525

Date_____

Name_____ Approx. Age_____

Address _____

Diagnosis _____

ORDERS:

Dr._____

Figure 17A. Referral form used to request visiting nurse service. (Courtesy of Washtenaw County Health Department and Affiliated Agencies, Ypsilanti and Ann Arbor, Michigan.)

"home care programs" are still registered with the hospital.[14] This scheme for extending hospital service and for making the best possible use of the home in total medical care was discussed in Chapters 2 and 3. In order that medical students should have some knowledge of the entire cycle of illness and the treatment of persons outside the hospital, Syracuse University set up a program of medical follow-up of the discharged hospital patient.[15] It is likely that in the next decade

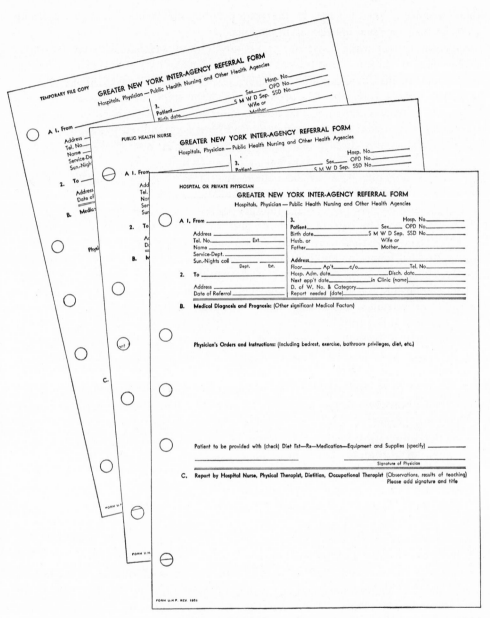

Figure 17B. Inter-agency referral form. The three sheets are identical except for color which indicates person or organization using form (yellow, hospital or private physician; pink, public health nurse and other health agencies; white, temporary file copy). Continuation sheets in corresponding colors for easy identification are also available. (Courtesy of The Greater New York Inter-Agency Referral Committee, New York City.)

there will be a great change in the responsibility the hospital and other health agencies take for rehabilitation of all patients.

Once in a great while a patient, or his family, is dissatisfied with the treatment given him in the hospital, and leaves against the advice of his physician. In such cases the patient, or his guardian, and a member of his family are asked to sign a statement before he leaves. This is a protection to the hospital authorities, who may be sued if the patient is convinced that he was maltreated or if he can prove that he was detained for treatment against his will. Unless he is a committed pyschiatric patient, has a communicable disease that limits his freedom, or is a prisoner of the law, a patient is free to leave the hospital at his discretion.[16] Every effort is made to resolve any difficulty between the patient and those responsible for his care and to prevent a premature termination of treatment.

It must also be mentioned that some people never leave the hospital alive, death being inevitable. The care of the dying and the dead is discussed in Chapter 35.

When those concerned have agreed on the time that a patient should leave a health agency for his home, or another institution, the doctor in charge of his treatment writes a discharge note on the chart and signs it. The person, usually the head nurse, responsible for the general management of the clinical unit notifies the financial office in advance, and arrangements are made for the payment of the patient's bill. His medical record is brought up to date, and as he leaves, the hour of departure and the mode of locomotion, whether on foot, in a chair, or on a stretcher are noted by the nurse. A medical summary is prepared by the physician, and the completed data sent to the medical records department to be filed. Except in illnesses that leave no temporary or permanent disability, discharge from the hospital should be preceded by a planned program of health guidance or teaching that extends over a large part, or the entire period, of hospitalization. Too often the patient is given explanation or instruction about treatments, diets, formulas, exercises, or medications just before he leaves the institution. This is no longer believed to be adequate. He should not be discharged until he has had a chance to demonstrate and practice his independence, if this is expected of him after he leaves the institution. The plan of care for the patient, as described in Chapter 4, indicates that medical services should aim at the complete restoration of the person's functions. It should provide for follow-up over a period of weeks, months, or even years and for whatever help he needs in getting employment suited to his physical and mental status. Directions for home care that the patient is to follow should be written. Illustrated and diagrammed directions often further the understanding of the patient and the family. Dates and hours for return visits to clinics should be put in writing. It cannot be said too often that all such plans should be made *with* the patient and his family in an unhurried and cooperative atmosphere.

Some hospital administrations attempt to improve their service by systematically soliciting criticism from patients. Administrative officers may visit patients and get such comments orally, or they may ask them to fill in questionnaires as they leave. Nurses could learn a great deal about the subjective aspect of illness if they kept a card file of significant comments made to them by patients. Periodically such comments could be summarized and valuable generalizations made.

In preparation for the patient's departure his belongings are assembled, checked, and packed. It is customary for the patient to sign a record indicating that the articles listed have been returned to him. The nurse gives the patient whatever help he needs in dressing. She makes every effort through cooperation with his family or the social service department to see that he has suitable garments for the journey to his next destination. The nurse is usually the person who, like a good hostess, speeds the parting guest and makes him feel that those he leaves behind wish him well and will be interested in seeing him again. She, or some other member of the staff, goes with him and his family to the front door, seeing that what baggage he has is delivered to him and that he has the necessary mode of conveyance. His welcome and farewell are major factors in the total impression made on the person by the institution. The nurse plays an important role on both occasions, and if it is possible, she should allow time to make these first and last services thorough, effective, and graceful. The attitude the patient acquires toward the institution may determine his willingness to return to the clinic, to keep up the suggested program, or to continue treatment in another agency.

REFERENCES

1. Pearse, Innes, and Crocker, Lucy H.: *The Peckham Experiment: A Study of the Living Structure of Society.* Yale University Press, New Haven, 1944.
2. Knight, Robert P.: "Why People Act the Way They Do," *Am. J. Nursing,* **38**:18, (supplement to April issue) 1938.
3. Robinson, G. Canby: *The Patient as a Person.* Commonwealth Fund, New York, 1939.
4. Hayt, Emanuel, and Hayt, Lillian R.: *Legal Guide for American Hospitals.* Hospital Textbook Co., New York, 1940, p. 256.
5. Lesnik, Milton J., and Anderson, Bernice E.: *Legal Aspects of Nursing.* J. B. Lippincott Co., Philadelphia, 1947, p. 213.
6. Gold, Harry (ed.): *Cornell Conferences on Therapy,* Vol. I. The Macmillan Company, New York, 1946, pp. 18-35.
7. Morrissey, Alice B.: *Rehabilitation Nursing.* G. P. Putnam's Sons, New York, 1951.
8. Newburgh, Louis H. (ed.): *Physiology of Heat Regulation and the Science of Clothing.* W. B. Saunders Co., Philadelphia, 1949.
9. Bates, Marston: *Where Winter Never Comes.* Charles Scribner's Sons, New York, 1952.
10. Gardner, C. M.: "Rehabilitation for Every Patient," *Canad. Nurse,* **45**:347, (May) 1949.
11. Committee on Inter-Relationships with Public Health Nursing Agencies of the United Hospital Fund, New York City: *The Greater New York Inter-Agency Referral Form.* The Committee, New York, 1946.
12. Frost, Harriet, and Lynch, Theresa I.: "From Hospital to Home Nursing," *Am. J. Nursing,* **48**:684, (Nov.) 1948.
13. Addams, Ruth, and Scott, Ruth B.: "The Unbroken Circle," *Am. J. Nursing,* **51**:181, (Mar.) 1951.
14. Cherkasky, Martin: "The Montefiore Home Care Program," *Am. J. Pub. Health,* **39**:163, (Feb.) 1949.
15. Jensen, Frode, et al.: *Medical Care of the Discharged Hospital Patient.* Commonwealth Fund, New York, 1944.
16. Hayt, Emanuel, and Hayt, Lillian R.: *op. cit.,* p. 372.

Additional Suggested Reading

Anonymous: "Was I Your Patient?" *Am. J. Nursing,* **51:**457, (July) 1951.

Cabot, Richard C., and Dicks, Russell L.: *The Art of Ministering to the Sick.* The Macmillan Company, New York, 1936.

Gilbert, Ruth: *The Public Health Nurse and Her Patient.* Harvard University Press (for The Commonwealth Fund), Cambridge, Mass., 1951.

Kogel, Marcus D., and Kruger, Alexander W.: "New York City's Long-Range Program for Extending Hospital Care into the Home," *Hospitals,* **24:**35, (Feb.) 1950.

Peplau, Hildegarde E.: *Interpersonal Relations in Nursing: A Conceptual Frame of References for Psychodynamic Nursing.* G. P. Putnam's Sons, New York, 1952.

CHAPTER 7. CONTROLLING THE SPREAD OF COMMUNICABLE DISEASE BY ASEPTIC MEASURES

1. DEVELOPMENT OF CONCEPTS AND METHODS

Old Practices and New Insight. Many effective methods of controlling communicable disease were known to the ancients, but we believe now that they were based on trial and error rather than on a knowledge of the underlying principles. The scientist of today considers that in order to understand thoroughly the prevention and control of a transmissible disease it is necessary to isolate the organism causing the disease and to learn at least some of the characteristics of the organism.

Some present-day practices have been known for centuries, and yet the scientific control of communicable disease is modern and, in a sense, in its early stages. The ancients were aiming in the dark, sometimes hitting their mark; but the scientists of the last few centuries have thrown a bright light on the target, and in the case of many diseases it is no longer necessary to shoot blindly. Not only is there a specific understanding of control measures for diseases of known origin but a working hypothesis has been furnished for research where the organism is unknown; therefore, it is possible to proceed more effectively now in dealing with any communicable disease than it was in the past.

Notwithstanding all the advances that have been made, however, about two million cases of communicable disease (not including gonorrhea, syphilis, and common colds) were reported in 1948 in the United States, and it is estimated that between 5 and 10 per cent of the world's population suffer from malaria.[1, 2] This high incidence of communicable disease is due partially to our failure to apply the findings of science and partially to the limitation of scientific discovery. The existence of diphtheria, smallpox, yellow fever, typhoid fever, malaria, and many other diseases is entirely the result of failure to use the preventive measures that are available; on the other hand, the means of preventing and controlling epidemics of virus diseases, such as the common cold and mumps, are not yet fully developed.

Ernest C. McCulloch[3] says that disinfection methods are a mixture of religious rites, empirical knowledge, and scientific discovery. Doctors, nurses, and sanitarians should constantly bear in mind that there is a great lag between scientific discovery and its application, and that our practices should be held up to scrutiny at frequent intervals to see whether they are consistent with the newer knowledge of microbiology.

It is conceivable that communicable diseases might be practically eliminated by an extension and application of what is now known about vaccines that produce immunity, diets that help to develop resistance to disease, sera and drugs that cure early cases, and methods of destroying pathogenic organisms that protect the well from those who are infected.

Changing Emphases.   It is an old story that, when bacteria were first discovered to be the cause of disease, physicians and sanitarians thought the secret of control lay chiefly in the use of strong chemicals. Disinfection of the air with chemicals was attempted. The public began to associate the smell of coal-tar products, such as carbolic acid and cresol, with safety from disease-producing bacteria, and hospitals were likely to reek of such drugs. A great variety of chemicals was manufactured, each one of which was believed to be effective in destroying practically every strain of microorganism. Fumigation with poisonous gases was used routinely in disinfecting rooms vacated by patients with communicable disease. Chemical disinfection was widely applied, and great confidence was placed in its efficacy.

Besides the emphasis on chemical disinfection, there was a general belief that bacteria thrived in dirty places, so that in attempting to control an epidemic of any kind a great effort was made to clean up cities, towns, and individual houses. Jenner demonstrated the effectiveness of vaccination with cowpox as a protection against smallpox in 1796, but the scientific principles of vaccination against any disease were laid down by Pasteur and his associates in what might be called the beginning of the modern program of communicable disease control. Shortly afterward came the knowledge that insects transfer infectious material from the sick to the well, and strenuous campaigns were launched against flies and mosquitoes.

Although none of these theories or practices has been discredited, some of them have been modified to the extent that control measures are becoming more specific as more is learned about the nature of the organisms causing disease, their portals of entry to the body, the ways in which they are transmitted from person to person, and their resistance to physical and chemical agents. At the present time emphasis is placed on the following preventive measures: (1) developing immunity to disease by general hygienic living, paying particular attention to an adequate diet; (2) the use of vaccines, particularly during periods of especial susceptibility; ③ isolation of the sick individual, using a technique adapted to the type of disease from which the patient is suffering; ④ destroying the breeding places of insects that spread disease; ⑤ general disinfection (with a physical agent, such as heat and light) of contaminated dishes, linen, toilet articles, and other objects used in common by persons in public places; and ⑥ reducing bacterial content of air by natural ventilation, oiling floors and bedding (see p. 204), treatment of room air with ultraviolet rays and disinfectant vapors, such as glycol. In item (6) is seen the swing of the pendulum back to an early and discarded practice. The value of light (particularly sunlight) in terminal disinfection of room air has been accepted for many years; the use of ultraviolet rays, disinfectant vapors, and oil treatment for floors and bedding is new. The results of numerous studies show that all these practices have promise but that they also have limitations.

Great advances have recently been made in the cure of communicable diseases by new drugs to which specific organisms or groups of organisms are peculiarly susceptible, and also by the rapid development of therapeutic sera. It is not within the scope of this chapter, however, to discuss the therapy of communicable diseases. The particular purpose here is to present the techniques and their underlying principles that the nurse applies in helping to prevent and limit the spread of transmissible diseases.

Responsibility of the Nurse. In Chapter 5 attention was called to the function of the nurse in organizing a safe environment. Of all the dangers in the surroundings none is more prevalent or more serious than the pathogenic microorganism. In both homes and institutions it is now considered chiefly the responsibility of the nurse to see that patients and other members of the household are protected, or understand how to protect themselves, from contact with disease-producing microbes. Whereas the nurse participates in other aspects of the communicable disease program, she is expected to take the initiative in instituting suitable measures for disinfecting and cleaning contaminated dishes, clothing, and bedding; for disposal of excreta, protection of the patient from droplet infection, cleaning and disinfecting contaminated hands, making a room safe to live in after it has been occupied by a patient with a communicable disease; and for all the other activities that go to make up what is usually referred to as *medical asepsis* or *surgical asepsis*.

In order to avoid confusion in discussing this subject it seems desirable to give the meanings of terms as they will be used in this text. The definitions are based on medical dictionaries and recently published standard texts dealing with bacteriology and communicable diseases. To facilitate the use of this section as a reference an alphabetical arrangement has been followed.

2. DEFINITION OF TERMS

Anaerobic Microorganisms. Microbes that can live in the absence of oxygen (air) as distinguished from aerobic microorganisms that require oxygen for life and growth.

Asepsis.   Literally, this means the absence of pathogenic bacteria. Since this condition is exceedingly difficult to maintain for any length of time, the term might be said to be used relatively in most cases. In *surgical asepsis* an attempt is made to render absolutely free from all microorganisms every object that comes in direct or indirect contact with a wound; in *medical asepsis* an attempt is made to prevent the transfer of pathogenic organisms from one person to another, but it does not mean that all equipment that comes in contact with the patient is sterile. Articles used in surgical asepsis are subjected to very high temperatures (sterilized), protected from air bacteria, and kept *sterile;* equipment used in medical asepsis is, at least theoretically, freed from pathogenic bacteria (sometimes called "sanitized") and not protected from air bacteria but kept clean, or *sanitary*.

Carrier of Disease.   This refers to a person who harbors and eliminates through some excretion of the body the organism causing a specific disease, although that person gives no evidence of having the disease himself. Obviously, he is a menace because he may spread the disease without any one knowing he is doing so. Carriers of diphtheria, streptococcus throat infections, and typhoid fever are not uncommon. Animals also may act as carriers, but the term as used ordinarily refers to the human carrier of disease.

Clean.   Free from discernible soil or dirt, sanitary, incapable of spreading disease.

Contact.   Individuals who are known or believed to have been exposed to a disease are referred to as *contacts*.

Contagious Disease.   Different writers give different meanings to this term. In some cases it is used to designate any disease that can be transmitted from one person to another by a living vegetable or animal organism. In other instances the term is applied to those diseases that are transmitted from person to person by direct contact or touching, as distinguished from those that require an intermediary host, such as malaria, which is spread by the bite of the mosquito. *Communicable diseases* and *infectious diseases* are terms that are now more commonly used than *contagious diseases* to designate all conditions that are transmissible by a living organism.

Contamination.   In surgery, where absolute freedom from microbes is the objective, contact with anything that is not free from living bacteria constitutes contamination; in medical asepsis contact with an object that has living pathogenic organisms on it from a person other than the person who is handling the object represents contamination; for example, the surgeon "contaminates" his sterile glove when he accidentally touches his cheek, and the glove must be changed before he proceeds with the operation; the physician "contaminates" his stethoscope when he places it on the chest of a child who has scarlet fever, and it must be sterilized before he uses it for another patient.

Disinfection.   This is the process of killing microorganisms by any means, physical or chemical. *Concurrent disinfection* refers to the disinfection of articles coming in direct or indirect contact with a patient during an illness, or while he is in an institution; *terminal disinfection* refers to the process of disinfecting the patient's skin, hair, and clothing, also his possessions and his habitation at the end of the period of isolation for a communicable disease, or after his death.

Infection. Although this term is ordinarily used with reference to a wound, it may mean the presence and growth of pathogenic microorganisms in any area of the body, giving rise to signs and symptoms of disease.

Inoculation. The purposeful introduction of the agent of a disease into the body of an animal or a human being is known as inoculation. The purpose is to produce a mild form of the disease, during the course of which the body develops within the blood substances or agents known as antibodies that protect the body from spontaneous inoculations of this or similar diseases.

Pathogenic Microorganisms. Microbes that are capable of producing disease.

Prophylactic Measures. Measures that prevent the development of a disease within an individual or the transmission of a disease from one person to another.

Pyogenic Microorganisms. Organisms that produce pus.

Quarantine. Derived from *quaranta* meaning 40, because at one time ships from ports where communicable diseases were prevalent were not allowed to dock in other ports until they had spent a period of 40 days outside the port. The period of quarantine now refers to the period of time during which public health regulations are enforced in order to prevent the spread of a communicable disease.

A Specific. A drug that seems to be particularly effective in destroying a particular organism. If a drug is highly destructive to the causative organism it is spoken of as a *specific* for the disease.

Sterile. An object is properly called *sterile* when it is free from microorganisms.

Sterilization. The destruction of microorganisms, the term ordinarily referring to destruction by heat.

Serum (Plural, *sera*). The fluid part of blood. *Immune sera* are taken from the blood of human beings or animals that have recovered from a specific disease. They may be introduced into the bodies of other human beings or animals to protect them from this same disease or to lessen the severity of an attack.

Vaccine. Any substance that is capable of stimulating the production of immunity to a disease within a living body. A vaccine may consist of living or attenuated microorganisms, a virus, or a toxin produced by microorganisms or proteins, such as foods or flower pollens that cause symptoms of hay fever, asthma, and anaphalactic shock.

Virus. A general term for the poison in an infectious disease. It is the name for a group of pathogenic organisms smaller than the previously accepted range for bacteria. Some can be seen with present-day microscopes; others cannot.

3. FACTORS MODIFYING METHODS OF CONTROL

Variation in Method. It is often puzzling to see one set of precautions taken in handling a patient with one type of disease and an entirely different set followed in caring for a person with another communicable condition. Certain measures may be used to prevent infections among infants that are not used for adults.

The nurse may notice that a practice followed in her own hospital is disregarded in an affiliated institution. Any nurse observing these variations in method naturally wonders which method is most desirable or whether one method is as good as another. All medical workers should be fortified with a knowledge of the underlying principles of bacteriology so that they themselves can judge the reliability of procedures and build up their own method based on reason rather than cut and dried rules taught them by someone else.

Rules are often inadequate guides because methods must be adapted to the conditions as they exist; it is impossible to make a sufficient number of rules to fit all the situations the nurse is likely to encounter. It is true that many of the differences in methods of communicable disease control are unjustifiable and represent confusion in the work and writings of those who should speak with authority, but certain differences in method indicate a thoughtful adaptation of practice to the demands of a particular set of circumstances.

The Seriousness of the Disease under Consideration.   When diseases are difficult to arrest or cure, as, for example, leprosy or meningitis, more drastic efforts are made to isolate the person having the disease than when the condition tends to be a mild one, such as epidermophytosis (ringworm) or the common cold. Leprosy is not highly infectious, and yet in some parts of the world lepers are segregated because the disease requires persistent treatment, is disfiguring, and on account of the public's horror of the disease; ringworm, although unpleasant and difficult to eradicate, is not considered a serious infection nor is it especially repellent in many of its forms; therefore, persons infected with ringworm are allowed to mix freely in society. In spite of its name, epidemic cerebrospinal meningitis is now believed to be transmitted only on intimate contact with the infected individual, but in many hospitals the patient with this disease is completely isolated; common colds, on the other hand, are highly contagious, but since the condition is often a mild one, many persons disregard methods of control and there are comparatively few who criticize them. These examples serve to illustrate the point that, whether it is sound reasoning or not, in practice we usually stress measures of control and follow a stricter regime for persons having dangerous conditions than for those having highly communicable but milder diseases.

Susceptibility of Groups or Individuals to Be Protected.   It is well known that certain precautions not considered necessary for adults are taken to prevent the spread of disease among infants and children. Workers in hospital nurseries regularly wear masks and gowns when handling infants who are peculiarly susceptible to infections, particularly of the skin. Since the protective nature of the vaginal secretions seems to be altered during the late prenatal, natal, and postnatal periods, special techniques are used in cleaning the genitalia of the mother to prevent contact with disease-producing microorganisms. There are many conditions that make individuals susceptible to communicable disease in general or to some special type of infection.

Malnutrition lowers the resistance to almost any disease invasion, and the same is true of conditions that interfere with normal circulation. Smoke and irritating gases, such as ether, predispose the lungs to pneumonia, and anything that destroys the integrity of the skin invites infection. The nurse should be familiar with such well-established theories and should be alert to the necessity for special protection of susceptible individuals and groups.

Mode of Transmission. The routes by which pathogenic organisms leave the body of the sick and enter the body of the well person are the two most important factors to consider in setting up measures of prevention and control. Communicable diseases and appropriate measures of prevention may be grouped into five classes according to the manner in which the causative organisms are transmitted from the infected person to another individual: (1) In *wound infections* disease organisms leave the sick through discharges from the wound and enter the body of a second person through a break in the skin or mucous membrane. It is obvious that measures of control consist in keeping infected wounds covered; handling used dressings with forceps or rubber gloves and immediately disinfecting or destroying them; disinfecting all instruments and articles of clothing that come in contact with the wound; and having the attendant take every precaution to prevent breaks in the skin, particularly those of the hands. When wounds are dressed it is possible for microorganisms to pass from dressings and linen to the air and for contaminated air to infect wounds. It is, therefore, important to use dust-suppressive measures and for workers to wear masks and gloves. (2) In *skin diseases* that are spread by material from the skin, the precautions are very similar. When it is not possible to cover the lesions, the discharges from which are a menace to the public, it is necessary to isolate the patient. Everything he touches—bedding, clothing, toilet articles, and dishes—is disinfected before it is handled by others. Workers who are obliged to handle any objects before they are disinfected are protected either by wearing gloves or by immediately scrubbing their hands with soap and water, depending upon the condition and the facilities available; gowns are worn also to protect the clothing from contamination; in rare cases masks are indicated. (3) Another group is the *infections of the alimentary canal,* diseases transmitted by discharges from the intestinal tract. These are controlled by disinfecting dishes, toilet articles, bedding, and clothing of the sick person that are contaminated by contact with the feces or anal region; and by disinfection of the excreta, including vomitus. The patient's attendants wear gowns and are careful to wash their hands after touching him or his belongings. (4) A similar type is the *communicable disease of the genital tract,* in which the danger lies in the discharge from this tract coming in contact with the mucous membranes of the well person. *The conjunctiva covering the eye* seems to be susceptible to infection from the same bacteria that invade the genital tract—for example, the gonococcus, streptococcus, staphylococcus, and other cocci forms. Precautions taken for diseases of both areas are similar. Attendants often wear goggles or eyeglasses when giving treatments, such as irrigations, where spattering of infectious material is likely to occur. Discharges from either the genitalia or the eyes are burned, disinfected, or disposed of in the sewerage system. As in skin and intestinal diseases, any clothing, bedding, and dishes or other utensils that may be soiled with discharges from the genitalia or eyes are handled with especial care and disinfected as soon as possible. The attendants wear gowns while in actual contact with the patient and wash their hands thoroughly after leaving him. (5) The last group includes many of the most common "children's diseases" and are usually classified as *communicable diseases of the respiratory tract*. These diseases are spread by discharges from almost any portion of the respiratory mucosa. The organisms may be discharged through the mouth, nose, possibly the eyes, and the ears if the latter become infected and the drums ruptured. Obviously, diseases of this class may be contracted by the well person if the causative organisms are deposited in the mouth, nose, or eyes. Special methods of control consist in putting up a barrier, in the shape of a mask, between the noses and mouths and possibly the eyes of the sick and the well. Either the sick or the well person may wear the mask, but it is rarely practical to mask the patient. Infected persons are taught to cover the nose and mouth with a handkerchief when coughing or sneezing; the handkerchief may later be disinfected or destroyed. The use of paper handkerchiefs, which can be burned or placed in toilets and hoppers, is rapidly spreading among sick and well. In addition to these precautions, especial care is taken to burn or disinfect discharges from the nose, throat, eyes, and ears; all dishes, toilet articles, bedding, and clothing are disinfected; attendants wear gowns and are careful to wash their hands after leaving the patient. Dust control by oiling floors and bedding and the reduction of air bacteria by sunlight, ultraviolet light, and disinfectant sprays are part of the program, although the use of some of these agents is still in the experimental stage.

In certain diseases there is some question of the route, or routes, by which the organisms leave the body. For example, the virus of poliomyelitis is found in the nasopharynx, in the intestinal tract, and in the nerves.[4] As long as the exact mode of transmission in this disease is unknown, it is logical to observe precautions used in the control of both respiratory and intestinal diseases until the mode of its transmission is established.

It is noticeable that one precaution is common to all groups; namely, that the attendants always wash their hands after handling anything contaminated by infectious material from the patient. As a matter of fact, it is pretty generally agreed that for sanitary reasons all medical workers should wash their hands after touching any patient or any objects that he has contaminated, whether he is believed to have a communicable disease or not. Actually, dishes and bed linen should be so handled in communal living, or in public places, that they are decontaminated after each use. Well-run kitchens and laundries are set up to accomplish this.

Although the mode of transmission determines very largely *what* shall be disinfected, it is the type of organism to be killed that influences the *selection of the disinfecting agent*.

Susceptibility of Different Microorganisms to Disinfecting Agents.   Extremes of temperatures, light rays, certain chemicals, and certain drying processes inhibit or destroy protoplasm. Bacteria respond differently to these destructive agents according to their strain and stage of development. For example, the thermal death point for the gonococcus is around 40° C (104° F); for the typhoid bacillus 62.8° C

(145° F); whereas staphylococci will survive a temperature of 82.2° C (180° F) for 30 minutes. The latter organism is also more resistant to drying and to many chemical disinfectants. Most vegetative forms of bacteria, however, are readily killed by boiling water.[5] In contrast, the disease-producing bacilli and clostridii, such as anthrax and tetanus, in their spore forms, are resistant to months of drying, to long exposure to chemical disinfectants, to freezing temperatures, and to boiling water. In order to ensure the destruction of spores, temperatures of 121° C (249.8° F) and over must be used. The more moisture present the more penetrating and effective the heat.

When an article is to be disinfected, the worker should first of all consider whether it is important or desirable to kill any spores that may be present on the object, for, if so, very high temperatures should be used. This question is not hard to decide because, with the exception of the botulinus bacillus, about the only spores that are pathogenic to man are those that infect wounds. David T. Smith lists the following as the most important (commonest) members of this group: the *Bacillus anthracis* (causing anthrax), the *Clostridium tetani* (causing tetanus), *Cl. septicum, Cl. perfrigens* type A or *Cl. welchii* A, and *Cl. novyi* or *Cl. oedematiens,* all gas forming and all found in wound infections.[6, 7] The common occurrence of many of these organisms in the intestinal tracts of sick and well animals and humans means that they are likely to be encountered almost anywhere. Apparently, the unbroken tissues are quite resistant to most, if not all, of them. Smith says that the organisms listed above, that under certain conditions form gas gangrene, are found in many wounds that seem to be healing normally. However, heavy contamination by these same organisms may be fatal.

From the evidence, it seems clear that spore-forming organisms pathogenic to man are common in nature. In small numbers and under certain conditions man is relatively resistant to them, particularly if the tissues are intact; in large numbers and in contact with impaired tissue they cause serious, often fatal, conditions. This means that *any object that is to come in contact with a wound of any sort should be sterilized in such a manner as to destroy spores.*

The consensus is that moist heat at a high temperature, which can only be secured by steam under pressure, is by all odds the most effective method of destroying spore forms. Spores are affected by chemical disinfectants if the latter are used properly, but the method is highly uncertain as compared with autoclaving (the use of steam under pressure). If most spores are exposed to boiling water for long periods of time, say for 1 or 2 hours, it is unlikely that any will survive; however, J. R. Esty and K. F. Meyer[8] reported that some spores survive 45 hours of continuous boiling. Even repeated boiling, however, is not as sure a method as a single exposure to steam at a temperature of 121° C (249.8° F) for 20 minutes. It is a generally accepted principle that, in order to prevent wound infections, all surgical supplies that withstand heat should be autoclaved, or subjected to hot air of even higher temperatures for longer time periods before they are used.[9]

Since practically all diseases, other than wound infections (with the exception of botulism), are caused by microbes that are thought to have vegetative forms only, medical asepsis is more easily attained than surgical asepsis. The organisms causing respiratory, intestinal, genitourinary, and skin diseases are readily killed by boiling water, many of them by temperatures below boiling, by light, some by drying processes, and practically all by chemical disinfectants if the latter are used properly. Heat and light are more universally effective, and also more readily available, than a suitable chemical; therefore, hospitals rely on physical rather than chemical agents. In medical asepsis, boiling water is used to disinfect all equipment that is not injured by moist heat. Mechanical cleaning with exposure to direct sunlight or ultraviolet rays is used for large surfaces that cannot be treated with boiling water. Chemicals are resorted to for materials, such as certain plastics, that are destroyed by heat. Chemical vapors are again being advocated for the destruction of bacteria suspended in the air.

The superiority of moist heat as a disinfecting agent can scarcely be over-emphasized, but it has its disadvantages. It destroys some articles and eventually injures almost anything. Generally speaking, high temperatures hasten chemical change; as, for example, oxidation. Because heat is injurious and destructive, and in some cases not available, there is a wide demand for chemical disinfectants. Before substituting a chemical disinfectant for heat, however, an attempt should be made to determine the risk and the relative cost. It may be less expensive, in the long run, to replace scissors and knife blades than to treat infected wounds; and the unnecessary death of one patient is a loss that no economy can justify.

To summarize, for surgical asepsis, if possible, employ temperatures above boiling to destroy spore forms.

Autoclaving periods range from 15 to 60 minutes, according to the temperature (pressure) used and the ease with which steam penetrates the material to be sterilized. When superheated air or steam is not available, use boiling water for periods ranging from 30 minutes to 1 hour, according to the barometric pressure and the pH of the water. If heat of any kind is impractical, employ the most effective chemical that can be found, determine the strength in which it is most powerful, and allow long periods of contact in order to ensure sterility of the object. In medical asepsis use boiling water for periods of from 5 to 30 minutes, and exposure to sunlight or ultraviolet rays for 6 hours or more when this is possible. Use chemicals only when physical measures are unavailable. Hot running water, detergents, and soapsuds may be relied upon to destroy and mechanically remove a large number of microorganisms from any object or surface.

4. TECHNIQUES TO PREVENT THE SPREAD OF DISEASE

Combating Communicable Disease by Controlling the Source. Everyone is in constant danger of contracting a communicable disease from contact with people, with animals, with insects, or with contaminated objects. Methods of controlling disease include making contact with both living and inanimate objects safe. Obviously, the former is more difficult than the latter. Tissue cells and microbes are both living protoplasm; therefore, a physical or chemical agent that is destructive to one is likely to be destructive to both. For this reason it is virtually impossible to completely disinfect the skin or mucous membrane without injuring them. Because disinfection of living human beings is so nearly impossible, the techniques used to prevent the transmission of the disease consist largely in putting up barriers between the well and the carrier of the disease—wearing masks and sterile clothing and reducing to a minimum the number of bacteria on the hands. Disinfection of inanimate objects can always be accomplished through the use of heat, light, drying, and chemical agents.

Skin Cleaning.   Of all the techniques for preventing the spread of disease, none is so important as handwashing.

Almost one hundred years ago Ignaz Semmelweis dramatically reduced puerperal fever in a Viennese hospital by merely insisting that physicians wash their hands before touching a patient. Children are taught at an early age to wash their hands after going to the toilet or before eating their meals, and all literate persons are now "germ conscious."

The practice of handwashing between contact with different patients or their belongings is expected in the pediatric, maternity, and communicable disease divisions of modern hospitals; and time is allowed for this.

A hospital that gives 3.2 hours of nursing care to general medical adult patients may give as much as 2.3 hours of nursing care to a newborn baby, 4.2 hours to the mother, and 4.7 hours to patients with communicable diseases.[10] A startling comparison between the number of times nurses washed their hands in the pediatric, maternity, and contagion units of the hospital and the general medical and surgical services was made by Blanche Pfefferkorn.[11] In the first case nurses washed their hands as often as 67 times in one day while those on the medical and surgical services in the same time period washed "only a few times."

It has been demonstrated repeatedly that those who have no symptoms of disease may have bacteria in their mouths that cause Vincent's angina, tuberculosis, pneumonia, diphtheria, or streptococci infections; also, in the intestinal tract there may be the welchii, or typhoid, bacilli, or the amebae that cause a form of dysentery. This is so well recognized that some communities require that the stools of all public food handlers be examined, to discover "carriers" of intestinal disease, and the practice of making throat cultures from all nurses assigned to maternity and pediatric divisions of hospitals is commonly observed. It is self-evident that from the standpoint of safety both to themselves and others and for esthetic considerations medical attendants should wash their hands before going from one patient to another, regardless of the diagnosis of patients. This is a time-consuming practice and it is useless to demand it without providing the personnel with physical facilities that make it possible.

Data on skin cleaning has been accumulating rapidly for many years, but studies in the past decade have been particularly numerous and fruitful. It is only possible in a text of this sort to point out what seem the most important steps leading up to present-day practice, much as one would like to cite more of the research that has contributed toward safer ways of skin cleaning.

An increased knowledge of the physiology and bacteriology of the skin has made it possible to control more effectively the epidermal flora. The acid reaction of the skin has been established and it is estimated that the average pH is 5.5.[12] It is generally conceded that normal skin tends to inhibit the growth of micro-organisms.[13] The mechanism by which skin (especially clean skin) prevents un-limited bacterial growth has not been established.[14] The "acid mantle," as it is called, varies from one part of the body to another and according to the amount of sweating. Eccrine sweat glands produce a more acid secretion than the apocrine glands. (The latter are found in the axillae, in the pubic region, and on the feet. Their secretions are particularly pungent and odoriferous. Activity of these glands is noticeable from puberty onward and decreases at the end of the child-bearing period.) Chemical analyses have so satisfactorily shown the composition of sweat that it is now given in medical dictionaries. Chemically it is like dilute urine and on decomposition it tends, like urine, to produce ammonia, which makes it alkaline and more favorable to bacterial growth. The composition varies with individuals, with the area of the body, with environmental conditions, such as heat and humidity, and with disease. It is affected by soap and other agents applied to the skin. In some skin diseases the "acid mantle" is lowered and in others it is raised, the range being, in one study, 4.5 to 9.5 pH. The tendency in diseased skin seems to be toward a less acid reaction.[15] All soaps reduce the acidity of the skin, sending it over on the alkaline side as high as 8 or 10 pH. A normal pH for the skin may be re-established in periods ranging from 15 minutes to 3 hours or more.[16] The free alkali and fatty acids released in the soap solution are believed to irritate the skin. Insoluble calcium salts, formed as the fatty acids combine with calcium in water (particularly hard water), are thought to harbor bacteria and to be a factor in skin irritation.[17]

In spite of the self-disinfecting powers of the skin, it is normal to find as many as 10,000 organisms to a square centimeter. The count is lower on the smooth surfaces and higher in the folds and under the fingernails.[18] Each person harbors his own particular flora. The majority of the organisms are not disease producing, but there are always pathogens present that will attack injured tissue. Skin organisms are divided into two classes—the resident and transient. The resident bacteria penetrate the hair follicles and sebaceous glands and, in contrast to the transient organisms, cannot be removed by any practical method of scrubbing. Philip B. Price[19] demonstrated that a 10-minute scrub would remove all transient organisms and most of the resident bacteria; it has been shown, however, that a surgeon's hand scrubbed for 10 minutes and covered with a sterile glove gives a high bacterial count at the end of a two-hour period. The deep-seated bacteria evi-dently work their way to the surface in this time. Although sweat is itself believed to be sterile, it appears to wash out the bacteria from the pits, crevices, and folds of the skin.

Carl W. Walter, citing Price's work, says that absolute sterilization of skin by scrubbing would, theoretically, take 2 hours or more. Since this is impracticable and any mechanical irritation of the skin is undesirable, it is important to foster and intensify the bacteriostatic action of normal skin. In medical asepsis it is desirable to go beyond ordinary handwashing, and a more rapid and effective means of ridding the hands of pathogenic bacteria is even more important in surgical asepsis.

Working on the assumption that the maintenance of the normal skin acidity is a factor in controlling bacterial growth and preventing irritation, detergents that do not change the pH of the skin were developed as soap substitutes, and so-called "neutral soaps" were also put on the market.

B. Thurber Guild lists nine groups of detergents (cleaning agents) as soap substitutes:

(1) Water, the greatest value of which is to aid in the detergent action of other agents; (2) substances that have an adsorbent action, such as wet corn meal and colloidal clays, or adsorbent abrasives, such as pumice and sand; (3) materials, such as liquid petrolatum, petrolatum and cosmetic creams, that partially emulsify and detach accumulated fat and soil; (4) so-called neutral soaps, that emulsify, saponify and disperse accumulated fat and soil; (5) superfatted soaps; (6) sulfated oils (commonly, but improperly, called sulfonated oils), that emulsify fats and when used with water disperse soil; (7) sulfated alcohols; (8) sulfated esters; (9) sulfonated ethers.*

The limitations of groups (1), (2), and (3) are obvious. Neutral and super-fatted soaps contain fatty acids and when mixed with water hydrolyze to give an alkaline reaction; they also react with water containing magnesium or calcium to form insoluble salts. Sulfated oils do not produce suds and have been reported as irritating and drying.[20] Sulfated alcohols and sulfated esters are effective, suds-producing detergents but they, too, are drying and irritating since they hydrolyze in water to produce sulfuric acid. Sulfonated ethers do not hydrolyze when mixed with water and can be adjusted to, and maintained at, the pH of the skin.

The detergent *pHisoderm*† meets the requirements set up by Guild for a good detergent:

(1) When worked with water it should emulsify and peptize the surface layer mixture of excreted and accumulated fats that have been adsorbed by particles of soil, so that it can be dispersed from the skin by rinsing, (2) it should not interfere with the normal functions of the skin or damage the protective layers of the epidermis, (3) the hydrolyzed product should have a pH value that corresponds to that of the average normal skin, (4) no undesirable residual layer should be deposited on the skin, (5) it should cause no discomfort and should be pleasurable to use, . . . and (6) it should produce suds.

pHisoderm is a "detergent cream composed of a sulfonated ether, petrolatum, lactic acid and wool fat cholesterols."‡ It is manufactured with more or less fat for dry and oily skins. Because it has a higher capillarity than soap (spreads more rapidly over surfaces) it penetrates pores and crevices of the skin more effectively

---

* Guild, B. Thurber: "Cutaneous Detergents: Experience with an Ether Sulfonate Compound," *Arch. Dermat. & Syph.*, **51**:391, (June) 1945.

† Winthrop-Stearns, Inc., New York.

‡ Guild, B. Thurber: *op. cit*

and cleans the skin more thoroughly. *pHisoderm* having the same pH as that of the skin does not interfere with bactericidal action; it is free from coloring matter and perfume, substances to which many persons are allergic. The constant use of this detergent is believed by most persons who have studied it to reduce skin irritation and to result in a consistently lower bacterial skin count.

Since it is impracticable, with even the best-known detergent, to remove all bacteria from the skin, the search for an "ideal skin disinfectant" continues. Methods of testing the efficiency of disinfectants have steadily improved.[21, 22] It is now possible to determine with some degree of accuracy the "degerming" power of a chemical applied to the skin and the duration of its effect. Some surgeons study the success of preparing operative sites by routinely culturing biopsies of skin from the areas of incisions. In many hospitals, cultures are made regularly of the surgeons' and nurses' hands. The accumulated data show that the use of a chemical disinfectant *in addition to* scrubbing is necessary for the best aseptic practice. Preparations of iodine have been the most widely used and reliable of skin disinfectants. The supremacy of iodine was challenged for a short period by mercuric compounds. Neither of these agents has been discarded entirely, but both have serious drawbacks. Iodine penetrates the skin and is a relatively effective disinfectant but, particularly in alcoholic solutions, is irritating to the extent of blistering the skin unless extreme care is taken. The mercuric compounds cannot be relied upon to kill microorganisms but tend to combine with protein to form a film over the wound that protects it from bacteria, just as the wound may be protected from contamination by varnishing the skin.[23] Mercuric disinfectants are mildly irritating to every user and cause a stubborn dermatitis in some persons. Chlorinated lime, which is still extensively used in sanitizing water and excreta, had a vogue in "degerming" the surgeons' hands. It was used in the form of a paste prepared with sodium bicarbonate and sodium carbonate. Even if the value were undisputed, the fact that it irritates the skin so markedly makes its use highly questionable.

Price[24] claims that 70 per cent alcohol, by weight, rubbed on the skin for 1 minute is as effective as 12 minutes of scrubbing, but concentrations above or below this figure are relatively less effective. Walter says that isopropyl alcohol can be used instead of ethyl alcohol. According to him, the dilution is not "critical," being effective in concentrations from 30 to 50 per cent. It is inexpensive, tax free, and pleasant to use.[25] Whereas the reliability of alcohol is frequently challenged, it is still widely used in preparing the skin for punctures and small incisions and, in conjunction with scrubbing, for the preparation of surgeons' hands.

A comparatively recent addition to the list of skin disinfectants are the quaternary ammonium compounds. *Roccal, Zephiran, Phemeral, and Ceepryn* are all trade names of disinfectants belonging to this group. *Roccal* is a less purified compound and is used to disinfect instruments, floors, etc.; the other preparations are more refined compounds that may be used for living tissues, as well as inanimate objects. *Zephiran* (a mixture of high molecular alkyl dimethylbenzyl ammonium chlorides) is a colorless, odorless, crystalline substance soluble in water and alcohol. It is available in aqueous solutions and in a tincture. Applied to the skin "it forms a tough invisible film which retains bacteria under it."* Unfortunately, most of the quaternary ammonium compounds react with soap, forming substances irritating to the skin, while losing some of their bacteriostatic properties. When used to "degerm" the skin, all traces of soap should first be removed. A color indicator is added to these preparations that shows the presence of an alkali on the skin.

The most recently developed skin disinfectant, _hexachlorophene_ (2,2'-methylene-bis or bis [3,5,6-trichloro-2-hydroxy-phenyl] methane), is a derivative of phenol. It is an odorless white crystalline powder soluble in alcohol, acetone, and dilute alkalis. The following characteristics make it a very desirable antiseptic. (1) It is quick acting and highly bacteriostatic to gram-positive bacteria (this includes the staphylococci, the chief among the _resident_ bacteria of the skin) and to gram-negative microorganisms in less degree. (2) It appears to penetrate and remain on the skin so that the bacteriostatic action persists. (3) It is compatible in soft, hard, and salt water with soaps and other commonly used detergents and may be combined with soaps and detergents. (4) It is said to be nonirritating locally (hypoallergenic) and relatively nontoxic internally.[26, 27, 28] Since its appearance _hexachlorophene,_ or G-11, has been widely investigated and enthusiastically endorsed by many who have studied it. In cake and liquid soaps and detergents it has been shown to reduce markedly the bacterial skin count. No harmful consequences have resulted in some institutions after two or more years of regular handwashing with these germicidal soaps, and appreciable reductions in skin infections with its use have been reported.[29] The Council on Pharmacy and Chemistry of the American Medical Association has endorsed it as a product to be used in medical practice and by the general public wherever it is desirable to maintain a low bacterial skin count.[30] (The bacteriostatic properties of _hexachlorophene_ give it deodorizing properties since bacterial action is largely responsible for the decomposition of skin excretions. Soaps containing _hexachlorophene_ are gaining popularity as aids in personal hygiene.)

The development of _pHisoderm, hexachlorophene,_ and the new _pHisoHex,†_ containing the virtues of the two, have revolutionized hand cleaning in both medical and surgical asepsis. Their daily use so markedly reduces the number of residual bacteria that it is possible to get as good results in less than half the time formerly spent in hand scrubbing. It is not likely to entirely replace other disinfectants of the operative site because a single application is not effective.

Reports of the successful clinical use of _hexachlorophene_ combined with various soaps and detergents are available from every section of this country and abroad, although Price does seem to fear undue dependence upon chemical action, and the writer has known individuals who believe _hexachlorophene_ to be the cause of skin irritation. Walter emphasizes the importance in surgery of mechanical removal of microorganisms from the skin by repeatedly scrubbing every aspect of the

---

* Walter, Carl W.: _The Aseptic Treatment of Wounds._ The Macmillan Company, New York, 1948, p. 28.
 † Winthrop-Stearns, Inc., New York.

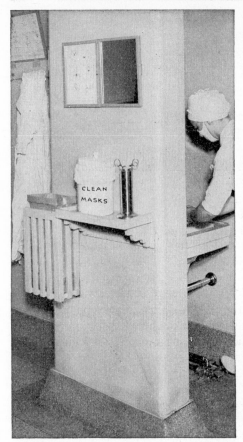
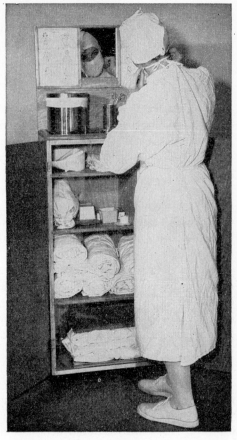

Figure 18. (*Left*) The gown-mask unit is placed next to handwashing facilities. Note graphic directions for gowning and masking and mirror for checking position of mask (two-string type of mask). The nurse is wearing glasses over the nose piece that absorbs moisture of the breath and prevents fogging of the glasses. (McNett, E. H.: "The Face Mask in Tuberculosis," *Am. J. Nursing,* **49**:32, [Jan.] 1949.)

(*Right*) Mobile isolation unit stocked with various items needed in the care of patients with tuberculosis in a general hospital. A nurse adjusting mask (conventional four-string type of surgical mask); mirror provided to facilitate correct position of mask. (Ulrich, Elizabeth: "The General Hospital as a Force in Tuberculosis Control Program: Education of Student, In-Service, and Graduate Nurses," *Transactions of the Forty-eighth Annual Meeting of the National Tuberculosis Association,* 1952.)

area with what he terms an "anatomical," rather than a timed, scrubbing. He says, however: "The disinfecting action of pHisoderm fortified with 3% G-11 is so rapid that a two-minute preoperative scrub is bacteriologically feasible."* [31]

It is generally agreed that with the use of *hexachlorophene* and a detergent that acts on *B. coli* and other gram-negative bacilli, the time period can be reduced. Recommended techniques differ in (1) the exact amount of time to be spent, (2)

* Walter, Carl W.: *op. cit.,* p. 185.

the number of strokes to be used, ③ the use of a brush and/or a file and orangewood stick, ④ the kind of brush—rubber, natural bristle, nylon bristle, and ⑤ the use of an additional chemical as a rinse after scrubbing with *hexachlorophene* and a detergent. No attempt will be made here to answer these questions with finality. It seems reasonable to continue to use a brush and orangewood stick to clean the nails when there is obvious soil under them and in preparation for surgery. The writer has concluded that they may safely be omitted from routine hand cleaning in medical asepsis. If *pHisoHex* or a soap containing *hexachlorophene* is used consistently, a low *resident* bacterial count is maintained and most of the *transient* microorganisms are removed with ordinary handwashing.

The control of the cleansing agent and water by foot levers is most desirable (see Fig. 18, *left*). Levers operated by the knees or elbows are to be preferred to faucets turned by the hand. With the latter a consistent technique must be adopted by those who use them. If they are considered contaminated they should be turned off with a clean paper square or the used paper towel; if they are considered clean they should be turned on with a clean piece of paper. Contaminated paper squares should be collected in a paper bag, preferably inside a covered container whose lid is operated with a foot lever. It is desirable that a sufficient number of autoclaved dry brushes be provided so that chemical sterilization is unnecessary. When this is not possible brushes should be kept in a nonirritating antiseptic, such as a 5 per cent *pHisoHex* solution. At best, the use of a common scrubbing brush is poor practice.

If a film of *pHisoHex* is left on the hands and arms a rinse seems unnecessary and actually undesirable, as it removes the long-acting *hexachlorophene*. For surgical skin preparation some authorities continue to recommend alcohol, *Zephiran,* or some other skin disinfectant in spite of the obvious disadvantage of removing the *hexachlorophene*.

The following procedure for the preparation of hands for surgery is recommended by the makers of *pHisoHex*. Slightly modified, this technique is advocated by a score of surgeons from various parts of the country who have studied *hexachlorophene*.

SURGICAL "SCRUB" WITH BRUSH

Suggested Procedure. *Preliminary Cleaning.* Wet hands and forearms; apply a few drops of *pHisoHex* or sufficient soap containing 3 per cent *hexachlorophene* to make a good lather. Clean under nails, which should be kept *very* short, with orangewood stick. Work lather into hands and arms, adding small amounts of water, but not enough to remove lather. At the end of 30 seconds rinse thoroughly. *Surgical "Scrub."* Apply to hands and arms 2 to 4 cc of *pHisoHex,* or soap containing *hexachlorophene*. Scrub with brush so that every area receives 15 to 30 strokes (about 2 to 4 minutes) according to the frequency with which the hands are exposed to this treatment. Use approximately twice this many strokes under the nails. Add small amounts of water frequently and use just enough detergent to maintain a lather. (Unlike soap, *pHisoHex* requires more water for more suds.) Rinse the arms and hands, but leave a thin film of *pHisoHex* on the skin. An additional disinfectant rinse is optional. In rinsing, keep the hands higher than the elbows, if possible, so that water does not run over the cleanest area from one that is less so. Dry the hands on a sterile towel moving from the hands upward. (For workers who cannot or do not wish to use *hexachlorophene* the scrubbing time should be increased to 10 minutes, and the effectiveness of the scrub may be increased with an alcohol rinse.) This same technique may be used to prepare or "degerm" the operative site if the area can be shaved 24 to 48 hours before the operation and if the cleansing process can be repeated on several successive days.[32] *Hexachlorophene* is not an effective skin disinfectant if used only once; its action is cumulative. Preparation of the patient for surgery is discussed in Chapter 38.

Gloves. Gloves are usually worn to prevent contamination of a wound by the micro-organisms on the hands of the attendant; or to prevent the contamination of the nurse's or surgeon's hands by discharges from a wound. They are also used to protect the physician in vaginal and rectal examinations and to lesson the hazard for any worker who is handling grossly infected areas of the skin or mucous membrane and danger-ously contaminated equipment.

1. *Suggested Procedure in Medical Asepsis.* Except when handling a wound post-operatively or the vaginal tract of an obstetrical patient, clean gloves are adequate and no special precautions need be taken in adjusting them other than to have the hands clean. Remove the gloves by grasping the cuff. If grossly soiled soak them in a disin-fectant before washing and sterilizing them, or wash them with gloved hands; or, better still, wash the gloves under running water before taking them off.

2. *Suggested Procedure in Surgical Asepsis.* Open the package of sterile gloves before washing or scrubbing the hands unless the operator has an assistant. The hands should be scrubbed if the worker is participating in a long-drawn-out or major surgical pro-cedure; for treatments, such as catheterization of the bladder, when there is no necessity for handling objects that come in contact with wounded tissues, it is only necessary to wash the hands in the ordinary manner. In any case sterile powder, put up with the gloves, is applied to the properly prepared hands. The first glove is drawn on by the inside of the glove cuff; the second, by placing the gloved hand under the cuff. The cuffs are turned up by manipulating only the sterile surface of the glove and not that which has come in contact with the hand. If a sterile gown is worn, it should be put on before the gloves, in order that the glove cuffs may be drawn up over its sleeves.

Use of Gowns. It has been pointed out that in the care of many communicable conditions it is essential to protect the clothing of medical workers by the use of a gown. Visitors to patients are also required to wear gowns. The type of gown most generally approved is one that entirely covers the wearer's clothing. It is wide enough to lap or be folded over in the back; it has tight cuffs on either long or short sleeves, is belted, and is of a closely woven, fairly heavy material like cotton twill. The simplest and most satisfactory technique is to have the wearer put on a clean gown each time, remove it, and place it in a canvas bag in which it is autoclaved before being worn again. When soiled, the gown is placed in a bag that is taken to the laundry, where the contents are carefully handled and sterilized in the laundering process. This is called the *discard technique* and is becoming more and more popular.

If it is impossible to supply the hospital or clinic with a sufficient number of gowns to allow for this practice, one gown is kept at the entrance of the patient's room or cubicle and as each medical worker enters he or she puts on the gown if the service required by the patient is such that the clothing is likely to become contaminated. This system necessitates putting on and taking off the gown in a way that will keep the inside clean and the surface of the gown near the fasteners as clean as possible; the manner in which this is attempted is shown in Figures 19 and 20.

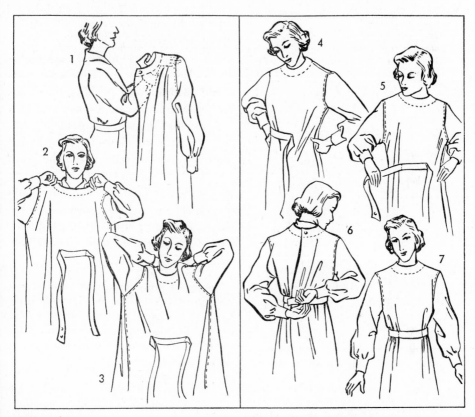

Figure 19. Putting on a gown in medical asepsis: (*1*) getting the hands and arms into the sleeves, touching only the inside of the gown; (*2*) drawing the neck of the garment into place, touching only the inside of the gown; (*3*) fastening the gown at the back; (*4, 5,* and *6*) lapping the back edges of the gown, drawing the belt ends into place and fastening them while the lapped edges are held in position; (*7*) the gown with back and belt fastened.

In order to make this technique even reasonably safe, it must be practiced in the same way by every one who uses the gown. Because of the probable difference in size, two gowns are usually kept for each patient—one for nurses and one for physicians. If small, medium, and large gowns are of different colors they are more easily differentiated. Philip Stimson[33] and other authorities condemn the prac‑ tice of wearing the same gown when caring for a group of patients with the same communicable condition. In the case of scarlet fever a dozen or more types of *Streptococcus pyogenes* may cause the characteristic symptoms, and cross infections among a group of such patients may lead to complications.[34] The so-called *group technique* is questionable in the care of patients with almost any one of the communicable diseases.

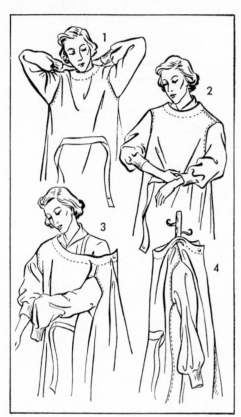

In surgical asepsis sterile gowns are used to protect the patient from the surgeon's and nurse's clothing. The design of the gown is very similar to that used in medical aseptic technique except that it always has long sleeves. The sterile gown is unfolded and put on after the hands are scrubbed, and care is taken to hold it high so that no portion of the outside surface is contaminated. The wearer must have an assistant fasten the gown and the belt ends in the back since the hands might be contaminated (surgically) in this process. In surgical cases the gowns are never used again until they have been laundered and sterilized by steam under pressure.

Suggested Procedure. In medical asepsis, *use a fresh gown each time,* or the *discard technique.* Equip each unit with a laundry bag in which to place contaminated gowns. (This bag may be kept just outside the unit in the corridor in order that the bags may be collected at any time by porters and sent to be autoclaved.) Provide another laundry bag for soiled gowns that require laundering. These two laundry bags should be of different colors so as to avoid mistakes. Keep an ample supply of gowns in a workroom convenient to the patient's unit. In one hospital where this technique is employed, it is estimated that if the gowns are collected and sterilized every 12 hours approximately 25 gowns will be required for each acutely ill patient having general nursing service; fewer gowns will be needed for convalescent patients. The gown should be put on before the worker's hands are contaminated; the sleeves of the uniform should be short or rolled above the elbow. If the discard technique is used, no special precautions need be observed in adjusting the gown except to see that it covers the clothing. A short-sleeved gown with a knitted cuff that comes just below the elbow is recommended; the belt

Figure 20. Removing a gown in medical asepsis: (*1*) unfastening the neck of the gown after washing the hands; (*2*) drawing off the first sleeve by slipping the finger under the cuff; (*3*) drawing the second sleeve off by grasping it through the first sleeve; (*4*) the gown hung on a standard with the shoulder seams together and only the contaminated outer surface exposed.

should be short enough to prevent the ends from touching the floor while the gown is adjusted. Snap fasteners are desirable because they may be opened without the fumbling at the neck that is often seen if tapes are used. The gown is removed by touching the outside surface only; it is then placed in the proper bag, and the wearer washes hands and arms as described under the technique for handwashing in medical asepsis.

The method in which the gown is worn repeatedly is much more complicated than the one just described because certain parts of the gown must be kept uncontaminated. A suggested method is illustrated in Figures 19 and 20. Surfaces of the gown will be referred to as contaminated and uncontaminated, but they are only relatively so. It is obvious that this method is much less safe than the discard method. It is the method, however, which must be used in homes and institutions where autoclaving facilities are not available.

Provide a standard on which to hang the gown inside the entrance of the patient's unit. Put on the gown with clean hands, touching only the inside of the gown. Fasten the neck at the back; put the back edges of the gown together and fold them over or lap the two sides. Fasten the belt and adjust the cuffs of the sleeves.

Controlling Air-borne Microorganisms. Alexander D. Langmuir, discussing "air-borne infection" in Maxcy's text, summarizes the changing attitudes toward controlling communicable disease by reduction in air bacteria, as follows:*

PERIOD	APPROXIMATE DATES	ATTITUDE TOWARD AIR-BORNE INFECTION	PREDOMINANT IDEAS
1	Prior to c. 1890	Popular	Miasma and malaria
2	c. 1890 to c. 1934	Apathy	Contact and droplet infection
3	c. 1934 to c. 1945	Expectation	Droplet nuclei and dust infection
4	c. 1945 to c. 1950	Disappointment	Failure of practical applications
5	Present	Guarded concern	Tuberculosis, laboratory infections, biological warfare

Microfilms have demonstrated that in coughing and sneezing a person discharges thousands of moist particles. These particles, or droplets, contain bacteria present in the respiratory passages. It has been repeatedly demonstrated that these particles dry out and leave microorganisms suspended in room air.[35] The bacterial air count rises in proportion to room occupancy. Dust particles, likewise, carry bacteria on them. Outdoors in city streets the air bacteria decrease from the ground upward. Sweeping, dusting, and bedmaking increase the number of organisms in room air. Techniques used to control air-borne microorganisms consist, therefore, in: (1) replacing contaminated air with fresh air by natural or artificial ventilation, (2) suppressing dust by oiling floors and bedding, and (3) killing organisms in the air by ultraviolet irradiation or disinfectant vapors.

Ventilation has played a large part in medical asepsis, particularly in recent years. The action of sunlight has been relied upon to disinfect contaminated mattresses and other large pieces of equipment. Rooms occupied by patients with

* Maxcy, Kenneth F. (ed.): *Rosenau's Preventive Medicine and Hygiene,* 7th ed. Appleton-Century-Crofts, Inc., New York, 1951, p. 154.

measles, mumps, etc., have been terminally disinfected by airing them and washing floors and furniture with soap and water. Air conditioning has been used to reduce the bacterial count in nurseries and operating rooms. Both natural and artificial ventilation can be effective in reducing the hazard of contaminated air; neither is entirely satisfactory since the rapid circulation of air creates unpleasant drafts and heating problems. When the air of occupied rooms is grossly contaminated, ventilating methods are usually reinforced by other methods of control.

Methods of suppressing dust have been described by Clayton G. Loosli[36] and other workers, the process having had wide usage in military hospitals and barracks during World War II. An emulsion of paraffin oil and a neutral detergent, such as *Triton NE,* is used to mop floors daily; saturating unvarnished floors with oil will suppress dust for several months. Painted or waxed floors, that would be injured by daily oiling, may be swept with an oiled sawdust compound. The stable oil emulsion with *Triton NE* is added to the rinsing water of blankets and other bedding in a concentration of 2 per cent by weight. This is said not to affect the appearance or feel of the material, and the dust-holding property is maintained for months by woolens even though they are washed repeatedly. Cotton fabrics must be treated more frequently.

Irradiation with ultraviolet requires expensive installation of equipment and the supervision of experts. Because bactericidal intensities of radiation are injurious to the skin, and particularly the conjunctiva of the eye, the lamps must be placed above eye level and special paint may be necessary to prevent reflection of the rays from the ceiling. In school buildings the radiation is sometimes operated at night only, when the rooms are vacant. The danger of using irradiation throughout an occupied room and the fact that the rays are not believed to penetrate bacteria embedded in suspended dust particles pose difficult problems. However, it has been demonstrated repeatedly that ultraviolet rays will bring about a 50 to 75 per cent reduction in the bacterial air count under controlled conditions.[37] Mildred W. Wells and William A. Holla[38] report that in two nearby and comparable towns, with similar school facilities and populations, the incidence of measles and chickenpox was 321 in the community where all places in which children congregate were treated with ultraviolet rays and 526 in the control town. They believe that a greater reduction might have been accomplished if the irradiated community had been surrounded by a protected zone. Reports such as this suggest that when methods are improved and financial support is available, air-borne infections can be substantially reduced with irradiation. It does not seem appropriate in a text of this sort to recommend a procedure. Nurses, as well as all health workers, should, however, be alert to, and further the development of, this promising agent.

Disinfecting Vapors.   In room air with a humidity ranging from around 20 to 50 per cent it is possible to get a high enough concentration of certain vaporized chemicals to penetrate and destroy an appreciable number of dust-borne particles in the air. It is thought that dried bacteria and those embedded in large dust particles are not affected by the vapors. Under favorable conditions of humidity and concentration, bacterial counts have been as successfully reduced in room air with the disinfectant vapors as with irradiation. They have the advantage over irradiation of penetrating every aspect of the room. Some of the chemicals used are the glycols, the halogens, hypochlorites, hexylresorcinol, lactic, and other hydroxy acids.[39] Commercial vaporizers are available. Many of them fail, however, to provide an effective concentration. It has been recommended that a slight but noticeable fog be maintained.[40]

While there is considerable hope that the use of bactericidal vapors may help to control air-borne infections, their use has not met with unqualified success. Saul Krugman and Robert Ward,[41] for example, were not able to achieve a reduction in respiratory cross infections in an infants' ward of a large hospital through the use of a triethylene vapor and dust-suppressive measures. It is possible that no methods of reducing air bacteria will greatly affect the incidence of disease in situations where the disease may be readily transmitted by direct and indirect contact.

Masks. A microphotograph shows only too clearly that thousands of moist particles are discharged from the nose and mouth in sneezing. Coughing and, to a lesser extent, laughing and breathing send droplets into the air. When a person has a communicable disease that may be transmitted through the respiratory passages, those who go near him may reduce the danger by putting up a barrier that will filter the air. At the present time the best-known barrier is a mask that will act as a filter. The mask may be worn by the patient, but in most cases it is more practical to mask the attendant or visitor. In surgical procedures where the object of masking is to protect the wound of the patient from contamination by droplets from the surgical team, the workers are masked.

The most effective mask that has been devised is close fitting, covering the nose and mouth. It is made of six layers of gauze with 42×42 threads to the square inch.[42, 43, 44] A piece of Canton flannel, substituted for four layers of gauze, is believed by some authorities to make an equally efficient mask. Washing reduces the space between the threads of these fabrics and therefore increases the value of the mask as a filter. When the mask offers *too much* resistance, the wearer is forced to rebreathe the warm air he has just expired, and great discomfort may result; there is a limit, therefore, beyond which it is unsafe to go in closing the spaces between the fibers of the mask.

Masks should fit the face closely to prevent the escape of air around them. Pliable metal strips may be run in a casing at the top of the mask so that it can be molded over the bridge of the nose.

Another comfortable but less close-fitting mask (Fig. 18, *left*) is made with the threads of the material running diagonally across the face and is held with one set of ties. Worn "on the bias" the mask has more give over the nose, and so the wearer feels less restricted. E. H. McNett designed this mask to be worn in medical asepsis. Walter advocates the mask made with a double set of ties for surgery.

It is still common to see masks pocketed by medical workers and worn a second or third time. This practice must be condemned. It is impossible to prevent contamination of the mask's clean surfaces, and the mask is progressively less effective as it is worn. A very large number of laundered (sanitized) masks must be available to workers, and they must be handled so that the clean masks are not contaminated and used masks not allowed to contaminate clean surfaces. "Expendable" masks would save time in handling and cost of laundering; so far,

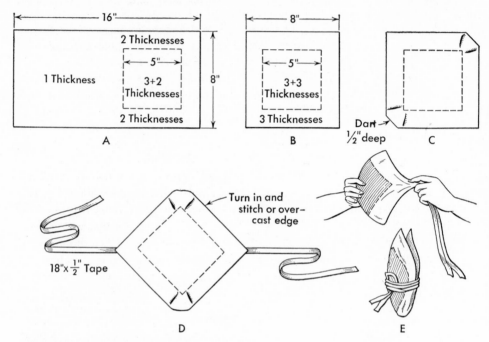

Figure 21.   Directions for making a face mask.

Material: Gauze, 42 × 42 threads per square inch (thread count *important*).

Pattern: Two straight pieces of gauze cut lengthwise; 8 in. × 24 in. and 5 in. × 15 in. (measurements must be *accurate*).

Procedure: (*A*) 8-in. × 24-in. gauze folded to make 8 in. × 16 in. Superimpose a 5-in. × 15-in. gauze, folded three times, and stitch in place. (*B*) Lap over one section; over-all size now 8 in. × 8 in. (*C*) Fold back diagonal corners as shown; sew in place. Make two darts each side. (*D*) Attach tapes (½ in. × 18 in.) to other corners. (*E*) Mask has been folded, prior to autoclaving.

(McNett, E. H.: "The Face Mask in Tuberculosis," *Am. J. Nursing,* **49:**32, [Jan.] 1949.)

no efficient mask has been designed at a low enough cost to make discarding after a single use economical.

Paper and cellulose film masks have been designed with low cost and transparency to recommend them. Desirable as are both of these attributes, the fact that they deflect, rather than filter, the air makes them virtually worthless as a protection to the wearer. It is possible that a low-cost, close-fitting paper mask designed to filter the air will eventually be produced. It is difficult to see how an efficient mask can be made transparent.

Suggested Procedure. (1) *In medical asepsis:* Keep clean masks in a suitable container in the clean area of a workroom near handwashing facilities. Take a mask from the supply with clean hands and adjust it before going into the contaminated area. When leaving the contaminated area, remove the gown, if one has been worn; wash the hands; *then* remove the mask, handling it by the strings. Place the used mask in a special laundry bag kept in a covered container, operated by a foot lever if possible. Another hand cleaning still further reduces the danger of transferring organisms from the mask to clean surfaces. Soiled masks should be transported and laundered by workers trained to protect themselves and others from contamination. (2) *In surgical asepsis:* Adjust the clean mask with clean hands, but before scrubbing the hands and putting on the gown. If a cap is worn, adjust that before putting on the mask. As worn in surgery, masks may be removed whenever the wounded area is protected by a dressing. Used masks are always contaminated by the wearer and should be treated as described under medical asepsis.

Aseptic Disposal of Discharges.   For esthetic reasons, as well as to prevent the possible transfer of disease organisms, body discharges from both sick and well persons are handled in an aseptic manner. Because the collection and disposal or disinfection of excreta are, or should be, carried out about the same way in all cases, the subject was discussed in Chapter 5. When there is a known communicable disease, even greater care should be taken to see that the suggested sanitary procedures are followed.

Aseptic Handling of Food Waste.   Collection and disposal of garbage also was treated in Chapter 5. The point was made that food or waste should be specially handled if it is believed to be contaminated by microorganisms that cause intestinal diseases. In communities where no provision is made for disinfection of the sewage, liquid waste should be disinfected with calcium chloride (lime) or some other suitable chemical before it is placed in the hopper; boiling may also be employed to kill the pathogenic microbes. Solid waste must be collected in waxed-paper bags, cartons, or newspaper containers, and then burned.

Cleaning and Disinfecting Dishes.   Any person or group of persons that serves the public is responsible for cleaning dishes and silverware so that they are comparatively free from pathogenic organisms. This is a problem of general sanitation rather than one confined to the care of the sick. Each hospital division, like any restaurant, should provide facilities for sanitizing dishes. Although there is much less danger of contracting communicable conditions in family groups an effective method of cleaning dishes should nevertheless be used, and if there is a known communicable disease in the house special precautions should be observed.

W. L. Mallman and David Kahler[45] after studying a variety of methods of dishwashing in food-handling establishments concluded that dishes should be (1) prewashed, (2) submerged in a detergent and water of 78° C (172.4° F) for at least 30 seconds, and (3) subjected to a double rinsing. They pointed out that if soiled dishes are put directly into the washing or sanitizing chamber much of the detergent combines with the organic matter and is lost as a cleansing agent. A dishwasher should be chosen that provides a prewashing period. Mallman and Kahler recommend placing ahead of the dishwasher a separate device known as a _"Salvajor"_ which combines "water scrapping" and soil collection. In situations where water of 78° C (172.4° F) is not available "chemical sanitizers" will give good results if the tanks, brushes, etc., are kept clean and if the method is carefully worked out. Chlorine preparations and quaternary ammonium compounds are often used for dishes, but they are not compatible with detergents. When chemical disinfection or sanitization of dishes must be resorted to, a substance that is not inactivated by detergents, such as _hexachlorophene_ or _diphenyl,_ should be used. Needless to say, odorless disinfectants should be selected, but in any event the dishes should be thoroughly rinsed with clear water after exposure to a chemical.

The sanitary codes in most communities require treatment of dishes similar to that recommended by Mallman and Kahler, although prewashing is not given so much emphasis. A low bacterial count for dishes is tolerated; no regulations insist upon disinfecting procedures that result in sterilized tableware. It is possible, however, by doubling or tripling the period of exposure to very hot water and detergents, to kill virtually all vegetative pathogens. (This is an objective in some communicable disease units.) Likewise, 1 to 2 hours of exposure to effective chemical agents will also reduce to a minimum the hazard of contaminated dishes.

Suggested Procedure. Have a clear understanding of what surfaces in the kitchen are to be considered clean and what contaminated; if possible, mark them so that there can be no doubt about it. In a hospital the contaminated areas are usually the inside of one sink and perhaps the shelf around it, a conveyor or rolling table for contaminated dishes, the inside of the garbage pail, and that part of the dishwasher in which contaminated dishes are placed. All other surfaces are kept clean. When such facilities are available, the following technique may be adopted: Bring the tray and dishes used by the patient into the kitchen, either in the hands or on the conveyor. Empty the dishes of liquid and solid waste, collecting this for immediate disinfection or destruction, as described. Place the dishes, utensils, and tray in the "scrapper" and prewasher or the dishwashing machine. Place soiled linen in the laundry container provided, or if paper substitutes are used place them in the waste container. Wash the conveyor or rolling table and allow it to air until the next meal. W. C. Cox[46] recommends an automatic control of machinery for dishwashing to ensure time periods of adequate duration. If dishwashing machines are not available or have been found to be ineffective, regular boiling-water utensil sterilizers may be used. They should be provided with a grease trap to prevent clogging of the sewerage system. In homes and in some institutions large covered vessels are used for boiling dishes and silverware.

The following technique is suggested for the home: Remove the food left on the dishes, using moistureproof containers for the collection of waste (such containers are kept just outside the room). Carry the dishes and silverware to the kitchen on a small tray and immediately place all of these in a pan of cool water containing soap or other detergent. (Protect the table with four thicknesses of newspaper if it is necessary to put the dishes on a table before placing them in the pan.) Remove them from this prewashing vessel to a second, having a cool detergent in it. Cover both vessels and allow the water to come to a boil, then boil vigorously for five minutes. Remove the decontaminated dishes and wash clean with soap and water in an uncontaminated pan or sink. The detergent, or soap, solution in both pans can be safely poured down the drain after this boiling period.

Distributing Trays to Patients.   In hospitals the same carts should not be employed for conveying clean and used trays unless the shelves are protected with paper. The distribution of clean trays may be accomplished without contaminating the worker if the patient and the furnishings of the unit are prepared in advance for the meal and if the patient is able to feed himself.

Disinfecting Bed Linen, Clothing, and Woolen and Silk Fabrics.   From the discussion of asepsis up to this point it must be clear that modern laundering processes in hospitals disinfect fabrics contaminated with microorganisms in vegetative forms. Therefore, washable articles may be collected in bags and sent to the laundry, care being taken to avoid contamination of the outside of the bag. The laundry operators who handle the contaminated linen may be protected with gowns, gloves, and masks. Clothing and bed linen used by persons with infections caused by spore-forming organisms (tetanus and gas gangrene bacilli) are sterilized by steam under pressure before being sent to the laundry.

In homes, contaminated linen is collected in a large covered kettle of cold soapy water, which is then placed on the stove; the contents are brought to a boil, and boiling continued for 5 minutes; at the end of this time the soiled linen is safe for handling. If pathogenic spore forms are known to be present, the boiling period should be extended to 1 hour or more. In such a case the safest procedure is to leave the linen in the container for 3 days and boil it each day, although this requires a large supply of linen and several kettles.

Textiles that are destroyed by moisture and heat can be made safe for future use by exposing all the surfaces to the sunlight for 6 hours. The dry-cleaning process is disinfecting to some extent, but articles used by persons with communicable diseases should not be sent to a cleaning establishment before they are disinfected in some other way.

There seems to be no reason for stripping bare the room in which a patient is sick with a communicable disease. Curtains and rugs should be considered contaminated if the patient was taken ill in the room, and these furnishings may just as well be left there to make the surroundings cheerful until the termination of the illness. Disinfecting vapors, laundering, sunning, boiling, autoclaving, and other appropriate and economical methods of decontaminating the contents of the room should then be used.

Disinfecting Mattresses and Pillows.   In some of the most trusted communicable disease hospitals, sunlight and air are employed in disinfecting pillows and mattresses. If large autoclaves are available for this purpose, they also are used. Hot-air sterilizers are not desirable because dry heat, which is sufficiently intense to kill the organisms in a reasonable length of time, is very destructive to the articles themselves.

Disinfecting Walls, Floors, and Furniture.   Washing the surfaces with a detergent and water and airing for about 12 hours are considered a satisfactory method of making safe for occupancy any room that has been used by a person with a communicable disease. An odorless diphenol, such as *diphenyl,* added to the detergent increases the bactericidal effect. *Roccal,* a quaternary ammonium compound, less refined than *Zephiran,* is used for furniture and floors. It is less compatible, however, with detergents than the phenol derivatives. If the walls are papered, airing the room for several days is believed to be adequate treatment. Since most vegetative forms of bacteria die readily in a dry environment, it is not likely that they will survive for any length of time on walls unless they are embedded in excreta or other kinds of moist organic material.

Floors are always considered a contaminated area in any part of a hospital or in a home. Because the shoe soles are constantly exposed to bacteria-laden dust, everyone should be wary of handling anything that comes in contact with floors. Babies' toys should be tied to their cribs to keep them from falling on the floor, and anything that is accidentally dropped should be disinfected before it is used again. In order to keep floors as clean as possible, mop heads that can be laundered should be used.

Books and Papers.   There is no satisfactory method for disinfecting books. Moisture and high temperatures are destructive to them, and it is difficult to expose all the leaves to sunlight, other sources of ultraviolet rays, and disinfectant vapors. When the patient has a highly communicable disease it is usual to limit the patient's reading to magazines or material that can be burned without distress to the owner. Speaking of books and furniture, however, Gaylord W. Anderson and Margaret G. Arnstein say: "Fortunately such articles require little if any treatment for their role in the spread of disease is insignificant if not actually nonexistent."*

Contaminated letters, if written in pencil, may be autoclaved. They may be safely handled if all sides are exposed to sunlight and air for 6 hours or more. To avoid the necessity of disinfecting books and letters, the nurse, or a member of the family, may read aloud and write letters in the room at a safe distance from the patient.

It is often necessary for a person with a communicable disease to sign an agreement or legal document of some kind. In this case the document is placed on a clean paper towel with another towel covering the part on which the patient's hand will rest. (See Fig. 22.) After the signature is affixed, the nurse, whose hands are not contaminated, removes the paper from between the towels and takes it from the room.

Enameled Ware, Stainless-steel Articles, and Glassware.   All contaminated basins, cans, mugs, and similar articles should be disinfected before they are stored or used for other patients. Exposure to boiling water is the preferred and most universally available method. Unless there is some reason to attempt spore destruction, a 15-minute boiling period is adequate. In preparing equipment to be used for surgical procedures, the time should be extended to 60 minutes. It cannot be

* Anderson, Gaylord W., and Arnstein, Margaret G.: *Communicable Disease Control,* 3rd ed. The Macmillan Company, New York, 1953, p. 53.

said too often that boiling water will not kill spores in any practicable length of time; steam under pressure should always be used in sterilizing surgical equipment. Soiled articles should be washed first in a sink, the basin of which is considered contaminated and is never used for clean articles. In communities where the sewage is not disinfected, if basin and drinking mugs have been used by patients with typhoid fever or dysentery, care should be taken to empty the contents of the vessels into a container of chloride of lime and then immediately disinfect the article before attempting to wash it clean.

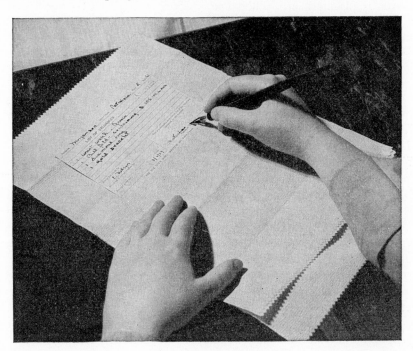

Figure 22. Patient signing a paper in medical asepsis. Contact between the paper and the patient, who has a communicable disease, is prevented by the use of paper towels.

In situations when boiling water is not available, a chemical disinfectant may be substituted.

Rubber Articles. It has been definitely established that heat and light and certain chemicals, especially mineral oil, are destructive to rubber. For this reason the sterilization of rubber by heat and sunlight should be reduced to a minimum. Draw sheets, treatment sheets, and hot-water bottles—all of which a patient uses more or less frequently—should be kept in his unit in order to avoid unnecessary concurrent disinfection. The practice of boiling articles for 15 minutes should be followed in disinfecting rubber tubing, bulb syringes, and similar articles, unless they are to be used in a surgical procedure in which case sterilization by steam under pressure is indicated. Methods of decontaminating and sterilizing rubber goods are discussed in Chapter 8. Rubber sheeting may be soaked in a chemical disinfectant or washed with a detergent and exposed to sunlight. The same precautions should be taken here as with other used and soiled equipment so as to avoid contaminating surfaces in workrooms that are supposed to be clean.

Instruments.   There are certain instruments (such as those for measuring blood pressure) that are destroyed or injured by heat. Articles of this class should be washed with a detergent and aired. Wiping with 70 per cent alcohol still further reduces contamination. To prevent the necessity for disinfection, a watch may be kept clean by placing it in a cellophane envelope (see Fig. 48) or holding it in a piece of paper and after use sliding it on to an uncontaminated surface in the room. The decontamination, sterilization, and care of instruments are given detailed attention in Chapter 8.

5. OPERATION OF STERILIZERS

Boiling-water Sterilizers.   Boiling-water sterilizers are metal tanks connected with the water supply and furnished with a gas, electric, or steam heating unit. The latter is more commonly used and is very satisfactory because it heats the water rapidly. The tank is furnished with a drain pipe that has a filter at its entrance. This device prevents clogging of the pipes by large objects, but care must be taken to keep the tank free from grease and dirt of all kinds. A sterilizer that is used constantly should be cleaned on the inside two or three times a day.

Water in the sterilizing chamber reaches boiling point, 100° C (212° F), in varying lengths of time, according to the temperature of the water introduced and the efficiency of the heating unit. Boiling water makes a characteristic sound, gives off vapor, and shows marked agitation at the surface. The writer has found, however, that all these signs are present before the water reaches the maximal temperature. The temperature of the water is lowered by placing cooler objects in the sterilizer. It is, therefore, a safeguard to have a self-recording thermometer attached to the sterilizer so that boiling periods can be accurately determined. This is especially desirable in surgical asepsis where sterility rather than decontamination of the object is the aim.

Nothing varies more in aseptic practice than the boiling period used in "sanitization," disinfection or sterilization as that process is described by different persons. Walter says:

> The safe minimum period for sterilization in boiling water at altitudes less than 300 meters is thirty minutes at 100°C for vegetative organisms. If the hydrogen-ion concentration is decreased by the addition of alkali, the period of exposure can be safely decreased to fifteen minutes. The fifteen-minute period is adequate for the destruction of certain spores, provided the pH is carefully controlled. At higher altitudes, the sterilizing periods must be increased. Boiling water is an inadequate germicide for preoperative sterilization and should not be used where steam is available.[*]

The findings of Esty and Meyer and many others back up such a recommendation; in practice a lower standard is commonly accepted. Contaminated dishes

* Walter, Carl W.: *op. cit.,* p. 53.

and bed linen are considered reasonably safe if treated with lower temperatures for briefer periods. Apparently, it is not thought necessary or practicable to enforce methods in *medical asepsis* that free equipment and supplies from all vegetative organisms. Fortunately, the majority of bacteria are destroyed at temperatures below the boiling point and few survive the first few minutes of boiling. Whenever it is possible, however, the boiling period should be extended to 15 to 30 minutes as advocated by Walter.

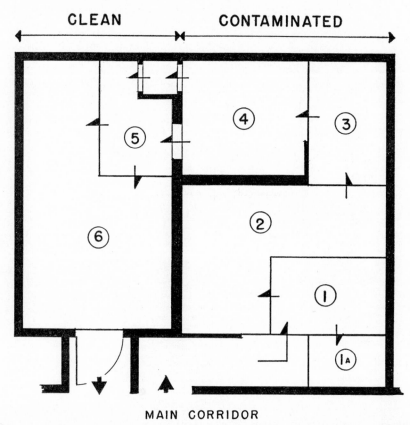

CLEAN   CONTAMINATED

MAIN CORRIDOR

Figure 23. Diagrammatic plan of a utility room. Arrows indicate direction of flow of equipment and materials: (*1*) collection for cleaning and disposal here; (*1A*) subcollection for cleaning and disposal elsewhere; (*2*) cleaning and disposal; (*3*) assembly for sterilizing; (*4*) sterilizing; (*5*) assembly for storage; and (*6*) storage and work. (Diagram by Jesse Orrick.)

All articles in the sterilizing chamber should be submerged. It may be necessary to weight certain pieces of equipment and to prevent trapping of air in tubing and bulbs.

The addition of sodium carbonate to make a 2 per cent solution, or sodium hydroxide to make a 0.1 per cent solution, is recommended to reduce the hydrogen ion concentration. A water softener, the nature of which is determined by the minerals in the water in each locality, should be added.

It is most logical to place boiling-water sterilizers in the workroom to which used equipment is taken for cleaning; or that portion of the room that is set aside for handling contaminated equipment. There should be a shelf beside the sterilizer that extends into the clean area. If the clean and contaminated areas are divided by a wall, or partition, an opening should be cut so that equipment,

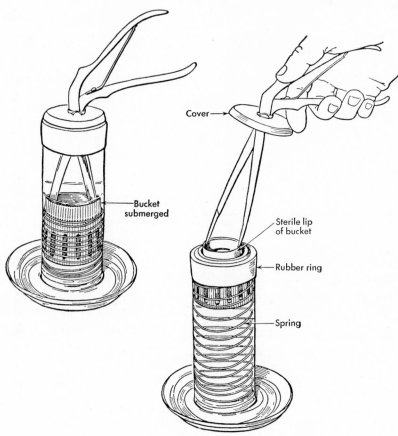

Figure 24. A safe transfer forceps. (Walter, Carl W.: *The Aseptic Treatment of Wounds.* The Macmillan Company, New York, 1948.)

as it is taken from the sterilizer can be passed directly into the clean area. (See Fig. 23.)

At least two sizes of boiling-water sterilizers should be available in each work-, utility, or treatment room; one for small objects, such as instruments, and the other large enough to accommodate the biggest pieces of equipment, such as treatment trays and foot tubs. There should be a common understanding about the type of article to be sterilized. When funds are available, every hospital division should be provided with an additional utensil sterilizer for bedpans, urinals, douche and enema apparatus. While it may be bacteriologically safe to sterilize all types of equipment in one chamber it is very unpleasant to think of cans for throat irrigations and drinking mugs coming in close contact with articles such as those just mentioned.

When large boilers or cooking utensils are substituted for boiling-water sterilizers the same rules of operation should be observed, although it is not possible to equip them with self-registering thermometers.

Sterile handling forceps, or transfer forceps, must be ready and nearby for the removal of objects from the sterilizer. Figure 24 shows a type recommended by Walter. The container and disinfecting solution in which the forceps rest are protected from air contamination by a lid attached to the forceps. A disinfectant should be chosen that is not irritating since a trace may be left on the object handled by the forceps. Ethyl propyl alcohol, 70 per cent by weight, or the more economical 50 per cent isopropyl alcohol is satisfactory. Potassium dichromate (one part to a thousand parts of alcohol) or sodium bicarbonate (one part to a hundred parts of alcohol) inhibits rust. According to Frank N. Speller[47] such electrolytes encourage the formation of a protective adherent film over the surface of the instrument. Forceps and containers should be boiled daily and the solution replenished.

Boiling-water sterilizers require frequent cleaning. Objects, such as rubber, that tend to leave scum in the tank should be wrapped in gauze before they are put in the sterilizer.

Streaming Steam Sterilizer. If steam is generated or held in a chamber under atmospheric pressure, it is said to be *streaming* or *free flowing,* and its temperature is that of boiling water, 100° C (212° F) at sea level. For the same unit of time this type of sterilizer is not as effective as boiling water, but for some materials, such as bottled liquids, it is practicable, whereas boiling water is not. Some bedpan sterilizers (so-called) and dish sterilizers operate with streaming steam. They cannot be relied upon to completely sterilize unless there is protracted and repeated exposure to the steam. Fortunately, diseases that may be transmitted by contaminated dishes and bedpans are, for the most part, caused by organisms that are readily killed by moist heat, so that dishes, for example, that have been thoroughly washed and then exposed to streaming steam are reasonably free from pathogenic organisms. If in laboratories streaming steam is depended upon for the sterilization of media, 1-hour periods repeated every 24 hours for 3 days are used. The first period kills the vegetative forms and encourages spores to germinate, or change into the vegetative stage, so that in the second and third heating periods all organisms may be killed. This method is less certain, however, than steam under pressure, and is rarely used if autoclaving facilities are available. Because any large kettle—for instance, a wash boiler—can be converted into a streaming-steam sterilizer, it is practicable in any rural situation and therefore of interest to nurses as a means of preparing certain types of surgical equipment in home nursing. A single exposure to superheated steam in a pressure cooker is, however, more effective.

Steam-pressure Sterilizers.   Autoclave is the name given to a sterilizer that utilizes saturated steam under pressure; "saturated" means that the steam exerts the maximum pressure for water vapor at the given temperature. Steam can be produced with a gas or electric heating unit or it may be delivered to the sterilizer through pipes from a central plant in the building. The latter system is ordinarily found in hospitals and is generally preferred. The sterilizing chamber is surrounded by an outer jacket into which the steam is first introduced. As steam enters the jacket it forces the air out, or should do so if the mechanism is properly

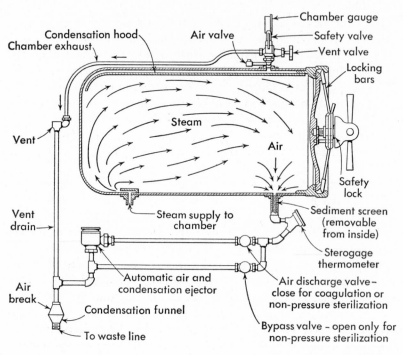

Figure 25A. Autoclave, single shell type. Diagram of a steam-pressure sterilizer showing the way in which steam enters the jacket and the sterilizing chamber and forces the air out. (Courtesy of Wilmot Castle Co., Rochester, N. Y.)

constructed and correctly operated. Steam is allowed to flow into the tightly closed outer jacket until the desired temperature is reached. At this point the steam is turned into the sterilizing chamber that has been packed with materials to be sterilized. The air from this chamber is forced out through valves opening outward as the steam under pressure rushes in. A supply of steam is kept flowing into the inner chamber until the desired temperature is obtained. (See Fig. 25A.)

Both the outer jacket and the inner chamber are equipped with pressure indicators; the inner jacket should be further equipped with a self-recording thermometer (see Fig. 25B). A pressure gauge was believed at one time to be the only indicator needed because the temperature should rise proportionately to the steam pressure. T. B. Magath,[48] McCulloch,[49] Walter,[50] and others have called attention to errors that may occur if the rise in pressure alone is used as an index of conditions in the sterilizing chamber. A rise in pressure may be due to compressed steam within a closed chamber, but it also may be caused by compressed air (or a mixture of the two); whereas a rise in temperature is the result of steam pressure only. Everyone who operates an autoclave should understand that it is the high temperature of compressed steam rather than the pressure effect that kills living protoplasm. In fact, the pressure gauge could be dispensed with if there is a safety valve on

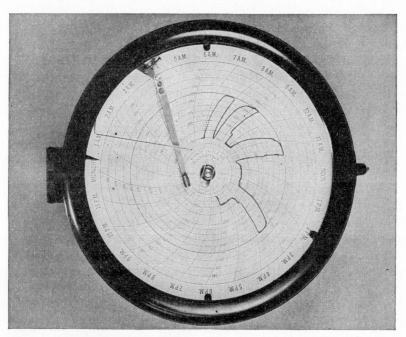

Figure 25B.   Temperature recording chart. Paper disk on which the temperature inside the sterilizing chamber is recorded automatically. Record shows repeated and regular sterilizing periods. (Courtesy of Wilmot Castle Co., Rochester, New York.)

the apparatus that prevents injury to the sterilizer from excessive pressures. Table 5 on page 218 gives the temperatures of the inner chamber when as much air as possible has been replaced by steam under varying pressures.

Efficiency of the autoclaving process depends upon complete penetration by the steam of all materials to be sterilized. The denser the materials and the more folds there are, the more difficult it is to get complete sterilization. The high temperature of steam under 10 to 20 lb of pressure kills most organisms immediately and even the most resistant spores in 20 to 30 minutes; in practice, however, autoclaving periods usually vary from 10 minutes to 1 hour, the time depending upon the nature of the materials to be sterilized. When a temperature as high as 133° C (271.4° F) is used, Walter claims that for mechanically clean surgical instru-

Table 5. Temperatures of Steam Under Varying Pressures
(Tests made at sea level)

	TEMPERATURE OF STEAM	
PRESSURE IN LB	CENTIGRADE	FAHRENHEIT
0	100.0°	212°
5	108.9°	228°
10	115.6°	240°
15	121.0°	249.8°
20	126.7°	260°
24	129.4°	265°
27	133.9°	273°
30	137.2°	279°

ments a sterilizing period of 2 minutes is adequate. He describes a method by which the entire process of sterilizing instruments may be carried out in 5 minutes. To ensure satisfactory cleaning and sterilization of contaminated instruments, he has designed a combination washer and sterilizer that cleans instruments with a superheated soap solution; the instruments are then exposed to steam at 133° C (271.4° F) for 1 minute, the whole process consuming about 10 minutes. (See Figs. 26 and 27.) Such a method eliminates the danger to the worker of handling dirty instruments and provides a high degree of safety to the patient. For all autoclaves Walter recommends a mechanical device that indicates the time at which the center of the densest bundle in the midst of the autoclave's load reaches the prescribed temperature. The process is further safeguarded by an automatic

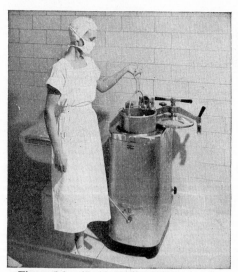
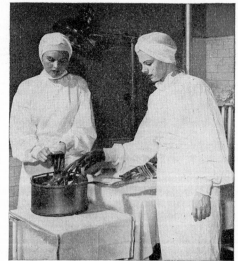

Figure 26. (*Left*) Worker lifting inside container from an instrument washer and sterilizer at the end of the period of sterilization. (*Right*) Workers placing used instruments and gloves in container prior to washing and sterilizing instruments. (Courtesy of Wilmot Castle Co., Rochester, New York.)

device which keeps the autoclave closed until this temperature has been maintained the prescribed length of time; if air enters the chamber, lowering the temperature, the sterilizing cycle is automatically repeated.

It might be assumed that the higher the temperature in the autoclave the more efficient and complete the process; this is not the case. Superheating chars, or burns, textiles and is destructive to all types of equipment. Very high temperatures are recommended only for sterilization of instruments in emergencies. There are

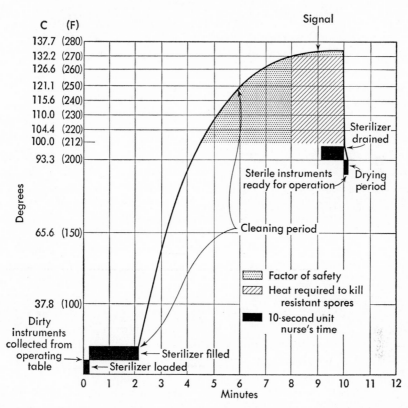

Figure 27. Graph showing that instruments may be cleaned, sterilized, and dried in 10 minutes when the "washer sterilizer" (Fig. 26) is used. (Courtesy of Wilmot Castle Co., Rochester, N. Y.)

many causes of superheating. Operators should guard against allowing the mercury gauge in the outer chamber to rise above 750-mm mercury (15-lb pressure) and other errors that produce temperatures in excess of 121° C (249.8° F) or thereabouts.

The efficiency of sterilizers is tested in a variety of ways. If a self-registering thermometer, or an automatic thermal timing device such as the one just referred to, is placed in the center of the load it checks sterilizing conditions satisfactorily. Perhaps the commonest method of checking the efficiency of the process is to place an envelope containing heat-resistant spores in the center of the load and then test their viability at the end of the sterilizing period. (See Fig. 28.) Controls that depend upon color changes in a chemical, due to the effect of moist heat at given temperatures, are not as reliable as either of the first methods mentioned.

Persons who operate autoclaves should thoroughly understand the mechanism and the sterilizing process. The inner chamber must not be too full, nor the contents arranged too compactly; bundles and drums must be packed loosely; cans or jars of dry goods must be opened and turned on their sides so that the steam can easily penetrate the contents; nothing should block steam inlets; also, care must be taken to avoid stoppage of openings for ejection of air; and a space must be left between the door and the load in the sterilizer.

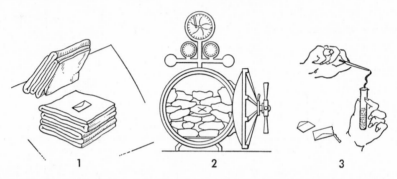

Figure 28. Bacteriological test for the efficiency of the autoclaving period: *step 1,* resistant spores are placed in the midst of the least penetrable item of the sterilizer's load; *step 2,* this article is placed in the center of the load (bundle marked *X*); *step 3,* the spores (on a short length of string) are removed from the envelope, with aseptic precautions, and tested for viability.

Walter[51] strongly recommends that a regular (not rotating) staff be employed to operate sterilizers, preferably in a central supply room. A highly trained personnel can make nice distinctions in relation to temperatures and periods of exposure to steam; he recommends, however, that a single safe process be adopted that provides a margin of safety for all types of equipment. He suggests that the temperature within the sterilizing chamber be held at 121° C (249.8° F) under a pressure of 15 lb or 750-mm Hg gauge for 30 minutes. At the end of the period the steam supply is shut off, but the door is not opened until the pressure gauge is at zero and the temperature has fallen to 100° C (212° F). This allows liquids to cool to a point where they will not escape from their containers with the reduction of pressure, and it also dries packaged goods.

Hot-air Sterilizers. Certain substances used in medical treatment—namely, oils and powders—must be sterilized with hot air because steam cannot penetrate them. Many bacteriologists call attention to the fallacy of trying to sterilize petroleum jelly and similar substances with moist heat at temperatures employed in autoclaves. Hot-air sterilizers are nothing more than ovens equipped with thermometers and, as a rule, thermostatically controlled. Dry heat is less effective than moist, and for this reason higher temperatures are employed in hot-air sterilizers. Walter recommends 1-hour exposure at 160° C (320° F) for instruments if they are free from oil, and 3 hours at this temperature for greasy instruments and petroleum jelly or gauze impregnated with it.

Obviously, temperatures as high as the figure just given are destructive to many types of materials; therefore, hot air can be used for only a limited number of articles. Glassware, needles, sharp instruments, and mineral oils and ointments may be sterilized in a hot-air sterilizer, but organic oils are decomposed by such intense heat and fabrics are likely to be charred.

Instruments are subject to corrosion if exposed to moisture, and this chemical change is accelerated by heat. In order to avoid corrosion and dulling of sharp instruments, *boiling-oil sterilizers* were designed. They are a form of hot-air sterilizer. The boiling points of oils are higher than that of water; but since there is no moisture present, this agent requires a much higher temperature and a longer sterilizing period. On the whole the boiling-oil method has not proved satisfactory. The oil must be removed from the instruments before they can be used, it is difficult to keep the sterilizer clean and in working order, and there is a fire hazard involved.

Of the various methods just discussed, steam under pressure is most effective and reliable. Dry heat is the method of choice for materials destroyed by moisture; boiling water should be used in preference to streaming steam. Less efficient sterilizing methods should be used only when the more reliable ones are unavailable or unsuitable for the materials to be treated.

6. GENERAL PRACTICES IN MEDICAL ASEPSIS

Universal Need for Precaution.   A number of isolated procedures have been discussed in this chapter and special precautions listed which should be observed in certain types of infections. By way of summary it might be helpful to enumerate the precautions that should be taken, in any hospital division, to prevent the spread of communicable disease, whether it is diagnosed or unrecognized. Many newly admitted patients, who are undergoing treatment for some other condition, have also tuberculosis, syphilis, gonorrhea, or streptococcus infections of the throat; or they may be carriers of diphtheria, typhoid fever, or amebic dysentery. When large numbers of persons are living under the same roof, sanitarians and epidemiologists recommend that a higher standard of cleanliness or asepsis be maintained than is usually considered essential in a home where exposure to communicable disease is more limited. For the protection of the *average patient,* it seems desirable that workers and patients recognize clean and contaminated areas in the hospital, that patients be furnished with at least a modicum of individual equipment, that attendants wash their hands after touching any patient or his belongings, that equipment used in common be disinfected each time it is used, and that rooms or ward units and the toilet equipment used by the patient be thoroughly disinfected after he leaves the hospital.

Identification of Clean and Contaminated Surfaces. In general the following are considered contaminated: the inside of toilets, hoppers, bedpan washers, and sinks over which hands are washed or in which contaminated objects are placed; the patient, his clothing, his bedding, his belongings that he handles from time to time, and any equipment that comes in contact with him. Workers in hospitals should try to keep uncontaminated objects separate and away from contaminated ones; when this is unavoidable, a disinfecting process should be used before the article is stored or used by another person.

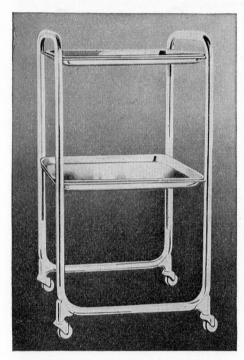

Figure 29. A conveyor for equipment with removable trays that can be sterilized with their contaminated contents. (Courtesy of Scanlon Morris Co., Madison, Wisc.)

In order to facilitate the handling of clean and contaminated equipment, it is suggested that workrooms be designed so that clean things are used and stored on one side of the room and contaminated objects are cleaned and disinfected on the other side. To illustrate the application of this principle: The worker collects equipment that has been used for giving a throat irrigation, carries it to the workroom, places it on the conveyor for contaminated equipment; she discards used paper covers, empties into the hopper any containers of fluid used in irrigating, washes the tray, reservoir, tubing, and all other equipment in the contaminated sink, and places them in the boiling-water sterilizer; she then washes the top of the conveyor or table, and lastly her hands over the contaminated sink. When the sterilizing process is completed, the worker removes the equipment from the sterilizer, places it on the clean table, shelf, or conveyor, washes it if necessary in the uncontaminated sink, dries it, and stores it for future use on the clean side of the room.

If two rooms are available, one for clean equipment and one for used equipment, it is much easier to prevent the transfer of infections by contaminated objects (see Fig. 23). Nonprofessional personnel should be regularly assigned to such rooms to conserve the time of nurses, doctors, and more highly trained workers who would otherwise have to process the equipment.

Figure 29 shows a freely moving lightweight table. The trays are removable and may be boiled with the used equipment. This type of conveyor is highly desirable from the standpoint of asepsis.

Individual Equipment for Patients.   To reduce the hazard of spreading disease and to prevent the necessity for constant disinfection of commonly used articles, it is suggested that each bed patient be provided with the following items: (1) Two bath blankets and one warm blanket in cool weather for use in chair or otherwise, in addition to the regular bedding; (2) as many pillows as are likely to be needed constantly and a rubber or plastic cover for each pillow that may perhaps become soiled by excretions from the body; (3) a small rubber or plastic sheet to protect the bed when the bedpan is in use or during certain treatments; (4) a bath basin; (5) a soap container; (6) a toothbrush mug; (7) a bottle of rubbing lotion;

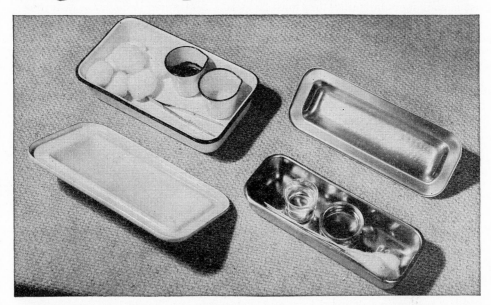

Figure 30.   Skin-cleaning trays. Supplies are taken to the patient's unit in the amounts needed to avoid contamination of stock supplies. Trays and cups are sterilized after use and left sterile until needed when solutions, sponges and a forceps or applicators are added.

(8) a container of powder; (9) a water pitcher, drinking glass, and tray; and (10) a thermometer and holder. If there is a private bathroom in which the bedpan and urinal can be emptied and cleaned, it is desirable to have each unit equipped with these articles; but when they are emptied and disinfected in the common bedpan washers and sterilizers, there is no point in storing these objects in the patient's unit.

When ointments or other applications are ordered to be applied at frequent intervals, small portions of the medication should be taken from the stock supply, put in a container of an appropriatae size, and then taken to the patient's room. Stock supplies should not be carried from unit to unit. Disinfectants used for skin cleaning, for example, should be transferred from stock bottles to small cups in the amounts required for each patient in order to avoid the possibility of contaminating stock supplies. (An individual skin-cleaning tray is shown in Fig. 30.)

The same principle applies to dressings, foods, linen, and all other supplies used in the care of patients.

Handwashing. It is generally agreed that medical workers should wash their hands after touching any patient or contaminated surface. Because the nurse often finds herself in situations in which the time factor limits the quality of the nursing care she is able to give, she should study ways and means of preventing unnecessary contamination of her hands.

Concurrent Disinfection of Equipment. There are many articles, such as dishes, bed linen, hot-water bottles, and therapeutic instruments of all kinds, that patients use in common. Ordinarily, they must be cleaned and stored in common workrooms because it is not practical to isolate this equipment with patients. It is necessary, therefore, to disinfect the equipment each time it is used, in order to prevent the transfer of disease organisms from one person to another. In hospitals where individual bath basins and other toilet articles are not provided, these articles also must be sterilized after use. When patients are sick with communicable diseases in homes, as much of the equipment as possible is isolated or kept in the patient's room, because concurrent disinfection presents a greater problem here than it does in the hospital. Fortunately, physical disinfectants are adequate in most cases and are nearly always available. Linen may be laundered in such a way that it is disinfected, dishes are easily boiled, and equipment that is injured by moisture may be sunned and aired.

In some cases it is possible to reduce the amount of concurrent sterilization by using disposable articles. Paper cups, for example, may be used for medications; paper dishes are also practical items; paper and cellulose sheets impervious to water and cellucotton pads may often be substituted for rubber sheets and bed linen that must be laundered.

Terminal Disinfection. After a patient has recovered from a communicable disease, at the time of his discharge it is usual to see that he has a shampoo as well as a bath, and that he is dressed in uncontaminated clothing. In case of death the body is prepared for the undertaker as described in Chapter 35 and carefully wrapped in a shroud, so that the outer surface is clean.

In modern institutions all rooms and ward units are treated almost the same way after the patient leaves, whether he had a communicable disease or not. Floors and furniture are washed and aired; the walls are rarely washed even in the communicable disease unit, unless they are obviously soiled. The mattresses and pillows are brushed and aired in all instances; in case of a communicable disease, they are treated with ultraviolet rays, sunned, or subjected to steam under pressure. All linen is laundered; blankets are either washed or dry-cleaned. Curtains are aired and sunned but not laundered unless soiled. All enameled ware, glassware, instruments, and rubber articles are boiled or disinfected in some other way. Anyone who is admitted to a well-ordered hospital should have a feeling of assurance that the equipment put at his disposal has been made safe for use by proper methods of cleaning and disinfection.

7. GENERAL PRACTICES IN SURGICAL ASEPSIS

Medical Asepsis for the Surgical Patient.   Every surgical patient is entitled to protection from respiratory, intestinal, skin, and other general regional infections, as well as being entitled to the special asepsis practiced in the care of wounds. When asepsis is referred to in the handling of surgical patients, it is assumed that they are provided with uncontaminated dishes, bed linen, clothing, and toilet articles, as well as with sterile surgical dressings. Operations are almost always debilitating; in addition, the conditions that necessitate the operation have often lowered the patient's resistance to infectious disease. Surgical asepsis, therefore, should be considered as supplementing the general plan for the protection of any patient from communicable disease.

Aseptic Care of Wounds.   One of the general principles that should be followed is that any object that comes in contact with a break in the skin or mucous membrane should be sterile, or as nearly free from bacteria as it is possible to make it. Since the air contains bacteria and the disinfection of the skin itself is only relative, absolute sterility of wounds is impossible. In order to reduce to a minimum the hazards of infection, however, all surgical supplies should be autoclaved if possible. Some of the most deadly wound infections are caused by spore-bearing organisms that occur very commonly in nature. Every person who handles wounds or surgical equipment should wear sterile gloves unless he can work satisfactorily with sterile forceps.

Many surgeons believe that the same precautions taken in the operating room should be used in dressing wounds in spite of the fact that a wound seems to be progressively resistant to infection. The use of masks for those changing dressings, dust-suppressive measures, and other methods of controlling air bacteria are recommended.

Preparation of the Skin or Mucous Membrane for Surgical Procedures.   In *major* operations the surgeon usually prescribes the way in which the skin is to be cleaned and disinfected and in most instances he carries out or supervises the procedure in the operating room; for minor operations the nurse is expected to assume a good deal of responsibility for preparing the skin. When she gives hypodermics she herself selects the cleaning and disinfecting agents unless there are "routine" techniques developed by a committee for the agency or institution. Certain treatments, such as catheterization and perineal care of a mother following a delivery, require surgical asepsis, because there may be a break in the mucous membrane and the tissues must therefore be treated as if there were an open wound. Relative merits of various skin disinfectants and detergents were discussed earlier in this chapter. The recommendations made there should be applied here.

Any hair on an operative site is removed since its presence makes cleaning of the skin difficult, and if left in a wound it acts as a foreign body. The skin is usually shaved the day before the operation and the area thoroughly cleaned with water and a detergent. If skin disinfectants with a cumulative action, such as hexachlorophene, are used, application may be started a day or more preceding surgery. Immediately before the operation the area is again cleaned, and a skin disinfectant applied under aseptic conditions. Sponges, preferably gauze to produce friction, should be sterile and held in sterile forceps. The area is scrubbed with a concentric motion, the actual site of the incision touched first while the sponge is clean. Figure 30 shows an individual tray of equipment for skin cleaning. It is recommended to prevent contaminating stock supplies. Specific techniques for various procedures and types of surgery are described in other parts of the text.

The preparation of sterile dressings, instruments, solutions, and all types of equipment may be, wholly or in part, the responsibility of the nurse, although there is a trend toward putting this in the hands of nonmedical personnel. The following chapter describes some of the more common procedures involved.

REFERENCES

1. US Department of Commerce, Bureau of the Census: *Statistical Abstract of the United States 1950*. US Government Printing Office, Washington, D.C., 1950, p. 90.
2. Maxcy, Kenneth F. (ed.): *Rosenau's Preventive Medicine and Hygiene*, 7th ed. Appleton-Century-Crofts, Inc., New York, 1951, p. 336.
3. McCulloch, Ernest C.: *Disinfection and Sterilization*, 2nd ed. Lea & Febiger, Philadelphia, 1945, p. 15.
4. Maxcy, Kenneth F. (ed.): *op. cit.*, p. 292.
5. Witton, Catharine J.: *Microbiology and Applications to Nursing*. McGraw-Hill Book Co., New York, 1950, pp. 103, 307, 404, 654.
6. Smith, David T., et al.: *Zinnser's Textbook of Bacteriology*, 9th ed. Appleton-Century-Crofts, Inc., New York, 1948, pp. 557-78.
7. Witton, Catharine J.: *op. cit.*, pp. 421, 654.
8. Esty, J. R., and Meyer, K. F.: "The Heat Resistance of the Spores of B. Botulinus and Allied Anaerobes," *J. Infect. Dis.*, 31:650, (Dec.) 1922.
9. Walter, Carl W.: *The Aseptic Treatment of Wounds*. The Macmillan Company, New York, 1948, p. 53.
10. Pfefferkorn, Blanche, and Rovetta, Charles A.: *Administrative Cost Analysis for Nursing Service and Nursing Education*. American Hospital Association, Chicago, and National League of Nursing Education, New York, 1940, pp. 55-63.
11. Pfefferkorn, Blanche: "Pray Let Us Wash Our Hands," *Am. J. Nursing*, 32:851, (Aug.) 1932.
12. Blank, Irwin H.: "Measurement of pH of the Skin Surface," *J. Invest. Dermat.*, 2:67, (Apr.) 1939.
13. Rebell, Gerbert, et al.: "Factors Affecting the Rapid Disappearance of Bacteria Placed on the Normal Skin," *J. Invest. Dermat.*, 14:247, (Apr.) 1950.
14. *The Story of G-11 (Hexachlorophene)*. Sindar Corporation, New York, 1950, p. 2.
15. Hudson, A. L.: "The H-ion Concentration of Normal and Diseased Skin," *Canad. M. A. J.*, 64:19, (Jan.) 1951.
16. Blank, Irwin H.: "Action of Soap on Skin," *Arch. Dermat. & Syph.*, 39:811, (May) 1939.
17. Jones, K. K., and Lorenz, M.: "The Relation of Calcium Soaps to Staphylococcus Infection of the Skin," *J. Invest. Dermat.*, 4:69 (Feb.) 1941.
18. Hirshfeld, John W.: "Bacterial Contamination of Wounds from the Air, from the Skin of the Patient," *Surg., Gynec. & Obst.*, 73:72, (July) 1941.
19. Price, Philip B.: "Bacteriology of Normal Skin; New Quantitative Test Applied to Study of Bacterial Flora and Disinfectant Action of Mechanical Cleansing," *J. Infect. Dis.*, 63:301, (Nov.-Dec.) 1938.

20. McCarthy, Lee: *Disease of the Hair.* C. V. Mosby, Co., St. Louis, 1940, p. 50.
21. Allen, William A., et al.: "A Bacteriological Appraisal of 34 Commonly Used Antiseptics," *Am. J. Surg.,* **23:**371, (Feb.) 1934.
22. Hufnagel, Charles A., et al.: "An In Vivo Method for the Evaluation of Skin Antiseptics," *Surgery,* **23:**753, (May) 1948.
23. Walter, Carl W.: *op. cit.,* p. 178.
24. Price, Philip B.: "Ethyl Alcohol as a Germicide," *Arch. Surg.,* **38:**528, (Mar.) 1939.
25. Walter, Carl W.: *op. cit.,* p. 25.
26. Gump, William: "The Development of a Germicidal Soap." *Soap and Sanitary Chemicals* March and April, 1945.
27. *The Story of G-11 (Hexachlorophene).* Sindar Corporation, New York, 1950.
28. Artz, Curtis P., et al.: "Clinical Uses of Hexachlorophene," *U.S. Armed Forces M. J.,* **2:**819, (May) 1951.
29. Traub, E. F., et al.: "New Cutaneous Bactericidal Agent Used in Soap," *Arch. Dermat. & Syph.,* **52:**385, (Dec.) 1945.
30. American Medical Association, Council on Pharmacy and Chemistry: "Hexachlorophene," *J.A.M.A.,* **143:**563, (Feb.) 1951.
31. Chisholm, T. C., et al.: "Disinfecting Action of pHisoderm Containing 3% Hexachlorophene on Skin of Hands," *Surgery,* **28:**812, (Nov.) 1950.
32. Artz, Curtis P., et al.: *op. cit.*
33. Stimson, Philip: *A Manual of the Common Contagious Diseases,* 4th ed. Lea & Febiger, Philadelphia, 1947, p. 442.
34. Maxcy, Kenneth F. (ed.): *op. cit.,* p. 77.
35. Wells, W. F.: "Air-borne Infection. II. Droplets and Droplet Nuclei," *Am. J. Hyg.,* **20:**611, (Nov.) 1934.
36. Loosli, Clayton G.: "Dust and Its Control as a Means of Disinfection of Air," *Am. J. Pub. Health,* **37:**353, (Apr.) 1947.
37. Moulton, Forest R.: *Aerobiology.* American Association for the Advancement of Science, Washington, D.C., Pub. No. 17, 1942.
38. Wells, Mildred W., and Holla, William A.: "Ventilation in the Flow of Measles and Chickenpox through a Community," *J.A.M.A.,* **142:**1337, (Apr.) 1950.
39. Bourdillon, R. B., et al.: "Studies in Air Hygiene," in *Medical Research Council, Spec. Rep. Series,* No. 262, His Majesty's Stationery Office, London, England, 1948.
40. Subcommittee on Air Sanitation of the Committee on Research and Standards, American Public Health Association: "Progress in the Control of Air-borne Infections," *Am. J. Pub. Health Year Book,* 1950, Pt. II.
41. Krugman, Saul, and Ward, Robert: "Air Sterilization in an Infants' Ward: Effect of Triethylene Glycol Vapor and Dust Suppressive Measures on Respiratory Cross Infection," *J.A.M.A.,* **145:**775, (Mar.) 1951.
42. Rooks, Roland, et al.: "Hospital Masks: Their Filtering Efficiency and Resistance to Air Flow. A Comparative Study," *Pub. Health Rev.,* **56:**1411, (July) 1941.
43. McNett, E. H., and Ellison, B. M.: *Basic Principles of Aseptic Technique.* Anti-tuberculosis League of Cleveland and Cuyahoga County, Ohio, 1942, p. 18.
44. Lurie, Max B., and Abramson, Samuel: "The Efficiency of Gauze Masks in the Protection of Rabbits Against the Inhalation of Droplet Nuclei of Tubercle Bacilli," *Am. Rev. Tuberc.,* **59:**1, (Jan.) 1949.
45. Mallman, W. L., and Kahler, David: *Studies in Dishwashing.* National Sanitation Foundation, School of Public Health, University of Michigan, Ann Arbor, 1949.
46. Cox, W. C.: "An Automatically Controlled Dishwashing Machine," *Am. J. Pub. Health,* **27:**865, (Sept.) 1937.
47. Speller, Frank N.: *Corrosion—Causes and Prevention,* 2nd ed. McGraw-Hill Book Co., New York, 1935, p. 185.
48. Magath, T. B.: "A Positive Inexpensive Method of Producing Sterile Goods," *Mod. Hosp.,* **41:**112, (Sept.) 1933.

49. McCulloch, Ernest C.: *op. cit.,* p. 76.
50. Walter, Carl W.: *op. cit.,* p. 68.
51. Walter, Carl W.: *op. cit.,* p. 292.

Additional Suggested Reading

Anderson, Gaylord W., and Arnstein, Margaret G.: *Communicable Disease Control,* 3rd ed. The Macmillan Company, New York, 1953.

Best, R. R., et al.: "Effectiveness of Soaps Containing Hexachlorophene for the Surgical Scrub: Special Reference to Bar Soap," *A.M.A. Arch. Surg.,* **61**:869, (Nov.) 1950.

Blank, Irwin H., and Coolidge, Mary H.: "Degerming the Cutaneous Surface, II: Hexachlorophene (G-11)," *J. Invest. Dermat.,* **15**:257, (Sept.) 1950.

Boeder, Paul: "The Effect of Ultraviolet on the Human Eye," *Am. J. Optometry,* **27**:437, (Sept.) 1950.

Bolle, A., and Mirimanoff, A.: "Antagonism Between Non-Ionic Detergents and Antiseptics," *J. Pharm. & Pharmacol.,* **2**:685, (Oct.) 1950.

Boyd, Mark F. (ed.): *Malariology: A Comprehensive Survey of All Aspects of This Group of Diseases from a Global Standpoint.* W. B. Saunders Co., Philadelphia, 1949.

Brandstadt, Wayne G.: "Air Pollution," *U.S. Armed Forces M. J.,* **1**:1195, (Oct.) 1950.

Broadhurst, Jean, and Given, Leila I.: *Bacteriology Applied to Nursing.* J. B. Lippincott Co., Philadelphia, 1945.

Buck, F. D.: "The Story of G-11," *Canad. Hosp.,* **27**:38, (Nov.) 1950.

Downes, Jean: "Control of Acute Respiratory Illness by Ultra-Violet Lights," *Am. J. Pub. Health,* **40**:1512, (Dec.) 1950.

Evans, Charles A., et al.: "Bacterial Flora of the Normal Human Skin," *J. Invest. Dermat.,* **15**:305, (Oct.) 1950.

Gill, Meyer J.: "G-11 Takes the Scrub out of Scrub-Up Procedures," *Mod. Hosp.,* **75**:67, (Oct.) 1950.

Silson, John E.: "Dust Inhalation in Relation to Pulmonary Disease," *Dis. Chest,* **18**:562, (Dec.) 1950.

CHAPTER 8. SELECTION AND PREPARATION OF STERILE SUPPLIES

1. STANDARDIZATION OF SUPPLIES

Variation in Practice. Surgical supplies vary widely in design as do the descriptive terms used for them. The sponge used to make pressure on the throat following the removal of a tonsil, or the dressing for an injured eye, may be made in a dozen different ways and may have different names in as many hospitals. Sterilizing agents and periods of exposure to the agent for an article, such as a forceps, differ in situations where all known agents and methods are available. A joint committee of the National Bureau of Standards, the American Hospital Association, and the American College of Surgeons,[1] has set up standards for surgical dressings, and progress has been made in standardizing sterile sutures and a few other products, but much remains to be done. It is difficult to show either standard or ideal practice. The procedures in this chapter are based on an attempt to apply recognized principles of physics, chemistry, bacteriology, and economics to the problems involved in selecting and preparing sterile supplies.

The writer has relied heavily on the findings and opinions of Ernest C. McCulloch[2] and Carl W. Walter,[3] both of whom have devoted years to the investigation of aseptic practice.

Standardization, Its Therapeutic and Economic Value.   One of the foundations of modern medical science is standardization of the weapons used to fight disease, and standardization is the cornerstone of industrial economy. Whenever artistry is involved, as in human relationships, painting, or music, standardization is to be avoided; in mechanical processes where the method or the product should be uniform, standardization is desirable. The preparation of antibiotics, narcotics, of anesthetics (indeed, all drugs), of diagnostic instruments, and of sterile supplies obviously falls into the second class. A drug whose potency is not known, an unsterile instrument and instruments that do not function accurately, may cost a human life.

In this chapter especial attention is given to standard nomenclature and standard methods of preparing sterile supplies. Danger and confusion result when the same kind of dressing is called a "compress" on one package and a "sponge" on another, when "clean" means free from all bacteria or decontaminated after use, when needles fit one syringe but not another, or when solutions in identical containers are both suitable and unsuitable for intravenous use.

Recognizing the need for uniformity, institutions are adopting *central supply services* that prepare and store all types of equipment, but particularly sterile items.[4] Supplies are ordered on standard forms. Articles are listed with the terminology used by supply houses rather than with local terms. Requisitions are made and supplies delivered at regular periods. Each division is charged with the material used, and records are kept. In this way the needs of the different services, and the institution as a whole, can be studied and anticipated. There are many advantages of a central supply service, but one that should be mentioned is that expensive equipment, such as a still or a mechanical washer may be made to serve the total needs of a hospital when they are placed in such a department. It was pointed out in Chapter 7 that asepsis, or the freedom from all microorganisms, is the ideal condition in surgery. This means that equipment and supplies coming in contact with wounds should be, if possible, sterilized with very high temperatures, the only sure means of destroying spores. It is economical to segregate autoclaves and hot-air sterilizers.

It seems quite clear that stocking, storing, and preparing supplies involve technical processes almost entirely. Except for the management of the personnel, operating a central supply service consists in manipulating inanimate objects. While methods should be worked out by physicians, surgeons, nurses, bacteriologists, chemists, and engineers, the full-time employment of medical personnel in central supply services, particularly nurses, is a waste of their potential medical value. The person in charge of the central supply service has need of managerial ability and enough knowledge of economics, physics, chemistry, bacteriology, and hospital management to enable him, or her, to use consultants wisely. When a blood bank is included in the central supply service and during experimentation with new procedures, medical personnel may be needed on a full-time basis.

2. METHODS OF WRAPPING, PACKING, AND MARKING SUPPLIES

Cotton Fabric and Paper Covers.   Making packages by covering articles to be sterilized with cotton fabric is probably the commonest method of preparing dry objects for steam sterilization. The fabric should be strong and closely woven, but permeable to steam. Drill and a high-grade unbleached muslin fulfill these requirements. Covers should be of new material, and a double thickness used. When the two layers are stitched together the cover lasts longer and is more easily handled. High temperatures discolor fabrics permanently, but even though laundering won't bleach them, covers should be washed frequently to remove soil. Covers of different colors offer a means of assorting, checking, and selecting supplies quickly.

Paper has within recent years entirely or partially replaced cotton fabrics for wrapping supplies in some situations. Kraft paper (brown wrapping paper) is the type most often used, but manufacturers are advertising clothlike papers that they claim to be both tough and highly permeable to steam.* Many laboratories use newspaper to wrap glassware and small articles, and medical supply houses sell a wide range of sterile supplies in glassine paper and cellophane wrappers.

There is a wide difference of opinion on the relative merits of fabric and paper covers. Walter states: "Paper-wrapped packages do not clear air promptly because the paper is impervious; they are too difficult to sterilize in the usual dressing sterilizer to justify their use."† Katharine Zorn[5] reports that tests made on paper-wrapped bundles indicate that sterility of the contents is achieved. She claims a substantial saving through the use of kraft paper that withstands eight or more sterilizing periods. It goes without saying that all covers should be examined before use. If paper is used there should be ample proof of its permeability and protective qualities. Since the wrapper must often serve as a sterile field from which the contents of the package are handled, it should be soft and tend to lie flat rather than to spring back over the sterile object.

Methods of fastening bundles vary greatly. Pins, clips, rope, string, bandage, cotton tape, gummed cellophane film, gummed brown-paper stripping, and adhesive are some of the agents used. Their high cost eliminates some of these from a list of desirable fasteners, but a variety of methods may be needed for the different kinds of supplies that must be packaged.

When pins are used they should be embedded to the head; otherwise, the exposed, or unsterile, portion of the shaft will contaminate the contents of the bundle when the pin is withdrawn. Bandage and adhesive are costly and unsuit-

---

* Meinecke and Co., New York City.

† Walter, Carl W.: *The Aseptic Treatment of Wounds.* The Macmillan Company, New York, 1948, p. 128.

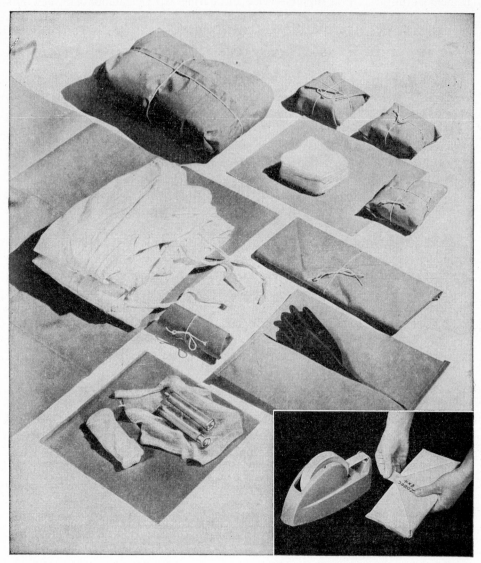

Figure 31. Packaging in paper or cotton wrappers is the most common and preferred method of preparing sterile supplies. The covers shown here are "Sterilwraps." (Courtesy of Meinecke & Co., New York City.) Inset illustrates use of Tyloc tape (courtesy of Johnson & Johnson, New Brunswick, N. J.).

able for tying bundles; tape can be used many times if properly fastened. Gummed paper has the advantage of offering a surface on which a description of the contents and the date of sterilization may be stamped.

Small articles are sometimes sterilized in cellophane or glassine-paper envelopes. When such coverings are used it is essential to ensure admission of steam to the contents of the envelope.

Regardless of the type of cover used, bundles must be packed so that steam can penetrate the entire contents. Some authorities recommend limiting the largest dimension of a bundle to approximately 30 cm, or 12 in.; Walter, on the other hand, describes a large bundle containing all the linen and dressings for an operation measuring 55 × 33 × 22 cm (22 × 13 × 9 in.) that he reports completely saturated with steam within 14 minutes after the temperature in the exhaust line rises to 121° C (249.8° F). He believes that proper arrangement and covering of material, and packing and operation of the sterilizer make it safe to use large bundles.

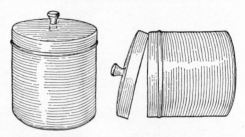

Covered Jars, Cans, and Trays. The practice of sterilizing dry surgical supplies in covered glass jars and in stainless-steel and enameled-ware containers of various sizes is not uncommon, although it is obvious that great care must be exercised to see that steam has access to the entire contents of the container. While in the autoclave the uncovered jars or cans

Figure 32. When upright, a metal dressing container pools air. To ensure rapid and adequate sterilization, it must be placed on its side in the sterilizer with the lid off (see *right, above*). (Walter, Carl W.: *The Aseptic Treatment of Wounds.* The Macmillan Company, New York, 1948.)

should be placed on their sides so that steam flows in readily. The sterilized lids are put on the cans at the end of the sterilizing process. (It must be recognized that any opening or closing of aseptic supplies, even under these circumstances, is undesirable.) If a collection of equipment for a certain treatment is assembled on a covered tray, or dish, the lid should be tied on at the termination of the autoclaving period. An uncovered deep tray, or dish, may be used for a "treatment set" if the whole is wrapped in a double fabric or paper cover. Cellucotton pads on the tray protect the equipment and reduce noise. Stainless-steel containers are most satisfactory for this purpose because they are less affected by heat than are glass- and enameled ware. Glass tubes of various lengths and diameters are recommended as containers for needles, syringes, rubber tubes, high-registration thermometers, and almost any small object. They may be fitted with screw caps that are adjusted at the termination of the sterilizing process. A gauze plug at the mouth helps to filter the air that rushes in as the sterilizer is opened. Commercial firms sterilize needles and dressings in closed containers that hold a measured amount of water which is completely used and evaporated as steam in the sterilizing process.

Drums. Metal containers with hinged tops and perforated sides that can be opened or closed are called *drums* because they are usually shaped like a drum.

Figure 33 shows the common round type; a rectangular box of similar structure may be used. Both styles are suited to the same purpose, but the round drum that economizes space in a cylindrical sterilizer is ordinarily used for large quantities of surgical dressings while the rectangular container is used for a single aseptic practice, such as an infusion. Drums are still used, but many authorities advise against them, and they are falling into disuse. Both McCulloch and Walter believe that they are usually packed too tightly, and that even when they are loosely packed it is difficult to replace the contained air by steam, a condition essential for proper sterilization. Drums have the additional disadvantage of being noisy and expensive.

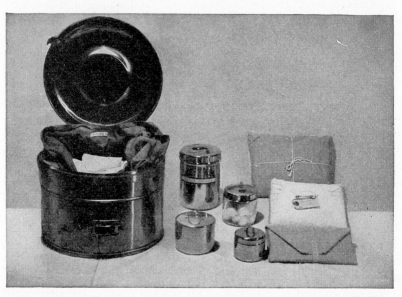

Figure 33. Preparation of dry dressings for sterilization (*Left to right*) A drum, stainless-steel containers of various sizes, and a glass jar. Two packages (*right*) are covered with paper; the middle package with a fabric wrapper. String, a safety pin, and a special tape are variously used to fasten the packages. (Jars are turned on the sides with the lids off during the sterilizing process.) (Courtesy of Columbia-Presbyterian Medical Center, New York City, and Clay-Adams Co., New York City.)

When drums are used they are lined with a cotton fabric, such as drill, that is permeable to steam and offers good protection. (Paper is employed by those who believe that it is easily penetrated by steam because it is more economical.) With some types of drums the perforations around the sides of the drum are left open while the drum is in the autoclave and closed when taken out. Acting on the principle that the lining of the drum filters the bacteria from any air that may enter through the perforations, manufacturers are now making drums without the mechanism that covers the holes.

The contents of unopened drums are considered sterile for two days to two weeks, or more, according to local rulings. Bacteriological tests indicate that it may be aseptic for months, or even years, if very well packed, sterilized, and stored.

Marking Surgical Supplies. A great deal depends upon legible and accurate marking of surgical supplies. Any bundle that is to be autoclaved must have the contents indicated on it before it is sterilized. While colored covers or tags may be used to simplify assorting supplies, color alone must not be depended upon. The names of articles inside must be printed or stamped on the tag or the cover. Waterproof ink may be used, or ordinary pencil; the former is more easily read. Indestructible metal tags with slits at each end may be run on tapes that tie bundles, or they may be attached by a chain to containers, such as flasks (see Fig. 34). Glassware may be etched, and stainless-steel containers are satisfactorily marked by plastering a printed label against the side of the vessel with a larger piece of Scotch tape. The latter, being transparent, leaves the label exposed. If cellulose film is used to cover the mouth of a flask, the identification label may be placed between layers of this material; thus the label is over the top of the flask, and is easily read. Whenever possible, handwritten labels should be replaced by a less time-consuming practice. The use of adhesive in labeling packages is wasteful and unattractive in appearance.

As sterile materials are removed from the autoclave a rubber stamp and brightly colored ink may be used to mark them "sterile," and the date of sterilization. Many agencies are finding it more satisfactory to indicate the date when the arbitrarily set period of asepsis expires. For example: "Do not use after December 15, 1955."

3. PREPARATION OF STERILE SOLUTIONS

Causes of Error. Improperly prepared solutions, if introduced into the blood stream, may cause mild or severe febrile reactions. Death has resulted from unsterile and chemically toxic solutions. Errors that may occur in the preparation of solutions are inadequate distillation of water, the introduction of a toxic substance during distillation or sterilization, the inaccurate measurement of substances that make up the solution, incomplete sterilization, contamination of the solution after sterilization, and mistakes in marking flasks. Reactions may result also from careless preparation of the apparatus through which the solution runs. So many accidents have occurred in connection with infusions that some institutions purchase all solutions used in such treatments from reputable manufacturers who guarantee the purity of their products. (For illustrations of ready-made solutions, see Fig. 34.) Very large institutions find it less expensive to employ the services of a highly qualified person to supervise the preparation of solutions, so that they are made with approximately the same degree of exactness that can be developed in a factory.

Removing Toxic Chemicals. All solutions introduced into the blood stream or under the skin, if in large quantities, must be prepared with *distilled water*. Any water that filters through the earth contains mineral salts and is unsterile. In addition to the microbes themselves, toxic products excreted by microorganisms may be present.[6] The pyrogenic factor in solutions, which is believed to be the commonest cause of unfavorable reactions to infusions, is a toxin produced by bacteria. Experiments have shown that when water is properly filtered and *freshly* distilled this danger is eliminated.[7] Air bacteria will grow in distilled water, producing a new supply of pyrogens that will pass through filters.

Apparently the secret of adequate distillation lies not in repeated distillations but in having the right type of still (one equipped with a baffle to prevent

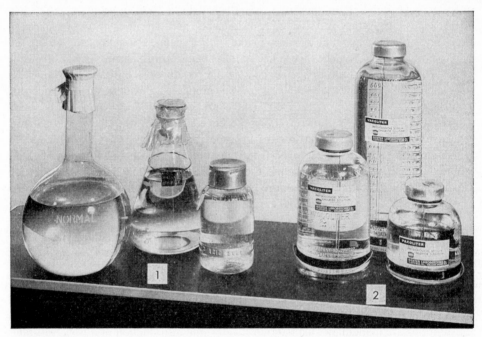

Figure 34. Sterile solutions: (*1*) solutions prepared in the hospital, capped and labeled in different ways; (*2*) commercial solutions in three sizes. (All commonly used intravenous solutions are also prepared by commercial firms.)

contamination of the distillate by droplets of boiling water during distillation) and in proper care and operation of the still. A single process is adequate if the still is efficient. Water should be collected from the still in alkaline-free and pyrogen-free glass bottles. Flasks in which solutions are sterilized also must be alkaline free. Forcible cleaning in mechanical washers with detergents, such as Calgonite (not soaps), and rinsing with distilled water are recommended. Sodium chloride, dextrose, and other chemicals used in preparing solutions must be chemically pure. Rubber, plastic, or other types of covers for flasks and bottles must be free from substances that might dissolve in the solutions during the sterilizing process.

Removal of Foreign Bodies. Filtration of solutions is essential for the removal of insoluble chemicals, lint, or dust that, in spite of the greatest care, may fall into the solution during the preparation. Small dust-free chambers, or hoods, in which the solutions are handled reduce the risk of air contamination.

It saves time to make and filter concentrated or "stock solutions" of saline, dextrose, etc. Distilled water may then be added to these stock solutions and no additional filtration is necessary. Concentrates are treated with activated charcoal that removes foreign bodies by adsorption; or they may be filtered through asbestos.

Caps, or plugs, must be lintless and free from all loose particles that might drop into the fluid. Although the contents of the flask should not boil up to the cap while in the autoclave, the best type of covering for the mouth of the flask is one that will do no harm to the solution if this occurs. Metal or plastic caps, cellulose films, and treated papers have been found satisfactory from this standpoint. Commercial firms employ rubber, plastic, and metal caps that cannot be punctured, and these are rapidly replacing the more perishable caps. To enhance their value as filters, and to prevent punctures, cellophane and paper, when used, should be reinforced with layers of muslin. If a good cover is bound tightly around the mouth of the flask there is little danger of air contamination.

The Fenwall flask is widely used for sterilizing and dispensing solutions. It is alkaline-free, heat-resistant glass; it is graduated and fitted with a rubber "bushing" and metal cap that facilitates sterilization, maintenance of asepsis, and administration of the solution from the flask. All parts have a long life, and each may be replaced without loss of the other parts.

Properly capped flasks and adequately sterilized solutions remain sterile for months, or perhaps years. However, most firms and health agencies indicate a date beyond which they do not recommend the use of the solution.

Preventing Undue Water Loss. Sterilization by heat almost inevitably results in water loss. Some authorities estimate a 5 per cent loss. With a nearly airtight cover, such as the Fenwall, there is a minimum tendency to concentration. (Zorn recommends two layers of cellophane with a cotton plug between them for small flasks.) The steam generated by the solution as it heats in the flasks drives out any air in the flask. The liquid will not escape from the flask and wet the plug if the steam pressure around the flask is maintained at 1536 mm of mercury during the sterilizing process. Walter recommends a period of 30 minutes at 121° C (249.8° F) for all supplies, including solutions. At the end of the period the steam supply is shut off, but the door is not opened until the pressure gauge is at zero and the temperature down to 100° C (212° F). When the metal cap on the Fenwall flask is pushed down into the rubber plug, or bushing, at the end of the sterilizing period a vacuum is created. Commercial solutions are equally airtight, and storage conditions should not affect them. If, however, there is access of air to the flask, storage at any temperature will eventually result in water loss. The higher the temperature the higher the rate of evaporation, or concentration.

Flasks are available in many shapes and sizes. The Florence flask is narrow-necked, fragile, and expensive. The Fenwall flask is a durable adaptation of this pattern. The Erlenmeyer flask is relatively cheap and as satisfactory for most medical purposes as the Florence flask. All solutions should, whenever possible, be sterilized in containers from which the solution may be administered.

Storage of Solutions.   At one time importance was attached to giving intravenous and subcutaneous solutions at body temperatures, and warming closets were devised for storage of such solutions on clinical services. It is now generally thought that the solution is rapidly warmed by the body and, if given slowly enough, it may be safely administered at room temperature, except in unusual circumstances.

If heated closets are provided they should be thermostatically controlled. A dummy flask with a thermometer resting in the solution can be used as a checking device to prevent the possibility of using overheated solutions. It must be borne in mind that heat produces concentration of the solution and chemical changes in carbohydrate and protein preparations; therefore, flasks should be left in such warming closets for brief periods only. To reduce the possibility of giving preparations unsuitable for parenteral therapy some communities have health regulations that require agencies to store solutions for intravenous and subcutaneous use in a separate closet. It is also desirable to use different types of containers for solutions given by injection.

4. CARE AND STERILIZATION OF INSTRUMENTS

General Principles.   Time, effort, and handling should be reduced to a minimum in sterilizing instruments. The worker and working areas should be so thoroughly safeguarded that the method can be used for all instruments no matter how dangerously contaminated. Used instruments should be dropped into a container in which they are decontaminated, and they should not be handled until this is accomplished.

Whenever possible a combination instrument washer and autoclave, such as that shown on page 218, should be provided. With this equipment instruments are washed and sterilized with minimum handling. Soiled instruments are unhinged and dropped into a bucket that is put directly into the washer sterilizer. A detergent and a water softener are added, the mechanism turned on, and within 15 minutes the instruments are washed and sterilized, ready for use or storage. The temperature of the water is raised to 132° C (269.6° F) which accounts for the rapid action. When such improved equipment is not available, soiled instruments may be unhinged (opened) with gloved hands and dropped into a deep basin or bucket to which is added a solution of 2 per cent sodium triphosphate. (This chemical dissolves blood clots.) The basin and its contents can then be decontaminated by moist heat. After this the instruments may be safely handled: cleaned and prepared for storage, or sterilized for the next operation or dressing. The objection to this method is that organic material is "cooked" on the instruments and the sterilizers coated with scum.

Before sterilizing decontaminated instruments, oily films, if present, should be removed with xylol or gasoline. All instruments should be examined; those that need it, soaked in detergents. Abrasives and soap tend to remove the protective film of corrosion-resistant metal put on by the manufacturer, and their use shortens the life of the instrument. The care and handling of all metals should be so designed that the removal of the outer protective layer is delayed as long as possible.[8, 9] The care and selection of instruments to prevent corrosion is a complex matter that cannot be treated thoroughly in a general text.

Steam under pressure should be used to sterilize instruments *whenever possible*. Walter recommends 15 minutes at 121° C (249.8° F), or briefer periods at higher temperatures when, as in operating suites, special instruments are needed in a hurry. To sterilize badly contaminated instruments he recommends 45-minute periods. (A pressure cooker is a good substitute for the hospital autoclave when instruments are needed for surgery in homes.)

When neither steam under pressure nor superheated water is available, boiling water is the best agency for sterilizing instruments. The longer the boiling period, the greater the likelihood that all organisms will be killed, but an arbitrary period of 30 to 45 minutes is commonly set in hospital practice. Even longer periods cannot be relied upon for the destruction of spores. The addition of sodium carbonate to the boiling water (to make a 2 per cent solution) increases the effectiveness of the boiling water.* Sterilization (more properly disinfection) of instruments with a chemical is the last resort and should be used only when other agents destroy the instruments. Walter states that formaldehyde solution will kill spores in 18 hours, vegetative forms in one-half hour, and he recommends the following solutions:†

Sodium tetraborate	50 gm.
Solution of Formaldehyde U.S.P.	100 cc.
Distilled water q.s. ad	1000 cc.

or

Sodium of Formaldehyde U.S.P.	130 gm.
Potassium nitrite	0.15 gm.
Sodium hydroxide	0.012 gm.
Ethyl alcohol (C.P.) (95%) q.s. ad	1000 cc.

Care must be taken to remove the solutions from instruments with sterile distilled water since formaldehyde irritates tissue.

Sharp Instruments. The cutting edges of knives and shearing edges of scissors are dulled in the sterilizing processes described for less sharp instruments. Electrically heated aluminum trays for the dry sterilization of knives, scissors, and needles are recommended by Walter. The instruments are held at a temperature of 160° C (320° F) for one hour. If an ordinary hot-air sterilizer (oven type) is used, a four-hour exposure is suggested.

---

* Sodium carbonate 2 per cent and sodium hydroxide in a concentration of 0.1 per cent in the sterilizer retard corrosion. This is also lessened if instruments are put into the sterilizer after the water boils.

† Walter, Carl W.: *op. cit.*, pp. 27, 34.

When sharp instruments are autoclaved, dulling of the edge can be lessened by submerging them in shallow trays containing diethylene glycol with a 10 to 20 per cent water content and exposing them to a temperature of 121° C (249.8° F) for 30 minutes. To decontaminate used sharp instruments place them on a soft material and boil them in a 2 per cent solution of sodium carbonate for 15 minutes. Chemical disinfection is always an undesirable substitute for moist heat, but it may be the only means at hand. Formaldehyde solutions such as those just mentioned are similar to commercial preparations sold for this purpose. For the destruction of spores an exposure of decontaminated and clean instruments to the solution for 18 hours is advocated. Since spore-forming organisms are found in the intestinal tracts of the majority of persons there is always the likelihood that spores are present on even the "cleanest" instrument. Many solutions formerly used for the disinfection of instruments are either ineffective or corrosive, or both. The merits of any chemical disinfectant should be carefully investigated before it is adopted.

Telescopic Instruments.   Proctoscopes, cystoscopes, bronchoscopes, and all instruments containing lenses must be disinfected in such a way that the lens and the substance used to hold it in place are not affected. In some such instruments the cement used is destroyed by heat, and the lens is affected by minerals in boiling-water sterilizers. Some of the newer "scopes" have been designed to withstand steam sterilization, but unless this is known to be the case such instruments should be disinfected with formaldehyde gas, an aqueous solution of formalin, or Zephiran, prepared in such a way as to discourage corrosion. The chemical must be removed with sterile water before the instrument is used, and this must be done with particular care when the solution is an irritating one, such as formalin.

Equipment for Injections.   The very considerable amount of time consumed in preparing and administering hypodermic injections has led to studies in the economics involved. A recent report by Robert R. Cadmus[10] (discussed in this text on page 720) demonstrates the advantage of using a presterilized and assembled syringe and needle, with, in some cases, the drug in the syringe. The entire unit is cheap enough to be disposable in the case of "Ampins."* Until such materials are adopted, the selection, care, and preparation of hypodermic equipment will represent a major problem of the hospital.

Needles.   Hollow needles used for the injection of fluids into the tissues are available in a wide range of sizes. They are scaled according to their length and diameter. Figure 35 shows the actual size of commonly used needles of this type. Points (or bevels) should be short or long, according to the purposes for which the instrument is used. Needles are made of platinum, iridium, gold, nickel, steel with chromium plate, and stainless steel. Platinum and gold needles are too costly for ordinary use; some metals are so soft that it is difficult to make and preserve a sufficiently sharp point. Stainless steel is relatively noncorrosive, takes a good point, is strong, moderately flexible, and probably makes the most desirable needle.

* Strong, Cobb and Co., Inc. (Professional Products Division), Cleveland, Ohio.

No instruments require more meticulous attention than needles. The bore is so fine that it becomes hopelessly clogged unless cleaned each time it is used; the points of needles are so delicate that the slightest contact with a hard surface may bend them backward, or produce a "burr."

After use, cold water and a hot detergent solution should be forced through the needle with a mechanical washer or a syringe. Alcohol, 95 per cent, or ether removes fats or oils and, since they evaporate readily, tends to leave the needle

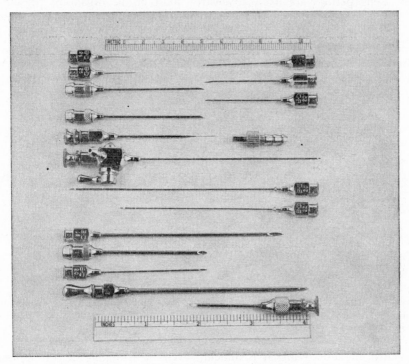

Figure 35.   Various needles of different gauges and lengths, and several adapters. (*Left, top to bottom*) Intradermal and hypodermic needles; two intravenous needles; Lindemann needle; needle and stopcock, used in venous pressure; three aspirating needles; trocar and cannula. (*Right, top to bottom*) Three intramuscular needles; adapter; two needles used in infiltration anesthesia; biopsy needle. (Courtesy of Becton, Dickinson & Co., Rutherford, N. J., and Clay-Adams Co., New York City.)

dry. If it is to be stored, however, the needle should be dried with motorized suction, a syringe, or a Brunet drier.

The temper of the needle is tested by flexing the shaft. If brittle, a break usually occurs at the junction of the shaft and hub. The point is examined with a magnifying glass, and if it is dull it should be honed on an oiled Arkansas stone, or in a sharpening device, with care to preserve the bevel. A cake of fine abrasive, such as Bon Ami, is a fairly satisfactory substitute for an Arkansas stone. A piece of chamois stretched over hoops is useful in testing the smoothness of needle punctures. By drawing the point over the skin the worker can also discover "burrs." After honing, needles should be cleaned with ether or alcohol to remove particles of the abrasive. Wire stylets are used in needles during storage periods to keep the bores open. The practice of oiling needles is undesirable, for, if the oil is not completely removed, it prevents the thorough penetration of bacteria by steam or water during sterilization.

Needles are frequently sterilized by boiling for periods varying from 5 to 20 minutes. Long periods are likely to destroy most of the organisms present, but more effective methods include the use of dry heat at high temperatures or

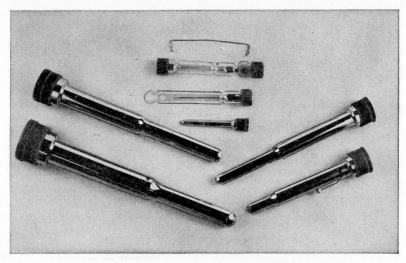

Figure 36. Various containers for sterilized needles that protect end of needle during sterilization and storage. (Courtesy of Becton, Dickinson & Co., Rutherford, N. J., and Clay-Adams Co., New York City.)

steam under pressure. While it is difficult, even by wrapping in soft fabrics, to prevent injury to the points of needles during the boiling process, this is easily done in an oven, or autoclave. One method of needle sterilization and storage is suspension of a needle in a glass tube made with a constriction near the top (see Fig. 36). The tube is covered with a cap that permits steam, or hot air, to enter the tube. An impervious cap may be used but this is put in place at the end of the sterilizing period. (It is convenient to store sterile needles in glass tubes because they are visible. This facilitates the selection of the proper size.) Sterile needles are prepared commercially in tubes with airtight caps applied before sterilization. A measured quantity of water is put into the tube, exactly enough to create sufficient steam for the sterilization of the needle and to be entirely evaporated in the process, leaving the needle dry.

It is common to see stylets left in needles during sterilization, but Walter thinks that the needle is weakened by an electrolytic action between the needle and the stylet. He, therefore, advocates removing the stylet before sterilization.

Even if an effective solution can be found, and there is sufficient time for soaking needles in it, chemical disinfection of needles is unsatisfactory because it is difficult to remove the irritating drug from the bore of the needle. Alcohol, still commonly used for sterilization of hypodermic and pricking needles used in collecting blood samples, is ineffective. The fear of spreading diseases, such as infectious hepatitis, by unclean needles has led some laboratory staffs to adopt the use of an inexpensive commercially sterilized dart, or needle, that is discarded after a single use.

Suture needles used in the repair of tissues are made in many shapes and sizes. In order to prevent undue trauma when taking stitches they must have sharp points; the shafts may be rounded or more or less triangular with cutting edges. The needle selected by the surgeon depends upon the nature of the tissue to be repaired, the size and position of the wound, and the kind of suture with which the needle is to be threaded. Suture needles are treated in the same manner described for other sharp instruments.

Devices for threading and holding needles are made so that all surfaces coming in contact with the needle, suture, patient, or surgeon can be autoclaved or boiled.

5. STERILIZATION OF SUTURES

Varieties. Catgut, silkworm gut, kangaroo tendon, horse hair, nylon, cellulose yarn (Fortizan), steel wire, linen, cotton, and silk thread and linen tape are some materials used for sutures.[11, 12] In the past, if a stitch was buried in a wound, an absorbable suture, such as gut suture, was used; today nonabsorbable sutures are frequently used internally. When sutures are placed in the skin, a fine suture, such as silk thread or horse hair, is employed, because it leaves only a small scar. The surgeon indicates the kind of suture he expects to use, but other workers prepare his materials in most situations.

Sterile sutures, put up in sealed tubes or vials, may be purchased from manufacturers. The tube contains a solution that helps to maintain aseptic conditions within the tube and also keeps the suture moist and pliable. In some cases suture materials are purchased unsterile, and later treated by the hospital staff with moist heat, or a combination of moist heat and chemicals.

Sterilization of Sutures. It is obvious that sutures, more than all other surgical supplies, should be absolutely sterile, because they are left embedded in all types of tissue.

If purchased in vials from reputable manufacturers, the sutures should be free from microorganisms. In order to make it possible to handle the vials with sterile gloves and to prevent contamination of the sutures when the container is opened, the outside of the tube must be sterilized immediately before the operation. Most suture material may be subjected to heat without destroying it, but chemicals must be used for some types. Tubes of suture material are marked boilable or nonboilable. To ensure sterility of the outer surface of the tubes of the latter type, after washing them with soap and water, they should be soaked in effective chemical disinfectants for several days, making sure that the tubes are immersed.

Tubes of suture material may be kept in labeled jars containing an alcohol and formalin solution as described on page 239.

Sutures, other than gut, are purchased untubed and are made ready for the surgeon in the hospital. The suture material is cut in convenient lengths, twisted into a hank, and laid in a glass tube that can be wrapped and autoclaved. Just before the operation the hank may be untwisted by the "scrub nurse" and laid in the folds of a sterile towel, with the ends protruding so that they may be seen and grasped easily. If the kinds of needles desired are known by the person who prepares for the operation they may be threaded and needles and sutures run loosely through a strip of bandage that is packaged and autoclaved. Almost every kind of suture is now available with a disposable needle fused or threaded on it, the whole presterilized.

Woven sutures should be hydrated, or run through moistened fingers before autoclaving. It is important to wax fine sutures for ease of handling by the surgeon. Beeswax is recommended because it adsorbs moisture and therefore does not interfere with sterilization of the suture by steam.

6. CARE AND STERILIZATION OF RUBBER, SHELLACKED, AND PLASTIC ARTICLES

General Rules. Articles made of natural rubber and its synthetic substitutes are so varied in kind and quality that it is difficult to make any rules that apply to all of them. They should be purchased only after their nature and durability have been investigated, and the use to which they will be put considered. Natural and synthetic rubber deteriorate with age, exposure to heat, light, moisture, and certain chemicals. Since hydrocarbons are soluble in each other, and natural rubber is a hydrocarbon, other hydrocarbons, such as benzene, kerosene, petroleum jelly, and mineral oil, literally dissolve rubber tubing, sheeting, and syringes. Cresols and the halogens, such as chlorine, are also destructive. While heat is harmful, many synthetic rubbers, as for example "Koroseal," "Cavolite,"* and "Neoprene," have been developed to withstand heat. Catheters made from them are usable after 75 to 100 autoclaving periods. Whenever possible rubber articles that survive high temperatures should be chosen since chemical disinfection is so much less reliable than sterilization with heat.

Heat is said to be more destructive if air is present. For this reason rubber goods should be so packaged and placed in the autoclave that air cannot be trapped in the package. Walter recommends the upper two thirds of the sterilizing chamber for rubber goods in order to avoid "residual air." Because rubber offers little resistance to penetration by steam, short periods of 15 minutes at 121° C (249.8° F) have been recommended by some authorities. Other writers take the

* Davis and Geck, Inc., Brooklyn, N. Y.

position that when a standard sterilizing period is adopted that is adequate for all materials fewer risks are involved.

When it is necessary to use chemical disinfection for rubber articles, Walter recommends an alkaline solution of formalin for two hours. Chemical disinfectants for synthetic products must be chosen with reference to their composition. Often, rubber articles must be decontaminated and always cleaned before they are packaged for autoclaving. Forcible cleaning with a mechanical washer is especially important for tubing. An attachment to the faucet and motorized suction may be used in the place of a mechanical washer to rinse tubing, to draw a detergent through the tubing, and to dry it. (See Fig. 37.)
It is difficult to get enough force with a syringe, which is the only tool available in some cases.

A few texts recommend the addition of salt as a preservative to the water in which rubber is boiled. The writer has not found this claim substantiated by chemical principles or laboratory tests.

Rubber surfaces in contact tend to adhere; it is, therefore, desirable to store rubber articles in such a way as to prevent folding, kinking, or flattening of rubber receptacles. Rubber equipment should be dried, powdered, and stored in cool dry closets. It should be purchased in quantities needed currently to avoid deterioration from aging. Dispensing rubber articles from a central supply service reduces the likelihood of overstocking. Because of its tendency to deterioration, rubber supplies should always be examined for defects before use. Needless to

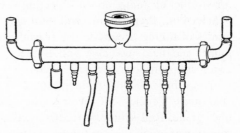

Figure 37. Tomac tube and needle cleaner to be attached to a cold-water faucet so that water is forced through eight items at the same time. The carefully ground spigots are tapered and grooved to accommodate any tubing up to ½ in. and to fit hypodermic needles as securely as a syringe. The 90-deg connections at the ends of the main tube make it easy to flush tubing or needles with saline or distilled water after pressure rinsing. When not in use, the spigots are protected by individual screw caps. (*Note:* Machines are now available that still further reduce the manual labor in cleaning tubing, needles, and syringes.) (Courtesy of American Hospital Supply Corp., Evanston, Ill.)

say, they should not be sterilized in a vessel with sharp instruments. Holes in rubber can be patched and vulcanized, but this is time consuming and the life of the article is shortened.

Gutta percha, a rubber-like substance, is destroyed by heat. Shellac, a natural resin, is used to make woven tubes stiff and waterproof. Such tubes, called "gum elastic," "woven," or "shellac catheters," are used in place of rubber catheters when a small stiff instrument is needed. Shellac is melted by heat and alcohol. Gutta percha and shellac tubes should be disinfected with aqueous solutions.

In many situations there is neither the personnel nor facilities for care of rubber supplies. Fortunately, many paper and plastic substitutes are available, often at such low cost that they can be considered "expendable." Plastics are developing rapidly—they and their derivatives—some of which are resins, proteins, and cellulose. Medical workers should be alert to the possibilities of improving procedures through the use of new equipment.

Walter tabulates 36 chief types of plastics used in hospitals and indicates that there are many more to be considered. In his table the resistance of each type to heat and solvents is shown.[13] Some plastics withstand temperatures of 160° C (320° F); others are distorted by a temperature of 50° C (122° F). Many are soluble in alcohol, esters, ketones, and acids. Alkalis attack a number of them. Before subjecting a plastic to a disinfecting process its reaction to the disinfecting agent should be determined. Most supply houses furnish with the articles directions for storing, cleaning, and disinfecting each item.

Selection, Preparation, and Storage of Tubing.   There are many types and grades of tubing. Ready-to-use plastic "expendable" tubing is convenient for office, home, and field medicine and is the type usually sold in the commercially pre-pared infusion sets. Sterile catheters and tubes for intestinal drainage and other purposes may be bought in plastic also. When a good sterilizing service is avail-able, most agencies still prefer to use rubber tubing. It is economical to purchase a high grade. Red synthetic rubber is used more than any other type, but the semi-transparent gum rubber tubing is preferred for parenteral therapy because it is more possible to see foreign bodies inside and it is flexible and resilient. Black rubber tubing gets hard and brittle most quickly.

Tubing is available in a wide range of sizes from less than 3 to 100 mm or more. Sizes of catheters in English and French scales are shown in Figure 38. The style of tubing is chosen according to the special need. When it is exposed to force, or suction, a heavy-walled tubing is desirable; when great flexibility is wanted a thinner wall is indicated. When a very small diameter combined with stiffness is required, a tube reinforced with a thread and shellac is chosen, or a plastic that answers these specifications. While rubber can be stiffened slightly by chilling it, plastics are very much affected by temperature and may, for this reason, prove very versatile in their uses, and less costly than woven, shellacked tubes.

Sterilization of tubes follows the general rules already discussed. *Rubber tubing to be used for parenteral therapy requires special handling.* It must be washed under pressure for one minute with detergents, such as "Haemosol," and distilled water allowed to "trickle" through it for ten minutes. Infusion solutions flowing through *new rubber tubing* have been found to contain products from the rubber that are believed to be toxic to the patient. Manufacturers of infusion sets are careful to purify the tubing they sell prepared for this purpose, but ordinary tubing must be treated to correct the toxic factor. The tubing is boiled in a 10 per cent solution of sodium hydroxide for 30 minutes, the chemical action being hastened by heat. Some authorities recommend autoclaving the tubing in the alkali. It is essential that the sodium hydroxide be thoroughly removed from the tubing. Water from a mechanical washer or the tap should be allowed to run over and through the tubing for several minutes, and distilled water used for the last 10 minutes. The neutrality of the tubing must be tested by adding a few drops of

French scale sizes	Approximate sizes in English scale	Actual diameter in millimeters
8	5	$2\frac{2}{3}$ mm
10	6	$3\frac{1}{3}$ mm
12	7	4 mm
14	8	$4\frac{2}{3}$ mm
16	9	$5\frac{1}{3}$ mm
18	10	6 mm
20	11	$6\frac{2}{3}$ mm
22	12	$7\frac{1}{3}$ mm
24	14	8 mm
26	16	$8\frac{2}{3}$ mm
28	17	$9\frac{1}{3}$ mm
30	18	10 mm
32	20	$10\frac{2}{3}$ mm
34	22	$11\frac{1}{3}$ mm
36	24	12 mm

Figure 38. Scale for rubber catheters; sizes in the French scale, approximate sizes in English scale, and actual diameters in millimeters are given. (Courtesy of Meinecke and Co., New York City.)

phenolphthalein to the rinsing water; if the alkali has been removed, the water remains colorless.

To prevent kinking and to facilitate selection of the proper type of tube, short lengths, such as catheters, may be sterilized in glass tubes by steam under pressure. In case the glass tubes are capped with a paper cap or other type of cover that protects the neck, they may be considered sterile for periods of a week or even longer. When it is not possible to see the caliber and length of the tube, packages of sterile tubing must be labeled. Standard scales of tubing are shown in Figure 38. Long lengths of rubber tubing should be coiled in a deep tray of adequate size to avoid kinking, or wound on a special rack designed to prevent sharp angles in the turns. Distilled and sterile (pyrogen-free) water should moisten the inside of the tubing to make steam for sterilization. Otherwise, trapped air is likely to fill the tubing. Decontamination by boiling is safe for medical asepsis and the method of choice for flexible rubber tubing.

Hard rubber tips used in cleaning and medicating body cavities, such as the nose and throat, vagina, and rectum, are molded into special shapes. It is essential that the original shape of these tips be maintained. Heat softens the rubber, reduces a curved to a straight tip, and roughens the polished surface. For these reasons, such instruments are disinfected with chemicals.

The selection of chemical disinfectants for woven, shellacked, and plastic tubing is influenced by the type of material from which each is made. The manufacturer usually indicates methods that will not destroy the instrument. Most plastic tubing is so cheap that it is "disposable" and is usually purchased in sterile packages.

Rubber Gloves. Since they are one of the heavy items of expense in hospitals, and a major factor in surgical asepsis, rubber gloves deserve special care. Gloves should be washed on the hands of the wearer just before they are removed to prevent the adherence of blood and other organic materials. The decontamination process should be reduced to the minimum time essential for safety since heat and handling shorten the life of gloves. Punctures are said to occur as often as once in every three times gloves are used. Holes may be patched and vulcanized, but the glove is still weakened. Tears and holes are discovered by submerging the glove, filled with air, in water. Bubbles will pass up through the water if the glove is not intact. Clean gloves are arranged on driers of various designs to drain, then turned and allowed to dry on the other side. Air in motion hastens drying, but hot air deteriorates gloves.

Steam under pressure is agreed to be the best method of sterilizing gloves. Boiling water or chemicals are used only when autoclaves are not available. When boiling water or chemicals are used, gloves are transferred from the sterilizing medium to a basin of sterile water. They are drawn on after the hands are thoroughly scrubbed and the excess water is forced out before the cuffs are turned up over the wrist. The use of dry gloves is obviously safer and pleasanter.

In order to prevent adherence of the opposing surfaces of gloves and the formation of air pockets, a piece of gauze is placed in the palms of the gloves. In the dry method gloves are powdered lightly to make it easy to draw them on. A special powdering chamber is available that protects the worker from inhaling the powder. Other machinery is now available to cut down manual effort in processing gloves.

C. Marshall Lee, Jr.,[14] and others[15] have reported that tissue irritation in wearers and patients has resulted from some powders used on gloves. "Bio-Sorb,"* a trade name for a mixture of amylase and amylase pectinates, is recommended as non-irritating although all powders should be used sparingly and/or rinsed from sterile gloves before the surgeon handles the patient. In addition to the powder on the gloves, the wearer will usually find it necessary to powder his hands before drawing on gloves.

Because steam cannot penetrate a mass of powder in a reasonable length of time the powder provided for the hands (about 1 gm or ¼ dram) should be distributed in the meshes of a gauze sponge. This is placed in a cuff and sterilized in each package of gloves.

The method of packaging gloves in cotton envelopes and outer covers is shown in Figure 31.

When gloves are placed in the autoclave they must be so arranged that the thumb is uppermost and that there are free horizontal paths for air clearance.

7. CARE AND STERILIZATION OF GLASSWARE

General Principles. The necessity of sterilizing glass articles used in medical care and all public services makes it important to select a hard glass that is resistant to heat and mechanical shock. This type is a borosilicate glass; Pyrex glass, an example. Glass used for solutions should be alkaline free; soft glass may change the pH of liquids in contact with it and start a series of chemical changes. To reduce to a minimum reactions between glass and other materials, and to facilitate cleaning, glass should have a hard smooth surface, or be properly annealed. Such a surface is relatively impervious to the action of water or steam and may be sterilized in the autoclave; ground glass as used in syringes is very susceptible to erosion by water or steam and should be sterilized with dry heat. Soaps and detergents erode the smooth surface of glass and attack ground-glass surfaces readily. Brushes and abrasives of all sorts are to be avoided in cleaning glass. *Immediate rinsing under cold running water to remove organic soil from glass articles is essential in prolonging their usefulness.* If blood or body discharges dry on glass they are dislodged with difficulty. Rinsing with force, as in a mechanical washer, is the preferred method of cleaning glass. Walter recommends "Haemosol," "Calgonite," or "Calgolac" as detergents in such washers. Contact with the detergent should be limited to the time essential for cleanliness. Glassware used for parenteral therapy should be rinsed in freshly distilled water and inverted on racks to drain. If a flask or a beaker is clean, distilled water leaves an unbroken film on the surface; if there is a greasy soil, the film will be broken and droplets form.

When foggy, cloudy glassware is caused by alkali earth soaps formed by the

* Johnson & Johnson, New Brunswick, N. J.

interaction of water, or soil containing calcium and manganese, and the washing agent (a soap or detergent), avoidance of the film depends upon: (1) prompt removal of soil with forcible rinsing, (2) the choice of high-grade glassware, and (3) a good "water softener" and detergent.

Porcelain and fritted glass filters are cleaned with a hot solution of 0.5 per cent of sodium nitrate and sodium chlorate in concentrated sulfuric acid. This is removed by running distilled water through the filter in the opposite direction from the acid, and until the rinse is neutral to litmus paper.

Heat-resistant glass will withstand steam under pressure used in sterilization and dry heat around 160° C (320° F). Flaming is tolerated and water may be boiled in Pyrex flasks, but exposure to sudden wide variation in temperatures is likely to crack even a high grade of glass. Soft glass breaks readily in extremes of temperature, or with rapid changes. Glass containers will be dry when taken from the autoclave if they are inverted during the sterilizing period and if they are preheated to reduce to a minimum condensation of steam on the glass. Leaving the door of the autoclave ajar at the end of the sterilizing period for 30 minutes dries the contents. If vessels must be sterilized in the upright position air trapped in them will prevent steam penetration of all surfaces. A small amount of distilled water in the vessel, which is converted into steam, will force out the air. One cubic centimeter of water will produce 865 cc of steam and will displace an equivalent amount of air.

Syringes.   Metal, glass, plastic, and rubber are all used alone, or combined, in syringes. There are standard designs with standard names. Medical workers should be able to differentiate between the common type of syringes illustrated in Figure 39 and know the commercial name for each.

In sterilizing *Asepto syringes,* remove the rubber bulb from the glass barrel. This facilitates penetration of the sterilizing agent and keeps the rubber from sticking to the glass, as it is likely to do when very hot. The bulb and the glass portion should be wrapped in the same package to avoid difficulty later in fitting them together, which is accomplished more easily if the neck of the rubber bulb is moistened. The woven plunger of the *Triumph syringe* also is difficult to fit into the glass barrel unless it is wet. In sterilizing this type of syringe, the two parts should be separated but wrapped in the same cover.

Luer syringes are costly and perishable because of their shape, the ground-glass surfaces, and the handling and high temperatures to which they are exposed. They must be made of alkaline-free and heat-resistant glass.

All tips to syringes should be of a standard size in order that they may be used with standard needles. Tips that are not centered in the end of the barrel are called *eccentric.* Syringes with eccentric tips are preferred by some surgeons for injecting veins. *Luer-Lok syringes* are distinguished by a metal tip made in such a way as to lock the needle on the syringe. Reputable firms have been careful to make tips and needles of standard patterns, so that all needles fit either the slip type of tip or the locking tip. A *Kaufman syringe* is one that has a second outlet on the side to which rubber tubing may be attached either for draining the syringe or for the injection of a solution.

Rinsing immediately after use is a big factor in lengthening the life of a syringe. If this is not done cleaning is difficult, and the barrel is likely to stick to the plunger. Stuck syringes may be forced apart with a special device. If such an instrument is not available, boiling the syringes for 10 minutes in a 25 per cent aqueous solution of glycerin is effective, if the parts are separated while they are hot. Soaking in a weak solution of nitric acid may be used also. If the needle is

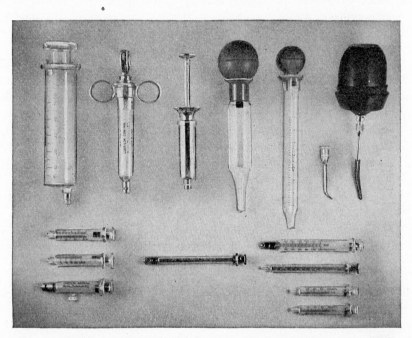

Figure 39. Various types of syringes. (*Top, left to right*) 50-cc eccentric tip, graduated glass syringe; Luer-Lok glass syringe with metal tip and metal finger rings; all metal irrigating syringe with flanged finger holder; Asepto glass syringe with detachable rubber bulb, 1 oz mark indicated; graduated irrigating glass syringe with detachable rubber bulb; curved irrigating needle; injection syringe with hypodermic needle and hard-rubber tip. (*Bottom, left*) Hypodermic syringe with center glass tip, 20 m; hypodermic syringe with center glass tip, 25 m; Luer-Lok hypodermic syringe. (*Bottom, center*) Insulin, long tuberculin type, blue plunger syringe with metal tip. (*Bottom, right*) Insulin, 125-unit glass syringe (3 cc); insulin, long tuberculin type, blue plunger syringe with glass tip; insulin, short type, glass syringe with glass tip (80 units); insulin, short type, glass syringe with glass tip (40 units). (Courtesy of Becton, Dickinson & Co., Rutherford, N. J., and Clay-Adams Co., New York City.)

stuck to the hub of the syringe, immersing it in boiling water will make the metal expand and leave the glass tip. Boiling in the glycerin solution is likewise effective.

Blood and organic matter may be removed with "Haemosol." Soaps and detergents are erosive to ground glass and should be avoided if possible.

Syringes have the same number on the barrel and the plunger in order that they can be easily matched. Some manufacturers make syringes so that the plungers of a given size fit any barrel of a corresponding size. In any case, if part of a syringe is broken the other part should be saved since most supply houses can replace the broken member through their repair service.

In cleaning and sterilizing syringes, barrels and plungers that are paired should be kept together to avoid wasting time later in matching parts. Some authorities say that the plunger and barrel should always be separated (but kept in the same package) during the sterilizing period; others maintain that if the glass has the same expansion coefficient the syringe may be sterilized with the plunger in place in a hot-air sterilizer. Steam, or chemical sterilization, is more effective if the parts are separated because the contact with the sterilizing agent is more complete.

Sterilization by hot air is the least destructive of the effective methods, according to Walter; chemical sterilization should be used as a last resort because it is the least reliable method. Walton F. Dutton and George B. Lake[16] state that a well-made syringe withstands 150 hours of continuous sterilization. They advise against boiling syringes in distilled water, calling attention to the chemical affinity of water for silicate. There is some silicate in natural waters, but none in distilled waters. If syringes are boiled in distilled water, silicate is taken from the glass; this results in a slow deterioration of the syringe.

James E. McCartney[17] reports his satisfaction with the use of a glassine-paper envelope in which an assembled syringe with a needle is autoclaved in large quantities for an active clinic. The point of the needle is protected with a piece of cellophane drinking tube. Glass or metal tubes that leave the needle hanging free offer better protection and are more easily opened, but the initial outlay for equipment is high.

All metal syringes should be cleaned by the same process described for glass syringes and should be sterilized with other metal instruments. While metal syringes have the advantage of being unbreakable, they are not widely used because they are expensive, are more difficult to keep clean, and the metal reacts with a greater number of drugs than does glass.

Thermometers.   Thermometry is based on the well-established physical principle that gases, liquids, and solids expand when heated and contract when cooled. Instruments for determining the temperature of the living body, water, drugs, foods, materials of all sorts, and for measuring the temperature of the air in rooms, oxygen tents, ovens, and sterilizing chambers usually consist of a scaled glass tube that has a liquid inside the bore of the tube. (Metal coils that expand when heated also are used, but the care of these is rarely one of the nurse's problems.)

Mercury, a liquid metal, is ordinarily used because it is very heavy and has a low coefficient of expansion, so that a short scale measures a wide range of temperatures. Lighter liquids are used in thermometers made to show temperatures of room air, because the variation in room temperatures is not ordinarily very great, and the reading is taken more easily when a slight change of temperature causes a marked fluctuation in the level of the liquid. The inner chamber or cavity that holds the liquid is larger at the bottom of the thermometer and acts as a reservoir.

Self-registering thermometers have a constriction in the bore above the reservoir that supports the column of liquid as it rises in the bore of the tube and keeps it from falling back into the reservoir as the instrument cools; vigorous shaking or jarring is required to make the liquid fall to the bulb or reservoir. This type of instrument is used for measuring body temperatures; chemical, dairy, and room thermometers are not self-registering and must be read while they are surrounded by the medium whose temperature they are employed to measure.

In using, cleaning, and sterilizing thermometers, the worker should remember that the instrument must not be exposed to temperatures above those which the thermometer is designed to measure because the liquid expands beyond the capacity of the inner bore and as a result may break the glass. Thermometers used to measure body temperatures have a short scale from 33.3° to 43.3° C (92° to 110° F), and therefore must not be washed in hot water or sterilized by heat. Some chemical thermometers and infusion thermometers register temperatures as high as 100° to 150° C (212° to 302° F). Such instruments may be sterilized by boiling, or in the case of a thermometer registering 150° C, it may be sterilized by steam under pressure. Infusion thermometers, for measuring the temperature of fluid flowing into body tissues, have been made with a high-registration point, so that they may be adequately sterilized for surgical procedures.

To clean used thermometers, rinse in cold water, wash in a tepid detergent solution, and sterilize with a suitable process. In medical asepsis, thermometers may be treated with exposure to sunlight or a chemical, preferably an aqueous solution of Zephiran 1:1000; for surgical disinfection of low-registration thermometers, soak them in Zephiran 1:1000 for several hours and rinse thoroughly in sterile distilled water. Thermometers that have sufficiently high-registration points to permit autoclaving may be placed in a glass vial or tube, capped, and sterilized. If boiling water is used, special care must be taken to wrap the instrument in a soft fabric to prevent breakage.

Hospital workrooms should be provided with a clean thermometer for testing the temperature of unsterile (but medically uncontaminated) solutions and a sterile thermometer for testing sterile solutions. The former may be kept dry, preferably exposed to the air in a clean area of the workroom; the sterile thermometer and its holder should be appropriately disinfected once every 24 hours and left standing in a chemical disinfectant. Alcohol is most commonly used for this purpose because it evaporates readily and therefore does not introduce a foreign substance into the solution to be tested; Zephiran and other chemicals are more effective, and if the disinfectant is drained from the thermometer it is not likely to affect materially the solution to be tested.

8. PREPARATION OF ENAMELED WARE AND STAINLESS STEEL FOR USE IN SURGERY

Enameled Ware. Many different qualities of enameled ware are on the market. The better grades are less affected by heat and mechanical blows than the poorer ones. The finish on all enameled ware is eroded by heat, mercuric salts, acids, alkalis, and many other chemicals. Even the best qualities are subject to chipping. Generally speaking, enameled ware is an unsatisfactory material for surgical procedures, because it is soon destroyed by the repeated exposure to high temperatures. Sterile forceps used for handling enameled ware should have the gripping ends protected by rubber; otherwise, there is danger of chipping the enamel.

Stainless-steel Utensils. Better grades of stainless steel are moderately heavy and are not easily dented; they are not visibly affected by high temperatures and are resistant to corrosion. Since mercury preparations react with most metals, it is wiser to use glass vessels for solutions of mercury salts; however, stainless-steel utensils are suitable for almost every other purpose. Because it is easily cleaned, heat resistant, and unbreakable, stainless steel is the material of choice for cups, bowls, and trays used in surgery.

Steam under pressure is the most desirable sterilizing agent for equipment of this type when it is used for surgical purposes. If autoclaves and hot-air sterilizers are not available, boiling water is the next best medium. Enameled and stainless-steel articles are packaged in cloth or paper covers, as discussed on page 233.

9. STERILIZATION OF SURGICAL DRESSINGS, CLOTHING, AND DRAPING FABRICS

Standardization of Dressings. A survey of hospital practice made under the auspices of the American College of Surgeons between 1928 and 1930 showed that 5000 designs of surgical dressings existed and that the same article was called by many different names. Dressings were frequently made by hand, and possibly three or more variations of the same article to comply with preferences of particular surgeons. The investigating committee recommended standardizations of the design of and nomenclature for surgical dressings. It further recommended machine-made products because they are cheaper and more uniform. No attempt was made to standardize all dressings, but specifications for the most common types were set up; the majority of manufactured products are now made according to these specifications.

Varieties of Dressings. Cotton, silk, wool, wood, and plastic fibers are used in making dressings. Wood fibers are cheap, and when made into a fluffy mass known as *cellucotton* they are absorbent, light, and satisfactory as compresses. Since it has little strength, cellucotton is usually covered with gauze to preserve the shape of the compress. By unit of weight, wood pulp absorbs more water than cotton and does not get so soggy or matted as absorbent cotton. For the sake of economy, this type of dressing should be used whenever it is adequate. Cotton fibers are absorbent if the natural oil is removed; if not, the fibers repel water.

Absorbent cotton is made into various sized sponges, and is a satisfactory material to use where friction is contraindicated. Absorbent cotton is wound around the ends of slender sticks to make applicators. Pads of absorbent cotton covered with gauze are used over draining areas if a softer material than cellu-cotton is needed. Generally speaking, absorbent cotton is cheaper than gauze, but since the fibers may be caught and held in crusts on wounds it is necessary to cover it with gauze when it is used for dressings.

Gauze is manufactured in various qualities, the price varying with the closeness of the weave. Sponges and compresses made of gauze are expensive, and there-fore, whenever possible, gauze is combined with wood pulp or absorbent cotton. Such dressings are sometimes referred to as *combines*. Gauze is folded to make dressings of many shapes and sizes. To reduce the cost of surgical dressings, used gauze may be "salvaged." This means that soiled dressings are sterilized, washed clean, and used again, perhaps for different purposes. In making gauze dressings, great care is taken to fold all raw edges inside since this material ravels easily. Ravelings may cling to wounded surfaces, may even get inside wounds and act as foreign bodies, delay the healing process, and foster infection.

Because the cotton fibers of gauze are harsh, slightly irritating, and tend to become matted in discharges of the wound, some surgeons place a layer of thin silk (usually China silk) directly over an incision. Silk is lintless, and since it is very soft and closely woven it can be removed with little damage to the new cells forming in the healing process. Some surgeons prefer to place a piece of aluminum foil directly over the wound.

Absorbent dressings (pads, "combines") are often made with an impervious paper, or cellulose layer, to protect bedding and clothing from discharges.

Drains for wounds are made of a fine mesh gauze, of rubber tissue and tubing, or of gauze in combination with rubber. The gauze may be impregnated with a chemical, such as iodoform.

Combinations of gauze and adhesive plaster made into sterile dressings in a great variety of shapes and sizes are available. They can be obtained in flesh color and are especially useful for face and hand dressings applied in offices and clinics.

Sterilization of Surgical Dressings. Attention has already been called to the importance of wrapping surgical dressings loosely, so as to allow free penetration of steam. Dressings may be wrapped singly, collected into small packages, and covered with paper or cotton wrappers, or they may be sterilized in cans and drums. The method of preparation depends upon the use to which the dressings will be put. If used in large quantities over a period of a few hours, drums and cans are appropriate; if used individually by a great number of persons, the contents of a can or drum are liable to contamination, and in this case small packages are more satisfactory. Dry dressings must be sterilized by steam under pressure. In emergencies outside hospitals, sponges are boiled and used wet, or wrung as dry as possible with sterile forceps or gloved hands. If a dry aseptic dress-ing is necessary in surgical emergencies in homes, a fabric may be made fairly safe by ironing it with a very hot iron. A pressure cooker is the best home substitute for an autoclave in sterilizing all types of surgical equipment, including dressings. Materials that hold water can be dried later in the oven.

Protection of the Operative Field. Sterile clothing is worn by the surgeon and his assistants in all major operations and in many minor surgical procedures. Protection of sterile equipment from unsterile tables is accomplished with sterile pads, towels, and sheets. The patient himself is covered with a large sterile sheet and the operative area surrounded with several thicknesses of sterile fabric. These articles, like all materials which come in contact with wounds, must be subjected to an effective sterilizing process.

Sterilization of Surgical Linen. The important points to remember in the sterilization of clothing, towels, and sheets are that bundles must not be too large or tightly packed and that all articles should be exposed sufficiently long to allow penetration of the steam throughout the bundle. It is not desirable to pack a drum with surgical linen because of the difficulty of securing complete penetration by steam. Articles should be folded so that corners and edges are visible when the package is opened; this facilitates handling sterile towels, sheets, and gowns in such a way that possibility of contamination of sterile areas is reduced to a minimum.

10. STERILIZATION OF OINTMENTS, OILS, AND GAUZE IN PETROLEUM JELLY

Containers. To prepare oily substances for sterilization, suitable containers must be chosen from the standpoint of size, appearance, efficiency in handling, and cost. Since large quantities of these materials are rarely used for one patient during a single dressing or operation, containers are ordinarily small. A container of sterile ointment once opened and exposed to the air is, theoretically at least, contaminated and the substance should be resterilized before it is used again. Small heat-resistant glass flasks covered with rubber or fluted paper caps are often employed for oils; tubes and small round metal boxes are used for ointments. Covered rectangular metal boxes are suitable containers for gauze in petroleum jelly (strips of gauze bandage, usually about 5 by 20 cm or 2 × 8 in. in size, covered with melted petroleum jelly). Each strip of bandage should be folded over at one end so that the corners can be easily grasped with sterile forceps in removing the preparation from the container.

Sterilization of Oils and Ointments. As steam does not penetrate oils and any bacteria present, if killed, are destroyed by dry heat, the importance of employing very high temperatures in sterilizing oily surgical supplies is obvious. A hot-air sterilizer should be used.

Walter says that it takes 230-minutes' exposure to dry heat at 160° C (320° F) to kill spores in shallow metal containers of gauze in petroleum jelly. This estimate includes the time required to bring the material to the sterilizing temperature.

While the filtration of bacteria from oils in pharmaceuticals is reported, the practice seems to be under question and does not seem to be a practical substitute for hot-air sterilization for surgical supplies.[18]

REFERENCES

1. American College of Surgeons: *Manual of Surgical Dressings.* The College, Chicago, Ill., 1930.
2. McCulloch, Ernest C.: *Disinfection and Sterilization,* 2nd ed. Lea & Febiger, Philadelphia, 1945.
3. Walter, Carl W.: *The Aseptic Treatment of Wounds.* The Macmillan Company, New York, 1948.
4. Nocka, Paul F., and Walter, Carl W.: "The New Central Supply Room at Peter Bent Brigham," *Hosp. Management,* **70**:37, (Sept.) 1950.
5. Zorn, Katharine: "Surgical Supply Service," *Am. J. Nursing,* **38**:643, (June) 1938; and personal communication, 1950.
6. Seibert, F. B.: "Fever-producing Substance Found in Some Distilled Waters," *Am. J. Physiol.,* **67**:90, (Dec.) 1923.
7. Walter, Carl W.: *op. cit.,* p. 276.
8. Lambert, John: "Control of Rust and Corrosion," *Canad. Hosp.,* **27**:72, (Aug.) 1950.
9. Walter, Carl W.: *op. cit.,* pp. 132, 143.
10. Cadmus, Robert R.: "Medication Cost Study," *Mod. Hosp.,* **75**:68, (Sept.) 1950.
11. Narat, Joseph K., et al.: "Fortizan (Regenerated Cellulose Yarn), A New Suture Material," *A.M.A. Arch. Surg.,* **60**:1218, (June) 1950.
12. Babcock, W. W.: "Metallic Sutures and Ligatures," *S. Clin. North America,* **27**:1535, (Dec.) 1947.
13. Walter, Carl W.: *op. cit.,* pp. 162-67.
14. Lee, C. Marshall, Jr., and Lehman, Edwin P.: "Non-Irritating Glove Powder," *Surg., Gynec. & Obst.,* **84**:689, (Apr.) 1947.
15. Postlethwait, R. W., et al.: "Talc Granuloma," *North Carolina M. J.,* **11**:247, (May) 1950.
16. Dutton, Walton F., and Lake, George B.: *Parenteral Therapy.* Charles C Thomas, Publisher, Springfield, Ill., 1936, pp. 12, 13, 55.
17. McCartney, James E.: "The Use of Transparent Film Envelope for a Syringe Service," *Lancet,* **1**:509, (Mar.) 1951.
18. Sykes, G., and Royce, A.: "The Removal of Bacteria from Oils by Filtration," *J. Pharm. & Pharmacol.,* **2**:639, (Oct.) 1950.

CHAPTER 9. OBSERVING, REPORTING, AND RECORDING OBSERVATIONS

1. **IMPORTANCE OF OBSERVATION IN ALL MEDICAL SCIENCES**
2. **RESPONSIBILITY OF THE NURSE**
3. **HOW AND WHAT THE NURSE OBSERVES**
4. **METHODS OF REPORTING AND RECORDING**

1. IMPORTANCE OF OBSERVATION IN ALL MEDICAL SCIENCES

In the whole realm of medical practice there is nothing so difficult as the diagnosis, and, obviously, nothing so essential to treatment. With all the modern laboratory aids at his disposal the physician finds no substitute for listening to the patient, for observation, and for analysis of his observations. The combination of these is "clinical judgment." Cyril M. MacBryde, in his text *Signs and Symptoms,* quotes a "master diagnostician" as saying, "Let me take the history and I will accept any good intern's word on the physical findings." Then he adds:

In other words, even today the accomplished physician can learn more in the majority of cases from what his patient says and the way he says it than from any other avenue of inquiry. . . . The physician today has many technics available to assist him in making accurate diagnoses. . . . However, without an understanding of the meaning of symptoms, how useless are these refined diagnostic technics! They are but tools which are only as valuable as the mind that directs them. . . . No mechanical measures can take the place of careful consideration of the patient's complaints.*

Clearly, this physician attaches great importance to what he can learn from the patient.

Diagnosis, prognosis, and therapy constitute the doctor's province. He carries this responsibility for observing accurately and developing a critical faculty or clinical judgment in treating the patient, but successful treatment usually depends on complementing the doctor's efforts with the work of others. So, likewise, must the nurse, the psychologist, the special therapist, the social worker, and all those who contribute to the total care of the patient develop the ability to learn about

* MacBryde, Cyril M. (ed.): *Signs and Symptoms: Their Clinical Interpretation,* 2nd ed. J. B. Lippincott & Co., Philadelphia, 1952, p. xi.

him by listening to him and studying his appearance and actions. The sum total of their findings and the continuous analysis of their observations are the basis for the initial and evolving plan of care.

2. RESPONSIBILITY OF THE NURSE

Of all the patient's medical attendants the nurse is with him most constantly. For this reason the quality of her observations and reports, written and oral, are of utmost importance. Her observations guide her primarily in assessing the patient's temporary and permanent limitations so that she may give adequate nursing care, but because nurses are in touch with the institutionalized patients around the clock, all other medical attendants have come to depend upon her observations. It is she who watches the patient in danger of hemorrhage, checking the pulse and blood pressure at brief intervals; she notes the signs and symptoms during labor, and it is she who gets the obstetrician there when he is needed; it is her vigilance and judgment that prevent self-destruction in the suicidal; it is the nurse who watches the heavily anesthetized postoperative patient. These examples suggest crises of a more or less exceptional nature; it is, on the other hand, impossible to enumerate the kinds of observations the nurse must make, nor can any limit be set to her value in the role of observer. Two nurses may be equally skillful with their hands; yet the first is outstanding in her clinical judgment and the other is a technician who, when she looks at the patient, notices only a small fraction of what the first nurse sees. Native ability and interest determine the quality of judgment, *but there is no substitute for experience in actual nursing.* The young nurse must reconcile herself to the idea that the capacity for detecting disabilities and perceiving slight changes in the patient's physical or emotional state, the ability to discriminate between the significant and inconsequential remark, and the art of reporting accurately and succinctly are built up gradually and increase with every year of nursing experience. She can add to the value of this nursing experience by going to medical and nursing clinics, when she can see highly trained and experienced observers at work, and by comparing her observations with those of veteran nurses and doctors.

Florence Nightingale, who probably saw the nurse's function more clearly than had any one before her, said, "Without the habit of ready and correct observation . . . we [nurses] shall be useless with all our devotion." She pointed out that otherwise nursing becomes a mechanical routine often inimical to the patient's interests. The nurse must be guided in everything she does for the patient by what she believes to be his needs; the estimate of the patient's needs is, of course, based on her observations. The nurse cannot carry out prescribed treatments effectively unless she observes intelligently. She does not, for example, continue ruthlessly to apply cold application when she sees signs of a circulatory stasis in the area, nor does she continue to give a prescribed drug when toxic symptoms appear. The nurse who can most nearly distinguish between normal and abnormal behavior— physical, emotional, and mental—and can describe such behavior contributes in largest measure to the physician's diagnosis. Obviously, this capacity knows no bounds. The physician is particularly dependent upon the nurse in treating infants and children, the irrational and unconscious, but the observations of an able nurse contribute toward effective medical care in any case.

The institutional nurse relies heavily on the other members of the medical team for a corroboration or correction of her judgment; the nurse working in homes has to depend more completely on her own observations. A great deal of the success of a community health program is the result of the nurse's ability to detect early signs of disease. The community nurse needs specific knowledge of "norms" in all ages so that she can recognize deviations. She should also be able to observe environmental conditions adversely affecting health since their correction by a health agency is often in response to a request from the nurse.*

Medical and nursing research is dependent upon observations accurately made and recorded. Such sciences as physiology, medicine, and nursing are built up on observations. Observing, recording, analyzing, and making deductions are the essential steps in so-called "scientific discovery." It is the typically human method of learning as distinguished from the trial-and-error method of animals.

A nurse learns to observe gradually and unconsciously. The technique of observation, like others used in nursing, is based upon knowledge, interest, attention, and the sympathetic understanding that enables the nurse to put herself in the position of the patient. The trained mind is essential. Pasteur said: "In the field of observation, chance favors only the mind that is prepared." A patient often will tell the nurse important facts which he "did not like to tell the doctor," "did not want to bother the doctor with," or "did not think it important enough" to tell him. Such symptoms should always be listened to attentively, and, if important, reported in the words of the patient as far as possible.

Symptoms may be misleading in various ways. They may be exaggerated by the patient's imagination, or minimized by his shyness and dislike of giving trouble. Often a patient is unable to describe his symptoms, or he may report those having little bearing on his condition and neglect to mention those most important. He may be too ill to concentrate on what the doctor is saying, or he may be confused by the questions asked and give answers that he knows to be misleading. Skillful questioning on the part of the doctor is often necessary to draw from the patient the subjective symptoms bearing on the case, and the answers must be supplemented by the observations of the nurse.

Moreover, symptoms may be misleading because they frequently manifest themselves in some part of the body remote or seemingly not connected with the seat of the disease; for instance, such symptoms as difficult breathing or coughing and expectoration may be caused not by disease of the lungs but of the heart; a cough

* Nervi Ahla, studying the cooperation between the visiting nurse and the social case worker, calls attention to the strategic position of the nurse in observing and reporting "family social disintegrations." She concludes that when many different nurses are assigned to one family, the referral of the family to social case workers is likely to be delayed. ("Briefs," *Nursing Research,* **1:**37, [June] 1952.)

may be the result of an abscess in the ear that is causing pressure on a nerve connected with that supplying the lungs, and so giving rise to a "reflex cough." Pain is often a misleading symptom, because it may be "referred" or felt in a spot far from the seat of the trouble. Physical signs must frequently be relied upon in making a correct diagnosis. The fact that certain symptoms may be misleading is all the more reason that they should be reported fully, accurately, and at the time of their occurrence; a symptom by itself may seem to be of no importance, but when associated with others, a group of symptoms may be very significant indeed.

Directed observations made by the patient or his family, as well as those by the nurse, contribute to the physician's diagnosis. For example, the doctor may ask the patient in his home to take his temperature once or twice a day and keep a record of it for a period of a week or more. Patients are sometimes taught to make estimates and records of their blood pressure. The American Cancer Society recommends that women over thirty-five make a monthly self-examination of the breasts and says: "The nurse should encourage women to examine their breasts once a month just after the menstrual period and, equally important, at regular monthly intervals after the cessation of menses."* This society is teaching every one the "seven danger signals of cancer": (1) Any sore that does not heal; (2) a lump or thickening in the breasts or elsewhere; (3) unusual bleeding or discharge; (4) any change in a wart or mole; (5) persistent indigestion or difficulty in swallowing; (6) persistent hoarseness or cough; and (7) any change in normal bowel habits. Likewise the National Tuberculosis Association, the American Heart Association, and other health agencies are educating the public to recognize signs of disease and to seek immediate medical aid. Nurses must be alert to the patient's particular need for guidance in making effective observations. Busy physicians rarely give full explanations or complete demonstrations of the procedures involved. In both hospitals and homes, nurses must assume the responsibility for teaching patients and their families to make certain health estimates.

To summarize: the nurse is responsible for observations that (1) guide her in constant adaptation of nursing care to meet the patient's changing needs; (2) serve as a basis for diagnosis, prognosis, and treatment by the physician; (3) guide others, such as social workers or rehabilitation officers, in their services to the patient; (4) contribute toward her own knowledge and the accumulation of data on which the development of medical science depends; and (5) assist the patient or his family to make effective observations.

3. HOW AND WHAT THE NURSE OBSERVES

While observation usually means what one sees, the term as used in medicine includes the discoveries made with all the senses. Certainly the nurse, like the

---

* American Cancer Society: *The Nurse and Breast Self-Examination.* The Society, New York. 1952.

physician, looks, listens, feels, and smells in making her continuous estimate of the patient's condition. Any impairment in the sense of sight, sound, touch, or smell would seriously handicap a nurse.

Symptoms are usually divided into the subjective—those felt or experienced by the patient, of which he may or may not complain, such as pain or itching; and the objective—those that may be seen, felt, heard, or smelled by others, as, for example, pallor, swelling, coughing, or fetid breath. Although the terms "physical sign" and symptom are often used interchangeably, the former is more properly used for objective symptoms detected by such special methods of examination as listening with a stethoscope, manipulating a part, or measuring body temperature with a thermometer.

The most effective nurse observes the patient in every aspect of his being. She realizes that "mind," "spirit," "intellect," and body of the person are interdependent and inseparable, even if disease is put by some persons into categories of mental, functional, and organic, as if "mind" might be separated from the body and an organ from its function. The experienced observer tries first to estimate the temperament, or the habitual pattern of moods, and the general appearance; in other words to get an over-all picture. No accurate idea of the patient's condition can be formed, however, without a long period of observation and study; even then our knowledge of others is always relatively incomplete. The necessity for continued observation cannot be overstressed.

The following is intended to suggest the scope of the nurse's observations and to serve as a limited guide in the terminology of reporting. Texts on psychiatric and physical diagnosis should be consulted for more detailed help. It is intentional that no separation is made here between psychic and physical behavior. By observation the nurse attempts to assess the general physical and emotional make-up. She tries to determine how normally the person functions in expressing his interests, needs, desires, and affection; how normally he functions in working, playing, learning, breathing, eating, excreting, regulating body temperature, moving, maintaining muscle tone and normal posture, resting and sleeping. She also tries to recognize indications that are, but may not seem, part of the abnormality of the functions just listed. Examples of such symptoms are pain, tenderness, itching, burning, tingling, swelling, hypertrophy, atrophy, discoloration of any visible tissues, the presence of a discharge from a normally moist or dry area, the presence of a growth, a lesion, and a rash.

1. General Appearance. It is natural to make an over-all estimate of a person by noting his physical make-up. Common terms used in describing a physique are tall, medium height, short, emaciated, thin, well nourished, fat, and obese. The description may indicate whether the person is symmetrically and normally developed for his age or the opposite. (A discussion of predominantly feminine or "gynic" and predominantly male or "andric" shapes is found on page 553.) The observer notes any missing members, prostheses (artificial parts), or obvious blemishes. The muscle tone, posture, and gait contribute to the general impression of personality and state of health. They may express excitement, vigor, interest, lassitude, acute

fatigue, dejection, depression, anxiety, and other emotions. Degrees of unconsciousness are also indicated by posture and muscle tone. Facial expression is no less a
part of the general appearance. The eyes are often referred to as the windows of
the soul, for with the mouth they are most affected by the emotions. Throughout
her association with the patient the nurse should be acutely aware of his general
appearance.

**2. Temperament, Mental or Emotional Life, Feeling, "Affect," or Psychic Con-
dition.** Temperament is an over-all term for the individual's usual emotional
reaction to life. It always involves moods that are passing emotional reactions.
Temperament is a pattern of moods. When a person is habitually interested in
others and expresses his interest and affection, he is said to have a warm temperament, or to be an *extrovert*; when he is habitually withdrawn and self-centered,
he is said to be cold, or to be an *introvert*. Stress may exaggerate both temperaments. The extrovert is more subject to variation in mood with "elated," "manic,"
"euphoric," or hyperactive phases followed by depressed or hypoactive periods;
while the introvert may become so withdrawn and egocentric that he suspects others
of wishing to harm him. The person whose mood swings are not apparent and
whose behavior suggests subnormal emotional development is said to have a
phlegmatic temperament. When a person's moods are of normal intensity but
usually under his control, and when his behavior is consistent, he is said to be "well
balanced" or "well adjusted." To form any reasonably accurate estimate of temperament, it is necessary to study a person's relationship to family, friends, acquaintances, and strangers; to note his behavior in work and play; and to take account
of his participation in the activities of his immediate environment, and those of
the larger community. The nurse can learn a great deal about the person's interests,
occupation and education, family and social life from the medical history, but
everything she does for, or with, him gives her additional opportunity to study his
personality. Nursing care and treatment are affected by her ability to recognize
varying states of alertness, interest, enthusiasm, excitement, apathy, aggressiveness, passivity, irritability, anxiety, fear, resignation, and acceptance.

3. Consciousness, Awareness of Surroundings, Sleep. Since the help the patient
must have from the nurse is so dependent upon his state of consciousness and his
interpretation of time, place, and people, it is especially important that she be able
to make an accurate estimate of his orientation. When a person is awake but
does not know those around him, where he is, or what time it is, he is said to
be *disoriented* with relation to people, place, and time. The sick man may be
hypersensitive to all stimuli of sound, sight, smell, or touch with a tendency to
sleeplessness, or he may be in a state of *unconsciousness*. If he cannot be aroused,
he is said to be in *coma*; if he can be aroused with difficulty, in contrast with
normal sleep from which he can be easily aroused, he is said to be in a *stupor*. The
depth and duration of unconscious states should be noted and recorded. Observation
of sleep should indicate the time of day or night and the duration. This is so important in some cases that a graphic sleep chart is kept so that the physician can

see the sleep pattern at a glance. The depth or soundness of the sleep should be noted.

4. Loss or Impairment of Special Senses. The patient who is handicapped in speaking or hearing, seeing, maintaining his equilibrium, or interpreting tactile sensations requires special help from the nurse; the loss of the sense of smell, or ability to differentiate common odors, is less serious but should be noted.

The condition of the eyes is particularly significant. When Uncle Remus spoke of an animal as "bright-eyed and bushy-tailed," he was picturing vitality. The patient's expression may be dull, fixed, or excited; the pupils may fail to respond to light or distance; there may be *photophobia* (sensitiveness to moderate light) and abnormal eye movements. *Nystagmus* is an example of the latter. Failure to interpret objects correctly should be reported. This may be a defect of vision or a misinterpretation.

Speech is affected by normal moods and almost always reflects the mental, if not the physical, condition. Common expressions are "mute with embarrassment," "speechless with astonishment," "screaming with rage," "whimpering with pain," "cooing with pleasure." What the person says and how he says it should be noted. Some disease conditions produce aphasia (inability to arrange words into a meaningful sentence); others produce mutism, tremulous speech, sub-speech (grunts), blocking (pausing), irrelevancy, echolalia (repetition of what others say), incoherency, and speech that is explosive, slurring, whispering, or hoarse. The mentally ill may go from one subject to another so rapidly and disconnectedly that they are said to have a "flight of ideas." In reporting the content of a patient's speech, samples of his exact words should be given.

Indications of deafness should be reported as they occur. Inattention to what is said may or may not be the result of deafness. Ringing in the ears or any tenderness in or around the ears should be noted. Impairment of equilibrium is often not apparent when the person can compensate by sight. Dizziness, swaying, and falling when the eyes are closed are serious symptoms.

Disease may affect the nerve endings in the skin or the centers in the brain that interpret sensation of touch or heat and cold. Complete failure to respond or failure to respond normally to such stimuli should be reported.

5. Abnormalities in Sensation or Interpretation of Stimuli; Abnormality in the Realm of Thought. A person is said to have an illusion when an object in his environment is incorrectly interpreted—a sick man may think his wife is sitting in a chair when it is only a coat thrown over the chair. When a woman with a high fever hears nonexistent voices or feels rats running over her while nothing is touching her but her own bedding or clothing, she is said to have hallucinations —sensations without external stimuli. Delusions are common symptoms of psychoses. The person holds a belief that has no basis in fact. He has what might be called pathological experiences in thought. He often thinks he is someone he is not, he is rich when he is poor, he holds a high office when he holds none; or he may believe he is being persecuted and that his friends, his family, or the medical personnel are menacing him. Often these ideas are systematically worked out, and in describing his grandiose position or his persecution he will be very convincing. It is important for the nurse to report *exactly what he says.*

Phobias—unreasonable fears and compulsions resulting in acts the person feels compelled to perform—are not uncommon, nor are obsessions—thoughts from which the person cannot rid himself. Sometimes the mentally ill will say they feel unreal or that an outside force controls their actions.

Loss of memory should always be noted, and a differentiation made between loss of memory for the immediate and distant past.

Fabrication is a term used to describe the practice of making statements contrary to fact if there is reason to believe that the memory is intact.

6. Motor Activity—Posture and Symptoms of Impairment of Motor Function. The physician and nurse are particularly interested in muscle tone as a health index. Posture is some indication of the general tone, but the condition of the muscle of the eyes, of swallowing, of respiration, of the urethral and rectal sphincters are studied in order to determine the normality of specific body areas. Disease, including highly emotional states, may produce hyperactivity or hypoactivity. The normal amount of activity differs with the personality so that the nurse should describe the behavior rather than designate it as hyper- or hypoactive. The gait should be noted in terms such as rapid, slow, hesitant, dragging, rolling, rocking, running, tottering, or staggering. Any rigidity, or tension of the whole body or part thereof, is significant, as are paralysis and difficulty or discomfort in moving an extremity, eyes or eyelids, in speaking, swallowing, breathing, defecating, or voiding. Rhythmic, stereotyped, or automatic motions, tremors, convulsions, and unnatural flexibility are motor symptoms that should be reported.

Posture is studied for signs of weakness, as when a patient continuously slips down from an erect sitting posture. Posture may indicate pain as when the legs are flexed to relax muscles over a distended abdomen, or when a side-lying position is assumed to limit the expansion of the chest as in pleurisy. When any position is assumed habitually, it should be noted, as should any unusual position.

7. Breathing. Respiration is an automatic function, but its rate and depth are nevertheless affected by emotional states, exercise, drugs, and anything that alters the body's need of oxygen. Mechanical interference with respiration also affects the rate and depth. The nurse should note the character of the respiration; the movements of chest, abdomen, and nose; the sounds accompanying respiration; the patient's position, his expression, and change in color; and actual complaints indicating difficulty in breathing. *Orthopnea* means difficult breathing. *Apnea* is a temporary suspension of breathing. *Cyanosis* is the term used to describe the bluish tint of the lips, nail beds, or skin resulting from inadequate oxygenation of the blood. Breathing with the mouth open habitually is abnormal and should be reported.

8. Eating and Drinking. It is obvious that health and recovery from disease are dependent upon food intake. Unless the patient is aware of his nutritional need and is able and willing to meet it, the burden of seeing that he gets adequate nourishment rests largely upon the nurse. She should observe signs of appetite or its lack, food likes, cravings, dislikes, idiosyncrasies, and phobias. If he does not enjoy his meals, she should try to discover the cause. Actually he may be hungry, but eating may be for some reason painful or uncomfortable. Sore mouth, ill-fitting dentures, difficulty in swallowing, or weakness may interfere with the satisfaction of eating. The mentally ill may think themselves unworthy of food, they may believe the food is poisoned, or it may represent an object that is unfit for consumption.

9. Elimination.   Reports on the amount, frequency, and nature of elimination are included in all nursing notes. If the patient is rational and ambulatory, he may assume the responsibility for reporting to the nurse or doctor any irregularity in defecation, urination, and sweating; if he is not able to assume this responsibility, the nurse notes the character of the excretions and the frequency of defecation and urination. If pain or discomfort accompanies these acts, the fact should be noted. Attention should be called at once to cessation of these functions. Sweating or abnormal dryness of the skin and the body areas affected should be reported. If the sweat has an unusual odor, as of urine, it should be noted. The balance between fluid taken in and eliminated cannot be too greatly upset without serious consequence. A record is therefore kept as a basis for estimating how nearly intake and output tally. Sunken eyes, dry mouth, loose skin, and concentrated urine are characteristic of dehydration and are danger signs. Any indication that fluid is held in the tissues is also significant. Puffy eyes, clubbed fingers, swollen hands and feet (edema), or accumulation of fluid in the tissues of the back when the patient is sitting should be noted. *Ascites* is the term used when free fluid distends the abdominal cavity. Occasionally, with the use of certain drugs, or in the case of poisoning, excretions are discolored or have an unusual odor. Drugs may be deposited in the tissues and give the mucous membranes, skin, or the sclera of the eye an unnatural appearance that should be noted and described.

10. Regulation of Body Temperature. With a thermometer the nurse can measure body temperature more accurately than in any other way. It is desirable, however, to observe and report the dry, hot, flushed, cold, or clammy skin; the obvious chill; or the sensation of which the person complains. If the patient has a dry nose and mouth, which makes swallowing difficult, the lips get cracked and parched and the tongue appears coated and discolored. All of these are signs of dehydration accompanying fever that the nurse can see and should record.

11. Noting Gross Disease Processes.   Abnormal functioning of the body constitutes disease, but there are pathological processes the nurse should note which have not been emphasized under the functional headings just used. For example, any signs of inflammation—redness, heat, swelling, discomfort, or pain—should be reported. Note and report any discoloration of the skin or mucous membranes, swelling, hypertrophy, any sign of a growth, break in the tissues, discharges from body orifices or lesions, abnormal odors, tenderness as the body is manipulated, and all subjective symptoms of which the patient complains. Examples are pain, tenderness, itching, burning, tingling, prickling, numbness, throbbing, chilliness or a sensation of being overheated, headache, nausea, dizziness, spots before the eyes, ringing in the ears (tinnitus), deafness, a sense of fullness, pressure, or a "gone" or weak feeling. All of these should be reported in the patient's own words with the sensation localized when it is local and characterized as the patient describes it. He may say that he has a "gnawing pain that comes and goes" in his stomach and that "it is relieved by food," or he "feels as if there is a heavy weight" on his chest, or he "can't get his breath." Since such comments may have a different significance for any two medical attendants, a verbatim report is desirable.

Feelings or emotions are expressed in such questions or statements as: "Isn't the doctor coming soon?" "Does the doctor think my condition is serious?" "I know it isn't cancer." "There's no danger in a blood pressure of 180, is there?" or "Do you think I'll get well?" When the nurse thinks that a question indicates any emotional state that markedly affects the patient's diagnosis, prognosis, or treatment, it is wise to record it in the patient's words. All symptoms are important, though not equally so; therefore, a selection must be made from the patient's acts, including speech, that seem significant. Everything he does is an indication of what concerns him, of the effectiveness or ineffectiveness of the care given him, and of the nature of his illness.

4. METHODS OF REPORTING AND RECORDING

Observation of the patient is continuous, as has been said repeatedly, and serves as a basis for the hourly and daily modification of nursing care. Since it is obviously impossible for the nurse to record all her observations, some guide is necessary in making a selection of items that may be helpful to other nurses, physicians, social workers, and special therapists.

She should report any signs of disorientation, unconsciousness, anxiety, fear, or any strong emotion and particularly instability of mood; deterioration of the patient's relationship with others or any marked change in the personality. She should report any handicap or limitation of function as soon as it is noted. In general, symptoms should be reported that meet any one of the following conditions: (1) intense or severe in character, as severe pain; (2) prolonged, even though not severe; (3) a departure from normal, as an increase or decrease in pulse rate; (4) tends to recur, as pain between meals; (5) shows progressive development, as loss of weight; (6) is a known danger signal, as a sharp abdominal pain in typhoid fever; (7) indicates a complication, as coughing following an operation; (8) points to the onset of a disease, as a rash; (9) cannot be relieved by nursing measures, as failure to eat or sleep, void, or defecate; (10) shows faulty hygiene or health habits that cannot be corrected by nursing care, as neglected teeth, the need of eyeglasses, or a more balanced diet; (11) indicates a disturbance in function of any organ or part of the body; and (12) shows a change for the better or for the worse.

Reports are made orally and/or by a notation on the patient's chart. Anything that is serious or that requires immediate attention should be reported promptly, both orally and on the medical record—the patient's chart. The written report must never be omitted for this helps to ensure notice of the condition and to protect medical personnel from accusations of negligence. Patient-centered conferences among nurses, doctors, nutritionists, social workers, rehabilitation officers, and special therapists offer an invaluable opportunity to exchange such observations and opinions as are difficult to report fully in writing. The nurse, particularly the student or inexperienced nurse, should err on the side of being overzealous in reporting orally to a nurse in charge of the service, or to the physician assigned to the patient, any observation that she thinks may even possibly have serious consequences. Ninety-nine times her caution may be unnecessary, her judgment questioned, but the hundredth time she may save a life.

The patient's record, or chart, is still the most commonly used medium for reporting observations (signs and symptoms of patient behavior). The value of the nurse's notations is a fairly good index of her nursing ability. Gradually she builds up a technique of observing and recording. Before going to the patient, she regularly reviews what others have written on his record and the treatment prescribed in the doctor's "order book." She gets whatever oral reports she can from others, she welcomes the opinions of the patient's family and friends; then, after observation made while she cares for the patient, she reports and records whatever she thinks is significant. Such records are made daily, hourly, or at less frequent intervals, according to the patient's needs and the time available for nursing care.

Observing, reporting, and recording are almost inseparable processes in the medical world, but a discussion of the nature of the medical record, or chart, is left for the following chapter since it merits detailed treatment.

Suggested Reading

Appel, Kenneth E., and Strecker, Edward A.: *Practical Examination of Personality and Behavior Disorders: Adults and Children.* The Macmillan Company, New York, 1936.

Cabot, Richard C., and Adams, F. Dennette: *Physical Diagnosis,* 13th ed. William Wood & Co., Baltimore, 1942.

Freeman, Frank S.: *Individual Differences: The Nature and Causes of Variations in Intelligence and Special Abilities.* Henry Holt & Co., New York, 1934.

Gesell, Arnold L., and Amatruda, C. S.: *Developmental Diagnosis: Normal and Abnormal Child Development: Clinical Methods and Practical Applications,* 2nd ed. Harper & Brothers, New York, 1947.

Houston, William R.: *The Art of Treatment.* The Macmillan Company, New York, 1937.

Hutchings, Richard H.: *A Psychiatric Word Book: A Lexicon of Terms Employed in Psychiatry and Psychoanalysis Designed for Students of Medicine and Nursing and Psychiatric Social Workers,* 7th ed. State Hospitals Press, Utica, N. Y., 1943.

Kalkman, Marion E.: *Introduction to Psychiatric Nursing.* McGraw-Hill Book Co., New York, 1950.

Major, Ralph H.: *Physical Diagnosis,* 4th ed. W. B. Saunders Co., Philadelphia, 1951.

Nightingale, Florence: *Notes on Nursing: What It Is, and What It Is Not* (facsimile of 1859 ed.). J. B. Lippincott Co., Philadelphia, 1946.

Sheldon, William H., and Stevens, S. S.: *The Varieties of Temperament: A Psychology of Constitutional Differences.* Harper & Brothers, New York, 1942.

Wiggers, Carl J.: *Physiology in Health and Disease,* 5th ed. Lea & Febiger, Philadelphia, 1949.

Woodworth, Robert S., and Marquis, Donald G.: *Psychology,* 5th ed. Henry Holt & Co., New York, 1947.

CHAPTER 10. TEMPERATURE, RESPIRATION, PULSE, AND BLOOD PRESSURE

1. THE CARDINAL SYMPTOMS
2. BODY TEMPERATURE
3. RESPIRATION
4. THE PULSE
5. BLOOD PRESSURE

1. THE CARDINAL SYMPTOMS

Temperature, pulse rate, and respiration rates are so constant and in health conform with such regularity to a standard that we speak of the "normal" temperature, pulse, and respiration. Mechanisms that govern them are so finely adjusted that any considerable change or departure from normal rates is looked upon as a symptom of disease; consequently, "taking" the temperature, pulse, and respiration is one of the first means of assessing a person's condition. As long as the patient is in the hospital or under nursing care in a home they are usually taken at least twice during each 24 hours, although in some cases this may amount to a meaningless and unjustifiable routine. If there is marked departure from normal, measurements are made and recorded every 4 hours. The pulse and respiration are watched constantly in critical conditions, and even though the temperature is not actually taken when it might disturb the patient, a nurse is on the alert to note signs of temperature elevation, such as flushing of the face; hot, dry skin; hot and tremulous hands; dry, parched, and tremulous lips; rapid breathing; and mental confusion.

Again, so important are changes in temperature, pulse, and respiration, so typical of certain diseases, and of certain stages in the disease, that a special "temperature sheet" is kept, indicating numerically and graphically by means of dots and lines the temperature and pulse curves and the relation of one to the other. (See Fig. 40.)

This temperature sheet is usually the first on the medical record so that the doctor sees it at a glance. From this alone in some diseases he is able to judge the patient's condition. The temperature is a symptom that may be accurately ascertained even by an inexperienced person. Since it is accompanied by and runs parallel with the other symptoms of injury to the nervous system not so easily recognized by the inexperienced, a record of the temperature over a 24-hour period may give the physician a valuable clue to the patient's condition during that time.

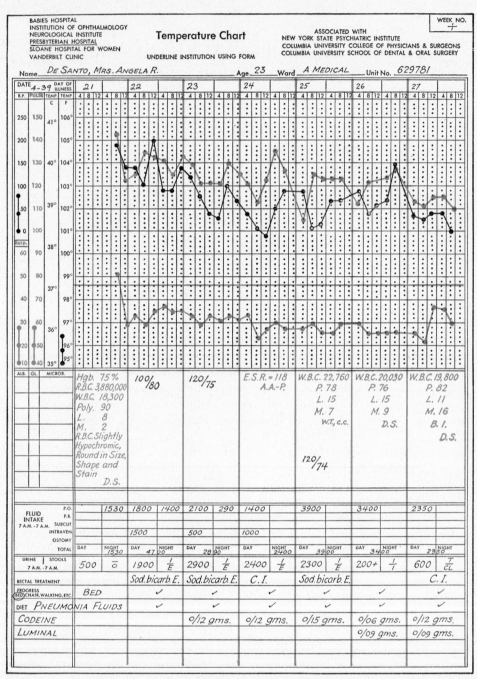

Figure 40. Graphic chart of temperature, pulse, and respiration. Because this is the first sheet of the record many other important items of information, to which reference is being made, are recorded here also. (Courtesy of Columbia-Presbyterian Medical Center, New York City.)

These signals of distress held out by nature must be closely and accurately observed; a nurse must never record a temperature, pulse, or respiration carelessly taken or one of which she is in doubt.

A full understanding of the temperature, pulse, and respiration as discussed in the following pages comes only with a thorough knowledge of anatomy and physiology and with wide experience. For a more complete treatment of these subjects the reader is referred to the texts listed at the end of this chapter.

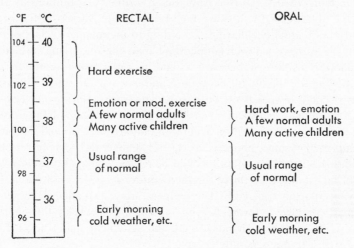

Figure 41. An estimate of the ranges in body temperatures found in normal persons. (DuBois, Eugene F.: *Fever and the Regulation of Body Temperature.* Charles C Thomas, Publisher, Springfield, Ill., 1948, p. 8.)

2. BODY TEMPERATURE

Normal Body Temperature. Body temperature is usually measured by placing a thermometer in one of the body orifices. This is usually a glass instrument containing a column of mercury that expands, or rises, as it is heated.* For each cavity there is a range of measurements that may be termed normal. Eugene F. DuBois suggests that thermometers should be made to show these ranges. (See Fig. 41.) At present they have arrows at 37° C or 98.6° F, and deviations from these points are unfortunately believed by the average person to indicate disease. DuBois emphasizes the range of temperatures in different areas of the body. In extreme conditions, he says, it may range from 38° C (100.4° F) (in the interior) to 0° C (32° F) (in the skin). "There is no one body temperature, but a series of gradients."† The liver, according to him, is the warmest part of the body. Charles

---

* An unbreakable metal thermometer is available with a spring mechanism and a dial face on which the temperature is read.

† DuBois, Eugene F.: *Fever and the Regulation of Body Temperature.* Charles C Thomas, Publisher, Springfield, Ill., 1948, p. 33.

H. Best and Norman B. Taylor[1] place the temperature of the liver at 37.8° C (100° F); the normal average mouth temperature at 37° C (98.6° F); the rectal temperature at 38° C (100.4° F); and the axillary skin temperature at 36° C (96.8° F). John H. Ferguson, writing in John F. Fulton's text,[2] says the blood of man is ordinarily about 38° C (100.4° F). Obviously, however, the blood in the liver is much warmer than the blood in the skin. Skin temperatures vary widely with climatic conditions, with the clothing covering the area, and with the structure of the underlying tissues. DuBois says under ordinary conditions it ranges from 34° C (93.2° F) to 37° C (98.6° F). Temperature varies during the day, and there are also individual peculiarities according to the manner of living. A sedentary person is likely to have a lower temperature than the one living an active outdoor life. Temperature is lowest between 2 and 6 A.M., rising gradually during the day and reaching the maximum between 5 and 7 P.M., and again falling during the night. This order is reversed in the person who sleeps during the day and works at night. The difference between the early morning and evening temperatures may be a fraction of 1° F or more.[3] For accurate comparison it should be measured for each patient at the same hours each day. The average temperature also varies slightly with age, that of an infant or child being less stable and usually 1° F higher than that of an adult. After thirty the temperature is said to fall about 1° F, while in very advanced age it rises 1° F. The temperature is also affected by temperament. Emotion may produce a fever. As the relationship between the endocrines and metabolism is more clearly demonstrated, the statement that a fever can have an emotional origin is more generally accepted.

Production of Heat.   Body temperature is maintained, according to Henry C. Sherman and Caroline S. Lanford, chiefly or wholly by the heat produced as a by-product of the work involved in the life process. Conservation of heat by constriction of skin blood vessels, by shivering, and other forms of exercise is called *physical regulation,* and burning foodstuffs for the direct purpose of producing heat is called *chemical regulation.*

The fact that physical regulation very nearly suffices for most of us . . . does not mean that the burning of foodstuffs for heat remains at complete zero for anyone. . . .

Need of heat as such for the maintenance of body temperature may at some times and for some people be a real factor in the energy requirement; but the body is not a heat engine, it usually gets enough heat in the course of doing its work, and one should not be misled by the fact that for convenience we count energy values in terms of calories.*

Body heat is nevertheless the result of cell activity, particularly contraction of muscle cells, and for this and all other metabolic processes food is essential. For this reason the body has been compared, perhaps erroneously, to a furnace where the foods we eat, if burned, will produce heat. Because the heat that food will produce is more easily measured than other forms of energy transformation, such

* Sherman, Henry C., and Lanford, Caroline S.: *Essentials of Nutrition,* 3rd ed. The Macmillan Company, New York, 1951, pp. 61-62.

as muscle activity or cell division, the value of food is reckoned in terms of the heat unit.

The calorie is the heat unit and is the amount of heat necessary to raise 1 gm of water 1° C. One large calorie (C) is the quantity of heat necessary to raise the temperature of 1000 gm of water 1° C. Each food has its own specific caloric yield. The following are averages commonly given:*

> 1 gm protein (heat value) =4100 calories (4.1 C)
> 1 gm carbohydrate (starch)=4100 calories (4.1 C)
> 1 gm fat   =9305 calories (9.3 C)

These figures therefore represent the amount of energy, either in the form of heat or mechanical work, these foods are capable of supplying to the body. In this way the quantitative value of any diet may be estimated.

Food in the body, however, will not produce heat without oxygen. Just as there are drafts in a furnace to regulate the oxygen entering according to the heat desired, so in the body in order to burn food and produce heat, we must have oxygen and a means of supplying it as needed. This is provided by the respiratory apparatus—air rich in oxygen is inhaled, and carbon dioxide, excess heat, and other waste products exhaled in air now poor in oxygen. Thus there is a definite relation between body temperature and respiration, and they should be considered together.

Production of heat in the body is the result of activity in all its cells, but most of the heat is produced in certain organs. The more active the organ, the more food it burns and the more heat it produces. This heat is distributed by blood vessels to cooler parts of the body so that while the temperature of both external and internal parts may vary, their temperature is nearly uniform. A cold environment, however, may bring the skin temperature which usually ranges from 37° to 34° C (98.6° to 93.2° F) as low as 0° C (32° F).[4]

The muscles and secreting glands are the furnaces where most heat is generated. Anyone knows that when he is cold, *exercise* warms him. Strenuous exercise is said by some authorities to raise the body temperature from 1° to 4° F or more.[5] *Shivering* is one of nature's methods of producing heat when the body is chilled. Infections are characterized by chills with subsequent fever. This production of heat by muscular activity is a matter of common experience, and we find in warm climates that people avoid exercise and diets rich in energy-producing foods— fats and carbohydrates. In cold climates the opposite conditions prevail.

It is generally known that eating increases body temperature. The maximal increase occurs about 1½ hours after meals. *Strong emotions,* which are the psychic response to glandular activity, also increase body temperature, and therefore we

* Sherman and Lanford say that technically a capital letter (Calorie) should be used to differentiate between the large and small unit, but that since only the large unit of measurement is used in nutrition, "calorie or the abbreviation C" is understood to mean the large "Calorie" as defined by the physicist.

have the familiar expression, "keep cool," when we really mean "don't get excited or angry."

A definite relation between body temperature and endocrine activity in health is demonstrated in women during the childbearing period. If a rectal temperature is taken daily in the morning before arising, most women show a characteristic variation during the menstrual cycle. Just before menstruation the temperature falls 0.5° to 0.75° F below its previous level and remains low until ovulation, which is about the thirteenth or fourteenth day of the cycle. After the rupture of

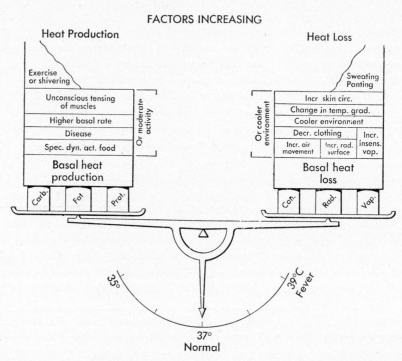

Figure 42. Balance between factors increasing heat production and heat loss. (DuBois, Eugene F.: *Fever and the Regulation of Body Temperature.* Charles C Thomas, Publisher, Springfield, Ill., 1948.)

the Graafian follicle and the escape of the ovum, the temperature rises 0.5° to 0.75° F and remains at the higher level until the next menstruation.[6] Parenthetically, this knowledge of temperature fluctuation is used as a means of controlling conception, since it indicates the time at which the ovum may be penetrated by a spermatozoon. Paul B. Beeson, writing in Cyril M. MacBryde's text,[7] says that adrenergic (sympathetic) phenomena are associated with a rise in body temperature; cholinergic (parasympathetic), with a fall. He calls attention to the cutaneous vasoconstriction, dilated pupils, and erection of hair that accompany the rise of temperature and the cutaneous vasodilation and constricted pupils associated with a fall. It is known that a shift in body fluids is associated with the menstrual cycle, some women gaining 5 lb or more just before menstruation. Some authorities attribute variations in body temperature to differences in the distribution of body water. Eventually, these relationships will be made clear.

Exposure to extremes of temperature in the surroundings—air or water—may also increase body temperature by radiation, convection, and conduction. *Brief exposure to cold* stimulates the body to produce more heat to protect itself. *A very high external temperature* upsets the balance of heat regulation by direct action on the heat-regulating center in the brain, it is thought, and may therefore produce a high temperature; for instance, a sunstroke may increase the body temperature to 41.7° or 43.3° C (107° or 110° F).

It is important for the nurse to have some knowledge of the physiology of heat regulation. It is not enough to take the temperature; she must know when the temperature is above normal, what measures will prevent a further elevation, when it is subnormal, and what measures will increase the temperature. For instance, when the temperature is above normal, the nurse should regulate the temperature of the surrounding air and the amount and kind of bedclothes; she should prevent all possible excitement or exertion on the part of the patient. The doctor will probably prescribe rest, a special diet, plenty of water to drink, and sponge baths if drug therapy does not remove the cause and control the fever.

When the temperature is markedly subnormal, it may indicate that the patient is in a state of collapse, and nursing measures must be instituted to increase heat production. Unless the decrease in the blood supply to the skin is a protective mechanism, as in shock, the nurse should try to warm the body by applying heated blankets, rubbing, and giving warm drinks. (Care of shock is discussed on p. 1053.)

Loss of Heat. If all the heat produced by cell activity were stored up in the tissues, such an accumulation would destroy the body. According to Best and Taylor:

The total quantity of heat lost in twenty-four hours must, of course, just equal the amount produced; otherwise, the body temperature would rise or fall. The heat production of an average man doing light work is about 3,000 calories. The proportions of this which are dissipated through the various channels at ordinary room temperature are given in the following table, in approximate figures.*

	CALORIES	PER CENT
(a) Radiation, convection and conduction	2100	70
(b) Evaporation from skin and lungs	810	27
(c) Warming inspired air	60	2
(d) Urine and feces (i.e., heat of these excreta over that of the food)	30	1
Total daily heat loss	3000	100

These figures correspond fairly well, though not exactly, with those given by C.-E. A. Winslow and Lovic P. Herrington.[8]

* Best, Charles H., and Taylor, Norman B.: *The Physiological Basis of Medical Practice,* 5th ed. Williams and Wilkins Co., Baltimore, 1950, p. 720.

The amount of heat lost by these various avenues varies with environmental conditions and the individual's physiology. Winslow and Herrington say that the minimum metabolism is observed at environmental temperatures of 20° C (68° F) to 25° C (77° F); above and below these figures the body tends to increase the metabolic rate. They say that a nude man in a semireclining position begins to sweat at 30° C (86° F). A clothed man in moist air starts sweating actively at an environmental temperature of 25° C (77° F). Activity lowers the temperature at which noticeable perspiration (sweat) starts.

Anything that reduces activity *decreases* heat production. The temperature falls during sleep, shock, and unconscious states. Sedatives lower body temperature; and vasodilators, such as alcohol, lower the temperature of the blood by bringing a greater blood volume to the skin, where it is cooled.

Heat Regulation.   Normal body temperature is the balance maintained between heat produced and heat lost. In warm-blooded animals this balance is set at a standard normal for that particular species. The so-called cold-blooded animals, such as the frog or fish, are those whose temperature varies with that of the surrounding air or water. The warm-blooded animals are those that maintain a relatively constant temperature summer and winter, practically independent of that of their surroundings. This is accomplished by a heat-regulating mechanism, and in man partly by clothing—an artificial means of preventing excess loss of heat through the skin by radiation and conduction.

The most important means of controlling loss of heat from the body is, therefore, by controlling that lost through the skin. This is accomplished by centers in the central nervous system that control the circulation of blood and the secretion of sweat. The arteries in the skin subdivide into an enormous number of minute capillaries and thus increase the amount of blood exposed to the influence of the surrounding cooler air. Through these vessels flows a very large volume of warm blood from the muscles and glands, giving off some of its heat to the cooler atmosphere before returning to the interior of the body. When the surrounding temperature is very cold, the nerve centers (the vasomotor centers in the brain, and possibly the spinal cord, that control the size of the blood vessels) cause the blood vessels in the skin to contract so that less blood flows through it and less heat is lost. The centers controlling the production of sweat also check its secretion in such a way that less heat is lost by evaporation. The effect of cold on the nerve endings in the skin stimulates the nerve centers that set at work the processes producing heat; shivering may result, and the appetite is stimulated so that more food is eaten. When the surrounding air is warmer, the opposite effect occurs: the blood vessels in the skin dilate, more blood flows through them, more heat is lost, sweating increases, and activity and appetite are diminished. DuBois says that "the skin can detect minute rises in temperature."* He, with other authorities, says that receptors for heat and cold have different structures and distributions.

It is thought that the regulating centers act, so to speak, like the regulator or thermostat connected with a furnace or oven. In health the thermostat is set for a temperature around 37° C (98.6° F). These centers will struggle against any

* DuBois, Eugene F.: *op. cit.*, p. 30.

marked change from the normal temperature until they themselves become exhausted. If there is an infection, the thermostat seems to be set at a higher figure. Fever and related nursing care are discussed in Chapters 22 and 41.

Variations within the limits shown in Figure 41 are ordinarily not significant. Mouth temperatures above 38° C (100.4° F) or below 36° C (96.8° F) usually indicate pathology of some sort. Temperatures above normal are called febrile; those below, subnormal. The elevation of temperature is not always an index of the seriousness of the disease, for it may be higher in the shorter, less serious infections than in the most fatal. For instance, the temperature in tonsillitis is frequently higher than in diphtheria, and in some fatal infections there may be no elevation at all. A prolonged high temperature is always serious.

Temperatures above Normal—Fever.   Beeson defines "fever" as "an elevation of the body temperature due to disease."* He makes it clear, however, that a person in health may have a rectal temperature of 40° C (104° F) as a result of exercise or an elevated mouth temperature from chewing gum. *Pyrexia* is another term for fever, and *hyperpyrexia* and *hyperthemia* for temperatures of 40.6° C (105° F) or above.

Fever is an imbalance between heat production and elimination. The origin of the imbalance is explained by several theories, but none has been established. Valy Menkin's[9] studies show that injured cells give off a chemical, named by him *pyrexin*, that produces fever. It is believed that substances causing fever act on hypothalmic centers in the brain and possibly other centers in the spinal cord. Some students of fever have attributed it to adrenal activity. Beeson says that this theory is disproven by the fact that animals without adrenals can be made febrile, while those without a hypothalmus cannot. He lists as causes of fever: infections; diseases of the nervous system; certain malignant neoplasms; blood diseases, such as leukemia and severe pernicious anemia; embolism and thrombosis; heat stroke from exposure to hot environments; dehydration; paroxysmal tachycardia and congestive heart failure, with and without known accompanying infections; surgical trauma and crushing injuries; possibly the gum injury in teething babies; peptic ulcer; skin abnormalities that interfere with normal heat loss; serums containing an irritating foreign protein and intravenous solutions containing pyrogens; and he lists some drugs that may cause fever. Beeson discusses "habitual hyperthermia" and cites Hobart A. Reimann's[10] study of rare persons, whose temperature seems to be set slightly above the average level. He thinks "most physicians are convinced that under certain conditions an emotional stimulus may induce an elevation of temperature."† He cites the slight rise of temperature so commonly seen in hospital admissions and army draftees, and Frank B. Wynn's[11] observation of 0.6° F average rise in body temperature among nurses about to write state-board examinations. Prolonged pain is believed to cause a temperature rise, which might be the result of tissue injury or of the fear that accompanies pain.

Treatment of fever (discussed in Chapter 41) depends upon the cause, its

* MacBryde, Cyril M. (ed.): *Signs and Symptoms; Their Clinical Interpretation*, 2nd ed. J. B. Lippincott, Philadelphia, 1952, p. 386.
† MacBryde, Cyril M. (ed.): *op. cit.*, p. 404.

severity, and duration. It is a symptom, not a disease. DuBois asks, "Fever—friend or foe?" and is inclined to say in most cases "friend." Extreme fever is always dangerous and should be reduced if possible. Reports of body temperatures above 46.1° C (115° F) are believed to be spurious. Ward J. MacNeil[12] gives 46° C (114.8° F) as the upper limit beyond which irreversible changes in tissues take place. Very high temperatures cause delirium and convulsions, showing injury of the central nervous system. On the other hand, syphilis, gonorrhea, and other infections have been effectively treated with brief periods of artificially induced moderate fevers, and experimentally it can be shown that many organisms are attenuated or killed by temperatures found in infectious disease. Fever is, therefore, believed to make the host less habitable to many invading organisms, and such efforts as are made to control fever are ordinarily used to stimulate the circulation, clean the skin, and give comfort. While moderate temperatures are not combated as they once were, the hyperpyrexia of heatstroke, which may well be fatal, is reduced by every available means. Convulsions often accompany a sudden onset of fever in children, whose heat-regulating mechanism is unsteady until puberty or thereabouts.

With every degree of body temperature there is believed to be a 7 per cent increase in the metabolic rate, just as all chemical reactions are speeded by heat. At a temperature of 40.6° C (105° F) metabolism is about 50 per cent above normal.[13] This suggests the danger of protracted temperatures where the food intake, for one reason or another, cannot be raised in proportion to the metabolic rate.

Course of the Fever, or Temperature Curve.   Fevers usually run a typical course, characteristic of a particular disease; so it is commonly said, "The fever must run its course." In some diseases the temperature curve, or the diagrammatic representation on the chart of the course of the fever, is so typical that the diagnosis is suggested at a glance. When the course of the disease is arrested by a drug as it so often is now, the fever curve will of course not be so characteristic.

The *onset* or *invasion* may be sudden, as in pneumonia and scarlet fever, or it may be gradual, as in typhoid. After the temperature has reached its maximum, it usually remains elevated for a few days to two or three weeks or longer unless the course of the disease is arrested by treatment. This period of high fever is called the *fastigium* or *stadium*. (*Stadium* comes from the Greek, a measure of distance in races, and *fastigium* from the Latin, the ridge of a roof.)

Fever may subside suddenly, the temperature falling 4° or 5° F within a few hours and reaching normal or below in from 12 to 24 hours, accompanied by a marked improvement in the patient's condition; or it may subside gradually. When the temperature subsides suddenly, as in unarrested lobar pneumonia, the drop is called the *crisis*. It is not so much the drop in temperature, but the lessened severity of symptoms that marks the true crisis. A sudden fall in the temperature not accompanied by an improvement in the general condition is not a true crisis. It may indicate the body's inability to combat the infection, or approaching death. In such cases the drop in temperature is a danger signal and not a sign of improvement.

Fever is said to subside by *lysis* when, as in typhoid, the temperature falls step by step in a zigzag manner for two or three days or a week before reaching normal. During this time the other symptoms also gradually disappear.

Types of Fever. (1) *Habitual hyperthermia* is a term used for the consistent elevation of temperature slightly above normal levels found in occasional individuals. (2) A *constant fever* describes one that remains near the same elevation throughout a period of days or weeks. (3) A *remittent fever* has wide variations in the temperature level morning and evening, but never falls to normal. (4) An *intermittent* or *quotidian fever* is one in which the body temperature rises and returns to normal daily. When the difference between the high and low points is very great, the fever is called *hectic* or *septic*. (5) A *relapsing fever* is one in which there are brief febrile periods followed by one or more days of normal temperature.

During convalescence from fevers there may be a recrudescence. The temperature elevation may be merely temporary, due to excitement, as from the visits of friends or to some unusual exertion. Such a recurrence, however, should receive careful attention, as it may mean a return of the infection that must again run its course, or it may indicate complications.

Subnormal Temperatures. The body must maintain a certain degree of heat in order to carry on vital processes. Subnormal temperatures may be caused by: (1) excessive heat elimination, as from profuse sweating, severe hemorrhage, or loss of other body fluids; (2) lessened heat production, as in starvation and lowered vitality; (3) extreme depression of the nervous system, as in shock or collapse; and (4) long exposure to cold environments. Studies within the last decade have shown that man can survive subnormal temperatures for a surprising length of time. Patients hopelessly ill with cancer have been treated in recent years with generalized applications of cold or exposure in cold rooms for days at a time. It was thought at first that the maintenance of body temperatures from 24° C (75.2° F) to 32° C (89.6° F) brought relief and arrest of that disease, but although the patients survived these temperatures, the value of the therapy is now questioned.[14, 15] Cold as a local anesthetic is discussed in Chapter 38.

Clinical Thermometer. The Fahrenheit self-registering clinical thermometer was the instrument commonly used in the United States, Canada, and Great Britain for measuring body temperature, but the continental centigrade scale is coming into general use in the United States. The clinical thermometer is a glass bulb containing mercury and a stem in which the mercury can rise. On the stem is a graduated scale representing degrees of temperature, the lowest registered being 35° C or 95° F; the highest 43.3° C or 110° F, because body temperatures below or above these points are exceedingly rare. The stem usually has a curved surface that magnifies the lines and figures on the scale and a flattened back with a sharp ridge that makes it easier to read the scale, prevents rolling, and lessens the danger of breakage.

Thermometers are made with bulbs of different sizes and shapes. The greater the surface of glass surrounding the mercury, the more rapidly the mercury heats and therefore the more rapidly the thermometer registers. Mouth thermometers with long, slender bulbs register more rapidly than rectal thermometers with short, fat bulbs. A slender bulb must not be used in the rectum as it is likely to injure the mucosa. Both mouth and rectal thermometers are made with short, fat bulbs and are probably less easily broken than the slender type, but it is esthetically important to have different instruments for these two methods of taking the temperature. Rectal thermometers often have colored bulbs. Pigment used in making the temperature scale is gradually removed with use, but manufacturers of high-grade thermometers will furnish pigment with which to replace the scale. Different shapes and methods of marking thermometers are shown in Figure 43.

The principle upon which the use of the thermometer is based is that mercury expands with heat, the height to which the column rises depending upon its intensity, which it therefore accurately registers, because in the self-registering

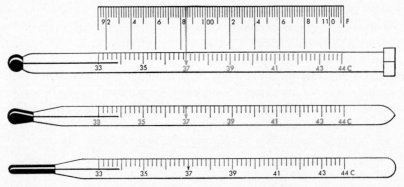

Figure 43. Clinical thermometers showing different types of tips, methods of marking, and comparative temperature scales. One thermometer has a hexagonal top to prevent it from rolling.

thermometer the mercury stays at this height until shaken down. Needless to say, the thermometer must not be used for anything hotter than 43.3° C (110° F), for the mercury would continue to expand and break the stem. Before using the thermometer, see that the mercury registers about 35° C (95° F). To shake the mercury down, grasp the thermometer securely by the upper end (never hold it by the bulb), flex the hand, and give a quick movement of the wrist as when snapping the fingers or cracking a whip. Do not shake the mercury below 35° C (95° F), as it may be difficult to get it up again. Be careful not to let the thermometer fall or strike against anything.

Instruments of special design are available for determining skin temperatures, a thermocouple giving the most accurate measurement. In a skin thermometer the same principles of construction are observed as those for the mouth and rectal thermometers except that the bulb is flattened to facilitate skin contact.

Suggested Method of "Taking Temperature." Body temperature may be determined by placing the thermometer in the mouth or rectum. Sometimes the axilla or groin is used and occasionally the vagina, but the last site is particularly undesirable.[16] The temperature sought is that of the interior of the body un-influenced by contact with clothing, air, or moisture. Therefore, the thermometer must be placed where it can be completely surrounded by body tissues and where there are large blood vessels near the surface. The nearer these conditions are approached, the more accurate the measurement.

In taking the *temperature by mouth,* place the end of the thermometer con-taining the mercury under the tongue, because here it will be close to large blood vessels. See that the lips are kept tightly closed. Leave the thermometer in position until the mercury reaches the maximum height, but do not leave it longer than necessary. Time required depends upon the thermometer used and environmental conditions; it varies from 3 to 10 minutes. High-grade thermometers are advertised to register in 1 minute, but as the mouth contains environmental air the lips must

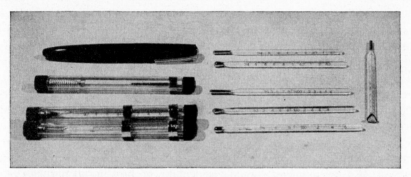

Figure 44. Various types of clinical thermometers and cases. (Courtesy of Becton, Dickin-son & Co., Rutherford, N. J., and Clay-Adams Co., New York City.)

remain tightly closed for at least 3 minutes to warm the air to body temperature. When taking temperatures of patients on cold porches, allow as much as 10 minutes for registration of the thermometer.

Katharine Brim and Betty A. Chandler studied the effects on oral temperature recordings of drinking hot and cold liquids, smoking cigarettes, and chewing gum. According to them:

Hot liquids caused a deviation from the control temperature for from twenty to eighty minutes, whereas following the drinking of cold liquids, the temperatures of the majority of test subjects returned to the original level in from five to ten minutes. However, in some cases, the temperature taken ten to twenty minutes after the drinking of cold liquids had not only reached the control temperature but had surpassed it by as much as 1.4° F. Ten minutes after drinking hot liquids, twenty-four individuals' temperatures were still one degree Fahrenheit above their control temperatures.

Both the chewing of gum and smoking may raise or lower the oral temperature, but the chewing of gum seems to have a more prolonged effect than does smoking.*

* Brim, Katharine, and Chandler, Betty A.: "Changes in Oral Temperature," *Am. J. Nursing* **48:**772, (Dec.) 1948.

These findings are similar to those of other investigators whose reports are listed at the end of this chapter.

It is far from simple to get an accurate estimate of the temperature of any body area. The nurse should be aware of and take into account the difficulties involved. Norman DeNosaquo et al. tested several thousand mouth thermometers from a number of manufacturers to determine the length of time necessary for accurate registration. They concluded that three minutes is the *minimum* period.[17]

Contraindications for Mouth Temperatures. The mouth is the most convenient place for taking the temperature, but should not be used immediately after the patient has smoked, chewed gum, or had hot or cold drinks or food, when he is breathing through the mouth or when having cold or hot applications to the face or throat. Do not use this method when the patient has difficulty in breathing from any cause or when the mouth cannot be closed for the required time: for instance, when the patient has an acute head cold or an inflamed obstructed respiratory tract; when he is sneezing or coughing; or when the mouth falls open from extreme weakness. It must not be used when the mouth is dry, parched, or inflamed; it must never be used for very young children or for restless, delirious, unconscious, or irrational patients because of the danger of biting and breaking the thermometer and swallowing the glass and mercury. Mouth thermometers are rarely used on psychiatric services. The mercury, if swallowed, would probably do no harm because in its metallic form it is almost inert.* If such an accident occurs, however, report it at once. The doctor may prescribe white of egg, milk, or another antidote for mercury. The broken particles of glass, if swallowed, might perforate the mucosa. If a thermometer should accidentally be broken, all particles of glass should be removed from the mouth. If any glass has been swallowed, eating bread or some other soft food may help to prevent injury to the lining of the esophagus.

Should the temperature taken by mouth seem unusually low, or should there be any doubt of its accuracy, take it over again, take it with another thermometer, or take it by rectum. While most studies of body temperature have been made with self-registering rectal thermometers and many clinicians favor this route, taking the temperature by mouth has many advantages. The chief argument for oral temperatures is that they are physically and psychologically so much more acceptable to the patient. They should be used unless the measurement is critical or conditions prohibit it.

The temperature is sometimes taken by axilla when it cannot be taken by mouth, because it is convenient, hygienic, and occasions little exertion for the patient, although many persons find it difficult to hold one posture for as long as is required. Before placing the thermometer in position see that the axilla is free from perspiration, but do not rub the part because friction may increase the temperature and make it inaccurate. Place the bulb securely in the axilla, surround it with body tissues by placing the arm over the chest with the fingers on the opposite shoulder,

---

* Several physicians report cases of broken thermometers with no ill effects from the swallowed mercury. Harry Gold says, ". . . the mercury released from the broken bulb of the thermometer may be ignored with impunity." (Gold, Harry [ed.]: *Cornell Conferences on Therapy*, Vol. 4. The Macmillan Company, New York, 1952, p. 5.)

and leave it in position 10 minutes. Do not allow the clothing to come in contact with the thermometer.

For infants the *groin temperature* is sometimes taken. The thigh must be well flexed over the abdomen. Ten minutes are required for registration.

Axillary and groin temperatures are usually about 1° F lower than that of the mouth.

The *rectal temperature* is generally used for the very ill, for infants, children, and irrational patients. Since exposure of the pubic and anal regions is generally distasteful, rectal temperatures should not be taken unnecessarily. This method must not be used after rectal operations or when the rectum is diseased, inflamed, or impacted with feces. Bacteria are always present in fecal matter, causing decomposition and consequent heat production. The presence of fecal matter therefore probably increases the rectal temperature and interferes with accurate measurement. DuBois says: "Although the rectal temperature usually changes in the same direction as the average body temperature, it may change in the opposite direction. . . . It is well to remember that in a man who exercises the rectal temperature rises while the oral temperature remains constant or falls."[*]

In taking a rectal temperature it is important to have the thermometer well lubricated not only because it is more comfortable but because irritation stimulates the muscles of the rectum to expel the instrument. Insert the bulb about 1½ in. Because the rectum is a closed cavity, less affected by external conditions than the mouth, its temperature is from ½ to 1° F higher.

Never leave children or irrational adults alone with a thermometer, no matter what method is used, for their restless movements are likely to displace or break it. Patients occasionally try to mislead the nurse into thinking that their temperature is elevated when it is not. They may have a second thermometer which they substitute for the one given them, or they may heat the mercury by friction in the hand, the mouth, or the rectum. Virginia Hale and Olga Evseichick report a case of "fraudulent fever," in which the patient made the thermometer register several degrees above the body temperature by "repeated contraction of the anal sphincter muscles."[†] MacNeil suggests the following procedure when it is suspected that the patient is using tricks to elevate the registration. Make "simultaneous observations of the temperature . . . by one or more thermometers in each axilla, another beneath the tongue, and another in the rectum, the stem of each instrument being held steadily by the hand of the observer and never entrusted to the patient."[‡] He believes that "reasonable agreement" of these readings indicates reliability. He suggests as a check testing the temperature of freshly voided feces and urine. Malingerers hope by running a fever to get more attention or to prolong hospitalization. They should always be considered and treated as psychiatric problems.

[*] DuBois, Eugene F.: *op. cit.*, p. 47.

[†] Hale, Virginia, and Evseichick, Olga: "Fraudulent Fever," *Am. J. Nursing,* **43**:992, (Nov.) 1943.

[‡] MacNeil, Ward J.: "Hyperthemia, Genuine and Spurious," *Arch. Int. Med.,* **64**:800, (Oct.) 1939.

Care of Thermometers.   Thermometers should be clean and free from infectious material when used or stored. They should be tested and compared at regular intervals with a standard thermometer, because, unless seasoned, the glass gradually contracts, and after a time the readings are inaccurate, being slightly high. Manufacturers of good-grade thermometers claim, however, that their instruments remain accurate until broken.

If individual thermometers are used and kept in the patient's unit, they should be washed with soap and water and dried after use. To prevent breakage, they should be kept in a covered box, cylinder, or other suitable container. There is no more reason for keeping the patient's individual thermometer in a disinfectant solution than there is his toothbrush. Before the instrument is used for another person, it must be disinfected chemically or in homes washed with soap and water and sunned from 6 to 12 hours. When the same thermometer is used from day to day by two or more patients, it is disinfected each time it is used.

Margaret Welsh and Martha E. Erdman[18] and Elisabeth Ryan and Virginia B. Miller[19] in two similar series of tests on disinfectants commonly used for thermometers found bichloride of mercury in a solution of 1:1000 the most efficient of the solutions tested. In both sets of tests, destruction of microorganisms was more nearly complete and rapid when organic material from the mouth or rectum was removed from the instrument by wiping and washing in soap and water before disinfection. A more recent study showed excellent results when, after thorough soap-and-water cleaning, thermometers were immersed for 10 minutes in 0.5 to 1.0 per cent aqueous or alcoholic solutions of iodine. Mercury compounds were not included in the study because, according to the authors of the report, "Previous work has demonstrated that its action is inhibited by organic material and it is a bacteriostatic rather than a bacteriocidal substance."* Soft paper squares in boxes are recommended for wiping thermometers. When in taking temperatures a group technique is used, it is desirable to have as many thermometers as there are patients so that all the instruments can be washed and disinfected at once. A flat dish, allowing immersion of the thermometers, should be provided for the disinfectant. Washing thermometers under tepid running water is desirable.

For esthetic reasons rectal and mouth thermometers must never be kept on the same tray. Petroleum jelly should be applied to rectal thermometers with paper squares. It must be wiped from the thermometer after use to keep it from interfering with the cleansing process. Obviously, the nurse should have clean hands when taking temperatures; otherwise, efforts made to provide a clean instrument are defeated.

Occasionally, skin temperatures are determined as a diagnostic measure in vascular disease. The technique is not described here since the procedure is rare and is usually performed by the physician or a special technician.

---

* Sommermeyer, Lucille, and Frobisher, Martin, Jr.: "Laboratory Studies on Disinfection of Oral Thermometers," *Nursing Research*, **1**:32, (Oct.) 1952.

3. RESPIRATION

Vital Importance of Cellular Respiration.   Respiration is the exchange of gases between an organism and its environment. It is one of the characteristics common to all living things in one form or another, because it is essential for the chemical changes of metabolism upon which life depends. The human body can survive for weeks without food (except that from its own tissues) but for only a matter of minutes without oxygen.

Oxygen and food are required by each body cell in order to maintain life and function. They must be carried to the cells, where they can be utilized in cell metabolism. Carbon dioxide is one of the resulting waste products; hence, it is important that the body be provided with a system that will not only supply the tissues with oxygen but rid them of carbon dioxide; otherwise, each cell would, in a sense, suffocate. When we speak of a person's strangling or smothering to death, we really mean that his cells are smothering. The greater the activity of the cell, the more oxygen required and the greater the amount of carbon dioxide eliminated.

Provision for this exchange of gases is made in man by the respiratory and circulatory systems. Air containing roughly 20 per cent oxygen and 0.4 per cent carbon dioxide is drawn into the lungs. Here oxygen is absorbed by and carbon dioxide given off from the capillaries. The expired air contains 16.3 per cent oxygen and 4 per cent carbon dioxide. By means of the circulatory system, the oxygen absorbed in the lungs is conveyed to the tissues, and carbon dioxide is conveyed from the tissues to the lungs to be exhaled. Both the respiratory and circulatory systems are a means to an end, the end being the absorption of oxygen by the cells, and elimination by the cells of carbon dioxide. Because the cells are so remote from the oxygen supply, the exchange of gases must take place both between the blood and the air in the lungs and between the blood and the tissue cells. The former is called *external or pulmonary respiration* and the latter, *internal or tissue respiration.*

Regulation of Respiration.   Rhythmical movements of respiration are regulated by the respiratory center, nerve fibers of the autonomic nervous system, and the chemical composition of the blood.

The respiratory center is in the medulla and coincides in position with the sensory center of the vagus. It was called the "vital knot" by its discoverer, Flourens, because he found that when it is destroyed, respiration ceases and death follows. This center sends out motor nerves that supply the muscles of respiration. It is essentially automatic—that is, it sends out impulses to the muscles independently of any impulses sent to it; however, it is also affected by sensory stimuli from all parts of the body. Sensory fibers travel to it through the vagus from the lungs and larynx. Sensory fibers also travel to it from the cerebrum so that stimulation of any sensory nerves in the body, through the cerebrum, may stimulate the respiratory center reflexively and thus affect the rate and character of the breathing. Because there is this connection between the cerebrum and the respiratory center and because the muscles of respiration are voluntary, a person can, to a limited degree, control respiration. When singing or speaking we regulate the depth and rate of respiration; most of the time, however, respiration is rhythmic and involuntary. The effort to "hold the breath" is soon overcome by exhaustion, accumulation of carbon dioxide, and lack of oxygen.

Stimulation of the sensory fibers of the vagus from the lungs and larynx is thought to regulate the respiratory rhythm; the center starts the respirations, but *the messages from the lungs regulate* them. This explains why a patient (when the respiratory center is not paralyzed) may often be revived by artificial respiration. (See pp. 1154 ff.) Stimulation of sensory nerves in the nose, pharynx, larynx, or bronchial tubes by foreign bodies will check respiration, and the glottis will close to protect the lungs.

The temperature and chemical composition of the blood regulate the rate and depth of the respirations by stimulation of the respiratory center. The rate and depth of respiration increases or decreases in relation to the increase and decrease in temperature and carbon dioxide content. David P. Barr, writing in MacBryde's text, says, however, that while chemical stimulation was once thought chiefly responsible for the rate of respiration:

. . . recent work has lent support to the belief of earlier investigators that reflex factors are of utmost significance. It must be realized that reflexes cannot be effective without mechanical mediation and that chemical factors may be less than adequate in the absence of reflexes. . . . It now appears that carbon dioxide acting directly upon the respiratory center furnishes the stimulus that adjusts pulmonary ventilation to meet the changing requirements of the body under ordinary physiologic conditions. This control includes the response to mild and moderate muscular exercise. In more strenuous exertion and in the common emergencies, such as severe anoxemia [low blood oxygen], asphyxia, shock and acidosis, adjustments are accomplished not entirely and perhaps not chiefly by chemical stimuli. In the case of anoxemia and perhaps in severe acidosis these reflexes can be identified with certainty as impulses from chemoreceptors in the carotid and the aortic bodies. . . .

It is entirely likely that both the mechanisms and the control of respiration are more complex than is now realized and that the factors mentioned here do not represent all that are concerned.*

Normal respiration consists in a rhythmical rising and falling of the chest wall and of the walls of the abdomen, occurring in a resting adult about 18 times per minute. It is quiet and effortless, or automatic.

Suggested Method of "Taking" the Respiration.   As in taking the pulse, the patient should be at rest. Allow any effect of exertion or excitement to subside, for these will increase the rate and alter the character of breathing. Even the consciousness of being watched will change the rate and rhythm; therefore, respirations should be counted without the patient's knowledge. After counting the pulse, with the fingers on the wrist as though still engaged in counting the pulse, watch the rise and fall of the chest or upper abdomen; or, better still, if it causes no discomfort to the patient, when counting the pulse, allow the patient's arm to rest lightly on the lower thorax so

* MacBryde, Cyril M. (ed.): *op. cit.,* p. 277.

that afterward and without watching him you can feel the chest and abdomen rising and falling. In this way you can count the respirations without a person's knowledge. In noisy breathing the count may be made by listening. There are certain characteristics, however, that can be noted only by watching the movements of the chest and abdomen. Counting for one minute is desirable although the half-minute count may be made and doubled.

What to Observe When Taking the Respiration.   A nurse must observe the *rate* and *character* of the respirations, *the movements and expansion of the chest and abdomen, the color of the patient,* and *the position* he may instinctively assume.

Rate and Depth of Respiration.   The average rate for a healthy adult is from 14 to 18 respirations per minute; it is more rapid in childhood (20 to 25) and in infancy (30 to 40). In health there is a fairly uniform relation between the frequency of the pulse and of the respirations in the proportion of one respiration to four or five pulse beats. In disease the respirations are usually increased with the pulse, but not always in proportion. In disorders of the lungs and air passages the respirations may increase out of proportion to the increase in the pulse, while in other diseases (and this is more common) the pulse increases out of proportion to the increase in respiration.

Conditions Affecting the Rate and Depth of Respiration.   *Certain changes in the atmospheric pressure increase the respiratory rate.* In high altitudes, such as are encountered in flying or in mountain climbing, the pressure of oxygen in the atmosphere is very low so that not enough oxygen is absorbed by the blood. The result is "mountain sickness," characterized by great weakness, and "air hunger" because the tissue cells have insufficient oxygen. At sea level, air is 20 per cent oxygen, and this is ample to meet the body needs and provide a sufficient margin of safety. When the proportion is reduced to 10 per cent, this margin of safety is removed. In high altitudes there is only a slight margin. It has been demonstrated that if the climb is sufficiently gradual, the normal respiratory and circulatory mechanisms can make the necessary adjustments. The altitude at which oxygen must be added to the atmosphere to make it safely habitable for man is discussed in Chapter 5.

Anything that increases the metabolic rate, or the oxygen used, and anything that interferes with an adequate supply *increase the rate and/or the depth of respiration.* As Barr says in discussing dyspnea, "Increased demand for oxygen by the tissues must be met by an increased supply." *Exertion of any sort* increases the metabolic rate and stimulates respiration. Dressing may increase metabolism as much as 60 per cent; swimming or housework, as much as 200 per cent above the basal level. There must be a proportionate increase in the oxygen supply. *Exposure to cold* increases the oxygen need as the body moves to keep warm, shivers, or goes into a chill; cold applied to the body may stimulate reflex centers affecting respiration. Fever increases metabolism and hence the respiratory rate. It is possible that the same chemicals in the blood, thought to set the temperature center at a higher level, may act in a similar fashion on the respiratory center.

Drugs increase the rate and depth of respiration in various ways. They may increase the metabolic rate, they may stimulate reflex centers, or they may be absorbed by the blood stream and act directly on the respiratory center. The exertion of eating and the *ingested food* increase metabolism, the need for oxygen, and hence the respiratory rate. Almost all emotion increases oxygen need. Everyone can recognize the smothering sensation that accompanies fright. Anxiety is really a low-grade and protracted fear that, like intense fear, stimulates adrenal activity, and increases metabolism and oxygen need. The air hunger of the neurotic state is one of its greatest afflictions. The long sigh of the anxious, depressed, fearful person is his effort to supply the needed oxygen. Elation, however, as well as fear, increases metabolism and oxygen needs.[20, 21]

Most diseases increase the respiratory rate. Endocrine disorders, particularly thyroid disease, raise the metabolic, pulse, and respiratory rates. *Anything that reduces blood volume or the oxygen-carrying elements of the blood* increases the respiratory rate. An example of the first is hemorrhage, and of the second, anemia, or carbon monoxide poisoning when the hemoglobin that ordinarily carries oxygen combines with the carbon monoxide. *Any condition that obstructs the air passages* mechanically increases the respiratory rate because less air is inhaled with each inspiration. A common cold, pneumonia, lung abscess, tuberculosis, bronchitis, fluid in the lungs, asthma, adenoids, or enlarged tonsils, all increase the respiratory rate. *Anything that cuts down the functioning lung area* increases the respiratory rate. A collapse of a lung or a part of it, inflammation of the pleura or covering of the lung, and fluid in the abdominal cavity that makes pressure on the diaphragm reduce lung expansion and force the person to breathe more rapidly in order to get an adequate oxygen supply.

Conditions that increase the carbon dioxide content of the blood increase the depth or rate of respiration, although the excessive stimulation of the respiratory center may finally exhaust and paralyze it. *Brain pathology* affects the respiratory rate and is most likely to slow it.

From the discussion of what increases the rate and depth of respiration it is comparatively easy to see what will *decrease* it. *Atmospheres rich in oxygen, lowering the metabolic rate, rest and sleep, warm (not overheated) environments, normal body temperatures, respiratory depressant drugs, a calm state of mind, normal blood, and normal conditions of the respiratory tract,* all reduce the rate and depth of respiration or keep it within the normal range for the individual. As has been noted, pathology usually results in an increased rate. The exception to this is brain pathology. When there is intercranial pressure from tumors, infections, or fractures, sufficient to affect the respiratory center, the result is usually a slow rate of respiration. Narcotics and sedatives, especially opium and its derivatives, are respiratory depressants, and morphine, for example, is sometimes fatal as a result of this action. It might be safe to say that most respiratory stimulants, such as carbon dioxide, can in too large doses overstimulate and so exhaust the respiration. When the respiratory rate falls below 8 or rises above 40 per minute, the outlook is grave.

Character of Respiration.   A normal average man at rest inspires and exhales about 500 cc of air with each respiration. If considerably more than this quantity of air passes in and out of the lungs, the respiration is said to be deep; if considerably less, it is called shallow. A normal sedentary man of average size has an estimated "vital capacity" of 4500 cc of air. (It must be estimated because he cannot force out all the air. If he did, his lungs would collapse.) An athletic person has a greater vital capacity than a sedentary one, and men's vital capacity is naturally greater than women's.[22]

Any disease that reduces the "vital capacity," that interferes with the exchange of gases by the blood, or that increases the need for oxygen beyond the body's capacity to supply it causes *hyperpnea* (Greek, *hyper* = beyond, above, over; *pnoia* = breath), hard or deep breathing; *polypnea* (Greek, *polys* = many), very rapid breathing; or *dyspnea* (Greek, *dys* = bad or difficult) faulty breathing. Violent exercise necessitates an increase in the depth and rate of respiration, but this is rarely called *dyspnea*. This term is reserved for pathological states. J. C. Meakins says, "Dyspnea is consciousness of the necessity for increased respiratory effort."* Whereas the need for more rapid or deeper respiration is felt briefly during health and easily met by compensatory mechanisms, oxygen need in sickness is likely to be protracted and fearsome to the patient because he senses that his compensatory mechanisms cannot cope with it.

Nurses should observe carefully for signs of *dyspnea*. The patient's position is telling. If the expansion of a lung is painful, he will lie on the affected side to splint it and to allow the unaffected side free movement. During abdominal pain the abdomen is held rigid, and the patient takes rapid, shallow breaths to prevent deep excursions of the diaphragm that make pressure on the abdomen. Shallow respirations must of necessity be rapid in order to pass sufficient air through the lungs. This type of respiration often heralds exhaustion of the vital centers.

Usually a dyspneic person has a rapid, labored respiration that makes a distinct sound; the lips are blue or dusky (cyanotic); the expression is anxious, and the eyes seem prominent. If the dyspnea is severe, unusual muscles are forced into action; the nostrils dilate, the upper chest is greatly expanded by the action of the neck muscles that stand out on either side of the throat, and as the diaphragm contracts forcibly, the abdominal walls protrude. Each breath is drawn with heavings of the chest and abdomen.

When respiration is very difficult, a person may instinctively sit up to relieve the pressure the abdominal content makes on the diaphragm and the organs of the chest. This condition, called *orthopnea* (Greek, *orthos* = straight), is typical of the dyspnea of heart disease.

When dyspnea is prolonged and severe and the patient weak and exhausted, the breathing is frequently irregular and gasping. Dyspnea may affect inspiration or expiration, or the whole act of breathing may be a struggle.

Dyspnea is often accompanied by generalized cyanosis. This bluish cast is

* Meakins, J. C.: "Dyspnea," *J.A.M.A.*, **103**:1442, (Nov.) 1934.

noticed first about the lips and in severe cases in the extremities, under the nails, and finally over the whole body.

Apnea (*a* = not) means absence or complete cessation of breathing. It occurs when there is an increase of oxygen in the blood and a decrease of carbon dioxide which is the normal stimulus to the respiratory center. *Cheyne-Stokes respirations* (named after the two men who first described them) consist of periods of dyspnea preceded and followed by periods of apnea and occurring in a rhythmical cycle, each paroxysm lasting from 30 to 60 seconds. The period of dyspnea begins with short, shallow, almost imperceptible respirations; but each respiration increases in rate, depth, and sound until a maximum of dyspnea is reached, when they gradually decrease in rate, depth, and sound until they finally cease altogether and the apneic period begins. It may last from 1 to 10

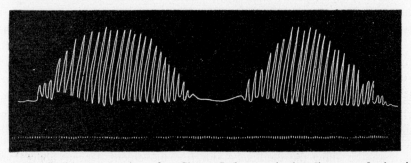

Figure 45. Stethograph tracing of a Cheyne-Stokes respiration [in a man]; the time is marked in seconds [in the lower white line]. (Kimber, D. C.; Gray, C. E.; Stackpole, C. E.; and Leavell, L. C.: *Textbook of Anatomy and Physiology,* 13th ed. The Macmillan Company, New York, 1955.)

seconds, when the whole cycle begins again. During the period of apnea, the patient may drop off to sleep for a few seconds, but during the period of dyspnea he is likely to be restless, even when he appears to sleep.

Although Cheyne-Stokes respirations may sometimes occur in healthy children and adults, when asleep, particularly when lying flat on the back, in disease it is usually a grave symptom. Patients in whom this symptom has been marked have recovered, but in acute illness it is usually a sign of approaching death. This form of breathing is most common in severe heart diseases, in uremia, and in cerebral diseases with increased intracranial pressure.

4. THE PULSE

Definition. The distention or pulsation of the blood vessels produced by the wave of blood forced into them as the heart's left ventricle contracts is called "the pulse." Ordinarily, the term refers to the pulsation of the arteries. Each time the heart beats, it more or less empties the vena cavae and forces approximately 3 oz of blood into the aorta and from there into the systemic arteries. The increased pressure within the arteries forces the column of blood onward, distending the vessels in a wave that extends into the capillaries. With proper instruments the pulse wave can be detected in these microscopic tubes. The wave of dilation and the recoil are felt in the elastic arteries at whatever point they can be compressed against a bone. An upward curve of the pulse wave is felt that corresponds to the contraction, or *systole* of the heart, and a recoil or downward curve that corresponds to the relaxation, or the *diastole,* of the heart. These two periods constitute "the pulse" and represent one heartbeat.

Nurses are rarely asked to note it, but the venous pulse is visible in the large veins of the neck and is the pulsation caused by the rhythmic partial emptying of these veins with each cardiac cycle. However, since these veins respond to the alternating pressure in the chest during respiration, it is difficult to get an accurate count of the venous pulse.[23]

Dependence of the Pulse on Heart Action, Blood Pressure, Volume, and Viscosity. No part of the circulatory system functions independently. Heart action, the tone of the blood vessels, and the nature and quantity of the circulatory fluids are in every case dependent upon all the others. The circulatory system is in turn affected by all the other systems of the body so that any discussion of its function is complicated. Knowledge of the physiology involved is incomplete, but the more understanding the nurse has of what is known, the more effectively she can care for herself and others.

Heart action and blood pressure are not under man's control. His behavior, however, is reflected in them just as it is

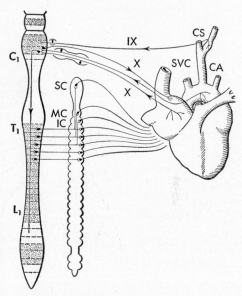

Figure 46. Nerve supply of the heart. *IX,* fiber of the glossopharyngeal nerve; *X,* vagus nerve; *C₁,* level of first cervical spinal nerve; *CA,* carotid artery; *CS,* carotid sinus; *IC,* inferior cervical ganglion; *L₁,* level of first lumbar spinal nerve; *MC,* middle cervical ganglion; *SC,* superior cervical ganglion; *SVC,* superior vena cava; *T₁,* level of first thoracic spinal nerve. *SC, MC,* and *IC* give rise to the superior, middle, and inferior cardiac nerves. (Kimber, D. C.; Gray, C. E.; Stackpole, C. E.; and Leavell, L. C.: *Textbook of Anatomy and Physiology,* 13th ed. The Macmillan Company, New York, 1955.)

in respiration and, to a less extent, the temperature of the body. This is partially understood even by those who have no knowledge of physiology as shown in the expressions: "My heart stood still," "My heart sank," "My heart leapt with joy," and "That made my blood pressure rise." The cardiac and vasomotor centers are in the medulla oblongata, and intercranial pressure affects the heart rate as it does the respiratory. There are nerve cells or ganglia outside the medulla that also influence the heart rate and the size of the blood vessels.

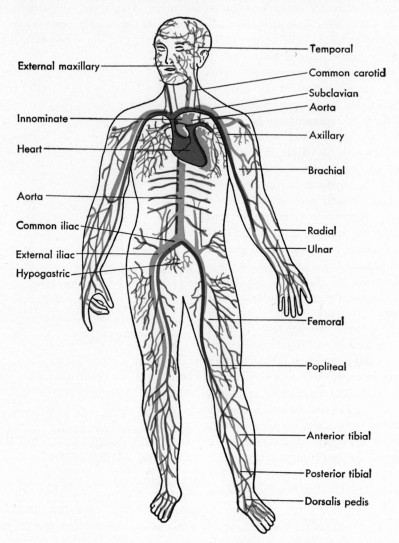

Figure 47. A general diagram of the circulation, showing the course of the major arteries and suggesting pressure points at which the pulse may be felt. (Kimber, D. C.; Gray, C. E.; Stackpole, C. E.; and Leavell, L. C.: *Textbook of Anatomy and Physiology*, 13th ed. The Macmillan Company, New York, 1955.)

Figure 46 shows the nerve supply to the heart. It diagrams two sets of motor nerves: the inhibitory fibers of the vagus that act as a check rein (the parasympathetic division of the autonomic system) and the accelerator nerve fibers that pass to the heart by way of the spinal cord through the cardiac nerves and through visceral branches of the five thoracic spinal nerves (the sympathetic division of the autonomic system).

These two antagonistic sets of motor, or efferent, fibers have their counterpart in two antagonistic sets of sensory, or afferent, fibers arising in the heart and blood vessels called *depressor* (inhibiting) and *pressor* (accelerator) fibers. With this complex nerve supply—that is, nevertheless, a simple system of checks and balances—the rate of the heartbeat and the blood pressure stay within a normal range unless the body taxes itself unduly.

Everyone knows that heart action, and therefore the pulse, is affected by emotion. Whereas the statement that every thought or emotion is reflected in the activity of the circulatory system is hard for many persons to grasp, exaggerated examples of the interaction of the psyche and the soma are recognized. Almost anyone, if alone in the house, reading a story of murder, and hearing an unexpected knock on the door, instantly feels his heart pound, and his respirations increase in depth and frequency, with a sense of weight in the chest. With the contraction of the smooth muscles in the skin, he can see goose flesh appear, and his skin will blanch. There are other indications that the medulla of the adrenal glands is sending adrenalin into the circulation to reinforce the action of the sympathetic system and to prepare this man for defensive action. His heart may have increased as much as 40 beats per minute, and the contractions are forceful; blood pressure has risen with the vascular changes associated with crisis —dilatation of vessels in the heart and voluntary muscles and vasoconstriction elsewhere; the blood sugar level has risen to supply fuel for muscular activity; respirations have increased in rate and depth, and the spleen has discharged more red blood cells to accommodate the increased oxygen needed; the pupils have dilated for far vision; and coagulation time of the blood has shortened for protection in case of injury.[24]

The reaction just described is an exaggerated one, characteristic of fear, but these changes in a less marked degree accompany other emotions. No medical worker can assess the vital signs intelligently or understand the psychic origin of pathology in the circulatory mechanism unless he has some understanding of its relationship to the interdependent endocrine and autonomic nervous systems. The rate and force of the heart, the caliber of the blood vessels, the character and quantity of the circulatory fluids, all vary with emotional, or glandular, behavior.

Muscles of the heart and blood vessels respond to chemicals other than endocrine secretions. The "chemoreceptors" are responsive to the most minute changes in the chemical composition of the blood. Other "thermoreceptors" are sensitive to temperature changes. Corneille Heymans, who has diagramed the regulation of heart rate, says: "The chemical and physical factors chiefly affecting the heart rate are adrenaline, nor-adrenaline, thyroxin, the O_2 and CO_2 content, ,d temperature of the blood."*

This sensitiveness of the heart makes the pulse a valuable index of the condition of the body. The sphygmomanometer, the electrocardiograph, and x-ray, all developed in the past century, enable the present-day physician to assess the condition of the heart and blood vessels far more accurately than could doctors in the past who had little more than the pulse and heart sounds to go by. It is still important, however, for the nurse, as well as the physician, to be able to form judgments on feeling the pulse. It is not practicable to detect by any other means the critical hourly or minute-to-minute changes that can occur in disease.

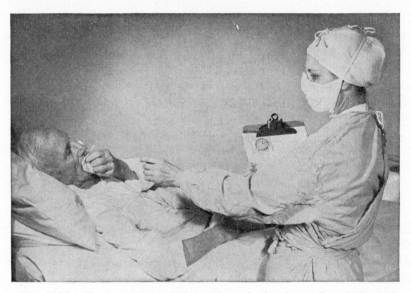

Figure 48. Taking the temperature, pulse, and respiration in a tuberculosis service. Note the watch is protected by a plastic sack and the way in which the patient is handling the thermometer to reduce its gross contamination. (McNett, Esta H.: "Face Mask in Tuberculosis," *Am. J. Nursing,* **49**:32, [Jan.] 1949.)

Frequency with Which the Pulse Is Noted. The pulse of a sick patient is usually assessed with the temperature and respiration twice during the 24 hours or every 4 hours in some cases; when the patient's condition is critical it should be noted almost constantly. The pulse may be taken before, during, and after many procedures requiring mental or physical strain or likely to overtax the heart.

Where the Pulse Can Be Taken. The character of the arterial pulse tracings taken from the aorta to the peripheral arteries varies considerably, but for practical purposes any large superficial artery that rests directly upon a bone against which it can be compressed is used for taking the pulse. (See Fig. 47).

* Heymans, Corneille: *Introduction to the Regulation of Blood Pressure and Heart Rate.* Charles C Thomas, Publisher, Springfield, Ill., 1950, p. 8.

The radial artery is most commonly palpated. It is convenient and compressible since it lies just underneath the skin of the inner surface of the wrist and directly over the radius. The temporal, facial, carotid, femoral, or dorsalis pedis arteries can be used when the wrist is covered by dressings, a plaster cast, or splint.

Sometimes the temporal artery may be used with least disturbance to the patient, and it must be used during packs, when the body is wrapped in blankets or sheets and when the patient is in a respirator. The carotid arteries, although not lying over bones, are large, near the surface, and quite close to the heart so that pulsations may be felt here when imperceptible at the wrist. In some diseases pulsations may be seen and counted in the temporal and carotid arteries without touching the patient. There may be a palpable pulse in the femoral artery

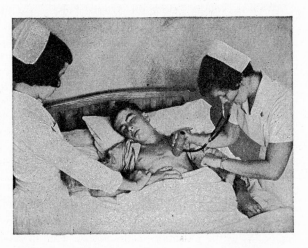

Figure 49. Two nurses taking the radial and apical pulse simultaneously. The Lectron-O-Scope makes the slightest heart sounds audible. It is particularly useful when the patient's circulation is failing and in taking the fetal heart rate. (Courtesy of Columbia-Presbyterian Medical Center, New York City, and Clay-Adams Co., New York City.)

when none can be felt in the radial. In shock or collapse and in approaching death, it may be possible to count the weakened cardiac contractions only by listening to the heart through a stethoscope. When the radial pulse is irregular, the physician may want the pulse taken by two persons simultaneously, one counting the pulsations at the wrist and the other listening to the heart sounds at its apex. (See Fig. 49.) The difference between the apical and radial counts, which must be made simultaneously, is called the *pulse deficit* and is the result of what Carl J. Wiggers terms "frustrate" heart contractions that fail to produce perceptible radial pulsations.

Slight differences in the pulse can always be detected most easily if the pulse is counted at the same place each time.

Suggested Procedure in Counting the Arterial Pulse.   See that the person is at rest and, usually, recumbent. If the pulse is assessed following exertion or excitement, the fact should be noted. In a fearful person the heart rate may be increased just because the pulse is being counted. The nurse should try to put him at ease and divert his attention if possible. Place the tips of the first, second, and third fingers on the artery, exerting such pressure as does not obliterate but makes the pulsation most distinct. With three fingers rather than one the character of the artery and the shape of the pulse wave are more easily felt. The thumb should never be used because the pulsation of its artery may be mistaken for the patient's pulse. A full-minute count should be made, and longer periods may be necessary to judge regularity in some cases.

When taking the radial pulse, support the forearm in a semipronated position. With a new patient check the pulsations in both wrists or verify the count at two pressure points. If there is any doubt about the count, get a more experienced person to repeat the procedure before recording the pulse.

The pulse count is graphed on the same sheet with the temperature and respiration. In hospitals this mechanical recording should be done by a clerk from figures given by the nurse, who in turn should write any necessary comments on the quality of the pulse under "Nurse's Notes."

What to Note in Taking the Arterial Pulse.   The most important measurement is the *rate* of the pulse, and the next, its *rhythm,* or regularity. In addition, and according to her ability, the nurse notes the *tension,* or compressibility, *of the artery* and the *volume of the pulse,* or the shape of the pulse wave. All of these qualities can be seen in the sphygmographic tracing of a pulse or by the trained eye in the electrocardiograph. The nurse will better understand what she feels in the arterial pulse and what she hears in listening to the heartbeat if she studies tracings similar to the one illustrated in Figure 45.

An electrocardiogram, called an ECG, is a graphic record taken from the body surfaces of the electric potential differences due to cardiac action. Record of a normal pulse shows 6 waves. The first, called the P wave, is due to excitation of the atria (auricles); Q, R, and S to excitation of the ventricles; T to repolarization of the ventricles; and U is a diastolic wave of unknown origin. (See Fig. 130.)

A sphygmographic tracing of a pulsation is made on a revolving drum by a stylus attached by a delicate spring to a mechanism that, when fixed over a pressure point, responds to the pulsation of the artery. The upward curve represents the expansion of the artery caused by the sudden inflow of blood during the contraction of the left ventricle. This measures the force of the heartbeat. A forceful heartbeat and a soft arterial wall give the upward curve height. An inelastic, or sclerosed, artery cannot be distended by a strong contraction of the ventricle. In hemorrhage there is less blood forced into the arteries with each heartbeat, and this lowers the height of the upward curve. While the upward curve is smooth, the broken line in the downward curve represents several pulsations of the artery. Normally these pulsations or waves on the downward curve are all imperceptible to the examining finger. In some diseases the middle, or dicrotic, wave is so pronounced, however, that the pulse is spoken of as the "dicrotic pulse," and it is necessary that nurses recognize and understand it.

It will be noticed that in the normal pulse the downward curve is much more gradual than the upward. This is because the upward curve is due to the forceful heartbeat, whereas the downward is brought about by the elastic recoil of the walls of the artery. The upward curve represents the systole of the heart when blood is streaming into the arteries and the artery rises against the finger; it is then the pulse is counted. The downward curve represents the diastole of the heart in which the semilunar valves are closed; blood has ceased to flow into the aorta; the elastic walls are returning to their original size, pressing constantly and steadily on the blood and sending it onward; and the artery seems to fall away gradually from the fingers. The dicrotic wave is caused by the closure of the semilunar valves. The elastic wall of the aorta as it recoils drives the blood in two directions—onward and back against the closed semilunar valves, which it strikes with considerable force, depending upon the original force of the heartbeat. From this wall of resistance and sudden check to its flow, it rebounds, and this rebound causes the expansion of the artery called the dicrotic wave. When the tone of the blood vessel is very low, it dilates abnormally at this point, and the dicrotic wave is felt almost as distinctly as the primary curve. This condition should be reported, but the dicrotic wave must not be counted as a heartbeat.

The "Normal" Pulse.   Since the heart rate and blood pressure vary in health with age, size, sex, and emotional and physical activity, there can be no one heart rate or blood pressure that is normal. On the other hand, measurements made of healthy persons of both sexes and all ages give averages that we tend to think of as normal. It would be more nearly correct, however, to think of a range in heart rate and blood pressure that seems characteristic of the healthy state.

The following are average resting *heart rates* for man at different ages.*

AGE IN YEARS	HEART RATE PER MINUTE
Fetus	150
0 (birth)	135
5	105
10	90
15	80
20	75
25–40	70
80	75

It is apparent that the heart rate, like the respiratory rate, decreases with size. The heart rate of a canary is about 1000; that of a mouse, 700; that of the elephant, around 25. Size partly accounts for the fact that a man's average heart rate is several counts lower than a woman's. Muscular exercise temporarily increases the pulse rate, but muscular development ultimately decreases the resting rate. Best and Taylor say that a healthy athlete may have a resting pulse as low as 50 or 60. A pulse rate of 55 to 60 is found during sleep in some healthy adults.[25] The pulse rate increases during health, however, from 20 to 60 counts or more to meet the needs of the body during physical and emotional activity. The heart is stimulated chemically by the endocrine secretions and by the effect of the endocrines on the blood vessels. It is now known that a normal heart rate is dependent upon the proportion of sodium, potassium, and calcium ions in the blood.[26]

* Heymans, Corneille: *op. cit.*, p. 8.

A normal pulse has a regular *rhythm*. The beats are felt by the fingers at regular intervals, and seem to be of equal force. The artery feels elastic, neither hard nor soft, under the fingers. Because even in health arteries tend to lose their elasticity, the judgment of normal tension, or *compressibility,* must take the person's age into consideration. The *volume* of the pulse is thought normal if the artery feels full to the touch and the pulsations strong with a normal interval between them.

Abnormal Conditions of the Pulse. Mental and physical disease, drugs, and exposure to harmful environmental conditions may result in abnormalities of rate, rhythm, tension, and volume of the pulse, as has been indicated in this chapter.

To judge whether a person's resting heart rate is rapid or slow, one must know the normal range for sex and age. The habitual pulse rate of the individual in health should also be considered. A resting pulse over 100 in an adult in comfortable environmental conditions, under no apparent emotional strain, is usually, but not always, an indication of disease; *tachycardia* (*tachys* = swift) is the term used for a heart rate over 150. The rate may rise to 250. When the rate is so fast that it cannot be counted it is described as "running." In organic and functional heart diseases the contractions of the heart may be so rapid and weak that the heart is said to "fibrillate," which means to quiver. Under such circumstances the pulse cannot be counted; a very low blood volume as in hemorrhage, and many other conditions, can result in such a weak and rapid pulse that it is even impalpable.

A pulse rate of less than 60 is usually, but not always, considered a sign of disease. *In certain conditions a pulse below 60 is a danger sign.*

Following brain injury or whenever there is a possibility of an increase in intercranial pressure, the pulse should be counted frequently, and *any slowing of the rate reported at once.* Under such circumstances a fall below 60 is a grave symptom that may indicate pressure on the nerve center in the medulla supplying the inhibitory fibers of the vagus nerve. Drugs given to slow the heart, such as digitalis, are discontinued when the pulse falls to 60. Occasionally, a very slow pulse (bradycardia; *bradys* = slow) indicates organic heart disease of a serious nature. Nurses who would report a rapid pulse at once often fail to understand that a decrease in the heart rate may be equally serious.

Irregularities of rhythm are called arrhythmias. The intervals between beats may be of different lengths, or the beats may be of unequal force. These conditions are seen in many apparently healthy persons, and in some cases the heart action is normal, but something interferes with its interpretation through palpation of the pulse. In some cases the symptom indicates a serious condition. It must always be reported and recorded. An electrocardiogram should be made to determine the origin of the irregularity.

Tension, or compressibility, of the artery is measured with the sphygmomanometer, and determination of blood pressure is a part of every medical examination. Softness and rigidity of the artery can be felt, however, and the nurse should note both conditions. A degree of softness is typical of the pulse in youth, but when that factor is taken into account, arterial pulsation that can be obliterated means very low blood pressure. This may occur when anything interfers with vasoconstriction, as in a sympathectomy, or when the blood volume is low, as in hemor-rhage. A hard artery that can be rolled under the fingers like a cord, sometimes called a pipestem, or one that feels torturous or knotted indicates disease of the vessels—arteriosclerosis. A tracing of such a pulse shows a shortening or straight-ening of all the curves seen in the normal pulse.

If the *volume* of blood is normal and the heartbeat strong, a very soft artery will give its pulsation a bounding quality. The tracing of such a pulse shows a high primary wave. Such a pulse is described as bounding, large, or full. If, on the other hand, there has been loss of blood as in hemorrhage, or redistribution of blood, as in shock, the decrease in volume is felt in the small, weak, or even flicker-ing pulse, a tracing of which would show a lower primary curve.

Any nurse who hopes to give maximum help to her patients will study the pulse and by specialized reading add to the limited information supplied by a general text of this sort.

5. BLOOD PRESSURE

Definition. Blood pressure is the lateral pressure exerted by the blood on the walls of the vessels. The term "blood pressure" usually refers to the pressure of blood on the wall of the artery. "Arterial blood pressure" is the more accurate term. Again, this is so general as to be misleading because the blood pressure with-in the artery varies during the cardiac cycle. So we should say the "systolic," the "diastolic," or the "mean" arterial blood pressure. Heymans describes these as follows:

The arterial pressure in the large arteries is characterized by a *systolic pressure*, an increase of pressure induced by the systolic contraction of the left heart ventricle, and by a *diastolic pressure*, a drop of arterial pressure occurring during the diastolic arrest of the heart between two contractions. The *mean arterial pressure* represents the average between the systolic rise and the diastolic fall of pressure.*

While in clinical practice blood pressure is usually measured in the arteries, it can be measured anywhere in the vascular system, and within recent years clinicians have used measurement of the venous pressure as a diagnostic aid.

Historical Note. Arthur M. Master et al.[27] credit Stephen Hales with the first actual measurement of blood pressure in 1733. The measurement was made on a horse. Hales, a minister with scientific leanings, found that the blood rose 8 ft in a tube inserted into the femoral artery. Since then, there have been many experi-ments and studies with animals and human beings leading to the development of more accurate instruments. The mercury sphygmomanometer (*sphygmos* = pulse), developed by Riva-Rocci in 1896, was based on the same principles as the instru-ment now in common use. Recent investigations have shown that when the width of the cuff of this instrument is not modified according to the diameter of the ex-tremity to which it is applied, its measurements are inaccurate. It is likely that other refinements of sphygmomanometry will follow.

* Heymans, Corneille: *op. cit.,* p. 1. (Italics are the writer's.)

The same general principles for measuring arterial pressure apply to the venous pressure. A more sensitive device than the air cuff must be placed over the vein and a water manometer substituted for a mercury scale. Mercury, being 13.5 times heavier than water, will not be lifted high enough in the manometer to be easily read. Clinical measurements of venous pressure have been used only within the past 25 years; present procedures require the introduction of a needle into a vein and considerable judgment in the use of such instruments as are available. Venous pressure measurements are therefore seldom made, and when they are, the physician makes them.

Physiology of Blood Pressure.   Blood is confined under pressure in the blood vessels. *Pressure varies from a positive pressure in the arteries to a gradually diminishing and finally a negative pressure just as the blood is returned to the heart by the large veins.* Blood pressure depends upon the force of the heartbeat, the elasticity or tone of the vessels, and the volume and viscosity of the blood. The pressure and also the velocity of the blood are highest in the aorta; from here to the smallest artery there is a drop of only 20 mm (mean pressure). On the other hand, as the blood passes from the arterial to the capillary end of the arteriole, there is a drop of from 50 to 60 mm of mercury. As the blood passes through the capillary into the venules, the pressure drops another 15 to 20 mm and the velocity of flow is greatly diminished.

As the arterioles divide into myriads of microscopic capillaries, their walls offer a resistance that slows the stream. Again the velocity increases as capillaries combine to form venules, and as venules are joined to form veins. With each beat of the heart the force of negative pressure is exerted on the veins emptying into it. Positive venous pressure is highest in the peripheral veins and lowest in those near the heart. Zero pressure is believed to be reached in the jugular veins at the base of the neck. Between this point and the right atrium (auricle), where the venae cavae empty, the negative pressure varies from about 2.5 to 6.1 mm mercury.

If the reader studies the figures just given, he can understand that the tone of the arterioles is very important since they act as a check or regulating force between the high pressure system of the arteries and the low pressure system of the veins. The heartbeat sends the blood into the arteries in great waves; the arterioles slow and steady the stream so that it flows into the vast network of capillaries as water flows from a river into a lake. While in the capillaries, some just large enough in diameter to accommodate a single blood cell, occurs the exchange of nutrients, regulators, and wastes between the blood and the other body elements. If the blood were said to run through the arteries, it would amble through the capillaries. It was formerly thought that normally pulsation was lost in the capillaries, but according to Best and Taylor, it is found in healthy young persons although it cannot be induced in the aged. Health depends upon keeping pressures in all parts of the vascular system within normal ranges.

Blood pressure may be measured in any accessible part of the circulatory mechanism at any moment in the cardiac cycle. To the physiologist "blood pressure" usually suggests the mean pressure; to the layman, the systolic arterial pressure; and to the clinician, the relationship between the systolic and diastolic arterial pressures. According to Veronica F. Murray,[28] the efficiency of the circulation is shown by the extent to which the heart raises the pressure of the stream of blood in systolic above the diastolic, or back pressure. This difference is known as the *pulse pressure* and represents the volume output of the left ventricle. Some physiologists say that the venous pressure gives the most reliable index of the efficiency of the heart.

Nothing could be more vital than normal capillary conditions, but estimates of their status are difficult to make and interpret. In discussing heart action (see p. 291) it was necessary to include *regulation of blood pressure* since the heart is only a specialized section of what might be diagramed as a continuous vascular tube. Anything that affects the heart also affects the blood vessels. Both are under the control of the autonomic system, and both respond to thermal and chemical stimuli. Both are safeguarded by a multiple nerve supply so that if one set of fibers or one group of cells is destroyed, other fibers and other cells eventually take on their function. Heymans says in speaking of the vasomotor center located in the floor of the fourth ventricle:

From this center vasoconstrictor impulses are distributed to the different segments of the spinal cord. These impulses pass over the sympathetic nerves to the various organs of the body. . . . When the vasomotor center in the medulla oblongata is destroyed, there occurs immediately a general vasodilatation with a fall of the arterial blood pressure to 30 to 60 mm. mercury. The blood pressure remains low for a considerable time but recovers slowly and progressively, owing to vasoconstrictor impulses arising from the spinal vasomotor centers. . . .

Experiments of Ransom and Billingsley demonstrate the existence of vasodilator centers in addition to the vasoconstrictor centers just described. A vasodepressor center has been described adjacent to the vasodepressor center in the medulla oblongata. Stimulation of this center induces vasodilation and a fall of arterial blood pressure. . . .

Finally chemical factors are also concerned in the control of vasomotor tone and peripheral resistance. Adrenaline, nor-adrenaline, pituitrin, histamine, CO_2, H-ions, O_2-lack and different metabolites may modify the peripheral vascular tone of arterioles, capillaries and veins and eventually induce a change in peripheral resistance and in arterial pressure.[*]

Since the caliber of blood vessels changes in response to the percentage of oxygen, carbon dioxide, salts of metabolism, and endocrine secretions in the blood, it is easy to see why blood pressure varies with emotional and physical activity. The exertion of eating probably has more effect on blood pressure than the absorbed nutrients, although blood vessel walls are believed to be modified by diet. Master and associates, in the report of an extensive study, say blood pressure tends to increase with weight. He attaches importance to the changes in blood pressure due to emotion but says the study of these changes is in its infancy. Homer Wheelon illustrates the effect of exercise on blood pressure with the following measurements made on a young person:[†]

[*] Heymans, Corneille: *op. cit.,* pp. 9-11.

[†] Wheelon, Homer: "The Interpretation of Blood Pressure Variations; with Observations on Normal Pressure Variations and Relation of the Adrenals and the Autonomic Nervous System to the Production of Blood Pressure." *New York M. J.,* **113**:505, (Apr.) 1921.

	BLOOD PRESSURE	PULSE PRESSURE
Lying down	116/75	41
Sitting..................	120/76	44
Standing................	122/82	40
After 5-minute exercise......	139/86	53

Since the diastolic pressure does not rise in proportion to the systolic, the pulse pressure, or the volume output of the ventricles, varies sufficiently to provide the adaptation of the blood supply necessary for the varying demands of the body. Blood pressure is lowered in health during periods of physical rest and freedom from emotional excitement. Master says the systolic blood pressure drops as much as 20 mm mercury during sleep. The diastolic drop is not so great.

Blood pressure, like heart rate, varies with sex but much more markedly with age. Henry I. Russek et al., studying about 5000 men, conclude that the old, but recently discredited, dictum that the systolic pressure should be 100 plus the age of the individual is fairly reliable. They say, however: "Essential hypertension cannot be defined solely in terms of the systolic pressure. It is the diastolic level alone that determines the existence of disease."*

Heymans gives the following averages for normal persons at five periods, or ages:†

AGE	SYSTOLIC PRESSURE	DIASTOLIC PRESSURE
Infancy...............	75 to 90 mm	Around 50 mm first
Childhood............	90 to 110 mm	5 years of life
About puberty........	100 to 120 mm	After that remains
Adults................	125 to 130 mm	fairly constant at
Old people............	140 to 150 mm	60 to 80 mm

Master and his associates, studying the records of 15,706 men and women between the ages of 16 and 65, taken by random sampling from 74,000 records, concluded that normal ranges for the middle-aged and elderly should be raised from the commonly accepted standards to the following figures.

Table 6. Average or Normal Blood Pressure in Middle and Old Age

AGE AND SEX	NORMAL RANGE		BORDERLINE HYPERTENSION	
	Systolic	*Diastolic*	*Systolic*	*Diastolic*
Males 55 years	115–165	70–98	165–180	98–108
Males 65 years	115–170	70–100	170–190	100–110
Females 55 years	110–170	70–100	170–185	100–108
Females 65 years	115–175	70–100	175–190	100–110

* Russek, Henry I., et al.: "The Influence of Age on Blood Pressure," *Am. Heart J.,* **32**:468, (Oct.) 1946.

† Heymans, Corneille: *op. cit.,* p. 1.

From this study the conclusion was reached that women tend to have a slightly lower blood pressure before the ages of 40, but after 50 it is slightly higher than men's. Master and his associates think that the limit of 150 mm of mercury that has been erroneously set on "normal" systolic blood pressure has aroused needless fear among healthy patients. They say: "There exists a high incidence of so-called hypertension in the normal population. . . . The need for upward revision of the commonly accepted limits of blood pressure . . . for each age group and for both sexes is, therefore, clear."*

Pathological Changes Affecting Blood Pressure.   Disease in any part of the circulatory system may cause abnormal blood pressure. Pathology of the endocrine glands, particularly the adrenals, whose secretions so greatly affect the cardiovascular mechanism, alters blood pressure. The kidneys secrete a pressor substance, it is believed, which is largely responsible for the cardiovascular involvement found in nephritis. This group of symptoms is akin to the uremia of abnormal pregnancy, characterized by blood pressure elevation. Drugs and bacterial poisons can constrict the arterioles just as these endotoxins do.

Most students of *hypertension* support the view that temperament can predispose to high blood pressure. The ambitious person who has drives perhaps beyond his capacity for achievement and who represses resentment against those who, in his opinion, thwart him is an oversimplified characterization of the type. Hypertension in such persons can often be relieved by severing the sympathetic (vasoconstrictor) fibers largely responsible for elevation of blood pressure seen in emotional states. Such a condition is called neurogenic hypertension and is a functional rather than an organic disease. Lewis Dexter, in the text edited by Russell L. Cecil and Robert F. Loeb,[29] says that there are as many classifications of hypertension as there are authors! He thinks also that the terms "mild" and "severe" mean substantially the same as "benign" and "malignant," terms in relation to hypertension that confuse many nurses.

The fact that certain peoples, such as the Chinese, who eat high-carbohydrate diets are generally free from hypertension has led to the theory that the American and European diet may be a predisposing factor in high blood pressure. Animal experimentation and clinical experience have, in some cases, substantiated this theory. Cholesterol, found in fats, is identified as the pressor substance, and many patients with hypertension are now treated with low-fat, high-carbohydrate diets.[30]

Some physicians are teaching their patients to "take" their own blood pressure and to control its range of elevation by diet, rest, and even vasodilating drugs. The value of this and other forms of the therapy is widely debated. William Goldring in the *Cornell Conferences on Therapy* says that neither the cause nor the cure of hypertension is known and that present treatment is essentially empirical.[31]

The danger of hemorrhage from a ruptured blood vessel is always present with an excessive blood pressure. Since there is less room for expansion of vessels in the cranial cavity than in any other part of the body, a hemorrhage is most likely

* Master, Arthur M., et al.: *Normal Blood Pressure and Hypertension; New Definitions.* Lea & Febiger, Philadelphia, 1952, p. 83.

to occur there. Intercranial pressure from any cause affects the vasomotor center in the medulla. A most important function of the nurse in the care of patients with cranial injuries or operations is the checking of blood pressure at intervals of 10 to 30 minutes. Marked deviations of any sort should be reported at once to the physician. Early recognition of blood pressure changes may save a life.

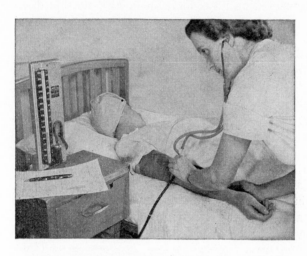

Figure 50. Taking the blood pressure with a mercury manometer. This instrument (Banker-Manometer) is mounted on its own free-wheeling stand and has a drawer in which cuffs and a stethoscope may be kept. (Courtesy of Columbia-Presbyterian Medical Center, New York City, and Clay-Adams Co., New York City.)

Hypotension, or low blood pressure, may be habitual, temperamental, or primary. Dexter says it can be "categorically stated" that there are no symptoms ascribable to this condition. He adds: "Therapeutically the patient may be congratulated."* Secondary hypotension following disease is a symptom that disappears with the condition if it is successfully treated. Hypotension is seen in Addison's disease

Figure 51. Various sizes and types of blood pressure cuffs. The largest are used over the adult thigh; the smallest is designed for an infant's arm. (Courtesy of Becton, Dickinson & Co., Rutherford, N. J., and Clay-Adams Co., New York City.)

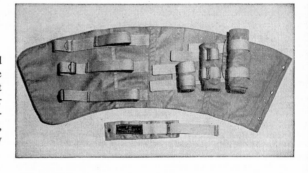

(chronic adrenal cortical insufficiency), in extreme malnutrition, and following acute and chronic infection. The marked drop in blood pressure accompanying anesthesia, traumatic shock, hemorrhage, insulin shock, and other crises is dangerous and should be corrected as quickly as possible. In some cases it is necessary

* Cecil, Russell L., and Loeb, Robert F. (eds.): *A Textbook of Medicine,* 8th ed. W. B. Saunders Co., Philadelphia, 1951, p. 1079.

to introduce blood or its substitutes continuously for several days. Saline and glucose are not effective because they rapidly filter out into the tissues.

The importance of making accurate estimates of blood pressure cannot be overestimated. Both systolic and diastolic readings must be taken and recorded. When the nurse is not sure of her findings, she should have them checked by a more experienced worker.

Types of Apparatus Used in Measuring Blood Pressure. For measuring *arterial blood pressure* the mercury manometer is usually employed because it is considered reasonably accurate and more easily kept in good condition than other devices. (See Fig. 50.) Some physiologists think the mercury manometer less sensitive than the aneroid type, which is an instrument with a dial on which pressure is shown by an indicator, or pointer, attached to a spring mechanism. Obviously, both these instruments must be connected by rubber tubing to a rubber cuff that is placed over an artery of the arm or leg. Reading the oscillation of the mercury column and the spring indicator is no longer thought to be a reliable means of estimating blood pressure. Listening to the sounds over the artery at the obliteration of pulsation and after pulsation returns is now thought essential; so a stethoscope is a necessary part of the equipment. A variety of cuffs should be available so that one may be chosen that is 20 per cent wider than the diameter of the arm or leg.

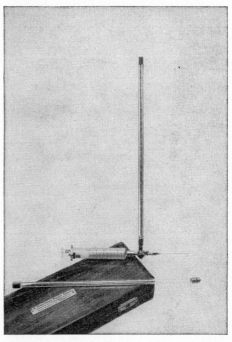

Figure 52. Manometer for measuring venous pressure. (Courtesy of Becton, Dickinson & Co., Rutherford, N. J., and Clay-Adams Co., New York City.)

For measuring *venous pressure*, a water manometer is used. Because mercury is a heavy liquid, the venous pressure may not be sufficient to make visible changes in the level of a column of mercury in a manometer. The manometer containing saline is attached by a stopcock to a venipuncture needle. The apparatus, because it comes in contact with the blood stream, should be sterile. The water manometer may be connected with a membranous tambour that is placed over the vein. This procedure is convenient because it does not involve asepsis, but measurements made in this way are not as accurate.

Capillary tension is judged by the changes in skin color following immersion of hands or feet in hot and cold water; or it may be assessed by the appearance of the skin during and after manual pressure with a glass slide.

When to Measure Blood Pressure.   Master contrasts the "basal blood pressure" —measurements following a 10- to 12-hour fast and rest—and the "casual blood pressure"—measurements made during an office visit or without special preparation. If the former measurement is used in order to rule out the effects of exertion and food, the operator may try also to eliminate the effect of fear by repeating the readings at 10-minute intervals for four or five times in order to accustom the patient to the test and to his presence. When "casual" measurements are made, they should also be repeated to minimize the effect of anxiety. If the tests are made in rapid succession, the reading is less likely to be distorted by a spasm of the artery, sometimes induced by the pressure of the cuff. James Bordley et al., in the report referred to (see footnote below), express the opinion that the "casual" blood pressure more nearly parallels the day-by-day level.

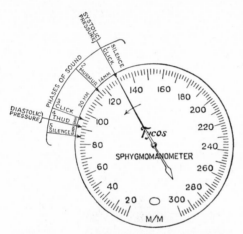

Figure 53. Dial of spring manometer. Shows the characteristic changes of tone and lengths of phases of sound as heard through the stethoscope in testing the average young adult. (Courtesy of Taylor Instrument Company, Rochester, N. Y.)

Suggested Procedure in Taking Measurements of Arterial Blood Pressure. Have the patient in a comfortable recumbent or sitting position, preferably the former, with the arm or leg to be used supported. Measurements may be made in either arm or leg, but repeated readings should be taken in the same extremity, since structural differences may affect the findings. Blood pressure is most often measured in the left arm.

Explain the procedure, and in every way try to prevent excitement and anxiety. The patient should be physically and mentally quiet. Expel any air in the cuff and adjust it comfortably around the arm above the elbow so that the tubes from it will not be over the point of the brachial artery where the stethoscope will be placed. When measurements are made on the leg, the cuff is placed above the knee and the stethoscope over the popliteal artery in the popliteal space. Before inflating the cuff, find the pulsation of the brachial artery (the inner aspect of the bend of the arm), and place the stethoscope exactly over this point. Inflate the cuff with the rubber bulb until the pulsation of the artery that has become audible during the inflation of the cuff is no longer heard. Then allow the air to escape very slowly until the sound reappears. This first reappearance of sound is the blood being forced through the partially compressed vessel during systole. The pressure in the cuff at this point (the reading of the manometer) is almost equal to the systolic pressure within the blood vessel, but the American Heart Association recommends that the systolic reading be made at the sudden disappearance of "the clear, faint tapping sound."[*]

* Bordley, James, et al.: "Recommendations for Blood Pressure Determination by Sphygmomanometers," Scientific Council of the American Heart Association, *Circulation*, **4**:503, 1951.

Having secured the systolic reading, further deflate the cuff until the sounds change from a loud to a soft thumping and then until it disappears. The compression of the artery is no greater now than the diastolic pressure, and the flow of blood is unimpeded. The American Heart Association recommends reading the diastolic pressure "at the point of complete cessation of sounds." Murray* gives the following description of the sounds to be heard following the distention of the cuff:

1. Silence. (Pressure in cuff higher than systolic pressure; no blood coming through.)
2. Sharp snapping or thumping. (Pressure [about] equal to systolic; blood coming through in spurts.)
3. Thumps get softer, swishing friction sounds. (Pressure still above diastolic; more blood coming through compressed artery.)
4. Thumping becomes loud again. (Pressure almost equalized by diastolic; blood just getting through during diastole.)
5. Sounds suddenly become much softer.
6. Silence. (Normal flow.)

Taking blood pressure readings accurately and expeditiously requires understanding and skill acquired through experience. Medical workers should practice this procedure with well persons before subjecting the ill to the risks of awkward manipulation of apparatus and uncertain interpretation of pulse sounds.

Suggested Procedure in Taking Venous Pressure by Direct Method. Since the nurse is never expected to make this measurement, the technique is not given here in detail. The nurse may be responsible for sterilizing the equipment, for preparing the patient psychologically and physically, and for working with the physician as he makes the test. The manometer, 3-way stopcock, syringes, and needle should be sterilized by steam under pressure. The manometer, a calibrated cylinder, is supported by a suitable stand. Sterile physiological saline must be provided for the manometer. The doctor, using a small pillow or a rolled bath blanket, adjusts the arm so that the vein is opposite and on the same level as the apex of the heart. The skin is prepared as for any needle puncture; the needle is inserted into the median vein of the forearm by the physician. The saline flows into the vein until the pressure within the vein stops the flow. The height of the column of saline above the level of the heart, after the saline ceases to flow, represents the venous pressure in millimeters of water if the scale is a linear scale.

After the doctor has ascertained the venous pressure, he may determine the circulation time by an injection of a drug such as sodium dehydrocholate (Decholin). He explains to the patient that he is to signal when he experiences a bitter taste in the mouth. The nurse times the interval between the beginning of the injection and the patient's signal.

REFERENCES

1. Best, Charles H., and Taylor, Norman B.: *The Physiological Basis of Medical Practice,* 5th ed. Williams & Wilkins Co., Baltimore, 1950, p. 608.
2. Fulton, John F. (ed.): *A Textbook of Physiology,* 16th ed. W. B. Saunders Co., Philadelphia, 1949, p. 1002.
3. Best, Charles H., and Taylor, Norman B.: *op. cit.,* p. 720.
4. DuBois, Eugene F.: *Fever and the Regulation of Body Temperature.* Charles C Thomas, Publisher, Springfield, Ill., 1948, p. 31.

* Murray, Veronica F.: "Technic of Taking Blood Pressure," *Am. J. Nursing,* **34:**1057, (Nov.) 1934.

5. Winslow, C.-E. A., and Herrington, Lovic P.: *Temperature and Human Life.* Princeton University Press, Princeton, 1949, p. 85.
6. Best, Charles H., and Taylor, Norman B.: *op. cit.,* p. 879.
7. MacBryde, Cyril M. (ed.): *Signs and Symptoms; Their Clinical Interpretation,* 2nd ed. J. B. Lippincott Co., Philadelphia, 1952, p. 391.
8. Winslow, C.-E. A., and Herrington, Lovic P.: *op. cit.,* p. 27.
9. Menkin, Valy: "Chemical Basis of Fever with Inflammation," *Arch. Path.,* **39:**28, (Jan.) 1945.
10. Reimann, Hobart A.: "The Problem of Long Continued, Low Grade Fever," *J.A.M.A.,* **107:**1089, (Oct.) 1936.
11. Wynn, Frank B.: "The Psychic Factor as an Element in Temperature Disturbance," *J.A.M.A.,* **73:**31, (July) 1919.
12. MacNeil, Ward J.: "Hyperthermia, Genuine and Spurious," *Arch. Int. Med.,* **64:**800, (Oct.) 1939.
13. MacBryde, Cyril M. (ed.): *op. cit.,* p. 393.
14. Smith, Lawrence W., and Fay, Temple: "Observations on Human Beings with Cancer Maintained at Reduced Temperatures of 75°-90° Fahrenheit," *Am. J. Clin. Path.,* **10:**1, (Jan.) 1940.
15. DuBois, Eugene F.: *op. cit.,* p. 38.
16. Tompkins, Pendelton S.: "Danger in Securing Vaginal Temperatures," *Fertil. & Steril.,* **1:**543, (Nov.) 1950.
17. DeNosaquo, Norman, et al.: "Clinical Use of Oral Thermometers; Report of Study to Determine Time Required for Reliable Registration," *J. Lab. & Clin. Med.,* **29:**179, (Feb.) 1944.
18. Welsh, Margaret, and Erdman, Martha E.: "Studies in Thermometer Techniques," *Nursing Educ. Bull.,* No. 11, Bureau of Publication, Teachers College, Columbia University, New York, 1929.
19. Ryan, Elisabeth, and Miller, Virginia B.: "Disinfection of Clinical Thermometers," *Am. J. Nursing,* **32:**197, (Feb.) 1932.
20. Dunbar, Helen F.: *Emotions and Bodily Change,* 3rd ed. Columbia University Press, New York, 1946, pp. 170, 239.
21. Stevenson, Ian: "Physical Symptoms During Pleasurable Emotional States," *Psychosom. Med.,* **12:**98, (Mar.-Apr.) 1950.
22. West, Howard F.: "Clinical Studies on the Respiration; 6: A Comparison of Various Standards for the Normal Vital Capacity of the Lungs," *Arch. Int. Med.,* **25:**306, (Mar.) 1920.
23. Wiggers, Carl J.: *Physiology in Health and Disease,* 5th ed. Lea & Febiger, Philadelphia, 1949, p. 670.
24. Best, Charles H., and Taylor, Norman B.: *op. cit.,* p. 801.
25. Best, Charles H., and Taylor, Norman B.: *op. cit.,* p. 243.
26. MacBryde, Cyril M. (ed.): *op. cit.,* p. 222.
27. Master, Arthur M., et al.: *Normal Blood Pressure and Hypertension; New Definitions.* Lea & Febiger, Philadelphia, 1952, pp. 11, 28.
28. Murray, Veronica F.: "Technic of Taking Blood Pressure," *Am. J. Nursing,* **34:**1057, (Nov.) 1934.
29. Cecil, Russell L., and Loeb, Robert F. (eds.): *A Textbook of Medicine,* 8th ed. W. B. Saunders Co., Philadelphia, 1951, p. 1068.
30. Contratto, Andrew W.: "Hypertension, Arteriosclerosis and Diet," *Am. J. Nursing,* **52:** 1235, (Oct.) 1952.
31. Gold, Harry (ed.): *Cornell Conferences on Therapy,* Vol. 4. The Macmillan Company, New York, 1951, p. 232.

Additional Suggested Reading

American Institute of Physics: *Temperature; Its Measurement and Control in Science and Industry*. Reinhold Publishing Corp., New York, 1941.

Goldblatt, Harry: *The Renal Origin of Hypertension*. Charles C Thomas, Publisher, Springfield, Ill., 1948.

Gray, John S.: *Pulmonary Ventilation and Its Psychological Regulation*. Charles C Thomas, Publisher, Springfield, Ill., 1950.

Griffiths, Ezer: *Methods of Measuring Temperature*, 3rd ed. C. Griffin, London, 1947.

Jonas, A. D.: "Variability of Blood Pressure Readings," *New York State J. Med.*, **50**:1249, (May) 1950.

Major, Ralph H.: *Physical Diagnosis*, 4th ed. W. B. Saunders Co., Philadelphia, 1951.

Master, Arthur M., et al.: "The Normal Blood Pressure Range and Its Clinical Implications," *J.A.M.A.*, **143**:1464, (Aug.), 1950.

Page, Irvine H.: *Hyptertension; A Manual for Patients with High Blood Pressure*, rev. ed. Charles C Thomas, Publisher, Springfield, Ill., 1951.

CHAPTER 11. THE PATIENT'S RECORD

1. NATURE OF THE RECORD

Contents. The medical record is a concise account of the health history of the patient and his family, a report of the findings on examination, the signs and symptoms occurring while the patient is under medical observation, the treatment, and progress of the disease, if one is involved. (A medical record is made for every patient who has a health examination.) Besides the data that bear directly on the medical problem, there is sociological information that may indirectly affect diagnosis and treatment and that is necessary for identification of the patient and the administration of the hospital or health service.

A record for each patient is kept by physicians in private practice and by all groups of medical workers associated with medical agencies. The hospital record is the one emphasized here, but it has many features in common with that used by private physicians, visiting nurse organizations, and other community health and medical services.

The *Manual of Hospital Standardization*[1] lists the following items that should be contained in a patient's record: (1) identification data; (2) complaint, reason for seeking medical aid; (3) present illness; (4) past history; (5) family history; (6) physical examination; (7) special examinations; (8) provisional diagnosis; (9) treatment, medical or surgical; (10) pathologist's report; (11) final diagnosis; (12) progress notes; (13) condition on discharge; (14) follow-up records; and (15) autopsy findings.

Parts of the hospital record in the usual order within the chart cover are as follows: (1) graphic chart of temperature, pulse, and respiration; other items of information, such as blood pressure, the number of evacuations, and volume of fluid intake and output may also be shown on this sheet; (2) orders for treatment written by the physician; (3) nurse's plan of care, record of care, and report of observations; (4) reports of laboratory findings and special examinations; (5) reports of anesthesia, operation, physical therapy, occupational therapy, social service, and any special treatment; (6) family history, record of present illness, and health habits, findings of the physical examination, medical progress notes, a summary made at the time of discharge, operative permit, autopsy permit, and a report of the autopsy (obviously, all these records vary according to the treatment and the outcome of a disease); and (7) statistical and social data. In many institutions this last sheet contains the medical summary. Examples of the forms used for the graphic chart, doctor's orders, nurse's notes, and statistical and social data are shown in Figures 40 (see Chapter 10), 54, 55, and 56 A and B.

The order as described above is the one found to be most convenient while the patient is in the hospital. After his discharge the chart is filed and the order is almost reversed, so that the record can be used more easily as a research tool.

If different colored papers are used for the various sections of the chart, it is much easier to locate them. An indexing device on the right-hand margin is a convenience.

It is likely that medical records will undergo a marked change in the near future. Those in current use do not make it clear to the medical worker that he should (1) provide the psychological or social aspects of care during illness; (2) treat the patient so that the best interests of his family or household are served; and (3) rehabilitate him through the combined resources of the community. Agencies that give a family health service, rehabilitation centers, and hospitals that have home care programs demonstrate the value of records such as those shown in Figures 56 A and B. If the present trend in emphasizing social aspects of medical care continues, all health agencies will develop records that, for the average patient, give a more complete picture of his living and working situations, his insight or understanding of his condition, and his independence or dependence in carrying out the essential activities of daily living. Forms will also be developed that will still further facilitate exchange of information between health agencies and pooling of services in the interests of a family. Jesse B. Aronson[2] points out that improvement in preventive medicine and "case finding" in syphilis, tuberculosis, and other diseases is dependent upon better family health records and exchange of data.

Making the Record. In private practice the record may be made by the physician or by physician, nurse, and clerical worker; in hospitals many persons contribute toward making the record. On the admission of the patient to an institution, an *admitting officer* records certain statistical, administrative, and social data, such as name, address, age, nationality, religion, and occupation. The *physician* prepares a history of the health of the patient and his family, also the history of the present illness. He records the physical findings on examination of the patient; he writes orders for care and treatment, which serve as a written record; he notes the patient's physical condition, progress of the disease, and success or failure of treatment.

On the patient's discharge, the physician writes what is sometimes called *a discharge note,* a summary report of the case. All these medical aspects of the record are made by medical students, or medical clerks, internes, medical residents, and attending and consulting physicians. Reports of special examinations, including autopsy reports, are made by physicians in charge of diagnostic laboratories and by *technicians* who act as their assistants.

Records of special treatments may be written by *dietitians, physical therapists, occupational therapists,* and *medical social workers,* as well as physicians and nurses. A relatively large part of the average patient's record is made by the *nurse.* Although *clerks* may be employed to assist her in some mechanical details, she is responsible for the graphic record of the temperature, pulse, and respiration, the report of other physical functions such as the amount of food and fluids taken, the elimination of feces and urine, or abnormal elimination by profuse sweating or vomiting. She is responsible for recording treatments and nursing care given by her and often by others and for making written reports of the patient's behavior that she thinks might affect diagnosis, medical treatment, nursing care, or rehabilitation.

In many cases the *patient* himself may contribute something toward the medical record. He may write portions of the social data, take psychometric tests, keep a diary, write a personal history, answer a questionnaire such as that referred to on page 552, sign statements signifying permission for operation or treatments involving risks, and in certain conditions his writing or drawing may be included in the record as evidence of symptoms or attitudes.

A standing committee on records composed of representatives of all departments concerned should exist in every health agency. The most useful medical record can be developed only through joint endeavor. Each professional group may have its own committee, but none of these can function satisfactorily without representation on the central committee. In many cases representatives of cooperating agencies should serve as consultants on the committee.

Nurse's Notes.   There is wide variation in nurses' records and in the value attached to them. In some institutions the nurse's notes are always filed for permanent reference with the remainder of the records; in some hospitals, only in special cases. Malcolm T. MacEachern[3] recommends the former, and this is undoubtedly the more common practice. Emanuel Hayt and Lillian R. Hayt say that "the accepted opinion" is that all data "pertaining to the patient," including the nurse's bedside notes, should be "preserved indefinitely for reference."*

A great effort should be made by the nurse to record *significant information* and to avoid producing a bulky report containing irrelevant material. The form for a plan of nursing care on pages 85 and 86 provides a space for checking, as they are given, items of daily care, such as baths and treatments that are administered at prescribed intervals and for which there are standing orders from the physician. The "running notes" made by the nurse, comparable to the medical progress notes made by the doctor, may then be devoted to recording the administration of drugs not on standing order and the observation of the patient's condition or behavior. Observation should be as specific and objective as possible. For example, record that the patient is talking incoherently and does not answer questions rather than "patient is irrational"; note that he appeared to sleep from 11:00 to 1:00 and from 3:30 to 5:30 rather than "patient slept badly"; or state that an infant lies on his

---

* Hayt, Emanuel, and Hayt, Lillian R.: *Legal Guide for American Hospitals.* Hospital Textbook Co., New York, 1940, p. 150.

DOCTOR'S ORDER SHEET

Patient **De Santo, Mrs Angela R.**

Floor **A**

Service **Medical**

Hosp. No. **629781**

Date	Time	Order	Doctor
4-21-39	P.M. 10:40	Blood Culture C.B.C. Sputum to Lab. Ice bag to Right chest. Codeine 0/09 Gm (H) Pneumonia fluids Measure Intake and Output	A.S. Livingston.
	A.M. 12:15	chloral hydrate 20/mls	R lochster
	4:25	Codeina 0/06 gm (h)	R Webster
4-22-39	9:30	Sod. bicarb Enema (1%) Colon Irrigation s.o.s. if exhausted by Enema	A.S. Livingston
	10-	Codeine Sulphate 0/06 Gm Pump Breasts. P.R.N.	A.S. Livingston
	10:10	Floxseed poultice to right chest for pain p.r.n. Discontinue ice bag to chest To X-ray for chest plate	L. Parks
	P.M. 1:30	Codeine 0/06 Gm (H)	A.S. Livingston
	3:30	Infusion 1500 cc 5% Dextrose in saline Blood Grouping Morphine Sulphate 0/016 Gm (H) Repeat S.O.S.	A.S. Livingston
	11:45 am	Chloral hydrate 20/mils Repeat S.O.S Morphine Sulphate 0/016 Gm (H)	A.S. Livingston
4-23-39	9:15 am	Codeine Sulphate 0/03 Gm. p.r.n.	A.S. Livingston
	P.M. 12:45	White Count and Differental 0.A. 5% Dextrose in Saline by infusion.	A.S. Livingston
	11:15	Morphine sulphate 0/016 gm (h) Repeat S.O.S	R Webster

U. of M. Hospitals
Form 190—4-38—5M

Figure 54. Doctor's order sheet. (Courtesy of University of Minnesota Hospitals, Minneapolis, Minn.)

313

right ear, groans from time to time, and puts his hand to his ear rather than "baby appears to be suffering from pain in ear."

Common flaws in nurses' notes are that comments tend to be confined to physical manifestations and that abnormalities and pathological signs are recorded, whereas moods, attitudes, favorable signs, and normal behavior are neglected.

Chapter 9 is a discussion of what and how to observe. The nurse's notes constitute a written report of the most significant of these observations.

The nurse, like the physician, should develop a simple, direct, and lucid style. A technical vocabulary is necessary, but the use of medical terms can be greatly overdone. Abbreviations and hospital slang are to be avoided. Symbols are convenient and proper in certain cases but are likely to be used indiscriminately. Only standard abbreviations and symbols, such as those given by Morris Fishbein,[4] should be used.

Notes, in practice, tend to be too brief rather than too full, and are often a monotonous listing of entries almost meaningless in their generality: for example, "breakfast," "morning care," "patient slept poorly," or "patient seems about as usual."

Each agency has its own regulations for nurses' records. In most places printing, or manuscript writing, rather than script is required. Notes by day and night staffs are often made in contrasting inks. Penciled notations are rarely permitted. Because the record may be used as a legal document, erasures should not be made. If necessary, a line is drawn through the error and the correction written above. If a portion of the record is recopied, a statement to this effect should be made, and the responsibility shared by the nurse who copies it and the nurse in charge of the unit, both nurses signing the statement. Some agencies require that notations on different topics be charted on separate lines; others attach more importance to spacesaving.

All mechanical aspects of record keeping, such as constructing forms, should be assigned to non-nursing personnel. A constant effort should be made to eliminate wasted time. The use of machine-made rather than handmade forms, rubber stamps for uniform entries, the use of color to make it easy to find parts of a record, and a good system of filing are helpful.

Adequate space in a quiet place should be provided. Effective recording requires concentration as well as other qualities of the mind. Above all else the record should be accurate; therefore, keen powers of observation and complete honesty are prime requisites in the nurse and in all medical workers who contribute to this document.

Accuracy in Medical Records.   It is so essential that medical records be exact and correct that each person who has a part in making them signs any notations he or she makes, using the full name rather than initials only. Insofar as possible, the record should consist of facts rather than opinions. The physician, the nurse, and others should report what they see, hear, smell, or feel, rather than what they deduce, although opinions cannot be avoided in some cases.

Name De Santo, Mrs Angela R.   Hospital Number 629781

Date	Hour	Nurse's Bedside Notes
4-23-39	A.M. 7:30	Nauseated; will take water but refuses nourishment.
	9:15	Respiration seems painful, wants to be quiet, dreads moving, is most comfortable on right side.
		Occasional cough, producing small amount of blood-tinged sputum Moderate amount yellow vaginal discharge.
		Enema given with good results but patient seemed exhausted from exertion.
		Breasts moderately full; 35 cc milk removed. No pain on expression of milk
	10:00	Drank 200 cc. lemonade with Cerelose and vomited almost immediately 225 cc.
	12:00	Nauseated, refuses any food by mouth.
	P.M. 1:00	500 cc. 5% dextrose by intravenous infusion (Dr. Livingston)
	2:30	Mrs De Santo seemed cheered by visit from sister who is helping grandmother to take care of De Santo infant. Mrs. De Santo told her sister that she thought she had pneumonia but that the doctors "believed she would get well."
	3:30	Less nauseated, retained 250 cc of ginger ale slept for an hour
	5:00	Drank 180 cc of broth without aversion but no relish Says that pain in chest "isnt as bad as it was" Is chilly; extra coverings used and hot water bottle kept at feet
	5:30	Breasts slightly distended; total amount of milk removed 20 cc
	8:00	Husband says his wife is worried about the cost of her hospitalization and the length of her illness; he thinks this is one of the things that is making her "feel so bad." He was assured that the Social Service Department would help them to work out their financial difficulties
	12:00	Has slept fitfully for past two hours; says pain in chest wakes her up, groans from time to time. Wants nurse with her
	A.M. 1:25	Morphine Sulphate /016 Gm (H) (E.W.)
	6:30	Has slept with little movement or other signs of discomfort since 2:00 A.M.

N. Notes

University of Minnesota Hospitals
Form 61—3-38—10M

Figure 55. Nurse's notes. (Courtesy of University of Minnesota Hospitals, Minneapolis, Minn.)

2. USES OF THE RECORD

As an Aid in Diagnosis, Treatment, and Nursing Care.   It was pointed out in Chapter 4 that a number of professional workers are usually coordinating their various services to the patient. It is essential that each one of these workers know what the others plan to do, are doing, and have done for the patient. The medical record is one means of making such information available to all concerned. *In any health organization all professional workers should have access to the record.* Some physicians keep a special file for confidential information to which no one else has access. This is highly desirable, but the material should not include data which other medical workers need in order to give intelligent, effective care. In some hospitals, social workers keep separate files, but, again, this is not justifiable except in the case of particularly confidential information. Nurses in psychiatric services, perhaps more than in any others, need the patient's medical and social history to give them some understanding of the patient's behavior and the psychiatrist's plan of therapy.[5] Any medical consultant is allowed to use the record for the benefit of the patient. It is filed so that during any subsequent illness members of the same institution, other institutions, or private physicians may refer to the record or secure a copy of the significant parts. Without this aid, effective treatment and nursing care are nearly impossible, for few have memories sufficiently accurate for matters of this kind; nor would it be practicable to try to secure verbal information about a patient from many persons concerned with his care.

As a Record of Data Essential to the Administration of a Health Service.   Items of information about the patient's age and occupation, the date of his admission and discharge or death, the nature of the medical treatment, and the space he occupied are the bases for computing charges for medical care and preparing annual reports of the work of the institution. While some of these data are reported elsewhere than in the medical record, the patient's chart is an indispensable item in the administration of a health service. Data taken from patients' records provide a base on which local, state, national, and international health services are planned.

As an Aid in Teaching Medical Students.   A large part of the education of physicians and other medical personnel is based on a study of patients' records. They are used in all case conferences and clinics. Students of medicine, nursing, dietetics, and social work would be immeasurably less well prepared if during their period of study they were denied the use of medical records. Not only do they study the history of the patients under their observation but also the records of those who have been discharged or those who have died. All *medical research* would be sadly hampered, and many kinds of research would be impossible without such sources of data.

As an Aid in Legal Justice.   Cases occur in which the patient, his family, the medical worker, or the administrative staff of the institution believe that they have received unfair treatment. A complaint may be brought against the hospital administration, or the physician or nurse may be charged with malpractice. Such cases are often settled out of court, but many of them are brought to trial. In either case the medical record is usually referred to, and if made by competent and conscientious workers, it may be a means of arriving at a fair judgment.

State laws differ with respect to the legal use that may be made of medical records.

Hayt and Hayt[6] say that most states in this country had adopted New York's 1928 "Confidential Communication Statute" in a similar or modified form. Such a statute makes "privileged" the relationships of physician-patient, man-wife, attorney-client, and clergy-parishioner. According to Milton J. Lesnik and Bernice E. Anderson[7] most states do not recognize the privileged relationship of nurse and patient. In the writer's opinion they should, since during illness the natural reserve of the individual is often broken down, and he may tell the nurse what he would ordinarily keep secret. To further effective treatment, he may confide the most personal details of his life to the physician or the nurse. In states that have a confidential communication statute the physician, and in some states the nurse, is not required by law to divulge such information, just as a wife is freed from obligation to testify against her husband, or a man against himself. In such states the patient's record cannot be subpoenaed into court; but if the subpoena is accepted by the authorities of the institution, they are then obliged to send a representative of the staff to court with the record. The person selected to do this should be someone who can interpret the record effectively.

Some state laws require public institutions to submit patients' records, or certified copies, for legal purposes, but exempt private institutions from this regulation.

In certain cases, such as claims for compensation, the patient may ask to have his medical history used as evidence. Leo P. Dolan[8] makes the point that the patient should read his record before he makes this request, because there may be facts in his history, of which he is unaware, that are detrimental to his interests.

Generally speaking, medical records are used legally to refresh the memory of the physician or nurse in testifying, but the data contained therein are not considered conclusive proof. It seems to be a common practice to call on living witnesses to give verbal testimony rather than to use written statements they have made as evidence. In case the observations of dead nurses or physicians are needed, the medical record is more likely to be used. A qualified person must identify the signatures of the deceased.

It is repeatedly stated that insurance companies have no legal right to demand access to medical records. On a written request from the patient, the hospital may give the company certain information from the record. If the case is taken to court, the laws of the particular state involved regulate the decision as to the use made of the record. The executors of an estate may be allowed to use the medical record to the extent that is necessary in their service to the patient and his legatees.

Hospital officers and medical workers should get legal advice before allowing anyone, other than a professional person in attendance upon the patient, to have access to his chart. While students and research workers in the medical field are allowed to use such records, they are bound by a strict ethical code to hold all

UNIVERSITY of MINNESOTA HOSPITALS
Minneapolis, Minn.

Name: Last De Santo — First Angela — Middle R. — Case No. 629781

Address 502 N. 16th Street — County Hennepin

Adm. date clinic — Adm. date hosp. 4-21-39 — Adm. Type Pay — Adm. No. 1

Referring Physician F. N. Nelson — Address 1801 N. Broadway

County Commissioner — Date of Papers — Co.

Age 23 — Sex F — Civ. St. M. — Race White — Religion R. Catholic

Birthplace Minneapolis — Birth Date 11-21-16 — Length of Residence (yrs.) U. S. — State — Co. — City Life

Service Medical — Station A — Classification Pay — Occupation Housewife

Father· Name Romano, John — Birthplace Naples, Italy

Mother: Maiden Name Bonjales, Nina — Birthplace Naples, "

Husband or Wife De Santo, Michael — Birthplace St. Paul, Minnesota

Relative or Friend to Notify Husband — Address 502 N. 16th Street, City — Tel. No. Cherry 1986

Brought by: Husband — Brought from:

Special Data — City Address of Relative

Provisional Diagnoses Staff — Pneumonia

	Adm. Date	Service	Station	Responsible Staff Member	Interne	Disch. Date
Admitted	4-21-39	Medical	A	Dr. Lucien Parks	R. D. Webster	6-2-39
Dept. Transfer						
Dept. Transfer						
Dept. Transfer						

Date	Consultant	Clinical, Surgical, Pathological Diagnoses to be Indexed.		CODE Major	Minor
4-21-39	A. S. Livingston	On admission thought to have lobar pneumonia.	1	(Used by	
		Sputum findings and X Ray negative for	2	Record	
		pneumonia.	3	Librarian	
4-22-39	L. Park	Considered physical signs more indicative	4	for filing	
	B. Simon	of lung abscess than pneumonia.	5	note.)	
5-20-39	F. Hansen	Interpreted series of chest plates made over	6		
		a four weeks period as showing a necrotic	7		
		area at the angle of the right scapula.	8		
		Taking into consideration all physical signs	9		
		and laboratory findings it seems most probable	10		
		that the patient had a pulmonary infarct	11		
		resulting in an abscess which ruptured	12		
		into the pleura and was drained through	13		
		the bronchus.	14		
		A. S. Livingston	15		
			16		

University of Minn. Hosps. Form 195
Minneapolis, Minnesota—5-38—5M

Surgery Yes (No) — Condition on Discharge (Recovered) Improved Unimproved Dead Left Against Advice

Figure 56A. Social and statistical data. (Courtesy of University of Minnesota Hospitals, Minneapolis, Minn.)

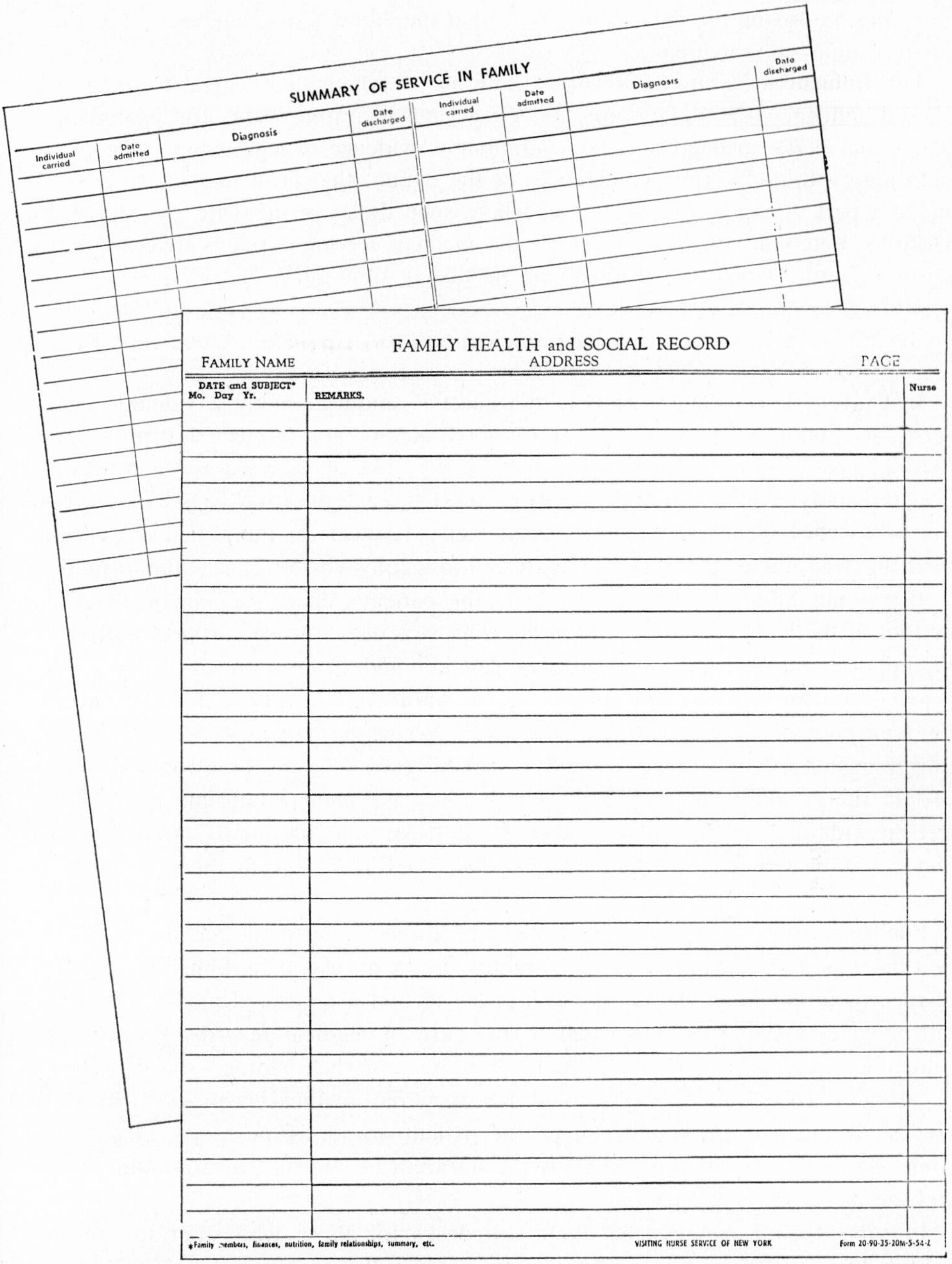
SUMMARY OF SERVICE IN FAMILY

Individual carried	Date admitted	Diagnosis	Date discharged	Individual carried	Date admitted	Diagnosis	Date discharged

FAMILY HEALTH and SOCIAL RECORD

FAMILY NAME ADDRESS PAGE

DATE and SUBJECT* Mo. Day Yr.	REMARKS.	Nurse

*Family members, finances, nutrition, family relationships, summary, etc.

VISITING NURSE SERVICE OF NEW YORK

Form 20-90-35-20M-5-54-Z

Figure 56B. Top form illustrates a family folder in which are kept records for all members of a family. Information on the family and notes of a social nature, including references to finances and family relationships, are recorded on "Family Health and Social Record." (Courtesy of Visiting Nurse Service of New York, New York City.)

such information in confidence. Some institutions codify medical records for filing purposes, removing the names entirely so that they may be used in research without identification of individuals.

Use Influences Nature of Record.   The use to which the medical record is put should influence the manner of collecting and recording data; for example, in states that make medical histories "admissible evidence in legal cases," the physician may withhold certain confidences of the patient that he would not hesitate to make a part of the record in a state where such data are inviolate. As shown by Dorothy Ketcham,[9] the use to which the medical record is put is determined by custom, statute, and the nature of the particular situation.

3. CARE OF MEDICAL RECORDS

In Current Use.   Since the patient's chart is unquestionably a valuable document, it should be made on paper of good quality and protected from soiling, tearing, and blurring. Hinged aluminum covers, like those used for a notebook, are commonly used in hospitals. Chart backs that leave the front page exposed also are used. They may be kept in a special rack on wheels or hung in a chart room near the head nurse's station and transferred to a conveyor for clinics and "rounds."

It was not unusual in the past to find the patient's chart hanging on the head or foot of the bed, particularly in wards. This practice is disappearing. Charting or recording at the bedside is more often than not undesirable. The recorder should be comfortable and the surroundings quiet. Another objection is that the patient, his family, or his friends can read the chart. While the patient may ultimately be told everything that his record contains, for his own sake the time for telling him certain things should be wisely chosen. In the case of a responsible adult, he is free to withhold any information about his illness from his family or his friends, and the institution has no right to make his chart accessible to them without his permission.

For Reference.   The American College of Surgeons has made recommendations that have tended to standardize and simplify the form, use, care, filing, and storage of records in hospitals and clinics. It is usual to find a registered medical librarian in charge of a department devoted to the care of medical records. Records are sometimes microfilmed after ten years or more to reduce storage space.[10] Briefs or abstracts also may be substituted for very old medical histories.[11] Records are usually filed by the number given the patient on admission to the hospital or clinic. An index system should enable the librarian to find the corresponding name and the diagnosis of the patient.

In some record departments there are desks for those who want to use the record. In some cases it is permissible to sign for the record and use it in other parts of the institution, but individuals are not allowed to take the record away from the hospital or clinic except under very unusual circumstances, as, for example, on an order from a court of law.

Since the welfare of a patient, even life itself, may depend upon the accessibility of a medical record, it is easy to see why such stringent regulations are made to protect it from destruction, loss, and injudicious handling.

REFERENCES

1. American College of Surgeons: *Manual of Hospital Standardization*. The College, Chicago, 1946.
2. Aronson, Jesse B.: "The Family Record in the Red Hook-Gowanus Health Center District," *Am. J. Pub. Health,* **40:**1230, (Oct.) 1950.
3. MacEachern, Malcolm T.: *Hospital Organization and Management*, 2nd ed. Physicians Record Co., Chicago, 1940, p. 581.
4. Fishbein, Morris: *Medical Writing,* 2nd ed. Blakiston Co., Philadelphia, 1948, pp. 98-106.
5. Kalkman, Marion E.: *Introduction to Psychiatric Nursing*. McGraw-Hill Book Co., New York, 1950, pp. 126, 159.
6. Hayt, Emanuel, and Hayt, Lillian R.: *Legal Guide for American Hospitals*. Hospital Textbook Co., New York, 1940, p. 150.
7. Lesnik, Milton J., and Anderson, Bernice E.: *Legal Aspects of Nursing,* J. B. Lippincott Co., Philadelphia, 1947, p. 298.
8. Dolan, Leo P.: "The Patient's Record—A Sacred Document," *Hospitals,* **11:**68, (June) 1937.
9. Ketcham, Dorothy: "Legal Side of Hospital Records," *Bull. A. Rec. Lib. North America,* **4:**19, (Dec.) 1932.
10. Jolly, Robert: "Record Librarians and the Movies," *Hospitals,* **13:**59, (Aug.) 1939.
11. Hayt, Emanuel, and Hayt, Lillian R.: *op. cit.,* p. 152.

Additional Suggested Reading

Crawfis, E. H.: "The Physician and the Privileged Communications As They Relate to Mental States," *Ohio M. J.,* **46:**1082, (Nov.) 1950.

MacEachern, Malcolm T.: *Medical Records in the Hospital.* Physicians Record Co., Chicago, 1937.

McPolin, J.: "Professional Medical Secrecy," *J. M. A. Eire,* **27:**64, (Oct.) 1950.

Meade, Agnes B.: *Manual of Clinical Charting Designed for the Use of Graduates and Students of Nursing.* J. B. Lippincott Co., Philadelphia, 1944.

Price, Alice L.: *A Handbook of Charting for Student Nurses.* C. V. Mosby Co., St. Louis, 1948.

Terenzio, Peter B.: "The Medical Record in Court," *Hosp. Management,* **70:**68, (Nov.) 1950.

CHAPTER 12. PERSONAL CLEANLINESS

1. THE MORNING TOILET

Importance of Personal Cleanliness. Habits of personal cleanliness are among the first requisites of hygienic living, and include daily care of the skin, nails, mouth, hair, clothing, and, under some conditions, the eyes and nose. Good grooming contributes to a sense of well-being, and the absence of it, in most cultures, suggests a low morale. This is even true in the animal world, where healthy creatures are seen to keep themselves clean by various means. Theodore Rosenthal, discussing personal cleanliness in relation to public health says: "No single article can compare with soap in respect to the amount of sickness and death prevented by its use."* He thinks that basic health truths are often treated so casually by doctors that patients overlook their advice on hygienic measures. Because hands act as tools in bringing food to the mouth, in cleaning body orifices, and in rubbing an itching part, it is particularly important that they are washed many times a day, but especially so after contamination with feces. This subject in relation to worm infestation and control of other communicable conditions is discussed in Chapters 5 and 7. Cleanliness is essential to a normal physical and mental state, as this is interpreted in our society, although "normal" persons vary greatly in their standards.

All that can be said about the physiological and psychological value of cleanliness in health has added significance in illness. The sick must be fortified with every weapon that will overcome disease and promote the zest for life. Many diseases inhibit physiological functions, such as lacrimation, salivation, or sweating, that, in a sense, clean the body. Therefore, cleansing processes, adequate in health, may require modification to meet the needs of the sick. The beneficial effects of

* Rosenthal, Theodore: "Personal Cleanliness: A Basic Problem in Hygiene and Public Health," *M. Times,* **78**:497, (Nov.) 1950.

hygienic measures on the appearance, emotions, and general condition of the patient contribute substantially to diagnosis and treatment. Florence Nightingale[1] wisely observed that a person whose hygienic care had been neglected might seem very ill when he was only hungry and uncomfortable and that such discomfort was often misleading to the doctor in diagnosis and therapy. In many cases the restless and sleepless need food and drink or a good bath rather than a narcotic.

Beginning a New Day. The average person in health begins the day refreshed by a night's rest; a sick man, although usually relieved to see the dawn, may be anything but refreshed. He may have had a sleepless night; he may dread what lies in store for him—a feared diagnosis, a painful dressing, an operation, or just another period of boredom. If the nurse does not irritate him by thrusting her morning cheerfulness in his face, so to speak, he will unconsciously absorb some of her strength and *joie de vivre*. While the wakeful hospital patient often says the sound of the day staff coming "on duty" is music to his ears, there is nothing about which there is more general complaint than noisy personnel beginning, only too early, the day's brisk round of activities. Hospital economy often demands that the patients' day begins early. There are seldom enough nurses to give highly individualized care, and it is thought desirable to have patients bathed and ready to see their physicians during the morning visiting hours. If reasonable hospital routines are explained to patients, such routines are less often resented.

At the beginning of each day the nurse who has a number of persons assigned to her care should try to determine who requires her attention first, which patients would like to sleep longer, and what, in general, are the needs of each. This analysis depends largely upon her powers of observation and sympathy.

In homes, where the nurse is freed from hospital routine, the sick person should normally be surrounded by quiet until he wakes naturally. If he must be waked, the hour should be determined by what is best for him, although in some cases the welfare of the household must also be considered. While a daily regimen is desirable in health, in sickness rest is usually more important than regularity.

Most persons, sick or well, are conscious of their appearance. Even the very ill may be favorably or unfavorably affected by it and dislike to be seen at their worst. The average patient likes to have his morning toilet completed before he has visitors, even his doctor.

Morning care usually includes taking the temperature, pulse, and respiration; then the morning toilet, changing the bed, and breakfast. It is wise in many cases to give the bath and make the bed after breakfast. If this is done, the patient should be prepared for the meal by having the teeth brushed, face and hands bathed, and hair combed.

The assistance the nurse gives a sick or helpless person with his toilet depends upon his condition. He may be so ill or so weak that she has to care for him as she would an infant, or he may need little if any help. The "good" nurse will prevent harmful exertion on the part of the sick but will also encourage children and invalids to develop independence. The hospital nurse who sends a convalescent home unnecessarily helpless has, to that extent, failed.

2. CARE OF THE SKIN AND NAILS

Hygienic Care of the Skin.   The appearance of the skin is not an accurate index of *general health,* but it often reflects the condition of the body as a whole. A clear complexion and a good color go a long way toward making a person look healthy. Skin, like all other tissues, is affected by its supply of the circulating body fluids and their quality. Changes in the caliber and condition of the vessels affect the quantity and quality of the blood and lymph they carry. Food and fluid intake affect available nutrients; whereas drugs, bacterial toxins, irritating proteins, and endotoxins may contaminate the fluids supplying the skin. Systemic diseases are manifest in the appearance of the skin. Dermatitis is one of the pathognomonic signs of pellagra, a nutritional deficiency; papules on the back are a common sign of continued use of bromides; fairly typical eruptions are the most prominent symptom of such systemic infections as scarlet fever, measles, and shingles (herpes zoster); "hives" are a common response to foreign protein in foods or to antibiotic drugs, and the discharge of bile into the skin gives the familiar discoloration and itching so characteristic of jaundice. This oversimplified list of systemic conditions that may affect the quantity or quality of the circulating fluids in the skin omits one of the most important. It is now generally accepted that intense or prolonged emotional stress, with the parallel effect on the endocrine system, may produce such marked changes in the caliber of the blood vessels and in the colloids of the skin that eruptions result.

Because the skin reflects the condition of the body as a whole (including what is called "the mind"), its hygiene involves a wholesome daily regimen in all its aspects. Obviously the skin must also be protected from environmental dangers: irritating chemicals, parasites, and microorganisms that may gain access to the deeper layers; mechanical irritation; and harmful temperatures. Age affects the kind and amount of attention to be given the skin. Infants have very delicate skin, easily injured mechanically and with relatively low resistance to infection. The newborn should have minimum handling, and all infants and children should be gently bathed, massaged, and protected from harsh and soiled clothing. After the first few weeks all babies and children should be bathed at least once a day. In hot weather several daily baths are desirable.

After puberty and up to middle age special care is needed to control odors from the secretions of skin glands, particularly active during the childbearing period. During the teens, eruptions are most likely to appear on the face; therefore, it should be kept especially clean and free from irritation. During the active hardworking span of life, the skin of the hands and feet need a great deal of attention. The necessity for repeated handwashing may require daily replacement of oils.

The aged need a different regimen from the young. With age the skin gets less moist and supple, and may lose some of its underlying fat that cushions it against injury. As glandular activity slows, the skin is less moistened by sweat and less lubricated by sebum. Moreover, the lowering of water content is said to be characteristic of aging cells, and the circulatory system may be less efficient in bringing nutrients and removing wastes. The elderly, sensing these changes, tend to bathe less often and may even find it necessary to use vegetable oil, cocoa butter, or lanolin to counteract dryness. The habit of oiling the finger- and toenails daily is especially desirable as they tend to get brittle. If neglected, the toenails may grow so thick and hard that it is impossible or unsafe for the person himself to cut them. Soaking the feet or applying pads saturated with warm oil softens the nails. Visits to podiatrists are a boon to the elderly, especially those with dim vision. Areas such as heels, toes, and elbows should be rubbed with oil. Because alcoholic lotions are drying, they are not good for the aging skin. Massage is beneficial but should be gentle, and an oil or fat should be used to lubricate the hands of the operator.

Neutral detergents are recommended in place of soaps that change the pH of the skin. Daily baths should not be urged upon the elderly. Any compulsion is damaging to the spirit, and frequent bathing still further dries the already dry skin. Incontinence of the bladder or rectum, discussed in Chapter 14, constitutes a special problem that may demand repeated baths.

Skin Diseases and Importance of Medical Treatment. Real skin pathology should be treated by physicians. No one should postpone medical help since the longer the duration of the disease, the more difficult the cure, the greater likelihood of scarring, and if the condition is communicable, the greater the danger of transmitting it. The physician always tries to remove the cause, but the etiology of some of the most familiar skin diseases is not established. Acne, for example, is being treated as an allergy by eliminating foods such as chocolate from the diet; as a vitamin deficiency by giving large doses of vitamin A or mixed vitamins; as an unbalanced glandular condition by giving cortisone or estrogens; and as a bacterial disease by chemotherapy or administering antibiotics.[2, 3, 4, 5, 6] Where systemic treatment fails in this, as in all skin diseases, the eruption is treated locally with preparations to clean, retard secondary infection, or relieve itching and burning. E. J. Moynahan[7] points out the danger of applying locally the chemotherapeutic and antibiotic agents which, themselves, may produce an "allergic sensitization dermatitis." He thinks there is less danger in oral medication and believes great strides have been made in controlling skin conditions with these two classes of therapeutic agents, with vitamins, the fungicide undecylenic acid, with antihistamines, and with cortisone and ACTH.

While the value of sunlight and of its substitutes is recognized in psoriasis and some other skin conditions, the medical profession is increasingly wary of any generalized application of radiation. The public should be educated to fear unlimited exposure to sunlight and "sun lamps" and even more the application of repeated doses of x-ray to large skin areas.

Age seems to affect the type of skin disorders to which the human being is susceptible. Infants and small children are most likely to contract diseases like impetigo, caused by microorganisms, and the so-called "children's diseases," characterized by rashes; adolescents and young adults who have not acquired an immunity during childhood may, of course, have all of these infections, but they seem peculiarly prone to acne and to dermatoses that are thought to have an emotional causation.* In the aged, eczemas, seborrhea, keratoses, and other skin tumors are common.[8, 9] Faulty diet is believed to be one of the chief causes of skin diseases in this group. Lessened activity of the glands of internal secretion and of the sweat and sebaceous glands and a low water content—all contribute to the wrinkled, dry, and sometimes scaly skin of the aged. J. R. Owen[10] thinks that this aging process, as it is often regarded, could be mitigated and the frank skin diseases of old people cured by improved diets, regular application of lubricants, such as lanolin, and the administration of estrogens. Neurodermatitis, while not so common in the aged, does occur. Correction of the emotional disturbance is then, as always in this condition, more important than local treatment.

Itching and burning should be relieved by removing the cause, but temporary relief is often necessary. David T. Graham et al. define the two aspects of itching: "(a) first pain: a sharp, superficial, well-localized pain of short latency, and (b) second pain: slower, diffuse, burning."† They think these sensations are induced by stimulation of two sets of nerves. Lotions that paralyze or reduce stimulation of cutaneous nerves relieve itching. When skin or mucous membrane is irritated by acid secretions of the body, a neutralizing lotion may be prescribed.

"Chapping" of the skin is an abnormal condition that plagues many, particularly workers who must wash their hands frequently. A serious and stubborn dermatitis is often the result of continued exposure to soap and water, disinfectants, and irritating chemicals, such as surgeons or hairdressers use. The outermost layer of the skin is composed of practically dead cells, whose protoplasm has changed to a protein called keratin, acting as a waterproof covering for the body. This *stratum corneum,* as it is called, is acid in reaction and is damaged by alkalis. The oil secretion (sebum) of the sebaceous glands lubricates the corneum; and sweat, which is acid, tends to neutralize materials that might injure it and also prevents drying of the waxy keratin. Because the glands of the skin are less active in cold weather, "chapped hands," with their characteristic dry, cracked, and reddened appearance are most common in winter. Any occupation in which the worker handles fabrics chaps the hands by constantly removing the secretions of the skin.

To prevent "chapping," cleansing agents should be neutral in reaction or should have the pH of the skin. I. B. Snedden says that when the hands are subjected to repeated washings, it is essential to waterproof them frequently with an oil or grease, or "barrier cream." He thinks that petroleum jelly and lanolin are effective but too greasy and recommends "*Aquosum* B. P. [U.S.P.] made by the addition of water to the B. P. ointment of wood alcohols. . . . A slightly less greasy application is *Ung. Emulsificans Aquosum,* the emulsifying agent of which is the B. P. emulsifying wax."‡ He attributes the effectiveness of glycerin in hand lotions to the fact that it is "hydroscopic" and so attracts water and keeps the skin moist. Snedden

* Irving Shapiro notes that acne usually makes its appearance at puberty and that it is not found in eunuchs. He says it is much commoner in males than females. (Shapiro, Irving: "Estrogens by Local Application in Treatment of Acne Vulgaris," *A.M.A. Arch. Dermat. & Syph.,* 63:224, [Feb.] 1951.)

† Graham, David T., et al.: "Itch Sensation in the Skin; Experimental Observations on the Neural Mechanisms Involved," *Tr. Am. Neurol. A.,* p. 135, 1950.

‡ Snedden, I. B.: "Chapped Hands," *Practitioner,* 165:452, (Oct.) 1950.

considers this action of far less value than the waterproof film made with oils or fats.

It is possible that when the hands are washed very frequently the fat-soluble vitamins are removed from the skin. At any rate, the writer has seen stubborn occupational dermatoses successfully treated with local application of vitamin A and D ointment and large oral doses of vitamin A. Some doctors and nurses regularly apply such ointments to the hands at the first signs of irritation.

Bathing and the Control of Skin Odors. While the skin reflects the condition of the body as a whole, external cleanliness is important. Physiologically speaking, the skin is bathed by sweat and oil from its glands, but even animals, fur-bearing and otherwise, contrive to help nature with this cleaning process. For persons, as for animals, there are many ways of doing this. Peoples with low hygienic standards, according to our customs, do not necessarily have a high incidence of skin disease, but it is safe to assume that other things being equal clean skin is less subject to disease than dirty skin.[11] Studies by Lloyd Arnold[12] and his associates, and by others since, have demonstrated that bacteria placed on the skin are killed in a period of 10 to 30 minutes. Acidity of sweat discourages bacterial life. If skin bacteria are heavily coated with the oil of unwashed skin, they are protected from the action of sweat and are therefore more likely to cause trouble when the integrity of the skin is destroyed.

Besides its cleansing value, a bath stimulates the circulation, and for the sedentary is particularly important since it is a substitute for exercise. Richard May,[13] discussing "The [many] Medical Hazards of [public] Bathing," enumerates infection of the skin, respiratory tract, sinuses, eyes, ears, and the intestinal tract; he includes the danger of allergy in pools, where some persons are sensitive to chlorine, loss of life from muscular cramps, and mechanical injury. Even so, he concludes that the advantages of bathing outweigh its dangers and thinks that if the hazards are known, they can usually be avoided.

Daily bathing for the normal person up to middle or old age should be stressed as an *esthetic* necessity rather than a health essential. Secretions of the skin, while they may clean it physiologically, contain waste products such as leucine and tyrosine that, particularly on decomposition by bacterial action, have ammoniacal and fetid odors distasteful to people of our culture. Anton J. Carlson and Victor E. Johnson[14] say that the chemical composition of sweat, the secretion of the eccrine glands, resembles that of dilute urine.

Secretions of the apocrine glands in the hairy body areas, such as the axillae and pubes, have a particularly strong odor which even daily bathing may not counteract. Young people should be prepared for this physiological change and helped to develop a regimen that controls body odors. Girls, particularly, should be taught that the apocrine glands are subject to stubborn infections and that the axillae and pubes should be kept very clean. Uncleanliness combined with the use of irritating drugs that stop or deodorize perspiration is particularly dangerous.*

* Theodore Cornbleet says, speaking of the apocrine glands: "The organs appear at puberty, a time too, when a growth of hair in connection with them is somewhat suggestive. . . . The apocrines are said to become smaller and secrete less after the menopause, but it is agreed that they enlarge and become more active just before and during the menses. For some unknown

(*Footnote continued on p. 328.*)

Application of astringents to control perspiration in the axillae is widely practiced. According to H. H. Hazen,[15] Charles Solomon,[16] and Mary C. Phillips,[17] these substances are usually harmless, unless the individual is peculiarly sensitive to the chemicals they contain. Aluminum or zinc salts, salicylic acid or tannic acid, are the astringent bases commonly found in commercial preparations. It is claimed by manufacturers that chlorophyll taken by mouth will deodorize virtually all body secretions. Joseph J. Seldin[18] says that 8 million dollars were spent on advertising chlorophyll in 1951. He quotes the Federal Food and Drug Administration as "skeptical concerning the effectiveness of the deodorant action," and says that the American Council of Pharmacy and Chemistry of the American Medical Association credits this substance as being effective when used on dressings in concentrations of 90 per cent. A number of studies support the claim that water-soluble chlorophyll promotes healing, controls bacterial growth, and has deodorizing properties.[19, 20] The council says: ". . . it does not exert a significant disinfectant action, and the mechanism of its deodorant effect on foul smelling chronic lesions is not clear."* Since raw chlorophyll costs about a dollar a pound, however, it is exceedingly doubtful whether many persons could afford to, or should depend upon, a sufficient intake outside their food to affect body odors.

John C. Brocklehurst in a thorough investigation of chlorophyll found that "mixtures of water-soluble chlorophyl and various strong-smelling solutions did not remove the smell of these solutions even after exposure for one or more months."†

Many chemicals control odors by oxidizing odoriferous materials or by inhibiting bacterial growth and delaying putrefaction. Sodium borate (borax) and zinc peroxide are the active agents in many skin deodorants. Borax is a cheap harmless powder that may be dusted on the skin after a bath. Hazen recommends as a skin deodorant a mixture of zinc peroxide and cold cream in proportions of about 1 to 8. Medicinal odors in such preparations are undesirable; to some persons they may be as unpleasant as those the deodorant is designed to destroy. Publications sponsored by the American Medical Association‡ and the Consumer's Research Movement§ expose false claims of manufacturers and give reliable advice on selection of cosmetics.

The skin may be cleaned by water and soap or soap substitutes. Studies by B. Thurber Guild,[21] A. L. Hudson,[22] and others have shown that soaps, having an alkaline reaction, destroy the protective acidity of the skin's secretions. For this reason they question the habitual use of soap and would substitute a sulfonated oil detergent (such as pHisoderm), which has a neutral reaction or a pH similar to

---

reason, diseases of these glands appear mostly in women." (Cornbleet, Theodore: "Pregnancy and Apocrine Gland Diseases: Hidradenitis and Fox-Fordyce Disease," *Arch. Dermat. & Syph.*, 65:12, [Jan.] 1952.)

   * American Medical Association, Council on Pharmacy and Chemistry: *New and Nonofficial Remedies.* J. B. Lippincott Co., Philadelphia, 1951, p. 420.

   † Brocklehurst, John C.: "An Assessment of Chlorophyl as a Deodorant," *Brit. M. J.,* p. 541, (Mar.) 1953.

   ‡ Cramp, Arthur J. (ed.) *Nostrums and Quackery,* 3rd ed. American Medical Association, Chicago, 1936.

   § Aaron, Harold: *Good Health and Bad Medicine.* The McBride Co.. Inc.. New York. 1940.

that of the skin. While allergic reactions to soaps are not uncommon, studies of pHisoderm, for example, have led to the claim that it is nonallergic.*

A cleaning process harmless to the rest of the body can scarcely injure the face. Because, however, the face and hands are more exposed to soiling and drying, fats such as lanolin, the base of cold creams, and vegetable oils are often used as a substitute for, or in addition to, other agents. Eskimos use oil and sun baths in place of soap and water, and physicians may prescribe oil baths for persons with excessively dry skins.

The consciousness of being clean and of wearing fresh clothing raises the self-respect. A person once accustomed to a morning bath is vaguely uncomfortable all day if deprived of it. No one should be more scrupulously clean than the nurse; she is often in close proximity to others, who are often hypersensitive to odors, and she teaches hygiene by her example. Besides daily bathing she should control axillary perspiration with an approved nonperspirant; if a hypersensitive skin prohibits controlling the secretion of sweat, a harmless deodorant should be substituted.

Removal of Superfluous Hair. Most of the body is covered with hair although, particularly in women, it is unnoticeable on large areas. Glandular activity influences hair growth; therefore, the location and quality of body hair is loosely associated with masculinity and femininity. Few persons have accurate knowledge of this relationship, but in each country custom dictates that noticeable hair on some parts of man or woman is superfluous. Those sensitive to public opinion, and few are not, should adopt a safe method of removing superfluous hair; its presence inevitably affects self-respect. Hair may be pulled out with tweezers, cut off with scissors, shaved with a razor, removed with depilatories, or the roots destroyed with an electric needle or radiation.

According to Hazen, *electrolysis* in the hands of a specialist is a safe and effective means of removing superfluous hair. The process is, however, lengthy and expensive. *Radiation* is unequivocally condemned.

Shaving is universally practiced by men and is recommended for both men and women. Hazen notes that a woman who shaves the legs or armpits shrinks from shaving the face. He believes this is because it increases her "feeling of masculinity." He thinks that if woman can work and play as man does, she might as well "shave" and says, "Possibly she will come to it."†

A popular misconception that it coarsens hair probably keeps many women from shaving. The stubble that appears a few days after shaving feels like coarser hair but actually isn't. The quality of a man's beard usually remains unchanged from maturity to old age even though he shaves daily or oftener.

* C. Guy Lane and Irvin Blank give an excellent list of soap substitutes, including trade names, in Fishbein's monograph. They are skeptical of the claims of the new detergents and suggest that with continued use of these detergents, as with the continued use of soap, allergies may appear. (Fishbein, Morris L. [ed.]: *Medical Uses of Soap: A Symposium.* J. B. Lippincott Co., Philadelphia, 1945, p. 152.)

† Hazen, H. H.: "Cosmetics," *Am. J. Nursing,* **38:**791, (July) 1938.

Shaving should be preceded by skin cleaning. The skin may be broken by the razor, allowing access of bacteria to the readily infected deeper layers.[23] If the waxy covering is emulsified by a shaving soap or cream, water can penetrate and soften the hair shaft; moreover, the razor is not so likely to injure the skin. Stretching the skin lessens the danger of nicking and gives a cleaner shave because it eliminates wrinkles and pits. The angle at which the razor should be held depends upon the make. Lester Hollander and E. T. Casselman[24] say that it should be at least 28–30 deg. Dull razor blades cause pulling but are not so likely to cut the skin. It is economical to get cheap safety razor blades and discard them often.

Cutting superfluous hair with scissors leaves a stubble. Hair *extracted with tweezers* is replaced by a new growth in about six weeks. Paste *depilatories* may soften and partially destroy the hair shaft or may harden around the hair and mechanically remove it when the dried paste is removed. Hazen says most depilatories consist of barium or sodium sulfide. He thinks their action identical with shaving except that the skin is more likely to be irritated.

After the climacteric, body hair gets straighter, finer, and sparse; while the eyebrows often coarsen, and superfluous hair appears on the face. The aged may need more encouragement and help than younger people in controlling undesirable hair growth. Hairs should never be pulled from moles, and, if they are cut, care should be taken not to prick the mole. Such disfiguring growths should be surgically removed.

Care of the Skin in Sickness.   Bathing and its stimulating effect on the circulation are even more important in illness than in health. The sick, especially those confined to bed, are deprived of exercise, particularly in the open, where air currents and changes in temperature may stimulate perspiration but also evaporate it and keep clothing dry. Bed patients suffer the necessity of living in garments and between sheets that as the day goes on get increasingly permeated with body excretions. In some cases they are sweating excessively; in others the skin is dry and failing to eliminate body wastes normally. In most illnesses of any duration skin care is of prime importance. The skin should be stimulated by massage, heat, light, and air motion; the body, kept clean and comfortably dry. Odors should be controlled with nonirritating preparations; some are so cheap that any hospital could supply them. Frequent change of clothing and bedding is essential.

Very sick persons should, in most cases, have at least one complete bath daily. In this country most patients, with the exception of the elderly, would enjoy and benefit from a daily bath. Unfortunately, few hospitals are equipped and staffed for this. When baths are limited, "routines" usually exist. Lists are kept so that all patients get at least two baths a week and partial baths on other days.

Ideally, baths would be given to each patient at the hour habitual to him. Actually, they must be given when there is adequate personnel and when they don't interfere with treatments, meals, and visiting hours. Rigidity should, however, be avoided here, as in all dealings with people. Kathleen Newton says:

How many aged patients have been made miserable in the hospital by such trivial rules as having to take showers instead of tub baths, and to take them in the morning instead of at night. Perhaps for fifty years the patient's routine has been to take a tub bath just before retiring. Such unimportant rulings often make the patient unhappy and resistive to important hospital procedures. Evidence of such inflexibility on the part of nurses is fortunately quite rare today.*

In hospitals the usual times for baths are early morning and bedtime. It is believed that a bath should not immediately follow a meal because it increases the volume of blood in the skin and thereby decreases the supply to the digestive organs.

Any doubts about the value of bathing are dispelled by seeing the effects on the very sick. The patient who in the morning after a sleepless night looks hopelessly ill may fall into a natural restful slumber after a warm bath, a massage, and a change of linen. His whole appearance is altered, and his pulse and respiration rates are nearer normal. If the doctor does not see the person before he is so refreshed, the nurse should be especially careful to note and record significant differences in his status before and after the bath.

The Cleansing Tub and Shower Bath. If the patient's condition permits (when the pulse is of good quality and there is no exhaustion or other contraindication), a tub bath or shower is usually allowed by the physician and preferred by the patient. A bed bath is at best a poor substitute for an immersion bath or shower. A nurse or some attendant should see that the bathroom is warm, that the bath is prepared at the right temperature, generally 37.8° to 40.6° C (100° to 105° F), and that everything necessary is in readiness. This includes soap, wash cloth, towel, nail brush, comb, nightgown or pajamas, bathrobe, slippers, and stockings in some cases. If the patient has no toothbrush or other requisite, it should be provided by those responsible for his care.

The patient should be given any necessary assistance. With sufficient help, and in tubs such as those shown in Figure 57, he can take a tub bath with comparatively little fatigue. In hospitals in this country attendants of the same sex as the patient help with tub baths, and most persons' sense of modesty would suffer if this were not so; on the other hand, medical workers consider unwillingness to give any patient needed help of this sort a form of prudery.

The patient should not be allowed to remain in the bathroom alone for any length of time if sick and never alone with the door locked. The attendant can keep busy close by, and, although not in the room with the patient, should be fully aware of his condition while bathing. The patient may become chilled or faint; he may be severely burned or fall and injure himself. Since patients have both purposely and accidentally drowned in bath tubs, the nurse who is responsible must take every precaution to prevent this by careful supervision. Patients often resent this supervision, and tact is needed to keep adults from feeling that their privacy is invaded. The amount of supervision needed varies considerably, and although hospitals must protect themselves by rules to prevent accidents, the individual is not to be treated in a routine fashion. After the bath, the patient should be warmly clothed and covered, according to the environmental temperature, to prevent chilling.

* Newton. Kathleen: *Geriatric Nursing.* C. V. Mosby Co., St. Louis, 1950, p. 87.

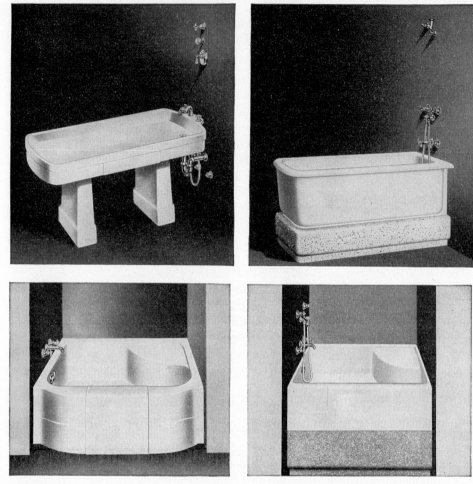

Figure 57. (*Top, left*) A bed patient may be put into a free-standing tub of stretcher height. (*Top, right*) A free-standing tub of this height makes it possible to give ambulatory patients assistance from both sides. (*Bottom, left*) A tub with a seat should be provided when chest or abdominal dressings prohibit immersion baths. (*Bottom, right*) A child's tub that prevents unnecessary stooping by the person giving assistance. (Courtesy of Crane Co., Chicago, Ill.)

Children should never be left alone while taking a bath. Tub baths and showers for infants and children are given at temperatures ranging between 32.2° and 37.8° C (90° and 100° F). (This temperature is one that feels comfortably warm to the elbow, which, because of its sensitivity, is used for testing temperatures when a bath thermometer is not available.) Well infants are given tub baths when cared for in homes. However, the problem of asepsis makes the use of tubs and showers for bathing infants and children in hospitals especially difficult. Decontamination of communal tubs and slabs on which babies lie for table shower baths is almost impossible. Babies and children are so much more likely than adults to contract skin diseases from contaminated tubs and showers that it makes such baths impractical for them.

Cleansing Bed Bath. The purposes of the bath are to clean the skin and refresh the patient. The nurse should see that the room is warm, that the windows are closed and the patient protected from drafts, that the bed is screened, and that everything necessary is at hand. The *technique* will vary in different hospitals and homes according to the facilities, but certain principles are the same for all bed baths.

A unit similar to that found in modern railroad trains is now available for hospital use. Without such a unit the articles needed include a large basin or foot tub of water at 43.3° to 46.1° C (110° to 115° F), a bath towel and face towel, wash cloths, soap, nail brush, comb and brush, rubbing lotion, talcum powder, protection for the bed, and covering for the patient. Each should have his own basin, or basins in general use should be disinfected by boiling. If his condition permits, the patient may be allowed to clean his mouth and teeth and sometimes to take his own bath; but the nurse is responsible for his preparation and for seeing that he does not tire himself and that the bath is adequate.

Preparation of the patient includes covering him with a blanket and removing the upper bedclothes. Sometimes a cotton bath blanket is placed under the patient for warmth and protection; in other cases a bath towel, under each part as it is bathed. In some hospitals a very large bath towel, almost the size of the bed, is used under the patient. Terry cloth bath blankets are used also to cover the patient in the place of a cotton or woolen blanket. In very hot weather cotton sheets may be substituted for blankets. One pillow is left under the head, unless this position is uncomfortable or contraindicated by the patient's condition. If necessary, a hot-water bottle is placed at the patient's feet for warmth; in most cases, except during warm weather, this adds greatly to his comfort. The mouth is then cleaned, and the gown removed.

In *bathing the patient* proceed in the following order—face, ears, neck, chest, arms and hands, abdomen, back, thighs, legs, feet, and pubic region. Give special attention to the ears, the skin between the fingers and toes, axillae, umbilicus, and pubic region. Work quickly, quietly, smoothly; and wash with firm but *gentle* pressure. It is almost necessary to have a compassionate feeling to get a sufficiently gentle touch for the very sick person who "hurts all over." Avoid the appearance of hurry, but if the bath is given slowly, the water becomes cold and the patient exhausted.

Make a mitten of the washcloth, holding the ends in the palm of the hand with the thumb. If the ends dangle, they will feel cold and uncomfortable to the patient. Washcloths made like thumbless mittens are very satisfactory. Expose, wash, and dry each part separately and thoroughly, covering the area immediately. Do not drip water over the patient. Change the water or add hot water sufficiently often to keep the temperature comfortably warm.

Place the tub or basin on the bed so that the patient can put his hands in the

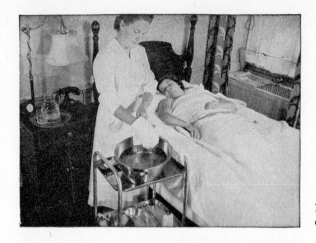

Figure 58A. Giving a bed bath. Note the thumbless mitten wash-cloth that reduces dripping.

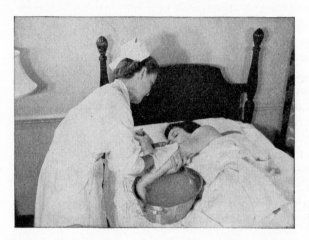

Figure 58B. The arm is supported and bathed while the hand rests in the water.

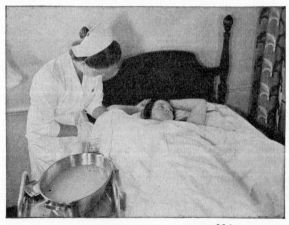

Figure 58C. The axilla, breast, and abdomen can be bathed with little exposure of the patient. Note the bath towel lining the bath blanket to prevent wetting the latter.

water while his hands and arms are being bathed. In washing the feet, place them in the tub and, if dirty, allow them to soak. The illusion of a tub bath is created somewhat by bathing the flexed leg and thigh while the foot is in the tub, allowing the water to flow over the parts from the cloth or sponge (see Fig. 58D). While the feet are soaking, the fingernails may be cleaned and trimmed. Remove the feet from the tub and dry them carefully, drying particularly well between the toes. Clean and trim the toenails.

After bathing and drying the back, massage or rub it thoroughly to stimulate the circulation. To rub the back, help the patient, if necessary, to turn on his abdomen or on his side with his back toward the nurse and his body near the edge of the bed so that he is as close to the operator as possible. If the prone position is used and the patient is a woman, a pillow under the abdomen and hips removes pressure on the breasts and favors relaxation.

In rubbing, use firm long strokes and kneading motions. (The amount of pressure to exert depends upon the patient's condition and his preference.) Massage with

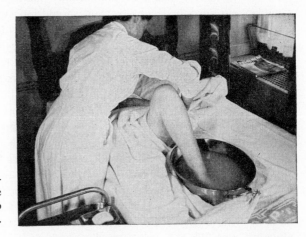

Figure 58D. The foot is soaking while the leg and thigh are bathed. Note care in draping to prevent exposure of the pubic area.

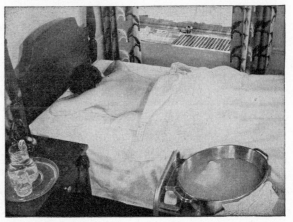

Figure 58E. The patient should be in a relaxed position while the back is bathed, rubbed, and powdered. Note the large pillow under abdomen and hips and the small pillow under the head.

(Figs. 58 A-E, courtesy of Columbia-Presbyterian Medical Center, New York City, and Clay-Adams Co., New York City.)

both hands and work with a stronger upward than downward stroke. Give particular attention to pressure areas in rubbing. Patients are especially grateful for massage of the neck and the lower part of the back. Lubricating the operator's hands with cocoa butter or talcum increases the comfort of massage. Alcohol is more generally used for its refreshing effect, but it is not a good lubricant for rubbing and it tends to dry the skin.* Powder the area at the completion of the process, which should consume from three to five minutes, or more.

Throughout the bath encourage the person to do as much of it as he can without tiring himself unduly. He nearly always prefers to wash his face, neck, and ears. Unless they are very ill or disabled, most persons also prefer to bathe the genitalia. The nurse may fold a bath towel and put it under the buttocks or place an empty bedpan under the patient so that plenty of water can be used without wetting the bed. She places what the patient will need where he can reach it and may leave him in privacy for a few minutes. It is routine in some hospitals to flush the genital area daily with warm water poured from a pitcher. When patients need assistance in bathing this area, they usually like to have a nurse or attendant of the same sex; no false modesty, however, should interfere with the performance of any nursing function on which the patient's comfort and welfare depend. When the nurse bathes the genitalia, it is important that she be both gentle and thorough.

Care of the nails is usually left until the gown is replaced. Cutting is said to make them brittle; so a fastidious patient usually prefers to have the fingernails filed. A daily application of an emollient, like cold cream, helps to keep nails and cuticles in good condition. The toenails are cut rather close to prevent scratching of the opposite leg and catching the bedclothes. Cutting the nails straight across rather than in a curve helps to prevent ingrowing toenails. Nails should be cleaned with an orangewood stick rather than with a metal instrument, which roughens the nail and makes it harbor dirt. Soaking in water and a detergent or in warm oil may be necessary if the nails are very dirty or thickened. After the bath, remake the bed (see p. 362), at the same time removing bath blankets. Whenever it can be done without tiring the patient, get him into a chair, on a stretcher, or on an "Invalift" (see Fig. 91) while making the bed. It is desirable to postpone *combing the hair* until after the bedmaking since this process disarranges the hair. If possible comb and arrange the hair while the patient is in a chair. If the hair is combed and brushed in bed, protect the pillow with a towel. Clear away all equipment used and see that it is cleaned and returned to its proper place. Put the patient's unit in order, and attend to his immediate wants, such as a drink or a hot-water bottle, so that he can at once get the benefit of rest that naturally follows a bath.

Bathing Infants and Children.   Bed baths for infants and children are essentially the same as those for adults. Until the infant's temperature-regulating mechanism is well established, he is particularly susceptible to chilling; therefore, the room should be kept warm and only small body areas exposed.

Baths for newborn infants have been eliminated in many hospitals. It is quite

* "Lubriderm" is a commercial skin lubricant containing vegetable oils that is very effective in skin care. (It is made by Ayerst Laboratories, Inc., New York City.)

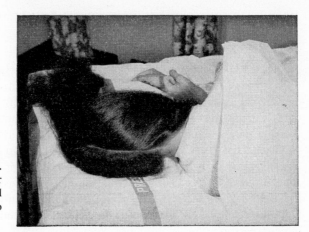

Figure 59A. To comb long hair. The head is turned so that the hair can be parted down the back, and access of the brush and comb to the entire scalp made possible.

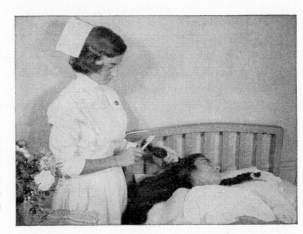

Figure 59B. The nurse has wrapped a strand of hair around her forefinger and is holding it slack between her hand and the scalp so that she can remove tangles without discomfort to the patient.

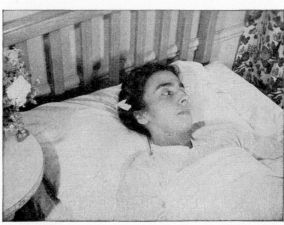

Figure 59C. The plaits are crossed and tied in front of the ears with ribbons. This is a becoming and comfortable way to dress the long hair of a bed patient.

(Figs. 59 A-C, courtesy of Columbia-Presbyterian Medical Center, New York City, and Clay-Adams Co., New York City.)

generally thought that the sebaceous material (*vernix caseosa*) covering the baby at birth is nature's protection of the delicate skin. This is allowed to wear off gradually, as nature doubtless intended. For the first week or ten days bathing is limited to cleaning the buttocks and genitalia with warm water or oil when the diapers are changed. Equipment for this purpose is kept in the infant's unit, the nurse's hands are clean, and she is often gowned and masked.[25, 26] In this way, it is thought, skin infections are reduced to a minimum.

The Partial Bath.   When a partial bath is substituted for a complete one, the face, hands, arms, and pubes are bathed. Morning care for bed patients should always include cleaning the mouth, rubbing the back, combing and brushing the hair, and making the bed. The most scrupulous attention should be given the mouth and pressure areas on the skin of the bedfast even though their condition or lack of nursing personnel prohibits a full daily bath.

3. SHAVING THE MAN PATIENT

Men accustomed to shaving daily are uncomfortable when illness interrupts the habit. An unshaven face makes a sick man look sicker. This lowers his morale and distresses those who love him. Hospital barbers, orderlies, and men nurses usually shave men unable to shave themselves. A woman nurse in the hospital often helps the bed patient by putting the necessary articles within his reach; in home nursing she may be more skillful in shaving a patient than anyone else available. Because a man, who practices daily, is likely to be more adept than a woman, the nurse may ask a man in the family to shave the very ill patient if a barber is not available.

If the patient is able to shave himself, he needs light and mirror, a basin of warm water, towel, squares of soft paper, waste receptacle, razor, special soap and shaving brush or a cream not requiring the use of a brush. An electric razor eliminates the use of shaving soap and brush. All these articles should be left within reach, and the patient put in a comfortable position for shaving. He will usually prefer to be left alone during the procedure if he needs no assistance.

To shave a helpless patient, collect the articles just enumerated and put them on a table near the operator's hand. See that the patient is in a position comfortable for him and convenient for the worker. Protect the bedding and clothing with a towel. Wash the face thoroughly before starting the process. Make a thin lather on the face with soap, warm water, and shaving brush or shaving cream. Allow a few minutes for the lather to soften the beard. Keep the razor and the skin wet while shaving. Hold the skin taut, use short strokes, and keep the razor at an angle of about 30 deg. In most areas shave against the direction taken by the hairs for a close shave. Shave very carefully around sensitive areas, such as the nose and lips. If able, the patient will prefer to shave these parts himself. The razor should be kept clean by frequent rinsing. Wash the soap off the face after the shave and apply a soothing lotion if the patient has one and requests it.

Hollander in Fishbein's monograph[27] recommends a lotion of 50 to 70 per cent ethyl alcohol containing salicylic acid in a 4 per cent concentration.

An electric razor is preferred by many men. Because it cannot be sterilized, it is not suitable for communal use in hospitals.

4. CARE OF THE MOUTH, TEETH, AND DENTURES

Importance of Mouth Care in Health and Illness. Because the mouth is the portal of entry for food and digestion is started here, the condition of the mouth directly affects health. Because the mouth is molded to some extent by the person's character, it can lend charm to the face. For physical and psychological reasons a healthy mouth is highly prized. In his text, *Patients Have Families,* Henry B. Richardson[28] attributes a series of family misfortunes to the father's failure to preserve his teeth!

Decayed teeth and sensitive gums cause such discomfort in eating that food is likely to be swallowed before it is thoroughly chewed and mixed with saliva, which contains the digestive enzyme ptyalin. Infected teeth, gums, and tonsils can infect other parts of the digestive and respiratory systems by direct extension; by contaminating the blood stream, they can cause joint or heart disease. An unpleasant breath can be attributed to the condition of the tonsils or the stomach, but it is often caused by diseased teeth, gums, or bony sockets.

The knowledge that one is offensive in appearance or odor is damaging to the self-respect. From this brief list of the dangers and disadvantages of neglecting the mouth, it can be seen that a person's general welfare is seriously affected by its condition.

Oral Hygiene. The development and maintenance of healthy teeth is dependent upon the constitutional factor, or the inherited quality of teeth and surrounding structures, and the environmental factor, or the condition of the tissues and fluids surrounding the teeth throughout life. The text of Russell W. Bunting[29] and his collaborators gives an excellent review of dental research. There seems to be general agreement that primitive peoples have better teeth than civilized peoples, and it has been suggested that in mixed races individuals may inherit a racially characteristic narrow arch from one parent and large teeth that do not fit into it from the other. The pure race and their unrefined and varied diet probably account for the relatively normal mouths of primitive people.

A person may have at birth teeth of poor quality because his mother had an inadequate prenatal diet. After birth, while the teeth are developing, the diet and general health of the individual are thought to affect the teeth. The relationship between the minerals and vitamins in the diet is not well established, nor is the relationship between dental health and general health entirely clear. Most authorities would agree, however, that an optimum diet and good general health are conducive to development and maintenance of a normal condition of the mouth and teeth. Since caries (the chief disease of the tooth itself) is a disease of civilization, its refined and often monotonous diet is thought to be the chief predisposing factor.

Dentistry is a comparatively new science, and until very recently it has dealt with treatment rather than prevention of disease. The last decade has marked the most striking advances in this field of knowledge. Old theories have been disproved, and a new era of therapy and oral hygiene is dawning. Even the most recent opinions are likely to be out of date before they reach the public. A rapidly extending program of public health dentistry, including research, is now in existence. With the passage of the Social Security Act in 1935, dental departments were established in public health agencies. The Dental Research Act of 1948 has enabled the United States Public Health Service to enlarge its program. Federal dental programs are administered through the United States Public Health Service, the Children's Bureau, the Office of Indian Affairs, the Veterans Administration, the Army, the Navy, and the Farm Security Administration. State and local health departments offer dental services of varying types. At present, public health programs concentrate on services to school children, health education, consultation service, and demonstrations of preventive methods. All types of services in the federal program are available to certain government charges and employees.

It is not possible with the existing number of dentists to offer adequate dental service to the entire population. In an effort to make dental care more universally available, Alfred C. Fones organized a school for dental hygienists. Prepared originally to work as health educators and to supplement the technical service of dentists in the schools, they are now employed to clean teeth and to serve as technicians wherever dental care is given. Markedly improved methods of disease prevention and control and the extension of dental services to all segments of the population are possible developments within the near future.

Diseases of the mouth fall into two main groups: diseases of the teeth themselves (the main one being caries) and diseases of the bony structures and soft tissues of the mouth, called periodontal disease.

Discovery of the means of preventing and controlling dental *caries* is one of the most dramatic medical accomplishments of this century. W. D. Miller is credited with laying the foundation on which modern treatment is based. He demonstrated the existence of a substance in saliva that converts carbohydrates to lactic acid and showed that this acid dissolves tooth enamel, permitting bacterial invasion and the development of caries. Since he found that sterile (or boiled) saliva will not convert carbohydrate, he concluded that the converting principle was a bacterial enzyme. This theory is now generally accepted, and the conditions essential to the development of caries are believed to be the presence in the mouth of the enzyme-producing bacteria (loosely referred to as the lactic acid bacilli group) + saliva in which the bacteria can function + carbohydrates (particularly sugars) + tooth enamel susceptible to caries. Alter any of these factors, and the chain of events known as caries formation is broken. Individuals who can eat sweets freely and remain immune to caries have been shown to be free from the lactic acid bacilli. It is thought that their saliva contains a substance that discourages growth of the microorganisms although the exact mechanism is not established. There is evidence that persons whose intake of fluorine is high (as in areas where the water contains relatively more fluorine) have few lactic acid bacilli in their mouths. It is also thought that fluorine has entered into the composition of the teeth during the formative period (during the prenatal period and the first eight years of life) and that the resulting enamel is more resistant to caries.

Research now in progress may prove that other substances, such as ammonia-liberating compounds and certain antibiotics, discourage the growth of lactic acid bacilli, either directly or by encouraging organisms antagonistic to the lactic acid bacilli. *The positive relationship between the intake of refined carbohydrates and the incidence of caries has been amply demonstrated.* Gullorm Toverad,[30] reporting on caries during World War II in Norway, concluded that the low intake of refined carbohydrates accounts for the lowered incidence of caries in that country. He says that similar reports came from England and Italy. It is conceded, therefore, that caries can be successfully controlled by two methods: (1) by diet, (2) by the use of fluorine (or some other inhibitor) to discourage the growth of lactic acid bacilli and/or to make enamel resistant to the action of the bacterial enzyme.

Philip Joy in Bunting's text says that good results may be expected with the reduction of carbohydrates to 100 gm daily for two weeks with the elimination of sugar, bread, potatoes, and other foods rich in carbohydrate. During the next two weeks sugar only is eliminated, and if the mouth is relatively free from lactic acid bacilli, no further dietary restriction may be necessary for months or, possibly, years. The dentist is guided by the bacterial mouth count. Obviously, this treatment is more successful if pursued with adults than with children, whose food intake is regulated with difficulty, but any treatment consistently adhered to yields richer rewards in the young than in the adult who has already suffered tooth damage.

Treatment based on inhibiting the growth of lactic acid bacilli by means other than diet has been most successfully demonstrated with fluorine. The low incidence of caries in certain areas of this country where drinking water is relatively high in fluorine content has led the health departments of Grand Rapids, Evanston, and other cities to experiment in treating the drinking water with sodium fluorine. It is estimated that the yearly cost is about 10¢ per person. (Sodium fluosilicate is cheaper and said to be less toxic.) One part of fluorine in one million parts of water is thought to be effective without causing noticeable mottling of the tooth enamel. The nature of the caries-inhibiting properties of fluoride water is not established, according to a number of authorities, but it is believed that children exposed to this treatment for the first eight years of life enjoy a high degree of immunity. Another method of control with fluorine is to apply it directly to the teeth of children. Mobile units in 35 states are demonstrating this simple process, and dentists all over the country are practicing it. Sodium or potassium fluoride solutions in strength from 0.1 to 3 per cent are applied after prophylaxis. How often the treatment should be repeated to confer immunity has not been clearly established, but dentists of the US Public Health Service say that topical treatment with a fluoride solution should be repeated every 3 to 4 years until the age of 13.[31, 32]

Signs of disease in the tissues surrounding the teeth include inflammation, swelling and tumors (hyperplasia or hypertrophy), lesions of various sorts, necrosis, and atrophy. The loss of teeth is more often due to disease of the periodontal, or surrounding, tissue than to disease of the tooth itself, so Hamilton B. G. Robinson states.[33] Herman Allington,[34] discussing the causes and treatment of dry mouth, says that a protracted diminution of saliva causes deterioration and finally loss of the teeth. Anything that traumatizes tissue predisposes it to disease; anything that interferes with normal metabolism is likewise an indirect cause. The conditions mentioned above are given names with which the nurse should be familiar. Inflammation of the gums is called *gingivitis*; inflammation of the deeper tissues surrounding the roots of the teeth (an extension of gingivitis) is called *periodontitis* or *periodontoclasia,* although many persons still use the term *pyorrhea*. Degeneration of the periodontal tissues, *periodontosis* (a rare condition), is a result of systemic disease. Atrophy of the tissues in which the teeth are embedded is common in the aged, although the fact that marked atrophic changes are not universally found in old age makes it doubtful whether this is a necessary accompaniment of the aging process. Inflammation that extends over the entire mouth, lips, tongue, and gums is called *stomatitis.* A gingivitis that progresses to a necrotic stage and is associated with the presence of fusospirochetal organisms in known as *Vincent's infection* or *trench mouth.*

Robinson, who treats the subject of periodontal disease in Bunting's text, lists improperly used toothbrushes and toothpicks as causative agents in periodontal inflammation. He also mentions acids, alkalis, and heavy metals, heat, x-rays, and atomic energy as possible sources of trauma. Gingivitis, however, is most often initiated by trauma from deposits, or calculi, at the gum margins. In normal occlusion, the force exerted by the bite is distributed over all the teeth, but with malocclusion this very powerful pressure of the jaw action falls on those teeth that hit; likewise, the teeth that have no contact with those of the opposing jaw lack the normal stimulation of the bite. Healthy periodontal tissue is therefore dependent upon the alignment of teeth, jaw structure, the inherited quality of the tissues themselves, diet and general health, and freedom from trauma by agents put into the mouth and from accretions on the teeth, either food or calculi, particularly at or near the gingival crevice or sulcus (the space between the gum and the tooth surface).

Admittedly, there is much to be learned about the prevention of periodontal disease, but what has been said about its cause suggests the means of prevention and cure. Leaving out the question of eugenics, or controlling structural factors through the genes, the mother can contribute something through the selection of an optimum prenatal diet; likewise, an optimum diet for the child throughout her guardianship. Dental supervision from early childhood prevents defective occlusion in many cases. Regular and frequent prophylaxis removes the traumatic deposits on the teeth, and, if the dentist is a teacher, he will help the individual to reduce the hazards of food deposits and calculi formation and, at the same time, to care for his mouth without traumatizing the tissues. It is now recognized that some persons most zealous in the care of their mouths have, by incorrect or too frequent brushing of the teeth, pushed the protecting gums away from the teeth, exposing an area of dentin that should remain covered. Improper habits of brushing may also wear away the enamel. It has been shown that primitive peoples have effective methods of cleaning the mouth and teeth, and the action of chewing their relatively rougher diet has a cleansing effect.

It cannot be urged too strongly that all persons from early childhood through old age visit the dentist at least twice a year. If more frequent visits are indicated, the dentist has an opportunity to advise accordingly. Dental prophylaxis, in its broadest sense, includes removal of all injurious deposits and stains on the teeth, reduction of bacterial action, repair of carious teeth, the correction of defective occlusion and misfitting dentures, smoothing of roughened surfaces, and instruction in oral hygiene.

There is sufficient evidence that certain vitamins are important in the prevention of periodontal disease. The role of vitamins is discussed more fully in Chapter 13, but it might be indicated here that those contributing most to healthy bone and mucous membrane elsewhere in the body and to bacterial resistance are of special significance. Periodontal diseases have been attributed to a lack of, and treated with, vitamins A and D, the B complex, and vitamin C. Gingivitis and its extension, periodontitis, are late accompaniments of many long-drawn-out illnesses, if diets used are not varied and are high in refined carbohydrates and low in the vitamin-rich foods.

Daily care of the teeth includes use of a toothbrush; a dentifrice or cleansing agent; dental floss; and, recommended by some authorities, interdental stimulators. A mouthwash is not thought necessary, although a number of writers mention its value in the control of *halitosis* (foul breath).* It is, of course, desirable to remove all causes of bad breath. Hydrogen peroxide (used in the strength of about 1 per cent) removes decaying food by its bubbling action and may reduce bacterial activity thereby, striking at a common factor in halitosis. Hydrogen peroxide if used improperly can injure the gums. It should be employed only on the advice of the dentist. Chlorophyll dentifrices are said by some to be deodorizing if the concentration is sufficiently great; William Bolton[35] says the American Dental Association reported recently that "as yet there is no scientific evidence" to support their use. A toothbrush small enough to reach all aspects of the teeth should be selected. Dorothy G. Hard, writing in Bunting's text, says that no one brush suits all persons, but she recommends in general that the head of the brush be 1⅛ in. long; the bristles, 7/16 in. in length; the tufts set in two or three rows of equal length and spaced far apart. Natural bristles are recommended because they are more flexible. Stiff bristles are best for most persons. Brushes should be rotated so that the

---

* Discussing a study of halitosis, P. P. Morris and R. R. Read report that saliva "putrefies rapidly," giving rise to objectionable odors. According to them, dilution with water does not materially affect putrefaction. They add: "Dentifrice helps materially up to 2 hours. Antiseptic rinse (a saturated 27% aqueous alcohol solution of thymol, menthol, eucalyptol, and methyl salicylate with benzoic acid and boric acid) helps three hours, also tobacco odors are reduced by the antiseptic rinse. . . . There are certain resistant types of odors, such as garlic, that are systemic in origin, and are not affected by water or antiseptic rinse." They also report that complete dental prophylaxis reduces mouth and breath odors, as one would expect. (Morris, P. P., and Read, R. R.: "Halitosis: Variations in Mouth and Total Breath Odor Intensity Resulting from Prophylaxis and Antisepsis," *J. Dent. Research,* **28**:324, [June] 1949.)

bristles may dry (and stiffen) and bacterial action inhibited by the drying process. Brushes recommended for children have the same characteristics, but should be proportionally smaller.

Dentifrices may take the form of a powder or a paste. Most authorities agree that, while they are not absolutely necessary to a thorough cleaning, they make the process easier and pleasanter. The value of ammoniated dentrifices was discussed under the heading of caries. There is reason to believe that it has value, but it should be selected on advice of the dentist. Most pastes, powders, and liquids for cleaning the teeth contain one or more of the following: an abrasive, soap, and flavoring. Pastes seem to have no advantage over powders except that they are controlled more easily. Powders may be insufflated by small children and irrational persons. Dentifrices that claim to remove stains may be injurious and are not recommended.[36] A homemade preparation of equal parts of sodium chloride, sodium bicarbonate, and prepared chalk, seasoned with oil of peppermint, is approved by the American Dental Association.

Flat dental floss is preferred to round. Interdental stimulants are pointed wooden or rubber instruments made to fit between the teeth. The rubber tip fastened to the handle of the toothbrush is used on the inner and posterior interdental spaces.

The motion used in brushing is important. The main object is to clean the surfaces of the teeth. Some authorities believe that a second object is to stimulate and harden the gingiva as fibrous food is thought to harden the gums of primitive peoples. This value is questioned by some students, who claim that the chewing of coarse foods, rather than their contact with the gums, is responsible for their beneficial effect. There is agreement that the motions used should be such as to produce no traumatic effect. Horizontal and rotary motions are discouraged, the former failing to remove material from between the teeth and both inclined to push the gums away from the teeth. Hard recommends for general use a downward stroke for the upper teeth and an upward stroke for the lower teeth, each process carried out in two parts. She says:

Instead of simply sweeping the bristles across the teeth, the stroke is done in two parts. First, the side of the toothbrush bristles is pressed against the gingival mucosa with sufficient force to blanch the tissues momentarily. Second, by rolling the wrist, the tips of the bristles are moved slowly and firmly lengthwise over the tooth surfaces.*

She suggests establishing a pattern and looking in a mirror to see that all surfaces are covered. The motion described does not reach the occlusal surface of the teeth; therefore, an additional motion across the grinding, or cutting, surfaces is used. Dental tape, or floss, should be slipped carefully between the teeth, avoiding any injury to the interdental gingiva. Friction with wooden or rubber stimulators between the teeth discourages the formation of tartar, or calculi, and promotes healthy gums. It is advocated that this thorough cleansing process be carried out three times

* Bunting, Russell W., and collaborators: *A Textbook of Oral Hygiene.* Lea & Febiger, Philadelphia, 1950, p. 190.

daily, and it is óbvious that it is most effective if it follows eating. For many people, however, brushing the teeth before breakfast is essential to a sense of well-being.

To summarize, the essentials of oral hygiene include the following: (1) an adequate diet containing enough coarse food to necessitate considerable chewing and (2) effective use of toothbrush, dental tape, dental "stimulators," and dentrifice two to four times a day, preferably after meals and at bedtime. Dental supervision is essential for the removal of irritating deposits, the early treatment of caries, and correction of malocclusion and other structural defects. Most dentists urge their patients to have a dental examination and prophylaxis at least twice a year. These visits should begin at the age of 2½ to 3 years and extend through the life span.

Care of Dentures.   Since most persons having artificial teeth are sensitive about it, nurses should be especially thoughtful in proffering and giving help in the care of the mouth when dentures are worn. Ambulatory patients will usually prefer to clean their mouths, plates, or bridges in the bathroom with running water; bed patients must have water, a dentifrice, brush, and a waste receptacle brought to them. If they are too ill for the effort required, the nurse must help them to rinse their mouths and must clean their dentures.

For the sake of morale the sick should be encouraged to wear their dentures unless their condition contraindicates it. Many persons sleep with false teeth in place. When not worn, plates and bridges made of plastic may be kept dry in an appropriate container; vulcanite dentures are said to be preserved by moisture and should be stored in a covered container of water. A few drops of peppermint essence in the water give them a pleasant odor. Wet dentures are more easily inserted than dry ones. Transparent containers should not be used for storage; false teeth exposed in a glass are grotesque and usually embarrass their owner. Plates are breakable; they must be kept in a safe place.

Plates and bridges should be cleaned when they are removed from the mouth for any purpose and after eating. The patient usually has a special powder recommended by his dentist, but any mildly abrasive tooth powder or ordinary soap may be used and applied with a brush. When the nurse gives this service to the patient, she should take the dentures to a source of running water, because they can be more satisfactorily cleaned if there is an abundant water supply. Water should be warm, never hot, since heat can distort the plastic or vulcanite. If the patient cleans the dentures, he should be given an ample amount of water and a large waste basin. He will ordinarily prefer to be unobserved. Vulcanite is porous and absorbs food debris that on deterioration gives plates a sour odor unless properly cleaned and treated. Soaking vulcanite plates in a 1 per cent ammonium hydroxide solution once a week is recommended by Fones.[37] Plastic has almost entirely replaced vulcanite in dentures. It is lighter and, being less permeable, can be kept free from odor.

Care of the Mouth during Illness.   High temperatures, mouth breathing, malnutrition, and other conditions accompanying illness cause drying and cracking of the lips and predispose all mouth tissues to infection. Salivary secretion is affected by many conditions and body functions that are likely to be disturbed in illness. John J. O'Rourke says:

Salivary flow is depressed during sleep. . . . There is also diminished flow in fever, profuse sweating, diuresis, diarrhea, and hemorrhage from lack of fluid intake. . . . Emotional factors have long been known to have definite effects on salivary secretion. . . . It is evident that any fall in water content of the tissues is reflected in the activity of the salivary glands, and the secretion is depressed.*

While he distinguishes between the salivary and mucous glands, he notes that the flow of mouth secretions is stimulated by appetizing sights and odors, by the presence of food in the mouth, by chewing, and by talking. Excessive flow may occur during pregnancy and is associated with lesions or irritation of the mouth, esophagus, stomach, and even the small intestines.

If the patient is too sick to brush his teeth and clean his mouth or does not know how to do it properly, someone must supply the needed energy and skill. In prolonged illness the examination and prophylactic treatment by the dentist, usually sought by the patient, should be provided by a dental service within the hospital, and at more frequent intervals in sickness than in health. Dental consultation should be available to the physician and nurse when the patient has bleeding gums or other signs of pathology. While gingivitis and pyorrhea during illness are often the direct result of an inadequate diet, they may be aggravated by the presence of tartar or other remediable conditions. The patient's food and fluid intake should be checked. Inadequate fluids or a deficient dietary essential can be the chief cause of mouth pathology. The diet should be adequate in calories and high in vitamins, particularly B and C, to prevent disorders of the soft tissues even though it may be necessary to give all or a part of the fluid and food needed by extraoral feeding.

When the mouth is dry, local treatment with fluids and emollients gives temporary relief. Even though the patient cannot or should not swallow foods or fluids, he will find it refreshing to rinse the buccal cavity frequently. The rinsing water may be flavored with peppermint, menthol, thymol, lemon juice, or any flavoring pleasing to the patient. Medicinal odors should be avoided. Most hospitals provide mouthwashes containing palatable aromatic substances. A mixture of lemon juice and glycerin (a trihydroxyalcohol) applied to the tongue and gums is a classic treatment for dry mouth. Louis S. Goodman and Alfred Gilman say: "Glycerin absorbs water and therefore in high concentration it is somewhat dehydrating and irritating to exposed tissue. Concentrated solutions, for this reason, are slowly bactericidal."†

The effectiveness of lemon juice and glycerin and its mode of action are open to analysis. Both are foods and harmless if swallowed, the lemon juice containing the much needed vitamin C and the glycerin having a sweet taste especially appealing

---

* O'Rourke, John J.: *Oral Physiology,* 2nd ed. (edited by Leroy M. S. Miner). C. V. Mosby Co., St. Louis, 1951, p. 274.

† Goodman, Louis S., and Gilman, Alfred: *The Pharmacological Basis of Therapeutics,* 2nd ed. The Macmillan Company, New York, 1955, p. 1018.

to children. Lemon juice stimulates secretion of saliva and so may be of definite value. Glycerin, being hydroscopic, attracts moisture and therefore softens dry tissue, but if too concentrated it is dehydrating and irritating. This mixture should be used critically, as should other empiric remedies. The nurse in charge of a large chronic disease hospital says that they regularly apply milk to sore mouths with excellent results. Carbonated drinks, such as ginger ale, also give comfort as a mouthwash. It is possible that the bubbles of gas break up tenacious mucus and make its expectoration easier. Plain or flavored oils are often applied with applicators or an atomizer to the inside of the mouth. The latter method is more effective. This treatment is not always acceptable to the patient, and there is the ever-present danger that the oil may run down into the lungs. If the oil is not absorbed, it acts as an irritant, or foreign body, and may cause a pneumonitis or an abscess.[38] Mineral oils are the most dangerous, and vegetable oils the least; P. H. Rossier and A. Bühlman[39] say that animal oils cause necrosis, or abscess formation. Lanolin and cocoa butter salves applied to the lips are of definite value. Petroleum jelly is effective, but is distasteful to most persons.

If the mouth is coated and lesions have developed and as a result the mouth is in a serious condition, the physician often prescribes some special application, such as sodium perborate, in addition to the general treatment suggested above, or he may combat the infection with systemic antibiotics.

In sickness teeth should be brushed at least as often as in health. Because many illnesses lower resistance of oral tissues, it is desirable to clean the mouth after each meal or feeding. *Hospitals should provide toothbrushes to patients who need them. Cotton applicators are no substitute; their inadequacy as cleansing agents accounts for the poor condition of many mouths during illness when they were substituted for the toothbrush.* Cotton when wet is slippery and doesn't clean teeth or a coated tongue. As a substitute for a toothbrush some nurses use gauze strips wrapped around the finger or a tongue blade. The sensation of gauze catching on the teeth is disagreeable, and if it is used, care should be taken to reduce this to a minimum. It is not an effective procedure.

It is more difficult to brush someone else's teeth than one's own, and nurses often practice on each other until they are skillful.

Suggested Procedure in Cleaning the Mouth of the Bed Patient. *If the person is able to brush his own teeth,* support him in a sitting position with a waste basin before him, if possible on a table, and protect his chest with a towel. If he cannot assume a sitting position, have him turn on his side with his face extending over the edge of the pillow. (Put a right-handed person on his left side and vice versa.) In this case, protect the bedding under his head with a towel and place the waste basin on the towel beside his cheek. Obviously, he will need more assistance if he is in a recumbent position than if he is sitting up.

Provide a cup of cool rather than hot water because the latter softens bristles and is not so refreshing. The patient will need toothbrush, dentifrice, dental tape, possibly dental stimulators, and a mouthwash. "Celluwipes" should be at hand. If the patient is lying down, a drinking tube is needed.

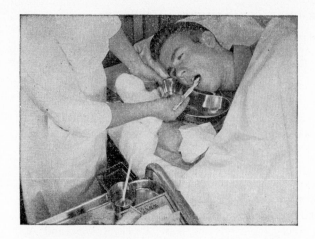

Figure 60A. Mouth care of the conscious patient who is unable to hold a toothbrush. The nurse is introducing the toothbrush into the open mouth.

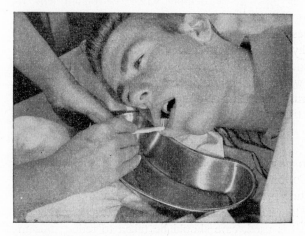

Figure 60B. The toothbrush is drawn out against the cheek.

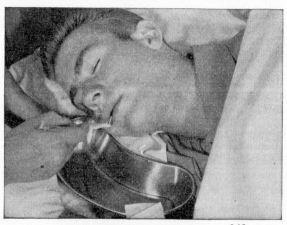

Figure 60C. The brush is in position for brushing the outer surface of the upper and lower right molars.

348

If the patient is unable to manipulate the toothbrush and the nurse is going to do it, place him in the side-lying position as described above. Wet (and rinse) the brush by pouring water over it, *not* by dipping it in the cup; this soils the water and makes it repellent as a rinse. Brush the central incisors first. Ask the patient to open his mouth; then while the mouth is open, insert the brush and bring it out against the cheek in position to brush the outer aspect of the right molars as the patient approximates the teeth. Repeat this process on the left side; then, while the patient holds the mouth open, brush the inner aspects of the teeth. Use a dentifrice of the patient's choice, or select the most appropriate one available. Let the patient rinse his mouth frequently, using the drinking tube and allowing the water to flow from the mouth into the emesis basin. When the patient is unconscious or likely to insufflate fluids that are in the mouth, use a suction machine throughout the cleaning process, if one is available. If the nurse places her finger over one end of a drinking tube, it may serve as a small siphon that enables her to place water in the mouth of the irrational patient who cannot, or will not, suck on the tube.

When cotton applicators saturated with mouthwash are used to clean the mouth, they are discarded into a paper bag as used.

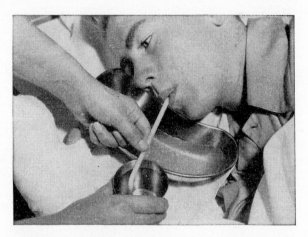

Figure 60D. With the water and tube held in the proper position, the patient does not have to raise his head to rinse his mouth or to drink.

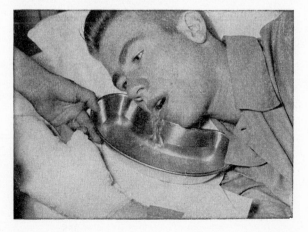

Figure 60E. Rinsing water will flow from the mouth if the head is in the right position. The bed will not be wet if the basin is placed at the edge of the pillow and the patient's face hangs over the basin.

(Figs. 60 A-E, courtesy of Columbia-Presbyterian Medical Center, New York City, and Clay-Adams Co., New York City.)

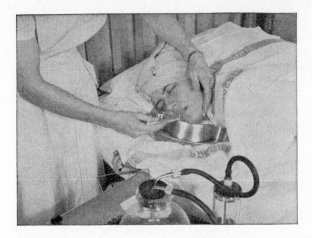

Figure 61A. Mouth care of the unconscious patient. The nurse is brushing the teeth with the same motions advocated for the person in health.

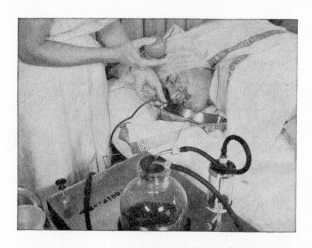

Figure 61B. Water is introduced with an Asepto syringe, and suction is maintained at the same time. (Note that tip is protected with a piece of rubber tubing).

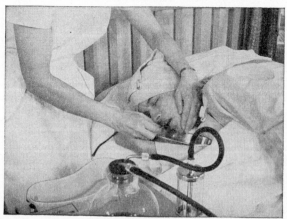

Figure 61C. Excess fluid is carefully suctioned from the mouth at the termination of the cleansing process.

(Figs. 61 A-C, courtesy of Columbia-Presbyterian Medical Center, New York City, and Clay-Adams Co., New York City.)

Throughout the procedure try to observe the wishes of the patient, at the same time using this as an opportunity, if the need is indicated and his interest can be aroused, to teach him the fundamentals of mouth care. Methods used by the nurse in either home or hospital speak more loudly, however, than anything she says. Instruction in oral hygiene is thought so important in some hospitals that specialists are employed to teach patients and to give them prophylactic treatment. There are dental clinics in hospital outpatient departments, and dental internes are found in a number of large institutions.

Discussing a "poll" of 41 general hospitals and their experience in a particular one, J. Orton Goodsell and R. E. Roper[40] recommend a dental department, or service, in every general hospital of 300 or more beds, this service to offer preventive and therapeutic care.

5. CARE OF THE NOSE

Care of the Nose in Health. The nasal secretions normally drain into the pharynx and are swallowed. The gastrointestinal tract is apparently able to destroy the nasal bacteria and those swept up from the lungs by ciliary motion into the bronchi and trachea. The habit of expectorating such secretions is unpleasant and unnecessary since they are of the same character as those which the individual is swallowing constantly and unconsciously. In health, blowing the nose gently is all that is necessary to keep the anterior nares free from dried secretions and dust that collects on the nasal mucus. Physicians discourage the use of nasal sprays and nose drops unless prescribed as treatment. The practice of snuffing water or salt solution into the nose to clean it is considered especially hazardous, the danger being that infectious material may be drawn up into the sinuses. Under normal conditions the nose drains itself. Medical opinion is against any unnecessary interference. Even blowing the nose is discouraged; if practiced, it should be done gently and with both nostrils open.

Cleaning the Nose in Sickness. Infants and ill persons are likely to have crusts form in the anterior nares. Being more or less helpless, they are unable to remove these without assistance. Patients who have nasal infections may also need instruction in cleaning the anterior nares. Paper handkerchiefs, that are destroyed as soon as soiled, are recommended in health and disease as a means of preventing infection of others and reinfection of the person using the handkerchief. A vegetable oil, such as cottonseed, is recommended for softening and removing dried nasal secretions, although water may suffice. The cleansing agent is applied with a cotton applicator. The end of the stick must be well covered. Experts in infant hygiene recommend removing the stick from the applicator before using it; because, even when the end is well covered, there is some danger of injury. If the skin around the nose is excoriated, petroleum jelly or cold cream usually relieves the condition. In cases where there are actual lesions, the physician may order some such medication as a mild mercurial, sulfur, or vitamin ointment.

6. HYGIENE OF THE EYES AND ARTIFICIAL EYES

Care of the Eyes.   When the lachrymal glands are functioning normally, the eyes are continuously washed with their secretion and need no additional cleaning; when the eyes are diseased, or when the neuromuscular mechanism that protects them by blinking is not functioning adequately, the nurse may have to protect and/or clean the eye.[41] Francis Adler[42] recommends a 1.5 per cent solution of sodium chloride as a cleansing agent because it approximates normal tears. Commercially prepared eye lotions for daily use are foisted on the public by high-pressure advertising. A pint bottle may contain nothing more than water and 5¢ worth of boric acid powder, a drug associated in the public mind with eyes. Boric acid has a low saturation point, and so undissolved crystals, that act as foreign bodies in the eye, are not uncommon. Clement Brooke and Thomas Boggs, reporting the death of a child from boric acid poisoning and a review of previously reported cases, comment on its toxicity and the readiness with which it is absorbed from injured surfaces. They say: "The therapeutic value of boric acid is doubtful and its antiseptic quality minimal. There are better and safer substances available for uses as antiseptics, irrigations, wet dressings, and ointments."*

Experts in the care of the newborn do not advocate daily bathing of the eyes. They recommend removing any crust that may form on the lids with a sterile eye cotton sponge wet with sterile water. The same method may be used for every one, or the eye may be flushed with an eye dropper or small syringe. It is a wise precaution to cover the tip of a glass syringe with a short piece of rubber tubing. Eye irrigations are discussed in Chapter 33, and removal of foreign bodies in Chapter 43.

When the blinking reflex is absent, as in the deeply unconscious, it may be necessary to keep a dressing over the eyes, such as that shown in Figure 220, until the reflex returns.

Care of Artificial Eyes.   Ocular prostheses vary greatly. They may be spherical, the size and shape of the normal eye, they may be a shell worn over a socket built up by plastic surgery, or they may fit into an implant. An implant is a spherical, nearly eye-shaped frame of tantalum or Vitallium or some other material that the tissues will tolerate. It is so constructed that the surrounding tissues and the muscles moving the eye may be attached to it permanently. The anterior visible portion, or the artificial eye, is held on the implant by some device that makes its removal possible. Newer artificial eyes are made so that the entire conjunctiva is in contact with the eye. This makes for greater mobility and comfort.

According to J. H. Prince, the trace of fluorine in tears roughens the surface of artificial eyes, and the slightest roughness irritates the socket or conjunctiva. For this reason ocular prostheses should be polished by the manufacturer at least yearly, and replaced when necessary. Charles A. Perera[43] says about every two

---

* Brooke, Clement, and Boggs, Thomas: "Boric Acid Poisoning; Report of a Case and Review of the Literature," *A.M.A. Am. J. Dis. Child.,* **82:**465, (Oct.) 1951.

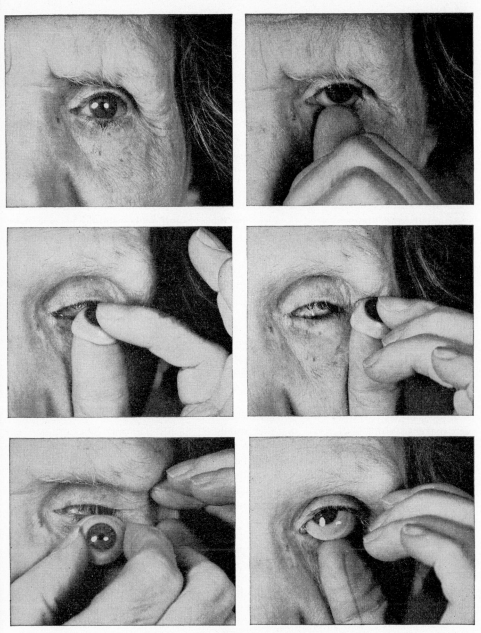

Figure 62. Removal and insertion of an artificial eye by a patient. (*Top, left*) Artificial eye in the socket; (*top, right*) with the thumb, patient dislodges eye slightly, prior to removal. (*Center, left*) As eye is removed, patient holds it firmly between the thumb and forefinger; (*center, right*) patient holds eye alongside the empty socket (note shell form of artificial eye). (*Bottom, left*) Patient places left hand on forehead to left of socket and exerts slight pressure to raise upper eyelid; artificial eye is held between thumb and forefinger prior to insertion. (*Bottom, right*) Final step in insertion of artificial eye; patient gently pushes eye in place with thumb. (Courtesy of Alfred Spitzer.)

years, but obviously many persons are unable to afford so costly a procedure. Prince suggests that the poor man should remove his eye nightly to prolong its life. He says, however, that "unless muco-purulent discharge is present to any degree, . . . there is benefit in an eye being retained at night if the patient is prepared to replace it frequently. Like a denture it assists in retaining better the shape of the cavity it occupies. . . ."* The eye socket must be watched carefully for signs of irritation.

If able, a person will prefer to care for the eye and socket himself, but the nurse must know how to do it for the very sick; she may also have to reinforce the doctor's teaching in hygiene. Prince describes some of the unsanitary ways in which patients he has known have handled their artificial eyes and stresses the importance of asepsis and the constant danger of infection. The hands of the operator and all instruments and material used for cleaning the eye and socket should be free from pathogenic organisms. After the eye is removed, the socket should be bathed or irrigated. Prince recommends eyecups, an undine, or a glass syringe with an emesis basin to receive the waste. A physiological saline solution (0.9 per cent sodium chloride) should be used if no other is prescribed by the physician. Prince suggests several mild antiseptic solutions.

Suggested Procedure. *To remove the eye* draw the lower lid down with the left hand, at the same time cupping it to receive the eye if it drops. Then, with the right hand, place the end of a small blunt instrument under the edge of the artificial eye, which is made to slip forward over the lower lid, when it will readily drop out. This maneuver must be carried out with care, as the eye can very easily be destroyed by dropping on a hard surface. *Clean the eye* before putting it away or returning it to the socket. Prince says it should be cleaned with "some weak germicidal solution or boiled (not boiling) water." One maker of artificial eyes says that they should be washed with mild soap solution and thoroughly rinsed with water. They caution that alcohol dims the luster of a plastic eye. For the same reason a plastic eye should be stored in water rather than left dry, while a glass eye should be kept in a box lined with soft material when not in use.†

Before inserting an artificial eye it should be moistened with physiological saline. Prince suggests dipping it in "pure castor oil." *To insert the eye* raise the upper lid with the tips of the two middle fingers, holding the hand flat against the forehead. Push the artificial eye beneath the upper lid with the right hand, and as it slips into place, allow the lid to fall over it. The eye must be supported by the left hand while the lower lid is drawn forward with the right hand over the lower edge of the eye. (See Fig. 62.)

Patients are naturally sensitive about the loss of an eye and anxious that attention should not be attracted to it. Their feelings should be respected, and precautions taken to safeguard their privacy.

7. CARE OF THE HAIR

Hygienic Care of the Hair. Authorities seem to agree that the condition of the hair is materially affected by the *general health*. This is easily understood when

* Prince, J. H.: *Ocular Prostheses.* Williams & Wilkins Co., Baltimore, 1946, p. 84.
† *Facts on the Care of an Artificial Eye.* Mager and Gougelman, Inc., New York.

one realizes that the visible portion, or shaft, is nourished by the root embedded in the scalp. The supply of nutrients to the root, the removal of wastes, and the lack of certain physiological substances, such as thyroxin, seem to affect the quality of the hair. Coarse dry hair is associated with hypothyroidism, falling of the hair is common in fevers of long duration, and there are many constitutional diseases that cause changes in its appearance.

In emphasizing the importance of general health, there is no intention of underestimating the beneficial effect of *local treatment* on the scalp and hair shaft. Stimulating the circulation of the scalp by massage and brushing is conceded to be desirable. Brushing the hair vigorously not only stimulates the circulation, but also, if the brush is clean, removes dirt particles and dead cells from the scalp.

Washing the hair every week or two is advocated by H. H. Hazen and Florence Biase.[44] There seems to be no adequate basis for the commonly expressed belief that shampoos at short intervals make the hair oily. On the contrary, oily hair should be washed more often than dry. Howard T. Behrman[45] says the oftener it is washed the better it is for the hair and scalp. He thinks a shampoo every five days is a good general rule; every two days, or every day, in very oily conditions of the scalp. Drying alcoholic lotions for oily hair are advocated by proprietors of beauty parlors, but physicians usually recommend cleanliness and stimulation of the scalp to make the oil glands function more normally. Dry hair may be treated by applying small amounts of oil to the hair and scalp. With age the sebaceous glands become less active, and the hair does not require as many shampoos.

No matter how medical workers regard *hair dyeing,* they should be accurately informed on its hazards. The basis of penetrating dyes, according to A. J. Reiches,[46] is *p*-phenylenediamine, "a potent skin sensitizer." He says that while there are surprisingly few cases of skin irritation due to hair dye reported, dye should be used with caution. He recommends making a patch test behind the ear 24 to 48 hours before each dyeing.

The body surface, including the scalp, is constantly shedding dead cells. Exfoliation is rarely noticeable on the body, but when the hair is neglected these cells produce a granular "scurf," or scale, which is caught and held by the unwashed, unbrushed hair. Agnes F. Savill[47] and Behrman in their respective monographs on the hair and scalp say this condition should not be confused with *dandruff,* which is a common but abnormal condition.

Pityriasis capitis is the medical term for dandruff. There are various types according to the appearance of the scale and scalp, as well as the organisms found. Pityriasis may occur alone or in conjunction with other scalp and skin diseases. It is often confused with other scaly eruptions.

Pityriasis simplex is believed to be caused by the *Pityrosporum*. This has been described as a bottle-shaped bacillus, but Savill says it is now classed under the group of *Monilia* or yeast organisms. This condition responds readily to treatment but tends to recur. It is rarely seen before puberty. Behrman thinks it is highly transmissible; Savill does not so regard it. She believes that many persons are immune to attack by the bottle bacillus. If this disease is neglected, a more stubborn form of infection follows in which the sebaceous glands appear irritated and hyperactive. This is known as *pityriasis steatoides,* sometimes less correctly called seborrheic dermatitis, of the simple type. A second organism, the *Micrococcus cutis communis,* or *morococcus,* is associated with the *Pityrosporum* in this oily dandruff. Severer forms of pityriasis may be associated with staphylococcal or streptococcal infections, or with an "eczematized form of seborrheic dermatitis."

All authorities consulted believe that good hygiene plays an important role in the prevention and cure of any pityriasis. When treated early a complete cure can be effected; in many cases persons susceptible to dandruff must maintain a vigilant hygienic program and use antiseptic lotions or salves at regular intervals. Behrman places more emphasis on the etiological part played by the endocrines than does Savill, but both recognize their relationship to this and other scalp disorders. Some dermatologists believe that the causative organisms are residents of the normal scalp and only cause trouble when conditions are especially favorable to their growth; Savill questions this theory. Behrman says that with visits to barber shops and beauty parlors, where disinfecting methods are almost never lethal to causative organisms, infection is almost inescapable.

Pityriasis is a disease that should be treated by a physician. Massage and thorough brushing several times a day are generally advocated. Shampoos every two or three days may be prescribed.

Savill says:

Innumerable are the combinations of drugs and the forms of spirit [alcohol] which have been recommended for pityriases. . . . The majority of these formulae are based on sulphur, tar and mercury, or phenol and salicylic acid, with spirit and water, together with an amount of oil or glycerine which has to be varied for the individual case. Only experience can teach the correct proportion of oil and spirits suitable for the individual scalp.*

She gives several formulas, and suggests frequency and method of application. The value of adequate diet, daily massage, and brushing and exposure of the scalp to air and sunlight are stressed. Hats and caps, which exclude light and air, should be worn as seldom as possible, until the condition is controlled; sunlight is beneficial.

The cause of *baldness* (idiopathic alopecia) is unknown. Its relation to pityriasis, or any other scalp disease, is not established although falling head hair may be associated with any severe scalp affection and it often follows a febrile disease. The quality, quantity, and placement of head and body hair are undoubtedly affected by the activity of the endocrine glands. The Committee on Cosmetics of the American Medical Association[48] cites the fact that "eunochoid and male castrates" do not develop baldness as evidence of the endocrine factor. The committee does not, however, suggest that endocrine therapy can or should be used to promote the growth of head hair, while admitting its value, in the hands of experts, as treatment for hirsutism and other conditions associated with abnormal personality

* Savill, Agnes F.: *The Hair and the Scalp.* Williams & Wilkins Co.. Baltimore. 1952. p. 169.

development. Men, who are far more susceptible to baldness than women, should follow the established methods of promoting healthy hair, and before using any "tonic" or "cure" for baldness should investigate its claims.

Shampoo preparations are usually liquid because such detergents are more easily rinsed from the hair than pastes or solids. Neutral detergents, such as the sulfonated ethers, are largely replacing liquid soaps. Potassium oleates (liquid soaps) are more expensive than sodium oleates (solid soaps), and where cost is important soap jellies and solutions can easily be made from flakes of sodium soap. Use of an acid, such as vinegar or lemon juice, in one of the rinsings helps to remove soap and possibly to improve the texture of hair.

Stiff bristles are recommended for *hairbrushes*. Nylon bristles are stiff, durable, and cheap; hair from the Australian boar makes excellent but costly brushes. Wire brushes are unyielding and tend to scratch the scalp. If tufts of bristles are set far apart, the brush is more readily cleaned. Public health regulations require manufacturers to sterilize all brushes to control transmission of disease, particularly anthrax from infected natural bristles.

Combs are usually made from plastics, hard rubber, or tortoise shell; occasionally from metal and pressed paper. Teeth should be dull so as not to scratch the scalp. Metal combs are likely to be injurious, and their use is discouraged in spite of their being unbreakable and resistant to sterilizing temperatures. Pressed-paper combs are very inexpensive and fairly satisfactory for brief use.

When more than one person uses a comb or brush, sterilization is essential to prevent possible spread of disease. In some hospitals when a patient has failed to provide himself with toilet articles, the institution supplies them and puts the cost on his expense account; in others the comb or brush remains the property of the institution, and is cleaned and sterilized after the patient is discharged. This process usually consists of washing in soapsuds containing a small amount of sodium borate (borax) or ammonium hydroxide and soaking for several hours in an odorless disinfectant, such as diphenyl or mercuric oxycyanide.

Care of the Hair in Sickness. Some illnesses demand such complete rest that a certain amount of neglect of the hair is inevitable, but in most cases it is possible to keep it in good condition. Generally, hair and scalp should receive the same treatment in sickness as in health. The hair should be brushed and combed twice a day and washed every few weeks or even weekly. A shampoo can be given to a bed patient with almost no exertion on his part, and the consequent improvement in appearance is cheering to a man, woman, or child.

In rare cases a regular shampoo requires too much exertion on the part of the patient; in such cases a "dry shampoo" may not. Dry shampoos are actually liquid dry cleaners but because they have alcohol or carbon tetrachloride as their solvent, instead of water, they evaporate rapidly and leave the hair and scalp dry in no time. The shampoo is applied to the scalp and hair with a large piece of cotton or gauze sponge. Hair oil, dissolved in the shampoo, is then removed with towels following the sponging. The scalp and hair should be treated in sections. Behrman says that repeated usage of dry shampoos may irritate the scalp and there may be toxic effects from inhaling the fumes. He recommends dry shampoos for "infrequent use only in special instances."*

Combing and brushing short hair presents no special difficulties, but during an illness that confines the patient to bed, care of long, heavy hair requires time and skill. Hair must be kept free from snarls, combed and brushed without hurting or irritating the patient, and should be arranged in a comfortable but becoming fashion. Appearance should always be considered; even when the patient seems indifferent to his looks, they affect the spirits of his family and friends.

Long hair is ordinarily parted down the middle of the scalp and plaited in two braids. They should not be very tight and should be started toward the front so that a patient lying on her back will not be conscious of them. Some patients like the braids pinned into a coronet; others prefer to have the unbraided hair tucked up on top; few are sufficiently vain to be willing to lie on hairpins; so even when the hair is ordinarily worn in a knot at the back, bed patients seldom want it arranged this way. Plaiting the hair keeps it neat and free from tangles, but the nurse should avoid seeming arbitrary about this detail of the toilet. Women are seldom indifferent to the arrangement of their hair, although they may hesitate to admit their distaste at seeing it slicked down and put into uncompromising braids.

In combing or brushing matted hair tackle it in small strands (see Fig. 59B). To prevent pulling and further tangling, hold the strand slack between the scalp and the part being combed so that the pull comes on the nurse's hand, not on the hair roots, and comb the tangles out progressively from the ends to the scalp. Comb gently but thoroughly. When the hair is so snarled, that it is impossible to disentangle it painlessly, it may be best to cut out the tangled parts. Applying oil or wetting the hair with alcohol as it is combed helps to remove tangles, but time and patience are also needed. Hair never mats when properly combed each day.

Braided hair should be held at the ends with ribbon, or if this is not available, with tape or rubber bands. Use of hair combings for this purpose is obviously unpleasant and would not be mentioned but that the practice is sometimes seen.

Washing the Hair of a Patient in Bed.   A shampoo may be given with the patient either sitting or recumbent if the proper equipment is available. Figures 63, 64, 65 and 66 illustrate how the hair may be washed in these positions and the use of three kinds of troughs for carrying off the cleaning agents.

The metal trough is the type seen in hairdressing parlors. It has a metal rod to hold it in position. In Figure 63 the rod is inserted between the end of the mattress and the footboard; in Figure 64 the rod is placed between the mattress and the patient's pillow. The pressure of the body against the rod holds it in place.

In Figure 63 the shampoo is being given in a treatment room. The patient has been placed so that the head is at the foot of the bed and the trough drains into a sink. The hose is attached to the water supply controlled by a pedal. If there is running water in the patient's unit, the shampoo may be given there, using this method. Of the two positions the recumbent is probably more comfortable, but

* Behrman, Howard T.: *The Scalp in Health and Disease.* C. V. Mosby Co., St. Louis, 1952, p. 128.

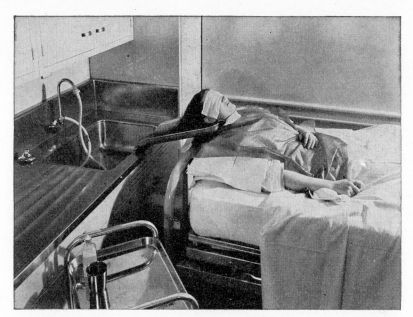

Figure 63. Shampoo in bed, using a metal trough and hose attached to faucet.

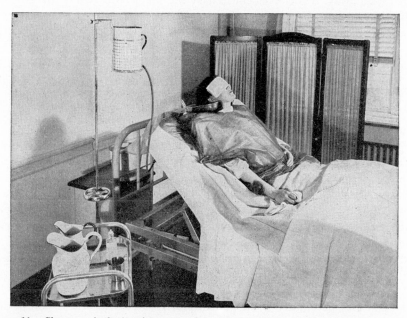

Figure 64. Shampoo in bed, using a metal trough to which a rubber sheet is attached that carries the water into a bucket on a table at the back of the bed. Water is delivered from an irrigator by means of a rubber hose and sprinkling nozzle.

there are some patients, for example, those suffering from certain types of heart disease or asthma, whose breathing is embarrassed except when the head and chest are elevated.

If a metal trough is not available, a Kelly pad may be used, or better still a trough made by rolling bath towels in the two edges of a rubber sheet or piece of oilcloth (see Figs. 65 and 66). The rubber sheet or oilcloth is more easily cleaned, and the method more adaptable to home nursing, since Kelly pads are not available except in institutions.

No matter what the trough is made of, it must be so arranged as to carry the water from the head. If this is done and the pillow and shoulders covered with a waterproof material, the patient's clothing and bedding need not even be dampened. To make the rubber trough drain properly, a very gradual incline should be built at the head of the bed so that it slants toward one side. It is well to place a board or ordinary tray under the top pillow on which the head rests in order to keep it from sinking into the pillows. While the trough should slope toward the edge, the patient must not have the sensation of falling out of bed. A small pillow under the shoulders will keep the body more or less straight while the head is on an incline.

An ample supply of water must be provided; otherwise the soap will not be entirely rinsed away. It is convenient to have the water flow from a nozzle, attached to a faucet where there is running water or to a large irrigating can. If pitchers are used, large ones should be provided for the general supply and a smaller one from which to pour. The soap solution or its substitute should be brought to the bedside in a convenient container. Any pure liquid soap may be used in strengths from 2 to 10 per cent. Liquids prescribed for treatment of the scalp should be applied with an eye dropper or a small syringe. All articles needed should be at the bedside before the shampoo is started so that it will consume no more time than necessary. A movable table or cart facilitates the nurse's work.

To get the hair clean, it is necessary to produce a good lather and rinse it off two or three times. If the oil of the hair is not thoroughly emulsified, it tends to hold the soap in the hair and makes its removal difficult. An unsatisfactory shampoo is in most cases the result of using too little soap. Massaging the scalp thoroughly with the balls of the fingers adds to the comfort and effectiveness of the shampoo.

If the juice of a lemon or an ounce of vinegar is used as a rinse, it should be applied in about 1000 cc (1 qt) of water before the last clear rinsing. The water used throughout should be comfortably warm. Rinsing with cool water at the end of the procedure is not necessary but may be done if the patient likes it. A wet cloth over the eyes gives reassuring protection from soap or drippings but is not essential and may be omitted if the patient prefers. Nonabsorbent cotton in the external orifice of the ear protects it from water, but a skillful operator can prevent the need for it.

At the completion of the shampoo, the trough is removed and the hair spread out on a bath towel over a rubber-covered pillow. The hair should be dried immediately by rubbing with towels, by warm air from an electric drier, or by

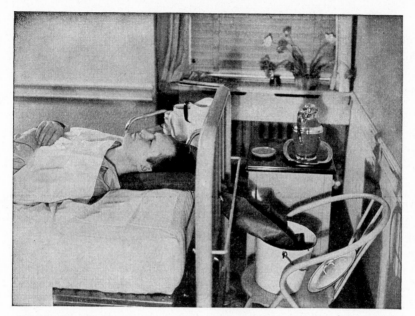

Figure 65. Showing the use of a Kelly pad in giving a shampoo in bed.

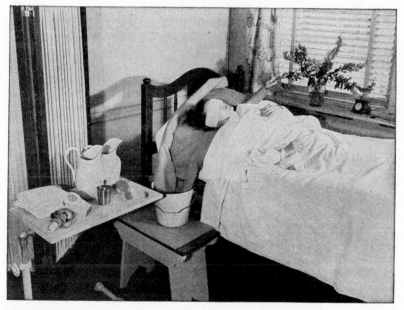

Figure 66. A trough made of rubber sheeting which drains into the bucket because the trough is placed on a slight incline. The incline is made with pillows.

a carefully regulated Thermolite (a lamp with a high-powered bulb). The room should be warm and free from drafts throughout the procedure to avoid the possibility of chilling the patient. Some hospitals have hairdressing departments, and patients are encouraged to use them or employ the personnel who will come to the patient. When patients are very sick, the nurse should assume responsibility for the shampoo, giving it herself or working with the technician.

Treatment for pediculosis is discussed in Chapter 5 (see p. 151).

8. MAKING THE PATIENT'S BED

In making a bed with the patient in it, observe the following principles: Screen the patient and allow no unnecessary exposure or drafts. Have everything at hand before beginning. Remove the upper clothing except one blanket—a patient should never be left without a blanket except in hot weather. Fold the spread, and place all the clothing on chairs to air; do not allow them to touch the floor. Remove the pillows also unless this is uncomfortable for the patient. One pillow may be left. Their removal provides a change of position, usually restful to the patient; it allows the pillows to cool and makes it easier for the patient to turn and the nurse to work. Loosen the lower bed linen. Shake out all crumbs from the patient's gown or change it if damp or soiled. Remove the rubber sheet and muslin drawsheet and allow them to air. Brush all crumbs from the lower sheet or change if necessary. Move the patient from one side of the bed to the other as occasion demands and his condition permits. Straighten the mattress and tighten or replace the under sheet. Replace the rubber sheet and muslin drawsheet or substitute a clean one. See that they are tight and smooth and in the proper position. Shake, turn, and replace pillows and upper bedclothes; be sure the latter are loose over the feet. This can be accomplished by having the patient keep his knees flexed while the sheet and blankets are tucked at the foot or by making a horizontal or vertical pleat over the toes (see Fig. 11D). Remove all articles used in the toilet, and see that the bed, table, and other furnishings of the unit are in order and that the whole has a finished appearance.

REFERENCES

1. Nightingale, Florence: *Notes on Nursing: What It Is and What It Is Not* (facsimile of 1859 ed.). J. B. Lippincott Co., Philadelphia, 1946, p. 6.
2. Kline, Paul R.: "Role of Parenteral Multivitamin Therapy in the Treatment of Acne," *Arch. Dermat. & Syph.,* **62:**661, (Nov.) 1950.
3. Savitt, Leonard E., and Obermayer, Maximilian E.: "Treatment of Acne Vulgaris and Senile Keratoses with Vitamin A: Results of a Clinical Experiment," *J. Invest. Dermat.,* **14:**283, (Feb.) 1950.
4. Ferguson, Bruce C., et al.: "Cortisone and Corticotropin in the Treatment of Diseases of the Skin," *Arch. Dermat. & Syph.,* **65:**535, (May) 1952.
5. Shapiro, Irving: "Estrogens by Local Application in the Treatment of Acne Vulgaris," *Arch. Dermat. & Syph.,* **63:**224, (Feb.) 1951.

6. Wrong, Norman W.: "Treatment of Acne with Sulphur Lotion," *Brit. J. Dermat.,* **62:**491, (Dec.) 1950.

7. Moynahan, E. J.: "Some Recent Advances in the Treatment of Skin Diseases," *M. Press,* **225:**187, (Feb.) 1951.

8. Ormsby, O. S.: "Skin Problems of the Aged," *J.A.M.A.,* **135:**831, (Dec.) 1947.

9. Hollander, Lester: "Care of the Skin in Older People," *Am. J. Nursing,* **47:**219, (Apr.) 1947.

10. Owen, J. R.: "Skin Diseases of the Aged," *M. Press,* **225:**178, (Feb.) 1951.

11. Rosenthal, Theodore: "Personal Cleanliness: A Basic Problem in Hygiene and Public Health," *M. Times,* **78:**497, (Nov.) 1950.

12. Arnold, Lloyd, et al.: "The Self-Disinfecting Power of the Skin as a Defense against Microbic Invasion," *Am. J. Hyg.,* **11:**345, (Mar.) 1930.

13. May, Richard: "The Medical Hazards of Bathing," *Practitioner,* **164:**545, (June) 1950.

14. Carlson, Anton J., and Johnson, Victor E.: *The Machinery of the Body,* 3rd ed. University of Chicago Press, Chicago, 1948, p. 358.

15. Hazen, H. H.: "Cosmetics," *Am. J. Nursing,* **38:**791, (July) 1938.

16. Solomon, Charles: *The Traffic in Health.* Navarre Publishing Co., Inc., New York, 1937.

17. Phillips, Mary C.: *More Than Skin Deep.* Richard R. Smith Publisher, Inc., New York, 1948.

18. Seldin, Joseph J.: "Chlorophyll: Fact or Fraud," *The Nation,* **175:**11, (July) 1952.

19. Combes, Frank C.: "Chlorophyll in Topical Therapy," *New York State J. Med.,* **52:**1025, (Apr.) 1952.

20. Westcott, F. H.: "Oral Chlorophyll Fractions for Body and Health Deodorization," *New York State J. Med.,* **50:**698, (Mar.) 1950.

21. Guild, B. Thurber: "Cutaneous Detergents: Experience with an Ether Sulfonate Compound," *Arch. Dermat. & Syph.,* **51:**391, (June) 1945.

22. Hudson, A. L.: "The H-ion Concentration of Normal and Diseased Skin," *Canad. M. A. J.,* **64:**19, (June) 1951.

23. Shallow, Harold: "Dermatitis from Use of Dry Shaves," *J.A.M.A.,* **110:**1748, (May) 1938.

24. Hollander, Lester, and Casselman, E. T.: "Factors Involved in Good Shaving," *J.A.M.A.,* **109:**95, (July) 1937.

25. Eastman, Nicholson (ed.): *Williams' Obstetrics,* 10th ed. Appleton-Century-Crofts, Inc., New York, 1950, p. 470.

26. Benz, Gladys S.: *Pediatric Nursing.* C. V. Mosby Co., St. Louis, 1948, p. 54.

27. Fishbein, Morris L. (ed.): *Medical Uses of Soap: A Symposium.* J. B. Lippincott Co., Philadelphia, 1945, p. 119.

28. Richardson, Henry B.: *Patients Have Families.* Commonwealth Fund, New York, 1945, p. 30.

29. Bunting, Russell W., et al.: *A Textbook of Oral Hygiene.* Lea & Febiger, Philadelphia, 1950.

30. Toverad, Gullorm: "Decrease in Caries Reported by England, Norway, and Italy," *J. Am. Dent. A.,* **39:**127, (Aug.) 1949.

31. Knutson, John W.: "The Nationwide Topical Fluoride Demonstration Program," *J. Am. Dent. A.,* **39:**438, (Oct.) 1949.

32. United States Public Health Service: *Better Health for 5 to 14 Cents a Year Through Fluorinated Water.* US Government Printing Office, Washington, D. C., 1951.

33. Robinson, Hamilton B. G.: "The Metabolism of Minerals and Vitamins and the Effect of Systemic Conditions on Dental Caries," *J. Am. Dent. A.,* **39:**51, (July) 1949.

34. Allington, Herman: "Dryness of the Mouth," *Arch. Dermat. & Syph.,* **62:**829, (Dec.) 1950.

35. Bolton, William: "That's a Good Question," *Today's Health,* **30:**2, (May) 1952.

36. "Tooth Paste and Powder; Ratings of 93 Brands, . . ." *Consumer Reports,* **14:**346, (Aug.) 1949.

37. Fones, Alfred C. (ed.): *Mouth Hygienists, A Textbook for Dental Hygienists,* 4th ed. Lea & Febiger, Philadelphia, 1934.
38. Schneider, Louis: "Pulmonary Hazard of the Ingestion of Mineral Oil in the Apparently Healthy Adult," *New England J. Med.,* **240:**284, (Feb.) 1949.
39. Rossier, P. H., and Bühlman, A.: "Oil Pneumonia after Use of Liquid Paraffin as Nose Drops over a Period of Years" (trans.), *Schweizerische medizinische Wochenschrift,* **79:**685, (July) 1949.
40. Goodsell, J. Orton, and Roper, R. E.: "The Place of Dental Care in the General Hospital," *Hospitals,* **25:**62, (Jan.) 1951.
41. Fox, Sidney A.: *Your Eyes.* Alfred A. Knopf, New York, 1944, p. 148.
42. Adler, Francis: *Gifford's Textbook of Opthalmology,* 4th ed. W. B. Saunders Co., Philadelphia, 1948, p. 439.
43. Perera, Charles A.: *May's Manual of the Diseases of the Eye,* 20th ed. Williams & Wilkins Co., Baltimore, 1947, p. 100.
44. Hazen, H. H., and Biase, Florence: "The Care of the Hair," *Am. J. Nursing,* **33:**123, (Feb.) 1933.
45. Behrman, Howard T.: *The Scalp in Health and Disease.* C. V. Mosby Co., St. Louis, 1952, p. 125.
46. Reiches, A. J.: "Skin Reaction to Hair Dyes," *Arch. Dermat. & Syph.,* **65:**619, (May) 1952.
47. Savill, Agnes F.: *The Hair and the Scalp,* 4th ed. Williams & Wilkins Co., Baltimore, 1952, p. 169.
48. American Medical Association, Committee on Cosmetics: "Hair and Scalp Treatments and Preparations, A Report of the Committee," *J.A.M.A.,* **139:**840, (Mar.) 1949.

Additional Suggested Reading

American Medical Association, Committee on Cosmetics: "Hair Dyes," *Hygeia,* **27:**318, (May) 1949.

Andrews, George C.: *Diseases of the Skin for Practitioners and Students,* 3rd ed. W. B. Saunders Co., Philadelphia, 1946.

Becker, Samuel W., and Obermayer, Maximilian: *Modern Dermatology and Syphilology.* J. B. Lippincott Co., Philadelphia, 1947.

Berens, Conrad (ed.): *The Eye and Its Diseases,* 2nd ed. W. B. Saunders Co., Philadelphia, 1949.

Bourne, T. I. H. J.: "Personal Hygiene and the Spread of Disease," *Lancet,* **1:**233, (Jan.) 1951.

Brain, R. T.: "Care of Skin in Newborn," *Practitioner,* **164:**45, (Jan.) 1950.

Brocklehurst, John C.: "An Assessment of Chlorophyl as a Deodorant," *Brit. M. J.,* p. 541, (Mar.) 1953.

Cady, F. C., and Knutson, J. W.: *Good Teeth.* US Public Health Service, Federal Security Agency, Washington, D.C., 1948.

Caro, Marcus R., and Szymanski, Frederick J.: "Seborrheic and Senile Keratoses," *M. Clin. North America,* **35:**419, (Mar.) 1951.

Cleveland, D. E.: "Psychogenic Aspect of Dermatologic Therapy," *Canad. M. A. J.,* **62:**122, (Feb.) 1950.

Conley, Veronica Lucey: "Deodorants," *Today's Health,* **29:**31, (Mar.) 1951.

Diehl, Harold S.: *Textbook of Healthful Living,* 4th ed. McGraw-Hill Book Co., New York, 1950.

Fabricant, Noah D.: *Modern Medication of the Ears, Nose and Throat.* Grune & Stratton, Inc., New York, 1951.

Fulton, John T.: *Experiment in Dental Care: Results of New Zealand's Use of School Dental Nurses.* World Health Organization, Columbia University Press, New York, 1951.

Garn, Stanley M.: "Hair Texture: Its Examination, Evaluation and Measurement," *Am. J. Phys. Anthropol.,* **8:**453, (Dec.) 1950.

Guy, W. B.: "Protein Deficiency in Cutaneous Disease," *Arch. Dermat. & Syph.*, **61**:261, (Feb.) 1950.

Henschel, Chester J., and Lieber, Leon: "Caries Incidence Reduction by Unsupervised Use of 27.5 Per Cent Ammonium Therapy Dentifrice," *J. Dent. Research,* **27**:714, (June) 1948.

Hirschfeld, Isador: *The Toothbrush: Its Use and Abuse.* Dental Items of Interest Publishing Co., Brooklyn, 1939.

Kesel, Robert G.: "An Appraisal of Various Methods for Caries Control," *Oral Surg. and Oral Path.,* **2**:670, (May) 1949.

Lerrigo, Marion O.: "Guard Those Baby Teeth," *Today's Health,* **30**:32, (Feb.) 1952.

Little, Robert P.: "What You Can Do about Acne," *Today's Health,* **30**:26, (May) 1952.

MacKenna, Robert M. B.: *Diseases of the Skin: A Manual for Students and Practitioners,* 5th ed. Williams & Wilkins Co., Baltimore, 1952.

Miller, Samuel C. (ed.): *Textbook of Periodontia,* 3rd ed. Blakiston Co., Philadelphia, 1950.

Ormsby, Oliver S., and Montgomery, Hamilton: *Diseases of the Skin,* 7th ed. Lea & Febiger, Philadelphia, 1948.

Pelton, Walter T., and Wisan, Jacob M. (eds.): *Dentistry in Public Health.* W. B. Saunders Co., Philadelphia, 1949.

Prince, J. H.: *Recent Advances in Ocular Prostheses.* Williams & Wilkins Co., Baltimore, 1950.

Reilly, Margaret G.: "Juvenile Acne," *Am. J. Nursing,* **50**:269, (Feb.) 1950.

Schwartz, Louis, et al.: *Occupational Diseases of the Skin,* 2nd ed. Lea & Febiger, Philadelphia, 1947.

Stokes, John H., and Taylor, Jane B.: *Dermatology and Venereology for Nurses.* W. B. Saunders Co., Philadelphia, 1948.

Stroud, Howard J., and Bramback, Clarence L.: "A Dental Health Program for Your Community," *Am. J. Pub. Health,* **40**:1423, (Nov.) 1950.

Sulzberger, Marion B., and Baer, Rudolf L. (eds.): *The Year Book of Dermatology and Syphilology.* Year Book Publishers, Chicago, 1952.

Thoma, Kurt H.: *Oral and Dental Diagnoses and Suggestions for Treatment.* 3rd ed. W. B. Saunders Co., Philadelphia, 1949.

Trotter, Mildred, and Duggins, Oliver H.: "Age Changes in Head Hair from Birth to Maturity," *Am. J. Phys. Anthropol.,* **8**:467, (Dec.) 1950.

Tylman, Standley D., et al. (eds.): *The Year Book of Dentistry.* Year Book Publishers, Chicago, 1952.

Volker, J. F.: "Caries Can Be Prevented," *Am. J. Nursing,* **50**:97, (Feb.) 1950.

Williams, Jesse F.: *Personal Hygiene Applied.* W. B. Saunders Co., Philadelphia, 1950.

CHAPTER 13. NUTRITIONAL NEEDS AND METHODS OF FEEDING

1. NUTRITION AND THE QUALITY OF LIFE

While devastating wars have overshadowed this century, and the development of laborsaving machines is its most obvious achievement, history may attach more importance to twentieth-century discoveries on the nature and needs of man himself. Of these none is more tangible nor more far reaching in effect than those of the physiological chemist in the field of nutrition. We know that human beings, like animals, can by what we call instinct select edible materials from their environment. By and large, superior individuals have always chosen their diet more wisely than inferior men, their parents' wise choice of foods being largely responsible for their superiority. In all previous centuries, however, man had little help in food selection except his cravings and the empiric wisdom of his elders.* Civilized man has lost much of this ability to recognize "hidden hungers," or food cravings, but a literate society can, if economically able, select a diet that will increase the average height, motor power, and capacity for intellectual achievement. Such a diet will at the same time eliminate scurvy, beriberi, pellagra, rickets, and a host of diseases not so generally recognized as nutritional deficiencies, which scourged all the societies of the past and still take heavy tolls. The food chemist of today can provide us with proof, lacking in the past, because he has watched the effect of controlled diets on hundreds of generations of small mammals whose behavior is in

* Josué de Castro contends that hunger is a "man-made plague," that it is the cause, not the result, of overpopulation and that many societies considered "primitive" have selected a varied and complete diet, producing a healthy people living in a balanced economy. (*The Geography of Hunger*, Little, Brown and Co., Boston, 1952.)

many respects comparable to that of persons. Scientific feeding of livestock and dietary studies made on human volunteers have added to our store of knowledge.

With increased communication between nations and literacy within, there is a growing realization that a large majority of the human race is underfed in quantity and quality. Hungry people who see and read about the more fortunate are not so willing to accept hunger philosophically as those who live unaware of the well-fed. Present even more than past governments will prosper or fall according to their ability to improve the national diet. Many students of the international scene maintain that peace depends upon recognition of this fact, the distribution of food and the dissemination of knowledge of how to produce and use it to optimum advantage. Texts such as Josué de Castro's *The Geography of Hunger*[1] and Stringfellow Barr's *Citizens of the World*[2] develop this theme. Julian S. Huxley's *On Living in a Revolution*[3] discusses the changing emphasis from the era of "economic man" to the future era of "social man." In *Our Plundered Planet*[4] Fairfield Osborn shows the necessity of conserving the land while raising the standard of living. If enough good food is to be produced, there must be what has been referred to as "a marriage of agriculture and health." Some might say there must be also a "marriage of nutrition and politics"—national and international.

Experiments with laboratory animals and livestock suggest that improvement of diet offers unlimited possibility for increasing the average life span and, more important, the quality of human life.* Titles such as *We Are What We Eat*[5] and *Climate Makes the Man*[6] (because climate affects his food) are the layman's attempts to popularize the findings of scientists. National governments through their Ministries of Health have extensive educational programs in nutrition. Many countries have improved the average diet by requiring food producers to enrich bread, milk, margarine, and other staples. Diet has been varied by better methods of preserving and distributing foods. In the United States, the Department of Agriculture and the Public Health Service through its various bureaus give educa-

---

* Josué de Castro says: "There is no doubt whatever that the low stature of tropical peoples is not a racial characteristic, but is the result of defective diet that is insufficient in protein. The average Chinese weighs 121 pounds and the average European 139, a difference due to hunger rather than to race. . . .

"On the Shetland Islands . . . grew the smallest horses in the world, hardly more than toys for children. It used to be thought that these Shetland ponies constituted a separate race of horses, stabilized by inbreeding. . . . The fact is, there are no separate races of ponies. Shetland ponies are descendents of English horses. . . ; the extreme proverty of the northern soil in certain minerals, and the consequent poverty of the pastures, led to a progressive deterioration of the species. Even after hundreds of generations, when the ponies were taken to areas with richer soil they regained the characteristics of their ancestors.

"Exactly the same sort of phenomenon takes place with certain human groups. The Chinese and Japanese may be considered 'human ponies,' their height and weight reduced by chronic malnutrition; . . . individuals of these races, emigrating to the United States, take only two generations to produce descendants with a significant increase of several inches in height. . . . The Pygmies of Equatorial Africa lose their Pygmy characteristics when transplanted to the plain's regions where agriculture and cattle raising provide much more varied alimentary resources than their . . . limited diet of wild products of the rain forest. Thus the so-called 'inferior races' turn out to be starved races; properly nourished, they are in all respects equal to the would-be superior races." (*Op. cit.*, pp. 38, 64, 65.)

tional and consultant services to state health departments. Nutritionists are regular members of such departments and are more and more consistently found in public and private agencies offering generalized health services. The Nutrition Foundation and other agencies are engaged in nutrition research, education, or service. Schools and hospitals of any standing in this country must provide specialists in nutrition who can plan and teach optimum dietaries. The effect of public education is seen in the improved use of the food dollar as reported in studies of the US Department of Agriculture over the last fifty years. We are slowly learning to buy the essentials first. For example, in 1942 we spent more than in the first quarter of the century on the following items: milk and cheese, fruits and vegetables. Less was spent on sweets, grains (bread), meat, fish, poultry, and eggs. While some of these differences are undoubtedly the result of wartime scarcities, it is generally believed that the national diet is improving.[7] We are still a long way from Henry C. Sherman and Caroline S. Lanford's recommendation that whatever the level of expenditure:

(1) At least as much should be spent for milk (including cream and cheese if used) as for meats, poultry, and fish; and

(2) At least as much should be spent for fruits and vegetables as for meats, poultry, and fish.*

The US Department of Agriculture in its 1939 Yearbook[8] estimated that 99 per cent of the people born in this country have sufficiently good heredity to enable them to become effective workers and useful citizens, but they conclude that half of them fail to "get enough in the way of dairy products, fruits, and vegetables" to enable them to realize their potential health and vigor.

Present-day food planners and providers have scientific and convenient guides for feeding families and larger groups. Examples are *Helping Families Plan Food Budgets,*[9] *Family Fare: Food Management and Recipes,*[10] both published by the US Department of Agriculture; *Feeding the Family*[11] by Mary S. Rose; *Essentials of Nutrition* by Henry C. Sherman and Caroline S. Lanford; and such specialized publications as *Infant Nutrition*[12] by Philip C. Jeans and William M. Marriott, and *Nutrition in Public Health*[13] by Lucy H. Gillett. Articles in the *Journal of the American Dietetic Association, Nutrition Review, Journal of Nutrition, Nutrition Abstracts Review,* and many other scientific journals provide the most up-to-date and accurate reports on current questions. Much of this information is simplified for general reading and published in popular magazines and texts. These are often reliable guides, but nurses, if they suggest such sources to patients, should use them critically.

Nurses especially should be prepared to choose foods according to the needs of those they serve. Much of the improvement in dietary habits in this and other countries is the result of the work of nurses, particularly "public health nurses." While community nursing services employ nutritionists as consultants, nurses carry the major part of the teaching program.[14, 15]

* Sherman, Henry C., and Lanford, Caroline S.: *Essentials of Nutrition,* 3rd ed. The Macmillan Company, New York, 1951, p. 352.

In hospitals, where diet is a vital part of the therapeutic plan for each patient, the physician prescribes the general nature of the diet, but he depends upon the nurses and dietitians to see that the patient is well fed—in fact, some physicians have, in the writer's opinion, taken too little responsibility for nutrition in health and sickness. Many persons under treatment for vague complaints are simply malnourished; many patients who seem to be making slow progress toward recovery in severe illness are suffering from weeks of incomplete dietaries. Eugene F. DuBois[16] demonstrated many years ago that a typhoid patient with a dietary requirement greater than that of the normal person could, if adequately fed, be brought through a six-weeks' illness with no loss of weight. He admits, however, that feeding a sick man 3000 calories daily requires great nursing skill.

The "good mother" and the "good nurse" must know how to provide for the nutritional needs of those in their care. This includes ensuring appetizing food and providing such assistance in eating as these persons require. Sherman and Lanford, summing up the "nutritional improvement of life," say:

Thus we are now in a new era of nutritional knowledge, in which this knowledge serves the improvement of life in two ways: (1) correctively, in the cure and prevention of deficiency diseases and of the less well recognized states of nutritional shortage or subnormality; and (2) constructively, in the improvement of already-normal health.*

2. DIETARY ESSENTIALS AND THEIR FUNCTIONS

Essentials of Adequate and Optimum Dietaries. Diets are measured quantitatively in terms of calories (see p. 273) and qualitatively according to how well they supply the essential elements: protein, carbohydrate, fat, minerals, and vitamins. Water is of course a most necessary element, but in health its availability is usually taken for granted. The role of each of the nutrients may be discussed separately, but the reader should realize that all are combined in most natural foods. A complete diet is one that provides (1) food fuel, the oxidation of which supplies energy for the varied, unceasing body activities; (2) what is needed for tissue building and upkeep; and (3) materials that regulate body processes of the components from which these regulators are formed. Since all of these processes are essential to life, nature has combined in our foods carbohydrates and fats, which are chiefly fuels; proteins, essential to tissue building and repair; and minerals, vitamins, and water, usually classified as regulators of body processes. Since none of these elements can act independently, such a statement may be a misleading simplification of a complex subject.

Carbohydrates. Sugar and starches are the chief *source* of carbohydrates. They are composed of carbon, hydrogen, and oxygen, the latter elements in the same relationship to each other quantitatively as in water; hence, the name. According to their molecular structure they are classified chemically as monosaccharides, disaccharides, and polysaccharides. All carbohydrates are hydrolyzed in digestion

* Sherman, Henry C., and Lanford, Caroline S.: *op. cit.*, p. 7.

into the monosaccharides or simple sugars, and when oxidized within the cells, their end products are carbon dioxide and water. Glucose, fructose, and galactose are simple sugars that are important nutritionally; sucrose, lactose, and maltose are disaccharides in common use; and starch, glycogen, cellulose, and hemicellulose are polysaccharides that must be hydrolyzed into many simple sugar molecules before they can be utilized by the tissues. Of all foods the simple sugars are most readily utilized; glucose infused into the tissues is available immediately for cell metabolism. Carbohydrate is stored largely in the liver but also in the muscles as the polysaccharide glycogen and is converted by the liver into glucose as needed.

The physiological *function* of carbohydrate is the production of energy. After its conversion by the digestive process into simple sugars, it is oxidized at once within the cells or carried to the liver, converted to glycogen, and stored there, in the muscles, or in traces throughout the body for future use. These processes keep the glucose concentration of the blood virtually constant, or from 0.08 to 0.11 per cent. The glycogen content of the liver fluctuates from 0.2 to 10.0 per cent of its weight in order to preserve this constancy of body fluids.[17] When carbohydrate intake exceeds the immediate needs of the body and its capacity or need for glycogen storage, it is converted into fat—a much more concentrated fuel that the body can accommodate in large quantity. Sherman and Lanford say that while the average adult human body stores only about ⅔ to 1 lb of glycogen in the entire body, a "well nourished individual carries in his body enough fat to serve him as fuel for a month or more."* Those who understand and accept these fundamental principles of carbohydrate metabolism can make two obvious applications to everyday living and medical practice: (1) simple sugars yield an immediate return in terms of energy, and (2) a diet with carbohydrate in excess of actual needs inevitably fattens the body.

Because sugars, starchy roots, and grains are palatable and relatively cheap, there is rarely a question of meeting the *need* for carbohydrate in the diet. Proteins and fats are, on the other hand, relatively costly. Ordinarily, diets should be planned to supply the necessary proteins and fats, leaving the remaining caloric needs to be met by carbohydrate. It is possible to reduce the carbohydrate intake too much. The fact that most natural foods combine fats and proteins with carbohydrates suggests that the metabolism of each is enhanced by the presence of the others. The saying, "Fats burn in carbohydrate fires" is an old warning against the too thorough elimination of starches and sugar from the diabetic diet. Charles H. Best and Norman B. Taylor say, however, that there is strong evidence that this incomplete fat oxidation may result from dysfunction of the liver and that we should keep an open mind on the subject. Some studies indicate that the interchange of potassium between the cells and the intercellular fluid is dependent upon the presence of glucose and that the oxidation of glucose depends upon the presence of potassium. As more is learned about nutrition, a greater number of such dependencies will undoubtedly be established.[18, 19]

When carbohydrate and fat intake is insufficient to supply the body's energy

* Sherman, Henry C., and Lanford, Caroline S.: *op. cit.,* p. 40.

needs, protein foods, and if necessary the tissue proteins, must be drawn upon. This results in wasting, or emaciation. Even when the process does not proceed this far, the utilization of protein as a major source of energy is uneconomical. When enough protein is eaten, the body actually meets the energy needs and stores fat. Carbohydrate can be synthesized from protein, and fats from the resultant carbohydrate. Best and Taylor say, "On an almost exclusively protein diet the fat formed was similar in composition to that synthesized from dietary carbohydrate."*

Fats and Lipids. Cream, butter, fatty meats and fish, and oils from vegetables and nuts are the chief *sources* of food fats and lipids. Fats and lipids are sometimes called lipins and lipoids. A true fat is in chemical nature a triglyceride, almost all of which during digestion is broken down into one glycerol and three fatty acid molecules. According to Best and Taylor, many steps in fat digestion and absorption are subject to debate. It is believed that fatty acids and glycerin pass across the intestinal mucosa and then recombine or combine with bile salts, sodium cations, phosphates, or other elements of the interstitial fluids, including plasma. Some investigators believe that virtually all of the resynthesized fat and fatty compounds find their way into the lymph vessels and are conveyed to the blood stream by the thoracic duct.[20] Blood plasma is reported to contain 0.598 per cent fat or fat-like substance (total lipid, 589 mg; total fatty acid, 353; neutral fat, 154; phospholipid, 196; free cholesterol, 47; and cholesterol ester, 192). These values vary, however, with the diet.[21] Physiological chemists believe that more knowledge of fat metabolism may enable us to control hypertension and other diseases in which unusual blood lipid values are observed. Fat metabolism is dependent upon secretions of the liver and pancreas as well as upon those of the small intestine.

Fats are ultimately oxidized to form carbon dioxide and water. During the process intermediary compounds are formed that are collectively named "ketone bodies." The blood normally contains minute amounts (1 to 3 mg in 100 cc blood or 0.001 to 0.003 per cent). When this value is markedly increased, as it may be in diseases of the pancreas or the thyroid, or when fever or starvation upsets the metabolic balance, "ketosis" or "acidosis" occurs. The blood does not actually become acid because if the pH of arterial blood, which remains remarkably constant around 7.4, rises above 7.8 or drops to 6.8, death occurs. However, the push toward the acid side given by these intermediate products of fat oxidization is dangerous and greatly dreaded.[22]

Lipids are fat-like substances that accompany fats. They are soluble in fat solvents or in fats themselves. Best and Taylor classify them as (1) phospholipids, examples of which are lecithin, cephalin, and sphingomyelin; (2) cerebrosides or glycolipids, to which group belong phrenosin and kerasin; and (3) waxes, important examples of which are the cholesterol esters. Sherman and Lanford classify *sterols* as lipids, but Best and Taylor list them separately, mentioning free cholesterol and ergosterol as examples. They also put the fatty *hydrocarbons,* such as squalene and carotene, into a separate category. In discussion of metabolism studies, blood chemistry, and

---

* Best, Charles H., and Taylor, Norman B.: *The Physiological Basis of Medical Practice* 5th ed. Williams & Wilkins Co., Baltimore, 1950, p. 685.

special diets, nurses will hear reference made to these fat-like substances. Diets are planned in some conditions to control the cholesterol and lecithin content.

Fats vary in character and food value according to their component fatty acids and vitamins. Like carbohydrates, fats are derived from carbon, hydrogen, and oxygen, but there is proportionately less oxygen in the molecule. The oxidation of glucose ($C_6H_{12}O_6$) is accomplished readily, while the oxidation of stearic acid ($C_{18}H_{36}O_2$), derived from the digestion of certain fats, is a far slower and more complex process.

Fats *function* chiefly as a source of energy. Like carbohydrates, they are stored for future use as adipose tissue. As fuel these two dietary elements are largely interchangeable, but some investigators have shown that a fat-free diet retards growth.[23] Cultural diets vary greatly in fat content. Americans consider a diet low in fats unpalatable. Sherman and Lanford say that in our diet and that of Europeans from one fourth to one third the total number of calories is furnished by fat. This means that a person on a 2400 calorie diet eats from 66 gm to 88 gm (roughly 2 to 3 oz) of fat daily. These authorities say that the nutritionally essential fatty acids are widely distributed in common foods and that everyday dietaries probably supply them in sufficient quantity without special planning. It is necessary, however, to supply special vitamin-carrying fats for infants as discussed on page 404.

Because fats are the least easily digested of the food elements and because animal fats, which are more digestible than the vegetable, are costly, many old people, particularly, reduce their fat intake below the optimum point. Lessened activity and a falling metabolic rate reduce the caloric need, and therefore the intake of carbohydrates and fats should be reduced proportionately, but if the reduction is made largely through fats, the diet is dangerously low in fat-soluble vitamins.[24, 25] Dietaries for the very ill are made up of foods quickly and easily digested, which are usually low in fats. Care is taken, however, during this limited period of illness to give vitamin supplements as indicated. The coating of foods by fats, as in frying, is believed to retard contact of the food with digestive secretions. Many dietary items well tolerated in other forms cause distress if so cooked.

Proteins. That element in the diet essential to tissue growth and repair is called protein from the Greek verb *prōteios,* to take first rank. The protein molecule is complex in *nature*. It contains nitrogen and sulfur in addition to carbon, hydrogen, and oxygen and is constructed of building units known as amino acids. According to Best and Taylor, 23 amino acids have been identified, and it is believed that some proteins contain almost all of these, making a very large molecule that can stretch or fold up. Protein is the basis of all living things, animal and vegetable; muscle is almost entirely protein. Some authorities believe that all protein molecules are essentially fibrous but that they vary enormously according to the number and arrangement of the building units, the molecular weight and shape, and chemical behavior.

Animals and plants are the chief *sources* of protein foods, as has been implied. Each animal or plant species is thought to have its chemically distinct protein.

The possible arrangements of the amino acids, or building units, is infinite since a protein molecule may contain a few or most of those known and there may be hundreds of links within the molecular structure. Plants can synthesize or build their characteristic proteins from materials in the soil and air. Animals are dependent upon their food for material with which to build their tissue proteins. They can synthesize some amino acids within their bodies, but others they cannot and are therefore dependent upon protein foods containing the amino acids they must have but cannot synthesize or perhaps cannot synthesize in sufficient quantities. Nutrients containing such tissue-building units are said to contain the indispensable, or nutritionally essential, amino acids.

Sherman and Lanford point out that only a small part of the evidence on the nutritional value of protein is in, but that according to our present knowledge, there are ten dietary amino acids essential to growth: (1) arginine, (2) histidine, (3) isoleucine, (4) leucine, (5) lysine, (6) methionine, (7) phenylalanine, (8) threonine, (9) tryptophane, and (10) valine. Apparently the animal organism cannot synthesize these amino acids from foods lacking them in sufficient quantities to meet the demands for normal growth. In order to maintain "protein balance" within the body, the adult's diet should contain all these amino acids except arginine and histidine. Apparently, he can produce those in sufficient quantity for maintenance needs. Sherman and Lanford classify proteins according to their nutritive value as follows:

(1) "Complete" proteins: those which maintain life and provide for normal growth of the young when used as the sole protein food. Casein [from milk] is the example of a complete protein. . . . [Some] other proteins in this group include lactalbumin of milk; ovalbumin and ovovitellin of eggs; glycinin of soybean; . . . and maize glutenin of the cereal grains.

(2) "Partially incomplete" proteins: those which maintain life but do not support normal growth. . . . gliadin is representative of this group.

(3) "Incomplete" proteins: those which, as sole dietary protein, are incapable of supporting either growth or life. Zein [from corn] clearly belongs to this class, as does also gelatin.*

Fortunately, almost all foods except gelatin contain more than one kind of protein. Animal protein is generally superior to vegetable. Whole milk and eggs take first place; animal tissues are next in importance, liver and kidneys being even more valuable than muscles. Whole grains provide important protein, particularly if fed with a diet containing milk. In the diets of children, pregnant or lactating women, or of emaciated invalids it is especially important to include abundant milk and eggs as sources of body-building proteins.[26, 27]

The *function* of protein is implied in its source. If protein is the chief component of protoplasm, it follows that its function is to build and repair living tissues. Both cells and intercellular substances contain protein; it is found in the complex molecular structure of hormones and other regulators of body activity. A diet

* Sherman, Henry C., and Lanford, Caroline S.: *op. cit.*, p. 94.

that does not supply the protein need affects every aspect of the body economy. It is such a threat to the future of a race or species that, according to some experts, nature responds to inadequate diets, but particularly to those deficient in protein, by increasing fertility. This is not just a theory. It is explained physiologically by studies showing that protein deficiency makes the liver less able to inactivate estrogens; excess estrogen raises the level of fertility in women. De Castro thinks that, while the scientific explanation is only partially available and the information even less widely known and accepted, the relationship between poverty and fecundity has been apparent for centuries. He cites the Latin expression, "The table is meagre, but fertile is the bed of misery," and the meaning of the Roman word for the poor and undernourished—"proletarian," he who has many *proles* or offspring. He goes on to say, "Cattle raisers have long known that animals which get too fat may become sterile and that reduced rations will re-establish fertility."* James R. Slonaker[28] studied 6 generations of rats and found that diets containing more than 18 per cent of the total calories in protein retarded the epoch of fertilization of the females, reduced the number of offspring in the litters and the number of litters. At the same time, the progeny, although fewer in number, showed a higher survival rate and a greater resistance to disease.

While substandard diets, particularly protein hunger, may increase the birth rate, starvation diets would not. The life of the starving individual rather than the continuation of the race is then at stake. He is actually ill, and his energy is concentrated on survival. Sex interest and, in fact, every aspect of the libido wane.[29, 30] In summary, the studies cited suggest the possibility of reducing to some extent the quantity of animal or human life and markedly improving the quality by feeding optimum diets, particularly with respect to protein.

The protein need in sickness is likely to be higher than in health, contrary to general opinion in the not so distant past. Whenever there is a breakdown in tissue, as with ulcers or abscesses, when there is hemorrhage or seepage from wounds and burns, or when fever raises the metabolic rate, dietary protein should exceed the individual's normal intake. Gone for good, we hope, is the once classic invalid's diet of toast and tea, baked potato, and rice with an occasional custard and a little beef extract. Such feeding inevitably led to protein hunger with all its ills and the avitaminoses and mineral deficiencies that almost routinely accompanied protracted illness. There is abundant evidence that healing takes place more rapidly with a high- than with a low-protein diet. This is so generally accepted that even in the critical stage of a self-limited illness, when it may be necessary to feed the patient through the veins, solutions of predigested proteins, whole blood, and plasma are given in sufficient quantities to meet the requirement. Liquid diets include milk, eggs, finely ground meats, poultry, fish or predigested animal protein, and even vegetable proteins according to the special demands of each patient. Protein supplements are used in all sorts of diets. Protenol is an example of such a preparation; sodium-free Lanolac is used in sodium-poor diets. These supplements can be given in orange juice, tomato juice, soup, or milk

* De Castro, Josué: *op. cit.*, p. 70.

(Chocolate-flavored Protenol is more palatable than the plain variety.) From the hundreds of studies published on this subject, a few are included in the references.[31, 32, 33, 34]

The amount and kind of protein required depends upon the immediate tissue needs for growth and repair. It is greater in periods of growth, during pregnancy and lactation, and following periods of malnutrition or diseases characterized by tissue destruction as in carcinoma, infectious diseases (owing to fever and toxins), exophthalmic goiter, and pernicious anemia, in which the cells are always poorly nourished. The amount required *by the adult* for tissue repair is relatively small and constant. The American Medical Association's Council on Foods and Nutrition and the Food and Nutrition Board of the National Research Council recommend the following: 70 gm of protein per day for a healthy man weighing 70 kg or 1 gm of protein for each kilogram of body weight; 60 gm of protein for a woman weighing 56 kg, or slightly more than 1 gm of protein to each kilogram of body weight; for the youth of 17, 2 gm of protein to each kilogram of body weight; and for a child from 1 to 3 years, 4 gm of protein per kilogram of body weight.[35] Some authorities recommend less; others, more than this. In order that about two thirds of this allowance be complete proteins, an adult's daily diet should include one moderate serving of meat, one egg, and two glasses of milk; the remainder may be furnished by cereals and vegetables. For *children* a relatively higher proportion of protein is required (about 15 per cent of the total calories), and at least two thirds of this allowance should be complete (animal) proteins. A quart of milk and an egg daily are advisable, with other foods providing the proper amount and kind of protein.

Physiologists have demonstrated that the body does not store amino acids; on the contrary, it maintains a nitrogen balance by increasing nitrogenous wastes when protein foods are eaten in excess of body needs. When the daily nitrogen intake equals the daily nitrogen output, the body is said to be in *nitrogen balance,* or equilibrium. Because the kidneys bear the brunt of excreting nitrogenous waste, a high-protein diet is believed by some physicians to injure these organs. The fact that Eskimos, who live almost entirely on meat, do not show a high incidence of renal disease has cast doubt on this theory. While 20 gm of protein may keep an adult male weighing 70 kg in nitrogen balance, the consensus is that the quality of life is improved by a higher intake.[36]

An idiosyncrasy to certain proteins is not unusual. For instance, some persons are allergic to eggs; others, to shellfish. Allergy is the term used for this sensitiveness to a food or an inhaled protein. The irritating factor in an article of diet, a pollen, feathers, or hair is believed to be a protein. Diets are restricted when idiosyncrasies are known or suspected, and attempts are usually made to desensitize the patient. Persons with severe food allergies are sometimes fed protein hydrolysates because the hydrolyzing process destroys the specificity of the protein to which the person is susceptible.

Mineral Elements.   Sherman compares the composition of the adult human body and the earth's crust. A study of his table shows that with the exception of the oxygen supplied by respiration the diet must provide most and possibly all of the elements of the earth in varying amounts. Our knowledge of the functions of these elements in the human body is incomplete, and it is not known whether all of them are physiologically significant. It has been established, however, that certain minerals present in minute amounts, such as iodine, are nevertheless essential dietary components. A varied diet of plants and animals grown in most habitable areas yields all the mineral elements. A monotonous diet or one taken from the products of depleted soils can fail to provide many of these minerals in sufficient quantity for optimum health. Pure carbohydrates and fats furnish no minerals, but man is dependent upon the sulfur that enters into the composition of proteins. Proteins also yield phosphorus, iron, and calcium, but, according to some authorities, an adequate supply of all minerals except sulfur can be supplied by other foods.[37] All components of the body are widely distributed in natural foods with the exception of sodium. De Castro says that although there are 13 metalloids and 16 metals always present in living matter, and "man may suffer sporadically from shortages of any or all of the mineral elements that go to make up his tissues, there are only a few whose deficiency may ordinarily be considered of social significance. They are iron, calcium, sodium, and iodine."[*] Diets should, therefore, be planned to include an adequate supply of these elements. Where the drinking water contains a sufficient concentration of iodine its provision is no problem.

Minerals *function* as constituents of rigid and soft tissues, and mineral salts in the body fluids act as regulators. A few of these functions are discussed briefly in the following pages. Nurses should, however, make a far more detailed study of the subject in such texts as those suggested at the end of this chapter.

Calcium is the most abundant mineral in the body; *phosphorus,* an element of every known cell. These two minerals are often considered together. Both function as constituents of hard and soft tissues and as regulators. Combined as calcium phosphate, they are preponderant in bone and tooth structure.

They are both widely distributed in plants; calcium concentrated in the leaves and phosphorus in the seeds, while they are present in equal amounts in roots and stems. Calcium deficiencies are therefore common in animals when leafy foods are eliminated, and phosphorus deficiencies when grains are omitted. Animal foods, including milk, are a rich source of both these minerals, but the meat of grazing livestock may be relatively poor in phosphorus. Sherman and Lanford think that regardless of its wide distribution in nature, "the phosphorus problem of human nutrition" should not be ignored.[†] Since phosphorus enters into the composition of all body tissues, any attempt to list its functions is obviously absurd. Because approximately 90 per cent of the body's phosphorus is in the skeleton, its deficiency, like that of calcium, is most apparent in abnormal bone structure.

Calcium deficiency is often said to be the most frequent and widespread dietary inadequacy. Because it is irregularly distributed in the soil and because its chief

* De Castro, Josué: *op. cit.,* p. 41.
† Sherman, Henry C., and Lanford, Caroline S.: *op. cit.,* p. 122.

sources—milk, egg yolk, and certain vegetables—are limited in supply, and therefore expensive, calcium hunger is one of the "hidden hungers." Length of life is increased and its quality improved by increasing calcium intake, even to surplus amounts.[38]

Infants are born "calcium poor" so that they will be flexible during the act of birth. Small wonder that the infant deprived of calcium or conditions favoring its assimilation develops a misshapen body. The daily recommended allowance of the National Research Council is as follows: 1.0 gm of calcium from infancy through 12 years; 1.4 gm for boys between the ages of 13 and 20; 1.3 gm for girls in this age span; for women who are lactating, 2.0 gm; for women in the latter half of pregnancy, 1.5 gm; and for other women and for men, 1.0 gm. Sherman says in his studies, ". . . optimal retention of phosphorus in the growing children of 3 to 13 years of age was not obtained until the intake reached from 1.16 to 1.46 gm of phosphorus per child per day. . . ."* It is generally agreed that the phosphorus requirement parallels that of calcium and that if the diet is so planned as to meet the calcium need, it will provide the needed phosphorus. Diets meeting such standards will go a long way toward increasing man's vitality and life span and toward preventing rickets in the young and fractures in the elderly. We may come to look upon the bowed legs of infancy and old age as a sign of the same dietary deficiency, although at present we tend to stress the needs of the young and ignore those of the aging.

Iron has such vital functions in the human body that, while the amount needed is small, the provision of an adequate quantity in the diet is essential to health. It enters into the composition of the oxygen-carrying hemoglobin and into the chromatin in the nucleus of every cell. It is therefore necessary for cell respiration, and deficiencies produce anemias with their widespread effects of oxygen want and other depletions. *Copper* enters into the composition of the hemoglobin molecule, but it is thought that most diets provide adequate amounts without special planning.[39] Lean meats are the chief source of iron in the adult diet of most Americans, Europeans, and others. Egg yolks are rich in iron as are certain grains and lentils. While whole fresh milk contains only 0.1 per cent iron as compared with lean beef, which has 3.0 per cent, the iron in milk is especially well assimilated, and therefore milk is valuable as a source. Potatoes, certain fresh vegetables, such as kale, and fruits, such as prunes and raisins, may be selected to meet the present recommended daily allowance of 6 mg during the first year of life, 12 mg for men and women, and 15 mg during adolescence, pregnancy, and lactation.[40] Enrichment of bread with iron has improved the American diet in recent years.

Iodine is essential in human physiology even though the entire body may contain as little as 25 mg. Traces are present in natural waters and plants, but the quantity varies markedly in different geographical areas. The iodine-poor lands are most often inland and mountainous. It is well known that goiter is endemic in such regions. Iodine deficiency decreases the amount of thyroxin secreted by

* Sherman, Henry C.: *Chemistry of Food and Nutrition*. The Macmillan Company, New York, 1946, p. 271.

the thyroid gland, and the gland enlarges in an effort to fulfill its function. Since all vertebrates depend upon a balanced endocrine activity for their normal development and emotional stability, a dietary deficiency that decreases the thyroid secretion has a profound effect. Most readers of this text will have some knowledge of cretinism and myxedema and the results of treatment with thyroxin. Even more important is the prevention of these deficiency diseases. In "goiter" regions there are public health requirements for the reinforcement of table salt (sodium chloride) with one part of sodium or potassium iodide to 5000 or even 200,000 parts of sodium chloride. This is harmful to no one and should be considered a replacement of an element that is normally in the dietary.[41]

Sodium and *chlorine* in the form of sodium chloride are the chief mineral constituents of the extracellular fluids, including the blood and lymph. Although both sodium and chlorine are widely distributed in foods and drink, man and some other vertebrates have developed an apparent need for more sodium chloride than is furnished by natural foods and water. The craving for what we call salt is so great that the people of India recovered it from sea water when, as a political protest against the English, they stopped buying taxed and manufactured products. A porcupine will gnaw through the thickest beams of a house, and buffaloes will travel miles, to lick salt.

In tropical countries where sweating is profuse and an excess of sodium chloride is lost in sweat, an adequate supply of salt is a serious economic and social problem as pointed out in Chapter 5. Because less salt is lost in sweat from the unclothed than the clothed body, natives of hot countries have learned to conserve sodium chloride by baring large skin areas. Fair-skinned Europeans living in the Tropics cannot compete with native laborers because they don't want to conform to this custom and could not tolerate the exposure. Colonizers tend to manage rather than those who labor manually. De Castro says:

> . . . the unavoidable deficiency of one mineral—sodium—played an extremely important role in the exploitation of a large part of the world's surface. There can be no doubt that this specific hunger, ever since the first colonization of tropical areas, has constituted a terrible handicap to these peoples' economic and social progress.*

According to Sherman and Lanford, the adult in our culture tends to eat and excrete "several grams of sodium chloride" a day, the amount varying with the individual's taste. Other authorities put the intake as high as 10 to 15 gm daily.[42] The average person in this country probably eats more salt than he needs under ordinary circumstances and neglects to increase his intake to compensate for losses in sweating. Some physicians believe that a high-sodium intake has some relation to the prevalence of hypertension in this country. William Dock says, "The salt-poor diet and the rice diet may be unappetizing, but they are physiological."† Sherman and Lanford think, however, ". . . most people at most times

* De Castro, Josué: *op. cit.,* p. 49.
† Dock, William: "Use of Sodium Depletion in Therapy," *Advances in Int. Med.,* 4:273, 1950.

may eat their food 'salted to taste' without anxiety in either direction; for the healthy body has power to adjust chloride output to chloride intake throughout a wide range."* Physicians who believe that a high-salt intake contributes toward hypertension would encourage us to salt our foods lightly, or not at all, as we grow older.

Potassium salts predominate in the fluid inside the cell as sodium salts do in the intercellular fluids. Magnesium is found chiefly inside the cells, while the calcium in solution is largely in the intercellular fluid. The constancy of these salts must be maintained to preserve the equalizing osmotic pressures inside and outside the cell wall that preserve the integrity of the cell. This is discussed more fully on page 718. Health depends upon a constancy of these minerals for other reasons. Acting as buffer substances, they preserve the neutrality of body fluids and maintain a normal state of muscle tone and irritability of nerves. Goodman and Gilman have stated that both a deficiency and an excess of calcium ions alter the function of cardiac muscle.[42a] The presence of sodium is essential to muscle contraction, and the normal function of all tissues seems to depend upon the antagonistic action between the substances that stimulate and those that inhibit their activity.

Vegetable foods are rich in potassium, and most diets contain an adequate amount. Magnesium is also adequately supplied by the nuts and grains in ordinary diets. It is now realized that persons fed parenterally must be given potassium as well as sodium salts. It is probably unfortunate that a solution of sodium chloride was ever called "normal" or "physiological" saline. Great advances are to be expected in parenteral therapy as the nutritional value of food elements is established.[43, 44]

Less is known about the functions of manganese, cobalt, and zinc. Although they are accepted as dietary essentials, so little is known about their functions that discussion of them is not believed to be profitable here.

It is not possible even to mention all the important known functions of minerals or to list the conditions attributed to their deficiencies. Perhaps enough has been said to suggest the importance of a varied diet and the danger of investing many calories in pure carbohydrates and pure fats, neither of which supply the essential minerals. Diets containing abundant vegetables, fruit, meat, eggs, and dairy products, unless grown on impoverished land, provide the needed minerals.

Vitamins. Through health education and commercial exploitation the importance of the so-called vitamins is familiar to most of us. Before the chemical nature of any of them was established, it was recognized that there were highly specialized substances in food, the lack of which produced specific disease. Some were believed to be soluble in fatty foods; others, soluble in water; and as knowledge of these increased, they were so designated. By 1920, vitamins A, B, and C were recognized in the science of nutrition. Because they were believed vital to health and in order to unify the rapidly expanding literature, it was proposed that they be called *vitamins*. The name was adopted, and they were divided into *fat-soluble* and *water-soluble* vitamins. Texts usually classify and discuss them under

* Sherman, Henry C., and Lanford, Caroline S.: *op. cit.,* p. 111.

these headings rather than in alphabetical order. (This distinction will disappear as manufacturers convert fat-soluble to water-soluble preparations.)

The term vitamins is so entrenched that the nutritionists now, 35 years later, find it difficult to get the public to adopt names that suggest their chemical nature. British and American terminology differ. Standardization of terminology and dosage is now in progress. Table 7A gives the present nomenclature and important sources for some of the vitamins and conditions resulting from their deficiencies. If the chemical nature of the vitamin is known, it is now possible to discover its concentration in the blood. Physical examinations may include such estimates. The blood level, in some cases also, may be computed from the amount excreted in the urine.[45] Only those vitamins whose function is best understood are discussed in this text. Again, nurses are urged to study nutrition in more specialized works.

Ascorbic acid (vitamin C) affects the body profoundly by entering into oxidation-reduction reactions and the formation and maintenance of intercellular material that keeps the cells in normal relationship to each other. Following its chemical identification in 1932 by Dr. King and his co-workers, the isolation and synthesis of ascorbic acid was accomplished by a number of laboratories. A deficiency of ascorbic acid is associated in the mind of the public with scurvy, and its name is designed to perpetuate this association. It is now thought, however, that a wide range of pathology may result from a very low vitamin C intake. To it one author attributes the following: structural changes in gums, teeth, bones, and cartilage, with displacement of bones, due to weakness of supporting cartilage; anemia, caused by interference with cell-forming bone marrow; degeneration of muscles, including the heart muscle; and even damage of the sex organs. This is not hard to accept when one sees the acute suffering of the person with scurvy and its fatal effect if unchecked. Sherman and Lanford say:

Medical surveys of nutritional status . . . have revealed in different parts of Canada and the United States relatively large proportions of people (especially in the low income groups) who are living at relatively low ascorbic acid levels, which, even if they do not show gross symptoms of scurvy, undoubtedly mean something less than optimal resistance.*

Charles G. King[46] lists among the symptoms of a vitamin C deficiency the decreased capacity to combat infections and to heal wounds.

Vitamin C is widely distributed in foods, but is concentrated in many fruits and vegetables. It is easily destroyed by oxidation, which is accelerated by heat. Ascorbic acid is also destroyed more rapidly in the presence of alkalies. It is recommended that exposure of foods to air and temperature be reduced to a minimum, and that no soda be added in cooking or processing. Most of the ascorbic acid in the American diet is provided by fruits and vegetables. Certain foods known to be rich in ascorbic acid are included in most dietaries, namely: tomatoes, citrus fruits, and cabbage. Young and sprouting vegetables are particularly valuable sources. Canned, frozen, dried, and stored fruits and vegetables have some of their ascorbic

* Sherman, Henry C., and Lanford, Caroline S.: *op. cit.*, p. 177.

acid destroyed, but they are protective if taken in sufficient quantity to compensate for the loss through oxidation. Estimates of the antiscorbutic value of foods are based on the processes to which they have been exposed.

King believes that long-term studies may change the present recommended values. Those given by the Food and Nutrition Board of the National Research Council are as follows: daily intake for children from birth to 12 years, 30 to 75 mg, depending upon their age and/or weight; for children over 12 years, 80 to 100 mg; for a man weighing 70 kg, 75 mg; for women in the latter half of pregnancy, 100 mg; for lactating women, 150 mg; and for all other women, if of average weight, 70 mg.

Vitamin B, accepted as an entity in 1920, has since been broken down into many vitamins with much more specific functions than those attributed to the original. The chemical composition of some but not all members of the B group, or B complex, is known. The isolation of all reported members has not been generally accepted. Walter H. Eddy and Gilbert Dalldorf in 1944 listed nicotinic acid, thiamine, and riboflavin, and as "lesser B vitamins pyridoxine [B_6], pantothenic acid, biotin, choline, inositol, and folic acid. Of these, the latter two have not been shown to be the cause of human disease, and relatively little is known of their morbid effects in other species."* In 1951, C. A. Elvehjem in the *Handbook of Nutrition* of the American Medical Association discussed the ten members of the "vitamin B complex" that have been "obtained in crystalline form," although he says at least a dozen factors are known to exist.† To those listed above he adds para-aminobenzoic acid and vitamin B_{12}. Both texts agree that inositol is not significant in human physiology. In recent years folic acid has proved effective in the treatment of types of macrocytic anemia. Only those members of the B group now thought to be most important are discussed in this text.

Thiamine, thiamine chloride or *hydrochloride* (vitamin B_1), was identified as the factor whose deficiency caused beriberi before it was isolated chemically in 1936 in the laboratory of Dr. R. R. Williams. It was first called vitamin B; recently *aneurin* has been proposed as a name that would suggest its therapeutic claim. While a marked deficiency of thiamine results in a multiple neuritis with cardiac symptoms and edema, its lack is manifested much earlier in a loss of appetite and, in the young, by retarded growth. It is believed to enter into carbohydrate metabolism, which explains its generalized symptoms. Studies with animals and human beings have shown that the capacity for learning and the actual performance in a wide range of skills is improved on an optimum thiamine intake. With a thiamine deficiency there is an abnormal accumulation of lactic and pyruvic acid in the brain. In such conditions the tissue is restored to normal by the administration of vitamin B_1. To what extent psychoses can be attributed to this and other vitamin deficiencies is debatable. Malnourished alcoholics and other cases of

* Eddy, Walter H., and Dalldorf, Gilbert: *The Avitaminoses.* Williams & Wilkins Co., Baltimore, 1944, p. 246.
† Council on Food and Nutrition of the American Medical Association: *Handbook of Nutrition.* Blakiston Co., Philadelphia, 1951, p. 162.

inanition show depression, irritability, insomnia, and hallucinations associated with the more typical neuritis.[47]

Thiamine is widely distributed in animal and vegetable foods. Processes that remove a part of the natural food, such as the polishing of rice or the separation of bran from meal remove a large part, and often most, of the thiamine. The nutritionist's advice to *"eat whole cells"* is particularly applicable here. Egg yolk, meats (especially liver and pork muscle), whole grains and legumes, including peanuts, are especially rich in thiamine. Most vegetables contain a fair amount of vitamin B, and if a total of 2 to 3 lb is eaten daily, they furnish one of the major sources of this vitamin.

Like ascorbic acid, but not to the same extent, thiamine is thermolabile and is more rapidly destroyed in an alkaline medium. Roasting is said to destroy almost half the thiamine present in meats.[48] Both vitamins are water soluble and are therefore partially lost when water in which they are cooked is discarded. Nurses as health teachers should encourage housekeepers to conserve the full value of foods by using cooking water for soups or vegetable "cocktails." In bakery products, vitamins are lost through oxidation in mixing and baking. When refined flours and/or soda is used, the loss is enormous. Public health regulations for the enrichment of flour by the addition of synthesized thiamine have to some extent offset these losses. Authorities, nevertheless, encourage the use of whole-grain products and discourage the use of soda.

The daily adult requirement of thiamine is estimated at from 1.2 to 3.5 mg according to size. This "optimal intake" should, according to Sherman and Lanford, aim at preventing not only beriberi but also the mild neurasthenia typical of this avitaminosis and should furnish a margin of safety for physiological variability of individuals.

Riboflavin (B_2) and *niacin, niacinamide* or *nicotinic acid,* are here considered together because their deficiencies are associated with pellagra and its related symptoms. Riboflavin was synthesized by Kuhn and his co-workers in 1935; pure niacin (nicotinic acid) is prepared in various ways, one being oxidation of nicotine with concentrated nitric acid.

Riboflavin is a heat-stable substance widely distributed in plants and animals. It is believed to be essential to growth and normal nutrition, and for this reason nature concentrates it in eggs and milk to ensure the health of the young. Riboflavin deficiency produces widespread tissue changes, including general weakness, dermatitis, fissures of the lips, and reddened eyes. A long-term deficiency in a culture shortens life, decreases the vitality of the people, and lowers resistance to disease. It is doubtful whether present knowledge of this vitamin enables the nutritionist to assess its value or to provide reliable human requirements. Its deficiency is widespread even in this economically favored country, but particularly among families with low incomes because their consumption of animal protein tends to be low. Some writers suggest that the health improvement noticeable after an increase of animal protein in the diet is due in large part to its riboflavin content. A quart of milk a day or a serving of liver will meet the daily requirement of 1.8 to 2 mg.

Other meats, eggs, and cheese together with wheat germ are valuable sources. Weight by weight, some leafy green vegetables, such as broccoli, kale, and spinach, have about one tenth as much riboflavin as liver and the same concentration as milk. Being economically available to many, they are important sources. Enriched bread must contain specified amounts of riboflavin as well as thiamine, niacin, and iron.[49, 50]

Niacin, or niacinamide (improperly termed nicotinic acid), is a heat-stable substance whose distribution in natural foods somewhat parallels that of riboflavin. While it is highly concentrated in yeast, dietary improvement results from emphasis on palatable and ordinary food in which it is abundant.

Severe niacin deficiency causes pellagra, the disease characterized by the three D's—dermatitis, diarrhea, and dementia. Some writers say four D's and add death. This disease occurs in areas where the land is given over to "cash crops," cotton and tobacco, for example. It is rare among peoples who raise their own food and who can therefore afford variety. Pellagra is cured by including milk, eggs, lean meats, fish, tomatoes, peas, and leafy green vegetables in the diet. In addition to that in foods niacin and riboflavin are usually given to hasten recovery. Niacin is produced within the body by some bacteria. Milk probably encourages the growth of niacin-producing organisms, for pellagra is not found among those children who live largely on milk. Sherman says that figures on the niacin content of food and daily intake standards must still be tentative. The National Research Council has set the daily requirement at ten times that of thiamine, or 12 to 35 mg, according to size. An optimum diet, as has been said, will usually provide an ample supply of this vitamin as a protective.[51]

Vitamin B_{12} is a cobalt-containing substance whose active principle has been named cobalamin. This vitamin has been broken down into several forms, but the effectiveness of all of them in treating pernicious anemia is due to the cobalamin content, and this refined substance is now used instead of the crude-liver extracts given for their B_{12} content. It is effectively given orally or parenterally. Innumerable studies have been made on this nutritional element, and much has been written because it so effectively controls a once fatal and fairly prevalent disease. There is still a great deal to be learned about it. The body apparently synthesizes adequate amounts under most circumstances. In anemias of unknown origin and when antibiotics and sulfa drugs destroy intestinal bacteria involved in synthesis of B_{12}, body stores are depleted. Cobalamin, or B_{12}, is used to combat this dangerous effect of some of the newer therapies. Liver is a rich source of vitamin B_{12}, and many years ago patients with pernicious anemia had to consume it in large quantities before concentrates were developed. While this vitamin is most abundant in animal protein, its presence has been demonstrated in the following vegetable sources: rice polishings, alfalfa, blue grass, and lettuce.[52, 53]

Vitamin B_{14} is another vitamin stimulating red-cell formation, but its value and use are not well established. Biotin belongs to the B vitamin group, but its distribution and function have not been thoroughly investigated.

Water-soluble vitamins, other than the ascorbic acid (C) and the B group, are pteroylglutamate, or PGA (the nutritional factor that has been called vitamin M, vitamin B$_c$, and *folic acid* by various investigators), *pantothenic acid, choline,* and *rutin* or *citrin* (vitamin P). Knowledge of all of these is very incomplete. To what extent they are synthesized within the body and to what extent they must be provided by the diet is undecided. Deficiencies in choline produce liver damage in animals. This information may lead to its clinical use in liver inpairment. Pteroylglutamate is thought to be synthesized by normal animals and human beings in sufficient quantities to maintain normal blood conditions to which its presence is essential. The occurrence of clinical deficiencies has led, however, to the emphasis on its chief sources: namely, highly colored vegetables, liver, white meats, milk, and whole grains. Folic acid itself is used in the treatment of certain anemias and widely used in sprue.[54, 55]

The first fat-soluble vitamin was A, but since 1920 the specificity of *fat-soluble vitamins D, E,* and *K* has been established. These may be further broken down, and the list might be still further enlarged in a full report of vitamin research, which is expanding so rapidly that any account of it is out of date before it can be published.

Vitamin A, found so abundantly in the liver oils of fresh- and salt-water fish, is also found in milk, eggs, and other animal fats. It has not been found in plants, but the yellow vegetables contain precursors, for convenience referred to as "the carotenes," that give rise to vitamin A in the body.

Deficiencies in vitamin A, even though slightly below the optimum intake, are believed to limit growth. The development and maintenance of normal eyes are also closely associated with this vitamin. While stunted growth, xerophthalmia, and night blindness as results of vitamin A deficiency have been repeatedly demonstrated with animal experimentation, authorities give dryness of the skin as the first indication of vitamin A shortage and list genitourinary, respiratory, and reproductive pathology, and lowered resistance to infections as other results. Vitamin A is essential to reproduction.

Unlike many nutritional elements, vitamin A can be stored for future use. Several months' supply may be accumulated, largely in the liver. Sherman and Lanford suggest that we don't yet know how greatly the span of "useful life" may be increased by feeding diets higher in vitamin A than are at present considered optimum. They advise readers to plan their dietaries to conform to present standards and then as a safety measure to take fish oils during the winter months. They imply that vitamin A is among the most important of the food elements.

The recommended daily allowances of the National Research Council are as follows: for children under 1 year, 1500 units; children from 1 to 3, 2000 units; children from 7 to 9, 3500 units; children from 10 to 12, 4500 units; young people from 13 to 20, 5000 to 6000 units; adults, 5000 units except during the latter half of pregnancy, when the allowance should be 6000 units, and lactation, when it advances to 8000 units. Some authorities believe that these values should be raised. Vitamin A itself has a higher nutritional value than carotene, the form in which it is sometimes administered. Both the International Unit (I.U.) and the United

States Pharmacopeia Unit (U.S.P.) of vitamin A have a value equal to that of 0.6 microgram of an internationally standardized preparation of pure beta-carotene.[56, 57]

Vitamin D (now known to occur in several forms) is another of the fat-soluble groups whose function in human nutrition is well established. It is essential to the utilization of calcium and phosphorus by the body, and its deficiency produces faulty bone and tooth structure. When calcification of growing bones is slowed up by insufficient minerals or vitamin D, the strain of supporting the body deforms the bones, and we have the bowlegs or knock-knees, enlarged joints, the beady processes at the cartilaginous junctions of the ribs, and the pigeon breast of rickets. Vitamin D is known as the "antirachitic factor," although a diet adequate in minerals and exposure of the body to sunlight are also antirachitic factors.

The activating effect of ultraviolet light, or direct sunlight, on the utilization of nutrients was recognized in ancient times although knowledge of its functions was less specific. Modern medicine has confirmed the theory that in the presence of direct sunlight the body can synthesize vitamin D from sterols found in plants and animals. In our culture and particularly in cold climates it is difficult to expose the body to a sufficient quantity of sunlight or artificial ultraviolet light to produce adequate amounts of vitamin D from its precursors. The only safe alternative seems to be a diet that includes liberal allowance of vitamin D in the form of activated sterols. This is generally accepted as essential in feeding infants and children. Emphasis in the past has been on development of normal bone structure in the young, but there is a growing tendency to stress the dietary prevention of bone disease in the aging. Irradiation of foods has not proved effective in the same way as has irradiation of the body. The emphasis is, at present, on exposure of the body to a reasonable amount of direct sunlight, use of foods reinforced with vitamin D, and the administration of fish oils. The latter is particularly important in infancy, childhood, and youth. Sherman and Lanford say:

> Vigorous adults, leading a normal life, are thought to require little if any supplemental vitamin D, and no dietary allowance is made for them in the National Research Council's recommendations. It is, however, suggested that: "for persons working at night and for nuns and others whose habits shield them from sunlight, as well as for elderly persons, the ingestion of small amounts of vitamin D is desirable."
>
> For women in the latter half of pregnancy and for nursing mothers, supplemental vitamin D is recommended, 400 units being regarded as "most likely adequate . . . on the basis of available evidence."*

Ability of the body to store vitamin D, like vitamin A, enables the mother, if properly fed, to provide the infant with a reserve of this protective element. The recommended daily allowance for infants and children through adolescence is 300 to 400 units; the need for adults has not been determined in more specific terms than just quoted.[58, 59]

The role of vitamin E is not thoroughly established although its deficiency in animal experimentation is characterized by sterility in both male and female. Other manifestations of the deficiency are muscular dystrophy, injury of the central

* Sherman, Henry C., and Lanford, Caroline S.: *op. cit.* p. 289.

(*Text continued on p. 391.*)

Table 7A. Vitamin Nomenclature Sources and Effects of Deficiences*†

WATER-SOLUBLE VITAMINS

VITAMIN GROUP	TERMINOLOGY	SOURCES	EFFECTS OF DEFICIENCY
Vitamin B	Other name: water-soluble vitamin B	*Animal :* Liver and other glandular organs Pork and other meats Poultry Fish Milk, liquid and powdered	Lowered resistance to infection Loss of appetite Nervous instability and depression Fatigue Gastrointestinal atony with constipation Polyneuritis Dermatitis Anemia Edema Cardiac failure
Vitamin B complex (includes all the B factors listed below and in Table 7B)	The B vitamins	*Plant :* Wheat germ Yeast Peanuts Whole-grain cereals Soy beans, legumes Green leafy vegetables Enriched foods	
Vitamin B₁	**Thiamine** Antiberiberi vitamin Antineuritic factor Other name: vitamin F		Marked thiamine deficiency results in *beriberi*
Vitamin B₂	**Riboflavin** Other names: vitamin G lactoflavin ovoflavin hepatoflavin		Marked riboflavin deficiency results in *cheilosis* (cracks at corners of lips); vascularization of cornea with photophobia; inflammation of lips and tongue
Vitamin B₆ group	**Pyridoxine** Other names: vitamin Y the pyridoximers		
Vitamin B₇	**Rice polish factor** Other name: vitamin I		

* Adapted from tables in: Proudfit, Fairfax T., and Robinson, Corinne H.: *Nutrition and Diet Therapy,* 11th ed.. The Macmillan Company. New York, 1955, pp. 142–45; and the Upjohn Company: *Vitamin Manual,* Kalamazoo, Michigan, 1953, pp. 4–5.
† Asterisks within table indicate official name; boldface type, common name.

Vitamin B$_{12}$ Group (B$_{12a}$, B$_{12b}$, B$_{12e}$, B$_{12d}$ believed to be identical)	**Vitamin B$_{12}$** Antipernicious anemia principle Other names: *cobalamin, a generic name *cyanocobalamin, synonym for vitamin B$_{12}$ *hydroxocobalamin, synonym for vitamin B$_{12b}$	Marked cyanocobalamin deficiency results in *pernicious anemia*
*Nicotinamide	**Niacinamide** Antipellagra factor Anti-black-tongue factor Other names: nicotinic acid amide PP factor (pellagra-preventing factor)	Marked nicotinamide deficiency results in *pellagra*
Nicotinic Acid	**Niacin** (converted to nicotinamide in the body)	
*Pantothenic Acid	**Pantothenic acid** Anti-gray-hair factor Other name: pantothen	
*Biotin	**Biotin** Other names: vitamin H coenzyme R bios II factor s factor w factor x	

Note: Certain foods in the above list are especially rich in one or more B factors. For example, liver is a particularly good source of cyanocobalamin and whole-grain cereals of thiamine

387

Table 7A—Continued

WATER-SOLUBLE VITAMINS

VITAMIN GROUP	TERMINOLOGY	SOURCES	EFFECTS OF DEFICIENCY
*Choline	Choline Other name: bilineurine		
Inositol	Inositol		
*Para-aminobenzoic Acid	PABA		

Folic Acid Group:
Pteroylglutamic Acid,
Pteroyltriglutamic Acid,
Pteroylheptaglutamic Acid,
  etc.
	Folic acid
	Growth-and-blood-formation
	  requirement
	Other names:
	  pteroylglutamic acid
	  PGA
	folacin, generic term for a group of
	  pteroylglutamates formerly
	  known as vitamin M, vitamin
	  B_c, factor U, *Lactobacillus casei*
	  factor, norite eluate factor,
	  vitamin R, vitamin B_{10}, and
	  vitamin B_{11}		

Folinic Acid (biologically active form of folic acid)			

Vitamin C	*Ascorbic acid
	Antiscorbutic factor
	Other name:
	  cevitamic acid
		Plant :
		  Citrus fruits
		  Tomatoes
		  Strawberries
		  Cantaloupe
		  Raw leafy vegetables
		  Broccoli
		  Kale
		  Potatoes
			Lowered resistance to infection
			Structural changes in bones, carti-
			  lage, and teeth with inhibition
			  of growth
			Degeneration of muscles
			Anemia
			Spongy, hemorrhaging gums
			Subcutaneous hemorrhages

Vitamin C_2	Other name: vitamin J		Marked deficiency results in *scurvy*

388

Fat-soluble Vitamins

VITAMIN GROUP	TERMINOLOGY	SOURCES	EFFECTS OF DEFICIENCY
Vitamin A Group Vitamin A$_1$ Vitamin A$_2$ Neovitamin A, etc. α-Carotene β-Carotene γ-Carotene Crytoxanthine, etc.	**Vitamin A** Antixerophthalmic factor Other name: axerophthal **Carotene**	*Animal:* Fish-liver oils Liver Butter, cream Whole-milk cheeses Egg yolk *Plant* (precursors): Yellow vegetables Yellow fruits Green leafy vegetables Margarine (fortified)	Dryness and keratinization of skin and mucous membranes Night blindness and *xerophthalmia* Arrested growth Lowered resistance to infection
Vitamin D Group Vitamin D$_2$ Vitamin D$_3$, etc.	**Vitamin D** Antirachitic factor Other names: calciferol viosterol irradiated ergosterol irradiated 7-dehydrocholesterol *cholecalciferol *ergocalciferol	*Animal:* Fish-liver oils Irradiated milk Activated sterols Butter, liver, egg yolk (contains small amounts) Note: Exposure to sunlight stimulates formation of vitamin D	Vitamin D deficiency causes faulty utilization of calcium and phosphorus resulting in: bony deformities poor posture carious teeth tetanic convulsions in infants Marked deficiency produces *rickets* in children and *osteomalacia* in adults

Table 7A—Continued

FAT-SOLUBLE VITAMINS

VITAMIN GROUP	TERMINOLOGY	SOURCES	EFFECTS OF DEFICIENCY

Vitamin E Group
* α-Tocopherol
* β-Tocopherol
* γ-Tocopherol, etc.
	Vitamin E
	Antisterility factor
	Other names:
	  the tocopherols
		Animal foods are poor sources
		
		Plant:
		  Oils of wheat and rice germ
		    and cotton seed
		  Green leafy vegetables
		  Nuts, legumes
		
		Intestinal synthesis doubtful
			Clinical evidence in humans of antisterility is doubtful
			Deficiency in male rats produces sterility; in female rats reabsorption of fetuses; in rabbits and guinea pigs there is muscular degeneration

Vitamin K Group
Vitamin K₁
Vitamin K₂
Menadione, etc.
	Vitamin K
	Blood-clotting factor or anti-hemorrhagic factor
	Other names:
	  Koagulation Vitamin (Danish
	    name)
	  phylloquinone
		Animal :
		  Liver
		
		Plant :
		  Alfalfa
		  Green leafy vegetables
		
		Synthesized in intestine
			Deficiency in mother's diet believed to be a factor in hemorrhage of the newborn
			
			Its use in the control of hemorrhage is tentative

390

Table 7B. Other Vitamin Groups*

WATER-SOLUBLE VITAMINS

VITAMIN GROUP	TERMINOLOGY
Vitamin B_3	Chick pellagra factor (pantothenic acid possibly)
Vitamin B_4	Riboflavin and pyridoxine (probably)
Vitamin B_5	Nicotinic acid (probably)
Vitamin B_8	Adenylic acid (rarely classified as a vitamin)
Vitamin B_9	An unused number
Vitamin B_{10}, vitamin B_{11}	Mixture of folic acid and vitamin B_{12} (probably)
Vitamin B_{13}	Protogen (probably)
Vitamin B_{14}	Related to folic acid (?) (unconfirmed)
Vitamin B_{15}	Pangamic acid
Vitamin B_o	Identical with folic acid
Vitamin B_p	Replaceable by manganese and choline
Vitamin B_t	
Vitamin B_w	Other name for biotin
Vitamin B_x	Other name for pantothenic acid
Vitamin F	Obsolete term for essential fatty acids and vitamin B_1
Vitamin G	Obsolete term for riboflavin
Vitamin H	Obsolete term for biotin
Vitamin I	Other name for vitamin B_7
Vitamin J	Postulated antipneumonia factor; other name for vitamin C_2
Vitamin L_1	Related to anthranilic acid; possibly a lactation requirement
Vitamin L_2	Related to adenosine; probably a lactation requirement
Vitamin M	Obsolete term for folic acid
Vitamin N	Obsolete term for factors reported to inhibit cancer
Vitamin P group; rutin (one of the P group)	A group of factors that decrease capillary fragility (no longer considered vitamins)
Vitamin R	Probably one of the folic acid group
Vitamin S	Biotin (probably); applied also to streptogenin
Vitamin T	Factor in rat and insect development
Vitamin U	Probably one of the folic acid group
Vitamin V	Probably diphosphopyridine nucleotide
Vitamin W	Biotin (probably)
Vitamin X	Biotin (probably)
Vitamin Y	Pyridoxine (probably)

* Adapted from a table in *Vitamin Manual* by the Upjohn Company, Kalamazoo, Michigan, 1953, pp. 4–5.

nervous system, abnormal heart action, and retarded growth. Because it is widely distributed in natural foods and/or because so little is definitely known about its function and the human requirements, it is not stressed nutritionally. Its clinical use in the treatment of muscular dystrophy and other diseases, including psychoses, is in the experimental stage[60, 61]

The K vitamins, the last of the fat-soluble vitamins to be mentioned, are not now included in dietary planning because they are widely distributed in natural foods and the consequences of their deficiency are not well established. Vitamin K given to the newborn raises the prothrombin level, and it has been called the "Koagulation Vitamin." Clinically, vitamin K has been used on a more or less tentative basis in the control of hemorrhage.[62]

Should vitamins be taken without the doctor's advice? This question often confronts the nurse. It is not easy to give an answer that would meet with general approval. Most physicians would probably say they should not; on the other hand, many nutritionists might say that under certain circumstances they should. Health experts agree that if we could get an optimum diet, animal and vegetable, from lands that had not been depleted, made up of foods neither stored, dried, frozen, nor canned, and if we could spend a reasonable time out of doors, we would need no additional vitamins for health maintenance. Because, however, many of us lead indoor, sedentary lives and eat many stale and processed foods, our health often demands vitamin supplements. Because they are foods and because it is doubtful whether quantities in excess of body needs can have harmful effects, their sale to the public is not regulated. Undoubtedly, we should work to make the use of vitamins outside food items unnecessary for the healthy individual.[63]

3. FLUID BALANCE

Critical Nature of Fluid Balance. Water is necessary for all the chemical and physical activity on which life depends. It is a constituent of all protoplasm. In it are suspended the circulating cells and the colloids, and in it are dissolved organic and mineral nutrients and wastes. Throughout this text there has been repeated reference to Claude Bernard's dictum that health depends upon the constancy of the fluids that constitute the "internal environment," or, in other words, the extracellular fluids. Their constancy depends upon the nature of the intercellular fluids, and since there is a continuous interchange of water between the cells and their environment, the fluids of each must be studied together. The water need is in direct relation to the concentration of solids dissolved in the body fluids. If their intake does not keep pace with the water ingested and eliminated, the cells drown— they are waterlogged. When the water intake does not keep pace with the intake and output of solids, the cells shrivel—they are dehydrated. Excretory organs, particularly the kidneys but also the sweat glands and the intestines, maintain this balance between water and solids as long as they can. When the tissues hold water in excess of their needs (edema), a positive water balance is said to exist; dehydration is referred to as a negative balance.

William E. Abbott[64] estimates that water composes two thirds of the weight of the body. A man weighing 70 kg (154 lb) has therefore 46.6 kg (102.5 lb, or 88 pt) of water within his system. Roughly, two sevenths of this fluid is extracellular (20 pt of interstitial tissue fluid and 6 pt of plasma), while five sevenths (62 pt) lies within the cells. H. L. Marriott says that in health the total body fluid fluctuation is only 3 to 5 pt (2 per cent of the body weight) although a man drinks a ton of water a year, and the ". . . constant to and fro movement of extracellular fluid, between capillaries and interstitial tissue spaces, amounts to hundreds of liters daily."* This ability of the body to maintain a fairly fixed percentage of its weight

* Marriott H. L.: "The Maintenance of Fluid Balance," *Ann. Roy. Coll. Surg.* (London), **7:**339, (Nov.) 1950.

as water depends upon the osmotic pressures of the intracellular and extracellular fluids. This in turn depends upon the protein molecules within the cells that tend to hold water within the cell membrane, upon the salts or electrolytes, and upon the water molecules in the fluids inside and outside the cells that regulate the passage of liquids, mainly, and solids across the membrane. Marriott and most authorities believe that the intracellular and intercellular fluids differ greatly in composition,

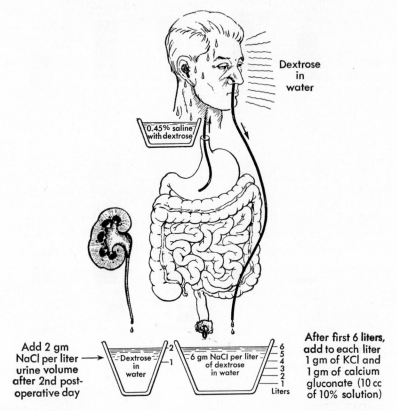

Figure 67.   Replacement requirements in terms of solutions and routes of loss. (Lyon, Richard P.: "The Prevention of Fluid Electrolyte Problem by Simple Means," *California Med.*, **73**:303, [Oct.] 1950.)

although the extent to which they differ is yet to be determined since the study of fluids within microscopic cells is extremely difficult.

The extracellular fluid surrounds the tissue cells. That part lying within the blood vessels and surrounding the blood cells is the plasma. It differs from the rest of the extracellular fluid in its high-protein content. Capillary walls are believed permeable to all the components of the extracellular fluid except the large protein molecules of plasma. The dissolved constituents are mainly salts of sodium kations and chlorine anions. There are also small amounts of potassium, calcium and magnesium, bicarbonate, phosphate, sulfate, and organic acids. Intracellular fluid electrolytes are chiefly potassium and magnesium kations and phosphate, sulfate, and bicarbonate anions.[65]

Abbott, summarizing the experimental data published up to 1946, says that the more recent studies show sodium and potassium ions not as confined to the extracel-

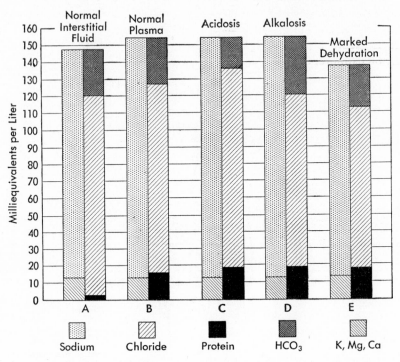

Figure 68. Composition of normal extracellular fluid (*A* and *B*) and possible structural changes that may occur in the plasma during disease (*C, D,* and *E*). (Abbott, William E.: "A Review of the Present Concepts of Fluid Balance," *Am. J. M. Sc.,* **211**:232, [Feb.] 1946.)

lular and intracellular fluids respectively as was once thought. Under certain circumstances, such as hemorrhage, shock, and anoxia, there is an increase of intracellular sodium and a decrease of intracellular potassium. Ordinarily, however, normal osmotic pressures are maintained by passage of water rather than the salt molecules across the cell membrane. Upon the constancy of body fluids and their dissolved salts, or electrolytes, depends the acid-base balance. An increase of bicarbonate, for example, pushes the body toward alkalosis; an increase in the chlorides toward acidosis.

With the rapid development in physiological chemistry within the last decades, there has been a shifting emphasis in fluid and electrolyte therapy.

In health, thirst and appetite regulate the fluid, electrolyte, and acid-base balance, if the individual has access to adequate food and drink. The balance is upset whenever shock, anesthetics, drugs, or any incapacitating illness dulls normal desires in eating and drinking or makes their satisfaction impossible. Infants and children are especially susceptible to upsets in fluid and acid-base balance because they have less freedom in satisfying their appetites and because the body chemistry is less stable. Now with the increased use of surgery and its accompanying anesthesia, loss of blood, interruption of diet, narcosis, and general incapacity, the problem of maintaining balance in body chemistry assumes major proportions. All effective medicine is highly dependent upon successful nutrition; modern medicine must often rely on extraoral methods, and the medical workers must assume responsibility for accomplishing what the appetites so effortlessly dictate in health.

As physicians learned to introduce fluid into veins and subcutaneous tissues, they learned that it is necessary to add salts to these fluids—or to give fluids with an osmotic pressure comparable to the body fluids. Recognizing sodium chloride as the major salt of the plasma, they first used this substance only. Later they learned the value of adding other salts, particularly those of potassium and calcium. The use of glucose as a parenteral food was discovered, and later the value of protein hydrolysates in parenteral solutions was established; the use of parenteral fat emulsions is under investigation. Now the physician can give a diet complete except for fats, using a wide variety of solutions from the standpoint of their chemical composition, any one of which has a physiological osmotic pressure. He must decide, therefore, whether the patient in addition to the food he can eat needs plain water, salt, sugar, or protein solutions; or if he cannot eat, which of these should be given extraorally.

The nutritionist attempts to keep the normal person in a state of water and electrolyte or acid-base balance by his recommended allowances of the various dietary elements discussed in the preceding pages. Most authorities contend that since many foods contain a high percentage of water, an ample diet, supplemented by drink as dictated by thirst, can be relied upon to maintain the fluid balance in health. Any marked deviation, however, from an adequate dietary intake, particularly a low-protein diet, can so disturb the fluid balance that edema (excess intercellular fluid) and excess fluid in the serous-lined cavities result. The protruding abdomen of the famine victim is a vivid demonstration of the derangement in fluid-electrolyte balance resulting from malnutrition alone. Eating in excess of body needs is harmful, but the fluid-electrolyte balance is not so drastically upset as in starvation. Sherman and Lanford say much more data are needed to enable us to say how far the nature of the diet affects the acid-base balance in the body. It remains essentially neutral with wide variation in the foods eaten.

In illness or surgery the physician tries to approximate the patient's normal nutritional needs, using the forms of food and the methods of feeding that are best suited to the conditions. When nausea and vomiting, suction of the intestinal tract, diarrhea, profuse sweating, hemorrhage, or drainage from wounds increases the output of fluids and electrolytes, and/or when nausea, unconsciousness, mouth lesions, or paralysis of the alimentary tract limits the intake, the maintenance of fluid-electrolyte or acid-base balance is difficult.

As the functions of sodium, potassium, and other minerals are better understood and as the harmful effects of chloride and protein losses are demonstrated in studies, the medical profession relies more and more heavily on analyses of their concentrations in samples of the patient's blood as a means of estimating his needs for water, electrolytes, and nutrients. While few nurses, and indeed few doctors, can know all that has been learned about fluid balance, they should understand the general principle that it depends upon *the total dietary intake, including water, and upon the capacity of the alimentary and excretory systems to function within a normal range.* Nurses as well as doctors should understand that re-establishing the balance following vomiting, diarrhea, seepage from burns, hemorrhage, and profuse sweating must be accomplished with different substances since the fluid lost in each case carries with it different solids or the same solids in varying concentrations.[66, 67] Richard P. Lyon says, "The content of the solution for replacement is dictated by the route of fluid output."[*] His diagram, as shown in Figure 67, illustrates this point, as does that by Abbott in Figure 68. Both writers urge the physician to depend on the over-all picture presented by the dehydrated or over-hydrated patient rather than on individual laboratory analyses. Abbott, reviewing the investigations of this complex subject, concludes his report with the following:

Thus, it becomes important to think in terms of total body water and salt rather than solute concentrations alone, since changes in the volume and concentration can occur in numerous different ways. . . . Changes in hydration can usually be demonstrated in the course of a physical examination (eyeball tension, condition of the tongue, elasticity of the skin, etc.) and an estimate of the severity of the disorder may be made from a careful history (type, severity, and duration of illness) and by observations of the response of the patient to therapy (changes in the amount and in the specific gravity of urine, in the turgor of the skin, in mental alertness, and in the weight and thirst of the individual in question).

The importance of these obvious and easily discernible findings ought not to be underestimated . . . often too much reliance is placed on single or isolated determinations of concentration of substances in the blood, especially chloride and protein. To be of value such data must be considered in relation to the general state of nutrition and hydration of the patient as indicated by the history, the physical examination, and the volume and specific gravity of the urine.[†]

Lyon's summary and conclusions are in general agreement, but because they give specific recommendation for method, they may be especially enlightening to the nurse, who often wonders why so many different kinds of parenteral solutions are used. His summary and conclusions are as follows:

[*] Lyon, Richard P.: "The Prevention of Fluid-Electrolyte Problems by Simple Means," *California Med.,* **73**:303, (Oct.) 1950.
[†] Abbott, William E.: "A Review of the Present Concepts on Fluid Balance," *Am. J. M. Sc.,* **211**:232, (Feb.) 1946.

Summary

Proper fluid balance may be maintained in patients after operations by the employment of simple inexpensive procedures which may be carried out even in the smallest hospitals.

Daily weighing of patients, measurement of fluid intake and output, and knowledge of the probable electrolyte content of fluid losses are adequate guides for replacement of fluids and electrolytes. An increase in body weight is a warning of overhydration.

The content of the solution used for replacement is dictated by the route of fluid output—whether from the gastrointestinal tract, the skin, or the kidneys. Insensible losses (by perspiration and respiration) are fairly static.

Except to replace extrarenal losses, parenteral administration of normal saline solution in the immediate postoperative period is contraindicated.

Mistakes in replacement methods, especially those causing overhydration are particularly hazardous for the elderly patient.

Conclusions

Adequate replacement of fluid and electrolytes requires the use of simple and easily available measures. They are measurements of body weight, measurement of intake-output, and knowledge of the probable electrolyte content of fluid loss.

Adequate replacement is made possible by—

(1) *a basic daily ration composed of 1000 cc. of dextrose in water and 1000 cc. of dextrose in ½ normal saline,* providing 800 cc. for insensible perspiration losses and 1200 cc. for urine formation with a salt concentration of 2 to 3 grams per liter. During the first 48 hours after operation, or until urine output reaches 2 liters, however, no salt is given and the two liter ration is met with dextrose in water.

(2) *replacement of gastro-intestinal losses volume for volume by a dextrose solution containing salt at a concentration of 6 grams per liter. After the first three liters have been replaced, further salt and water replacement is supplemented by the addition of one gram of KCl per liter.* If losses continue beyond the six liter mark, two grams of KCl are added to each replacement liter.

(3) *replacement of visible perspiration with dextrose in ½ normal saline,* the volume of loss being measured by changes in body weight beyond that expected from the intake-output calculation.

Use of normal saline solution parenterally in the early postoperative period is contraindicated in the absence of extrarenal salt losses.*

Nurses render invaluable service by observing and reporting the signs of plus-and-minus fluid balances as just listed. In many cases this balance depends on their skill in feeding patients. Nurses' records of intake and output of fluids and solids are essential to the doctor's estimate of the patient's needs. This topic is discussed further in Chapter 14.

Water is so essential to body economy and the demand for it is so insistent that drinking water should always be within the patient's reach unless the physician has restricted his intake. While there are no hard and fast rules for the amount that

* Lyon, Richard P.: *op. cit.,* and personal communication, March, 1953.

should be drunk in a 24-hour period, it should be sufficient in the case of adults to ensure the elimination of at least 1000 to 1500 cc (1 to 1½ qt) of urine.

4. FOOD SELECTION AND THE OPTIMUM DIET

Factors Affecting the Caloric Requirement. The amount of food required per unit of body weight depends upon the rate at which the body utilizes nutrients. DuBois[68] lists the following factors as affecting this rate, or the basal metabolism: sex, age, sleep, exercise, diet, temperature, climate, clothing, athletic training, disease, and physiological states such as puberty, menstruation, and the climacteric. Temperament or glandular make-up and/or the psychic state also affect the metabolic rate. For example, the hyperthyroid person may have a metabolic rate of +30 which will fall within the normal range (+10 to −10) after a thyroid-ectomy. In 1929 George W. Henry[69] called attention to the difference between the caloric needs of the same individual in the hyper- and hypoactive phases of a manic-depressive psychosis.

To estimate scientifically the caloric requirement of a subject it is necessary to measure the metabolic rate and then to take into account the factors just listed. Such estimates are complicated and impracticable for everyday use, but the average caloric needs of persons of all ages with typical builds and in various occupations, usually shown in tabular form, are arrived at by such exact calculations made on hundreds of subjects. A study of such data shows that the caloric need per unit of body weight gradually diminishes from youth to old age. Activity and the rate of growth decrease with the years, and hence we need less food as we grow older. Those who fail to change their habits of eating as they pass from young adulthood to old age get fat.

For young adults the caloric need per kilogram of body weight varies from 33 calories per day for a sedentary woman to 70 calories for a laborer who needs strong muscles.[70] The caloric needs of all other adults fall between the two extremes.

Maintenance of Normal Weight. It is not possible to determine *the normal weight* for anyone. Averages for normal males and females of all ages and body builds have been adopted as "norms." Mortality statistics prepared by life insurance companies have influenced medical opinion to set the normal weights at lower figures than were used in past decades. The findings of animal experimentation have been popularized in such articles as "The Thin Rats Bury the Fat Rats."[71] Thorstein Veblen, however, in his *Theory of the Leisure Class*[72] shows the relationship between the cultural pattern and what we consider normal weight. In societies, for example, where "the ideal woman" can labor all day and bear many children without much interruption of her work, normal weights in relation to heights are higher than those in a culture where the "ideal woman" does little with her hands and is cherished as an ornament to the man's household. Height-weight tables should therefore be used with reference to a specific people, their body build, and the kind of life they lead. Even then standards should not be applied too arbitrarily.[73]

The Energy Requirement of Adults*

ESTIMATE OF ENERGY REQUIREMENT FOR ONE DAY

I Activity	II Time, Hrs.	III Factor (Cal. per Kg. per Hr.)	IV Cal. per Kg. II × III
Lying still, awake	0.50	0.1	0.05
Sitting	1.25	0.4	0.50
Standing relaxed	0.75	0.5	0.38
Sitting, writing, or eating	8.00	0.4	3.20
Standing at attention	0.25	0.6	0.15
Dressing and undressing	1.75	0.7	1.23
Light exercise	1.00	1.4	1.40
Walking (3 mi. per hr.)	1.00	2.0	2.00
Dancing	1.00	3.8	3.80
Skating	1.00	3.5	3.50
Walking up stairs (4 flights)		0.036	0.14
Walking down stairs (4 flights)		0.012	0.05
	16.50		16.40

Body weight, 56 kg.
Total calories for activities per kg. (sum of column IV), 16.40 cal.
Total cost of activities (56×16.40 cal.), 918 cal.
Saving in sleeping 7.5 hrs. (0.1×56×7.5), 42 cal.

TOTAL FOR DAY

	Calories
Basal metabolism for 24 hours (see p. 24)	1,313
Saving in sleep, to be deducted	42
Corrected basal metabolism	1,271
Cost of day's activities	918
Total cost of metabolism	2,189
"Tax" for influence of food (6 per cent)	131
Day's requirement	2,320

Daily Energy Requirement According to Occupation*

TYPE OF OCCUPATION	TOTAL CALORIES PER DAY		CAL. PER KG. PER DAY
	Men	Women	
At rest but sitting most of day	2,000–2,200	1,600–1,800	30–33
Work chiefly done sitting	2,200–2,700	1,900–2,200	34–37
Work chiefly done standing or walking	2,800–3,000	2,300–2,500	38–42
Work developing muscular strength	3,100–3,500	2,600–3,000	43–50
Work requiring very strong muscles	4,000–6,000	—	55–70

* MacLeod, Grace, and Taylor, Clara M.: *Rose's Foundations of Nutrition*, 4th ed. The Macmillan Company, New York, 1944, pp. 59 and 60.

Undernourishment and malnutrition are the great plague of mankind. Hunger with its far-reaching effects has been discussed in the introduction to this chapter. Its prevalence in all countries, even the economically favored, is recognized by the experts. Many of us eat an adequate diet in terms of calories but suffer from "hidden hungers" because our food is unwisely chosen or diseases may interfere with its assimilation. Fashion often dictates a figure, and some cults influence their followers to adopt a diet incompatible with good nutrition. The weakness, irritability, inability to concentrate on given tasks, and the general inertia characteristic of underfeeding are such universal experiences that the ills of malnutrition would seem self-evident, needing no emphasis in a text for health workers. It may, however, be necessary to keep reminding ourselves that what we eat is conditioned more by habits and custom passed from one generation to another than by intelligence. Some one has said, "We like what we eat," rather than eat what we like. Nutritionists find repeatedly that the diet of most persons in certain large geographical areas is inadequate in kind, quantity, and quality. Anyone can become so habituated to a low-vitamin, low-calorie diet that appetite loses its protective function.

A healthy, normal person suddenly deprived of food may be crazed by hunger. To get food, crimes are committed by the starving, even murder and cannibalism. This acute state differs, however, from that of the chronically and habitually undernourished. The latter assume that their incapacity for sustained effort is normal. It is not easy to change the eating habits of such persons or, in fact, to stimulate them in any way. The beneficial effects of vitamins as a means of increasing desire for food has been mentioned. Insulin, which speeds up the metabolism of carbohydrates, and produces acute hunger, has been used as an artificial whip to the appetite in extreme cases. Adoption of adult diets that include the basic seven food groups would eliminate gross malnutrition. Modifications according to special needs will eliminate more elusive forms of underfeeding.

Malnutrition, where the person's food supply is adequate, often has its origin in an emotional disturbance. Indigestion and aversion to food often accompany stress, although many neurotics seek comfort in food and get very fat. Malnutrition in children is a common symptom of unhappy family relationships. For all these and other reasons, nurses soon find how difficult it is to change eating patterns.

Overeating and the resulting *obesity* is a common nutritional disorder in the economically favored countries. Anton J. Carlson says, "The obese may enjoy a good diet, but they do not use it wisely. Apart from pellagra, perhaps obesity is the most serious aspect of malnutrition in this country."* The danger of excess weight is now generally accepted, but it has not always been looked upon as detrimental to health to the same degree. A physician in 1913 wrote as follows on "The Advantages of Adipose":

Nine times out of ten it is a mark, not of disease, but of health. It is an indication that the system, by good management and good housekeeping, has brought its expendi-

* Carlson, Anton J.: "Some Obstacles in the Path Towards an Optimum Diet," *Texas Rep. Biol. & Med.,* **1:**5, (Spring) 1943.

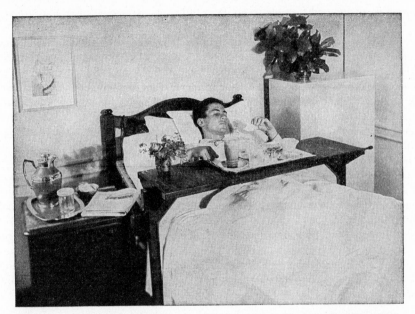

Figure 69. An adjustable table that fits over the bed is ideal for holding food trays.

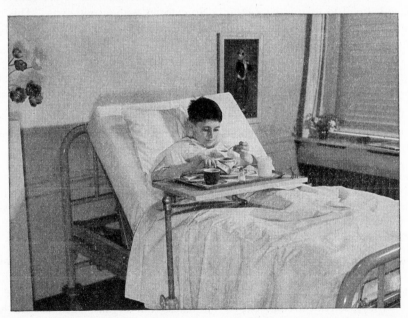

Figure 70. Another type of overbed table that allows the tray to be placed in a position which is convenient for the patient.

tures within its income and is able to lay by a little, against a rainy day. Fat is Nature's savings bank, a hoard which can be drawn upon in times of scarcity or of need. . . .

One of the most successful methods of treating neurasthenia and nervous bankruptcy the celebrated Weir Mitchell treatment, consists chiefly of rest and overfeeding, and its object is to make the patient fat. So that a growth of healthy fat up to or even slightly in excess of twenty per cent of your former weight is a protection against disease, a buffer against the shocks, and a shield against the darts and pin-pricks of fortune, a lubricator of all the frictions of life; it adds beauty to the beautiful and favor to the plain, and, in short, is an advantage in every way and a thing to be desired instead of dreaded, to be proud of instead of ashamed of.

My advice, therefore to the vast majority of those who are anxious to lose weight, to get thin, is like "Punch's" famous advice to those about to get married: *"Don't."* Your balance in the body bank may be a trifle unpoetic in the matter of waist-line, may show a regrettable preference for accumulating where the miners used to carry their gold,—under the belt,—but do not worry about it. You will have a good time spending it before very long, and most of the means that you can adopt to get rid of it will do you far more harm than it ever will or can. Moreover, unlike the gold [money] it will float, and in the extreme emergency of shipwreck will act as a life preserver instead of dragging you down to destruction, as so thrillingly described in the Shilling Shockers.*

Most persons in this country must change their eating habits after young adult-hood or suffer a weight increase. This may not be necessary for future generations who have learned to follow the dictum, "No calories without vitamins." This auto-matically eliminates most concentrated fats and carbohydrates or processed foods, in contrast with natural foods.

The overweight like to think that their metabolism is abnormal, and they often claim to eat less than their thin friends and relatives. While a low basal metabolic rate does lower the number of calories a person can eat without gaining, no dis-agreement has been found with W. N. Mann's statement:

An increase in weight is always due to eating more than the body needs; it depends therefore upon an appetite disproportionate to the body's needs. . . . There is . . . no evidence that the obese utilize food differently from the spare. . . .

Although obesity may be associated with endocrine disorders, it is incidental to the general state. No endocrine preparation is of value in the treatment of obesity as such, and diminution of an "endocrine" obesity following specific treatment will only occur if attention be paid also to diminishing the intake of food to a quantity commensurate with the energy output.†

In the article quoted, Mann outlines reduction and maintenance diets in weight control. They are similar to diets prepared in nutrition clinics of hospitals, schools, and industries. Life insurance companies distribute lists of *Weight Control Ma-terials*.[74] They, convinced that excess fat taxes vital organs, such as the heart, interferes with body mechanics, and in various ways undermines health, find it

---

* Hutchinson, Woods: *Common Diseases.* Houghton Mifflin Co., The Riverside Press, Cambridge, Mass., 1913, pp. 48, 53, 54.
† Mann, W. N.: "Obesity and Its Treatment," *Practitioner,* **164:**436, (May) 1950.

profitable to give away pamphlets, charts, and diagrams that spread the facts of weight control.

The Optimum Diet.   The best diet for each person is one which provides him with all the food elements he needs in that quantity and in those proportions that will keep him in optimum health. Obviously, our concept of the optimum diet must be influenced by each major discovery in the field of nutrition. People complain because what the doctors tell them one year they refute in the next. This will continue until man loses his capacity to learn. There is, then, no such thing as the optimum diet, but nutritionists have furnished us some general rules epitomizing present-day knowledge.

It isn't possible in a text of this sort to discuss all considerations in feeding any individual. Many have been suggested in the pages on dietary elements: carbohydrates, fats, proteins, minerals, vitamins, and water. For the reader's convenience, however, and because these topics are so important, some major questions on the feeding of infants and the aged are given special treatment.

Infant Feeding.   The first question the young mother will want answered about infant feeding is the relative value of breast and bottle feeding. During the first half of this century, as sanitation made clean milk available to babies, there was a tendency even among medical workers to think that artificial feeding was a good substitute for the baby's natural food—breast milk. There were always some physicians who disagreed, who did all they could to promote breast feeding, but in recent years obstetricians, pediatricians, and psychiatrists have combined to bring the value of nursing the baby to the attention of mothers. Custom so far prevails, however, that many women are convinced that bottle feeding is as good, if not better, for the child and more convenient for them. Benjamin Spock[75] takes the reasonable stand that at least two persons are concerned and that the woman should not be made to feel that she is a failure as a mother if she cannot or will not nurse her infant. He, of course, advocates *breast feeding* because he thinks it (1) makes the mother feel close to the baby emotionally, (2) gives the baby a sense of security or oneness with the mother, (3) saves the mother's time in preparing a formula, (4) saves money, (5) protects the child from communicable diseases because breast milk is sterile, and (6) the mother's nipple satisfies the sucking reflex more adequately than the artificial nipple, and the infant is less likely to be a thumb sucker. To these advantages should be added the protection offered the baby in the antibodies of breast milk.

Nurses who are convinced of its value can greatly encourage breast feeding. Without this conviction it is hard to help mothers keep trying until the flow of milk is established. The nurse who does not make this effort for the mother desiring to nurse her baby has a great deal to answer for, as has the doctor who discourages or is neutral to breast feeding.

Generally speaking, artificial feeding and the preparation of formulas have been simplified. Whole milk, condensed milk, and dried-milk preparations are commonly used. The pasteurization or boiling of mixtures made of fresh milk is usually advocated to protect infants from bovine tuberculosis, dysentery, and other communicable diseases. Establishment of human milk bureaus in which breast milk is collected under aseptic conditions, packed in ice, or frozen, has made this food available for many sick or premature infants.

Formulas for infants, sick or well, are usually prepared in a central laboratory or kitchen, from which the bottles, labeled with names of the babies for whom they are intended, are sent to the clinical services. The clinical staff is responsible for warming the mixtures so that they are at the proper temperature—38° C (100.4° F)—when given to the infants. The nurse may judge the temperature by shaking a few drops on her wrist. If nipples have been put on in the laboratory, they are covered with a paper cap. If nipples are applied by the clinical nursing staff, they are so handled as to keep the whole nipple as clean as possible and the part coming in contact with the baby's mouth uncontaminated. With both breast- and bottle-fed babies, other foods are added to the milk diet within the first few months of life. Orange juice and cereals are usually the first additions, but by the sixth month many infants are getting puréed fruits, vegetables, and meats. Vitamin supplements (particularly the fat-soluble A and D vitamins) are also added to the diet soon after birth. This is thought to be particularly important for infants in cold climates.

Regularity has been especially stressed in the feeding of infants. One reason is that their stomachs are small and the baby's total needs will not be met unless he is fed frequently. Feedings are usually spaced at 3- or 4-hour intervals, being less frequent at night. A typical schedule is 6-9-12-3-6-10-2. After the child is a few months old, he will usually sleep through the two o'clock feeding and will demand food at longer intervals. A few physicians may have hard and fast rules for the spacing of feedings, but most now believe that each child should establish his own rhythm. Even this, however, implies regularity. Such texts as those of Spock and Milton J. E. Senn and Phyllis K. Newill[76] have revolutionized the feeding of children. Some psychiatrists believe that rigidity in feeding infants builds up hostility and insecurity since the baby may interpret the withholding of food he craves as an expression of dislike or rejection by the mother, or "the big person." Actually, if the baby is fed on his demand—which means those signs of hunger he makes—he soon establishes regular habits of nursing every three or four hours.[77, 78]

The infant's position while he is fed with a bottle is perhaps still open to question, but most pediatrists advocate holding him in the arms. Contact with the mother's or the nurse's body gives him the reassurance his nature demands. No matter what position is used, the nurse should remain with the child throughout the feeding period. Strangulation and death have occurred from leaving a baby sucking a bottle of feeding mixture. Holes in the nipple should be such as to allow the food to pass through neither too rapidly nor too slowly. The feeding of an infant should take from 10 to 20 minutes.

Air swallowed with the food from the bottle or the breast may fill the stomach before the child has had enough. In order to prevent this the infant should be held with the head higher than the abdomen while nursing, a position said to make the gas rise toward the cardiac opening of the stomach. Some physicians recommend that at least once during the feeding period and at the end the infant be held over the shoulder for several minutes. Gentle pressure exerted by patting the baby while he is in this position helps to produce eructations.[79]

Premature infants, because of their extreme delicacy and sensitiveness to chilling and infection, are not removed from their warm surroundings for feeding periods.

There are a number of *devices* designed to facilitate feeding infants. The infant feeding bottle can be used effectively whenever the sucking reflex is present. A *Breck feeder* is a glass cylinder with a nipple on one end and a bulb on the other that can be squeezed to exert pressure on the contents. This feeder is used for premature infants when they do not have sufficient strength to suck the nipple. It is easy to strangle the baby by giving him more milk than he can swallow; an eye dropper with the tip protected by rubber is perhaps a safer instrument.

Mothers and guardians of infants and children are often in need of guidance in preparing and serving their foods. Visiting nurses all over the country are giving such help. In some hospitals it is customary for the nursing staff to teach the parents whatever is necessary about the preparation and administration of feedings before the infant or child is discharged. Conferences, demonstrations, moving pictures, and written directions are used as teaching methods.

Feeding the Aged.   People differ so greatly in the rate at which they age that it is hard to generalize about their nutritional needs. A. L. Vischer[80] shows a chart on which are graphed the curves of mental capacity, procreative power, physical fitness and capacity, and metabolism of a hypothetical, or standard, person. The curve of mental capacity reaches maximum height around the age of 60; procreative power at 30; physical fitness at 20; and metabolism at birth. After the age of 20 the metabolic rate remains nearly constant, falling less than 5 per cent. This suggests that metabolic needs, at least in quantity, are not, after adulthood, materially altered by age itself. Between the ages of 20 and 90 there is a gradual decline in physical capacity and fitness—about 20 per cent. This decline in vitality usually too reduces the activity of the individual, and for this reason he needs less food. If, however, the older person continues to be a very active person, he may need many more calories than is generally believed to be the case. The maintenance of normal weight and particularly the avoidance of overweight are stressed. Some physicians believe the control of obesity would markedly reduce the incidence of chronic disease.[81] Diabetes mellitus is said to occur two and a half times as often, and cardiovascular-renal disease one and one-half times as often, in the obese as in those of average weight.[82]

No authorities have been found advocating a diet for the aged differing materially from the optimum diet in younger adulthood. Geriatrists repeatedly say that the protein, mineral, and vitamin needs are little altered by age. Occasional reference is made to the diminished secretion of the digestive enzymes and the difficulty some elderly persons find in digesting fats in particular. While no one advocates trying to force on the elderly a diet better than the one they are eating, it must be recognized that a fixed and unwholesome habit of eating can be the cause of the poor appetite and the inability to take care of the meager fare that is eaten. Edward L. Bortz summarizes the "primary requisites of those growing into the later decades" as "restriction in total calories plus extra fortification with protein, certain essential vitamins, and minerals (iron and calcium) and an adequate, indeed, a generous, fluid intake."*

The faulty teeth and poor posture so often seen in the aged contribute to poor nutrition. Marked improvement may be impossible until these conditions are corrected. Food should be of a texture that the person can masticate until the dental

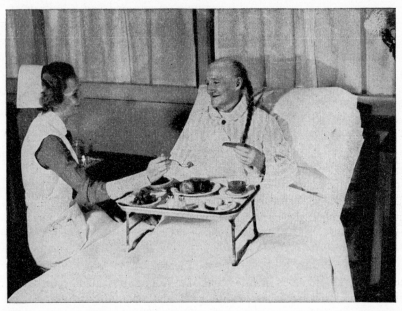

Figure 71. Nurse feeding a cardiac patient who is not allowed to feed herself. Note the comfortable position of the patient and the nurse. (Courtesy of the Yale University School of Nursing, New Haven, Conn.)

problems are solved. The constipation that accompanies faulty body mechanics must be treated until the cause can be removed, because a poor appetite is one of the effects of constipation.[83, 84, 85, 86]

Loneliness and a feeling of uselessness dull the latter part of many lives, while economic want is a common source of stress. When the relative security of a home for the aged is sought, years of boredom are usually the price exacted. Vischer makes a plea for keeping the aged in the current of life. He believes that they need its stimulation and that without a consideration of the psychic causes of premature aging the correction of the physical conditions is to a large extent futile.

Changing Food Habits. Young nurses, filled with a desire to share their enlarged concepts of nutrition, soon learn that it is difficult to change dietary patterns.

* Bortz, Edward L.: "Nutritional Deficiencies and Premature Aging," Second International Gerontological Congress, St. Louis, 1951, *J. Gerontology*, Supplement No. 3, **6**:44, (Sept.) 1951.

If we are honest with ourselves, we will admit that we apply a small fragment of what we know about health, including food needs, in our own life.

Agnes M. Erkel, discussing "The Human Side of Eating," quotes a bulletin prepared by Margaret Mead for the United Nations:

". . . . First of all, we eat that which is available within the confines of the community; how it is prepared is dependent upon the equipment available for cooking. The ultimate result in any home, in any society, is a set pattern of food habits. . . ."

Erkel goes on to say:

In every community there are patients, young and old, whose dietary habits we are trying to change. It does take time to individualize one's teaching, . . . progress will be slow . . . until we recognize the fact that eating habits are an expression of a pattern of living and . . . change must be built upon . . . the patient's economic and social background.*

Both authors sound a warning and give advice which, in the writer's opinion, most inexperienced health workers need. Successful nutritionists, including the nurse when she can qualify under this title, must be students of their subject and of society as well. They must be able to help individuals plan normal diets and follow diets prescribed by the physician; they must be prepared to help housewives plan meals for healthy families and invalids, and all of this within the cultures and economic resources of those they serve. The tables on page 399 in this text are helpful in the solution of such problems, but the more specialized sources listed at the end of this chapter should be consulted.

5. CONDITIONS THAT FAVOR DIGESTION AND ASSIMILATION

Sight and Smell of Savory Food.   Walter B. Cannon[87] cites his experiments and those of Pavlov, Richet, and others showing that the smell and sight of appetizing food stimulates digestive juices and muscular movement of the alimentary tract. This knowledge should be applied in health and sickness. A person may not be hungry, or if questioned may say that he does not want anything to eat, and yet have his appetite aroused by seeing and smelling a tempting dish. Bed patients who are too ill to feed themselves should see the food that is fed them for the psychic effect on digestion, if for no other reason.

Food Preferences.   Close kin to this idea is that expressed by Sir Walter Langdon-Brown and Reginald Hilton's *Physiological Principles in Treatment:*

The nervous factor in gastric digestion affords a scientific explanation of the old adage, "Hunger is the best sauce." Indeed, as we have seen, it is the sauce which will greatly increase the rate of digestion. This should lead us to attach great importance to the personal equation in dieting a patient. Too rigid a dietary, albeit compiled on

* Erkel, Agnes M.: "The Human Side of Eating," *Pub. Health Nursing,* **42**:606, (Nov.) 1950.

an admirable chemical basis, may prove distasteful and upset the appetite, thereby preventing all the good that might be expected.*

It is often surprising to see the ill unable to tolerate simple bland foods and yet able to eat without discomfort some dish ordinarily considered indigestible but which they especially relish. Medical workers learn to study the likes and dislikes of patients and to provide them with foods meeting their needs but also appealing to their palates.

Freedom from Pain, Stress, and Fatigue.   It is well known that strong emotions, even though pleasurable, interfere with digestion. Experiments have shown that pain, excitement, worry, fear, anger, passion, depression, irritability, nervousness, homesickness, or distress of any kind inhibits the flow of saliva, gastric juice, intestinal and pancreatic juice, and also the motor activity of the alimentary tract. Pain or violent emotion involves the autonomic nervous system which also controls alimentation.

Eating should be postponed, if possible, until excitement of any sort has abated. Infants and children should not be excited even by play immediately before or after a meal. Pleasurable emotions and sensations, however, if not too exciting, aid digestion, and so one hears such expressions as "Laugh and grow fat," and "Joy never kills." The beneficial effect of pleasure and laughter on the digestion was recognized in the custom of having a jester present at the evening meal or in our own day by soft music with meals.

Excessive fatigue is close kin to pain. Insofar as possible everyone, sick or well, should avoid eating when very tired or hurried. Physical exhaustion can usually be relieved by resting before the meal, and mental fatigue overcome by substituting a pleasant train of thought for exciting or disturbing ideas. Hurried eating is likely to inhibit digestion because the food is neither adequately ground by the teeth nor thoroughly mixed with the saliva.

A Pleasant Environment.   Attractive surroundings and a cheerful atmosphere add greatly to the enjoyment and hence the digestion of a meal. The environment should be free from anything offensive to the senses, such as noise, disorder, confusion, dirt, unpleasant odors, excessive heat or cold, or anything to arouse unpleasant associations. Those with whom one shares a meal, who serve the meal, or even the company in the room can contribute much to creating an atmosphere conducive to digestion. Visitors who demand attention from the patient should be excluded tactfully while a sick person is eating, but an agreeable and understanding companion should be encouraged. The mildly sick should eat in groups rather than in solitude except under special circumstances. Many hospitals are now designed to foster communal meals.

Regularity in Eating.   Periodic recurrences of hunger demand that human beings and animals eat at regular intervals. Cannon concludes that hunger is a result of contractions of the empty stomach, indicating that it is again ready to

---

* Langdon-Brown, Sir Walter, and Hilton, Reginald: *Physiological Principles in Treatment,* 8th ed. Williams & Wilkins Co., Baltimore, 1943, p. 60.

receive food. He compares intense hunger to pain and implies that it is a sensation to be avoided as unwholesome and not necessarily conducive to digestion, because the very hungry are likely to bolt their food. Habit and other factors affect the rhythm so that individuals feel the need of food at different intervals. Regularity is probably desirable for everyone, sick or well, since meals too close together may overload the stomach and too far apart decrease effective effort in work and play.

Rigid feeding schedules versus self-demand feedings for infants are discussed under "Infant Feeding" on page 404. Because their stomachs hold so little, it is obvious that they must be fed frequently and with some degree of regularity.

The elderly are often psychologically dependent upon regularity. Since their activities and interests tend to be curtailed, they have a keener anticipation of their food than do busy young adults. Their habits, also, are more fixed, and a delayed dinner can be a serious annoyance. With the decreased vitality of age they may also feel a more acute need of refueling.

Meal Spacing.   Through a study of variations in muscle power, believed by Howard N. Haggard and Leon A. Greenberg[88] to be an index of the individual's efficiency, they have shown that meal spacing affects efficiency. They believed the American custom of three meals a day to be the result of an industrial system that allowed one rest period during the working day, rather than consideration of body needs. They demonstrated that motor power is lowest in the morning before breakfast in spite of the long preceding rest, and that feeding individuals five meals a day instead of three resulted in a more uniform state of efficiency. Prevention of fatigue is highly important in health and even more so when the body is fighting disease.

It is customary to feed the very ill at frequent intervals, and in some cases nutrients are injected continuously into the veins. In most hospitals midmorning and midafternoon nourishments are served to patients, and in many cases are available to the staff. Meal spacing is of great interest to nurses, for, while the physician prescribes the diet, in many instances he leaves its administration to the nurse.

6. DIET IN SICKNESS

Special Feeding Problems in Illness.   All forms of illness affect digestion and assimilation, either directly as a result of organic disease or indirectly from poor circulation, lack of exercise, or the worry and depression that often accompany illness. Lack of exercise lessens muscle tone and reduces the metabolic rate, so diminishing the food requirement. As less food is needed, and eaten, bulk is decreased unless the diet is wisely chosen. This diminishes the stimulation of the muscular walls of the intestines brought about through distention. Constipation is the natural result, and sensations evoked by it retard appetite. Muscle tension characteristic of emotional states is favorable to action but unfavorable to the process of digestion. Bacteria and other toxins act directly on digestive glands and muscles as chemical poisons and in this way alter digestion; or they may produce nausea and vomiting or diarrhea. A dry mouth, a bad taste, and even more distressing symptoms may accompany fever and discourage eating.

Illness limits variety in a person's life and turns his thoughts inward. With too much time to think about details, he exaggerates the importance of what he eats. The limitation of his diet, due to the nature of his illness, may be a source of irritation and make it difficult to plan his meals. Acute illness and conditions that limit motion may make feeding himself or even eating an effort. He must in many cases be fed, and unless this is very skillfully done, it detracts greatly from the pleasure of the meals.

These are only a few of the many problems involved in feeding the sick. Their solution may be the main factor in the patient's recovery. No one can live for many days without water. The omission of food for the same length of time is much less harmful, but even short periods of starvation produce discomfort and lessen the powers of resistance. D. M. Dunlop in an article, "Modern Trends in Therapeutic Diets," decries the old methods that rarely included all dietary essentials. Referring to the surreptitious drinks from flower vases and hot-water bottles, he says patients deprived of food and water were often "wiser" than the doctor. He advocates complete diets individually planned and says: "There can be few instances in dietetic out-patient departments in which the giving out of printed diet sheets is justifiable. Advice on diet should be individual. . . ."*

In spite of Dunlop's recommendation, it is common practice for physicians to prescribe the patient's diet on admission in some such terms as the following: General diet, high-caloric, low-caloric, light, soft, low-fat, low-cholesterol, high-vitamin, low-protein, high-protein, or liquid diet. If there is a good working relationship between the physician, dietitian, nurse, patient, and his family, modifications are made consistent with Dunlop's recommendations. Too often these diets are rigidly planned and administered and far too often deprive the patient of basic food needs either because they don't include them or because the diet, being unpalatable, is only partially eaten.

Responsibility of the Nurse. Although the physician prescribes the diet and it may be prepared and served by a dietary staff, there is still much expected of the nurse in the matter of feeding the patient. She, it may be repeated, is responsible for his being served the prescribed diets. She observes his likes and dislikes. This observation will guide her if she is preparing and serving the food herself, or she may report it to the dietary department if the patient is in the hospital. It is essential that the physician know whether the sick person is eating the food served to him. The nurse, who is with the patient almost constantly, is in the best position to estimate and report what he eats. She should be given and should accept the responsibility for his getting concentrated dietary supplements through some channel when his needs are not met by what he eats at meals. In some cases where the amount consumed must be accurately determined, as in metabolic disorders such as diabetes, food left on the tray is often weighed and measured. The

---

* Dunlop, D. M.: "Modern Trends in Therapeutic Dietetics," *Brit. J. Nutrition,* 4:225, (Feb.) 1950.

nurse is responsible, as far as possible, for making the patient comfortable and the surroundings pleasant at meal times. In some situations where there is no one who can do it so well as she, the nurse must plan, prepare, and serve the food. She may even have to select and purchase food supplies. Often the spacing of feedings is left to her. In many cases she is the person most able and best qualified to guide the planning of diets consistent with the doctor's orders, general health needs, and the family budget. She may also be the most experienced in selecting, buying, preparing, and serving foods and in modifying habits of eating. When the patient is helpless or acutely ill, it is her responsibility to feed him or to teach some member of the family to do so.

7. NURSING MEASURES IN ORAL FEEDING

Preparation of the Environment. The *room* should be well ventilated, quiet, and in order during meals and the patient undisturbed by treatments, dressings, visitors, or doctors' rounds. Also, in homes the atmosphere should be conducive to enjoyment of the meal. All disturbing sights should be removed, insofar as possible. In a ward, for example, disturbing patients are screened. In most institutions bedpans are offered at regular intervals between or half an hour before meals.

The patient's *bed* should be comfortable and orderly. All unappetizing objects (for example, a sputum container) should be out of sight, and the bedside stand made as attractive as possible.

The *table holding the tray of food* should be cleared except for flowers, which, if not overpowering, add to the pleasure of the meal. In every case the food is in front of the patient, who is in a comfortable position. When overbed tables are available, bedside stands should not be used, because the patient has to turn on his side, support himself with one elbow, and eat with one hand. A sick person will often give up the struggle before he has eaten as much as he would relish if he were more comfortable.

A return to normal habits should be encouraged; therefore, as soon as the patient is able to be up for part of the day, it is a good thing to draw a suitable table up to his chair and let him eat one or more meals sitting up. Patients are encouraged to eat in groups around a table when facilities are available.

Many very sick patients prefer not to have *visitors* during meals. While it is pleasant to share a meal with another, it is tiring to have to attend to a meal and a visitor at the same time. A member of the patient's family or an intimate friend may in some cases be a pleasure and, moreover, improve his appetite. Friends and volunteer workers are often asked to help nurses to feed patients. No hard and fast rule can be made for all situations. Because hospital regulations are made in the interests of the majority, however, in wards, visiting sometimes is restricted during meal hours. In private rooms and homes the visiting periods should be regulated according to the special demands of the patient.

The Patient's Diet. Since in many cases the patient's recovery depends largely upon his getting the prescribed diet, and errors may have far-reaching and serious results, hospitals usually have a rigid schedule about serving food. Lists of patients with the diets prescribed for each are posted in the divisional kitchen; trays are plainly marked with the names of the patients and often with the type of diet. Some terms used for diets are *regular* or *full, high-caloric, light, soft, liquid* or *fluid, strict* or *moderate low-sodium, nonconstipating,* and numerous others. (The general nature of some of them is suggested by the foods of which they are composed. More detailed information may be found in any textbook on dietetics.) Often colored cards are used to differentiate diets.

There is a great deal to learn about the successful feeding of persons on liquid diets. The inexperienced nurse thinks that any liquid may be given. Actually, this may not be intended, and she should determine, for example, whether milk is included in the liquids to be given a particular patient. C. J. Speas,[89] decrying the common tendency to omit some essential nutrients from liquid diets, has published one which he, with Milla Newland, has worked out. An analysis of this diet shows that it meets the present recommended daily requirements for fats, carbohydrates, proteins, minerals, and vitamins. When milk is eliminated from the diet, other nourishing fluids must be substituted. Eggs are an item in most high-caloric liquid diets. Sugars, such as lactose, and preparations, such as Cerelose, which are not as sweet as cane sugar may be used in fairly large quantities. Drinks that are neither sweet nor heavy are generally more easily tolerated in nausea than others. Ginger ale, although it has little food value, is often refreshing. (See Appendix VI.)

Preferences of the patient should be considered insofar as possible, and there are various ways of making them known to the person in charge of planning and serving diets. There is considerable disagreement as to whether patients should be asked what they want to eat, since this robs the meal of the pleasant element of surprise, pleasant to everyone, sick or well. The selection of dishes is often a bore and a person will name the first thing he thinks of, whereas there may be many he would enjoy more. To avoid both difficulties, hospitals have adopted the practice of printing advance menus. The patient chooses from a variety of dishes on Tuesday, for example, what he would like for dinner on Thursday and Friday. Checking a printed list requires little effort, and by the time the meal is served, the patient has usually forgotten what he selected. This system is expensive; therefore, simpler, if less effective, methods are ordinarily used in ward service. For example, dietitians on visits to patients may ask their likes, dislikes, and idiosyncrasies; or the nurse may make such notes and send them to the dietary department. Forms may be used indicating the beverage, or the cereal preferred, or how to cook eggs.

All medical workers should have specific knowledge of *racial, religious,* and *national habits of eating.* Having learned general customs, such as that Italians use olive oil rather than lard or butter in cooking, that the Chinese have rice and tea with all meals, that the orthodox Jew does not eat dairy products and meat in the same meal, nurses have some basis on which to plan meals for these people. In guiding patients in their homes in food selection and when discussing specific therapeutic diets, the nurse will find her suggestions much more likely to be followed if they do not run counter to the family's established dietary habits. It isn't possible

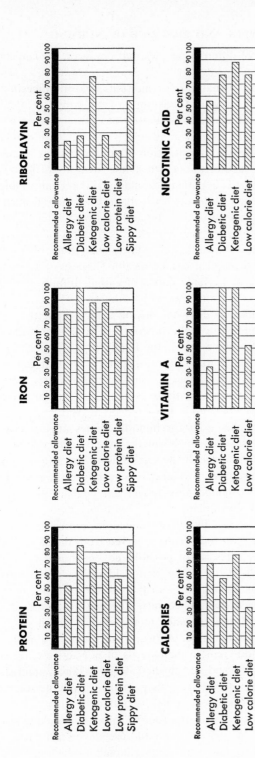

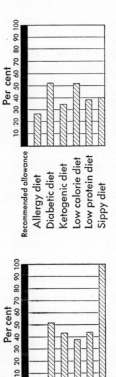

Figure 72. Comparison of nutrients in special therapeutic diets with recommended allowances. (Spies, Tom D.: "The Birmingham Study," *Rehabilitation through Better Nutrition.* W. B. Saunders Co., Philadelphia, 1947.)

413

to discuss here the characteristic diets of different peoples, but books on the subject are listed at the end of this chapter.

Preparation of the Patient for Meals.   Analysis of conditions favoring digestion indicates that in preparing anyone, sick or well, for eating, a calm frame of mind and a body free from pain and discomfort are important. Not even the most accomplished nurse can make every patient easy in mind and body, but that should be her aim. The means she uses will vary with the situation. Painful dressings or any upsetting event should be so scheduled as not to occur near the meal hour. Serious or upsetting topics should be avoided. The patient should be in a comfortable position and helped to feel fresh by having his hands washed and his mouth cleaned, or other steps taken according to the demands of the case and his own wishes. Some fastidious persons will demand more preparation than the distribution of nursing time provides; others will not realize until shown that cleanliness adds to the pleasure of meals and at the same time helps to control communicable diseases. Children, especially, require help in the practice of hygienic habits of eating. Infants should be changed, if necessary, and made comfortable before feedings.

Serving Diets.   The service has much to do with making a meal appetizing— or the reverse. Trays should be large enough to hold the contents without crowding. Linen covers are probably the most attractive, but if the family or institution cannot provide a sufficient number, it is better to substitute paper covers that can be fresh for each meal. The same observation applies to napkins. Silverware, glass, and china should be spotless, its arrangement on the tray similar to that used on the dining table. (See Fig. 73.) If the patient is left-handed, he will appreciate the thoughtful attendant who reverses the order for him. In homes an attractive and matching set of dishes should be selected; in hospitals there is a tendency to get away from institutional types of china. Gaily flowered dishes are often seen. A child will sometimes drink from a pretty cup when he would refuse the nourishment from an ordinary one. Chromium coffee pots and cream pitchers are good looking and easily cared for although silver plate is still commonly used.

A nurse, caring for one patient can usually serve a meal in courses. This is likely to make it more appetizing, since hot foods can be served from the stove and cold dishes from the refrigerator. When this is not possible, covers should be provided for hot dishes and every effort made to see that cold dishes are chilled. Hospital kitchens often serve trays on moving belts so that all food items can be put on them by a line of workers in a matter of seconds. The belt moves the tray onto elevators that take them in a few more seconds to the clinical division.

Small servings are more appetizing than large. A heaped-up plate is appalling to the sick, who are in many cases indifferent to their meals, if not actively averse to eating. It is wise to serve dainty meals and add to the caloric intake by nourishment between meals. Frequent feedings, however, if they spoil the appetite for the more substantial foods offered at mealtimes, should be discontinued.

A liquid diet *must* be fed at frequent intervals in order to get an adequate caloric intake. If the choice of fluids is left to the nurse, she should use some such guide as that developed by Speas and Newland. This should be adapted to each patient's needs and, of course, to the resources at hand. Ordinarily, hot drinks are most acceptable in the morning when the patient wakes up; warm, nourishing drinks are given to encourage sleep. If the patient has a fever, it is usually at its height in the afternoon; then cold drinks are particularly appealing. In feeding infants and very ill persons on liquid diets, punctuality is especially important. Since concentrated foods cannot so easily be used to make up the 24-hour food requirement, the loss of even one feeding is serious. Infant feedings are largely liquid, but the major aspects of this highly specialized subject are brought together for brief treatment on pages 403-5.

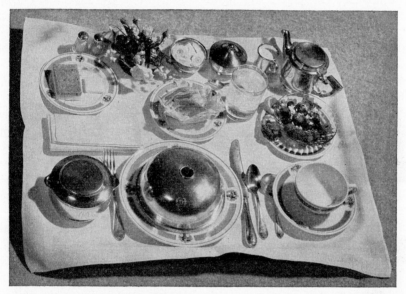

Figure 73. Dinner tray showing proper arrangement of dishes and silverware. (Courtesy of St. Lukes Hospital, New York City.)

Assistance in Eating and Rehabilitation of the Handicapped. Every normal person prefers to feed himself. Illness or disability may, however, reduce him to the helplessness of infancy. The need for assistance in getting food to the mouth is usually temporary; in rare cases it is a permanent handicap. It should be the aim of the nurse in every case to establish independence as soon as possible.

Brief and temporary help is usually needed when severe illness prostrates or weakens the patient or when burns and wounds make it impossible to use the hands or when the patient is in a respirator. Permanent help is required by anyone who loses the use of his arms and hands and who cannot be fitted with a functioning prosthesis. Some form of assistance is needed by many patients until they can adjust to their handicap and learn new techniques of eating.

The following are *general recommendations*: Help the patient into a comfortable position. Unless contraindicated by the nature of his disease, his head should be elevated and supported by pillows or a back rest. The tray of food should be within his range of vision; the sight of it whets his appetite and gives him the opportunity to suggest the rotation in which he wishes his food. The nurse should see that clothing and bedding are well protected so that the patient will not be afraid of soiling them.

If the nurse is seated, the patient loses his sense of hurry and some of his embarrassment over "causing so much trouble." A high stool that brings the nurse on a level with the patient is illustrated in Figure 71. Liquids are most easily taken through tubes. Glass tubes are seldom used, because expendable tubes of waxed paper, cellophane, or plastic are more satisfactory. (See Fig. 158.) Irrational patients and young children who may break glass tubes might possibly swallow a piece. If the nurse sees herself as the patient, she can usually feed him more naturally. He may occasionally suggest what he would like next, but if he has to do this often, it is tiring. No hard and fast rule can be made as to whether or not the nurse should talk during the meal. In some way she should convey the impression that she is glad to give this service and above all is not feeling hurried or bored. Friendly remarks every now and then certainly contribute to a pleasant atmosphere, while stories to which the patient must give close attention are likely to be a bore.

The patient will prefer to wipe his mouth himself if he possibly can. If he cannot, the nurse keeps him "neat." If the regular napkin is spread over his chest, an extra, small napkin that he can hold in his hand should be provided. Sometimes the patient cannot manipulate utensils but can hold bread and butter or celery in his hand. He should be encouraged to help himself up to the point of fatigue or frustration. An attempt should be made to judge the size of the mouthful to which he is accustomed. The nurse should avoid imposing on the patient her own eating habits. Any health teaching at mealtimes must be done skillfully; otherwise, it may irritate the patient and set up a psychological state inhibiting appetite and retarding digestion.

A sick or weak person can often feed himself if everything is within reach, bread buttered, and other foods cut into bits. Some sensitive individuals will leave food untasted rather than ask help.

The *blind* need special help in eating. Juliet Bindt,[90] blind herself, makes these suggestions: Help the person to use ordinary table appointments so that he acquires increasing independence. Place utensils in conventional positions, for this is where he expects to find them. Help the newly blinded to acquire the technique of locating what is before him with careful movements of his hand. It should be held half closed, palm down, and the little finger used as a feeler. Tell him in a low tone what foods are served him and give their location by imagining that the plate is a clock. For example, "The beef is at one o'clock, the potato at five, and the spinach at nine; celery and pickles are beside the plate at ten, and coffee at two o'clock." If there are shells, artichoke leaves, or bones to be discarded, provide an empty plate to separate waste from foods to be eaten. Try to treat him in every possible respect like a normal person, giving the help he needs inconspicuously rather than solicitously.

Persons with motor disabilities can usually feed themselves if they have devices and utensils suited to their handicap. Use of special devices and foods of special textures, however, should be reduced to a minimum because dependence upon them is itself a handicap in visiting or traveling. The child with cerebral palsy, the adult with an injury to the motor area of the brain, or with a disease such as paralysis agitans or muscular dystrophy that affects motor power, coordination, or both, needs special help. Everything possible should be done to enable him to feed himself, but his rehabilitation should be so gradual that he is never discouraged by his failures. When a meal becomes a physical struggle it ceases to be a pleasure, and he is likely to eat less than he needs. Marjorie Abel[91] points out

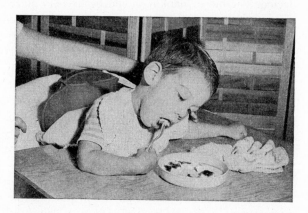

Figure 74. The child with cerebral palsy can learn to feed himself with help and encouragement from the nurse and his parents. (Abel, Marjorie: "Feeding the Child with Cerebral Palsy," *Am. J. Nursing,* **50:**558, [July] 1950.)

that a 12-year-old child with cerebral palsy may require 6000 calories daily because tension and muscle spasm set his energy expenditure at such a high point. The child and the mother must be helped to relax and enjoy mealtime; otherwise, it is difficult to get him to meet his nutritional needs. Foods are selected primarily to meet nutritional requirements, but they should be chosen also for the ease with which the patient can eat them. Those with motor handicaps may be able, for example, to grasp a banana, a hard-boiled egg, or celery. Food textures must be considered, especially when the muscles used in swallowing are affected.

The child should sit in a chair that gives him optimum support at a table of the right height. Ethel D. Patterson[92] and Alice B. Morrissey[93] show a number of mechanical aids for those with motor disabilities. These include: a table with depressions into which dishes can be set to keep them from sliding out of place; utensils with cylindrical or built-up handles, designed to give maximum contact when grasped; forks and spoons with short handles to help those with poor coordination; others with lengthened or bent handles to serve those whose motion is limited; cups with handles; drinking tubes in cartons, and glasses with crocheted jackets to help prevent spilling liquids; bands, into which a fork or spoon can be fixed for those who lack the muscle power to hold one; plates with rims to prevent food from being pushed onto the table by the hand with limited control; and lastly the rocker splint that supports the arm in an elevated flexed position while allowing a range of motion that enables the patient to get his food to his mouth.

While in some cases it may be easier to teach the handicapped more independence in eating when he is alone with the medical worker, communal eating should be the goal in most cases. Patients can sit at the table in wheelchairs and can come on crutches. A sufficient number of trained persons should be present to give them whatever help they may need. Music is conducive to a relaxed atmosphere for most, but it must be unobtrusive; otherwise, it will distract or irritate.

Whenever there is poor control of table utensils, the clothing should be protected. The bib or napkin should be fixed in place. It should have a top absorbent layer and a waterproof lining. Disposable protectors are best, economically and esthetically.

Feeding the Moribund and Unconscious.   Although it is more and more common in hospitals to nourish the very ill extraorally with intravenous infusions and with intubations, these methods may be impossible in homes, and most people can be successfully fed orally if their attendants have sufficient time and patience. The touch of a spoon on the lips or the presence of food in the mouth elicits the swallowing reflex even when all cerebral activity seems to have ceased, as in severe illness. In such cases food must be given very slowly, very frequently, and in small amounts. Eye droppers, cups with spouts, and tubes of various kinds are used in the care of both children and adults, according to their condition and the particular demands of the case. Food put into the mouth of a deeply unconscious patient may, however, be sucked into the lungs instead of the esophagus. Paralysis or dystrophy of the muscles of swallowing makes oral feeding hazardous, and food must be put into the patient's mouth with extreme care. Many unconscious patients die from lung infections as a result of oral feeding or of the drippings from tube feedings. A weak cough reflex and inactivity contribute toward the development of pneumonitis and lung abscess. When a patient with weakened reflexes is fed by mouth, a suctioning device should be at hand if possible. Motor-driven suctioning machines may, in some situations, be rented from hospital supply houses for home use.

Records and Charting in Oral Feeding.   All medical workers rely upon the nurse's reports on the amount the patient eats, his appetite, likes and dislikes, and any resultant discomfort from feeding. The nature of these reports varies according to the patient's condition and the importance of diet in his treatment. Detailed reports are made, for example, on the feeding of babies and young children because so much depends upon their getting the proper amount and kind of food and because they are unable to describe their needs and difficulties. In acute illness careful reports must be made because the physician prescribes other methods of feeding if insufficient food is being taken by mouth. In diabetes and other metabolic diseases it is sometimes necessary to weigh and measure and record the food left on the patient's tray in order to make a sufficiently accurate estimate of the food intake to serve as a basis for the prescribed therapy.

Written reports on diet and feeding may be incorporated in the nurse's notes, as her daily running comments are usually called, or special forms may be provided.

8. EXTRAORAL METHODS OF FEEDING

Indications for Extraoral Methods of Feeding.   There are some conditions that make oral feeding impossible, ineffective, or undesirable. Examples of such conditions are disease, with or without surgical treatment, of the alimentary tract, persistent nausea and vomiting, or refusal of food. In such cases the physician may prescribe nutritive infusions (injections into the veins), oral or nasal gavage (the administration of liquid foods through a tube inserted into the esophagus and stomach by way of the mouth and/or nose), and less frequently the administration of nutrients by rectum. This last method is believed almost totally ineffective. Operations on the upper alimentary tract may necessitate temporary or permanent feedings through an opening made from the stomach or small intestine to the abdominal wall.

Nutritive Infusions.   The practice of administering nutrient solutions into the veins during *brief periods* of illness has been referred to earlier as the preferred substitute for oral feeding. With modern asepsis and improved knowledge of needle injection, there seems to be comparatively little danger from infection, mechanical injury, or chemical poisoning. It is difficult to use this technique in homes, however, and with very active or irrational patients. The veins of infants are so small that introduction of a needle presents a problem. In some cases physicians introduce the nutritive solution by needle injection through the abdominal wall into the peritoneal cavity.

Dextrose or glucose, which can be given in 2 to 10 per cent solutions, or in even more concentrated forms, is similar to blood sugar, so that the food is immediately made available to the tissues through the circulating fluids. Salts of sodium, potassium, and calcium; chlorides; and phosphates are introduced alone or in combination with dextrose. Predigested proteins and vitamins are also given by infusion, while plasma and whole blood constitute an important part of intravenous feeding. When fats and fat-soluble vitamins can be given parenterally, the patient can get a complete diet extraorally as long as the veins will carry it.[94] Because the method of giving nutrients by infusion differs in no respect from the administration of drugs given this way, the technique is described in Chapter 26 (see pp. 741 and 746).

Rectal Feeding.   Nutritive enemas and the drop-by-drop method of rectal feeding known as proctoclysis were used extensively at one time. There is great doubt that an appreciable amount of nutrient is absorbed from the colon. It is generally agreed that the only foods that could be absorbed this way are dextrose, a simple sugar, and salts. Since both the distention of the colon and the presence of a foreign body in the anus can stimulate the defecation impulse, it is difficult to use this method of feeding with any degree of success. The techniques of rectal feeding and medication of the colon are so much alike that they are treated together in Chapter 30.

Gastric and Nasal Gavage. The word *gavage* comes from the French *gaver*, meaning to gorge fowls. In medical practice gavage is associated with the idea of forcible feeding, since it is most often used for psychiatric patients who refuse to eat. Gavage is a method of introducing liquid food into the stomach through a tube that has been passed into the esophagus and stomach through the nose and/or mouth.

Gavage is often employed in the practice of medicine. It has an advantage over other unnatural methods of feeding in that it allows the administration of a complete

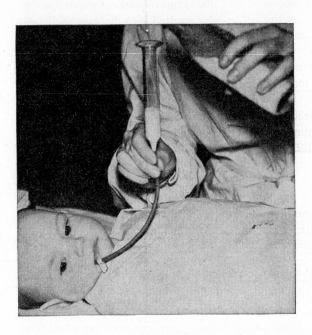

Figure 75. Gavage of an infant, showing mummy restraint. (Courtesy of Bellevue Hospital School of Nursing, New York City, and Clay-Adams Co., New York City.)

diet. Its common uses are as follows: (when the patient refuses food; when conditions of the mouth or esophagus make swallowing difficult or impossible; when operations on the mouth make it desirable to keep it as clean, dry, and as inactive as possible; and when the patient is unconscious.)

The feeding must be in liquid form, but the mixture may contain a wide variety of ingredients. Electric grinders and blenders reduce almost any foods to particles small enough to pass through a tube. Most texts on psychiatry deal with this subject in detail. The liquid diet of Speas and Newland is suitable for gavage. No single formula should be taken as a standard. The diet administered by gavage should be calculated for each child or adult with even more care than that given by mouth, since the patient's appetite does not control what he eats.

Among the *articles* of equipment required for this procedure is a feeding tube, the length and caliber of which depend upon whether the oral or nasal route is used and upon the size of the individual. In general, small tubes cause less irritation than large ones, but unless the food mixture is thin, there is some danger of their clogging. It is desirable to use a tube marked off in centimeters or inches so that it is not necessary to indicate the length of insertion with an adhesive strip. A bowl of ice to cool and stiffen the tube is usually advocated. A lubricant for the tube should be used. Oil softens the tube and may be disagreeable to taste and touch. Glycerin is believed by some authorities to be the most satisfactory substitute. An ideal lubricant for this purpose has not been found. It is possible that sterilized milk or cream might be the best choice.

The lubricant should be applied to the tube with a "Celluwipe" (paper square). If the tube is dipped in a liquid, such as milk or glycerin, make sure that the blind end is not left filled with the fluid, because this may drop into the larynx during the passage of the tube. A drop of mineral oil, because it is not absorbed by the lung tissue, acts as a foreign body. Water-soluble lubricants dropped into the larynx can strangulate and might carry infectious organisms, but on the whole they are not so dangerous as the hydrocarbons. The tube should be open at the side rather than at the end. A funnel or syringe is inserted in the open end. An effective clamp must be provided. If the tube is brought to the bedside in a covered container on a tray with the feeding beside it in an attractive pitcher, the patient is less likely to be offended and his appetite destroyed by a method of feeding, unesthetic at best. Because the food is not warmed by chewing and swallowing, it should be heated to body temperature.

There is some question whether gavage is a medical or nursing procedure. In some institutions it is performed by the medical staff; in others by the nursing staff. Certainly, there are dangers of mechanical injury to the tract, of strangulation, and of lung infections, from allowing the tube or some part of the feeding to enter the respiratory passages. Such dangers can be prevented, and, since there are many situations in which there is no physician available to give this service, it seems important that the nurse at least know how to carry out the procedure. When she must assume responsibility for gavaging the patient, she should insist that a physician give the first feeding in order to determine whether there is any obstruction to the passage of the tube. The patient should be *protected* by a large waterproof bib, and paper handkerchiefs are needed to wipe mucus from the mouth and to wrap the tube where the operator holds it. The operator usually wears a waterproof apron as vomiting sometimes occurs. There is also, with resistant disturbed psychotic patients, considerable danger of soiling the clothing.

Gavage is performed with the patient in either a lying or sitting position. While the passage of the tube may be facilitated by the sitting position, nausea is less likely to occur when the patient is recumbent.

Some *restraint of the patient may be necessary* if he is an infant, is irrational, or is resisting gavage. His cooperation should be gained if possible, since physical and psychic resistance interferes with digestion and may even cause nausea and vomiting, greatly increasing the danger of strangulation and mechanical injury.

If restraint is necessary, it should be limited to essentials. The operator should be calm, quiet, and reassuring. In the case of the patient who has refused to eat, there should be no implication that he is being punished, although the dread of the tube feeding often acts as an incentive to eat. In such case the gavage should not be administered until the patient has refused the food served to him, and he should be given to understand that the treatment will be discontinued as soon as he resumes normal eating.

Passage of the tube through the nose is probably less irritating and less likely to cause nausea and gagging than that through the mouth. Nasal gavage must be employed when the patient is likely to interfere with the treatment by biting the tube or when there has been an operation on the mouth. The procedure should be thoroughly explained to him, and directions given to breathe deeply as the tube is passed. This tends to relax the voluntary muscles and to divert the person from his discomfort. The operator should tell the patient to swallow as the tube reaches the mouth of the esophagus; this act is intended to carry the tube into the opening and inhibit gagging. Directions to swallow should be repeated every few seconds and the tube pushed downward immediately afterward, each time the esophagus relaxes.

There are several methods of *determining whether the tube is in the alimentary or the respiratory tract*. If the tube has been passed through the larynx, it will be impossible for the patient to speak; if the funnel or syringe barrel is inverted in water, bubbles of air will appear, and there will be hissing breath sounds at the open end of the tube. Gurgling noises from the stomach may be mistaken for breath sounds, however; so one of the first two means of determining the position of the tube should be used.

After the tube is in place, it is desirable to wait for a few minutes until persistalsis has subsided before *introducing the feeding,* which should be allowed to flow in slowly. Nausea and vomiting seem more likely to occur if the food is given rapidly. At the end of the feeding, allow some water to pass through the tube to remove food particles and thereby lessen the danger of insufflation of the feeding as the tube is drawn through the pharynx.

To remove the tube, adjust the clamp securely before all the fluid flows from the tube and it is filled with air. Remove the tube gently but quickly to shorten a disagreeable process, to prevent passage of air into the stomach, and to lessen the danger of the entrance of some of the feeding into the trachea.

Clamping the tube is most important. If this is not done, the liquid will run out as the tube is withdrawn and almost certainly cause insufflation. The patient should remain as quiet as possible after the *treatment* in order to lessen the tendency to nausea and vomiting.

In recording nasal or oral gavage it is usual to state which method was used, the time of administration, the kind and amount of food, and the patient's reaction.[95]

Gastrostomy and Enterostomy Feedings. When tumors or operations on the upper alimentary tract make it impossible for food to reach the intestine by the normal route, it may be necessary to bring a part of the stomach or the small intestine to the abdominal wall and make an artificial opening, or mouth, through which food can be passed into the part of the alimentary tract remaining. In malignancies of the esophagus an artificial gullet is sometimes made on the outside of the body after an esophagectomy has been performed so that food can be eaten and swallowed. While it is possible to maintain life without the pleasure of eating, this loss makes any semblance of normal living difficult. It is therefore desirable to make gastrostomy or enterostomy feedings as much like an ordinary meal as possible.

Nutritional needs are estimated as with any patient. These may be supplied by intravenous feedings until the operative site has begun to heal, but within the first week after surgery, fluids will be passed through a tube left by the surgeon in the false mouth opening, until its patency is established. The nature of the feeding will be prescribed by the physician, but the formula for a liquid diet as given in the nutrition texts is usually used. It is, of course, necessary for the food to be ground sufficiently fine to pass through the tube; on the other hand, it need not be of so thin a consistency as that used for nasal feedings. The mixture should be carried to the bedside on an attractive tray and in a glass or china pitcher, preferably the latter unless the mixture is appetizing in appearance. The funnel and tubing, which must be attached to the tube in the artificial mouth, should be of glass or plastic and carried on the tray in a paper napkin. An effort should be made to make the tray look like a feeding and not an irrigation.

As one can imagine, the patient doomed to this unnatural way of eating is suffering a profound psychic shock. In cases where the esophagus or stomach has been cauterized by poison or where accidents have destroyed their integrity, the patient's life may not be threatened, but usually he faces death in a few months or years. He must be given time in which to grieve and learn to accept his fate. As he does, normal desires and appetites return. He will long to taste food, and the longing will usually overcome his repugnance to the way in which this desire may be partially satisfied.

When the patient is ready for it, he should be encouraged to take food into his mouth, taste and chew it, and then spit it into the funnel. It may be necessary to wash it down into the tubing with water poured from a pitcher. The process of tasting and spitting out the entire meal is too time consuming for most patients, but they should decide how much food they want to put through this process. The saliva mixed with the food is conducive but not essential to its digestion.

Obviously, the individual will want privacy for this procedure, or the presence of the necessary helper only. As soon as possible he should learn to feed himself. Although the nurse, relative, or friend who is helping him should try to allay his fear that his condition repels others, the person with a permanent gastrostomy must learn to accept the idea of "eating" alone.

Almost any item of diet that the patient relishes is usually allowed him, although he should progress slowly from a simple to a general, or full, diet before he tries out less easily digested foods. If the small intestine is intact and healthy, there is no reason why he cannot take care of his ordinary diet when it is reduced to the suitable consistency. If his former diet has been incomplete, however, he should be helped to recognize and correct this condition.

REFERENCES

1. De Castro, Josué: *The Geography of Hunger.* Little, Brown and Co., Boston, 1952.
2. Barr, Stringfellow: *Citizens of the World.* Doubleday and Co., New York, 1952.
3. Huxley, Julian S.: *On Living in a Revolution.* Harper & Brothers, New York, 1944.
4. Osborn, Fairfield: *Our Plundered Planet.* Little, Brown and Co., Boston, 1948.
5. Tranter, G. A.: *We Are What We Eat.* Currawong Publishing Co., Ltd., Sydney, Australia, 1945.
6. Mills, Clarence A: *Climate Makes the Man.* Harper & Brothers, New York, 1942.
7. Sherman Henry C., and Lanford, Caroline S.: *Essentials of Nutrition,* 3rd ed. The Macmillan Company, New York, 1951, pp. 318, 351, 353.
8. Sherman, Henry C., and Lanford, Caroline S.: *op. cit.,* p. 346.
9. US Bureau of Human Nutrition and Home Economics: *Helping Families Plan Food Budgets.* US Department of Agriculture, Misc. Publ., US Government Printing Office, Washington, D.C., 1948, No. 662.
10. Bureau of Human Nutrition and Home Economics: *Family Fare: Food Management and Recipes.* US Department of Agriculture, Home and Garden Bull., No. 1, US Government Printing Office, Washington, D.C., 1950.
11. Rose, Mary S.: *Feeding the Family,* 4th ed. The Macmillan Company, New York, 1940.
12. Jeans, Philip C., and Marriott, William M.: *Infant Nutrition,* 4th ed. C. V. Mosby Co., St. Louis, 1947.
13. Gillett, Lucy H.: *Nutrition in Public Health.* W. B. Saunders Co., Philadelphia, 1946.
14. Parran, Thomas: "Nutrition in Public Health Programs," *Nutrition Rev.,* **4:**129, (May) 1946.
15. Downes, Jean, and Barandvsky, Anne: "An Experiment in Nutrition Teaching by Public Health Nurses," *Milbank Mem. Fund Quart.,* **23:**227, (July) 1945.
16. DuBois, Eugene F.: *Fever and the Regulation of Body Temperature.* Charles C Thomas, Publisher, Springfield, Ill., 1948.
17. Best, Charles H., and Taylor, Norman B.: *The Physiological Basis of Medical Practice,* 5th ed. Williams & Wilkins Co., Baltimore, 1950, p. 659.
18. Weller, John M., and Taylor, Isaac M.: "Some Problems of Potassium Metabolism," *Ann. Int. Med.,* **33:**607, 1950.
19. Retterbush, William C.: "Potassium Metabolism," *M. Arts & Sc.,* **4:**9, (first quarter) 1950.
20. Best, Charles H., and Taylor, Norman B.: *op. cit.,* p. 690.
21. Boyd, Eldon M.: "A Differential Lipid Analysis of Blood Plasma in Normal Young Women by Micro-Oxidative Methods," *J. Biol. Chem.,* **101:**323, (June) 1933.
22. Best, Charles H., and Taylor, Norman B.: *op. cit.,* pp. 134, 694.
23. McAmis, Avor J., et al.: "Growth of Rats on Fat-Free Diets," *J. Biol. Chem.,* **82:**247, (May) 1929.
24. Vinther-Paulsen, N.: "Investigations of the Actual Food Intake of Elderly Chronically Hospitalized Patients," *J. Gerontol.,* **5:**331, (Oct.) 1950.
25. Community Service Society, Nutrition Service: *Foods for Health—As We Grow Older.* The Society, New York, 1949.
26. Lewis, Howard B.: "Problems in Nutrition," *J.A.M.A.,* **138:**207, (Sept.) 1948.
27. Ohlson, Margaret A., et al.: "Studies of the Protein Requirements of Women," *J. Am. Dietet. A.,* **24:**744, (Sept.) 1948.
28. Slonaker, James R.: "The Effect of Different Per Cents of Protein in the Diet in Successive Generations," *Am. J. Physiol.,* **123:**526, (Aug.) 1938.

29. Jacobs, Eugene C.: "Effects of Starvation on Sex Hormones in the Male." *J. Clin. Endocrinol.*, **8:**227, (Mar.) 1947.
30. Keys, Ancel: "Human Starvation and Its Consequences," *J. Am. Dietet. A.*, **22:**582, (July) 1946.
31. Schaeffer, Alexander J.: "Effect of Certain Amino Acids on Healing of Experimental Wounds of the Cornea," *Proc. Soc. Exper. Biol. & Med.*, **61:**165, (Feb.) 1946.
32. Elman, Robert: *Parenteral Alimentation in Surgery with Special Reference to Proteins and Amino Acids.* Paul B. Hoeber, New York, 1947.
33. Lund, Charles C., and Levenson, Stanley M.: "Protein in Surgery," *J.A.M.A.*, **128:**95, (May) 1945.
34. Sherman Henry C.: *Food and Health.* The Macmillan Company, New York, 1947, p. 73.
35. American Medical Association, Council on Food and Nutrition: *Handbook of Nutrition.* Blakiston Co., Philadelphia, 1951, p. 15.
36. Cuthbertson, D. P.: "Quality and Quantity of Protein in Relation to Human Health and Nutrition," *Nutrition Abstr. & Rev.*, **10:**1, (July) 1940.
37. MacLeod, Grace, and Taylor, Clara M.: *Rose's Foundations of Nutrition*, 4th ed. The Macmillan Company, New York, 1944, p. 146.
38. Sherman, Henry C., and Lanford, Caroline S.: *op. cit.*, p. 125.
39. Sherman, Henry C., and Lanford, Caroline S.: *op. cit.*, p. 142.
40. Sherman, Henry C., and Lanford, Caroline S.: *op. cit.*, p. 150.
41. Kimball, O. P.: "Endemic Goiter—A Food Deficiency Disease," *J. Am. Dietet. A.*, **25:**112, (Feb.) 1949.
42. Maxcy, Kenneth F. (ed.): *Rosenau's Preventive Medicine and Hygiene*, 7th ed. Appleton-Century-Crofts, Inc., New York, 1952, p. 588.
42a. Goodman, Louis S., and Gilman, Alfred: *The Pharmacological Basis of Therapeutics*, 2nd ed. The Macmillan Company, New York, 1955, p. 809.
43. Smith, Francis H.: "Potassium Deficiency in Gastrointestinal Disease," *Gastroenterology*, **16:**73, (Sept.) 1950.
44. Randall, H. T., et al.: "Potassium Deficiency in Surgical Patients," *Surgery*, **26:**341, (Mar.) 1949.
45. Sherman, Henry C., and Lanford, Caroline S.: *op. cit.*, p. 205.
46. King, Charles G.: "Vitamin C," *J.A.M.A.*, **142:**563, (Feb.) 1950.
47. Eddy, Walter H., and Dalldorf, Gilbert: *The Avitaminoses.* Williams & Wilkins Co., Baltimore, 1944, p. 212.
48. Sherman, Henry C., and Lanford, Caroline S.: *op. cit.*, p. 211.
49. American Medical Association, Council on Foods and Nutrition: *op. cit.*, p. 166.
50. Jolliffe, Norman, et al. (eds.): *Clinical Nutrition.* Paul B. Hoeber, New York, 1950 p. 512.
51. American Medical Association, Council on Foods and Nutrition: *op. cit.*, p. 217.
52. Bethell, Frank H., et al.: "Cobalamin (Vitamin B$_{12}$) and the Intrinsic Factor of Castle," *Ann. Int. Med.*, **35:**518, 1951.
53. Yamamoto, R., et al.: "Further Studies on the Absorption of Vitamin B$_{12}$ Following Oral and Parenteral Administration," *J. Nutrition*, **45:**507, (Aug.) 1951.
54. Jolliffe, Norman, et al. (eds.) *op. cit.*, p. 420.
55. Jukes, T. H., and Stokstad, E. L. R.: "Pteroylglutamic Acid and Related Compounds," *Physiol. Rev.*, **28:**106, 1948.
56. Bogert, L. Jean: *Nutrition and Physical Fitness.* W. B. Saunders Co., Philadelphia, 1949, p. 261.
57. Guilbert, H. R., et al.: "Minimum Vitamin A and Carotene Requirement of Mammalian Species," *J. Nutrition*, **19:**91, (Jan.) 1940.
58. Krestin, D.: "Prophylaxis of Rickets by Single Massive Doses of Vitamin D," *Brit. M. J.*, **1:**78, (Jan.) 1945.
59. Jolliffe, Norman, et al. (eds.): *op. cit.*, p. 449.
60. American Medical Association, Council on Food and Nutrition: *op. cit.*, p. 219.
61. Sherman, Henry C., and Lanford, Caroline S.: *op. cit.*, p. 295.

62. Shemiakin, M. M., et al.: "Studies in the Vitamin K Group," *J. Am. Chem. Soc.,* **65:**264, (Nov.) 1943.
63. Bogert, L. Jean: *op. cit.,* p. 286.
64. Abbott, William E.: "A Review of the Present Concepts on Fluid Balance," *Am. J. M. Sc.,* **211:**232, (Feb.) 1946.
65. Gamble, James L.: *Chemical Anatomy, Physiology and Pathology of Extracellular Fluid,* 5th ed. Harvard University Press, Cambridge, 1947.
66. Shindler, Frederick P.: "Considerations of Postoperative Electrolyte and Fluid Replacement," *California Med.,* **73:**309, (Oct.) 1950.
67. Darrow, Daniel C., and Pratt, Edward L.: "Fluid Therapy," *J.A.M.A.,* **143:**432, (June) 1950.
68. DuBois, Eugene F.: *Basal Metabolism in Health and Disease,* 3rd ed. Lea & Febiger, Philadelphia, 1936.
69. Henry, George W.: "Basal Metabolism and Emotional States," *J. Nerv. & Ment. Dis.,* **70:**598, (Dec.) 1929.
70. MacLeod, Grace, and Taylor, Clara M.: *op. cit.,* p. 61.
71. Rorty, James: "The Thin Rats Bury the Fat Rats," *Harper's Magazine,* **198:**28, (May) 1949.
72. Veblen, Thorstein: *The Theory of the Leisure Class.* Modern Library, New York, 1923.
73. Dublin, Louis I.: *The Facts of Life from Birth to Death.* The Macmillan Company, New York, 1951, p. 355.
74. Metropolitan Life Insurance Company: *Weight Control Materials.* The Company, New York, 1951.
75. Spock, Benjamin: *The Common Sense Book of Baby and Child Care.* Duell, Sloan and Pearce, Inc., New York, 1946, p. 33.
76. Senn, Milton J. E., and Newill, Phyllis K.: *All About Feeding Children.* Doubleday, Doran and Co., Inc., New York, 1944, p. 6.
77. Senn, Milton J. E. (ed.): *Problems of Infancy and Childhood. Transactions of the Fourth Conference, New York, March, 1950.* Josiah Macy, Jr. Foundation, New York, 1951.
78. Aldrich, C. Anderson, and Aldrich, Mary M.: *Feeding Our Old Fashioned Children.* The Macmillan Company, New York, 1941.
79. Nelson, Waldo E. (ed.): *Mitchell-Nelson Textbook of Pediatrics.* W. B. Saunders Co., Philadelphia, 1950, p. 143.
80. Vischer, A. L.: *Old Age; Its Compensations and Rewards.* The Macmillan Company, New York, 1947, p. 31.
81. Vilter, Richard W., and Thompson, Carl: "Nutrition and the Control of Chronic Disease," *Pub. Health Rep.,* **66:**630, (May) 1951.
82. Vilter, Richard W., and Thompson, Carl: *op. cit.*
83. Rynearson, E. H., and Gastineau, C. F.: *Obesity.* Charles C Thomas, Publisher, Springfield, Ill., 1949.
84. Bureau of Human Nutrition and Home Economics: *Food Guide for Older Folks.* US Department of Agriculture, US Government Printing Office, Washington, D.C., 1952.
85. Spies, Tom D.: *Rehabilitation Through Better Nutrition.* W. B. Saunders Co., Philadelphia, 1947.
86. Community Service Society, Nutrition Service: *Foods for Health—As We Grow Older.* The Society, New York, 1949.
87. Cannon, Walter B.: *The Wisdom of the Body.* W. W. Norton & Co., New York, 1939.
88. Haggard, Howard N., and Greenberg, Leon A.: *Diet and Physical Efficiency.* Yale University Press, New Haven, 1935.
89. Speas, C. J.: "The Liquid Therapeutic Diet," *J. Tennessee M. A.,* **43:**321, (Sept.) 1950.
90. Bindt, Juliet: *A Handbook for the Blind.* The Macmillan Company, New York, 1952.
91. Abel, Marjorie: "Feeding the Child with Cerebral Palsy," *Am. J. Nursing,* **50:**558, (Sept.) 1950.

92. Patterson, Ethel D.: "The Public Health Nurse's Role in Feeding the Handicapped Child," *Pub. Health Nursing,* **43:**559, (Oct.) 1951.
93. Morrissey, Alice B.: *Rehabilitation Nursing.* G. P. Putnam's Sons, New York, 1951, p. 70.
94. Stare, Frederick, and Geyer, Robert P.: "Fat in Parenteral Nutrition," *Surg., Gynec. and Obst.,* **92:**246, (Feb.) 1951.
95. Henry, George W.: *Essentials of Psychiatry,* 3rd ed. Williams & Wilkins Co., Baltimore, 1938, p. 325.

Additional Suggested Reading

Bland, John H.: *The Clinical Use of Fluid Electrolyte.* J. B. Lippincott Co., Philadelphia, 1952.

Boudreau, Frank, et al.: *International Approaches to the Problem of Undeveloped Areas.* Milbank Memorial Fund, New York, 1948.

Chatfield, Charlotte, et al.: "Changes in World Consumption of Calories and Proteins Over the Last Decade," *Milbank Mem. Fund Quart.,* **28:**103, (Apr.) 1950.

Chitre, R. G., et al.: "Nutritive Value of Canned Foods," *J. Nutrition,* **42:**207, (Oct.) 1950.

Clark, G. W.: *A Vitamin Digest.* Charles C Thomas, Publisher, Springfield, Ill., 1951.

Eddy, Walter H.: *Vitaminology.* Williams & Wilkins Co., Baltimore, 1949.

Elman, Robert "Fluid Balance from the Nurse's Point of View," *Am. J. Nursing,* **49:**531, (Aug.) 1949.

Follis, Richard H.: *The Pathology of Nutritional Disease.* Charles C Thomas, Publisher, Springfield, Ill., 1948.

Gaunt, Robert, and Birnie, J. H.: *Hormones and Body Water.* Charles C Thomas, Publisher, Springfield, Ill., 1948.

Hawley, Estelle E., and Carden, Grace: *The Art and Science of Nutrition,* 3rd ed., C. V. Mosby Co., St. Louis, 1949.

Homann, R. E., Jr.: "Fluid and Electrolyte Therapy in Surgical Patients," *Am. J. Surg.,* **81:**10, (Jan.) 1951.

Keys, Ancel, et al.: *The Biology of Human Starvation.* University of Minnesota Press, Minneapolis, 1950.

Krause, Marie V.: *Nutrition and Diet Therapy in Relation to Nursing.* W. B. Saunders Co., Philadelphia, 1952.

Lee, Frank A.: "Nutritional Value of Frozen Foods," *Nutrition Rev.,* **9:**1, (Jan.) 1951.

McDougall, Frank L.: *Food and Population.* Carnegie Endowment for International Peace, New York, 1952.

Moyer, Carl A.: *Fluid Balance.* Year Book Publishers, Chicago, 1952.

Ohlson, Margaret A.: "Dietary Requirements of Aging Women," *Am. J. Nursing,* **48:**706, (Nov.) 1948.

Pollack, Herbert, and Halpern, Seymour L.: *Therapeutic Nutrition.* National Academy of Sciences—National Research Council, Washington, D.C., 1952.

Proudfit, Fairfax J., and Robinson, Corinne H.: *Nutrition and Diet Therapy,* 11th ed. The Macmillan Company, New York, 1955.

Royce, Stephen, et al.: "Indwelling Polyethylene Nasogastric Tube for Feeding Premature Infants," *Pediatrics,* **8:**79, (July) 1951.

Sherman, Henry C.: *Chemistry of Food and Nutrition.* 8th ed. The Macmillan Company, New York, 1952.

————: *The Nutritional Improvement of Life.* Columbia University Press, New York, 1950.

Shoun, Frances N., and Jones, Jana W.: "Nutrition Education and Public Health Nursing," *Am. J. Nursing,* **48:**430, (July) 1948.

Stone, Simon: "Evaluation of Vitamin E Therapy in Psychiatric Disorders," *Dis. Nerv. System,* **11:**355, (Dec.) 1950.

Turner, Dorothea F.: *Handbook of Diet Therapy,* rev. ed. University of Chicago Press, Chicago, 1952.

Vitamin Manual. The Upjohn Company, Kalamazoo, Mich., 1953.

Watt, Bernice K., and Merrill, Annabel L.: *Composition of Foods—Raw, Processed, Prepared.* Bureau of Human Nutrition and Home Economics, US Department of Agriculture, Washington, D.C., 1950.

Weng, Lorraine: "Establishing Good Food Habits," *Am. J. Nursing,* **50:**155, (Mar.) 1950.

Wood, Bertha M.: *Foods of the Foreign-Born.* M. Barrows & Co., Boston, 1929.

World Health Organization: *Prevention of Severe Malnutrition in Times of Disaster.* Technical Report No. 45, Columbia University Press, New York, 1951.

CHAPTER 14. PROVISION FOR ELIMINATION

1. IMPORTANCE OF ELIMINATION
2. ELIMINATION OF WASTE FROM THE INTESTINES
3. ELIMINATION OF WASTE BY THE KIDNEYS
4. INCONTINENCE OF BOWEL AND BLADDER
5. RECORDING ELIMINATION

1. IMPORTANCE OF ELIMINATION

Elimination in Health and in Disease.   As seen in the previous chapter, the quality of life depends upon diet, digestion, and assimilation; but equally important is elimination of metabolic waste products.

The excretory organs are the kidneys, bowels, skin, and, of course, the lungs as a means of eliminating carbon dioxide. So important is their function that urinalysis is included in all physical examinations, the patient is always questioned on bowel habits, and the feces often examined. The function of the skin and lungs as organs of elimination is not discussed in this chapter.

So important is elimination in disease that if the kidneys and bowels can be kept active so that waste is eliminated as fast as formed, the patient will have a good chance of recovery. There is always great danger, however, that excessive wastes of metabolism or bacterial or chemical toxins may be so irritating to the organs of elimination (especially the kidneys) that they break down. Constipation can cause discomfort and even injury, but when the kidneys "shut down," death occurs within a matter of hours or a few days. Elimination of water and dissolved substances in the form of sweat is physiological, but when this function is partly destroyed, as with burned patients, the kidneys can often compensate. The critical nature of elimination of carbon dioxide by the lungs was discussed in Chapter 10. We all know that death follows respiratory failure within a few minutes, although resuscitation is possible if instituted soon enough.

Responsibility of the Nurse.   In her capacity as *health teacher*, a nurse has many opportunities to teach healthful habits of elimination, and to prevent disease by encouraging periodic health examinations.

In her *care of the sick* the nurse helps to provide conditions that promote proper elimination. For infants, and for all those too sick to assume the responsibility for themselves, the nurse notes the number, quantity, and character of eliminations

429

from the bowels and kidneys. In answer to a critic of present-day nursing, who thought giving and emptying bedpans waste of a "professional" nurse's time, Sally Johnson, the teacher and leader of nurses, said that the macroscopic examination of excretions by the nurse is just as "professional" a function as the microscopic or chemical examination by the physician. Nurses should cultivate the habit of noting the appearance and odor of body discharges as indexes of the patient's condition.

Before emptying a bedpan or urinal, the nurse, or any other attendant, should see whether the urine is to be measured and charted, whether it is to be sent for examination, whether all the urine voided is to be saved for examination, and whether a specimen of the stool is to be saved for examination. The diagnosis, treatment, and recovery of the patient may depend upon these precautions. Metabolic studies are based largely on dietary measurements and analysis of excretions.

It is largely the responsibility of the nurse to provide patients with the proper facilities and the privacy people desire during elimination from the bowel and bladder. For those unable to judge the adequacy of these functions and to get the needed help, it is the nurse's responsibility to make such estimates and to get the necessary medical advice. She works with the physician in the rehabilitation of those such as paralytics whose loss of bladder and bowel control represent their major social handicap.

2. ELIMINATION OF WASTE FROM THE INTESTINES

Physiology of the Intestines As It Affects Elimination. *"The length and complexity"* of the alimentary tract of vertebrates is affected by the nature of their diets, according to Walter C. Alvarez.[1] When it consists chiefly of meats, the tract is relatively short, especially the distal portion, the colon; and digestion is nearly completed within the small intestine. When the diet is composed of plant foods, the tract is longer and more complex, particularly the distal portion, and the digestion of herbaceous foods is continued in the large intestine by the fermentive action of the resident bacteria. Alvarez thinks that the usual estimates of the length of the alimentary tract are too long because they are made on cadavers. Having lost their tone, the muscular organs from the dead body may stretch to many times their length in the living body. Alvarez cites the work of R. J. Noer and C. G. Johnson, who concluded that the tract from mouth to anus might be about 2.4 to 3 meters (8 to 10 ft). They had healthy adult subjects swallow strings in order to make their estimates. It is possible, however that the intestine may have been plicated or pleated on these strings. Meyer O. Cantor[2] reports that the swallowed end of intubation tubes approximately 130 cm (52 in.) in length have repeatedly worked their way through the anus within 48 hours. This means, of course, that the small intestine was gathered on them as the casing of a curtain is on a rod.

Joel E. Goldthwait and his associates point out structural and physiological differences in the slender, intermediate, and stocky types of men and women. They say:

Not only are the mechanics of the body and the potentialities of strain different in the various types of body structure, but the physiologic processes differ also.

Probably the greatest variation lies in the functioning of the gastro-intestinal tract. In the slender type it is short, as in carnivorous animals; here, a more concentrated kind of diet is indicated, since the ingested food passes quickly through the tract, and therefore assimilation must be rapid. In the stocky type there is a long intestinal tract, as in the herbivora; here, a less concentrated type of diet is indicated, since the passage of food is slower, and assimilation can be carried on for a longer time. The result of this differentiation in the length of the tract is shown by the protest of the digestive system of slender children to a high-caloric, high-fat diet in large amount when this is given in an attempt to obtain the weight specified in height-weight tables.*

While there seems to be some doubt as to whether man's alimentary tract is more typically herbivorous or carnivorous, most authorities would probably say the latter. Alvarez says an herbivorous animal has a digestive tract 25 to 75 times the length of its body. In man the small intestine is the essential organ of digestion and absorption; the colon's function is chiefly that of absorbing water and eliminating waste from the alimentary canal. Man can live for years deprived of the stomach or the colon, but he could not exist for many weeks without the small intestine.

Digestion, started in the mouth and carried a little further in the stomach, is virtually completed by the time the contents of the tract reach the cecum. This is particularly true if the diet is a mixed one or largely animal foods. The breakdown of cellulose is believed to depend upon the action of bacteria in the large intestine; therefore, when diets high in cellulose enter the colon, they are not so completely digested.

Absorption of solid nutrients is accomplished within the small intestine, whereas water is absorbed by the colon. Alvarez says it acts like "the condenser of a steam engine." The liquid content of the small intestine is held in the colon until, under normal circumstances in the human being, it is dejected in a soft formed mass, although in some vertebrates, for example, the rabbit, the feces is so dry it will float on water. Alvarez suggests that constipation and diarrhea might be considered disturbances of the condensing mechanism, but such a mechanical interpretation is limited and, in a sense, misleading.

Movements of the alimentary tract churn and break up the contents and keep it moving from the mouth to the anus. Charles H. Best and Norman B. Taylor[3] say that the following affect the rate at which a meal passes through the tract: (1) the character of the food; (2) the individual's intestinal motility and rate of absorption, affecting the consistency of the contents; (3) the "fullness" of the bowel; (4) concurrent muscular exercise; and (5) emotional states.

In health an ordinary mixed meal leaves the stomach in 3 to 4½ hours. Its progress through the small intestine is progressively slower. It passes in spurts

* Goldthwait, Joel E., et al: *Essentials of Body Mechanics in Health and Disease,* 5th ed. J. B. Lippincott Co., Philadelphia, 1952, p. 26.

into the large intestine anywhere from 4 to 8 hours after it leaves the stomach and may stay in the colon from a few hours to days according to individual differences in the irritability of the colon and habits of elimination. Barium increases motility of the intestinal tract, and because most estimates cited are made from barium test meals and x-rays, they do not show the normal progress of food through the alimentary canal. Alvarez and F. L. Burnett estimate that part of any given meal may remain in the tract as long as a week if no purge is used in this period. Apparently, the small intestine empties only part of its contents into the cecum daily, and a certain proportion may be held back as much as a week. The gross appearance of stools after certain foods like cranberries are eaten is evidence of this, but controlled experiments have demonstrated it even more convincingly. Tiny colored beads were mixed with a normal diet and fed to healthy young men. Using different colored beads on different days, the experimenters found that the average subject eliminates only 75 per cent of a given color bead in 4 days.[4]

Food is propelled from the mouth through the anus by (1) the voluntary muscles used in swallowing and defecating, (2) by the involuntary muscles of the alimentary canal, and (3) by waving movements of the villi (microscopic fingerlike projections on the surface of the intestine). The movements of the walls of the tract vary according to the structure of its component organs and according to the function of each. The movements are not described by all authorities in the same terms, but the following are commonly used: (1) *peristalsis,* a band of contraction beside a band of relaxation in a muscular organ which pushes the contents forward toward the anus; (2) *antiperistalsis,* a band of relaxation followed by a band of contraction forcing the contents backward toward the mouth; (3) *segmenting movements,* described by Walter B. Cannon as simultaneous restrictions spaced regularly along a bowel; (4) *pendular movements,* described by Best and Taylor as simple annular constrictions that travel rapidly up and down short lengths of the bowel; and (5) *mass peristalsis,* sweeping the contents of the bowel for considerable distances. This last peristaltic rush is the movement that pushes segments of fecal matter into the rectum, compared by Alvarez to pushing cars off on a siding.

It is probable that normal alimentary motility decreases from the mouth to the anus. Best and Taylor, discussing "the metabolic gradient theory of Alvarez," say that the vomiting of fecal matter, occurring in some disease conditions, can be explained as a reversal of this normal condition accompanied by peristalsis. E. Leonard Posey, Jr., and J. Arnold Bargen studying the subject conclude that "intestinal motor function is a complex form of activity made up of three basic components: tone, motility of various types, and the intersegmental relationships including coordination and incoordination."

They think:

. . . the intestinal tract is heir to a variety of motor derangements which are only dimly perceived and generally unappreciated. Until these abnormalities are brought to light in various functional and organic conditions, therapeusis will continue to rest upon the insecure background of "spasmolysis." It has recently been pointed out that the majority of so-called antispasmodics are ineffective when administered orally and that the rationale for their administration should be seriously questioned.*

Whatever the nature of the movements, food is normally propelled from the mouth to the anus but held in each part until that organ has performed its functions. The sphincters of the stomach, the ileocecal valve, and to some extent the transverse constrictions throughout the colon slow the progress of the contents through the digestive tract. There is evidence that in health the colon, particularly, reverses the movement of its contents. If feces deposited in the rectum is not expelled, it is in some cases carried back to the transverse colon. This is called *retrotransport*. Movements of the colon are reported to be powerful enough to break a steel clamp. Vomiting, a reverse peristalsis, or spasm, can be so forceful that the contents of the stomach are shot across a room. It is difficult to find a definite answer to the question, "Is the rectum normally empty?" There is considerable evidence to support the theory that the presence of feces in the rectum usually gives rise to the *defecation impulse* and that this act empties it. There is also some reason to believe that if the person does not obey the impulse, the stool in the rectum ceases to act as an irritant, although the irritability of the rectum varies markedly in different persons, and so the stool may stay in the rectum. There it gets smaller, drier and harder, and therefore more difficult to expel. In some cases, as has been noted, it may be "retrotransported" into the upper parts of the colon.[5, 6, 7]

The bulk of evidence supports the view that mass movements that push segments of the contents of the colon into the rectum occur, usually after eating, once, twice, or oftener during a 24-hour period. When this happens the person has an "urge to stool." This more or less automatic rhythmic activity of the colon, and/or rectum, is apparent in paralyzed animals and human beings, who usually establish regular habits of defecating once or twice a day. When the voluntary control of the anus is lost, it apparently relaxes to empty the rectum whenever feces is deposited there.

The psyche can stimulate mass peristalsis just as eating and drinking do. Alvarez tells about a patient with an incompetent anal sphincter who had a bowel movement after each meal. Between times he did not dare think of eating or even pass a restaurant because the thought or sight of food caused an involuntary bowel movement. Pleasurable excitement, such as that accompanying the purchase of a desired object, acts as a cathartic on a woman whom the writer knows. A person with a colostomy (an artificial anus, but lacking a sphincter, made by surgery into the abdominal wall) who has a regular daily evacuation under ordinary circumstances may have his routine completely upset by any unusual or exciting event. The nerve supply is too complex and controversial to be included in this brief discussion, but the severance of sensory pathways is said to affect the rectum more than injury to the motor nerves.

It is common knowledge that diet affects the rate at which food progresses through the alimentary canal. Foods that are completely absorbed, or nearly so,

* Posey, E. Leonard, Jr., and Bargen, J. Arnold: "Observations of Normal and Abnormal Human Intestinal Motor Function," *Am. J. M. Sc.*, **221**:10, (Jan.) 1951.

leave no residue, and therefore do not distend and stimulate the walls of the intestine to contract and force its contents onward. Low-residue diets are used to control diarrhea; and high-residue diets, to combat constipation. Alvarez says there is reason to believe that diets with a high-cellulose content are laxative not because they make bulk in the colon but because in their breakdown through bacterial action an irritating substance is released.

Regular and Adequate Bowel Elimination. Healthy persons tend to have a soft, formed stool at approximately the same time daily. Equally healthy individuals empty the rectum twice a day, or every other day. When evacuations are regular and the stool is soft and formed, we say that bowel elimination is *normal*. When the stools are frequent and liquid the person has *diarrhea,* and this means that the contents of the colon are ejected before the usual percentage of water has been absorbed from it. Premature defecations are the result of "an irritable colon." When the stools are irregular and excessively dry, or hard, the patient is *constipated*. A stool of this consistency can cause fissures (slitlike ulcers) of the anus, and Harry E. Bacon[8] lists constipation as an indirect, traumatic cause of a fistula (a pathologic tract or abnormal communication between the anorectum and some adjacent tissue, viscus, or skin surface).

The correction of protracted diarrhea and constipation is difficult, and no pretense is made to present the subject thoroughly in this text. Nurses should realize, however, that the *emotions* affect all visceral activity and that most psychiatrists, pediatrists, psychologists, and anthropologists believe that bowel function and mental health have a very close relationship. George P. Murdock and John W. M. Whiting, studying forms of marriage and parental behavior, arranged their data around a very few activities. During the child's infancy they studied the behavior of parents in relation to (1) nursing and (2) dependency; subsequently, they studied the parents' behavior toward (1) weaning, (2) toilet training, (3) independence training, (4) aggressive training, and (5) sex training.[9] These studies were made in the hope that they would lead to a clearer understanding of the effect of early training on adult behavior. It is significant that the parents' treatment of the infant and child in relation to his bowel and bladder evacuations was included. About 30 social scientists from numerous professions, discussing these studies at a conference, accepted the thesis that adult personality is profoundly affected by early experiences connected with elimination. Too early or too rigid bowel training with punishment for lack of control or excessive approval for control changes a normal natural function into something that involves an emotional upheaval. This association between elimination and the individual's relationships with those he loves and/or hates becomes a part of him and is expressed in ways that are now only partially understood. Dorothy Baruch tries to show some of this in the story of *One Little Boy*.[10] Thomas P. Almy, reporting experiments on "the irritable colon," in which he contrasted the behavior of 50 healthy persons with 100 persons suffering with some form of colitis, concluded that:

When under stress induced by experimental stimuli, both healthy persons and patients with irritable colon may show disturbances. . . . Two patterns of altered sigmoid motility have been recognized: the one an increase in tone and/or wave-like contractions associated with overt moods of hostility and aggression; the other a decrease in tone and/or contractions associated with overt behavior symbolizing hopelessness and defeat.

. . . . We therefore conclude that in most instances irritable colon is a bodily change accompanying emotional conflict in response to environmental stress.*

William J. Grace and his associates offer visible proof of this theory in their monograph. They were able to observe the response to stress in the colonic mucous membrane of four patients, parts of whose large intestines had herniated through abdominal fistulas (openings from the abdominal cavity). Their thesis that the "threatened" individual responds with the ejection-riddance reaction (vomiting and diarrhea) and the "holding fast" reaction (constipation) is so convincingly presented that Allen Gregg, in the Foreword, suggests that this almost irrefutable demonstration of the relationship between the psyche and the soma may influence the whole field of preventive medicine and therapy. He and the authors believe that stress may affect other organs as it is shown here to affect the colon. All medical workers would find a study of this report profitable. The following summary of material in Grace's book gives the reader an idea of its value.

The ejection-riddance reaction, Grace and associates believe, is a protective pattern of defense that involves the stomach, duodenum, and large bowel. The reaction varies in intensity and pattern with the age and temperament of the individual. A feverish, fretful child who is teething may try to protect himself by the bodily reaction of vomiting and diarrhea, even though the gastrointestinal tract is not primarily involved. As the child approaches adolescence, he usually abandons this nonspecific reaction to "assault," unless there are noxious agents actually present in the gastrointestinal tract. Some adults in stressful situations in which they feel inadequate and thwarted may experience a similar body reaction. "Thus, a person who has 'taken on more than he can handle' or feels inadequate to the demands of his life situation, or a thwarted and passive person filled with hatred, defiance, contempt, and the unconscious aim to eject a threatening or overwhelming situation may have diarrhea. However, the riddance pattern being integrated through unconscious processes, the subject exhibiting violent diarrhea may be calm, sweet mannered, and seem serene."

The "holding fast" reaction, also a protective pattern of defense, involves the skeletal muscles and the large bowel. Various body postures of alertness or abjection associated with states of tension or despair are examples of sustained skeletal-muscle patterns that give rise to complaints. Such skeletal-muscle and pressor cardiovascular responses are often associated with constipation. During bodily preparation for violent exercise or competitive sports, the urge to defecate does not occur. In addition to prolonged periods of active exercise, situations evoking sadness, dejection, or cheerless striving may inhibit the gastrocolic reflex, induce nonpropulsive phasic contractions in the sigmoid, and interfere with the mass reflex. It is as though the person facing an immediate "assault" reacts by "holding on."†

* Almy, Thomas P.: "Experimental Studies on the Irritable Colon," *Am. J. Med.,* **10:**60, (Jan.) 1951.

† Grace, William J., et al.: *The Human Colon; An Experimental Study Based on Direct Observation of Four Fistulous Subjects.* Paul B. Hoeber, New York, 1951, pp. 209 ff.

Not all physicians subscribe to the theory that many colonic disorders have a psychic origin. Bacon, although citing the work of those who have found certain personality traits occurring repeatedly in the patient with ulcerative colitis, says that the findings in such studies are not yet convincing. Whether he is right or wrong, the incidence of colitis is high in this country, and it is possible that the same stresses in our culture that have led to an increase in frank psychoses are producing such somatic conditions as ulcers of the stomach, the irritable, hyperactive, ulcerative colon, and even the atonic hypoactive colon with its associated constipation.*

Causes of constipation as listed in many sources include: (1) emotional disorders, (2) self-medication, (3) restricted diets, (4) restricted fluids, (5) congenital weakness of muscles, (6) abdominal positions with kinks in the bowel, and possibly (7) excessive utilization of food.

For those who have no serious psychological or structural handicap, normal bowel movements can usually be accomplished by: (1) reasonable freedom from stress, (2) making an effort to empty the rectum at the same time or times every day, (3) sufficient exercise to maintain a normal tone of the muscles used in defecation, (4) a squatting posture or the one that makes pressure on the bowel contents possible, (5) a diet containing foods that leave sufficient residue in the bowel, and (6) a sufficient fluid intake.

Regularity in defecation is clearly important as shown by the fact that the person who has lost voluntary control eliminates rhythmically. Moreover, we cannot fail to see that if the feces is not ejected as it is deposited in the rectum by movements of the colon, it shrinks, dries, and hardens, making the act of defecation painful and even injurious to the mucous membrane of the anus. Children, fearing this discomfort, often postpone defecation. A simple explanation may help them to realize that this will only increase their difficulty. Everyone must learn that ignoring the stimulus finally weakens it, so that the rectum becomes habituated to the presence of feces.

Since the powerful intestinal contractions that push small masses into the rectum usually occur after meals, it is logical to select this time for having the daily bowel movement. This may not be desirable if the person is hurrying then to get to school or to his work, for stress interferes with relaxation of the anal sphincter and with normal vegetative functions in general. The contractions elicited by breakfast may also result from drinking several glasses of water. Many people accomplish a daily evacuation before breakfast in this way. John L. Kantor and Anthony M. Kasich say constipation is the "most common of all disorders of digestion."†

* J. Clark Maloney compares the 400 mentally ill per 100,000 population in this country in 1949 with the 80 mentally ill per 100,000 in 1880. He also compares figures for this country with the 49 mentally ill per 100,000 in Japan in 1940. The suggestion is that the rigid infant toilet training in the United States may be a contributory factor. (Report of the Sakuraga-Oka, Hoyoin or Cherry Hill Asylum, Tokyo.) (Senn, Milton J. [ed.]: *Problems of Infancy and Childhood; Transactions of the Fourth Conference, New York, March, 1950.* Josiah Macy, Jr. Foundation, New York, 1951.)

† Kantor, John L., and Kasich, Anthony M.: *Handbook of Digestive Diseases.* C. V. Mosby Co., St. Louis, 1949, p. 313.

Constipation often develops as the person grows older. This may be the result of a less active life; also, the tendency to stoop seen in the aging relaxes abdominal muscles used in defecating. Invalids weakened by inactivity are constipated as a result of poor muscle tone, a less bulky diet, and other conditions. Exercise for the aging and the sick helps to maintain muscle tonicity. The best use can be made of the muscles involved in defecation in the squatting position. The height of toilets should be given more attention. The infirm find it difficult to get on and off very low seats, and the high seat is disadvantageous to the "bearing down" act. An adjustable footstool may be the best solution of the problem until an adjustable toilet seat is developed.

There is considerable misunderstanding about high- and low-residue diets. Many persons, for example, think that milk is completely absorbed and therefore a low-residue food. If this were true, infants, largely milk fed, could never have their typically full and regular evacuations. Many foods favor multiplication of bacteria which make up 30 per cent or more of the bulk of feces. Alvarez lists the following foods as high residue: milk, cheese, cabbage, black bread, and carrots; and these foods as low residue: lean meat, rice, hard-boiled eggs, sugar (except lactose), small amounts of fruit juices, tea and black coffee. White bread and butter, noodles, macaroni, and white of egg are mentioned by him as reported by other authorities.

Kantor and Kasich[11] list the following causes of constipation: (1) anomalies of the colon (malformation), (2) diets that are irregular or restricted, (3) psychic and nervous disorders, (4) endocrine disease, specifically thyroid deficiency, (5) associated organic digestive disease such as gallstones, and (6) the cathartic or enema habit.

Treatment depends upon the established cause. It is clear that nurses should not initiate but can participate in the physician's program of therapy. Emphasis should be placed on regular movements, normal in consistency, rather than a specific time interval. Anxiety over the failure to defecate daily sends many persons to the corner drugstore for cathartics, and soon a vicious habit is established.*

A patient may or may not have formed good bowel habits. If he has them, a nurse must see that no neglect on her part interferes; if he has not, the importance of regular adequate elimination should be discussed (if his condition permits) and special efforts made to see that it is established. Irregular and inadequate elimination should be a matter of real concern. In many cases his helplessness and his lowered vitality make the nurse responsible, but to the extent that his condition permits, the patient should be encouraged to feel that he too is responsible. Often he is able to go to the bathroom, to exercise, and to use his discretion in food selection. No rehabilitation program is complete until the person can manage all aspects of elimination. This includes, of course, getting medical help when he needs it. The most modern hospital construction provides ample facilities so

* In a discussion of cathartics Martin Kirby reported that a healthy 17-year-old boy had a 14-day rhythm for defecation. He was free of symptoms, and an x-ray examination showed a normal alimentary tract. (There are reports that some persons have suffered no dire results from going 6 months without a bowel movement.) (Gold, Harry [ed.:] *Cornell Conferences on Therapy*, Vol. III. The Macmillan Company, New York, 1949, p. 298.)

that patients who cannot walk may wheel themselves or be wheeled to toilets. Movable commodes are now available (see Fig. 76). Bedside units have been constructed to make the patient confined to bed independent of his attendant and the usual bedpan; the high cost and the present emphasis on ambulation have delayed its adoption.

In order to retain or develop regular elimination in bed patients, bedpans must be given at regular intervals. With the majority of people, the impulse to defecate is felt immediately or shortly after breakfast. The bedpan should therefore be given at this time unless the patient has the habit of defecating at another hour,

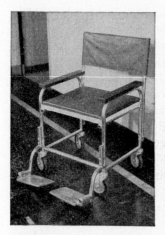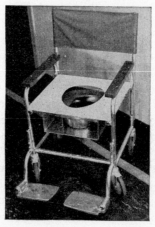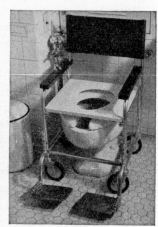

Figure 76. A commode that has many uses. (*Left*) In this view it looks like an ordinary wheelchair with a solid top over fenestrated seat. (*Center*) A stainless steel tray containing a bedpan has been suspended on runners under the seat. (*Right*) Tray and bedpan have been removed, and the commode is in place over the toilet. (N. B. The toilet seat should be raised to prevent soiling.) (Courtesy of Columbia-Presbyterian Medical Center, New York City, and Clay-Adams Co., New York City.)

in which case the bedpan should be given to him then. The impulse to urinate is felt at more frequent intervals. For this purpose, the bedpan or urinal should be given before bedtime, on waking in the morning, and before each meal. Except when the patient has had a cathartic or has diarrhea or some disease of the urinary tract, which makes frequent voiding a necessity, the irregular use of bedpans should be avoided. Every consideration, however, should be shown the patient, who cannot conform to this regimen. If regularity is observed, it not only benefits the patient but also eliminates the use of the bedpan during mealtime, visiting hours, doctors' rounds, and at other undesirable moments.

Regularity may also make the use of cathartics unnecessary. Such a result may be quite rightly a satisfaction to the nurse; the frequent need for cathartics by patients for whom she is responsible should give her pause.

Method of Giving a Bedpan to a Patient.   A bedpan should always be completely covered and carried to and from the patient as unobtrusively as possible, although false modesty should never be allowed to interfere with its use. The bed should be screened. The bedpan should be warm and placed gently under the patient in the proper position. Avoid the use of a bedpan with enamel chipped off because of the danger of injuring the skin, or cover the seat with a pad. This should always be used when the skin is tender. Cushions made of sponge rubber with a smooth outer covering are now available for this purpose and are very satisfactory.

In placing the bedpan, if the patient requires assistance, direct him to draw his knees up and press his heels against the bed. At the same time, slip your left

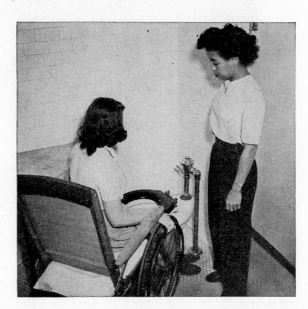

Figure 77. Instruction and supervision of a wheelchair patient so that she can move from the chair to the toilet without assistance. (Courtesy of National Foundation for Infantile Paralysis, New York City.)

hand under the pelvis, raise the hips, place a waterproof pad or protector on the bed and the bedpan in the proper position, and gently lower the patient. (The nurse uses not merely her arms and shoulders but the large trunk muscles and gets leverage with her elbow.) When the bedpan is in use, place the cover on the bar of the bed out of sight, so that the patient need not be embarrassed should someone come behind the screen. Leave the patient alone unless he is very ill or weak and likely to faint or to become fatigued. Give him plenty of time, but do not leave any patient longer than necessary on the bedpan.

In removing the bedpan, support the patient as before. Turn him on his right side. Cover the bedpan immediately. If the patient is able to complete the toilet, see that toilet paper, basin of water, and washcloth or sponges are within easy reach. If he is unable to do this satisfactorily and without fatigue, the nurse must do it for him. In hospitals there are generally a sufficient number of orderlies to give men any assistance they need in the use of the urinal and bedpan. The bedpan should be removed as soon as possible and washed first with cold running water, then cleaned with a brush, a detergent, and hot water. When automatic bedpan washers are available, as they are in most hospitals, the pan is put directly in this apparatus. (Sterilization of bedpans is discussed in Chapter 8.) In some hospitals all equipment is processed in a central supply service. While the inclusion of bedpans and urinals in such a service might save equipment and personnel, it will make observations of excreta by the attendants concerned very difficult.

Women nurses should not attempt to put helpless adults on the bedpan, for they may injure themselves and hurt the patient. A trapeze makes it possible for

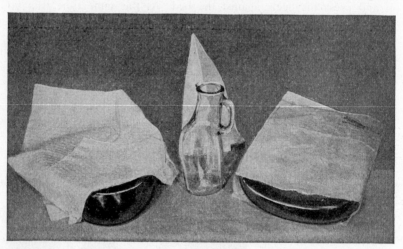

Figure 78. Disposable paper covers for bedpans and urinals. (Courtesy of Clay-Adams Co., New York City.)

many disabled persons to lift themselves. A turning sheet should be used when the patient cannot help himself or when his condition makes it important that he maintain all segments of the body in the same plane. Figures 79 A and B show the use of the turning sheet for this purpose.

Toilet Training and Changing the Infant's Diaper. In the Conference on Problems of Infancy and Childhood, where the discussion centered on the mid-century White House Conference theme, "How Can We Rear an Emotionally Healthy Generation?" there was a consensus that toilet training is one of the main areas affecting personality development (see pp. 434 and 442). The child whose mother expressed disgust when he soiled his clothes or who punished him for it will have associations with defecating that make it difficult to develop normal, much less unconscious, habits of elimination. Worse still, his self-confidence will be shaken and he will learn to fear the person he loves best. On the other hand, a child whose mother shows undue concern over his eliminations may learn that he can please or punish her with them, and so an emotional association is set up that, operating on the unconscious level, can lead to psychosomatic disease in later life when he may punish himself or others with alimentary disorders.

In the cultures described by the anthropologists of the Child-Care Conferences, parental behavior toward the child's elimination varies from no effort to train the child in adult habits to the rigid chamber training in our culture as described in pediatric texts 25 years ago. Most peoples wait until the baby can walk and

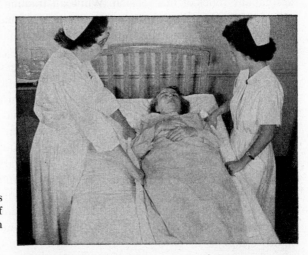

Figure 79A. Moving a helpless patient is facilitated by the use of a turning sheet that extends from the occiput to the knees.

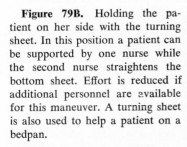

Figure 79B. Holding the patient on her side with the turning sheet. In this position a patient can be supported by one nurse while the second nurse straightens the bottom sheet. Effort is reduced if additional personnel are available for this maneuver. A turning sheet is also used to help a patient on a bedpan.

(Figs 79 A and B, courtesy of Columbia - Presbyterian Medical Center, New York City, and Clay-Adams Co., New York City.)

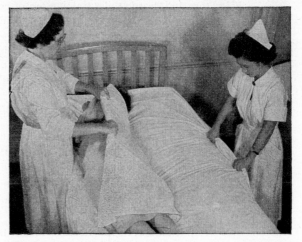

talk. John W. M. Whiting reported only the Madagascan, Japanese, and American middle class as training in bowel habits before this time. The Knoma people did not understand what toilet training meant. One parent said "What do you mean, toilet training? I don't understand. I don't see any problem. We wait until the child can walk and talk and we say, 'This is where you go,' and the child does it." Whiting adds "This was indeed the case."*

* Senn, Milton J. (ed.): *Problems of Infancy and Childhood: Transactions of the Fourth Conference, New York, March, 1950.* Josiah Macy, Jr. Foundation, New York, 1951, p. 16.

Even though we recognize the limitations of our knowledge and understanding, it is nevertheless agreed that emptying the rectum and the bladder are physical satisfactions in the same class as eating or giving and receiving expressions of love. Tension is the result of unsatisfied hunger, or drives, and pleasure should accompany relief of this tension. While all training or education consists of a discipline of native drives, a discipline which is beyond the capacity of the individual substitutes frustration and failure for the satisfaction or pleasure that comes with normal tension-relief activity.

It is doubtful whether a healthy, loving mother would ever have forced a rigid toilet training on her baby had she not been taught to do so by her elders. There is general acceptance of Lawrence K. Frank's insistence that society must trust and respect the dictates of maternal (and paternal) affection. As applied in this instance no rule should be set for toilet training at a chronological age. Milton J. Senn thinks that toilet training, like weaning, should be influenced by the child's total development. Since rates of maturation vary, a range of toilet behavior should be accepted for children of the same chronological age. Some pediatrists believe, however, that the child is more easily "trained" between the ages of 8 and 12 months than either earlier or later.[12, 13] Benjamin Spock and Mabel Huschka more than ten years ago made the following recommendation to parents on training in cleanliness:

. . . . Premature and drastic toilet training are often important contributing factors in the development of emotional difficulties . . . training should not be started until the child spontaneously begins making his toilet wants known, for this means he is psychologically ready to accept training. This he will do by grunting, wriggling, putting his hands to his genitals, or by such signs as . . . a slight tension in the legs. He may begin making his wants known as early as eight months; more often he will do so after fifteen months. . . .

In the long run the mother benefits . . . as well as the child.*

Parents and nurses will find conflicting opinions to confuse them, but few persons will recommend rigid training or punishment. Most experts in child care believe that a normal and happy child as he begins to walk and talk will want to imitate the toilet customs of his parents and his siblings, if a good relationship exists between them. Chambers or toilet seats, adapted to his size, must be provided so that defecation, and, later, voiding will be physically comfortable. Periods free from excitement, particularly following meals, may be arranged for the baby so that his attention is not diverted from the stimulus provided by intestinal movements likely to follow eating. Many babies, even at 6 months, have a single daily bowel movement after their first feeding; many continue to defecate more frequently. Regularity and normal consistency are the more important criteria for judging whether or not the infant's elimination is healthy.

Discomfort from soiled diapers differs in infancy with the age and, of course,

* From Spock, B., and Huschka, M.: *The Psychological Aspects of Pediatric Practice,* in Blumer, G. L.: Practitioners Library of Medicine and Surgery, Vol. 13. Appleton-Century-Crofts, Inc., New York, 1938, p. 757.

with the individual. Urine, however, is irritating to the skin, and stools, particularly liquid stools, are likely to be excoriating. To prevent chafing, rashes, or frank skin lesions, it is necessary to change a baby's diapers frequently. The practice of "waterproofing" him so that adults are protected from his soiled diapers should be discouraged. The skin in such cases is not only macerated by the wet cloth but is also deprived of the healing and drying power of air. Beds, furniture, and clothing should be protected by waterproof fabrics, but pants made of them should not be put on the baby except for special occasions.

Opinions vary greatly on skin care of newborn and older infants. There is a growing tendency to reduce handling and treatment of the skin to the absolute minimum for the first week. In some hospitals, however, oil is still used for skin cleaning; in others, plain water and water with detergents. Robert A. Lyon[14] discussing physical hygiene in Waldo E. Nelson's text says, "If the skin is soft and smooth, no oil or powder is necessary," although he thinks powder can do no harm if it isn't caked in the folds. Dry skin may be cleaned lightly with a vegetable oil. Nina A. Anderson, discussing infant care in the same text, mentions bacteriostatic ointments, but says some infants may be sensitive to them. She thinks bland or neutral soaps may be used. Collections of secretion should be removed from the genitalia with water or oil on cotton applicators. A rash on the buttocks may be the result of neglect or improperly laundered diapers. The latter should be thoroughly washed with a mild soap and boiled to kill bacteria that might reinfect the skin. Rinses (such as Diaparene*) have been developed that discourage urea-splitting and therefore ammonia-producing bacteria. Soft and loosely woven diapers dry quickly. Many layers should be used. The most satisfactory type are more bulky toward the center, or can be folded to give this effect. Rectangular or kite-shaped diapers are thought to make less pressure over the genitalia, to be less restricting, and to provide better protection than triangles.

If cleanliness and proper diapers do not prevent irritation, it may be necessary to use a bland ointment or to expose the buttocks to the warmth and light of the sun or an electric light suspended from a cradle over the bed. Chemicals that retard bacterial action may also decrease the irritating alkaline ammonia. Cleanliness, however, has the same effect, and when there is time for this, drugs of any sort are rarely necessary.

Soft expendable paper diapers are a convenience in traveling or whenever laundering service is unavailable.

What to Observe about the Feces. The principal points to be observed are the number of movements in 24 hours and any accompanying pain or straining; the consistency, shape, color, and odor of the stool, and the presence of unusual matter. The expulsion of gas, or flatus, should always be noted.

Although the *number of movements* varies in adult life, there should usually be one satisfactory daily movement; with some, two daily movements are normal unless cathartics have been given, in which case the intestinal tract is so completely emptied that it may require 48 hours or more for the deposit of sufficient

* Pharmaceutical Division, Homemakers Products Corp., New York, N. Y.

feces in the colon to stimulate contraction. As Alvarez says, the empty colon will not contract. The stool should be formed, but not hard, and molded to the shape and size of the rectum. R. B. H. Gradwohl[15] says the usual amount of stool is from 100 to 200 gm (3½ to 7 oz) a day. The significance of small, dark, hard stools has been discussed as has the more common explanation of diarrhea, or frequent fluid stools. Often, but not always, fluid stools contain an irritating substance that makes their elimination uncomfortable, or even very painful. The nurse must note and record this if she observes signs of it, or if the patient complains of it. Changes in bowel habits, even of short duration, are said to be one of the early signs of cancer. Specialists are constantly urging people, particularly as they grow older, to have x-rays of the colon after a few weeks of diarrhea or constipation.

The *color* of feces is normally a greenish brown, due chiefly to the bile it contains. Pale or clay-colored stools indicate its absence. This usually means either that the liver is not secreting bile or that there is some obstruction to its passage into the intestines. In the latter case bile passes into the blood stream, and the patient is jaundiced. Light-colored stools may also be due to undigested fat. When the stool is dark and of a tarry consistency, one suspects the presence of partly digested blood. The red cells have been broken up, freeing hematin. A dark, tarry stool therefore indicates that a hemorrhage into the intestines occurred sometime previously, probably high up in the intestines or coming from the stomach. Bright red undigested blood is a sign of either a very recent hemorrhage or one from the colon. Blood from the rectum appears on the surface of the stool, while blood from the stomach or small intestines is mixed throughout. Every person who passes a bloody stool should have a careful examination. Wendell G. Scott concludes an article on rectal bleeding with the following:

(1) Cancer of the colon is common. (2) The best protection . . . is the complete periodic health check-up. (3) The surgical treatment of cancer of the colon has progressed ahead of consistent ability to diagnose it in the early stages. (4) The most urgent phase in the problem . . . is the education of people over 35 to seek medical attention for minor changes in their bowel habits and the elimination of self-medication. (5) The most important step is the education of physicians to institute examinations of the colon for suggestive symptoms and not to wait for the appearance of the advanced signs of cancer.*

Any bloody discharge from the body should be treated as a grave symptom. Bloody stools may be the result of rectal fissures or fistulas, of varicosities of the rectum or intestines, of ulcers or malignancies in any part of the tract, and of hemorrhage from other causes. The nurse should describe the appearance of the stool exactly, indicating whether the bright red color is on the outside of the stool or whether it is distributed throughout; whether the entire mass is of a dark, tarry consistency or whether only a part of it has this appearance, and so on. When the patient is menstruating it should be noted, since this may be the source of bright red blood on the surface of the stool.

* Scott, Wendell G.: "Significance of Rectal Bleeding and the Importance of Diagnosing Early Cancer of the Colon." *J. Nat. M. A.* **42**:352. (Nov.) 1952.

When the presence of blood is suggested by the appearance of the stool, laboratory tests are made. These are described briefly in Chapter 19. Color and odor vary with foods eaten and with some drugs. For instance, a green color may be due to the chlorophyll from vegetables, and black stools to iron and bismuth preparations. Stools discolored by beets may suggest the presence of fresh blood.

Although the *odor* of the stool, as a rule, has no particular significance, any unusual odor should be noted. It may be caused by food or drugs, but is usually the result of bacterial action producing odoriferous gases, such as hydrogen sulfide. Alvarez thinks excessive gas formation, especially if associated with reverse peristalsis, may account for the foul breath characteristic of intestinal stasis.

The *presence of any other unusual matter* such as pus, mucus, and worms should of course be reported.

Irritation of mucous membrane results in increased secretion of mucus. Excessive *mucus* gives the stool a *slimy* appearance. In severe forms of inflammation, as in dysentery, the stool may consist of nothing but mucus and blood and its passage is accomplished by pain and tenesmus (an urge to evacuate the bowels or the bladder, without result.)

Pus in the stool results from suppuration in the intestines, liver, or pancreas, or an abscess in the intestinal tract. Pus is hard to see in any but a fluid stool.

Intestinal parasites most commonly found in the stools are the pinworm or threadworm (*Enterobius vermicularis* or *Oxyuris vermicularis*); the roundworm (*Ascaris lumbricoides*); the whipworm (*Trichuris trichiura*); the hookworm (*Ancylostoma duodenale* and *Necator americanus*); the various tapeworms of pork and fish (*Taenia solium, Taenia saginata,* and *Diphyllobothrium latum*); and in another classification, the protozoan amebae. (See Fig. 80.) Worm infestation is far more prevalent than most people realize, as was pointed out in Chapter 5. In human beings sufficiently well nourished to feed themselves and the parasites, some of them may produce no disease symptoms, but they are a serious menace to the undernourished. Control lies chiefly in sanitation, and in thorough cooking of foods through which certain parasites are transmitted. The person whose intestinal tract is infested is given a drug believed to kill or paralyze the particular parasite. Such drugs are usually accompanied by a cathartic so that the worms will be removed and so that the absorption of the drug, usually toxic to the patient as well as the parasite, is reduced to a minimum. In *Diddie, Dumps and Tot*, a story of plantation life, there is a vivid description of dosing the children with "vermifuge" each spring, a necessary precaution in the last century. Some modern vermifuges or anthelmintics are: medicinal gentian violet for pinworm; oil of chenopodium, tetrachloroethylene or hexylresorcinol for roundworm and whipworm;* antihistamine compounds for hookworms; pelletierine, carbon tetrachloride, or quinacrine for beef, pork, or fish tapeworm. Gilbert F. Otto, writing in Maxcy's text,[16] says that no effective treatment for the whipworm is known. The patient, his family, laboratory technicians, nurses, and others will have to examine stools to determine the effectiveness of treatment.

* Success with "Hetrazan" (1-diethylcarbamyl-4-methyl piperazine dihydrogen citrate) is reported by James N. Etteldorf and L. Crawford: *J.A.M.A.*, **143**:799, (July) 1950.

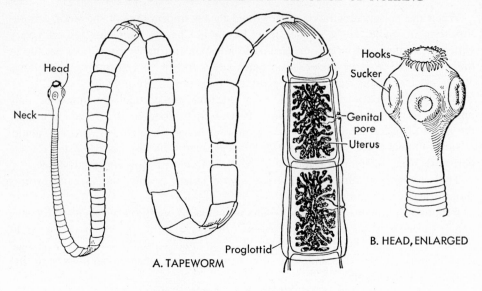

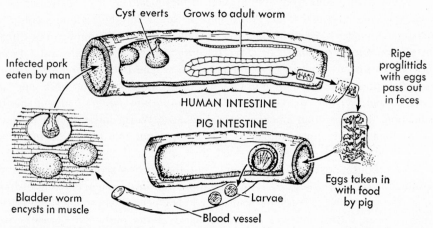

Figure 80. (*Top*) The pork tapeworm, *Taenia solium.* (*Left*) Specimen about 8 ft. long, consisting of about 900 proglottids, with four sections omitted. The uterus filled with eggs is shown in the last two proglottids. The portions of the work are shown about four times natural size. (*Right*) Head, enlarged about 40 times. (Hegner, Robert W., and Stiles, Karl A.: *College Zoology,* 6th ed. The Macmillan Company, New York, 1951.)

(*Bottom*) Diagram of life cycle of the pork tapeworm, *Taenia solium.* (Storer, Tracy I.: *General Zoology,* 2nd ed. [After Bucksbaum.] McGraw-Hill Book Co., New York, 1951.)

The *pinworm* or *threadworm* occurs quite frequently in the rectum and colon. Its presence causes itching, irritation, restlessness, loss of sleep, anorexia, and, finally, anemia. It appears in the stools as fine threads, usually moving actively.

Roundworms and *whipworms* are very common parasites occurring chiefly in children. They cause restlessness, irritability, twitchings, and convulsions. They are easily recognized in the stool.

When pinworms, roundworms, or whipworms are found in the stools, the greatest precaution must be taken to prevent spreading the infection to others and also to prevent the patient (usually a child) from reinfecting himself by contaminating his hands. These parasites enter through the mouth. The anus and surrounding parts must be carefully washed and also the hands of both patient and nurse. Infected persons should never be allowed to handle foods.

The *ameba* is the cause of amebic, or tropical, dysentery, which is characterized by inflammation and ulceration of the intestines and abscesses in the liver. The stools contain amebae and so are highly infectious. Strict precautions must be taken to prevent the spread of the infection. (See Chapter 7.) The ameba is a one-celled organism that can be seen only under the microscope.

Tapeworms are taken into the alimentary tract usually in infected pork, beef, or fish which has not been thoroughly cooked. They lodge in the intestines and cause pain, nausea, diarrhea, and anemia. Infected with worms in the larval stages, cysts may form in the nervous system with such serious effects as epilepsy. These worms may be from 5 to 20 ft or more in length. Segments may be passed frequently in the stool, but until the head is removed the worm will continue to grow. When treatments are given, therefore, to expel the tapeworm, the minute head, about the size of a pinhead, with a very fine neck like a thread must be found, difficult as it is.

A stool to be examined for a tapeworm should be received in a bedpan containing water at body temperature and every bit examined. All segments should be burned, never thrown into the toilet.

When a stool has an unusual appearance, indicating the presence of mucus, blood, pus, or worms, it should be saved, undisturbed, for inspection by the doctor, who will decide whether a specimen should be sent to the laboratory for further examination. In any case, when it is suspected that the stool contains any abnormal substance, and an examination will aid in diagnosis, a specimen is required for examination. Usually, a small amount is adequate, but sometimes it is necessary to save the whole amount undisturbed.[17, 18, 19]

The character and number of the stools of an infant differ in some respects from those of adults. A normal breast-fed infant ordinarily has two or three stools daily during the first week. It is very important for the nurse to watch the number and character of the stools during this period. An absence of bowel movement may be caused by some congenital malformation of the anus, rectum, or colon, which should have the immediate attention of a surgeon. After the first month, there are usually two stools each day; there should be at least one daily bowel movement.

The stool of a breast-fed infant is orange yellow in color, soft, smooth, mealy, or stringy in consistency, having a pungent odor and acid reaction. The stool of an artificially fed infant changes in appearance with the food given.

The character of the stool indicates whether the infant is getting the proper feeding or not. If there is any abnormality in the color, odor, or consistency of the stool, the nurse or mother should save it for the doctor's inspection.

Recording Observations. The number and character of the stools are often recorded routinely on infants' charts. The number of stools daily are recorded for adults. A patient able to judge reports the effectiveness of his bowel function to his nurse or doctor; if for any reason he is not able to assume this responsibility, the nurse, or her substitute, must report the number and character of his eliminations so that his diet may be modified, and drugs or other treatments instituted, as needed.

Treatments for Abnormal Bowel Elimination.   When the number or character of the stools indicates constipation or diarrhea, the physician, the mother, the nurse, or the adult patient may himself try to discover the cause. The condition is often of such short duration that it can be explained on a dietary basis and as easily corrected. Some mothers, for example, regulate their infants' movements by increasing or decreasing the intake of fruits and vegetables, and many adults are equally successful with such simple means. Regulation of exercise and fluid intake are other harmless measures. When the condition is so serious that drugs, colon injections, or psychotherapy is indicated, the physician should take over. Alvarez, Alfred J. Kantor,[20] and all enterologists decry self-medication for alimentation. They speak of the "vicious cycle" set up by the cathartic habit and the even more dangerous practice of taking enemas frequently. Cathartics that irritate the intestinal wall are likely to cause fluid stools and hurry the food through the alimentary canal before optimum food absorption has taken place. Mineral oil, a hydrocarbon, has been considered harmless by many persons in the past. It is now believed, however, that it absorbs calcium, removes this essential nutrient from the intestinal contents, and interferes with absorption of the fat-soluble vitamins.[21] Used over a long time, this can be injurious. Substances that attract water and increase bulk in the intestines, such as agar, gum tragacanth, bran, and psyllium seeds, are probably the least injurious cathartics since their effect is similar to that of a bulky diet. They must be taken with plenty of water. Cascara, senna, and licorice powder are relatively mild in their action. The usefulness of saline cathartics is limited to special conditions. Most cathartics lose their effectiveness if the underlying cause of constipation is not removed. Even if not harmful, they are a waste of money when the bowels can be regulated without them.[22]

During illness when exercise must be reduced to a minimum and a low-residue diet is necessary, the physician may find it necessary to prescribe cathartics or enemas. In the convalescent stage of illness, however, the patient should be helped to regulate elimination physiologically. A thoroughgoing rehabilitation includes bowel and bladder control with noninjurious procedures.

3. ELIMINATION OF WASTE BY THE KIDNEYS

Hygienic Measures to Promote Elimination by the Kidneys.   Best and Taylor, discussing the secretion of urine, refer to "theories of renal function." This suggests that our knowledge of kidney physiology is incomplete, and indeed it is. Perhaps there is now a greater realization of what we don't know than there was in the past, for we seldom find dogmatic statements in current texts about diet and fluid intake in relation to kidney functions.

It is believed that urine is manufactured by the kidney through a filtration of the blood with a selective reabsorption within the kidney of substances from the filtrate. The effectiveness of the artificial kidney has proved that this theory is somewhere near correct. The conditions under which the kidney functions normally are not entirely understood, but it is known that anything increasing the rate of filtration or reducing the rate of reabsorption increases the volume of urine. The reverse actively decreases the urine volume.

Conditions that affect the rate of filtration and reabsorption are: (1) the number of functioning units in the kidney structure; (2) changes in the rate of capillary and renal blood flow and in the general circulation; (3) changes in pressure within the kidney capillaries and in the general circulation; (4) changes in the protein content of the plasma because this so greatly affects its osmotic pressure; (5) the concentration of other solids (such as salts of sodium, potassium, calcium, magnesium, chloride, sulfur, and phosphorous), glucose, and urea and uric acid; and (6) the hormones, particularly the secretions of the pituitary and adrenal glands.

Upon the kidneys fall a large share of the work of keeping the circulating fluids constant. They not only eliminate waste, largely that of protein digestion, but also maintain the neutrality of the blood by eliminating acid or base in the urine as demanded by the intake of preponderantly acid or basic diets. Kidney function can adapt itself to a wide range of conditions. When one kidney is removed, the other, if it is healthy, can take care of the body's ordinary needs; the kidneys function normally with remarkably high and low blood pressures and blood volumes; the same is true of varying concentrations of protein, glucose, electrolytes, hormones, and nitrogenous wastes. We must realize, however, that when any one of these conditions exceeds the limits tolerated by the kidneys, they break down; when this happens the acid-base balance is disrupted, nitrogenous wastes and water accumulate in the tissues, and death follows rapidly.

Normal kidney function is encouraged by living a sane life with respect to food and drink, exercise, rest, and sleep. Since the emotions affect blood pressure, digestion, and in fact the entire body economy, mental health is part of this sane life. It is no longer believed that simple rules for drinking water and avoiding protein, or any other dietary element, are the answer. Avoidance of irritating chemicals, particularly those eliminated by the kidneys, and freedom from bacterial poisons help to maintain the kidneys in a normal state.

What to Observe about Urine. A nurse should note the amount of urine voided in 24 hours and the amount at each voiding; the frequency, any urgency, effort, discomfort, or pain that accompanies voiding; also the transparency, color, and odor of the urine. According to standard texts on physiology, the *amount of urine* voided by the average adult in a 24-hour period varies from 1000 to 2000 cc (1 to 2 qt). All authorities, however, comment on the very wide range in health according to the intake of fluids, the diet, and the amount of water excreted by sweat or feces.[23, 24] Averages given by Nelson for healthy children appear on page 450.

The amount, either in children or adults, may be greatly increased by disease, or temporarily by physiological conditions. In acute nephritis, the amount may be

Average Daily Excretion of Urine in Childhood*

AGE	FLUID OUNCES	CUBIC CENTIMETERS
1st and 2nd day	1–2	30–60
3rd to 10th day	3–10	100–300
10th day to 2 months	9–15	250–450
2 months to 1 year	14–17	400–500
1–3 years	17–20	500–600
3–5 years	20–24	600–700
5–8 years	22–34	650–1000
8–14 years	27–47	800–1400

only 200 to 500 cc, while it has been reported that in diabetes insipidus (caused by a lesion in the midbrain) 43 liters or quarts of urine were passed in 24 hours.[25] The voiding of a large amount of urine is called *polyuria*; when the amount voided is scanty, the condition is called *oliguria*; when there is a total absence or marked deficiency, the condition is called *anuria*.

Failure to void the normal amount of urine should be reported immediately. In diseases marked by either an increase or decrease in urine it must be carefully measured and the amount recorded.

Transparency is a characteristic of most normal urine. Cloudy urine or the deposit of a sediment may indicate disease or may be due to such simple causes as a change in the reaction of the urine on standing or to a change in its temperature. Normal urine is acid in reaction and always contains phosphates which are held in solution in an acid medium. Under certain conditions, for example, an herbivorous diet, the urine is alkaline, with the result that the phosphates are no longer held in solution but are precipitated out. This makes the urine very cloudy, and when it stands a sediment is formed. Even acid urine will turn alkaline and cloudy in a few hours because normal waste products in it (urea) are decomposed by bacteria, setting free ammonia, which is highly alkaline. This will again precipitate the phosphates. People are sometimes needlessly alarmed, thinking they have "kidney trouble" when the urine is cloudy. Adding a little acid to the urine will determine whether the cloudiness is caused by phosphates. If it is, the cloud will disappear. Sometimes, also, people may be needlessly alarmed by a brick-red sediment in urine that has been in a specimen bottle for some time. This sediment consists of normal waste products, urates and uric acid crystals. Urine when voided is warm, and this heat keeps the urates, etc., in solution; when cooled, particularly if concentrated, they are no longer held in solution. To test the urine, heat it; if the cloud of sediment is caused by urates, it will disappear.

When a cloud or sediment cannot be removed but is increased by adding acid or by heating, it is always due to abnormal substances—albumin, pus, blood, epithelial cells, or casts. (Urine tests are described briefly in Chapter 19.)

The *color* of urine depends upon the amount and kind of pigment, concentration of the urine, the amount and kind of solids, decomposition of the solids, the

*Nelson, Waldo E. (ed.): *Nelson's Textbook of Pediatrics,* 6th ed. W. B. Saunders Co., Philadelphia, 1954, p. 1048.

presence of abnormal constituents, and the action of drugs. *The color of urine is not of any great importance in diagnosis of disease, but it is an important guide for the nurse. A pale urine is a dilute, low specific gravity urine and shows that the patient is drinking enough water; amber-colored urine is concentrated, and of high specific gravity, indicating that the patient is not getting sufficient water.* Some clinicians think the color and specific gravity of the urine a more helpful guide than the record of intake and output. The latter can mean very little unless fluid intake in the diet is measured and unless the fluid lost by sweat can be estimated.

The *odor* of newly voided urine is characteristic. This odor is caused by its volatile, aromatic components. When urine stands it smells of ammonia, liberated on the decomposition of urea by bacteria. When freshly voided urine has this odor, it shows that decomposition has already taken place in the bladder; and this suggests cystitis. In diabetes the urine may have a sweetish odor, due to the presence of acetone. The odor of ammonia or of acetone should therefore always be reported, as either one indicates disease. Drugs and foods may also alter the odor of urine.

Some Causes of Increased Urine. A marked increase in the amount of urine voided may be caused temporarily by drinking a large amount of fluids, by excitement, cold baths, by food, and by diuretic drugs. In winter, urine is voided more frequently because less water is eliminated by perspiration. Because, however, less water is drunk in cold weather, this may not follow.

The amount is usually increased in conditions such as hysteria, chronic nephritis, diabetes mellitus, and diabetes insipidus. In chronic nephritis without edema, the diseased kidney has difficulty in eliminating solid wastes; so it eliminates a small amount of solids and, to dilute them, it at the same time eliminates a very large amount of water; the urine will be pale and of a low specific gravity. In uncontrolled diabetes mellitus, the blood sugar rises, and this makes the patient thirsty just as eating candy does. He drinks quantities of water in order to dilute the sugar and eliminate it through the kidneys.

Some Causes of Decreased Urine. A marked decrease in the amount voided may be caused (1) *temporarily* by drinking small amounts of fluid, by the loss of body fluids by perspiration, by vomiting, diarrhea, and by the action of drugs, such as opium, that check the secretion of urine; (2) by *suppression* of urine, failure of the kidneys to secrete urine; and (3) by *retention* of urine, failure of the bladder to expel urine contained in it.

It is very important to know whether failure to void urine (anuria) is caused by *suppression* or *retention,* as the effect on the body and the treatment required differ greatly.

Suppression of urine, or anuria, is a very grave condition, indicating that the kidneys are failing. Waste products in the blood, normally eliminated through the kidneys, are held in the body, and it must find another means of getting rid of them. Part will be eliminated by the bowels and the skin, but combined they cannot do the work of the kidneys; some of the waste products will of necessity accumulate, and give rise to serious symptoms. The symptoms of *retention* are largely local—that is, confined to the region of the bladder, but those of *suppression* are general.

Death from drug poisoning is often due to *suppression*. This is particularly likely to happen when the drug is eliminated by the kidneys. Francis G. Harrison and Herbert L. Warres clasify some common causes of anuria as follows:

A. "Prerenal causes" due to (1) shock; (2) dehydration from diarrhea, vomiting, excessive perspiration or inadequate fluid intake; (3) cardiac decompensation; (4) vascular spasm or abdominal surgery, abdominal distention and other conditions.

B. "Renal causes": (1) acute nephritis; (2) acute nephrosis caused by heavy metal and phosphorous poisoning, liver damage, the toxemia of pregnancy, and accidents involving crushed tissues; (3) destruction of renal tissue in tuberculosis, trauma, or the necrosis that sometimes follows childbirth.

C. "Post-renal causes": (1) blockage of tubules from crystalline materials following transfusions, chemotherapy with the sulfonamides and from other causes. (2) blockage of ureters.*

Absence of urine can result from obstruction in the urethra but this is retention rather than suppression.

Harrison and Warres say:

Though patients tolerate uremia well the mortality rate in anuria is 46 per cent, death usually resulting from pulmonary and cerebral edema. In other words, treatment by forcing fluids in all cases is worse than the disease.*

They divide treatment into early and late phases. Early treatment is aimed at preventing the causes just listed, and they mention BAL as an especially helpful agent in metal poisoning and alkalinization with forced fluids when sulfonamides are the toxic agents.

Late treatment consists of determining the existence and nature of obstructions by the passage of instruments into the pelvis of the kidney. After this, the problem is one of trying to get the patient into a state of fluid-electrolyte-acid-base balance. Limiting fluids to 1000 to 1500 cc daily is usually indicated. The kinds of salts needed are determined by blood and urine analyses. Other therapeutic measures include the use of the artificial kidney; lavage of the alimentary tract to remove waste, and to apply heat to the kidney; exchange transfusions; and, in some cases, surgery.

Symptoms of suppression are dizziness, nausea, headache, dimness of vision or the appearance of bright spots before the eyes, puffiness under the eyes, or a general swelling. In suppression, no urine flows from a catheter inserted into the bladder, because there is none; whereas in retention the urine immediately flows from the instrument. Every nurse should be alert to the preceding symptoms and realize the importance of reporting them at once.

Retention means that urine secreted by the kidneys is retained in the bladder. *Retention with overflow* sometimes occurs; that is, some urine is voided but the

* Harrison, Francis G., and Warres, Herbert L.: "Present Day Therapy of Anuria," *Am. Pract. & Digest Treat.*, **1**:584, (June) 1950.

bladder is not emptied. The distended bladder can often be felt through the abdominal wall.

The symptoms of retention are failure to void; fullness and discomfort, sometimes severe pain; and a distended bladder.

Any of these symptoms should be reported immediately. If voiding cannot be induced by nursing measures, catheterization must be resorted to. This is accompanied by some risk to the patient, and should be avoided if possible. It is discussed in Chapter 31.

Nursing Measures to Stimulate Micturition. The nurse can most effectively relieve retention if to some extent she understands bladder physiology. While there is much more to learn about it than is now known, a great deal of data have been accumulated through cystometry (estimates of intervesicular pressure) in recent years.

Micturition, urination, or voiding is initiated by the stretching of the bladder walls, or by the pressure of urine. The stretching, or the pressure required to elicit the desire to empty the bladder, varies with the person and with his condition. Under stress a very small amount can give rise to an urgent desire to urinate, while the same person, under other circumstances, can store a large volume of urine without discomfort. Physical and psychic factors affect bladder function, which is for normal children and adults a reflex act under voluntary control. Best and Taylor describe it and the conditions affecting it as follows:

> Micturition . . . presents a very unusual feature in that movements inervated by autonomic nerves can be controlled by voluntary impulses. The higher centers from which the inhibitory impulses emanate are situated in the hypothalamus and cerebral cortex. . . .
>
> Contractions set up by a distended bladder by sudden increases of intra-abdominal pressure acting upon the viscus, as in coughing, sneezing, defecation, etc., may, by forcing a little urine past the sphincter into the urethra, cause micturition unless a strong effort of the will is exercised. Psychic influences may also induce bladder contractions which evoke the act unless opposed by restraint. The lifting of voluntary inhibition, unless the bladder is fully distended, may on the other hand be prevented and the power to micturate be temporarily lost, as when a shy or nervous examinee is asked for a specimen of urine in the presence of another person.*

By cystometry (described in Chapter 31) it has been learned that in the average adult the bladder adapts itself by periods of contraction and relaxation to its contents until 450 to 500 cc of urine have accumulated. Up to this point it maintains its tone; when it is distended beyond the physiological point, it tends to lose its muscular character and behave more or less like an elastic bag. While there are great individual differences in bladder function, it empties most normally at that point when it is, physiologically speaking, full—rather than partially filled or distended. Voiding occurs most easily when nothing interferes with the removal of the voluntary inhibition. Reflex acts are dependent upon the sensitivity of the

* Best, Charles H., and Taylor, Norman B.: *Physiological Basis of Medical Practice,* 5th ed. Williams & Wilkins Co., Baltimore, 1950, p. 46.

nerves and muscles involved; therefore, anesthetics, narcotics, hypnotics, or anything that depresses neuromuscular mechanisms may interfere with micturation.
Some such drugs retard the formation of urine; some delay emptying of the bladder; while large doses may remove the voluntary control and cause incontinence.

When the patient is not voiding and there is reason to believe that he is storing
urine, the nurse may encourage micturation by (1) promoting mental and physical
relaxation through such measures as the particular case demands; (2) removing
any distracting sources of physical discomfort; (3) suggesting the act by the
sound of running water; (4) relaxing the urethral sphincter in women by pouring

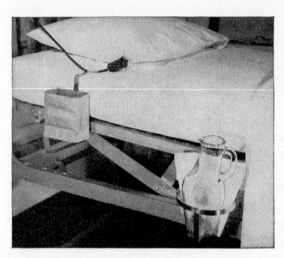 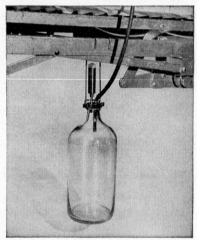

Figure 81. (*Left*) In many cases it is necessary to leave a urinal within reach of the
patient. A metal holder, as illustrated, is a desirable type. A disposable paper cover is placed
over, or beside, the urinal. (Courtesy of Columbia-Presbyterian Medical Center, New York
City, and Clay-Adams Co., New York City.)

(*Right*) Tomac deodorizing drainage bottle. (Courtesy of American Hospital Supply Corp.,
Evanston, Ill.)

warm water over the vulva; (5) stimulating the bladder walls by gentle massage
and pressure on the abdominal wall above the symphysis pubis; and (6) seeing
that patients are put, as nearly as possible, into the position in which they normally
urinate. Even immediately after an operation the surgeon may prefer having the
patient sit up, in or out of bed, to void if this makes catheterization unnecessary.
Many persons find it difficult to micturate or defecate in the presence of another.
Unless the patient is very ill, the nurse should try the effect of leaving him alone.
If there is reason to believe that the bladder is not distended, the patient should
be encouraged to drink water, but this is unsuccessful when the bladder walls are
already stretched beyond the point where they function effectively. Physicians ask
that patients be catheterized rather than to allow them to suffer from retention for
any length of time. Thinning of the walls, with its effect of decreasing the blood
supply is believed to predispose the bladder to infection and to be as much of a

hazard as the introduction of a catheter. With skillful nursing most patients can avoid both these dangers.[26] (Catheterization is described in Chapter 31.)

4. INCONTINENCE OF BOWEL AND BLADDER

Causes of Partial and Complete Loss of Bladder Control—Enuresis and Incontinence. In most cultures the child starts controlling bowel and bladder evacuations between 8 and 14 months of age. Spock[27] says a child usually becomes dry during the day between 1½ and 2½ years. He thinks most children are ready to stay dry at night between 2 and 3 years. Making these reflex acts voluntary ones is easier for the child when he is awake than when he is asleep; therefore, reflex night voiding, or bed wetting, persists in childhood beyond the age when he wets his clothing by day. *Enuresis,* which means literally "incontinence of urine," is the medical term for bed wetting after the age at which the child usually acquires complete control over the bladder (about 2½ years). In our own culture bed wetting often persists throughout childhood and occasionally into adult life.

Pediatrists, psychologists, and psychiatrists almost universally believe that enuresis is a symptom and should never be treated as a disease entity. Spock and Huschka say: ". . . as a rule enuresis is psychological in origin rather than physical. . . . Enuresis is usually only one of a group of emotionally determined symptoms in a given child and . . . to attack this one symptom alone is as unwise as to concentrate on reducing temperature in a case of physical illness. . . ."* Ralph Townsend[28] expresses the same idea in virtually the same words. He thinks enuresis in a child can often be corrected by psychological guidance for him and his parents; when it persists to adult life, he thinks the treatment is "essentially psychiatric." Experts agree that the cause must be determined; any physical irritation of the genitalia corrected, and emotional disturbance identified and its cause removed or modified through identification and understanding. This cannot be accomplished unless the therapist gains the friendship and cooperation of the patient. Punishment is not effective. Control is made less difficult if the fluid intake in the late afternoon and evening is reduced.[29, 30] While *incontinence* is synonymous with enuresis in the dictionary, it is used in medical parlance for the loss of control over the sphincters guarding either the bladder, the rectum, or both during the day and night. The term is not applied to infants since sphincter control is actually abnormal in babies.

After infancy, control of elimination by bowel and bladder depends upon a normal neuromuscular mechanism. Many otherwise healthy and normal persons are incontinent or "spill urine" in emotional states. "Stress incontinence" is fairly common, particularly in women.[31]

In John C. Brocklehurst's study of incontinence in about 3000 old people in hospitals he says: "The incidence has proved to be twice as common among females as among males." He suggests the following as possible explanations:

* Spock, Benjamin, and Huschka, Mabel: *op. cit.,* p. 779.

(1) women live longer than men, and senile changes are therefore more often seen; (2) mental confusion was twice as common in the women as in the men, possibly for the same reason as in item one; (3) men can keep some sort of urinal in position, which may relieve the anxiety about wetting; and (4) the difference in anatomical structure. He cites the conclusion of William T. Kennedy, based on surgery and dissection, that the female urethra opens as the result of muscle contraction rather than relaxation, as is generally believed. As Brocklehurst says:

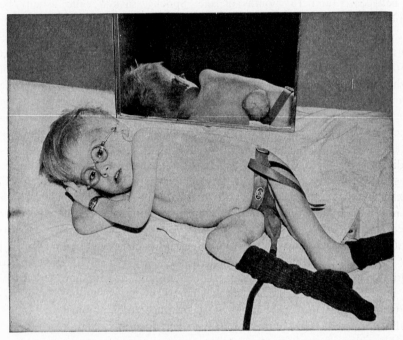

Figure 82.   Rubber urinal worn at night by a spina bifida child who is incontinent. (Courtesy of Eastern New York Orthopedic Hospital-School, Inc., Schenectady, N.Y.)

The short female urethra does make the woman more liable to stress incontinence, . . . the external sphincter may take the form of a Muscle of Micturition [Kennedy's] in the female, and any increase in the tone of the muscle . . . would tend to open up the urethra, instead of closing it more tightly as a true external sphincter would do.*

Injuries, growths, spontaneous hemorrhages, and poisoning by chemicals or bacterial toxins may temporarily or permanently destroy the nerve pathways. The nerve supply to the bladder or rectum may be interrupted, or its function destroyed by disease in the central nervous system (brain and spinal cord) or in the nerves leaving and entering the cord to and from the bladder and rectum. Sometimes the abnormal condition, therefore the incontinence, is curable; sometimes it is

---

* Brocklehurst, John C.: *Incontinence in Old People.* E. and S. Livingstone, Ltd., Edinburgh, 1951, p. 102.

permanent. Whether of long or short duration, it is a major nursing problem. Any accident, growth, or disease severe enough to interfere with the function of the pelvic organs is likely to interfere with the blood supply, hence nutrition, of the skin and often to limit motor activity. Pressure sores or bedsores (discussed more fully in Chapter 15) are the inevitable result of lying in one position too long. Their formation is hastened by poor nutrition and by maceration and irritation of the skin by moisture and chemicals in the urine and stool. It is imperative that the patient be kept clean and dry. Pressure sores can be cured only by correcting the conditions that provoke them; it is therefore wise to institute these measures early enough to prevent the breakdown of the skin.

In rare cases, congenital defects or growths make storage and discharge of urine by the bladder impossible. The surgeon will then make a permanent or temporary opening from the bladder to the skin; he will attach the ureters to the rectum, or he will attach their outlets to the skin surface of the trunk. Under the latter circumstances the person is saddled for the rest of his life with a type of incontinence difficult to manage, since there is not even an incompetent sphincter to guard the outlet.

Treatment of *incontinence* of the urinary bladder depends upon its cause and the supposed duration; a temporary condition will be treated differently from a permanent one, but all methods are aimed at (1) preventing contact of urine with the skin or (2) removing it as quickly as possible. Rehabilitation is the ultimate aim in all but a few cases.

To prevent contact between the urine and skin, a catheter is inserted and held in the bladder, the ureter, or even the pelvis of the kidney. This is called an "indwelling catheter," and the procedure is described in Chapter 31. Another means of diverting urine from the skin in the male patient is to attach a bag to the penis or to clamp the penis.[32, 33] All of these procedures have serious disadvantages. Catheters invariably irritate and infect the cavities in which they lie; and the meatus is excoriated by a penile bag with a rapid extension of the irritation to the bladder. The use of a penile clamp is perhaps the most traumatic of the three procedures, and although a few physicians recommend it as a very temporary measure, it is generally condemned. Indwelling catheters, accompanied by several types of irrigation, to stimulate bladder function and combat infection, are extensively used until the degree of bladder disability is determined, and for patients whose condition limits life. In such cases the low-grade bladder infection accompanying so-called "catheter-life" may be more tolerable than the struggle with wet and foul clothing and bedding.

For persons with intact urinary tracts but incompetent sphincters, treatment is always aimed at restoration of function until the bladder can be evacuated with external pressure by massage of the lower abdomen and by "bearing down" as in defecating or coughing. With persistence the paralyzed bladder can be made to function automatically. After an injury to the central nervous system producing incontinence, an indwelling catheter is used for days, weeks, or months, according to the rate of recovery and the judgment of the physician. During this time a record is made of the intake and output of body fluids, and the capacity of the bladder is studied as discussed in Chapter 31. Then the catheter is removed and habit training instituted. It is usually necessary to continue daily catheterization and measurement of urine that remains in the bladder after the patient's effort to void. Opinion differs as to whether one or more daily irrigations should be continued. Patients should understand such treatments and should participate in them to the extent that they are able. By the time the catheter can be discarded they know a good deal about bladder physiology. Throughout this treatment, but particularly after the removal of the catheter, the patient's fluid intake should be regulated. V. H. Youngblood and C. A. Fort suggest that they drink measured amounts of fluid three times a day at meals and at bedtime. From one half to one hour later the patient should try to void; Youngblood and Fort say:

. . . using as many aids as may be necessary, such as pressure over the bladder, straining, stimulation of "trigger points," and stretching the anal sphincter or external urethral meatus. The patient will usually be able to suggest changes in his individual schedule that may help him in emptying the bladder. . . .

Except in patients with very spastic bladders of small capacity, habit control works satisfactorily, whether the bladder paralysis is reflex, atonic or autonomic in type.*

Obviously, this habit training is easiest with young, otherwise healthy persons. Alice B. Morrissey points out the patient's psychological handicap; he is naturally embarrassed that he cannot control elimination, and after a few "accidents" he may "take refuge in withdrawal behavior and refuse to cooperate with further attempts towards rehabilitation."

Therefore, the first step . . . is on the psychological level. . . . The nurse must approach the problem with realism, tact, patience and knowledge. She must gain the patient's co-operation and confidence. . . . Sometimes, simply extending the hope that it is possible to overcome these difficulties is sufficient. . . . In urinary and bowel rehabilitation, as in other rehabilitation procedures, the disabled person must learn to do most of the work himself. When success is finally achieved, the rewards and satisfactions are great.†

Embarrassment is reduced if the nurse and patient are of the same sex but the fact that they are not should never keep the nurse from giving the patient the help he needs.

George G. Deaver,[34] Morrissey, and others suggest that after the removal of the catheter, the patient try to void every hour. When this schedule can be maintained with no leakage, the time interval is gradually increased to a three-, four-, or even five-hour schedule. The intervals are the same day and night; so the patient must be waked as many times as necessary. Eventually, he may accustom the bladder to holding its contents during a normal night's sleep.

Morrissey quotes a report of a patient who said that by limiting his intake in the

---

* Youngblood, V. H., and Fort, C. A.: "A Practical Method of Handling a Paralyzed Urinary Bladder," *North Carolina M. J.,* **11**:557, (Oct.) 1950.

† Morrissey, Alice B.: *Rehabilitation Nursing.* G. P. Putnam's Sons, New York, 1951, p. 104.

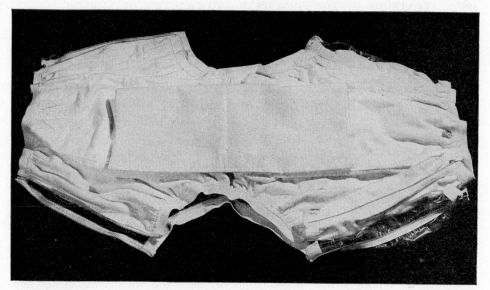

Figure 83A. Protective pants for the incontinent showing absorbent pad, cotton jersey lining, and outer plastic garment.

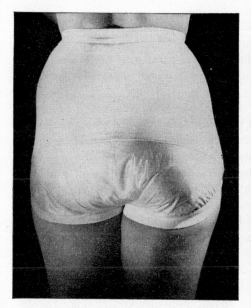

Figure 83B. Garment for ambulatory girls or women who are incontinent.

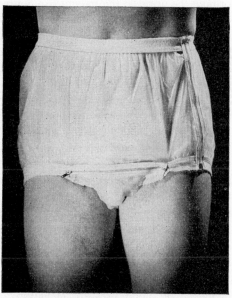

Figure 83C. Plastic outer garment for daytime wear, children or adult sizes, male and female.

(Figs. 83 A-C, courtesy of Ferguson Manufacturing Co., Grand Rapids, Mich.)

afternoon and keeping the 24-hour total around 1900 cc he could go from 10:30 at night until 8:30 in the morning without voiding or "spilling." He also said that he was then able to empty the bladder at a normal rate while at first it had been a slow process.

Achievement of an automatic bladder—one that empties at periodic intervals— may take weeks or months. During this time, there may be leakage between void- ings. (Persistent "spilling" or leaking means that rehabilitation is not entirely effective.) As long as there is leakage the clothing and bedding must be protected. During the day an ambulatory patient should be fitted with a pad that is not noticeable under the clothing. Figure 83 A shows an outer plastic garment with a cotton jersey lining and a zippered compartment into which is fitted an absorbent pad.* They are available in all sizes. Some men prefer to use a rubber urinal (see Fig. 82) during the day. Worn at night or too steadily, it is likely to macerate the glans penis. The meatus must be examined daily for signs of irritation. It should be kept clean and dry. This is difficult when using a rubber urinal. Control of odor from a urinal is also difficult.

Thomas S. Wilson [35] has succeeded in helping those with *senile urinary in- continence* to control the desire to void. He fills the bladder very slowly with an antiseptic solution. The very excitable bladder responds with waves of contraction, which the patient interprets as a desire to micturate. It may be urgent enough to seem painful to the subject. The physician asks the patient to bear this discomfort or hold the urine. If the patient can control the impulse to void, the contractions will cease and the patient will be relieved. Wilson believes that if the patient can be convinced that relief follows inhibiting the impulse, as well as giving in to it, that he can reduce the excitability of the bladder, or train it to hold more urine. This same sort of retraining applies to any patient who has habituated his bladder to holding only small amounts.

Brocklehurst, comparing incontinence among comparable populations of old people in different institutions, concluded that morale had a direct bearing on the incidence. He says: "There is no doubt that the status of the nurses in charge of these old people, and the nursing methods they use have a direct bearing on the incidence of incontinence."† It was highest in a hospital staffed with untrained personnel; it was lowest in that giving what he believed to be the best nursing care. Old people who are occupied and encouraged to "keep on their feet" are not nearly so likely to be incontinent as the bedfast. Ability to go to the bathroom is a great stimulus to keep dry, and this privilege should be maintained as long as it is possible. Brocklehurst found little difference between the incidence of in- continence in the age groups 60-69, 70-79, and 80 years and over. He did not find that organic disease of the nerves played a part although he noted a high incidence of blood pressure elevation and spastic muscular contraction. The in- cidence was high in the mentally confused if they were inactive and confined to bed.

---

*"Drico" garments are manufactured by Ferguson Manufacturing Co., Grand Rapids, Mich.

† Brocklehurst, John C.: *op. cit.,* p. 100.

A hopeless attitude toward incontinence in the aged is inconsistent with high standards of medical and nursing care. In most cases it can evidently be controlled and certainly not allowed to take the old man or woman "out of circulation."[36]

When rehabilitation of bladder function is impossible, the patient's incontinence must be treated as it is in infancy. When the patient is in bed the mattress is protected with a full-length waterproof cover. The usual bottom sheet is then adjusted. On top of this another waterproof rectangle covered with a cotton sheet is placed so that it extends from the neck to the knees and is tucked in at the sides. On this and directly under the buttocks is a waterproof rectangle, covered with a heavy absorbent material like cellucotton. Smaller absorbent pads should be placed between the legs and over the rectum. If the cellucotton pads are changed often enough, the larger sheets are never soiled, but there must be several layers of protectors for the mattress. When they are inefficient, control of odor is impossible.

Brocklehurst has designed a padded plaster shell molded to the person's form, in which the completely incontinent and senile patient lies. It is suspended over the bed frame and has an opening for the escape of urine and feces. While it may equalize pressure on all supporting parts of the recumbent body and *may* also reduce the time and linen needed for custodial care, it has obvious disadvantages. The shell is unesthetic and difficult to clean, and since the occupant is practically immobilized, he must approximate a vegetative existence.

A sawdust bed is also used for bedfast mental defectives, the senile, and others whose incontinence does not respond to treatment. A box 15 in. deep and the width and length of the bedspring is filled with sawdust. It can then be mounted on legs with rubber casters. A head- and footboard make it look like a bed, which is desirable. A half sheet and pillow are placed under the head and shoulders and the usual covering over the patient. When the patient urinates or defecates, he is dried and bathed, and the foul sawdust replaced with clean. Such beds are said to be surprisingly comfortable and offer considerable protection from pressure sores. One report mentions a patient whose skin is "like velvet" after 12 years' use of such a bed.[37]

Completely incontinent patients may be ambulatory if they wear waterproof garments and change the absorbent pads often enough. A great injustice is done many persons with this difficulty when they are not gotten into wheelchairs or encouraged to lead as normal a life as possible.

Alkaline, or ammoniacal, urine is believed to be more irritating than acid; the diet should therefore be one that fosters formation of acid urine, although Best and Taylor say that it is the function of the kidney to excrete ammonia combined with acids, and George Nagamatsu et al.[38] believe that urea-splitting, ammonia-producing organisms are present in the normal genitourinary tract. This means that all urine is to some degree ammoniacal and for this reason excoriating. The antiseptic methylbenzethonium chloride (Diaparene), said to inhibit the action of urea-splitting bacteria, is recommended in the care of incontinent adults as it is for infants. Diapers and pads are impregnated with the powders.[39, 40]

Frequent skin cleaning is, of course, indicated. A neutral detergent such as pHisoderm is recommended, especially since it replaces some of the fat that is removed in bathing. Vegetable oils, lanolin, or the commercial preparation "Lubriderm" should be applied after using nonfatted detergents. Deodorizing powders are helpful esthetically and in drying the area but must not be allowed to cake in skin folds. "Keradex,"* a coating for the skin, waterproofs it, or protects it to some extent from the urine and feces.

The same therapeutic principles as just discussed underlie the treatment of *bowel incontinence.* If the rectum and anus are intact, rehabilitation can usually be effected. The internal anal sphincter, controlled by the autonomic nervous system, can be trained to take over the work of the external sphincter whose function is temporarily or permanently lost along with that of other voluntary muscles.

For the paralyzed patient all conditions that regulate bowel movements under ordinary circumstances are even more important; namely, (1) freedom from stress, (2) a regular time for defecation, (3) a diet that results in a soft, formed stool, and (4) exercise to strengthen abdominal muscles used in defecation. Patients should be taught exercises they can carry out in bed and encouraged to get up and move about as soon as possible.

Medications should be used only when more natural means of encouraging evacuations are ineffective. The gums such as tragacanth or senna leaves that produce bulk are probably the most desirable. Cascara, mineral oil, milk of magnesia, and other preparations will, however, be prescribed. Impactions are not uncommon. In such case the injection of oil followed in several hours by an enema or an irrigation may remove the impaction; often it must be removed with the gloved hand.

Unless the patient can be helped to train the bowel function, his independence and usefulness are sadly curtailed. If he cannot accomplish regular and more or less normal bowel habits with diet, exercise, position, and manual pressure over the lower abdomen as he bears down in defecation, he may find that glycerin suppositories will stimulate an evacuation. He should be taught to insert from one to three suppositories about one-half to three hours before the usual time for defecation, depending upon the sensitivity of the colon. Glycerin is mildly irritating and stimulates contraction of the colon by drawing fluid into the rectum, increasing and at the same time softening the bulk of the stool. The physician may prescribe small, evacuating enemas until regularity is established.

Brocklehurst found that 70 per cent of the old people who had bladder incontinence also suffered from incontinence of the rectum. He believes rectal incontinence in the aged has a physiological basis, but, like bladder incontinence, the chief causes are (1) paralysis, (2) bedfastness, and (3) confusion.

The writer's summary presents Brocklehurst's opinion on senile incontinents.

Incontinence is commonly described by neurologists as "loss of sphincter control." It would appear, however, that the function of the sphincter is a subsidiary one, certainly less important than the tonus and movements of the bladder and large bowel. Between intervals of defecation the presence of a constantly filled rectum suggests

* Made by Texas Pharmacal Co., San Antonio.

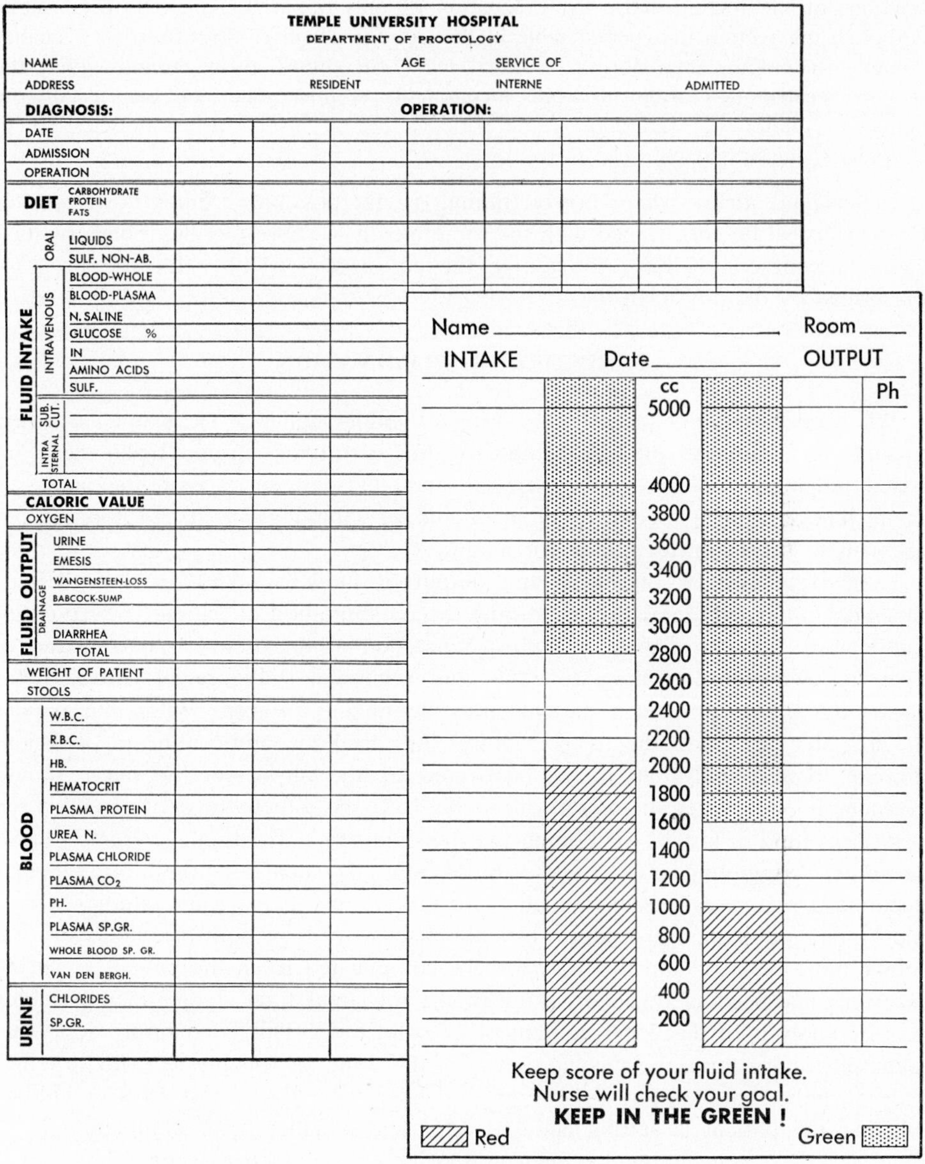

TEMPLE UNIVERSITY HOSPITAL
DEPARTMENT OF PROCTOLOGY

| NAME | | AGE | SERVICE OF | |
| ADDRESS | RESIDENT | INTERNE | ADMITTED |

DIAGNOSIS: **OPERATION:**

DATE									
ADMISSION									
OPERATION									
DIET CARBOHYDRATE PROTEIN FATS									

FLUID INTAKE
- ORAL — LIQUIDS / SULF. NON-AB.
- INTRAVENOUS — BLOOD-WHOLE / BLOOD-PLASMA / N. SALINE / GLUCOSE % / IN / AMINO ACIDS / SULF.
- SUB. CUT.
- INTRA STERNAL

TOTAL

CALORIC VALUE
OXYGEN

FLUID OUTPUT
- URINE
- EMESIS
- DRAINAGE — WANGENSTEEN-LOSS / BABCOCK-SUMP
- DIARRHEA
- TOTAL

WEIGHT OF PATIENT
STOOLS

BLOOD
- W.B.C.
- R.B.C.
- HB.
- HEMATOCRIT
- PLASMA PROTEIN
- UREA N.
- PLASMA CHLORIDE
- PLASMA CO_2
- PH.
- PLASMA SP.GR.
- WHOLE BLOOD SP. GR.
- VAN DEN BERGH.

URINE
- CHLORIDES
- SP.GR.

(Inset)

Name _____ Room ____

INTAKE   Date _____   OUTPUT

| cc | Ph |
| 5000 |
| 4000 |
| 3800 |
| 3600 |
| 3400 |
| 3200 |
| 3000 |
| 2800 |
| 2600 |
| 2400 |
| 2200 |
| 2000 |
| 1800 |
| 1600 |
| 1400 |
| 1200 |
| 1000 |
| 800 |
| 600 |
| 400 |
| 200 |

Keep score of your fluid intake.
Nurse will check your goal.
KEEP IN THE GREEN !

///// Red   Green ░░░░

Figure 84. Laboratory sheet on which can be summarized data for fluid intake and output, blood, and urine. (Courtesy of Temple University Hospital, Philadelphia, Pa.)

(*Inset, right*) Fluid intake and output record which the patient fills in with the help of the nurse. (Copyright, 1944, American Hospital Supply Corp., Evanston, Ill.)

463

at once senile incontinence as well as colonic overactivity; but the uninhibited contractions of the rectum cause the evacuation of only a part of the intrarectal mass.
Although the rectum is hyperexcitable in this condition and empties itself at a smaller
volume of contents than normal, residual feces are almost always found within the
rectum because defecation in senile incontinents is precipitate and can usually be
neither facilitated nor retarded by the patient's use of his accessory muscles (recti,
abdominis, diaphragm, etc.).

In terminal illness where bowel training is not possible, regular bowel movements can still be encouraged with the same means as those just described. In such
cases the nurse may have to assume the entire responsibility for the program
prescribed by the physician.

5. RECORDING ELIMINATION

When one considers the critical nature of kidney function, it is not surprising
to find great emphasis put on accurate records of urinary output. Upon these are
based judgments on the fluid-electrolyte and acid-base balance in the body. In
many illnesses single specimens of urine and/or samplings of the 24-hour output
are sent to the laboratory daily for analysis.

Concurrent records of intake and output of fluids are kept in most serious
illnesses, in chronic illnesses, and during the rehabilitation of patients where elimination is a problem. The person most concerned—the patient—is encouraged to
keep his own record to the extent that this is possible.[41] Figure 84 (inset, right)
shows a daily form, which patients may be taught to keep. When the patient
is not able to take the responsibility for drinking and eating a sufficient
amount to accomplish an intake advocated by the physician, the nurse should
consider it one of her major obligations to help the patient to do this. With the
very sick, fluid is lost by suctioning the intestinal tract, by drainage from wounds
or burns, by vomiting or diarrhea, or by sweating. In such cases the nurse keeps as
accurate a record as possible of all these losses, and in metabolic studies it is a
meticulous and skilled procedure. Equally exact records of both oral and extraoral
intake must be kept, and this may also be complicated when the patient is getting
infusions and feeding through a tube in the intestinal tract. Exact measurements
require analysis of the water content of all solid food. This is so rarely done that
some physicians think the specific gravity of the urine, or roughly its color, whether
pale or amber-colored, and the presence of edema are the easiest ways of judging
whether the patient is getting enough water and whether he is eliminating it. A
daily record of defecation is a regular item of every patient's record. The nature
of the stool should be recorded unless the patient is able to assume responsibility
for adequacy of bowel function. Fluid-electrolyte, acid-base, and protein balance is
discussed in Chapter 13. Nutrition and elimination cannot be completely separated. These two chapters should be studied as a unit.

REFERENCES

1. Alvarez, Walter C.: *An Introduction to Gastro-enterology.* Paul B. Hoeber, New York, 1948, p. 607.
2. Cantor, Meyer O.: *Intestinal Intubation.* Charles C Thomas, Publisher, Springfield, Ill., 1949, pp. 112, 133.
3. Best, Charles H., and Taylor, Norman B.: *Physiological Basis of Medical Practice,* 5th ed. Williams & Wilkins Co., Baltimore, 1950, p. 583.
4. Burnett, F. L.: "The Intestinal Rate and the Form of the Feces," *Am. J. Roentgenol.,* **10**:599, (Aug.) 1923.
5. Best, Charles H., and Taylor, Norman B.: *op. cit.,* p. 579.
6. Alvarez, Walter C.: *op. cit.,* p. 574.
7. Brocklehurst, John C.: *Incontinence in Old People.* E. S. Livingstone, Ltd., Edinburgh, 1951, p. 133.
8. Bacon, Harry E.: *Anus, Rectum and Sigmoid Colon,* 3rd ed. J. B. Lippincott Co.. Philadelphia, 1949, pp. 137, 169.
9. Senn, Milton, J. E. (ed.): *Problems of Infancy and Childhood; Transactions of the Fourth Conference, New York, March, 1950.* Josiah Macy, Jr. Foundation, New York, 1951, p. 22.
10. Baruch, Dorothy: *One Little Boy.* Julian Press, Inc., New York, 1952.
11. Kantor, John L., and Kasich, Anthony M.: *Handbook of Digestive Diseases.* C. V. Mosby Co., St. Louis, 1949, p. 314.
12. Senn, Milton J. (ed.): *op. cit.,* pp. 57, 59.
13. Fries, Margaret E.: "The Child's Ego Development and the Training of Adults in His Environment," *Psycho-analytic Study of the Child II,* 1946, p. 85.
14. Nelson, Waldo E. (ed.): *Mitchel-Nelson Textbook of Pediatrics,* 5th ed. W. B. Saunders Co., Philadelphia, 1950, p. 318.
15. Gradwohl, R. B. H.: *Clinical Laboratory Methods and Diagnosis.* C. V. Mosby Co., St. Louis, 1948, p. 1097.
16. Maxcy, Kenneth F. (ed.): *Rosenau's Preventive Medicine and Hygiene,* 7th ed. Appleton-Century-Crofts, Inc., New York, 1951, pp. 227, 242.
17. Chandler, Asa C.: *Introduction to Parasitology,* 7th ed. John Wiley & Sons, New York, 1950.
18. Seaton, D. R.: "Anthelmintics—Current Therapeutics XXXV," *Practitioner,* **165**:64, (Nov.) 1950.
19. Gold, Harry (ed.): *Cornell Conferences on Therapy,* Vol. I. The Macmillan Company, 1946, p. 224.
20. Kantor, Alfred J.: *Ambulatory Proctology,* 2nd ed. Paul B. Hoeber, New York, 1952, p. 412.
21. Steigmann, Frederick, et al.: "Influence of Mineral Oil Ingestion on Plasma Vitamin A Level," *J. Lab. & Clin. Med.,* **36**:993, (Dec.) 1950.
22. Gold, Harry, (ed.): *op. cit.,* pp. 282, 298.
23. Fulton, John F. (ed.): *Textbook of Physiology,* 16th ed. W. B. Saunders Co., Philadelphia, 1949, p. 893.
24. Carlson, Anton J., and Johnson, Victor: *The Machinery of the Body.* University of Chicago Press, Chicago, 1948, p. 638.
25. Houssay, Bernardo A., et al.: *Human Physiology.* McGraw-Hill Book Co., New York, 1951, p. 545.
26. LeComte, Ralph M.: *Manual of Urology,* 4th ed. Williams & Wilkins Co., Baltimore, 1948, p. 205.
27. Spock, Benjamin: *Common Sense Book of Baby and Child Care.* Duell, Sloan & Pearce, New York, 1946, p. 201.

28. Townsend, Ralph: "Etiological Aspects of Enuresis," *J. Tennessee M. A.*, **43**:328, (Sept.) 1950.
29. Nelson, Waldo E. (ed.): *op. cit.*, p. 1188.
30. Glicklich, Lucile B.: "An Historical Account of Enuresis," *Pediatrics*, **8**:859, (Dec.) 1951.
31. Royal Society of Medicine: "Discussion on Stress Incontinence of Urine of the Female," *Proceedings*, **43**:255, (Apr.) 1950.
32. Campbell, Meredith: "A New Incontinence Clamp," *J. Urol.*, **64**:821, (Dec.) 1950.
33. Rowe, Albert G.: "Enuresis in the Comatose Patient," *M. Technician's Bull.*, **1**:10, (Nov.–Dec.) 1950.
34. Deaver, George G.: *Evaluation of Disability and Rehabilitation Procedures of Patients with Spinal Cord Lesions.* Institute for the Crippled and Disabled, New York, 1947.
35. Wilson, Thomas S.: "Incontinence of Urine in the Aged," *Lancet*, **2**:374, (Sept.) 1948.
36. Howell, Trevor H.: "Treatment of Incontinence in the Elderly," *Practitioner*, **164**:467, (May) 1950.
37. Hoffman, H. Marguerite, et al.: "Sawdust Bed Therapy," *Am. J. Nursing*, **49**:654, (Oct.) 1949.
38. Nagamatsu, George, et. al.: "A New Skin Treatment for the Incontinent Patient, A Preliminary Report," *Geriatrics*, **4**:293, (Sept.-Oct.) 1949.
39. Silverstein, Martin A., and Gips, Claudia D.: "Skin Care for Incontinent Patients," *Am. J. Nursing*, **52**:63, (Jan.) 1952.
40. Council on Pharmacy and Chemistry (New and Nonofficial Remedies): "Methylbenzethonium: Diaparene chloride," *J.A.M.A.*, **144**:548, (Oct.) 1950.
41. Morrissey, Alice B.: *Rehabilitation Nursing.* G. B. Putnam's Sons, New York, 1951.

Additional Suggested Reading

Cook, Edward N.: "A New Clamp for Use with a Bag Catheter," *Mayo Clin., Proc. Staff Meet.*, **26**:14, (Jan.) 1951.
Davis, David M.: *Urological Nursing*, 4th ed. W. B. Saunders, Co. Philadelphia, 1946.
Dwyer, Sheila M.: *Modern Urology for Nurses.* Lea & Febiger, Philadelphia, 1945.
Etteldorf, James N., and Crawford, Lloyd V.: "Treatment of Ascariasis in Children," *J.A.M.A.*, **143**:799, (July) 1950.
Gershenfeld, Louis: *Urine and Urinalysis*, 3rd ed. Romaine Pierson Publishers Inc., New York, 1948.
Grace, William J., et al.: *The Human Colon; An Experimental Study Based on Direct Observation of Four Fistulous Subjects.* Paul B. Hoeber, New York, 1951.
Kennedy, William T.: "The Muscles of Micturition," *Am. J. Obst. & Gynec.*, **52**:214, (Aug.) 1946.
Lattimer, John K.: "A Plan for the Management of Anuria," *J. Urol.*, **54**:312, (Sept.) 1945.
Lowsley, Oswald S., and Kirwin, Thomas J.: *Clinical Urology*, 3rd ed. Williams & Wilkins Co., Baltimore, 1956.
"Plastic Panties for Adults" (The Trading Post), *Am. J. Nursing*, **51**:37, (Jan.) 1951.
Prather, George C.: *Urological Aspects of Spinal Cord Injuries.* Charles C Thomas, Publisher, Springfield, Ill., 1945.
Rolnick, H. C.: *The Practice of Urology.* J. B. Lippincott Co., Philadelphia, 1949. (2 vols.)
Schwartz, M. S., and Staunton, A. H.: "A Social Psychological Study of Incontinence," *Psychiatry*, **13**:399, (Nov.) 1950.
Sunderman, Frederick, and Boerner, Frederick: *Normal Values in Clinical Medicine.* W. B. Saunders Co., Philadelphia, 1949.

CHAPTER 15. BODY MECHANICS—TRANS-PORTATION, REST, SLEEP, AND PRE-VENTION OF PRESSURE SORES

1. BODY MECHANICS AND ITS RELATION TO DISEASE

Body mechanics is an over-all term defined by the White House Conference on Child Health and Protection as ". . . the mechanical correlation of the various systems of the body with special reference to the skeletal, muscular and visceral systems and their neurological associations. Normal body mechanics may be said to obtain when this mechanic correlation is most favorable to the function of these systems."* The nurse is likely to think of it as including posture and the use of the body in moving and lifting, but it encompasses more than this. Joel E. Goldthwait and his associates[1] attribute many chronic ailments to poor body mechanics, for the function of bones, joints, muscles, viscera, and nerves naturally falls under general physiology. They point out that posture affects the size and shape of the thoracic, abdominal, and pelvic cavities and that this in turn affects the position of, and pressure on, the viscera. Posture also determines the distribution of weight and pull on the joints. Lack of balance or poise may create tension throughout the body, affecting the vascular, nervous, and muscular systems. Discussing muscular

* White House Conference: *Body Mechanics.* Appleton-Century Co., New York, 1932, p. 5.

467

dystrophies, arthritis, diabetes, constipation, heart disease, and hypertension, to name a few of the chronic conditions covered, they reported marked improve- ment or complete relief of symptoms chiefly by correction of defective body mechanics. Pictures of patients showing postural changes over many years are convincing evidence of the success of those orthopedists.

Goldthwait et al. take the position, attributed to George Draper and William Sheldon in Chapter 18 (see p. 553), that mankind can be divided into structural types. They recognize three: the slender, the intermediate, and stocky figures. The intermediate is probably nearest to normal, while the slender and stocky figures have characteristic temperaments, and each group seems subject to characteristic disorders. That these disorders might be explained on a structural basis is not too farfetched since the viscera of the slender and stocky figures differ in size and shape and in the position they assume in the body cavity. Goldthwait et al. make this comforting statement, however:

. . . while the type of the body cannot be changed, the manner in which it is used can be modified greatly. The health of the individual depends largely on this, as well as whether or not he will succumb to one of the diseases of which he is a potential victim. Good health is possible in all the variations from the so-called normal, or intermediate, body type.*

Titles such as *Lumbar Breakdown Caused by the Erect Position in Man*[2] sug- gest that had man continued to walk on all fours, the need for hundreds of articles and books such as Philip Lewin's *The Back and Its Disorders*[3] might not exist. Mabel E. Todd says:

At that stage of the evolutionary process when man assumed the upright posture, he secured freedom of motion and a larger command over his environment than is possessed by any other creature. There are, however, mechanical disadvantages and points of weakness in his structural provision that threaten the stability of his support and the protection of his vital processes.†

This is a widely accepted point of view, but some students of the subject main- tain that the upright body is an efficient mechanism, that its difficulties are the result of misuse, and that if good posture is once established little effort is required to maintain it. They think that postural faults originate in the misuse of our capacities rather than in the structure of the body.[4] Adults often suffer from mistakes made in infancy. For example, they may have been forced to sit, stand, or walk before they were developmentally ready. It is believed that an infant will spontane- ously do all these things when the structures involved are strong enough. If he does them earlier, faulty relationships in body segments are started that tend to be exaggerated in later life unless a great effort is made to overcome them. The spine is admittedly the fundamental basis of support and movement in vertebrates, and

---

* Goldthwait, Joel E.: *Essentials of Body Mechanics—In Health and Disease,* 5th ed. J. B. Lippincott Co., Philadelphia, 1952, p. 8.

† Todd, Mabel E.: *The Thinking Body; A Study of Balancing Forces of Dynamic Man.* Paul B. Hoeber, New York, 1937, p. 8.

abnormal spinal curves profoundly affect the entire body. Nutritional status affects the body's mechanical efficiency. A starved child with his protruding abdomen maintains his balance by increasing the lumbar curve. Less severe stages of malnutrition at any age are characterized by a musculature too weakened to hold the body erect. We are born in a bow and if we live long enough, most of us will return to it. We learn to stand erect, but the maturing process brings changes in cartilage and bone that make the maintenance of this carriage difficult. David E. Morton found by dissection of the cadavers of persons past middle age that 28 showed "brown degeneration of intervertebral discs that resulted in exaggeration or decrease in normal vertebral curvatures."[*] He considered them sufficiently marked to have produced not only poor posture but also considerable discomfort. The point here, however, is that without being facetious we might say that our life represents an effort to stay erect—at least physically.

That bodily attitudes affect our outlook on life is almost undisputed. Todd puts it overstrongly perhaps when she says:

> We sit and walk as we think. Watch any man as he walks down the avenue, and you can determine his status in life. With practice, a finer discernment will have him placed socially and economically. . . . We judge our fellow man more by the arrangement and movement of his skeletal parts than is evident at once.[†]

By the development and maintenance of good body mechanics we may hope to make possible our optimum physical effectiveness and prevent many chronic ailments, but we can expect with equal assurance that the mental and emotional aspects of life, if they can be said to be separated from the physical, will likewise be affected. Goldthwait and his associates believe that efforts to develop good posture should begin at birth and that children should be universally taught the right way to stand, walk, run, lift, and so on. With their methods of re-education they are able to help the cooperative patient of almost any age. Henry O. Kendall, Florence P. Kendall, and Dorothy A. Boynton assume that nature takes a more aggressive role in developing good posture. They say:

> Most postural deviations in the growing individual fall in the category of developmental deviations; when patterns become habitual they may result in postural faults. . . . A young child is not very likely to have habitual faults and can be harmed by corrective measures that are not needed. Over-correction may lead to atypical faults more harmful and difficult to deal with than the ones which caused original concern. . . . [‡]

While there may be points of disagreement among orthopedists, most would agree that with an adequate diet and minimum supervision by experts almost everyone in this country could avoid the now-prevalent structural defects with their threat of concomitant ailments. It is hard to think of a preventive program more far reaching in its effects. The nurse should learn as much as she can about

[*] Morton, David E.: "An Anatomical Study in the Human Spinal Column with Emphasis on Degenerative Changes in the Cervical Region," *Yale J. Biol. & Med.*, 23:126–46, (Feb.) 1950.

[†] Todd, Mabel E.: *op. cit.*, p. 1.

[‡] Kendall, Henry O.; Kendall, Florence P.; and Boynton, Dorothy A.: *Posture and Pain*. Williams & Wilkins Co., Baltimore, 1952, p. 167.

body mechanics in order to practice what she learns for her own benefit; she will soon realize, however, that not only is she able to influence others by her example but also that almost every activity of patient care offers an opportunity to foster good habits in her patients or improve poor ones. As far as this topic is concerned, we are all trainees subject to stress and strain, and should be constantly alert to danger. A nurse will often leave her patient beautifully "postured" to promote rest and sleep and then herself lie down to rest in an atrocious position; or she will lift a prostrated patient to spare him effort, not considering that she may incapacitate herself for further service. The writer suggests that the nurse study this chapter for its value to her as an individual and as a worker. In many cases no effort will be made to differentiate these values since it is assumed that a principle of body mechanics is as applicable to one person as another. School and industrial nurses are in a particularly good position to contribute to the prevention of structural defects and so-called orthopedic illness. They can help to select and design chairs, stools, ladders, tables, and desks that make good body mechanics for students and workers possible.* Clothing and particularly shoes affect posture; their choice is especially important during infancy and childhood, and in pregnancy. Many industries present special orthopedic hazards as, for example, those that require workers to maintain one posture or that necessitate wearing heavy equipment. It may take the combined efforts of the industrial physician, the nurse, the industrial engineer, and the workers themselves to control fatigue and prevent disease in the occupations concerned.

No attempt has been made to cover the treatment of orthopedic conditions. Nurses should develop the habit of consulting articles and texts in the fields of body mechanics, neurology, and pediatrics as they are faced with complex orthopedic problems in patient care.

2. GOOD POSTURE—STANDING, SITTING, AND LYING

Standing Posture. "Ideal," "normal," and "standard" postures as described usually refer to the standing position. The terms are often used interchangeably and refer to skeletal alignment. In *Posture and Pain,* the Kendalls and Boynton[5] say that standard posture as shown in texts usually refers to an ideal which they have never seen matched "in all respects." The drawings of standard postures show two symmetrical halves when the body is divided through the midline of the pelvis, spine, sternum, and skull. The other midline divides the body into the anterior and posterior sections of equal weight. The intersections of these two midplanes form a line which is analogous to the gravity line. Around this line the body is hypothetically in a position of equilibrium. Goldthwait et al. describe the torso of the intermediate body type, which they say represents "the standard,"

* I am forcibly reminded of this obvious need at the moment. Working in a beautiful *medical* library where the only seats are the traditional Windsor chairs, whose arms keep them at a respectful distance from the table on which I write, I must use a pad in the seat to keep from being thrown backward and a foot stool made from my materials to keep my feet from dangling.

giving the normal angles of from 70 to 90 deg at the subcostal border, the comparative measurements of the thorax and abdomen, and other details too numerous to list here. They also describe the slender and stocky figures whose typical measurements will vary considerably from each other, but of course less from those of the intermediate type. In the physical education of these various types it is obviously useless to try to make all achieve the same results.

A good standing posture is characterized by poise or balance without tension or rigidity. Goldthwait et al. give a more complete description of the following requirements for good body mechanics:

(1) The curves of the spine shall not be exaggerated; (2) the subcostal angle of the ribs shall be at least a right angle; (3) the circumference of the chest at the xiphoid process in the habitual standing position shall be approximately halfway between the girth at full inspiration and that at full expiration; (4) the abdomen above the umbilicus shall be larger and bigger than that below the umbilicus and it shall show firm, resistant structures; and (5) the line drawn through the patella and the middle of the ankle shall strike the base of the second or third toe.*

The authority just cited compares the present emphasis on pulling in the abdomen and the old admonition to "throw the shoulders back." It is now believed that the older method of maintaining "good" posture was detrimental because the person generally assumed a position of extreme lordosis and prevented correct use of the lower abdominal muscles. To maintain correct trunk alignment which is the basis of good posture, it is important that the lower abdomen is pulled in and up, the back flat, the head up and the chin in, and that the weight is thrown well forward on the outer borders of the feet. The body is then stretched tall but without rigidity. Only with such a posture can correct weight-bearing lines be maintained. When the lower abdominal muscles only are pulled in, there is no interference with normal breathing.

No posture is a good one if it is taut. Directions to "hold" any position is not only wrong but impossible to follow for any length of time. When it is necessary to stand for long periods it helps to separate the feet and thus to broaden the base supporting the body; this is done instinctively when standing in a moving vehicle. If the weight is shifted from one leg to the other by flexing one knee, the transverse axis of the pelvis should be kept horizontal with the floor to prevent lateral spinal curvatures. Because it is almost impossible to stand correctly in the wrong shoes it is advisable, before describing sitting and lying posture, to discuss their selection and emphasize the position the feet should assume.

Foot Posture and Selection of Shoes. A well-balanced body is only possible if the feet are in the relationship to it described in the preceding paragraph and shown in Figure 85 B. Likewise, the most normal feet are found in those whose bodies are in good alignment. Orthopedists warn against treating the back, for example, without considering the feet or trying to correct a foot disability or without attempting to modify an accompanying spinal curvature. Minor structural foot

* Goldthwait, Joel E., et al.: *op. cit.,* p. 268.

defects often disappear when body mechanics in other parts of the body is improved, although many conditions require local treatment.

Most persons are born with potentially efficient feet; a few have congenital defects such as flatfoot or clubfoot, missing or extra toes. In flatfoot the connective tissues holding the bones together (ligaments and fascia) are too relaxed to preserve the arched arrangement of the tarsals and metatarsals seen in the average foot. The condition appears in both feet whereas it is rare to find more than one clubfoot—a condition of inversion and rotation with abnormally short tendons, or contracted fascia, in parts of the foot producing and maintaining this abnormal position. Normal feet in a normal standing posture are parallel with each other; inverted feet are called *talipes varus,* while feet turned outwards, or everted, are called *talipes valgus.* Inversion is more likely to be a congenital defect; eversion is more likely to be acquired as a result of faulty posture of the entire body. A short Achilles tendon is sometimes present at birth but is usually found in those who habitually wear high heels. Other acquired foot deformities associated with poor body mechanics are pronation of the foot (eversion of the heel with depression of the longitudinal arch) and the changes that result from wearing high-heeled shoes over a long period of time. Besides shortening the tendon of Achilles (the tendon of the gastrocnemius muscle) this practice thickens the muscles above the ankle and spreads the forefoot which bears the weight of the body. Short shoes, especially if pointed and coupled with high heels, turn the big toe away from the midline of the body and enlarge the metatarsophalangeal joint (*hallux valgus*). Over this joint a protective cushion soon forms which we call a bunion. When the weight of the body is thrust on the point of the foot the second toe is often elongated (a "hammer toe") and calluses form on it. Calluses (corns) form on any area of the foot where irritation is constant. Nature develops them, like bunions, to protect underlying tissues.

It seems quite obvious that training in body mechanics will prevent many of these difficulties. The child with a well-balanced body will stand and walk with the feet parallel. Stressing this position of the feet helps to promote good posture throughout the body but correcting only this aspect of posture is rarely enough. Shoes should be chosen with utmost care, and the child helped to understand why certain features of their construction are important. The points stressed by most orthopedists are shown in Figure 85 A: (1) a straight inside line, (2) adequate space for the forefoot without undue spreading, (3) sufficient length to prevent pressure on the end of toes, and (4) a low heel as broad as the foot itself.

Persons who suffer from foot defects should seek the advice of an orthopedist who may correct the posture, the gait, and the selection of shoes. Occasionally surgery is indicated.

Sitting Posture. The same objectives should be kept in mind for sitting that have just been implied in the discussion of standing. Spinal curves should not be exaggerated, but the trunk held or supported in an upright position with the lower abdomen in, the back flat, and the chin in. To "sit tall" is just as important as to "stand tall." The chair should be long enough to support the buttocks

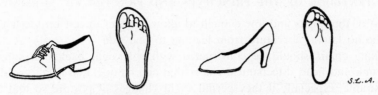

Figure 85A. (*Left*) Correct style of shoe, and toes in natural position; (*right*) incorrect style of shoe, and toes cramped. (Based on Krusen, Frank H.: *Physical Medicine*. W. B. Saunders Co., Philadelphia, 1941.)

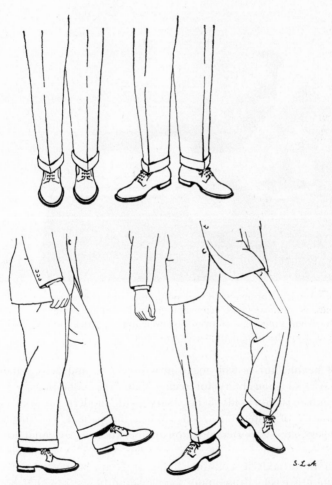

Figure 85B. (*Top, left*) Correct standing position; (*top, right*) incorrect standing position. (*Bottom, left*) Correct walking posture; (*bottom, right*) incorrect walking posture. (Based on Krusen, Frank H.: *Physical Medicine*. W. B. Saunders Co., Philadelphia, 1941.)

and most of the thighs and low enough to allow the feet to rest on the floor. There should be no lateral curvature from leaning to one side.

Reclining chairs should be constructed with a straight back that supports the entire trunk and head. Mechanical chairs that can be operated by the occupant are very desirable, especially if they permit slight changes of posture so that the pressure on the supporting body surfaces can be modified at frequent intervals. A concave back rest results in a spinal flexion that crowds the thoracic viscera, relaxes the abdomen, and displaces its contents. Everyone should observe these rules for

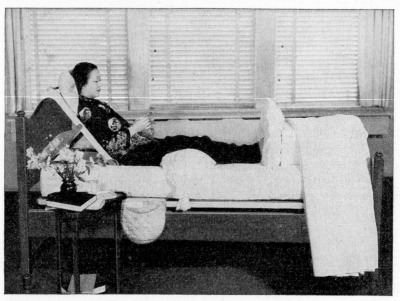

Figure 86. Devices for maintaining comfortable sitting posture in bed that are available in most homes. Note inexpensive removable back rest, pillow wrapped in a sheet and tied to bedsprings for knee support, a wooden box weighted by bricks to support the feet, prevent foot drop, and keep the weight of the covers off the toes.

the sake of health; nurses who make provisions for, and help, patients into sitting postures have a responsibility for seeing that these conditions are met. In some situations improvisation will be necessary; with modern hospital equipment it is merely a matter of using it correctly. When the patient is sitting up in bed, the thighs and legs are supported. Flexion of the knees is essential for comfort. The back should be straight from the coccyx to the occiput. A small pillow to fill in the cervical curvature adds to comfort. If the arms are supported with pillows, as in an armchair, it is easier to maintain the elevation of the ribs that prevents pressure on the thoracic organs. A footboard in bed takes the place of the floor when sitting in a chair. It helps the patient to maintain erectness of the spine and it prevents "foot drop."

Goldthwait makes the point that there are many ways of sitting correctly and incorrectly. A good sitting posture is one that prevents crowding of the viscera, exaggeration of normal vertebral curves, fatigue from lack of support, or contractures. Ralph M. Barnes,[6] discussing industrial fatigue, emphasizes the importance of good posture in sitting, properly constructed seats, and frequent changes of position. No matter how comfortable it is at first, any position is tiring if maintained for any length of time.

Lying Posture.   A firm bed is essential to good alignment of body segments in a horizontal position. Too many springs and mattresses allow the heaviest part of the body (the hips usually) to sink far below the level of the head and shoulders, which results in a marked lateral, posterior, or anterior spinal curvature according

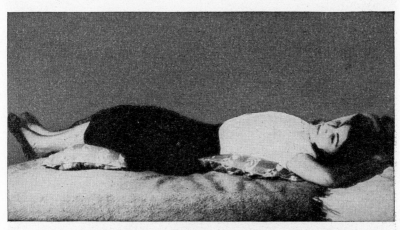

Figure 87.   Recumbent position used for anyone during a rest period. Hyperextended dorsal spine, arms outwardly rotated and abducted, knees flexed to relax abdominal muscles and flatten lower back. A postural rest position for the prenatal patient, arthritic, or person with round shoulders. It elevates the chest, brings the diaphragm higher, and makes more room for abdominal organs. (Courtesy of Joint Orthopedic Nursing Advisory Service, New York City.)

to whether the person is lying on his back, side, or abdomen. Orthopedists are discouraging the use of inner-spring mattresses, and there is such a general demand for firm beds that some hotels will supply patrons with "bed boards" on request. Back ailments seem to be increasing. Inner-spring mattresses, automobiles that discourage walking, and all the laborsaving mechanisms that replace muscular activity are contributing factors.

Figures 87, 88, and 89 show what is believed to be correct *supine, side-lying* (lateral), and *prone* positions. In each, the following principles are observed: (1) the back is straight, or its normal curves unexaggerated, from the coccyx to the occiput; (2) the legs are flexed to relieve the strain on the lumbar spine, the abdomen, and the legs; (3) the ribs are elevated and the "rib cage" enlarged, or constriction prevented; (4) the legs are supported so that the weight of one does not fall on the other; and (5) excessive ankle extension is prevented.

Many modifications of these positions are used according to patients' special needs. For example, weak or paralyzed muscles require more extensive support from pillows, sandbags, and other devices; pain in the back or the abdomen may call for increased flexion of the legs, and in spastic conditions contractures are prevented with splints, sandbags, bivalved casts, and other devices. Texts on orthopedic and neurological nursing should be consulted for amplification of the subject.

Cradles.   The weight of the bedclothes may often cause pain or distort posture. In such cases a device called a cradle is placed on the bed to support the covers. A

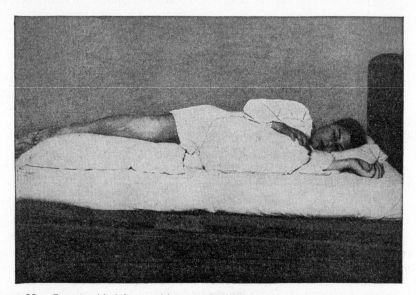

Figure 88.   Correct side-lying position. A small pillow or pad under the head preserves alignment of cervical spine. Pillows to support upper arm and thigh prevent strain on ligaments and on joint capsules of shoulder and hip. (Courtesy of Joint Orthopedic Nursing Advisory Service, New York City.)

great variety is available. Equipment used in hospitals should be light so that it can be transported easily, and collapsible so that it can be stored in a small space. It should be possible to use it on any part of the bed and to fix it in position. Figure 90 shows an aluminum cradle made in two parts and having these qualifications. It can also be equipped with a removable thermostatically controlled light bulb, which may be a means of warming the air under the cradle or furnishing heat prescribed for therapy. Cradles may be improvised in homes from a variety of materials. In Figure 86 the box used as an improvised foot rest serves also to keep the weight of the covers off the toes. A suitably shaped carton or wooden box with the bottom and one side removed makes an excellent cradle to put over a leg or arm.

Terms Used in Faulty Postures.   The orthopedist uses the following terms in

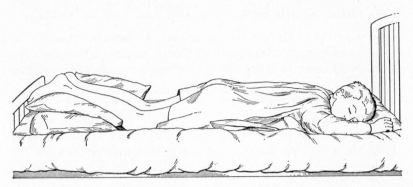

Figure 89. Diagram to illustrate prone position. Pillow under abdomen preserves alignment of spine. Pillows permit knee flexion, prevent pressure on toes, and allow good position of feet. If knees are straight, feet should hang over end of mattress at right angles, and a small pad placed under ankles. Small roll under shoulders maintains shoulder girdle in correct alignment. (Courtesy of Joint Orthopedic and Nursing Advisory Service, New York City.)

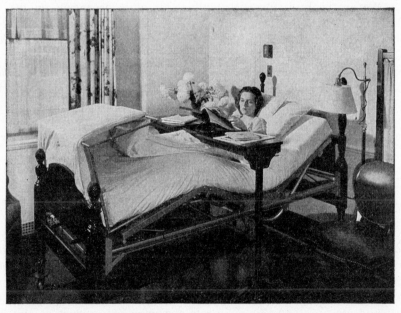

Figure 90. Devices for maintaining a comfortable sitting posture that are available to hospital patients. Note Gatch frame providing support for the back and knees, cradle to take weight of the covers off the feet, and an adjustable table to hold books, writing materials, and so on. (Courtesy of Columbia-Presbyterian Medical Center, New York City.)

describing common postural faults or deviations: An anterior, posterior, or lateral *tilt* of the pelvis or *rotation* of the pelvis or thorax; *lordosis,* a forward curve of the spine used with reference to an increase in the lumbar curve; *kyphosis,* a backward curve of the spine most commonly seen in the thorax; *round shoulders,* abduction of the scapula associated with a forward position of the shoulders; "bowlegs," lateral outward curvature of the legs from postural or structural causes; *knock-knees,* touching of the knees when the feet are separated; *pronation,* weight-bearing on the inside of the sole; and *supination,* weight-bearing on the outer side of the foot.

3. EXERCISE IN HEALTH AND SICKNESS

Life is a series of actions and reactions. Living cells have rhythms of increased and decreased activity. Contraction followed by relaxation, the "specialty" of muscle cells, is the most conspicuous cell activity. The 434 muscles of the body constitute about one half of the body weight. Their contraction and relaxation give the face its expression, produce voice sounds and movements of the body characteristic of species and individuals. There is some form of movement in every part of the body. When we speak of exercise we usually refer to activity of voluntary or striated muscle. We are likely to forget that life is far more dependent on the smooth muscles of the viscera. Because they are involuntary, not under the control of the cerebral cortex, we are likely to forget that normal visceral activity depends indirectly on the tone of the voluntary musculature. The condition of the striated skeletal muscle determines the size and shape of the thoracic, abdominal, and pelvic cavities and the pressures brought to bear on excretory and circulatory organs.

It is a safe generalization that physiological use of an organ maintains it in a normal state: excessive use causes hypertrophy; disuse, atrophy. This is conspicuously demonstrated in muscle tissue. Exercise is therefore essential for the maintenance of normal and for the re-education of abnormal muscles. Splints and braces that assume the supporting function of normal muscle and connective tissue are used only as temporary measures or to take the place of organically unsound tisues whose function cannot be re-established with exercises.

Thomas L. Delorme, writing in William Bierman and Sidney Licht's text,[7] lists and discusses the following effects of active exercise: (1) increased respiratory rate and oxygen consumption; (2) liberation of heat with increase of body temperature; (3) increase in the number of active capillaries; (4) increased venous return to the heart resulting in (5) larger output of blood with each stroke; (6) rise in blood pressure; and (7) pulse rate and increased production, distribution, and elimination of lactic acid and carbon dioxide. Any increase in metabolism is attributed to circulatory stimulation and is therefore an indirect effect.

Analysis of these reactions suggests that exercise has a beneficial effect as long as it is moderate and does not overtax the compensatory mechanisms. With exercise the oxygen need may increase from 250 to 4000 cc, and the pulse rate may rise from 20 to 40 beats or more per minute. An abnormal heart or lungs cannot adjust to such excessive demands, nor can hypertensive arterioles adjust to an increased blood volume that raises the systolic blood pressure 60 to 70 mm of mercury. For these reasons exercise in health and sickness should be adapted to the body needs of all ages and under varying conditions. Regular and appropriate activity results in physiological development and in improvement of every function, including thought. It stimulates the brain by increasing through the circulatory system its supply of oxygen and food and by removing metabolic wastes; movement also increases messages received through the sense organs. Just as the mobility of man has enabled him to control his environment to a greater degree than any other creature, the exposure of the individual to a variety of stimuli enlarges his outlook. Bodily motion is in itself a satisfaction. This engagement of rhythmical movement through suitable occupations and diversion is among the most beneficial effects of exercise.

In health we take for granted the free movement in all parts of our anatomy and the freedom of our person. An analysis of Table 1 on page 22 shows that a large part of the national income is spent on transportation and on games involving motion. Medical workers, usually active persons, should continually remind themselves of the psychological and physical handicap of any illness that limits free movement—either of a part or of the whole person. Emphasis has shifted within the last two decades from the emphasis on rest—bed rest—as a panacea for all ills to emphasis on ambulation. Since the first warnings that continuous recumbency favored the formation of kidney stones, of thrombi, the development of pulmonary edema, and other complications of illness, literature on bed rest and ambulation has steadily grown. In reporting his own investigation, G. Donald Whedon lists more than fifty such articles and summarizes current opinion. Nurses will find his report very helpful. In an effort to rule out the confusing factor of illness, Whedon and his associates studied the effect of recumbency on the metabolism of four normal, healthy young men who spent six to seven weeks lying in bivalved plaster casts extending from the umbilicus to the toes, in fixed and oscillating beds. Because the findings on nitrogen and calcium metabolism, creatine retention, and other physiological factors followed the same curve, they are significant even though there were only four subjects. A parallel study of patients and patients' records contributed to the value of the investigation. Dr. Whedon and *Medical Clinics of North America* have generously granted permission to include his summary in the following pages.*

Summary

The place of recumbency or bed rest in treatment of disease and in convalescence has been of increasing concern in recent years. Criticisms of bed rest have generally relied upon observations of patients bedridden by illness in which effects of recumbency

---

* Whedon, G. Donald: "Management of the Effects of Recumbency," *M. Clin. North America,* **35:**545, (Mar.) 1951.

per se could not be clearly differentiated from those of the underlying disease. Studies designed to clarify these effects by immobilization of healthy young male subjects have shown significant mineral losses and derangements in physiologic functions. These studies provide a basis for assuming little danger to the average patient from two to three weeks of unrestricted bed rest, but indicate that for patients immobilized for many weeks there are certain hazards; these include urinary tract stone formation, osteoporosis, altered circulatory response to gravity, and loss of muscle mass and strength. These experiments also indicate that disturbances in function due to recumbency are sluggishly reversed by ambulation and that metabolic and physiologic function will be maintained in the best possible state by keeping patients mobile, as shown by the beneficial effects of oscillation.

Review of reports of early postoperative ambulation considered in conjunction with the immobilization studies of normal subjects suggests that ordinary postoperative bed rest, whether of few or many days' duration, bears little relation to postoperative vascular and pulmonary complications. While the experience with normal subjects does not preclude the possibility that ordinary recumbency is a contributing factor in the development of vascular complications in decompensated cardiacs or in others whose circulation may be seriously deranged, no evidence is available that a few days of ordinary recumbency is particularly harmful to the average patient. It is emphasized that the extreme degree of immobility during the day of operation plus certain factors from the operation itself may offer the maximum risk of postoperative complications.

Various measures with respect to position, sedation and exercises in bed have been suggested for the management of recumbency of brief and moderate duration. For patients recumbent for a prolonged period measures designed to minimize the metabolic and physiological effects of immobilization have been presented; these included among others the use of the oscillating bed and of aluminum gels.

During illness the physician should take the initiative in planning the patient's activity; in most cases, however, his directions are limited and stated in general terms. For example, he says that the patient may go to work, use stairs, be up a whole or part of the day, sit in a chair, or stay in bed. Very often he prescribes a certain amount of walking or specifies passive movements, massage, or pressure devices as substitutes for exercise. But there are many other ways in which the patient's energy may be expended or conserved, and these must be regulated by the nurse, who is with the patient constantly. It may be highly desirable for the patient to have the exercise of turning, moving about freely, of feeding himself, or assisting with his bath; in rare cases it is harmful. Many patients have prescribed exercises to be repeated every few hours or every day. They may be the most important part of the therapeutic program. When the patient cannot have *active* exercise, *passive* exercise in the form of massage may be given to supply the benefits of exercise.

When exercises are the chief means of re-establishing normal function, as in the treatment of skeletal deformities and disease conditions, the patient is usually under the supervision of a physical therapist. Nurses who specialize in orthopedic nursing also may be prepared to give massage, special types of manipulation, and expert assistance in carrying out prescribed exercises. Physical therapists and orthopedic nurses should, however, be available for consultation on the problem of body mechanics presented by any patient. Chapter 23 deals briefly with the techniques of massage, pressure mechanisms, and therapeutic exercises. Its contents may be studied in conjunction with this chapter. Postoperative ambulation and exercise are discussed in Chapters 38 and 39.

4. HELPING THE SICK AND HANDICAPPED TO MOVE

Importance of Moving Frequently. A healthy person has an almost unlimited choice of posture, and most of us change it every few minutes. The charm of repose is actually rare, and nothing is more foreign to average behavior than the stillness imposed, for example, during photography, or the fitting of clothes. Yet helpless patients are thought to be adequately nursed, if a major change is made in their positions every hour. This is probably the minimum in activity a person can tolerate. The chronically ill who are unable to move themselves and those who have nothing more than custodial care may be suffering very largely from the baleful effect of far less than hourly changes of posture.

Everything possible should be done to make patients independent of others in moving. Any mechanical aid that is always within reach is preferable to human aid that must be summoned and that cannot be constantly at hand. When men workers are available, their services should always be used in moving adult patients. One nurse should never try alone to lift an adult because of the danger and strain on both nurse and patient. Few patients have confidence in the strength of a nurse; and while

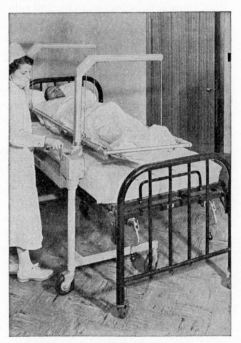

Figure 91.   Equipment used in moving patients; with an "Invalift" one person can transfer a patient to a wheelchair with ease by using a special sitting sling. It is also used to move patients effortlessly from room to room or from one floor to another. (Courtesy of Invalift, Inc., Seattle, Wash.)

they may laugh during the effort, they may really be excited and alarmed, and this is injurious. Two nurses at least are required to lift a small person. To spare medical personnel, hoists, such as that shown in Figure 91, should be supplied. While similar equipment might be rented for home care, this is rarely practical, and nurses must depend upon the help of families and neighbors, the use of lifting sheets, and their knowledge of body mechanics to protect themselves from injury.

Nurses should bend their efforts toward developing independence and should move patients "log fashion" only when patient participation is prohibited. A nurse may be able to move a small helpless child; two to four persons may be required to move such an adult. Margaret C. Winters[8] suggests that the weight of objects to be lifted not exceed 35 lb and that when several persons lift a heavy object together each person's share not exceed this amount. Heavy patients and objects should be transported on carriers equipped with casters or wheels.

Patients are likely to lie on their backs much of the time because in this position they can eat their meals, read, and talk to visitors. While the strain on the muscles of the legs, abdomen, and back can be relieved with pillows and pads, contractures of the knees result if the patient is in this position too constantly. Pressure on the calf muscle is thought also to be a contributing factor in the formation of thrombi and phlebitis. Change of position is most important in all cases, but especially so when the position is one of marked flexion. Jessie L. Stevenson[9] shows how necessary it is for those doing general nursing to be alert in noticing symptoms that indicate skeletal disease and in preventing deformity. She describes the serious plight of a patient who recovered from typhoid fever, but who had contractures of both hips and knees because the legs had been kept flexed throughout the illness. A variety of pads and pillows can be used to maintain the body in the alignment, discussed on page 475. In each position the patient must be studied to see that the weight of the arms is not dragging the shoulders forward, that the straight line of the back is maintained, and that no muscles are stretched or strained. Pillows at the back or against the abdomen give a comforting sense of warmth and support.

When patients can turn themselves without injury, and they can in almost all cases, the nurse encourages them to do so. For instance, when movement causes pain, as after an abdominal operation, the patient can turn himself with greater ease and comfort than the nurse. He will turn very slowly, first one part of the body, then another, instinctively making those adjustments which cause the least pain. A nurse may gather many useful hints by observing his movements.

Winters, in her discussion of lifting and moving heavy objects in *Protective Body Mechanics in Daily Living and in Nursing: A Manual for Nurses and Their Co-workers,* discusses ways to conserve effort. The writer's summary of her material includes a number of Winters' suggestions.

1. Roll or slide rather than lift an object whenever possible.
2. Remove all causes of friction (such as a wrinkled sheet) before rolling or sliding the object.
3. Roll or slide a heavy patient on a level rather than a sloping surface if possible (keep the patient who requires help on a firm bed).
4. Keep the weight to be moved as near the worker's hip level as possible (elevate a low bed or stand on a fixed platform in moving a patient).
5. Stand near the weight to be moved in order to maintain balance and use the large muscles.
6. Separate the legs to get a broad base and to enable the worker to shift the weight of her body as the object is moved.
7. Move an object toward rather than away from the worker.

8. Keep the back as straight as possible, flexing the hips or the knees rather than bending the back to get on the proper level to move an object. In this way the large muscles of the trunk and thigh are used in lifting rather than those of the arm.

These recommendations are based on the principles of simple machines or leverage. Their application to nursing is discussed in the manuals by Winters, by Bernice Fash,[10] and Juliette T. Lee and Anna M. Sewall,[11] and in the pamphlet *Posture and Nursing,* published by the Joint Orthopedic Nursing Advisory Service. Such sources should be studied for a more thorough treatment of moving and lifting than can be given in the following suggested procedures.

Moving a Patient to the Side of the Bed and Helping Him to Turn on His Side. When one nurse moves the patient, she puts her forearms under the body, sliding first the head and shoulders, next the hips, and then the legs across the bed. This requires more effort than rolling him over, log fashion. A turning sheet as shown in Figure 92 A-F requires the least effort.

When the patient has effective arm and trunk muscles and is encouraged to use them, he is taught to turn on his side. Patients with completely paralyzed lower extremities learn to do this with ease.

Turning the Patient into a Prone Position. Turning from the supine to the prone position is accomplished with three steps if the person is in a single bed. He moves or is moved to one side of the bed while supine; he then turns on his side or is turned; and in the third stage he tips over on his face by a slow rotation of the hips and shoulders. In this process, it is important to adjust the arms and legs so that they will not be pinned under the body and so that their weight is used to help rather than hinder the movement of the body in the desired direction. The person with paralyzed legs learns to turn over without assistance by manual placement of his legs in the proper position for each phase of the move.

Approved prone posture and the use of supports are shown in Figure 89. For patients who must spend a major part of their time in a prone position the Stryker frame (see p. 1126) is a boon because it is mobile and its structure makes occupation in the prone position more possible.

Moving the Mattress and the Patient Up in Bed. There is a constant tendency for the mattress and the patient to slide toward the footboard with any elevation of the head of the bed. To correct this condition begin, if possible, by making the springs level; it is wasted effort to pull or push a weight uphill. If the patient's condition permits, he can help bring the mattress up by grasping the headboard and pulling upward as the nurse moves the mattress into position. He can often push himself up in bed by flexing the knees and pushing on the mattress with both feet. Grasping the head of the bed or rope handles attached to the head of the bed also helps. If the patient is allowed to stand up or sit in a chair, the mattress should be adjusted while the bed is unoccupied. If a mechanical hoist is unavailable, it is often desirable to move a patient who must remain horizontal to a stretcher while his bed is remade.

Helping the Patient into a Semireclining or Sitting Position. Before elevating the upper part of the body, the patient must be far enough up in bed so that the

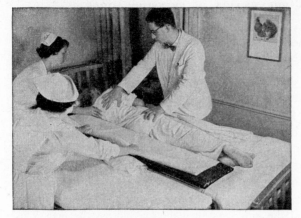

Figure 92A. A roller is used to move a patient who is unable to cooperate from bed to stretcher. Roller in place on bed with the lifting sheet over it and under the patient. Note the pillow placed so that the roller cannot get wedged in the crack between the bed and the stretcher.

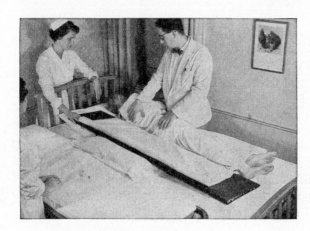

Figure 92B. Workers are easing the patient over onto the roller.

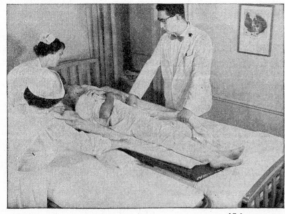

Figure 92C. One nurse is pulling the lifting sheet, the second nurse is supporting the head, and the aide is elevating his rolled edge of the lifting sheet.

484

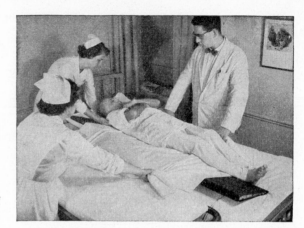

Figure 92D. Another phase of the passage from bed to stretcher.

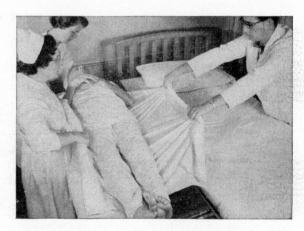

Figure 92E. The shift has been completed.

Figure 92F. The aide is removing the roller while the nurses steady the patient who has been rolled on his side with the lifting sheet.

(Figs. 92 A-F, courtesy of Columbia-Presbyterian Medical Center, New York City, and Clay-Adams Co., New York City.)

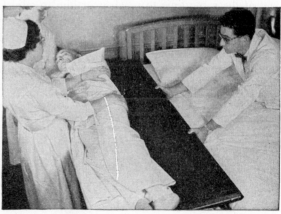

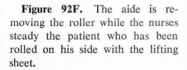

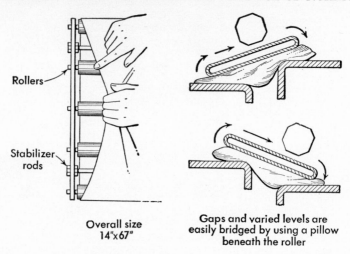

Rollers

Stabilizer
rods

Overall size
14"x67"

Gaps and varied levels are
easily bridged by using a pillow
beneath the roller

Figure 92G.   Diagram to show construction of the Davis patient roller. (Courtesy of Gilbert Hyde Chick Co., Oakland, Calif.)

back is straight from the coccyx to the occiput when the Gatch, or back rest, is raised. This upward movement must be made while he and the mattress are horizontal.

With a Gatch bed, sitting postures are accomplished with the turn of a crank or pressure on a button; some are made to be operated by the patient. When such equipment is not available and pillows or improvised back rests and knee rests must be used, several workers are needed; one or more to support the patient in a sitting position while another worker adjusts the back rest. Most patients can lift themselves with an overhead trapeze (Fig. 93, *right*), which should always be provided for those who are expected to be partially helpless for any length of time. A patient may lift himself, using the nurse as an aid as shown in Figure 94, but weak and heavy persons are likely to put too much weight on the woman nurse in this maneuver. Too often she attempts to support the patient in this way and at the same time to reach over him to adjust his pillows. This is likely to unbalance her, with disastrous results to the nurse and patient. It is far better in most cases to call a second worker, but when adjustment of pillows is attempted by one nurse, she can remember that she is less likely to be unbalanced if she draws a pillow toward her than if she pushes it away from the central axis, or center of gravity, of her body. Figures 86 and 90 show patients in semireclining and sitting positions with modern hospital and improvised equipment. The principles emphasized on page 475 have been observed, and the arms and shoulders protected.

With the present emphasis on bed exercises and walking as soon as the patient's condition permits, change of position rarely causes the circulatory symptoms so much dreaded in the past when complete bed rest and virtual immobility were advocated as treatment for many conditions. Nurses should, however, be observant and forestall accidents by noting the pulse before and after the assumption of each new exertion of the person who has been ill or has undergone surgery. Faintness and/or nausea are indications for a return to the horizontal position.

The Use of a Bedside Table in Dyspnea. Patients obliged to sit up in order to breathe with comfort may want to lean forward for a change of position. Sometimes they breathe more easily so, because the pressure of the mattress against the posterior chest is removed, and it can expand more freely. To support the head and arms place a table with one or more pillows on it over the bed in front of the

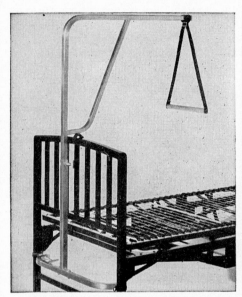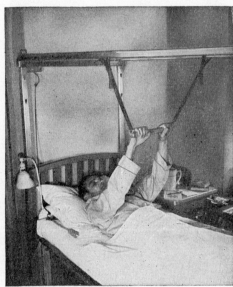

Figure 93. (*Left*) An exercise bar is a desirable attachment for the bed in almost any long-term illness. The patient can lift himself when indicated during nursing care and treatments. This gives him needed exercise and reduces moving and lifting by the staff. A sponge-rubber grip for the cross bar is available, if its use is indicated. (Courtesy of Simmons Co., New York City.)

(*Right*) Another type of exercise bar. Such equipment should be provided for any patient on a Balkan frame. Its use strengthens the patient's muscles and gives him needed exercise. (Courtesy of Columbia-Presbyterian Medical Center, New York City, and Clay-Adams Co., New York City.)

patient for him to lean upon, and press pillows against the lower part of the back for support. Protect the back and shoulders with a light blanket or jacket, according to the room temperature.

Because it is difficult to eliminate strain on the legs and loin muscles sitting in bed in such a position, it is usually better to get the patient into a chair. "Cardiac beds" are so made that the bedspring can be converted mechanically into the same angles as a chair. An adjustable chair is well suited to the needs of the person with chronic circulatory disorders.

Helping the Patient into a Chair from the Bed. Select the most suitable chair available, consider its size, the support it gives, and whether it is mobile, if movement of the patient in it is desirable. See that it is in good repair, protected with cushions or pillows, and placed conveniently (at right angles to the bed) for lifting, or helping the patient in and out. The arrangements of two blankets to protect the patient in cool weather is shown in Figure 95.

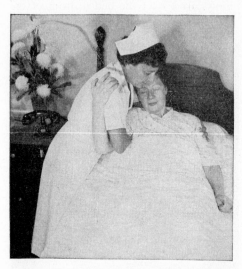

Figure 94. A nurse helping a patient to sit up. Note that the patient is cooperating by pulling herself up, using the nurse's shoulder as a fixed point. The nurse is cradling the patient's head with her left arm. (Courtesy of Columbia-Presbyterian Medical Center, New York City, and Clay-Adams Co., New York City.) ·

Protect the patient with dressing gown, stockings, slippers, and blankets to suit the weather and his condition. He may be dressed while he is lying down, if this is indicated, with little exposure of the body. With the patient near, but not on, the edge of the bed, elevate the head and trunk, and at the same time swing the legs over the edge. For a short patient on a high bed, provide a very stable footstool. Ask the patient to support himself, if he is weak or unbalanced, by grasping the nurse's arm, or arms, firmly. Move slowly until the seat of the chair is immediately behind the patient's thighs, and direct him to grasp the arms of the chair as he lowers himself into it with the nurse's steadying support. When he is in the chair, see that he is well supported, with no hollows in the back; that the head is comfortable; that in a cool environment the feet and legs are snugly and neatly wrapped in the blanket; that a footrest keeps the feet from the floor, and that even a hot-water bottle is provided for the feet if necessary, and that the arms are free and supported with armrests. If the legs are edematous or ulcerated, or the joints painful, keep the limbs elevated.

Watch for signs of fatigue and don't wait until the patient is exhausted before putting him back to bed. A patient is seldom allowed to sit up the first time for more than half an hour. While he is in the chair, the mattress may be turned and the bed aired and remade. If the patient is in a wheelchair and when his condition permits it, an effort should be made to give him a change of scene by rolling him outdoors, into a sun porch, on the roof, or into almost any other environment than the one he must so constantly occupy.

In order *to put the patient back to bed,* observe the same care as when lifting him into the chair, reversing the steps taken in getting him up. Undress him without exposure; make him thoroughly comfortable and allow him to rest, quiet and undisturbed. Chart the rate and character of the pulse, the time allowed in the chair, and the effect on the patient. The chair must be made stationary by an assistant worker, a mechanical device, a sandbag or heavy piece of furniture, or some other means.

If this is the patient's first change from a reclining or semireclining position, there is some danger that the stimulation of the circulation may dislodge a clot

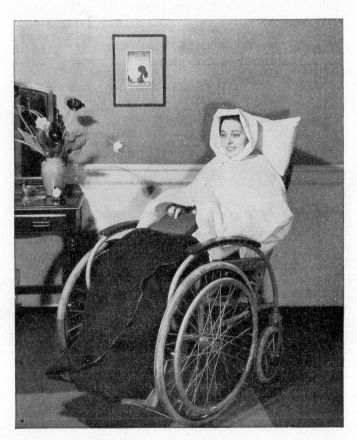

Figure 95. Patient prepared to go on porch or roof. Note the warm blanket around the patient, hood for protection of head and neck, and folded blanket pinned around shoulders leaving the hands free.

that has formed in a blood vessel (*a thrombus*), setting it in motion (*an embolus*), and causing death if the clot obstructs a vital artery in the heart, lungs, or brain. For this reason nurses have been cautioned to move the patient with great gentleness and to count the pulse before and after getting the patient into the chair. With bed exercises and early ambulation this accident is increasingly rare.

Teaching a Patient to Move from the Bed to a Chair and from One Chair to Another. One of the activities in the rehabilitation of the person with motor paralysis of the legs is moving from the bed to a chair without assistance. Medical workers help the patient to progress to complete independence as rapidly as possible. A patient eventually learns to adjust his brace lying in bed and to move freely from bed to wheelchair and from wheelchair to another chair or a toilet seat.

The bed must be the right height or the move is too difficult. In one method the seat of the chair is placed against and at right angles to the mattress at the level of the buttocks. (The patient learns to leave the chair at this spot with the brake on or with the wheels stopped by sandbags.) In a sitting position, the patient

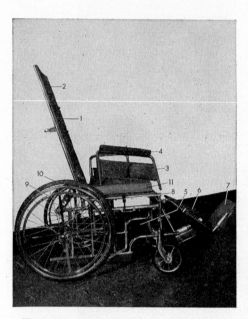
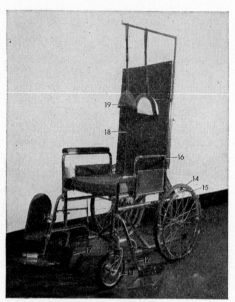

Figure 96. Two views of an up-to-date wheelchair. This chair can be folded and lifted into an automobile after the occupant gets in.

1. Reclining back
2. Extension headrest
3 & 4. Detachable arms and upholstered arm-rests
5. Adjustable leg rest
6. Leg rest panel, wooden (leather panel not shown)
7. Swivel footboard
8. Brakes
9. One-hand drive
10. 24-in. wheel
11. Airform cushion
12. Swivel footrest
13. 8-in. casters
14. 20-in. wheel
15. Hand rim with propelling knobs
16. Desk arm (detachable)
17. Heel strap
18. Zipper back (not used in reclining back—shown here for purpose of illustration only)
19. Arm sling

(The following are not shown: 5-in. casters, foot block, bridgeboard.)

(By permission from *Living with a Disability,* by Howard A. Rusk, M.D., and Eugene J. Taylor, in collaboration with Muriel E. Zimmerman, O.T.R., and Julia Judson, M.S. Copyright 1953. Doubleday and Company, New York.)

pushes himself off the bed with his arms and swings the legs around until they are across the bed with the buttocks hanging slightly over the seat of the chair. He reaches behind, one hand at a time and grasps the arms of the chair; he can then

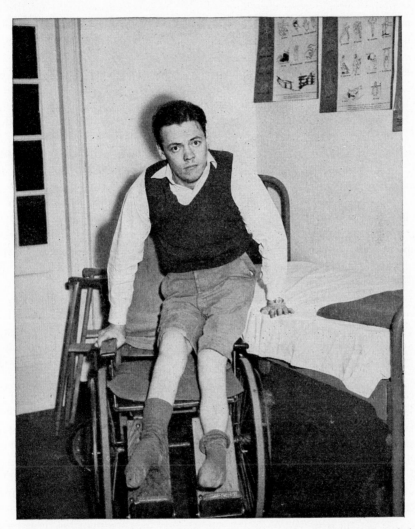

Figure 97.   Patient moving from wheelchair to bed. (Courtesy of National Foundation for Infantile Paralysis, New York City.)

pull himself into the chair seat. Releasing the chair brake, he wheels it backward until the ankles are resting on the mattress; he then lowers each flaccid leg to the footrest, holding it with both hands around the calf.

In the second method the chair seat is placed parallel with the length of the bed and slightly above its center. The patient hitches to the side of the bed, reaches over the chair and grasps the far armrest. Then, pushing on the bed with his other hand, he slides the buttocks over the near chair arm and into the seat. The legs are then grasped with the hands and one after the other swung from the bed into position. Getting from the chair into the bed is accomplished by reversing these processes.

Figure 77 shows a patient being taught to move from a wheelchair to the toilet seat, and Figure 97 a patient moving from a wheelchair to a bed.

In all these moves it is essential that the patient have strong arm and trunk muscles together with confidence in his powers. It is essential that the bed and chair brakes be locked. (In the home these pieces of furniture must be braced securely.) If either rolls out from under its occupant, he may be badly injured, and it will almost certainly destroy his self-confidence.

Teaching the Patient to Move from a Wheelchair into a Tub and Back to the Chair.   The seat of the chair is covered with a waterproof square and a large turkish towel. The patient, dressed in a bathrobe, is directed to bring the chair as close as possible to the tub, facing it. After braking the chair, he lifts each foot into the tub. Pushing up on the arms of the chair, he moves toward the tub so that the buttocks are partly on the edge of the chair and partly on the rim of the tub. Leaning forward and grasping the tub on each side, or a handle on one side of certain tubs, the buttocks can be lowered into the water. A paralyzed leg can be lifted and flexed so that the foot and lower part can be bathed. Bracing the foot against one end of the tub or resting against the back steadies the body.

To get out the process is reversed. With the body braced against the back of the tub, it is brought out of the water by pushing up on the rim. The buttocks rest first on the edge of the tub and with another push are moved over on the seat of the chair. After unlocking the brakes, the chair is moved out 6 in., and the legs are removed singly from the tub. The body is dried and the gown replaced.

Turning the Mattress with the Patient in Bed.   When the patient is in bed for a long time, the mattress may become uneven or uncomfortable, so that it is necessary to turn it, to change it, or to move the patient to another bed. The mattress may be easily turned or changed with no discomfort to the patient. *One method* is to remove the pillows and all the top bedclothes except the sheet and blanket, which are folded back neatly over the patient. The under linen is rolled toward the patient, making a firm roll on either side. The patient is lifted to one side of the mattress, which is drawn from the side partly off the springs. Pillows are placed on the springs, the patient is moved on to the pillows, and then the mattress turned (from the head toward the foot), after which the patient is lifted on to the mattress, the pillows are removed, and the mattress placed in position. The bed is then remade. If the mattress is to be changed, the procedure is essentially the same. A *second and far simpler method* used in the hospital is placing the patient on a stretcher or another bed while his mattress is turned.

Moving the Patient from One Bed to Another.   Put a lifting sheet under the patient. Place the beds (if of equal height) close together, and draw the patient to the fresh bed by pulling him on the lifting sheet. When the beds cannot be placed together, the upper sheet and blanket may be rolled snugly around the patient, who may then be lifted and carried to the fresh bed prepared for him. All those who lift him stand on the same side, one supporting the head, shoulders, and back; the other, the back, thighs, and feet. First draw the patient to the edge of the bed, and together lift gently, the patient holding himself stiff.

5. TRANSPORTATION IN ILLNESS AND TRAVELING WITH PATIENTS

Moving the Patient from One Room to Another.   In hospitals a patient can be transferred from one room to another simply by moving him on his bed, on a stretcher, or, if his condition allows it, in a wheelchair. In homes it may be necessary to improvise a stretcher or litter from a table top or a stoutly woven cloth with poles through hems on each side. If three strong persons are available, they can move the patient log fashion; or strong individuals who make a packsaddle of their hands can carry a person who is able to sit up. Patients may be carried in an armchair if it is well built and can be firmly grasped on each side by the rungs. No matter how the patient is to be moved, the method should not be discussed before him, because he himself is likely to be fearful and even uncooperative if those moving him fail to proceed with confidence.

Moving the Patient from House to House.   If ambulances are available, the transportation from one house to another is easy. When such facilities are lacking, moving the patient may present so many hazards as to be contraindicated while he is acutely ill. Children and small adults may be made fairly comfortable if stretched out on the seat of an automobile and carefully supported with pillows. The greatest difficulty is encountered in getting the patient in and out of the conveyance. In every case the services of a strong man should be secured, and he should be shown how to lift and carry the patient so that there will be as little jarring as possible.

Collapsible wheelchairs are very useful in the case of those with motor disabilities; such chairs can be folded and put in an automobile or stored on a train. The patient may be wheeled from his room to an automobile, taken to his destination, and when there wheeled into the house. This saves effort on the part of those assisting him, and makes him feel less dependent and generally more comfortable. In all large cities and many other communities, wheelchairs may be rented, and welfare organizations are often prepared to lend them to persons unable to pay.

Traveling with Patients.   The responsibility of a nurse when she travels with a patient varies with the nature and severity of his illness. Her preparation for the trip will be modified accordingly, but in any event she should be well informed and prepared for emergencies. An attempt should be made to relieve the patient of all anxiety; he should feel that the nurse is capable of solving the problems connected with the journey, and, unless he will benefit by assisting her, that nothing is expected of him.

A suitable means of taking the patient to the railroad station, dock, or airport should be provided. This depends upon his condition. Wheelchairs and elevators are available in most large stations. The nurse should learn by telephone well in advance of starting the journey what facilities are available and to what entrance the sick person should be taken. The patient is often sensitive and nervous, and will be grateful to the nurse for providing as much privacy as possible. The average person dislikes undue notice in public, and the nurse should try to see that the sick person is not made conspicuous during his travels.

Contraindications for air travel are discussed on page 121. In some cases the necessity for getting the patient to a treatment center may override the dangers of altitude. Medical personnel are rarely found on any but hospital planes. Commercial airplane and railroad companies have medical services prepared to advise passengers and to give medical attention at large terminals, although the latter is usually confined to first aid. The physician in charge of the patient should furnish the nurse with careful instructions about drugs to be used in an emergency. If the journey is to be a long one and the patient's own doctor therefore not available, the nurse should ask him to supply her with names of physicians or hospitals en route should the patient need medical attention.

There are customs in relation to tipping, making reservations, protection of luggage, and similar matters with which the nurse should familiarize herself if she hopes to avoid difficulties and embarrassment in traveling.

The art of companionship plays an important part in traveling with convalescents and those who are mildly ill. When a trip is part of a plan for rehabilitation, the nurse's problem may be largely that of tactfully limiting activity or suggesting diversions and occupations that will help to bring about a return to health.

Whether the journey is long or short, the patient acutely or mildly ill, it is the function of the nurse to see that he is as comfortable as circumstances permit, that hygienic care and diet are disrupted as little as possible, and that he gets an adequate amount of exercise, rest, and sleep.

6. LIMITING MOVEMENT TO PROTECT THE PATIENT FROM INJURY

Regulations Governing Limitation of Movement.   While many sick persons tend to be quiet and even need encouragement to move as much as is good for them, with some conditions movements may be irrational and injurious. In such instances protective devices must be employed. Almost always, restraint of motor activity is distasteful. Many sick persons limit their movements voluntarily for comfort, but limitation of movement enforced by another person nearly always meets with mental if not physical resistance. The restrained individual feels frustrated mentally and physically, and if kept in one position very long, begins to suffer from physical fatigue. The natural reaction to restraint is so violent and in some cases so injurious that laws have been passed in many states to protect the patient from its injudicious use. The word *restraint* is seldom heard because of its distasteful connotation, and a sincere effort is being made to limit motion only when this is necessary for the *protection of the patient*.

Devices limiting movement cannot be used legally in many states without a physician's orders. In some mental hospitals the physician is required to fill in a form, stating why a restraining sheet, a strait jacket, or solitary confinement is necessary. In general hospitals as well as psychiatric institutions, physicians and nurses try to gain the patient's cooperation, thus making restraint unnecessary. Protective devices should be as unnoticeable to the patient as possible and should allow as much motion as can be permitted without injury to him. Whether the patient is rational or irrational, the physician or the nurse should tell him why his movements are restricted.

Patients often struggle against a device that limits motion, and care must be taken to prevent skin abrasions. Metals and rough materials should not be used in the construction of such equipment, and any surfaces likely to cause friction or pressure should be padded with absorbent cotton, lamb's wool, or some other soft material.

Some Conditions That Necessitate Limitation of Movement.   Patients, particularly children, who have itching *skin conditions* must often have their hands restrained to keep them from scratching, removing crusts, and exposing the skin to mechanical injury and infection from the many organisms on the hands and under the nails. Even cooperative patients will scratch the skin when half asleep. In some *surgical conditions where disturbance of the dressing* would be very disastrous, as, for example, in the operation for cataract or harelip, devices may be used that keep the patient from touching it.

In the treatment of *fractures,* the two broken ends of bone must be immobilized to allow nature's process of repair to take place without interference. Local infections and areas of inflammation—such as that seen in phlebitis—may require immobilization to promote healing.

Paralysis, and temporary conditions like anesthesia, may result in a *limitation of motor power or muscular coordination.* Conscious or semiconscious, the patients may fall out of bed while trying to get something from their table or while trying to change position. Such patients may require the protection of restraining sheets or side rails on the bed when continuous nursing care is unavailable.

Irrational states from any cause may make the patient's movements dangerous to himself or others. High temperatures, anesthesia, diseases, injury, operations on the nervous system, and functional mental diseases are some conditions in which movements must occasionally be restrained.

Devices Used to Limit Movement.   When it is necessary to limit motion of the entire body, as, for example, in irrational states, canvas, wooden, or metal side boards may be attached to the bed.* If the person is very active, these are not adequate. A body pack, in which the patient is wrapped tightly in sheets and

---

* Unwisely used, side rails can be dangerous or futile. A very elderly, confused patient was found not long ago padding barefooted and in his nightshirt down a hospital corridor with his side rails in his hands. Meeting the night nurse, he said, "Miss, couldn't you find some place to store these things? People keep putting them on my bed and they get in my way." It was fortunate that he was neither hurt by climbing over them nor exhausted by the effort of bringing them to the nurse.

blankets, may be used. Folded sheets laid across the thighs and upper part of the body and tucked tightly around the side rods of the bed are used with and without packs to keep a patient from falling out of bed. Stout restraining sheets which cover the patient more completely are applied in some cases. A jacket, having straps attached to the shoulders that can be tied to the head of the bed, will give adequate protection unless the patient is conscious and makes an effort to remove it. Anklets and wristlets made of leather and folded cloths, the latter called a *clove hitch,* might keep a patient from falling out of bed, but are ordinarily used to limit motion of the hands and feet. Wristlets prevent scratching of the body and interference with head dressings. A jacket, with sleeves closed at the end, also may be used to prevent scratching, whether the patient is in or out of bed.

Immobilization of an inflamed area, a fractured bone, or a dislocated joint, for example, is accomplished through the use of splints, plaster casts, or sandbags placed on either side of the leg; or an arm may be immobilized by binding it to the body with bandages or supporting it with a sling. Binders also may limit motion of an area to some extent, but are usually applied for other purposes.

The importance of careful and considerate nursing of patients who are in any way restrained can scarcely be overemphasized. No matter how well selected or skillfully constructed, these protective devices tend to irritate the skin and stimulate resistance in the conscious or semiconscious patient. Any type of restraint that causes pressure on underlying tissues should be removed at intervals and normal circulation re-established before it is again applied. Appliances likely to be soiled by body secretions must be protected with moistureproof materials. Excoriation of the skin occurs most often in the groin, the buttocks, the neck, or the axillae, where skin surfaces, moist with perspiration or other excretion, touch. Pressure sores, or necrotic areas, generally appear over bony prominences, such as the end of the spine, the hips, shoulders, heels, and elbows.

Limitation of motion predisposes the patient to pressure sores (bedsores), and since their prevention is one of the main reasons for changing the position of the bed patient at frequent intervals, they may very well be discussed in connection with posture and limitation of motion in the sick.

7. PREVENTION AND TREATMENT OF PRESSURE SORES (BEDSORES OR DECUBITUS ULCERS)

Nature of a Bedsore. Pressure on the skin can interfere with the circulation to such an extent that the tissue, deprived of nourishment, literally dies and becomes gangrenous or necrotic. Skin areas lying between bony prominences and the bed are most subject to pressure sores. An area of discoloration (reddened, bluish, or mottled appearance of the skin) is an incipient pressure sore. When the process develops to the point in which a break in the skin occurs, a true pressure sore results and the wound is soon infected with *Staphylococcus aureus,* hemolytic streptococci, colon bacilli, procyaneus bacilli, diphtheroids, and others.

Predisposing and Direct Causes of Pressure Sores. Bedsores, pressure sores, or *decubiti* are caused by an *interference in the circulation* in a part, owing to pressure. This may result from the body's lying too long in one position, or from splints, casts, bandages, or bedclothes. The effect of pressure is frequently aggravated by heat, moisture, and decomposing and irritating substances on the skin, such as perspiration, urine, feces, or vaginal discharge. Wrinkles in the undersheet, crumbs, friction from restlessness, rubbing of the bedclothes or of two surfaces of the skin in contact, all predispose to bedsores.

Anything that interferes with the circulation or nutrition of a part, especially if the nerve supply is deficient (as in a broken back, in some fracture cases, and after operations in which nerves have been severed), is likely to result in a pressure sore. Inadequate diets have played a larger role than is generally thought. Great emphasis is now placed on high-vitamin and high-protein diets for patients in danger of developing decubiti.

The *danger points* on the body are the bony prominences (where there is no rich supply of blood to nourish, and over which there is only a thin layer of skin) —the coccyx, hips, elbows, heels, shoulder blades, knees, and inner malleoli (inner surfaces of the ankles), and the back of the head in infants. The obese are in danger because they exert so much pressure on each square inch of the supporting body surface; the emaciated are especially prone to bedsores because their bony prominences are uncushioned by fat. Paralysis, more than any other condition, predisposes the subject to pressure sores because he cannot feel the effect of pressure or respond as the normal person does with a change of position.

Preventive Measures and the Responsibility of the Nurse. Prevention of bedsores is the responsibility of the nurse. As a student she should learn how to take care of a patient in such a way as to prevent bedsores, for with sufficient nursing care they can be prevented. The carelessness, neglect, and ignorance of one nurse may in a few hours undo the most skilled and painstaking care of another. "An ounce of prevention is worth a pound of cure." Development of a pressure sore is a reflection on the nursing care the patient has received. Hospital nursing staffs make such an effort to prevent their occurrence that student nurses may have little if any opportunity in some situations to see the treatment of a well-developed lesion unless patients come to the hospital with this condition from homes where skilled care was not available.

Pressure sores are dreaded by the patient and medical attendants because they are painful and very difficult to heal. After the skin is broken, the area almost inevitably becomes infected. Considerable difference of opinion and variability in practice exist in the prevention of bedsores; everyone agrees, however, that the most important measure is the relief of pressure on bony prominences.

When the patient is in danger of developing pressure sores, keep him on an alternating pressure mattress or on an air mattress that distributes the weight evenly on the entire supporting surface. A Stryker frame (see p. 1126) may be used for many patients and is even more effective in distributing the weight since the patient is first supine and then prone. It is recommended especially for the paraplegic whose range of voluntary motion is limited at best. When such equipment is not available, support the weight of the body and protect all bony prominences by the use of air rings and sponge-rubber rings and by the use of padding and bandaging joints. Be careful not to put too much air in rings—that is, not enough to make them hard and unyielding, as this causes pressure and may do more damage than the bed; they should be inflated with just enough air to relieve pressure. (Inflatable rubber rings and mattresses have been almost entirely replaced by sponge rubber.)

Turn the patient frequently—the position may have to be changed every hour or oftener. Avoid careless use of the bedpan, such as using a chipped pan or leaving the patient on it too long; cover the pan with a pad when there is danger of a bedsore. When the patient has involuntary passages of feces or urine, protect the bed as described in Chapter 14. When a patient has a vaginal discharge, watch the back carefully as the discharge is likely to moisten the back under the dressing or pad and excoriate the skin. Next to an adequate diet and the relief of pressure, absolute cleanliness is the most important preventive measure. Bathe the pubic area and buttocks frequently to remove decomposing urine and other discharges; apply olive oil or cocoa butter to prevent the urine from coming in contact with and irritating the skin. A neutral detergent should be used. Ordinary soap changes the pH of the skin, which is believed to be a protection against bacterial growth. (See p. 195.) See that the patient's gown, bed linen, and coverings of pillows and rubber rings are clean, dry, and free from wrinkles or crumbs. It is customary in most nursing services to rub the skin and surrounding tissue frequently with alcohol—morning and evening, three times a day, every four or two hours, or every hour, as the case demands. The alcohol cools, refreshes, and is believed to harden and dry the skin. There is great question, however, as to whether this is desirable. The writer believes that drying increases the tendency of the skin to break or crack, and recommends an emollient such as "Lubriderm" and a protective waxy coating such as "Keradex" (see Chapter 14). Whatever lotion is used, however, there is benefit from the rubbing accompanying its application. When the skin is broken, rub only around the lesion and with a circular motion away from the part so as to stimulate the outflow of venous blood and the inflow of arterial blood. Exposure of the reddened area to electric light and radiant heat from a metal reflector is an effective means of improving the circulation and preventing further tissue damage. Keep the skin dry and prevent friction by the use of powder, but do not use enough to cake or roll into hard particles.

Symptoms of a Bedsore.   The first symptoms are heat, redness, tenderness, discomfort, and smarting. Heat and redness show that nature has come to the rescue with an increased supply of arterial blood to nourish and revive the injured tissue. At this point it is damaged and congested but still living, and the chances of recovery are good with immediate and constant care.

If pressure is not relieved, the tissues become more congested. The superficial veins first feel the pressure so that the outflow of blood is reduced and the veins engorge, which mechanically prevents an inflow of arterial blood. This congestion makes the part blue, purple, or mottled, like a bruise; it is also cold and insensitive. If the pressure is not immediately relieved and normal circulation restored, true gangrene results. The physician's attention should be called to the first signs of a pressure sore since he may want to prescribe something other than routine preventive measures.

Treatment of Pressure Sores. The great variety of methods used in treating an established pressure sore indicates that none is entirely satisfactory. There are many reports advocating the surgical removal of the gangrenous area with the usual sutured closure of the wound when the area is small or with application of skin grafts to large areas. Bradford Cannon and his associates[12] say that in this practice ". . . surgical closure of the ulcers has become an established procedure" and they attribute successful treatment to improved surgery and emphasis on nutrients—particularly fluids, proteins, and vitamins. Dead tissue cannot be restored to life, but remains as a slough (dead flesh in living flesh) that must either be absorbed and carried away by the circulation or removed externally before healing can take place. Ferments or enzymes liberated from the dead and dying cells gradually decompose or soften it so that it may more easily slough away, or be absorbed by the blood and later eliminated. When the slough is removed, an open raw surface or ulcer remains. Only the physician should attempt to separate the dead from the living tissue because of the danger of hemorrhage.

When surgery is not used, a "bedsore" may be treated by sealing it off under a waterproof dressing. Theoretically, the exudates from the lesion form a water cushion that protects the granulating surface. Cellulose film and waterproof adhesive dressings have been used with some degree of success. A great variety of ointments has been advocated as wet or dry dressings, including zinc oxide, boric acid, vitamins A and D, balsam of Peru, and ichthyol; antiseptic powders and liquids including sulfonamides, antibiotics, horse serum, sodium hypochlorate (Carrell-Dakins solution), and Aveeno (a colloid) paste. Some clinicians recommend leaving the ulcer uncovered and exposed to sunlight, if available, or more practically to light bulbs suspended from a cradle over the pressure area. Keeping patients in sawdust beds (see p. 461) is said to prevent bedsores, and relieving pressure by suspending the body by Kirschner wires through the shoulder and hip girdle has been reported as successful, but it seems heroic treatment. Patients threatened with pressure sores are often placed on Stryker frames (see Chapter 42). Any management of decubiti is successful if at the same time pressure is relieved and a high nutritional status maintained. Any therapy fails if the underlying causes are not removed.

A pressure sore must be cleaned and the dressing applied with the same care as with any wound. Depending upon the nature of the treatment, the physician may do the dressing himself or at times delegate it to others. Since pressure sores usually occur on the supporting surfaces of the body, their dressings are likely to be soiled by body excretions, and it is necessary, in many cases, to change these dress-ings frequently unless they are well protected. Methods of treatment that demand frequent dressings, however, tend to remove and injure the delicate granulating tissue formed in healing. Additional data on care of wounds and surgical dressings are found in Chapters 36 and 37.

8. REST AND SLEEP

General Value of Rest in Health.   Rest, mental and physical, is a physiological necessity, as everyone knows. Even a few minutes of complete relaxation, here and there throughout the day, will go a long way toward conserving mental and physical energy, relieving tenseness, and preventing accumulation of fatigue products in the body. A great volume of literature is growing up around the effects of "stress," which is the opposite of relaxation. The Kendalls and Boyton[13] in their text, *Posture and Pain,* define stress as "any force that tends to distort a body"; "tension" as a force that lengthens a body; and "strain" as injurious tension in contrast to tautness, which they use for tone or noninjurious tension. Physical and mental fatigue produce strain and would be eliminated in an ideal state. Actually, few people succeed in regulating their lives so as to avoid fatigue. Industrial health programs are aimed very largely at reduction of fatigue. Workers' tools and their environment are studied for their effect on fatigue; work schedules are tried out for the duration and spacing of work periods. For example, telephone operators are found to make more mistakes and machine workers have more accidents if their concentrated service is not interrupted by frequent and regularly spaced rest periods. More accidents are said to occur during the latter part of the afternoon when workers are fatigued and fewest in the early morning after a night's rest. When a person habitually wakes rested after a night's sleep, his occupation cannot be said to cause "stress."

Sleep is recognized as rest par excellence. The ability to fall asleep and stay asleep for an unbroken period is a measure of mental and physical health. The psychotic and psychoneurotic suffer as acutely from want of sleep as from any other aspect of their condition. Some psychiatrists ask that charts be kept showing the pattern of sleep because this helps them to assess therapeutic progress. As depression or anxiety lessens, for example, the subject sleeps for longer periods, and instead of waking at 2 or 3 in the morning he will sleep until 4 or 5, or until finally he re-establishes his normal pattern. "Neural vigilance," as one writer terms consciousness,[14] is so exaggerated in these disturbed patients that hypnotics may not overcome the wakefulness for any length of time. Those who have attempted suicide will often say that they could not face any more sleepless nights and the accompanying physical symptoms. Herbert Hendin, studying 600 cases of attempted suicide, says:

A number of patients, particularly those with neurotic depression, gave sleeplessness as a major cause and precipitating event in their suicidal attempts. While the dynamics of the individual personality are responsible for the insomnia, once sleeplessness becomes a symptom, it in turn would then act to lower the "threshold" with regard to suicide.*

Nurses as individuals must face the fact that broken sleep from which we wake fatigued is a disorder, and as nurses we must realize that unless our patients have natural and relatively unbroken and restful sleep, their rehabilitation is incomplete. The medical team should consider their work incomplete when they discharge a patient who has very abnormal habits of sleeping, or who is dependent upon drugs. It can be said unequivocally that no hypnotic has been discovered that is not habit forming, that does not have harmful side effects, and that does not require larger and larger doses to be effective. Doctors and nurses should hesitate to induce an unnatural loss of consciousness except for acute pain whose cause cannot be removed by any other means. A continued use of hypnotics and narcotics with the associated reduction of muscle tone results in depression of the respiration, circulation, digestion, and elimination; appetite and thirst are often so inhibited that the acid-base balance is seriously upset. The normal stimulation of all these processes that comes from mental and physical activity is also lessened by the sluggish consciousness of the "doped" individual. Henry K. Beecher,[15] discussing the resuscitation of wounded military personnel, emphasizes the harmful effects of morphine even in emergencies where its need is believed most urgent. Paul Barringer, writing his memoirs at the end of a long and distinguished medical career, says:

. . . none of us [medical students] appreciated for a moment the profound change in medicine that an accurate thermometric record [thermometer] would bring any more than we foresaw the evils that could follow the foolish and indiscriminate use of the hypodermic as a "pain reliever."†

One of the major aims of nursing care, and one of the measures of its success, is the induction of normal sleep and the re-establishment of what is for each individual a normal pattern of sleeping. Closely allied to this is the acceptance of a regimen that eliminates fatigue, or certainly the exhaustion unrelieved by a night's rest.

If this concept is correct, namely, that we are kept awake by the stimuli that on reaching the thalamus are relayed to the cerebrum, our clue for inducing sleep is to reduce the stimuli to a minimum. Edmund Jacobson[16] believes that it is largely the stimuli from contracted muscles that keep us awake, and his text, *You Must Relax,* is based on this thesis. Hans Kraus, discussing therapeutic exercise, says:

Since the mind's only outlet is the striated muscle, whatever disturbs a person is reflected in muscle action. If emotional irritations recur daily and establish similar patterns of response, it can be readily understood that an habitual pattern of muscular reaction is formed.

* Hendin, Herbert: "Attempted Suicide; A Psychotic and Statistical Study," *Psychiat. Quart.,* **24:**39, 1950.

† Barringer, Paul: *The Natural Bent.* University of North Carolina Press, Chapel Hill, North Carolina, 1949, p. 226.

. . . . Once the state of tension has reached the borderline of physiology, it can become either more localized, for example, in the shoulder girdle, in the respiratory muscles, neck muscles, etc., or generalized as evidenced by sleeplessness, hyperirritability, or poor general health. These symptoms may be part of the whole complex called "nervousness." It has been shown that by teaching a person how to relax, this complex can be immensely relieved, and that muscular relaxation may in addition lead to a lesser degree of nervousness.*

There are many theories on the causes of sleep but it is neither practical nor possible to review them. Some investigators believe sleep is an active, others, a passive, process; chemical change is believed to be a major factor by certain physiologists, physical stimuli, or their inhibition, by others; sleep is thought to be a function of the central nervous system and conversely of the autonomic system. Many of the older theories are at variance with more recently demonstrated physiological changes during sleep. These findings have definite implications for the nurse and suggest ways in which she may promote normal sleep for herself and others regardless of the causation theory she accepts as most reasonable.

The Nature of Sleep and Theories of Sleep Induction.   Stanley Cobb in his *Borderlands of Psychiatry* says sleep is the "most common variant of consciousness," but in spite of the fact that we spend almost a third of our lives in this state, and it is much discussed by "poets, essayists and scientists," we know "almost nothing" about its nature. He goes on to list the few physiological facts that have been established: (1) that there is no anemia of the brain during sleep and probably an increased blood supply; (2) that the body temperature falls; (3) that muscular relaxation roughly parallels the depth of sleep; (4) that there is "periodic breathing," an increase of carbon dioxide with slight acidosis; and (5) the nerve cells of the central nervous system are less irritable, and there are characteristic changes in the electroencephalogram. The last finding more accurately parallels variation in sleep. Cobb thinks that these variations in the electric potentials of the brain together with the fact that sleeping subjects can dream and discriminate between stimuli, all show that a sleeping person is partly conscious. A mother will wake from deep sleep to a squeak from her baby when much louder sounds fail to disturb her. A city dweller will sleep through the roar of "the elevated," but will wake to the click of an opening door. We remember dreams, which Cobb refers to as mental activity "less censored by repressive conscience" than those of our waking moments.

A discussion of the brain centers concerned with a more or less discriminating awareness is of considerable interest and should be studied by the nurse.

Experiments with animals show that with the cortex of the brain removed they can discriminate between stimuli in a simple way. A barking dog, for example, will enrage a decorticate cat.

Cobb believes that:

The function of the thalamus in man in relation to consciousness . . . is probably much greater [than in animals]. A stimulus reaching the thalamus may be relayed to the cortex

* Kraus, Hans: *Principles and Practice of Therapeutic Exercise.* Charles C Thomas, Publisher, Springfield, Ill., 1949, pp. 276, 278.

and set up an acute alertness that is continued for some time. The original stimulus may be visual, or tactile, or any sensation, but it gets its meaning through cortical associations and its ability to continue by the thalamic circuits. An important precursor is stimulation of the thalamus by the hypothalmus. Ranson and Magoun have shown that here lies a "waking center" that probably bombards the midbrain nuclei and higher thalamic centers with stimuli. As soon as these stimuli are shut off, sleep is likely to supervene. Thus the vegetative centers below have a marked effect on the whole mechanism, and such factors as metabolism, fatigue, sleep rhythm, and circulation have a means of affecting consciousness profoundly. This is not the only means of keeping an organism awake and alert; any of the afferent tracts from peripheral sense organs to the thalamus can equally well bombard the thalamus with exciting stimuli. Chief among these are the proprioceptive stimuli from tense and contracting muscles, for nothing puts one asleep so fast as complete relaxation, and muscular exercise is the best thing to keep one awake.*

Inducing Sleep. Since the state of relaxation parallels the soundness of sleep, nurses may well approach sleep promotion primarily through inducing relaxation. Jacobson and Josephine L. Rathbone[17] describe techniques of relaxation and breathing exercises that the nurse might study and teach her patients. Everyone could profit by the neuromuscular control that enables him to make his body feel heavy, loose, and relaxed as if it were melting into the bed. Even without this special technique, however, the nurse can see that the body is in a posture favoring relaxation, such as those illustrated in Figures 87, 88, and 89, or in the special positions demanded by the patient's peculiar needs. It seems obvious that the relief of emotional disturbance, insofar as this can be accomplished by the nurse, will eliminate one source of tension. Diverting occupation during the day promotes sleep, but exciting activities of all sorts should be avoided at bedtime. The accumulation of lactic acid from muscular exercise is possibly a chemical state conducive to the normal state of semiconsciousness; a marked acidosis results in coma. Reducing the stimuli or message from the eyes, ears, nose, and tactile sense organs induces sleep. A dark, quiet cool room, free from disturbing odors, a smooth bed, and soft, loose sleeping garments all invite sleep. A neutral bath is a classic treatment for psychotic excitement. Hyperactive patients will nearly always sleep if supported in a tub of water that is kept at body temperature.

Whenever possible the patient should be prepared for sleep at a regular hour, according to his sleeping habits. The latter is not easily accomplished in an open ward where it is necessary to establish an arbitrary hour for dimming lights. Serious illness that necessitates treatment during the night interrupts the normal regimen, but this should be reduced to a minimum. Conditions likely to interfere with sleep, if noted early, can often be corrected before bedtime. Sometimes the nurse can relieve them; in many cases medical help is necessary.

Massage is a form of passive exercise and if skillful is very soporific. Stroking motions should predominate when massage is used to induce sleep. The patient

* Cobb, Stanley: *Borderlands of Psychiatry.* Harvard University Press, Cambridge, 1946 pp. 95, 96, 98, 99.

must be in a relaxed position. The back, neck, arms, and legs may be rubbed, although for patients who have had recent surgery massage of the legs is contraindicated, particularly if they complain of leg pain. Following operations blood clots may lodge in the vessels, and in the past the leg was a common site for a thrombus. With the emphasis on postoperative exercise and ambulation, blood clots and inflamed vessels are infrequent accidents, but nurses must be alert to this danger.

While the room air should be cool, body warmth induces sleep. Muscles respond to cold by contracting, and this bombards the central nervous system with messages from the proprioceptive sense organs. A hot-water bottle or an electric pad to the feet or abdomen is often more conducive to relaxation and sleep than a hypnotic drug.

Methods of inducing sleep must, like most aspects of care, be individualized to be effective. Treatment that is relaxing and soothing to one person may be disturbing and exciting to another. The very young and the very old require more warmth than the vigorous person as a rule. Both are very sensitive to the effect of narcotics and hypnotics. Such drugs must be given with great caution, and nurses should ask elderly people whether they have ever noticed untoward reactions to drugs of this sort. Doctors often leave very general orders for hypnotics and narcotics. The nurse must often rely on her own judgment and discretion in following these orders. All preparation for the night should be finished before sedatives are given so that the patient will derive the full benefit. Drugs are given to induce sleep when other measures fail. Nurses, and doctors too, should avoid this too easy solution for one problem that creates others more difficult to solve.

Amount of Sleep Needed.   Charles H. Best and Norman B. Taylor[18] say that the sleep requirement of individuals varies widely, and that it varies with age. They give the following averages: Newborn infants require 18 to 20 hours; growing children, 12 to 14; adults, 7 to 9; and old persons, 5 to 7.

There have been many investigations of man's tolerance for sleeplessness, but the lethal dose has never been established. D. B. Tyler[19] worked with 600 subjects, some of whom went without sleep for 112 days. He found no significant effect on blood chemistry, hemoglobin, red or white cells, body temperature, or weight, and only slight changes in the respiratory rate, pulse rate, and blood pressure. There were, however, marked psychological changes; notably, irritability, hallucinations or illusions, inattention, and loss of memory. The behavior of some subjects suggested mild schizophrenia.

It has been repeatedly noted that the young suffer most acutely from loss of sleep. Nature protects them by making them sleep long and soundly. An infant, if he is moved gently, will scarcely wake when his mother turns him. Although an infant is not very sensitive to his surroundings, sudden noises, a bright light, and any physical discomfort that might wake him should be avoided. Good sleeping habits should be formed early. An infant should be put to bed at a regular time each day and night. (Putting to bed should not be used as a punishment.) Mental excitement, nervousness, and fear of the dark should be prevented. A child should not be told bedtime stories that excite him; in fact, anything should be avoided that may cause sleeplessness or a dislike of going to bed.

The quality as well as the quantity of sleep determines its value. Human beings acquire a daily sleep rhythm; infants and some animals have frequent periods of sleep within the cycle of night and day. Adults tend to get all their sleep in one stretch. The soundness of sleep varies from hour to hour. Best and Taylor say it deepens rapidly toward the end of the first hour, lessens "sharply," and then more slowly until the subject wakes. Children have two periods of deep sleep, at the end of the first or second hour and between the eighth and ninth. Deep sleep is dreamless and restful. Dreaming precedes waking during light sleep. The deeper the sleep, the more complete the relaxation. This partly explains why a short period of sound sleep can be more restful than a long period of fitful slumber. Another explanation lies in the fact that many somatic functions are greatly affected by the quality of sleep. For example, while the volume of urine is decreased in sleep, the excretion of urinary phosphate is increased, as is the secretion of sweat and gastric juice. A person's general appearance and outlook on life are in some cases dramatically improved by an uninterrupted period of deep, natural sleep.

9. PREPARATION OF THE PATIENT FOR THE NIGHT

The *purpose* of the preparation is to refresh the patient after the discomforts of the day and to remove or minimize causes of restlessness and sleeplessness. Ward patients are in many hospitals wakened early; the day is long and may be monotonous and dreary. Or the patient may have passed through ordeals and be exhausted by pain, discomfort, the long hours in bed with hot, aching, cramped limbs, by visitors, by worry or excitement, and by the active and sometimes trying scenes around him.

The Evening Toilet. Screen the patient and bring to the bedside the necessary articles, a basin of water, rubbing lotion, powder, comb and brush, and requisites for cleaning the mouth, clean linen, if necessary, and whatever may be required for his special needs.

The patient should use the bedpan if he cannot go to the toilet. If the upper bedclothes are loosened and turned back at the foot (without exposing the feet), the clothing will be aired and cooled, and the feet given more freedom. A bath blanket is of course used to replace the upper bedclothes. If the patient can sit in a chair, the unoccupied bed can be more easily made.

Clean the mouth, face, hands, and back. To dabble the hands in water is refreshing, soothing, and restful to the patient. Rub the back with lubricant or lotion and powder, giving particular attention to parts that are red or in danger of becoming a bedsore. The patient should be in a relaxed, prone position, if his condition permits. If he is wearing a binder, loosen it when washing or rubbing the back. Inspect dressings for bleeding or discharge and see that they are reinforced if necessary. Replace a soiled gown or binder with a clean one. Remove all crumbs from the gown or bed linen. Loosen the drawsheet and pull it through to give the patient a cool place to lie on. Tighten the bottom bed sheet so that it will be smooth. Remove, shake, turn, and rearrange the pillows. Brush and comb the hair. Straighten the upper bedding. If the patient has a hot-water bottle, an icecap, or a water pitcher, see that it is refilled. Give any special attention he may require and attend to all requests. While giving this physical care, show an equal consideration for the patient's psychic or emotional needs. Indications of interest or sympathy cannot be formalized or stereotyped. The patient senses them, however, and if the interest and sympathy are genuine, he will talk to the nurse about fears that she may be able to dissipate or problems that solve themselves in the telling.

Report and record the condition of the patient. Note any physical change or any expressions of anxiety or disturbing emotion. The night nurse should be warned of the patient's condition and possible developments. The day nurse should see also that all supplies that may be required for the patient during the night are on hand.

REFERENCES

1. Goldthwait, Joel E., et al.: *Essentials of Body Mechanics—In Health and Disease,* 5th ed. J. B. Lippincott Co., Philadelphia, 1952.
2. Thieme, Frederick P.: *Lumbar Breakdown Caused by the Erect Position in Man.* University of Michigan Press, Ann Arbor, 1950.
3. Lewin, Philip: *The Back and Its Disorders.* McGraw-Hill Book Co., New York, 1948.
4. Kendall, Henry O., and Kendall, Florence P.: *Muscles, Testing and Function.* Williams & Wilkins Co., Baltimore, 1949.
5. Kendall, Henry O.; Kendall, Florence P.; and Boynton, Dorothy A.: *Posture and Pain.* Williams & Wilkins Co., Baltimore, 1952.
6. Barnes, Ralph M.: *Motion and Time Study,* 3rd ed. John Wiley & Sons, New York, 1949.
7. Bierman, William, and Licht, Sidney (eds.): *Physical Medicine in General Practice,* 3rd ed. Paul B. Hoeber, New York, 1952.
8. Winters, Margaret C.: *Protective Body Mechanics in Daily Life and in Nursing: A Manual for Nurses and Their Co-workers.* W. B. Saunders Co., Philadelphia, 1952.
9. Stevenson, Jessie L.: *Posture and Nursing.* The Joint Orthopedic Nursing Advisory Service of the National Organization for Public Health Nursing and the National League of Nursing Education, New York, 1942.
10. Fash, Bernice: *Kinesiology in Nursing.* McGraw-Hill Book Co., New York, 1952.
11. Lee, Juliette T., and Sewall, Anna M.: *A Manual of Selected Physics Topics for Students of Nursing.* Burgess Publishing Co., Minneapolis, Minn., 1949.
12. Cannon, Bradford, et al.: "An Approach to the Study of Pressure Sores," *Tr. Am. S. A.,* **68:**439-57, 1950.
13. Kendall, Henry O.; Kendall, Florence P.; and Boynton, Dorothy A.: *op. cit.,* p. 103.
14. Head, H.: "The Conception of Nervous and Mental Energy," *Brit. J. Psychol.,* **14:**126, 1923.
15. Beecher, Henry K.: *Resuscitation and Anesthesia for Wounded Men.* Charles C Thomas, Publisher, Springfield, Ill., 1949, p. 115.
16. Jacobson, Edmund: *You Must Relax,* 3rd ed. McGraw-Hill Book Co., New York, 1948.
17. Rathbone, Josephine L.: *Corrective Physical Education,* 5th ed. W. B. Saunders Co., Philadelphia, 1954.
18. Best, Charles H., and Taylor, Norman B. (eds.): *The Physiological Basis of Medical Practice,* 5th ed. William & Wilkins Co., Baltimore, 1950, p. 1051.

19. Tyler, D. B., et al.: "Effect of Experimental Insomnia on Rate of Potential Changes in the Brain," *Am. J. Physiol.*, **149**:185, (Apr.) 1947.

Additional Suggested Reading

Barringer, Paul: *The Natural Bent*. University of North Carolina Press, Chapel Hill, 1949.

Bartley, S. Howard, and Chute, Eloise: *Fatigue and Impairment in Man*. McGraw-Hill Book Co., New York, 1947.

Bender, James F.: *How to Sleep*. Coward-McCann, Inc., New York, 1949.

Bender, M. B.: *Disorders in Perception: With Particular Reference to the Phenomena of Extinction and Displacement*. Charles C Thomas, Publisher, Springfield, Ill., 1952.

Buchwald, Edith, et al.: *Physical Rehabilitation for Daily Living*. McGraw-Hill Book Co., New York, 1952.

Cobb, Stanley: *Borderlands of Psychiatry*. Harvard University Press, Cambridge, 1946.

Diehl, Harold: *Textbook of Healthful Living*, 4th ed. McGraw-Hill Book Co., New York, 1950.

Flitter, Hessel H.: *An Introduction to Physics in Nursing*. C. V. Mosby Co., St. Louis, 1948.

Freeman, W., and Watts, J. W.: *Psychosurgery in the Treatment of Mental Disorders and Intractable Pain*, 2nd ed. Charles C Thomas, Publisher, Springfield, Ill., 1950.

Gesell, Arnold L., and Amatruda, C. S.: *Developmental Diagnosis: Normal and Abnormal Child Development: Clinical Methods and Practical Applications*, 2nd ed. Harper & Brothers, New York, 1947, Chap. 15.

Gold, Harry (ed.): *Cornell Conferences on Therapy*, Vol. 1. The Macmillan Company, New York, 1946. "Use and Abuse of Bed Rest," pp. 18-35.

———: *Cornell Conferences on Therapy*, Vol. 5. The Macmillan Company, New York, 1952. "Use of Sedatives and Narcotics," pp. 99-115.

Knocke, Frederick J., and Knocke, Lazelle S.: *Orthopaedic Nursing*. F. A. Davis Co., Philadelphia, 1951.

Kraus, Hans: *Principles and Practice of Therapeutic Exercises*. Charles C Thomas, Publisher, Springfield, Ill., 1949.

Krusen, Frank H. (ed.): *Physical Medicine and Rehabilitation for the Clinician*. W. B. Saunders Co., Philadelphia, 1951.

Leithauser, Daniel J.: *Early Ambulation: And Related Procedures in Surgical Management*. Charles C Thomas, Publisher, Springfield, Ill., 1946.

Lewis, Sir Thomas: *Pain*. The Macmillan Company, New York, 1942.

Livingston, W. K.: *Pain Mechanisms*. The Macmillan Company, New York, 1943.

Metheny, Eleanor: *Body Dynamics*. McGraw-Hill Book Co., New York, 1952.

Morton, Dudley J.: *Human Locomotion and Body Form*. Williams & Wilkins Co., Baltimore, 1952.

Ogilvie, Sir Heneage, and Thomson, William A. R.: *Pain and Its Problems*. Blakiston Co., New York, 1951.

Olson, Lyla M.: *Improvised Equipment in the Home Care of the Sick*, 4th ed. W. B. Saunders Co., Philadelphia, 1947.

Prosser, Edith M.: *Manual of Massage and Movements*, 3rd ed. J. B. Lippincott Co., 1951.

Slocumb, Charles H., et al. (eds.): *Rheumatic Diseases*. W. B. Saunders Co., Philadelphia, 1952.

Stone, Eleanor B., and Deyton, J. W.: *Corrective Therapy for the Handicapped Child*. Prentice-Hall, New York, 1951.

Tracy, David F.: *How to Sleep without Pills*, rev. ed. Sterling Publishing Co., Inc., New York, 1951.

Wiggers, Carl J.: *Physiology in Health and Disease*, 5th ed. Lea & Febiger, Philadelphia, 1949.

Williams, Jesse F.: *Personal Hygiene Applied*, 9th ed. W. B. Saunders Co., Philadelphia, 1950.

Wolff, H. G., and Wolf, S.: *Pain*. Charles C Thomas, Publisher, Springfield, Ill., 1951.

CHAPTER 16. REHABILITATION AND RELATED THERAPIES

1. REHABILITATION AS AN ASPECT OF COMPREHENSIVE
   MEDICAL CARE
2. SPECIAL THERAPIES IN REHABILITATION
3. THE ROLE OF THE NURSE IN REHABILITATION

1. REHABILITATION AS AN ASPECT OF COMPREHENSIVE
MEDICAL CARE

Modern Concepts of Rehabilitation.   When Ambrose Paré operated on a French nobleman in the sixteenth century he sometimes stayed with him until he could resume his normal life. He provided medical attention, nursing care, occupation, and entertainment in various forms. Although he didn't use this term he was *rehabilitating* his patient. It seems strange that an idea, demonstrated throughout the ages by great practitioners, should be considered new. As far as we know, however, the modern concept of rehabilitation has only recently been clearly stated and generally accepted. Herbert Whiting says: "Of comparatively recent origin is the harnessing of the separate forces—of physical medicine and the psycho-social and vocational counseling services—into a . . . team, and the projection of this concept into dynamic activities that will restore the individual to a self-sufficient, self-supporting, and self-respecting individual."*

About rehabilitation there are two prevailing viewpoints: the first, that it is the restoration of *certain categories* of handicapped persons to their optimum physical, mental, social, vocational, and economic usefulness; the second, that this restorative process is a part of the comprehensive care which should be available to everyone. In other words the disabling effects of illness should be assessed with each patient and his program of therapy designed to minimize, and eliminate, when possible, every crippling effect, early or late, mild or severe, physical or emotional.

The writer believes the first persons in this country to make the concept of rehabilitation crystal-clear were Mary E. Brown, George G. Deaver, and John N. Smith, Jr. They accomplished this by developing a record for an adult, based on one designed for child care by Marjorie P. Shelton, that listed the essential daily

---

* Whiting, Herbert: "Classification of Rehabilitation Potential," *J. Rehabilitation,* **16:**7, (Nov.–Dec.) 1950.

DAILY ACTIVITY RECORD OF

BY MARY ELEANOR BROWN

RECORD OF: *Doe, John, Jr.*

INVENTORY DATE (S)	*1/9/48*
TOTAL TIME	*1 hr. 30 min.*
EXAMINER'S SIGNATURE	*Ellen Diller*

This Daily Activity Record is for a disabled person of any age who has motion difficulties of any origin hampering everyday living.

Its purpose is to serve as a basis for a rehabilitation program by providing a record of daily activity achievement.

It follows the disabled person through his medical and education periods until he has reached the height of his progress from bed to job.

These Record Blank Forms:
Supplied by Eastern New York Orthopedic Hospital-School, Inc., 124 Rosa Road, Schenectady 8, New York.
Instructions for Use:
"Daily Activity Inventory and Progress Record for Those with Atypical Movement," by M. E. Brown. In The American Journal of Occupational Therapy, beginning with Vol. IV., No. 5, September-October, 1950. (Reprints available: M. E. Brown, 124 Rosa Road, Schenectady 8, New York.)

COPYRIGHT 1950 BY MARY ELEANOR BROWN

(6) GRAPH KEY

INVENTORY	
WITHIN TIME	BLACK
WITHIN TWICE TIME	BLACK
NOT WITHIN TIME OR TWICE TIME	
NOT APPLICABLE	

PROGRESS			
WITHIN TIME	RED		DATE
WITHIN TWICE TIME	RED		DATE
WITHIN TWICE TIME; LATER WITHIN TIME	BLACK	RED	DATE
WITHIN TWICE TIME; LATER WITHIN TIME	RED	RED	DATE DATE

(11) SCORES

1/9/48 54 1st	2/14/48 61 2nd	3/14/48 68 3rd
4/15/48 92 4th	5/15/48 97 5th	6/23/48 100 6th

(1) CLASSIFICATION	(2) INVENTORY LIST	(3) TIME ALLOWANCE	(4) NO.	(5) GRAPH	(7) SYMBOL	(8) TIME	(9) DATE	(10) NOTES
XII. TRAVELING, UPRIGHT	Public vehicles, upright.	Traffic	100	red		not timed	6/23/48	
	Crossing dummy street on green light, upright.	22"	99	red		22"	6/9/48	this tires him greatly
	Floor to standing.	1'	98	red		10"	5/19/48	
	Standing to floor.	1'	97	red		4"	5/12/48	
	Automobile to standing.	1'	96	red		28"	4/7/48	
IV. DRESSING & UNDRESSING	Putting on and adjusting necktie.	1'	25		ON			
	Fastening shoes or tying shoestrings.	1'	24			24"		
	Dressing except for fastening shoes or tying shoestrings and putting on and adjusting necktie.	15'	23		DRESS	7'40"		
III. BATHING & GROOMING	Shaving or applying cosmetics—(motions).	30"	22			30"		
	Washing body—(motions).	30"	21		WASH	30"		
	Brushing teeth—(motions).	30"	20			30"		
	Combing hair—(motions).	30"	19			30"		
TOILET, BED	Cleansing after bedpan use, bed—(motions).	10"	18			10"		
	Off bedpan, bed.	30"	17		OFF	4"		
	On bedpan, bed.	30"	16	red	ON	37¾"	2/10/48	this is hard for him. Practice
	Readjusting clothing as if after bedpan use, bed.	30"	15		CLO	11"		
	Adjusting clothing as if for bedpan use, bed.	30"	14		CLO	10"		
	Urinal, bed—(motions).	10"	13			10"		
II. BED	Sitting to lying (not falling), bed.	10"	12			7"		
	Lying to sitting, bed.	30"	11	red		59¼" 15"	2/10/48	comes up sidewise uncomfortable week
	Edge to edge, bed.	30"	10			5"		
	Left side to back, bed-lying.	20"	9		L → B	1"		
	Abdomen to left side, bed-lying.	20"	8		A → L	2"		
	Left side to abdomen, bed-lying.	20"	7		L → A	3"		
	Back to left side, bed-lying.	20"	6		B → L	2"		
	Right side to back, bed-lying.	20"	5	red	R → B	1"	1/13/48	
	Abdomen to right side, bed-lying.	20"	4		A → R	2"		
	Right side to abdomen, bed-lying.	20"	3		R → A	3"		
	Back to right side, bed-lying.	20"	2		B → R	1"		
I. SPEECH	Speech.	10"	1			10"		
CLASSIFICATION (1)	INVENTORY LIST (2)	TIME ALLOWANCE (3)	NO. (4)	GRAPH (5)	SYMBOL (Z)	TIME (8)	DATE (9)	NOTES (10)
						PERFORMANCE		

Figure 98. Record of daily activities, prepared for handicapped persons during the period of rehabilitation. (Brown, Mary E.: "Daily Activity Inventory and Progress Record for Those with Atypical Movement," *Am. J. Occup. Therap.*, 4:195, [Sept.] 1950.)

activities of an independent person.[1] (See Fig. 98.) Using this as a guide they evaluated the degree of disability of those who applied to the Institute for the Crippled and Disabled in New York City, which has been in operation since 1917 when it was organized as a vocational training center. Observing the individual in such functions as walking, getting in and out of a chair, eating a meal, or dressing himself they discovered which of his daily activities he could perform unaided, those with which he needed assistance, and those which were beyond him. His program from then on was designed to develop independence. The person

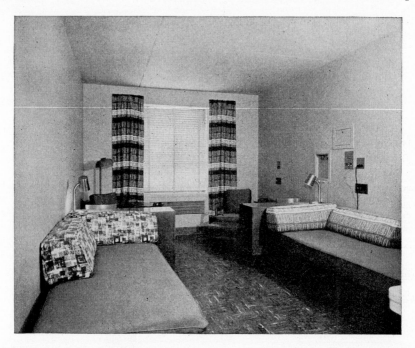

Figure 99. A typical room in the Clinical Center of the National Institutes of Health to which ambulatory patients are assigned. (Courtesy of National Institutes of Health, Bethesda, Md.)

might have had sufficient motor power and coordination, but might lack confidence. Assessment included the latter as it did the person's insight into his condition. As its name implies, this institute was devoted to the rehabilitation of those with neuromotor disabilities. The activity record, therefore, stresses motor function but it includes the essential daily activities, and, in a modified form, the record can be used for anyone: the person who has a loss of vision, a colostomy, or a metabolic disorder. At first glance it may not seem to apply to the psychotic patient whose major problem is a breakdown in human relationships; however, on the psychiatric service, as on the orthopedic, the person who independently performs the daily activities listed on this record is rehabilitated. In other words the mentally ill demonstrate emotional stability through physical acts.

Two world wars have undoubtedly accelerated the adoption of the methods used at such civil centers as the Institute for the Crippled and Disabled. Reconstruction hospitals were established during World War I, and medical care during the World War II was organized around the concept of returning the soldier to "normal" activity as soon as possible. In 1918 New York passed the first state compensation law for the orthopedically handicapped, and since that time public funds have been made available to an increasingly varied list of categories of handicapped persons.[2] The federal health services have better resources, generally speaking, than civil

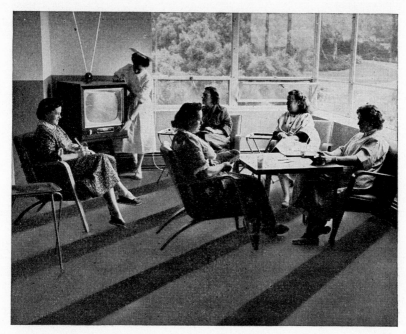

Figure 100. A group of convalescent patients enjoying a recreation room. (Courtesy of Kaiser Foundation Medical Center, Los Angeles, Calif.)

services, but the patient's prospects of restoration to a state of optimum well-being and usefulness are brightening wherever modern medicine is practiced.

Most rehabilitation is accomplished in special centers; some are independent agencies, others are a division of a hospital. In either case these units are different from most hospital divisions in their design and furnishings. Efforts are made to dispel the "sickroom" atmosphere. Sleeping rooms are sometimes furnished to look like sitting rooms as in Figure 99. Dayrooms are provided with books, games, radios, televisions, and whatever might stimulate normal interests and activities. Communal dining is encouraged for all who can feed themselves, or who need minimum help. Workrooms offer patients an opportunity for sewing and laundering. All kinds of household equipment such as stoves, refrigerators, and vacuum cleaners are provided so that patients may learn to use them in spite of motor handicaps. Practice buses, curbstones, and traffic lights are found in some centers. Departments of physical, occupational, and recreational therapy are essential. A few rehabilitation units include shops in which prostheses (artificial legs, arms, etc.) are built and adjusted. They may include shops in which patients learn occupational skills. If not, they usually furnish transportation to such workrooms, for vocational training is essential when a handicap prevents a man's employment in his former occupation.

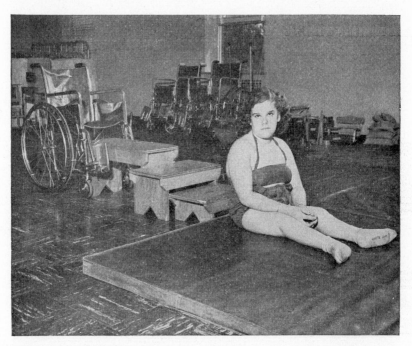

Figure 101. A physical therapy unit for rehabilitation of handicapped persons. Note the progression of footstools from plastic-covered mat to the wheelchair. (Courtesy of Eastern New York Orthopedic Hospital-School, Inc., Schenectady, N. Y.)

Rehabilitation centers are staffed with physicians, including such specialists as the psychiatrist, internist, orthopedist, and pediatrician; with nurses, and physical, occupational, and recreational therapists; with social workers, clinical psychologists, vocational advisers, and special teachers for those who have impairments of sight, speech, and hearing. Makers of prostheses, who are experts in their adjustment and use, may be employed part time. Full-time instructors are employed in the vocational workshops. In some programs, personnel trained to perform a combination of some of these functions are called "rehabilitation officers." Rehabilitation centers may be organized to give 24-hour service to patients or function as day centers only.

While these highly specialized units have clarified concepts, developed methods,

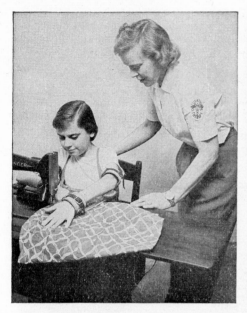
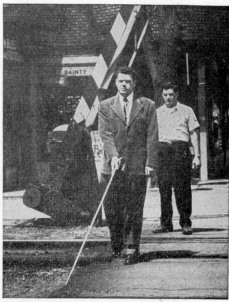

Figure 102. (*Left*) *An* occupational therapist instructing a cerebral palsy patient to make a suitable attractive skirt, which the patient can put on easily with a minimum of assistance or by herself. (Courtesy of Eastern New York Orthopedic Hospital-School, Inc., Schenectady, N. Y.)

Figure 103. (*Right*) Orienting the blind patient for independent foot travel. (Courtesy of Veterans Administration, Washington, D. C.)

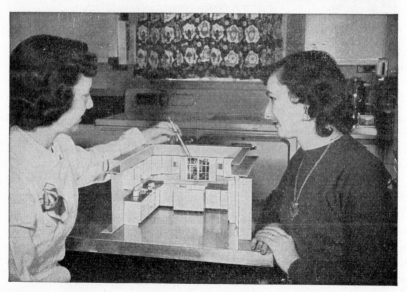

Figure 104A. Model of a cardiac kitchen being discussed with a patient by a member of the hospital staff. (Courtesy of University of Buffalo Chronic Disease Research Institute, School of Medicine, Buffalo, N. Y.)

and trained personnel, the movement they initiated will never reach its full expression as long as they are relied upon to serve all who need rehabilitation.

Most general hospitals can, or could, command the services of the essential personnel and have, or could have, the essential facilities. Too often the hemiplegic is discharged almost completely dependent, whereas his rehabilitation might have begun immediately and been well on its way when he left the general hospital. The same is true for the amputee, the laryngectomized patient, or the person with atrophic arthritis. Where the hospital staff has the concept of bringing each patient

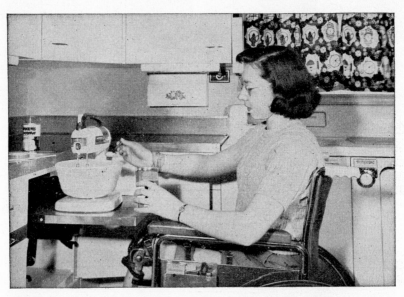

Figure 104B. A rehabilitated person working in her home. (Courtesy of University of Buffalo Chronic Disease Research Institute, School of Medicine, Buffalo, N. Y.)

to a state of optimum independence with each stage of his illness, it is not necessary to send patients to, so-called, rehabilitation centers. We must learn to think of rehabilitating the person with circulatory disease, with glandular deficiencies, with mutilating surgery, with impairment of any special sense, with an emotional disorder, or, in fact, any condition that interferes with his previous way of life or his independence. Howard A. Rusk, an international authority on this subject, said that in 1952 there were an estimated 28,000,000 persons in need of rehabilitation.[3] Until the general practitioners in medicine, nursing, and the allied arts accept their responsibility for each patient who comes to their attention, this waste in human usefulness and happiness cannot be eliminated. A daily activity inventory, such as that shown on page 509, could be the basis of all medical care; its use need not be reserved for the fortunate few who find their way to special centers.

Because the writer believes rehabilitation is an inseparable part of the best, or comprehensive, medical care, it has been discussed in relation to every aspect of basic nursing. This chapter may seem to deal briefly with a very important subject unless the reader notices that restoration of independent function is discussed in chapters devoted to planning nursing care, to eating, eliminating, body mechanics, sleeping, and, in fact, all body functions. While some consider the idea of rehabilitation for all patients as impractical and "idealistic," Samuel S. Sverdlik, reporting a symposium on this subject, says that "hospitals must be made institutions of opportunity."

Hospitalization can be a constructive experience instead of a morbid period overloaded with idleness and boredom, introspection and anxiety. Medical care can be based on a recognition of the universal needs of man, and the patient can learn in the hospital to lead a fuller richer life. Because it often involves the co-operation of many specialists, rehabilitation is said to be too costly for general adoption. A humanitarian might consider this objection invalid; an economic experiment, on the other hand, might easily prove that it costs less to restore a person to optimum function than to provide custodial care for the remainder of the person's life. This is a common claim by those who plead for reform in state psychiatric programs.

2. SPECIAL THERAPIES IN REHABILITATION

Generalizations. Although the doctor, the nurse, the patient, and his family must still make up the rehabilitation team, in many situations the modern medical institution provides the services of many specialists, as was mentioned on page 512. Physical therapists seem to have taken a leading role, possibly because the emphasis has been on rehabilitation of the orthopedic patient up to the present time; occupational and recreational therapists and clinical psychologists have been prominent in rehabilitation of the psychiatric patient. The vocational adviser, the speech expert, and the teacher of Braille are of primary importance to the aphasic and the blind. Illness and its handicapping consequences are viewed more and more as a social dilemma. The kinds of workers brought in to help the patient out of his dilemma and the suggested methods of dealing with his problem are varied and unlike the traditional patterns of therapy.

If stress is recognized as a factor to be dealt with in sickness, either as its underlying cause or as an accompaniment, the therapist will turn to those who can give him the most help in recognizing the forces producing stress. For this reason the psychiatrist's contribution to rehabilitation is often reinforced by help from the clinical psychologist. More recently the anthropologist and sociologist are joining the therapeutic team because they have, for many years, studied the effects of restraints imposed on man by his nature, society, and culture. The psychiatrist and the various social scientists are saying that in order to help the patient the therapist must learn, and help him to learn, what situations exert the stress that breaks down his defenses.[4] This recognition of stress-producing situations is a step in the emotional rehabilitation of every patient. With understanding, the patient may learn to avoid undue stress, and to accept irreversible disabilities and limitations. It seems obvious that when sources of stress, hidden in the realm of the dimly lit unconscious, are brought into the light of reason, or consciousness, there is a good chance that the victim can deal with them effectively. The anthropologist and sociologist have come to this study of stress or anxiety by a different route from that of the therapist but they are also in a position to help the patient to understand and combat the forces that are exerting pressure on the defenses of his personality. Leo W. Simmons, an anthropologist, and Harold G. Wolff, a physician, discuss this in their monograph *Social Science in Medicine.*

From various social science approaches, the individual has become the center of attention. He is now, in much more than a figurative sense, the *bug* on the social science pin. It is recognized that stamped upon his personality, built into his reaction patterns, and sometimes deeply embedded in his bodily structures are the impact of his culture and the scars of his society, inflicted as a consequence of his particular place in life. Moreover, his personal history, more than anything else we can call upon, reveals the conflicts and stresses, the processes of conditioning by achievements and defeats, and some of the dynamics that have gone into the shaping of his adaptations to his total milieu. As a "whole person," the individual has, indeed, come into his own for scientific study.*

In some medical schools and service agencies the social scientist and the medical worker are pooling their knowledge for the benefit of the patient, as have the two authors of the text just quoted. The process of rehabilitation challenges the best efforts of persons in many fields. Re-education of the patient, so successfully accomplished in part through group activity, may bring the social scientist into the medical agency as a regular member of "the team" or as a consultant to staff and patients.

Regardless of whether the medical worker is deeply religious, agnostic, or atheistic, he can accept the position taken by the social scientist that the patient's religion is part of his culture and the source of many, sometimes most, of his ideas and attitudes. These may come through the religion of his forebears and associates, and he may be relatively unconscious of their source and influence. To understand the patient, however, some knowledge of his ethical values is essential; therefore, the representative of his faith, the minister or priest, may be, even in a scientific sense, an essential member of the therapeutic team. To its members he can function as interpreter whether or not he serves as a priest to the patient. Where the patient's stress originates in religious conflicts the counsel or intervention of the minister can be therapeutic. This latter concept especially is influencing increasing numbers of the clergy to join hospital staffs on a full-time basis, and it is encouraging medical workers to seek the participation of the clergy in patient-centered clinical conferences.[5] Rehabilitation, in the sense used in this text, should be the ultimate goal of such conferences. Little has been said about the role of the physician in rehabilitation, but only because it can be assumed that he is, or should be, the prime mover in the program. Unless the physician is aware of the means of restoring the patient to optimum function other medical workers are

* Simmons, Leo W., and Wolff, Harold G.: *Social Science in Medicine.* Russell Sage Foundation, New York, 1954, p. 45.

usually unable to activate such ideas as they may have. It is also evident that unless pathological processes are being brought under control by effective therapy the re-education of the patient holds little promise.

Because the nurse so often substitutes for the physical, occupational, and recreational therapists their functions are discussed briefly in this chapter. The nurse should have some of the skills of these therapists because, in the first place, their numbers are so small that few patients have the benefit of their specialized services, and, in the second place, the nurse must be able to reinforce or follow up programs (prescribed by physicians) instituted by these therapists. Nurses give a 24-hour bedside service whereas the special therapy departments usually close at five and the workers, for the most part, serve patients within their departments rather than in the clinical division. Since the nurse is with the patient more constantly than any other medical worker she may also, if she has good working relationships with the physician and the physical therapist, be able to contribute toward the plan they make for him.

Physical Therapy. When a man with a motor disability refers to "my therapist" he usually means the physical therapist. In rehabilitation centers these workers are assigned to patients and treat them day after day. With the physician they test the degree of muscle function and with him plan a program of treatment. They use heat, cold, pressure, light and electricity, active and passive exercise, massage, and manipulation. Less and less is the physical therapy program something that is done *to* the patient; on the contrary, it may consist of re-education with the patient cast in a very active role. In certain cases all the patient may need is knowledge of how to use his crutches, walk with an artificial leg, or strengthen the muscles of the back through corrective exercise. Physical therapists of today are prepared in a collegiate program and are well equipped to participate effectively in plans for comprehensive medical care. They occasionally say that nurses do not yet know how to work with them for the greatest possible benefit to the patient.

Occupational and Recreational Therapy. During the acute stage of an organic disease instinct seems to dictate to the patient that he concentrate his energy on self-preservation. It has often been remarked that physically ill or starving men, women, and children seem to lose interest in family and friends; they are indifferent to everything but the bodily processes concerned with survival. At such times occupations, diversions, and recreation, as we understand them, are usually suspended although some rare persons manage to maintain their interests in people and their environment.* Except in periods when life itself is threatened, occupation and diversion are essential aspects of the well-planned therapeutic program.

* It might be helpful to state the meanings attached here to the following terms:
Diversion, play, and recreation are used more or less synonymously as the opposite of work. Activities that have no serious motive and from which there is no material gain are thought of as play or diversion. Recreation, or an activity that "re-creates" the individual, has a slightly deeper meaning. The distinction between work and play, however, lies in the mental attitude. Baseball can be play, diversion, recreation, or the work by which the professional ball player makes his living.

The term *occupation* is applied to an activity yielding tangible results, or products, and is usually done with serious intent and for material gain.

(*Footnote continued on p. 518*)

Before prescribing a drug or a diet it is necessary to study the individual. It may be just as important in some cases to assess his need for occupation and diversion. Special institutions for the care of the psychotic, the defective, and the physically handicapped have made a science of recreational and occupational therapy; the general hospitals are less well prepared to give this service, and many doctors seem to overlook these therapies. The rehabilitation movement is emphasizing them, however, and there is growing conviction that facilities for occupation

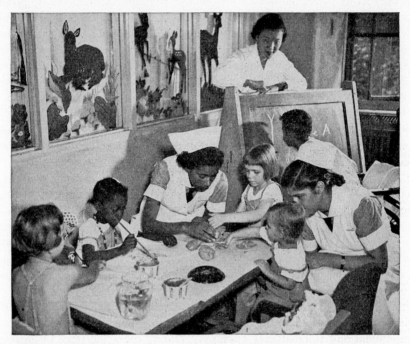

Figure 105. Play teacher and two student nurses supervising recreational activities of hospital patients. (Courtesy of Yale University School of Nursing, New Haven, Conn.)

and recreation must be made available in all hospitals. They should have a place in the plan of care for each patient, and all medical workers should be aware of their value. (This was discussed in Chapter 4.) In planning occupations and recreation with and for the patient, the following are taken into account: age (chronological and intellectual), sex, tastes, interests, experience, cultural prejudices, the physical condition, and the mood, emotional slant or attitude.

As very small children girls and boys have the same interests and may con-

---

Play therapy has a slightly different connotation, which may be confusing to the nurse. To psychologists, psychiatrists, and teachers of children it means a process by which a child acts out, or expresses, his unconscious personal relationships through play. Watching him, the play therapist learns to understand him better, and eventually to help the child understand himself. Such uninhibited, yet subtly directed, play has the added, or primary, value of releasing tension and relieving the anxiety of the emotionally disturbed child.[6],[7]

tinue to do so unless taught that certain interests are "sissy" for boys or "too rough" for girls. In our culture this distinction is made early, is fixed, and cannot be ignored. Nurses of children, just as teachers of children, must learn the toys, the games, the types of stories, and, in general, the range of interests of each sex at different ages.

In adults the differentiation between recreation and occupation for men and women is quite marked, but in the more cultivated strata of society there are perhaps fewer prejudices. Also if the patient's masculinity is evident, as in the case of a soldier, he is less likely to object to an activity because it is "effeminate."

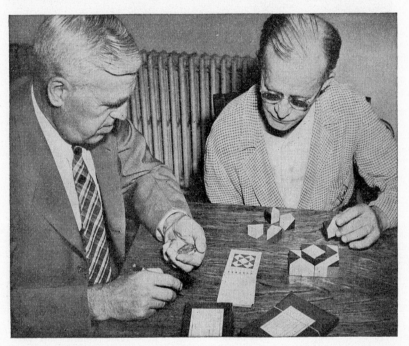

Figure 106. Aptitude testing is one of the functions of vocational counseling. (Courtesy of Veterans Administration, Washington, D.C.)

With the growing emphasis in occupational therapy on developing interests and skills that will persist beyond hospitalization, many of the handicrafts that yielded a product of doubtful beauty or value have disappeared. It is likely that with the tendency for women to enter more and more occupations there will be less and less differentiation in the occupational therapy offered the sexes. In recreational therapy the same general trends are apparent. Perhaps the most interesting change is that of encouraging men and women patients to work and play together in health institutions. This alone will help to develop a greater mutuality of tastes and interests although this is only one of the desirable outcomes.

The mental age is a better guide in selecting occupation and recreation for an individual than his chronological age. Very retarded adults will play with an infant's toy, and very gifted children have the interests of normal adults. Psychometric and aptitude tests are helpful, but a great deal can be learned about the patient's "I.Q." simply by observing and talking with him.

A person's interests are, of course, affected by his experience, and this should be taken into account. While novelty has its charm new skills, games, exercises etc., should be introduced gradually. Many persons are self-conscious in a learning situation and until they feel at home with the therapist or the nurse will prefer

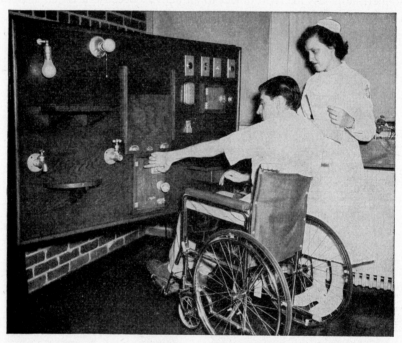

Figure 107.   Training in activities of daily living is important. (Courtesy of Veterans Administration, Washington, D.C.)

a familiar activity. A knowledge of national customs and mores is of great value to all medical workers.

The physical status, of course, limits the choice of occupation and recreation as does the patient's mood. During a prostrating physical illness exertion and emotional tax are contraindicated, and only the thoughtless or ignorant try to amuse or occupy the patient. Gradually as strength increases and interest returns diversional and occupational activities are introduced. Nothing requires more sensitivity and imagination on the part of the nurse than the management of this phase of illness. She can do a great deal to prevent the dependence, depression, or anxiety that often accompanies convalescence. Selection of occupational and recreational therapy for the psychotic patient is both difficult and critical. When the emotional disturbance is so marked that the person is said to have a mental illness his mood, or attitude, is the primary consideration in prescribing therapy. The silent withdrawn, depressed, hypoactive person cannot be expected to take part in games that require concentration and quick response; on the other hand he should be encouraged to participate in group activity, for the ultimate aim of psychotherapy is to bring the person into satisfying relationships with others. Anything that diverts him from the anxiety underlying his depression, anything that

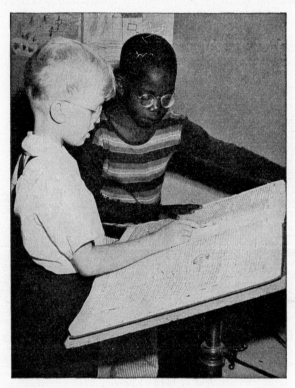

Figure 108. Children with impaired vision enjoy reading an enlarged edition of a book. (Courtesy of Michigan State Normal College, Kalamazoo, Mich.)

brings him back into normal life situations, is therapeutic. Activities for the hypoactive should be stimulating and interesting but they cannot require too much from him; activities for the euphoric and hyperactive should, on the other hand, be quieting. A manic patient who works alone at a painting or making a toy finds a constructive expression for the impulses that otherwise drive him to tear his clothes or rip his mattress to shreds.

Between these extremes of moods there are many degrees of introversion and extroversion, depression and elation. Shyness, suspicion, timidity, aggressiveness, arrogance, and so on can be modified by occupational and recreational activities. However, the mentally ill have no corner on these attitudes that make for unhappiness. Principles on which activities are prescribed for the "psychotic patient" apply as well to the patient in the medical and surgical division of the hospital. We are all "emotionally disturbed" during illness. Some of us manage to hide it more successfully than others; some of us express this disturbance in socially acceptable behavior, others do not. The mood or attitude of the patient is to be considered in planning the program of every patient. This does not imply that there is a specific activity for a given diagnosis; each prescription must be suited to the particular needs of the patient. It goes without saying that he should be encouraged and invited to participate rather than forced into the activity.

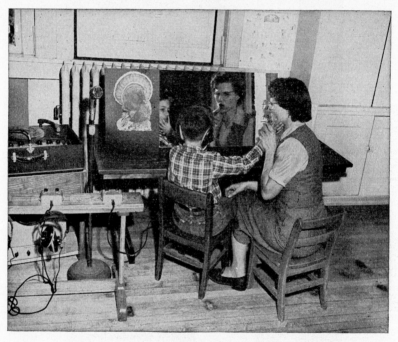

Figure 109. Children who are deaf or hard of hearing need specialized speech instruction. (Courtesy of Champaign Community School, Champaign, Ill.)

Rehabilitation may include preparing the patient for a change in his gainful occupation. Chronic illness or a physical handicap may necessitate this. Vocational guidance of this type should be based on the findings in aptitude tests and a study of the patient's social history. Psychologists, vocational advisers, physicians, social workers, nurses, and special therapists usually confer with each other, with the patient, and his family. The training program may be available within the medical agency. Often the medical agency arranges transportation for the patient to a training center. Some industries give preference to the handicapped. It has been shown that some handicaps can be converted into assets. For example, the tactile acuity of the blind may be utilized in examining ball bearings for defects, and persons with motor disabilities of the legs tolerate long hours of sitting required in watch-making more readily than active persons. Possibly the handicapped who are employed make an extra effort to satisfy; whatever the reason, there are many encouraging reports from the workshops for the handicapped but, better still, from industries where the rehabilitated worker can feel that he is once again a part of the stream of life.[8, 9]

3. THE ROLE OF THE NURSE IN REHABILITATION

Generalizations.   If throughout the care of each patient the nurse bears in mind the goal of helping him to retain or regain his independence in breathing, eating, eliminating, sleeping, moving, dressing, communicating and establishing satisfactory human relationships—in other words carrying on his daily activities—she is taking a leading role in his rehabilitation. This process of assessing, teaching, and encouraging is not to be confused with the all too prevalent practice of allowing the prostrated patient to take his own bath, of letting a person, unaided, grope his way toward an effective use of crutches, or the insistence that an overprotected child dress himself. Nor does it mean turning over physical care to the untrained worker. It is rather an attempt throughout all nursing care and treatment to decide what part of the procedure the nurse should do herself and what part she should encourage, or teach, her patient to perform. She must assess his physical strength, his understanding, his desire or will to do it. Obviously this is a more difficult process for the nurse than to give the entire bath, inject the hypodermic, or irrigate the wound herself. The nurse is traditionally one who gives service. The patient may enjoy his dependence, and, who knows how often, the nurse may revel in "being needed."* In contributing toward his rehabilitation she may be working against strong emotional drives. She may also be combating the patient's determination to get all the service he can for what he may consider exorbitant fees. This is rare but an attitude the private duty nurse may encounter. More often the nurse is coping with a breakdown in morale, a sense of futility which is both the cause and the accompaniment of so much illness. Betsy Barton, a paraplegic following an automobile accident, describes in *And Now to Live Again*[10] the utter hopelessness she faced. In her case rehabilitation was delayed unduly and did not begin until months after her accident. A doctor began the restoration of normal functions by teaching her how to breathe so that she strengthened the abdominal muscles. (Something, by the way, any nurse might have done.) In describing her gradual return to a full and useful life helped by the program at the Institute for the Crippled and Disabled in New York City, Barton comments on the failure of nurses and doctors in the general hospital to set her on her way as soon as

* While it may not be necessary to make this comment let no one suppose that the positive aspect of dependence is overlooked. It is appropriate and desirable under some circumstances to do things for patients that they are entirely able to do themselves. This is a normal expression of our interest and feeling for others. At certain stages of his illness the patient may need the assurance that he is liked by the nurse, the doctor, or the therapist more than he needs his physical independence.

they might. She makes a generous allowance for her own bitter detachment and psychological rejection of her disability but then concludes that she need not have wasted so much time had the staff been more prepared to help her. Hundreds of similar cases might be cited. The concept of rehabilitation has not fully penetrated our thinking, nor have we learned what we must know in order to (1) identify ourselves with the patient so that we can understand the psychological blocks, (2) assess his comprehension and his physical ability, and (3) teach him the new skills involved in caring for his disabled body. Too few nurses have these skills. For example: manually expressing urine from an atonic bladder, irrigating the colon following a colostomy, keeping the stump of an amputated leg in good condition, using crutches, or planning a diabetic menu. All of these are common procedures in the rehabilitation of certain patients. To be an effective member of a rehabilitation team the nurse must be able to promote the patient's full participation in his daily hygienic regimen. This may involve simple procedures but it may also include skills that are quite foreign to normal living—and for the nurse may involve hundreds of procedures with almost as many modifications.

The nurse's role in rehabilitation varies greatly according to the number of specialists available in the situation. She may have to substitute for a variety of therapists or, when they are "off duty," she may have to encourage the patient to continue the program that therapists have instigated. In private duty nursing, in homes, in doctors' offices, industrial nursing, and in some visiting nurse agencies the nurse is the only person at all prepared to work with the doctor in his efforts at rehabilitation. This will continue to be so until there are sufficient physical, occupational, and recreational therapists, psychiatric social workers, clinical psychologists, teachers of the blind, and so on to staff health services.

What has been said applies to the role of the nurse in rehabilitation of any and all patients. The reader should consult texts by Alice B. Morrissey, Rusk and Eugene J. Taylor, James F. Garrett, and others suggested at the end of this chapter for a more detailed discussion of this subject. An attempt is made in the following pages to suggest some of the emphases in certain clinical nursing services.

The Psychiatric Nursing Service.   Rehabilitation in psychiatry will assume different patterns according to the psychiatrists' school of thought. Increasingly, however, we are coming to look upon mental illness as a failure on the patient's part to establish and/or maintain satisfying relationships with others. The corollary is that rehabilitating the patient means helping him to accomplish this. If the last sentence is a simple statement the process referred to is not, and putting it so simply may be misleading.

Whatever the school of psychiatry, the nurse is likely to be working with a team of experts. In the private institution the numbers may be adequate; in the average state hospital they are so inadequate that their presence may be almost unknown to some inmates who can go for days, even weeks, seeing no one but self-taught attendants.

Just how effective in the rehabilitation of the psychiatric patient a well-prepared nurse in a favorable setting *can* be is shown through such case reports as those of Gwen E. Tudor's.[11]

In well-organized and adequately staffed psychiatric services patients have prescribed programs of physical, recreational, and occupational therapy. They go to these departments daily, and specialists may work with them on the clinical services. Patients also have access to psychologists, psychiatric social workers, and others prepared to give special help. If, however, a therapeutic community is to exist throughout the hospital, or wherever we find the psychiatric patient, nurses must be able to participate in most aspects of the program. In a psychiatric service described by Gwen Tudor Will, hospital patients have much of the freedom of a good home. They determine the hour at which lights will be put out at night; they have their meals with the medical personnel and use first names in addressing them. Nurses do not wear uniforms and by various means they try to establish the atmosphere of friendliness and acceptance that promotes therapeutic relationships. Each patient assumes increasing responsibility for planning his day as he progresses, and the entire staff helps him to make it as "normal" as possible.*

The nurse in psychiatry has greatest need for psychological knowledge and skill although the same art can be used in preventive psychiatry elsewhere. Musical, dramatic, and other social talents are an asset in work with the psychotic. It is difficult for a person to enter enthusiastically into any social activity if she is inept.† For this reason, as well as for her own sake, the nurse should cultivate a wide variety of interests. Student nurses usually spend several weeks in the occupational and recreational therapy departments while they are studying psychiatric nursing, but this gives them only the barest introduction to the work of these specialists. A more extended experience is desirable for the graduate nurse student who can continue almost indefinitely to cultivate new skills and interests. Those who work with disturbed children profit by study with the play therapist.

While the psychological aspects of psychiatric nursing have been emphasized, the physical rehabilitation of the patient goes hand in hand with the emotional and intellectual, and this is apt to be left even more largely to the nurse. Although it requires a different approach it is as important and as difficult to bring the depressed patient to the point where he can and will eat, dress himself, sleep normally, and take adequate exercise as to do this for the physically handicapped. After psychosurgery the nurse may have to teach personal hygiene to the patient as she would to a child. Those with brain damage sometimes withdraw in anxiety and frustration. Joe K. Brown,[13] discussing their retraining, says this "catastrophic reaction" makes *any* experience an overwhelming threat.

The Orthopedic Nursing Service. In hospitals designed for the convalescent

---

* Will, Gwen Tudor: personal communication.

† Francoise R. Morimoto,[12] who made a study in the Boston Psychiatric Hospital under an American Nurses' Association grant, concluded that most of the nurses' social skill can be used in patient activity, that nurses tend to let patients initiate activity, and that they gravitate to patients who share their own interests and skills. If typical, this study suggests the importance of a catholicity of tastes on the part of the nurse.

orthopedic patient there are usually physical and occupational therapists and ample facilities for these therapies. Even more carefully than in psychiatry the physician prescribes the program—daily activities, exercises, games, and crafts are selected to exercise the whole body, or groups of muscles and joints affected by disease or injury.[14, 15, 16, 17] Because, however, the majority of orthopedic patients are found in general hospitals, where special therapists are few—sometimes nonexistent—doctors and nurses are often responsible for the entire rehabilitation program. The graduate nurse studying advanced orthopedic nursing is often given the chance to

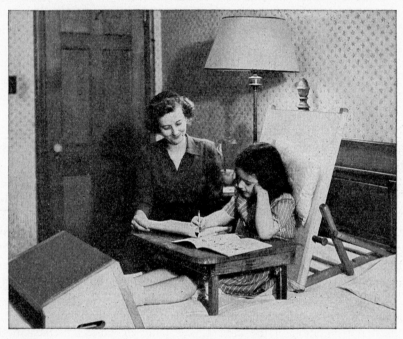

Figure 110. A convalescent (rheumatic fever) child being given classroom instruction by a visiting teacher in her home. (Courtesy of Department of Health, Commonwealth of Virginia, Richmond. Photo by Whitaker Studio, Richmond, Va.)

acquire a fair amount of skill in muscle testing, massage, therapeutic exercise, and heat, cold, and light therapy. Occasionally nurses complete the program designed for physical therapists. Crutch walking, how to measure patients for crutches and wheelchairs, the adjustment of braces, and the preparation of the stump for a prosthesis are some of the special skills needed by all orthopedic nurses. Helping the patient to accept his disability demands even more of the nurse, but is part of her responsibility toward every handicapped person.

Whether or not special therapists are available for initiation of a program, the nurse has an active part to play. She is with the patient constantly; and if she cannot help him to move from his bed to a chair, to get up from the floor if he falls, or to climb stairs, his rehabilitation will be greatly delayed.

. **Neurological nursing** requires a combination of the qualities demanded in psychiatry and orthopedics. Rehabilitation in this service is as difficult as in any, and makes heavy demands upon the nurse.

The Pediatric Nursing Service. To achieve any degree of success in the rehabilitation of the sick child the nurse must be something of a "play therapist," an occupational, recreational, and physical therapist. In fact to be acceptable to children at all she must know something about the interests of age groups and be able to provide them with suitable occupation or diversion. In a study of toys for hospitalized children Claudia D. Gips[18] concluded that painful treatments at the hands of doctors and the nurses are far less traumatic if the child associates these workers with play experiences. She also points out that the child provided with play materials is not so aware of his physical discomforts as one who is unoccupied.

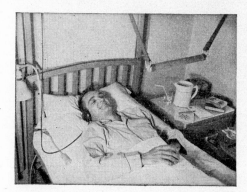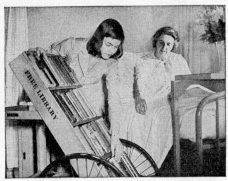

Figure 111. (*Left*) Patient with earphones listening to one of six programs available in the hospital. A pull on the black cord changes the station. (Courtesy of Columbia-Presbyterian Medical Center, New York City, and Clay-Adams Co., New York City.)

Figure 112. (*Right*) Volunteer with book cart in patient's room so that patient can select a recent publication for recreation. (Courtesy of St. Lukes Hospital, New York City.)

It is now a common practice in the education of nurses to give them some experience in nursery schools where they work with well children and have at least an introduction to child development. Nursery school teachers often comment on the tendency of the nursing students who come from the hospital environment to dress, feed, or manipulate a toy for a child instead of encouraging him to do these things for himself. In all child training, but particularly in the rehabilitation of handicapped children, the nurse should encourage independence and should analyze each service she gives in these terms.

Many pediatric services employ play teachers, full time, who are actually recreational therapists with special training in child care. They may work with the children in a specially equipped room or they may bring play materials to the child's bedside, or do both. Student and graduate nurses may participate full time or part time in this program. The most effective pediatric nurse is one who gives the child's play the same continuous interest and supervision that she gives his personal hygiene and prescribed treatment. Whether or not there is a planned program, a pediatric unit should be furnished with toys, games, books, and play materials suited to the ages and interests of the patients. Occupations that give the child a chance to make something, or to take an active part, are more constructive than those that the child merely looks at or handles; however, these also have their value. Play materials may be prescribed in some cases for restoration of func-

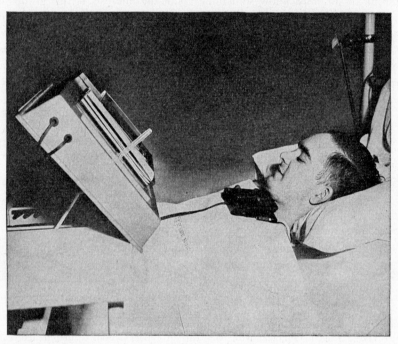

Figure 113. An electro-mechanical page turner molded from laminated plastics, light in weight but strong and durable. Thin metal clips tied by a series of knots on a thread are slipped on the edges of successive pages of a book. When a switch adjusted under the chin is depressed by the patient, a motor-driven rotating cylinder automatically pulls the metal clips and a page is turned. (Courtesy of General Textile Mills, Inc., New York City.)

Books that can be shown on a ceiling with a projector are available through Projected Books, Inc. (nonprofit agency; 313 North Street, Ann Arbor, Mich.).

tion, and it may require considerable imagination to interest the child in their use. Teachers from the public school system are assigned to hospitals in large centers. When possible, schoolrooms should be set up for their use since it is difficult for the children to concentrate if they are in an open ward.

The effects of separating children from parents and familiar surroundings are under investigation. After seeing the research film, *The Three-Year-Old Goes to the Hospital,* a nurse is reminded that the most one can do for an institutionalized child cannot compensate him for the loss of parental and sibling companionship. In one British hospital mothers are admitted with all children under four years and give much of the nursing care to their child.[19] Child care, and particularly that directed toward rehabilitation, is more and more designed to minimize institutionalization, and, when this is necessary, to bring the family into the re-education program for the sick or handicapped to the fullest possible extent. Increasingly the nurse must learn to guide not only the child but the parents, and to work with groups as well as individuals.

Diversions and Occupations Available in Most Situations.   In making the daily plan of care for most patients the nurse should realize that rehabilitation is fostered by providing the variety that people in our culture expect in a "normal day." Most of us like to spend part of the day alone with some interesting occupation, but the average person seeks company for many of his activities. We look upon reading as a daily diversion, or duty, and music in some form enters into the daily pattern of many lives. Games are a standard form of recreation, and, to the creative individual, the day is lost if he doesn't make something—or work on some productive task.

Congenial companionship is of course a source of recreation and the one most lacking in the sick man's day. The potential therapeutic value of the medical worker's personality is often discussed. Whereas we have just come through a "scientific" era in which nurses were taught that it was "unprofessional" to sit and talk with patients, we now realize that the provision of a listening, interested companion is one of the most important forms of therapy. The patient may be in greater need of the nurse's unhurried attention than of any aspect of physical care.

Most patients have *visitors* to provide company and affection. Ideally the amount of visiting should be determined by the effect upon the patient. Because there is limited visiting on the ward services it should not be assumed that the under-privileged person has less need for his family and friends than the person in the private service. "Visiting hours" are an administrative device to regulate activity in treatment areas. Some hospitals have instituted unlimited visiting, and, according to some observers, the increased well-being of the patients more than compensates for the extra demands made on the staff.[20] Indeed some people believe that the visitors help with the care of the patient and incidentally are prepared to promote the patient's rehabilitation at home in proportion to their opportunity to serve and participate in the hospital. Occasionally visitors have an unwholesome effect; in such cases it is the responsibility of the doctor and the nurse to control their visits or at least to help the patient solve this problem.

Visitors should be made comfortable. They should be within the patient's sight and hearing. They should not sit on or jar the bed. It often tires the patient less to have two visitors who talk to each other than to have one demanding his full attention. About such individual matters, however, few rules can be made.

Letters, flowers, and other gifts are means of preserving personal relationships. For patients who can't write, the services of a nurse or a volunteer worker should be provided if possible.

The satisfaction of making purchases to supply daily needs and desires is taken for granted until one is deprived of it; therefore, carts containing such items as magazines, bouquets, soaps, candy, tooth paste, writing paper, and stamps are a pleasure to bed patients who have no access to shops within the hospital.

Reading is an unending source of diversion. Patients may visit a library in the hospital or books may be brought to them on carts (see Fig. 112). Bibliotherapy is often discussed as a means of altering a mood or an attitude. The use of specific books as therapy is, to the writer's knowledge, rare, but reading as recreation and for educational rehabilitation is well established. Nurses should be able to read aloud so that it gives pleasure since volunteer workers, who might do this, are rarely available. The American Library Association, the Child Study Association, and other agencies can provide lists to those who need help in selecting books according to age and interest.

Radio and television have put music and drama within the reach of the sick population. Music therapy has been discussed since David soothed Saul with his harp and his songs and probably long before that. Recently there have been some experiments with the use of music in psychiatry.

Music for and by the sick is certainly receiving an increasing amount of attention. Active participation in concerts and theatrical entertainment undoubtedly helps to re-establish the patient's self-confidence and enables him to have a normal group interest, for diversion is most satisfactory in a form that allows the patient a choice.[21, 22]

Variety in dress and provision of suitable clothing is a part of every rehabilitation program. Children and adults enjoy deciding what they will wear. Even in otherwise poor state hospitals, uniforms have been discarded because of their depressing effect. A hundred years ago Florence Nightingale suggested that nurses wear different colored uniforms and that pictures be changed in "the sick room" from time to time to combat monotony. Normal dress is encouraged in a rehabilitation program, and patients may be taught how to make suitable attractive clothing (see Fig. 102).

Meals can be pleasurable events if appetite is present. Enjoyment depends upon a combination of good food, attractive service, and companionship. Communal dining is encouraged for patients who can feed themselves and who will not be tired by company. The psychological effect of eating alone is admittedly bad, and it should be avoided in institutions and homes unless the patient's condition indicates it. In these circumstances the nurse and the dietary service should use every means at their disposal to make the solitary event a pleasurable one. This was discussed in Chapter 13.

A change of scene is possible for all patients who aren't critically ill. Beds and their occupants can be wheeled to roofs or porches. Helpless persons can be lifted into wheelchairs, and taken almost anywhere. Motorized wheelchairs have been available for years.[23] As soon as patients are ambulatory they may be moved to parts of the hospital where normal living is the order of the day. Some military and civil hospitals are classifying patients according to their independence, or the type of service they need. As the acute stage of the illness passes the patient is moved to a unit operated more like a club or a hotel and equipped and staffed differently from the acute service. Properly managed this will certainly promote rehabilitation. The average hospital could adopt certain aspects of this program.

Most of the facilities mentioned in this section are generally available. The use made of them depends upon the interest, imagination, and talents of medical workers. For many patients no other activities are needed for their rehabilitation; for others, organized programs of games, entertainment, and handicrafts are indicated.

SUMMARY

Rehabilitation is not a new concept. The organization of specialists into a "rehabilitation team" is, apparently, a modern accomplishment. The daily activity inventory against which any sick, or incapacitated person's dependencies can be checked is a modern tool that has made the rehabilitation program specific. Publicity, health legislation, and economic support are making rehabilitation available to an increasing number of persons. The position taken in this text is based upon: (1) that the restoration of the patient to optimum independence and self-respect is a part of comprehensive medical care; (2) that it should be available to everyone in "the ideal state"; and (3) that rehabilitation can begin with treatment and that all medical workers can practice it as soon as they have the concept. While specialized workers and departments can usually give the most effective care, these are so limited in number that general practitioners in medicine and nursing must assume responsibility for the rehabilitation of most patients. Programs are geared to the specific disabilities, sex, age, intelligence, and interests. Since sickness is never wholly mental or wholly physical, the nurse needs the same abilities regardless of the clinical service, although the rehabilitation of a psychotic patient may make greater demands on her psychological skill, and the rehabilitation of a paraplegic on her ability to redirect motor activity. While the nurse must learn to follow up, and in some cases initiate, the specialized programs, her particular task is to encourage optimum independence of the patient throughout his illness, and to make his hourly existence as constructive as it is possible to make it. If for no other reason than that she spends so much time with him, the nurse, of all medical workers, is in a position to contribute most to the patient's rehabilitation.

REFERENCES

1. Brown, Mary E.: "Daily Activity Inventory and Progress Record for Those with Atypical Movement." *Am. J. Occup. Therap.*, **4**:195, (Sept.–Oct.) 1950; **4**:261, (Nov.–Dec.) 1950; and **4**:23, (Jan.–Feb.) 1951.
2. Sverdlik, Samuel S., et al.: "Fifty Years of Progress in Physical Medicine and Rehabilitation in New York State," *New York J. Med.*, **51**:90, (Jan.) 1951.
3. Buchwald, Edith (in collaboration with Howard A. Rusk, George G. Deaver, and Donald A. Covelt): *Physical Rehabilitation for Daily Living*. McGraw-Hill Book Co., New York, 1952, p. v.

4. Grayson, Morris: "Psychiatric Aspects of Rehabilitation." *J. Nerv. & Ment. Dis.*, **112**:453, (Nov.) 1950.
5. Schorr, H. A., et al.: "The Patient's Spiritual Needs," *Am. J. Nursing*, **50**:64, (Feb.) 1950.
6. Axline, Virginia M.: *Play Therapy; The Inner Dynamics of Childhood.* Houghton Mifflin Co., Boston, 1947.
7. Rogers, Carl: *Client-Centered Therapy; Its Current Practice, Implications and Theory.* Houghton Mifflin Co., Boston, 1951.
8. Lane, Ronald E.: "The Patient and His Job." *Guy's Hosp. Gazette,* **65**:9, (Jan.) 1951.
9. Rusk, Howard A., and Taylor, Eugene J.: *New Hope for the Handicapped.* Harper & Brothers, New York, 1949.
10. Barton, Betsy: *And Now to Live Again.* D. Appleton-Century Co., New York, 1944, pp. 13, 32.
11. Tudor, Gwen E.: "A Socio-psychiatric Nursing Approach to Intervention in a Problem of Mutual Withdrawal on a Mental Hospital Ward," *Psychiatry,* **15**:193, (May) 1952.
12. Morimoto, Francoise R.: "The Socializing Role of Psychiatric Ward Personnel," *Am. J. Nursing,* **54**:53, (Jan.) 1954.
13. Brown, Joe K.: "Retraining Patients with Brain Damage," *Lancet,* **70**:455, (Dec.) 1950.
14. Morrissey, Alice B.: *Rehabilitation Nursing.* G. P. Putnam's Sons, New York, 1951.
15. Knocke, Frederick J., and Knocke, Lazelle S.: *Orthopaedic Nursing.* F. A. Davis Co., Philadelphia, 1952.
16. Willard, Helen S., and Spackman, Clare S.: *Principles of Occupational Therapy.* J. B. Lippincott Co., 1947, p. 177.
17. Pratt, Marian: "Integration of Physical Therapy in a Generalized Public Health Nursing Program," *Pub. Health Nursing,* **43**:319, (Aug.) 1951.
18. Gips, Claudia D.: "A Study of Toys for Hospitalized Children," *Child Devel.,* **21**:149, (Sept.) 1950.
19. "Mothers Go to Babies' Hospital" (editorial), *Am. J. Nursing,* **54**:582, (May) 1954.
20. Flores, Florence: "Visitors Unlimited," *Am. J. Nursing,* **53**:1351, (Nov.) 1953.
21. Van de Wall, Willem, and Liepmann, Clara M.: *Music in Institutions.* Russell Sage Foundation, New York, 1936.
22. Wenger, Paul: "Value of Music in Successful Psychotherapy of Schizophrenic Patients," *Psychiat. Quart.* (Suppl. 2), **26**:202, 1952.
23. Johnson, Marilyn: "Magic Carpet," *Crippled Child,* **25**:8, (Oct.) 1947.

Additional Suggested Reading

Ashbrook, James B.: "Not by Bread Alone," *Am. J. Nursing,* **55**:164, (Feb.) 1955.
Barckley, Virginia: "They Go to School in the Hospital," *Am. J. Nursing,* **54**:328, (Mar.) 1954.
Bindt, Juliet: *A Handbook for the Blind.* The Macmillan Company, New York, 1952.
Campbell, Latis, and Davis, Larcie: "Nursery School Experience," *Am. J. Nursing,* **53**:1448, (Dec.) 1953.
Galioni, Elmer F., et al.: "Group Techniques in Rehabilitating Back-Ward Patients," *Am. J. Nursing,* **54**:979, (Aug.) 1954.
Gardner, C. M.: "Rehabilitation for Every Patient," *Canad. Nurse,* **45**:347, (May) 1949.
Garrett, James F.: *Psychological Aspects of Physical Disability.* Office of Vocational Rehabilitation, Washington, D.C., 1952.
Grayson, Morris, et al.: *Psychiatric Aspects of Rehabilitation.* Institute of Physical Medicine and Rehabilitation, New York, 1952.
Jans, Paul: "Meals on Wheels," *Nursing Outlook,* **3**:130, (Mar.) 1955.
Kessler, Henry H.: *The Principles and Practices of Rehabilitation.* Lee & Febiger, Philadelphia, 1950.

Kiefer, N. C.: *Present Concepts of Rehabilitation in Tuberculosis*. National Tuberculosis Association, New York, 1948.

Molyneux, Molly: "A Rehabilitation Program in Canada," *Am. J. Nursing,* **54:**41, (Jan.) 1954.

Olsen, Guhli J.: "The Observation Study," *Am. J. Nursing,* **54:**589, (May) 1954.

Pinner, Max, and Miller, Benjamin F. (eds.): *When Doctors Are Patients*. W. Norton & Co., New York, 1952.

Rennie, Thomas A. C., et al.: "Vocational Rehabilitation of the Psychiatrically Disabled," *Ment. Hyg.,* **33:**200, (Apr.) 1949.

Treister, Bert A.: "Physical Medicine and Rehabilitation in Geriatrics," *Phys. Therap. Rev.,* **30:**411, (Oct.) 1950.

Veterans Administration: *Rehabilitation of the Chronic Neurologic Patient*. US Government Printing Office, Washington, D.C., 1949.

Whitehouse, Frederick: "Vocational Training at a Rehabilitation Center," *J. Rehabilitation,* **17:**3, (Jan.–Feb.) 1951.

CHAPTER 17. RESPONSIBILITY OF THE NURSE FOR HEALTH TEACHING

1. **EFFECTIVE HEALTH GUIDANCE**
2. **METHODS OF TEACHING USED IN HEALTH EDUCATION AND IN CARE OF THE SICK**
3. **ASPECTS OF HEALTH EDUCATION TAUGHT BY THE NURSE**
4. **OPPORTUNITIES FOR TEACHING IN HOMES, HOSPITALS, CLINICS, AND SCHOOLS**

1. EFFECTIVE HEALTH GUIDANCE

Teaching is an art, and there is no more justification for assuming that one is a "born teacher" than that one is a "born nurse" or a "born doctor." The best teachers, like the best nurses and doctors, are those who not only have aptitude for teaching but who, in addition, have studied the underlying principles and methods used by masters of the art. By trial and error a fairly satisfactory technique may eventually be evolved for almost all skills, but it is intelligent to adopt a more economical way of learning.

The teaching or guiding function of the nurse is now generally recognized. More emphasis is given, both in basic and postgraduate courses, to the nurse's preparation for teaching. Nursing services are in some cases organized for the sole purpose of giving health guidance.[1, 2] Actually, every practicing nurse is and always has been some kind of teacher—good, bad, or indifferent. Even when unaware of her obligation, she unconsciously teaches by reaction to what the patient says to her and by her behavior as a person and a nurse. A flaw in this argument may be that by the same token everyone teaches health by the example he sets, but actually this is not true. No other persons are expected to understand and apply the principles of healthful living to the same extent as medical workers. Any nurse teaches when she answers the questions patients ask. Those who have studied the functions of the graduate or student nurse have noticed that these questions cover a wide range of subjects, and that even the student cannot avoid this incidental type of teaching. She cannot refer all inquiries to someone else or avoid showing attitudes of some sort in her manner. Whether the nurse likes it or not, *teaching is inherent in her profession,* and her position makes health guidance one of her obligations. The nurse's choice is not whether she will teach but whether she will be a successful, an average, or a poor health teacher.[3, 4, 5]

The general preparation of the nurse should include some instruction and practice in conscious teaching. The qualifications of the effective teacher of health are analogous to those of the teacher in other fields. She should have some conception of the psychology of the learning process; she should understand that her relationship to the patient is an influence in itself; she should be able to stimulate interest in those she teaches and impart what she knows; she must like people, be able to enter into their difficulties, and speak the language of those she hopes to teach; she should recognize teaching opportunities, have some idea of how to measure the success of her teaching, and above all she must have a thorough familiarity with her subject and yet realize the limitations of her knowledge.[6, 7, 8]

It is now recognized that nurses engaged in preventive health work must have specific information about nutrition, child care, mental hygiene, social hygiene, communicable disease control, and health legislation if they expect to be of real service. Assuming, however, that they have acquired a fund of useful and accurate information and an ability to find reliable data, they still have to learn that they cannot force this upon individuals, that the most they can do is to help the patient to understand his problem and then let him make his own choice. The interest of the learner must be aroused, or he is unreceptive to new ideas. He must indicate a need for assistance; otherwise, the teacher's efforts are likely to be futile.

Health organizations are rapidly changing their approach to the public to comply with accepted educational principles; for example, before trying to institute a program of treatment for any disease or condition, general interest in the health problems involved is aroused by newspaper publicity, audio-visual presentations, and group meetings. More and more attention is given to individual and family guidance in recognition of the psychological principle that what the teacher has to say is of greatest interest to the learner when it is selected with reference to his personal problems. This type of teaching is illustrated in the consultation services in many health centers. The patient alone or with members of his family comes to the center with definite questions in mind and often talks as much or more than the nurse or doctor, the psychologist or social worker. It is only through listening to and studying him that they can give assistance. Medical workers attempt to help the patient to arrive at a reasonable solution of his difficulty rather than to force a solution upon him. They try to speak his language, begin where he is, and proceed at his pace. This same concept of teaching is illustrated in small group meetings where, for example, persons meet to discuss problems of child care, diabetes, alcoholism, drug addiction, or where patients with the same disorders discuss their common difficulties. The health teacher may act as chairman, but those most concerned are encouraged to talk freely, exchange opinions and information, and to work things out together.[9, 10, 11]

Patients who have made a good adjustment to their handicap are in many cases most helpful. A person rehabilitated after blindness, an amputee who is skillful in the use of a prosthesis, and a person who has learned to take care of a colostomy without interruption of his former occupation can give invaluable encouragement and instruction to persons just faced with these problems. In the rehabilitation process, guidance is given by many persons. A list of them might include the following: the doctor (both general and specialist); the nurse; the minister; the physical, occupational, play, and speech therapist; the psychologist; the social worker; and teachers of various subject matters or trades, according to the age and needs of the individual. Many other specialists may be brought in. For example, the man who makes the artificial leg can help the one who wears it, the manufacturer of wheelchairs can instruct those who operate them, and so on.[12, 13]

The effective health teacher is never patronizing. She listens attentively to those she hopes to help; she shows respect for their views even if they are at variance with her own. She tries to get at the real difficulties, the inner significance of what the patient tells her, knowing that destructive or abnormal behavior, either mental or physical, has some cause, and that only by recognizing its origin and helping the person to recognize its source can she help the individual or he help himself.

The generally accepted principle that learning should be accompanied by satisfaction is applied in various ways. In teaching either skills or facts, the student is encouraged by commendation, or other forms of recognition of accomplishment. In teaching skills to a patient such as the method of giving a baby a bath or the calculation of a diabetic diet, an attempt is made to simplify the procedure so that it is never beyond the learner's grasp and to limit the amount to be learned each time in order that he will not be fatigued and his satisfaction correspondingly decreased. Failure to comprehend is frustrating, and the learner feels awkward and unhappy; unless he is very much interested he spares himself further embarrassment by giving up the struggle to learn.

2. METHODS OF TEACHING USED IN HEALTH EDUCATION AND IN CARE OF THE SICK

Almost every known method of teaching is used in health work at the present time. Lectures are given in hospitals, clinics, industries, schools, clubs, and over the radio and television; moving pictures on a wide variety of health problems are available and extensively used; demonstrations are considered essential whenever skills are taught to individuals or groups, and every effort is made to have the students, young or old, practice the skills under the supervision of an expert. The discussion method is generally used in group meetings. Individuals in the group are often encouraged to prepare themselves to discuss certain topics by reading material on the subject chosen by themselves or recommended by the leader. Individual conferences and the incidental, indirect, or unconscious teaching that is accomplished through example and through listening to and talking with patients about their problems are, however, the most universal and probably the most effective methods used. When the nurse is misinformed, superficially educated, or prejudiced, she may do a great deal of harm.

The nurse cannot escape being an influence. She must teach through some method, and the more nearly the method she selects is suited to the particular situation in which she finds herself, the more effective her efforts. A high development of teaching skill is not expected of the average practicing nurse. She should, however, be alert to the importance of trying to discover the meaning that sickness has for the patient and the opportunities she may have to make the experience less unhappy or even to make it a constructive one. Any graduate nurse should be able to guide individuals toward sounder health practices, but only in certain positions is the nurse expected to teach groups either formally or informally. Inevitably, she will do the incidental and unconscious type of individual teaching inherent in her work.[14, 15, 16, 17, 18]

3. ASPECTS OF HEALTH EDUCATION TAUGHT BY THE NURSE

To define the nurse's responsibility for health teaching is difficult. Attention has frequently been called to the overlapping of the functions of health workers. There is as much confusion with relation to their teaching activities as there is in distinguishing between nursing procedures and medical treatments.

The hygienic care of patients and the home care of the sick are the particular responsibility of the nurse, although a disability may make any ordinary daily activity so difficult that the patient will need the combined efforts of a rehabilitation team to solve the problem. The nurse through her teaching may help patients to organize and maintain a healthful environment when it is obvious that they need and want her help. The nurse should be able to give to some accurate information about matters of personal cleanliness and habits of elimination; she may help others in selecting and preparing normal diets; still others with habits of sleep, rest, and exercise and problems of mental hygiene related to these questions. She should also be able to give advice in securing competent medical care and in making use of the health services in the community. The nurse should be able to recognize and give some guidance to the psychological or emotional aspects of all these questions. She must be able to differentiate between a deep-seated and serious disturbance that is interfering with appetite or sleep, for example, and one less serious that the patient may be easily helped to recognize. In psychotherapy the nurse is one member of a medical team with a common plan for the patient.[19, 20, 21]

Because the science of hygiene and medical treatment is developing so rapidly, there is rarely a final answer to any problem. The nurse is of greatest service to the patient when she helps to arouse his interest, guide his study, and then develop health practices based on the knowledge and insight he has acquired.

During her care of a patient, questions such as the following will come up which the nurse should refer to the physician: questions related to the physician's reasons for employing the prescribed therapeutic measures; the significance of symptoms; and the probability of recovery. The physician usually prefers to explain the purpose of the prescribed treatment to his patient. He is certainly the best interpreter of this as he is best fitted to discuss the causes of pain and other symptoms of disease;

and it is his obligation to discuss with the patient his general health status, as shown by a physical examination, or his hope of recovery.

Under the circumstances, the physician may ask the nurse to interpret the prescribed treatment or to amplify his directions; for example, a patient visiting a skin clinic may be found to have scabies (itch). In this case the treatment is clear cut and definite, and if the patient understands it thoroughly, the relief is immediate and the cure certain. Since the physician may have to see many persons during the course of a few hours, he will not have time to explain thoroughly the nature of the disease or the treatment, and may therefore ask the nurse to do this for him.

The physician often asks the nurse to teach a pregnant woman how to treat varicose veins or inverted nipples; the pediatrist may leave the management of feeding problems of children in the hands of a competent nurse. Under all these circumstances, if the nurse discusses the diagnosis, the symptoms, the treatment, and the prognosis, she is not infringing on the doctor's field but merely acting as his agent. Whenever she acts as the agent of a particular physician, the nurse should be certain that she complies with his wishes and that her interpretation is similar to his. If she believes that he is dangerously misinformed or incompetent, she cannot conscientiously assume the responsibility of carrying out his wishes, and will not be willing to act for him.

Rules, however, must never take the place of reason or common sense, and although these general principles may be used to help the nurse in the practice of health guidance, occasions will undoubtedly arise when, as in emergencies, she may find it necessary to assume some of the functions of the physician or other medical specialist.

Student nurses need a great deal of help in dealing with patients' questions. They must learn which they should be able to discuss, which should be referred to an experienced nurse, and which should be referred to a physician. Student nurses should be encouraged to talk about these problems with instructors capable of making constructive criticism of the way in which the teaching opportunity was handled. Students profit by listening to conferences between patients and graduate nurses who can teach effectively. Afterward, students and graduates should discuss the experience. Throughout their period of preparation for nursing, students need as careful supervision of the health guidance they give as of the manual skills used in the care of the sick.[22]

4. OPPORTUNITIES FOR TEACHING IN HOMES, HOSPITALS, CLINICS, AND SCHOOLS

Almost every contact that the visiting nurse or the one in private practice has with a *patient in a home* offers teaching opportunities. Nell V. Beeby's analysis of "nursing situations" in obstetrical nursing shows the wide range of human experience encompassed in just one of the clinical services.[23] This is paralleled in every

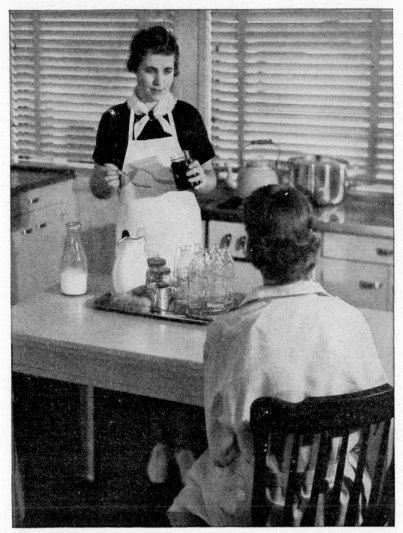

Figure 114. Visiting nurse showing young mother how to prepare the feeding prescribed by the doctor for her baby.

other such study. It is impossible to enumerate the problems that nurses help their patients to solve, but a few examples may be given.

Figure 114 shows a visiting nurse teaching a young mother to prepare her baby's diet formula, including the aseptic handling of the food, bottles, and nipples. When the mother is able to nurse the infant, the nurse shows her how to keep the breasts clean; she discusses the value of breast feeding from the emotional and physical standpoints and helps her to overcome any difficulties in this connection. (See Fig. 115.) Later, if problems arise in relation to the child's eating habits, the nurse may be called upon to help the parents analyze the causes, to understand their or the child's difficulties, and to overcome them. (Some feeding difficulties, however, are the result of such deep emotional disturbance in the mother that the psychiatrist's help may be needed.) Infants' and children's baths are often demonstrated to the parents in the hospital and home, and they practice this procedure under the nurse's supervision. The equipment for the care of the baby may be selected with the help of the nurse, and the room in which the baby sleeps arranged after consultation with her.

When a communicable disease occurs, a nurse from the official health department, a visiting nurse, or a nurse in private practice is expected to show the family

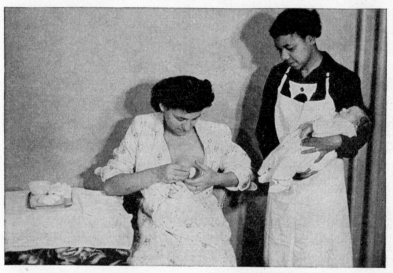

Figure 115. Nurse teaching mother breast care. (Courtesy of Visiting Nurse Association of Brooklyn, Brooklyn, N. Y., and Clay-Adams Co., New York City.)

how to control the spread of the disease. She explains and demonstrates methods of handling dishes, linen, excreta, and all objects contaminated during the patient's illness, and methods of terminal disinfection after his recovery or death. If members of the family are helping her to take care of the patient, she may have to teach them to give medications, sponge baths, and other treatments and, in fact, to take the patient's temperature, to clean the mouth, and to perform all those services required by febrile patients.

Since many patients with orthopedic conditions may need protracted treatment, the care they require is frequently given in the home; in such cases the nurse's supervision may be important in hastening recovery and rehabilitation. For orthopedic conditions, the nurse may show the patient and his family how to maintain prescribed postures in lying, standing, or sitting; she may be asked by the physician to teach the mother of a sick child corrective manipulation and massage; she can often help in the arrangement of the room and in the provision of facilities for moving the patient about so that his life will be more nearly normal. Unless there is a physical therapist and an occupational therapist in attendance, she must to some extent fulfill the functions of both of these specialists. Most health agencies employ such specialists who advise the nurse.

Chronically infected wounds and inoperable cancer are other types of disease often treated outside hospitals. When a surgical dressing is required that must be changed frequently, the nurse usually teaches the patient or some member of the family to dress the wound. The patient may be hospitalized for a short period of observation, at which time a great deal of help may be given him; but it is always more satisfactory to teach a technique of this kind in the home than in the hospital, because it is so difficult to visualize the home conditions, no matter how vivid the patient's description is of the facilities available.

Besides the problems involved in the physical care of extra-institutional patients, there are the many and varied mental adjustments to be made by the person who is sick and by members of his family. The depression, the sense of futility, the nervousness or irritability that often accompany illness may be more difficult to deal with than the physical limitations imposed by disease. The nurse may be able to do nothing more than listen sympathetically, but in many cases, if she is skillful, she can relieve the patient's discouragement or irritation by helping him to understand the source of it and to substitute constructive for destructive ideas.

In the *care of patients in the hospital,* the necessity for teaching is not so obvious as it is in homes when the visiting nurse or the hourly nurse leaves the sick person most of the day in less skilled hands. Under such circumstances it requires little imagination to see that the patient must be taught how to take care of himself or that some member of the family must be shown how to attend to his needs. When the patient is in the hospital, however, the care he requires is provided by the hospital staff, and nurses and doctors may lose sight of what will happen to him after he leaves. This failure to recognize the patient's need of assistance in the period following his discharge from the hospital results in many incomplete cures and unnecessary complications during convalescence. There is a growing recognition of the importance of discovering how much and what kind of assistance the person should have, and of providing as much of this as possible while the patient is in the hospital where doctors and nurses are available to teach him the fundamentals of nursing and medical care needed in his particular case. Although it is possible for patients to learn a good deal simply by being in the hospital, observing its operation, and asking questions, nevertheless planned programs of guidance for each patient should be more highly developed in the institution. The necessity for cooperation among medical workers is as important here as in any other part of the patient's program of care. (Schemes for fostering cooperation have been discussed in Chapters 4 and 16.)

Conspicuously successful programs of teaching in hospitals have been carried out for certain types of patients, such as, for example, diabetics. Persons having diabetes, or suspected of having it, are usually sent to the hospital for a thorough physical examination. If they show evidence of the disease, a diet is worked out that alone, or in combination with insulin, leaves them free from the symptom of sugar in the urine. All this work is in vain if the patient is not taught subsequently to regulate his diet, to test his urine, to take insulin if prescribed, to recognize the symptoms of insulin shock, and to treat this latter condition effectively. Diabetics must also be taught special care of the skin and nails, which are abnormally susceptible to infection. These patients must be encouraged to take an optimistic attitude toward their condition and, in general, to follow a hygienic daily regime.

In order to educate the diabetic patient, he is given demonstrations of testing the urine for the presence of sugar, administering insulin, and calculating diets.

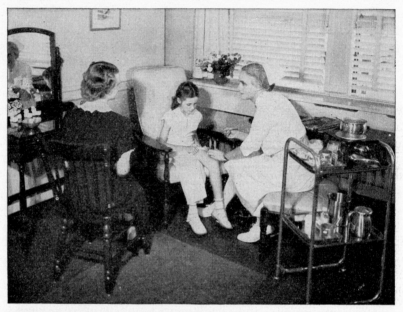

Figure. 116. Nurse teaching diabetic child and her mother how to administer insulin and carry out steps of a urine test.

Figure 116 shows a graduate nurse demonstrating some of these techniques to a diabetic child and her mother. Later, the patient practices these skills under the supervision of the nurse. A dietitian teaches the patient and her family food values and methods of calculating diets. The physician explains the prescribed treatment and goes over the significance of symptoms. He not only teaches individually, but in many diabetic clinics holds a series of conferences. Patients in the hospital, as well as those who return to the clinic after discharge from the clinical division, attend such group meetings. Nurses may discuss general hygiene, and chiropodists, the care of the feet and the particular danger to diabetic patients of injudicious treatment of calluses, ingrowing toenails, and other abnormalities. Explanatory literature is given to the patients, and they are shown, and urged to buy, a manual prepared especially for the diabetic. There is no doubt that many hospitals, by a carefully organized program of teaching, prepare the diabetic to take care of himself successfully after he goes home.

Another type of patient whose need of instruction has been generally recognized in hospitals is the pregnant woman. Maternity clinics in hospitals have set up demonstrations of suitable clothes for mother and infant, the equipment needed for the baby's bath, and the care of the mother's nipples. Classes are organized in which the process of reproduction is explained and problems of mental and physical hygiene during pregnancy and the care of the newborn are discussed with prospective mothers and fathers. Where natural childbirth is stressed, the teaching program

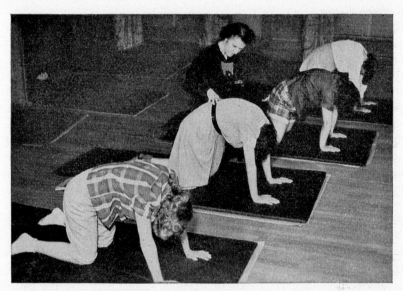

Figure 117. Nurse teaching principles of posture to the prenatal patient; pelvic rocking exercise, quadruped position, and humped back exaggerated. (Courtesy of Visiting Nurse Association of Brooklyn, Brooklyn, N. Y., and Clay-Adams Co., New York City.)

is especially thorough and includes special exercises and discussion, designed to help the woman and her husband understand the mechanism of labor.

Individual instruction is given to patients according to particular needs. Opportunities are made for conferences with medical workers at regular intervals. Advisers try to uncover the fears so common during pregnancy. Often these fears are groundless and disappear if given expression or if shown to be without basis. Even when there is some cause for anxiety, the patient is relieved by knowing the best way to face it and by feeling that the medical workers recognize that the danger exists and are prepared to give the assistance required. Many patients have physical difficulties, such as varicose veins, and need instruction in relation to treatment by posture and the elimination of tight clothing; others have abdominal discomfort, and benefit from advice on the selection and adjustment of supports. The incidence of eclampsia and other complications of pregnancy is greatly reduced by teaching women the danger signs and symptoms and the importance of early treatment.[24, 25]

In some hospitals the staff helps the cardiac patient work out a plan for regulating the daily regimen in accordance with his condition. He is taught the importance of limiting exercise, of resting at well-spaced intervals, and of eating frequent simple and light meals. In some cases he is encouraged to cultivate occupations that do not make too great a demand on his strength. Tuberculous patients also are taught to modify their manner of living sufficiently to arrest the disease; they are shown how to control coughing as much as possible, to dispose of discharges in such a way as to protect others, and to practice other precautions designed to prevent the spread of the disease.

Teaching is likely to be stressed for amputees, and persons with permanent colostomies or tracheostomies.

Every attempt should be made to see that not only these but each and every patient who needs help is learning throughout his hospital experience how to take care of himself so that his recovery will be complete or, when this is impossible, his condition no more disabling than it need be. Incidentally, the patient sees and may learn to appreciate during his stay in a well-run hospital the value of order and cleanliness; he may acquire a knowledge of some of the characteristics of a well-balanced and well-cooked diet; he should gain confidence in the benefits of medical treatment; and he has an opportunity to learn a good deal about the personal cleanliness and nursing measures that are a part of his care. The sum total of this planned and incidental teaching should be no small part of the service given the average patient in the hospital. Chapter 16 emphasizes the value of *rehabilitation for every patient*.

The fact that *persons admitted to clinics* are, as a rule, assuming responsibility for their own health problems makes their need of guidance apparent. The clinic staff usually realizes that the weekly or monthly service they give the patient will not affect his health nearly so much as the daily care he gives himself. Medical workers in clinics understand that their chief service to the patient is the help they give him in working out a regimen that he can carry out.

Clinics may be associated with, or separate from, hospitals. They may be set up to give health supervision to well persons, to diagnose and/or treat disease. The type of teaching done depends upon the nature of the clinic. Examples of clinics for health supervision include prenatal, well baby, mental hygiene, and nutrition. In such places guidance is given in diet, exercise, rest, personal relations, and other problems of mental and physical hygiene. Instructions may be given to individuals or groups or to both. In Figure 118, the nurse in a clinic is discussing suitable toys with the mother of a small boy. Maternity centers are conducting classes to teach fathers, as well as mothers, the principles of child care, and parent education classes are a part of the programs conducted by many health services.

In diagnostic clinics, if abnormalities are discovered, the patient is advised to undergo treatment; and, if necessary, assistance is given in securing proper medical attention. In clinics conducted for therapeutic purposes, the professional staff attempts to teach the patient enough about the nature of his ailment, the purpose of the treatment, and the way in which it is carried out to enable him to cooperate to the fullest extent; for example, to the patient with syphilis, the physician explains its nature, mode of transmission, the plan of treatment, and the prognosis or probable outcome. The possibility of transmitting the disease is freely discussed, and an effort made to gain the patient's cooperation in reaching the person infecting him and persons he may have infected, for they also should be treated. The nurse may be asked to amplify the directions given by the physician or to see that the patient understands them thoroughly.

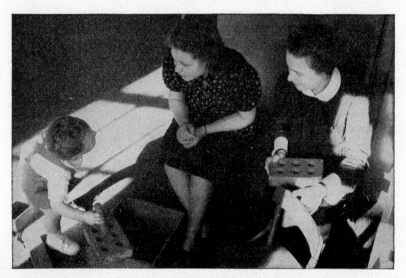

Figure 118. Nurse in a clinic discussing suitable toys with the mother of a small boy. (Courtesy of East Harlem Nursing and Health Service, New York City.)

Many social problems arise in treating the syphilitic, problems that require as skillful handling as the physical manifestations of this disease. If the social worker is not available, the nurse and the physician must assume his responsibility.

In the management of ambulatory patients with nutritional diseases, medical workers spend the greater part of their time in teaching. Each patient is guided in the selection and preparation of his particular diet, and regular lectures, discussions, and demonstrations for groups of patients are given on subjects of food selection and preparation. There are many audio-visual aids on this subject.

The sole treatment of many patients with psychiatric disorders consists in helping them to establish more constructive relationships with others. The psychiatrist analyzes the person's difficulties and decides upon the therapeutic approach to use. The nurse who works with the doctor cooperates in his plan, which may consist chiefly in encouraging the patient to make his own decisions or, in another case, to face realities; however, the problem is rarely so simple, and few medical personnel are as well prepared to give psychiatric guidance as they are to help those with physical problems. The great need for a general knowledge of psychiatry and psychiatric nursing has been stressed throughout this text. It has been pointed out that mind and body cannot be separated and that in every illness there are psychic problems. Attention has been called to a number of studies showing that approximately half the persons who apply to medical clinics have conditions caused by emotional stress.

It is unusual to find any patient attending a therapeutic clinic who does not need or would not profit by some sort of instruction. There are few if any cases in which a patient should be kept in ignorance of his condition. Patients, including medical workers when they are sick, are more and more insistent that they be told exactly what is wrong and that they be given some choice, if there is a possible choice, in treatment. Although much of this teaching is done by the physician, the cooperation of the nurse is usually essential. When the nurse is aware of and makes use of the opportunities a clinic affords for teaching, this is her most important service. [26, 27, 28]

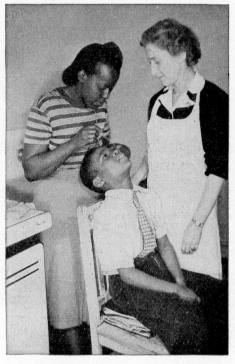

Figure 119. Instruction in eye care of a school child. (Courtesy of Visiting Nurse Association of Brooklyn, Brooklyn, N. Y., and Clay-Adams Co., New York City.)

Industrial nurses who interpret their functions broadly are health counselors to management and labor. Industrial health services function as clinics, but since the physician is rarely present full time, the nurse carries a particularly heavy burden of responsibility.

Emphasis on health education is steadily increasing in schools throughout the country, from the primary grades through college. In many of the more recent curriculums, health subjects are a large part of the social science content. They are integrated with the physical sciences, languages, and history. When treated as an aspect of living and when subject matter is organized around questions asked, or problems stated by students, the interest is marked. The traditional hygiene course is rarely popular although much depends on the instructor. Some states have set up examinations in health education that every teacher must pass. It was hoped when this ruling was made that it would ensure more thorough health teaching throughout the schools and better supervision of the pupils' health. Although a large part of the health teaching and supervision is in the hands of nonmedical groups, most schools have doctors and nurses employed either on a full-time basis or as consultants.

In some schools annual medical examinations of all students are made, and in addition there is inspection by the physician at more frequent intervals or whenever the need is indicated. In such services an effort is made to teach the students the significance of tests used, the value of health examinations, and to build up pride in physical fitness. When the physician thinks the person needs treatment, he notifies the parents, if the student is a minor; or in college health services, he discusses the abnormality with the student. Some colleges have morbidity services and provide treatment; others refer students to their own or local physicians.

In school health services the nurse works with the physician, assisting in periodic examination and inspection; she gives first aid and teaches the protection of slight injuries from infection, and the importance of treatment of colds and other mild diseases; she demonstrates and explains communicable disease and discusses many kinds of health problems with individuals. School nurses conduct health courses in some institutions. They visit day pupils who are sick in their homes, and when assigned to school infirmaries, nurses have the same opportunities for teaching as have been suggested in hospital nursing.

Health education is believed by many to be one of the major functions of the school. The Office of Education in the Department of Health, Education, and Welfare has made extensive studies of the subject, and is working toward improvements in the education of children and adults. State health departments are likewise developing methods of health teaching. In most states there is a division of school health supervision and public health education (not always given this title), which sets up state programs of health education.

With growing recognition that treatment of disease is costlier than prevention, in terms of money and human suffering, more and more attention is given to the dissemination of health knowledge. As in most aspects of education, it seems wise to begin with the child in order to prevent the formation of habits and prejudices that interfere with learning later on. The incidence of disease could be reduced enormously, if health education in schools were as thorough as it might be.[29, 30, 31]

SUMMARY

Teaching is a part of nursing just as it is a part of the practice of medicine. Because nurses and physicians are health advisers, teaching is unavoidable for them. Patients constantly ask questions, and the nurse as well as the physician should strive to give accurate information and adequate help. One of the commonest criticisms of members of the medical professions is that they so often give equivocal answers or vague and incomplete explanations and fail to take the responsibility for the patient's rehabilitation through adequate instruction.

Federal, state, and local governments have organized health-education programs; some private organizations function solely for the purpose of teaching health, and many agencies that have morbidity services put equal emphasis on health-teaching programs. Even when there is no organized program, an incidental type of teaching is carried on. All health workers teach by demonstrating health practices in their daily living and in their care of the sick, by answering questions, and by giving directions to patients and their families in relation to home care. This informal type of teaching is the most universal and probably the most effective one, but planned programs of health guidance and rehabilitation are essential.

The nurse, like the teacher in any other field, profits by having some knowledge of the art of teaching. Many nurses are placed in positions where they must instruct groups as well as individuals. Without some practice in teaching under the guidance of a trained and successful instructor, they may find it difficult to organize their material or to select and use the most effective method of presentation; they may not know how to stimulate the interest of the persons they want to teach or to elicit the participation of the student. During the basic education of the nurse, she should be helped to recognize teaching situations and obligations, and carefully selected opportunities should be provided for her to give health guidance to patients under competent supervision.

The tendency at the present time is to place more responsibility for the practice of health upon the individual and to make him independent through health instruction. It is generally accepted that effective health guidance is accomplished only when the patient is stimulated to seek advice or help. Programs of public instruction that build up an interest in the control of diseases, such as tuberculosis or syphilis, are followed by the establishment of advisory services and therapeutic clinics that deal with the problems of the family and individual. Every nurse who is taking care of the sick has an opportunity to do effective teaching of some sort, because the very fact of illness creates health problems that stimulate the patient to seek assistance from those who have a wider knowledge of medical questions than he has.

The nurse must learn to distinguish between matters on which she can advise patients and those that she must refer to other medical workers, to sense situations in which her help is needed and welcome. She can do harm by injudicious teaching, just as she can fail to do good by neglecting legitimate opportunities. Wherever she practices nursing—in the home, hospitals, clinics, schools, and industrial plants—the nurse is teaching directly or indirectly, consciously or unconsciously. When nurses recognize teaching as one of their major functions, they will be more concerned about preparing themselves to teach effectively.

REFERENCES

1. *An Experience in Health Education.* W. K. Kellogg Foundation, Battle Creek, Mich., 1950.
2. Shetland, Margaret: *Family Health Service; A Study of the Department of Educational Nursing of the Community Service Society.* Community Service Society, New York, 1943.
3. Blackburn, Laura: "Unconscious Teaching," *Am. J. Nursing,* **41**:526, (May) 1941.
4. Leahy, Kathleen M., and Bell, Aileen T.: *Teaching Methods in Public Health.* W. B. Saunders Co., Philadelphia, 1952.

5. Streeter, Virginia: "The Nurse's Responsibility for Teaching Parents," *Am. J. Nursing,* 53:818, (July) 1953.

6. Johnson, Jean E.: "Students Teach Their Patients," *Nursing Outlook,* 2:319, (June) 1954.

7. Wandelt, Mabel A.: "A Planned Program of Education Versus Incidental Instruction for Patients in Tuberculosis Therapy," *Nursing Research,* 3:52, (Oct.) 1954.

8. Ferguson, Marion, et. al.: "What Does the Consumer Want," *Nursing Outlook,* 2:571, (Nov.) 1954.

9. Murphy, F. D.: "The People Can Solve Their Problems," *M. Social Work,* 3:133, (Oct.) 1954.

10. Moir, Berta H.: "A School Health Program Is a Community Enterprise," *Nursing Outlook,* 3:342, (June) 1955.

11. Neal, Ernest E.: "Health Is What You Think It Is," *Nursing Outlook,* 2:478, (Sept.) 1954.

12. Wilma, Irene R.: "As a Blind Nurse Sees," *Am. J. Nursing,* 55:205, (Feb.) 1955.

13. Secor, Sophia M.: "New Help for Colostomy Patients," *Nursing Outlook,* 2:642, (Dec.) 1954.

14. Hollingsworth, Helen, et al.: *Health Programs Digest.* US Public Health Service, US Government Printing Office, Washington, D.C., 1952.

15. Spangler, Romayne: "We're on T.V. Every Week," *Am. J. Nursing,* 55:592, (May) 1955.

16. Crenshaw, Virginia P.: "Teaching Patients," *Am. J. Nursing,* 50:666, (Oct.) 1950.

17. Ehling, Charlotte L.: "School Health Records in Health Counseling of Children and Parents," *Nursing Research,* 3:125, (Feb.) 1955.

18. Shimberg, Benjamin, and Aird, Ellen L.: "Effectiveness of Television in Teaching Home Nursing," *Nursing Research,* 4:28, (June) 1955.

19. Frost, Harriet: *Nursing in Sickness and in Health; The Social Aspects of Nursing.* The Macmillan Company, New York, 1939.

20. Hargreaves, Anne G., and Robinson, Alice M.: "The Nurse-Leader in Group Psychotherapy," *Am. J. Nursing,* 50:713, (Nov.) 1950.

21. Barton, Walter E.; "The Nurse as an Active Member of the Psychiatric Team," *Am. J. Nursing,* 50:714, (Nov.) 1950.

22. Hudson, Bernice C.: "The Nursing Process Record," *Nursing Outlook,* 3:224, (Apr.) 1955.

23. Beeby, Nell V.: "Where and What Shall We Teach," *Am. J. Nursing,* 37:64, (Jan.) 1937.

24. Carney, Ruth: "Guidance Programs for New Mothers," *Am. J. Nursing,* 51:699, (Nov.) 1951.

25. Jackson, Edith: "New Trends in Maternity Care," *Am. J. Nursing,* 55:584, (May) 1955.

26. Lennon, Sister Mary Isadore: *Teaching in the Outpatient Department.* G. P. Putnam's Sons, New York, 1954.

27. Bulla, A. C., et al.: "Case Finding in Early Syphilis by the Public Health Nurse," *J. Ven. Dis. Inform.,* 32:122, (Feb.) 1951.

28. Wolf, Ilse S.: "Should the Patient Know the Truth?" *Am. J. Nursing,* 55:546, (May) 1955.

29. Koos, Earl L.: *The Health of Legionville, What People Thought and Did about It.* Columbia University Press, New York, 1954.

30. Heinz, Irma C.: "Health Teaching for Employees," *Nursing Outlook,* 3:340, (June) 1955.

31. Anderson, Agnes: "The Changing Emphases in Industrial Nursing," *Am. J. Nursing,* 55:39, (Jan.) 1955.

Additional Suggested Reading

Alfano, Genrose J.: "What Rapport Means to Me," *Nursing Outlook,* 3:326, (June) 1955.

Brown, Martha M., and Fowler, Grace R.: *Psychodynamic Nursing.* W. B. Saunders Co., Philadelphia, 1954.

Coffin, Margaret A.: "Visiting Hours for Parents," *Am. J. Nursing,* 55:329, (Mar.) 1955.

Corbin, Hazel: "Changing Maternity Service in a Changing World," *Pub. Health Nursing,* 42:427, (Sept.) 1950.

Dunlap, Mary M.: "The Tape Recorder as an Aid in Evaluation," *Nursing Outlook,* **3:**338, (June) 1955.

Educational Film Library Association: *Health Films Catalog; An Annotated List* (with supplements). The Association, New York, 1947.

Ford, Marie, and Wilson, Alberta B.: "Testing a Public Health Nursing Pamphlet," *Nursing Outlook,* **3:**289, (May) 1955.

Gregg, Dorothy: "Reassurance," *Am. J. Nursing,* **55:**171, (Feb.) 1955.

Jones, Margaret L.: "How Effective Is My Teaching?" *Am. J. Nursing,* **51:**135, (Feb.) 1951.

Law, Stanley: *Therapy Through Interview.* McGraw-Hill Book Co., New York, 1948.

Moak, Frances L.: "Audio-Visual Aids in the Nursing School Library," *Am. J. Nursing,* **49:**356, 1949.

Morgan, Mary L., and Lloyd, Barbara J.: "Parents Invited," *Nursing Outlook,* **3:**256, (May) 1955.

"Motion Pictures Move into Hospitals; A Carefully Planned Visual Program Serves Many Purposes for the Sick" (editorial), *Nursing World,* **124:**365, (Aug.) 1950.

Murphy, L. B.: *Emotional Factors in Learning.* Columbia University Press, New York, 1945.

Patterson, Raymond S., and Robert, Beryl J.: *Community Health Education in Action.* C. V. Mosby Co., St. Louis, 1951.

Porter, E. H., Jr.: *An Introduction to Therapeutic Counseling.* Houghton Mifflin Co., Boston, 1950.

Reid, Mabel: "Nursing in New York City's Home Care Program," *Nursing Outlook,* **2:**591, (Nov.) 1954.

Rogers, Carl R.: *Client-Centered Therapy.* Houghton Mifflin Co., Boston, 1950.

Rosenthal, Helen, and Rosenthal, Joseph: *Diabetic Care in Pictures,* 2nd ed. J. B. Lippincott Co., Philadelphia, 1953.

Turner, Clair E.: *Community Health Educator's Compendium of Knowledge.* C. V. Mosby Co., St. Louis, 1951

CHAPTER 18. MEDICAL EXAMINATION

1. TYPES OF EXAMINATIONS
2. METHODS OF EXAMINATION
3. EXAMINATION OF BODY AREAS, ORGANS, AND SENSES
4. FUNCTIONS OF THE NURSE IN THE MEDICAL EXAMINA-
   TION
5. POSITIONS AND DRAPING USED FOR PHYSICAL EXAMI-
   NATIONS

1. TYPES OF EXAMINATIONS

Periodic Health Examinations. With increased emphasis on prevention, more and more importance is attached to a periodic health appraisal. This examination differs very little from one made to determine the cause of pathological symptoms except in its purpose, which is to detect disease in its embryonic stage as a basis for early, and consequently more successful, treatment. It is the foundation stone of preventive medicine when made by competent physicians who combine it with health instruction. If disease is detected, the saving in human life and happiness are obvious; if the findings are negative, the person usually profits by an increased sense of well-being. The nurse is in a position to promote its use by her own example and by discussing its value with others.

The more complete the examination the greater its value as a preventive measure. It should include a medical and social history, or written data on the person's development, his family, his occupation, his manner of living, and history of illness. It should include inspection of the entire body, examination of the organs in the chest, including x-ray pictures, examination of the abdomen and the pelvic organs. Measurements of pulse rate, blood pressure, body temperature, vision, and hearing should be made. Laboratory tests on blood and urine are essential. For example, blood tests for hemoglobin, cell count, and syphilis are routine; the urine is always tested for sugar and albumin. Tests for the presence of certain microorganisms in the sputum and stool are indicated for those persons in occupations where there is a special danger of disease transmission. Body weight should be considered in relation to the bony structure, age, habits, and physical condition.

Health appraisals used in vocational placement may include psychometric tests and efforts to measure emotional maturity and stability. Such measurements are desirable in all health estimates.

Keeve Brodman[1] and his associates describe the "Cornell Medical Index-Health Questionnaire as a Diagnostic Instrument." The patient is given a four-page sheet containing 195 questions, stated in simple language. The questions are designed to uncover physical and emotional disorders of all sorts. Those who designed, and have used, this questionnaire believe that it is an extremely useful instrument that brings to light many conditions that are likely to be overlooked in the ordinary medical examination. Patients seem to take satisfaction in filling in the form, and this has the added advantage of saving the physician's time. A brief study of the patients' answers to such questions as "Do you often feel unhappy and depressed; keyed up or jittery? Do you cry easily? Do you have frightening thoughts?" shows emotional disturbances that otherwise might only be discovered after a long period of observation. The use of this form with the physical measurements and tests listed above would go a long way toward the "multiple screening" that A. L. Chapman[2] thinks every physical examination should include. He points out that the wholesale adoption of thoroughness in medical examinations is the most effective means of combating the vast problem of chronic illness, in such forms as heart and kidney disease, syphilis, and diabetes. He might well add our most expensive chronic condition—mental disease. It is urged in many quarters that the general practitioner and the general hospital accept more responsibility for diagnosing and treating conditions like tuberculosis and mental disease, which in the past have often gone unrecognized and when diagnosed have been treated in special hospitals.[3, 4] The New York State Health Department lends x-ray equipment to hospitals and gives them $0.50 for each chest x-ray of employees and adult patients. The Hospital Council of Greater New York says: "There is no question . . . that the general hospital can serve as a focal point in the campaign to detect, isolate, and treat cases of tuberculosis."*

Examinations for Diagnosis of Disease. When illness occurs the physician modifies the medical examination according to the patient's symptoms. Diagnostic examinations, therefore, vary considerably even though all of them should include the general examination just described, unless the physician knows the patient and has just made some such appraisal. Diseases are not always limited to the area in which the pain, or discomfort, appears. In an extensive text edited by Cyril M. MacBryde,[5] entitled *Signs and Symptoms,* a chapter is devoted to "Backache and Back Pain." It is noted that this symptom may indicate disease in the chest, abdomen, or pelvis; or in the legs or feet; or it may be caused by fatigue resulting from any number of systemic diseases as well as from diseases of the spinal column itself.

A thorough diagnostic examination is a long procedure, often requiring the

* Hospital Council of Greater New York: *Bulletin,* **6:**2, (Mar.) 1950.

services of different physicians and technicians and including many tests. In some instance the patient may go to a clinic where physicians practice in a group, giving the patient the advantage of their varied preparations and combined judgments. In other instances the entire examination is made by one physician in a home, or in a hospital. Physicians of the present day, practicing in and outside institutions, depend heavily on help from laboratory technicians and pathologists in making diagnoses.

Medical practitioners who are convinced that mind and body cannot be thought of separately, and certainly not studied independently, make an analysis of the personality development of the patient. They record data on his relationships with family, friends, and associates, and the way he lives and works; they note his behavior and his general appearance.[6, 7] George Draper, who with Ernst Kretschmer,[8] William H. Sheldon and S. S. Stevens,[9] and others has written extensively on genetics and medicine, believes that the person's appearance, shape and size are, in themselves, a clue to his ailment. A chapter is devoted to the "Mosaic of Androgny" in the book by Draper and his associates, *Human Constitution in Clinical Medicine.*[10] He says:

So far as one knows, the actual phenomenon of reproduction is achieved through the genital organs alone. A person's other task of survival depends upon adequate adjustment to a complex environment, which includes human relations. The impulse to survive is expressed extragenitally by the man in manly fashion, and by the woman in womanly ways. The opposite and special endowments for these purposes are in general well known, and are displayed by differences between man and woman in morphology, physiology, immunity, and psychology—or as cellular sex in the total organism. This composite structure of masculine and feminine characters has been called "the mosaic of androgny" ($\alpha\nu\delta\rho\sigma\varsigma$ = male; $\gamma\upsilon\nu\bar{\eta}$ = female).

The term is used because the nongenital qualities appropriate to each sex are never complete in a given man or woman to the exclusion of some evidence of the counterpart. Thus, traits that are ordinarily judged to be the man's may appear in the woman to form kaleidoscopic patterns with her own; the reverse is likewise true. The contrasting qualities have to do not only with outward design, structure and function, but even more significantly with the extragenital dynamics of the whole person. *So far as the relation of human constitution to disease is concerned, the androgynous phase of sex seems to be of greater significance than the genital.* And it is for this reason that the terms "andric" and "gynic" (adjectives formed from the joint word's component parts) have been chosen to designate the divergent organismal aspects of man and woman.†

Sheldon and Kretschmer use different terminology to designate structural types, but both believe that there is a characteristic emotional make-up associated with each of the following: the stocky figure with a large visceral cavity and a tendency to fat; the contrasting type, the asthenic, whose trunk is slender; and the athletic type, whose skeletal and muscular systems are well developed. These constitutional patterns are predisposed to different kinds of emotional disorders or so-

* The italics are the writer's.

† Draper, George, et al.: *Human Constitution in Clinical Medicine.* Paul B. Hoeber, New York, 1944, p. 75.

called "mental disease." According to some psychiatrists they have different interests, capacities, and need for affection, approval, and so on.

Physicians are not in agreement on the relationship that has just been suggested between constitution and disease; nevertheless, the "gallbladder type" with feminine or "gynic" characteristics predominating and the "ulcer type" with the pronounced "andric" characteristics are a part of medical language.

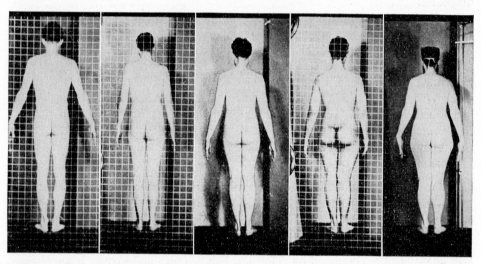

Figure 120A. Comparison of the male morphology when male, or andric, factors predominate (*left*) and when female, or gynic, factors predominate (*right*.) (Sheldon, William H., and Stevens, S. S.: *The Varieties of Temperament: A Psychology of Constitutional Differences.* Harper & Brothers, New York, 1942.)

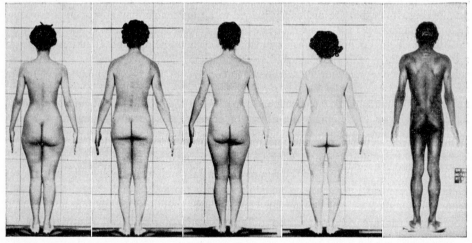

Figure 120B. Comparison of the female morphology when female, or gynic, factors predominate (*left*) and when male, or andric, factors predominate (*right*). (Courtesy of Dr. William H. Sheldon and associates.)

The point of view suggested in the preceding paragraphs is in harmony with the concepts of the much bandied term "psychosomatic medicine," another way of saying that organic, or somatic, disease may have psychic or emotional origin. The physiological explanation is that strong emotion and anxiety states either affect the endocrine system or in fact are actually our interpretation of their activity. It is easy to see that organic disease can result from a lack of balance in glandular physiology with its all-powerful and pervasive influence over the rest of the body. The wise family doctor has in all ages recognized a relationship between temperament and illness. Our present concepts are more scientific, and their application more necessary as the patient often finds himself treated by a group of specialists, none of whom know him or his family. Draper and his associates say that the medical history holds the key to diagnosis. Any thorough diagnostic examination takes into account the psychological, or emotional, aspects of disease. If the symptoms suggest a marked emotional disturbance, the examination may include an extensive psychiatric investigation or a psychoanalysis. A description of these procedures is found in the psychiatric texts listed at the end of this chapter.

A psychiatric examination varies according to the school to which the examining psychiatrist belongs. Edward A. Strecker[11] says it has two aspects—the physical and the mental, or psychic; others would hesitate to make this clear-cut division. He lists the "parts" of the examination in the traditional pattern: (1) chief complaint, (2) present illness, (3) past history, and (4) family history. The physical aspects of the examination differ in no particular from those of any complete medical examination. Discussing the psychic aspects, Strecker includes the following: (1) *general appearance and behavior,* embracing such signs as catalepsy (fixed position), stupor states, negativism, and echopraxia (tendency to repeat gestures of the examiner); (2) *stream of thought and speech activity,* noting such characteristics as incoherence, dissociation of ideas, or garrulousness; (3) *content of thought and special preoccupation,* under which heading would fall illusions, hallucinations, delusions, obsessions, and compulsions; (4) *mood-emotions, affective reactions* as determined by what the patient says and how he says it, his tone of voice, facial expression, and accompanying physical changes, such as sweating, flushing, or trembling; (5) *sensorium and intellectual reaction,* including orientation, memory of remote, intermediate, and recent events, ability to retain and recall, to count, calculate, to write from dictation, to attend to what is said, to discuss current events and other subjects; and (6) *insight,* or the patient's capacity to see himself as others see him, and to assess his condition or recognize that he is mentally sick. In addition, Strecker says that the psychiatrist may use special examinations, such as psychometric tests, word-association tests, the Rorschach test, hypnosis, and dream analysis. The psychoanalyst would not disregard any of the items included in Strecker's listing but would use an analysis as the foundation stone of both diagnosis and treatment.

Oscar Diethelm[12] warns against thinking of a psychiatric examination in the narrow terms of "mental status." He describes an examination that is a study of a patient over a period of days which he calls a group of experiments. He attaches little importance to the findings from psychological tests made when the person is under the strain of anxiety.

The physician attempts through the patient's own story and through observation of the patient in various situations to gain some understanding of his life development and his present behavior. By direct observation and interpretation, the psychiatrist tries to gain some understanding of psychopathological reactions, if they exist. He studies the dream life, and he may give the person a drug, such as amobarbital (sodium Amytal), that makes the patient not only more communicative and responsive to questions, but actually able to recall repressed emotional reactions and events.

Emotions produce measurable physiological reactions; therefore, the psychiatrist learns a great deal about the emotional basis of disease by the measurement of pulse rate, blood pressure, leukocytes, adrenergic and cholinergic substances, and sugar in the blood during the psychiatric examination. The psychiatrist bases his conclusions on the combined findings from the psychophysiological experiments, the total physical findings of the usual medical examination, the developmental medical history, the analysis of the patient's environment, the knowledge he gets through direct observation, and in some cases the insight gained by listening to the person under the influence of a drug.

Howard F. Hunt, discussing psychodiagnostics, says that the clinician is learning to interpret handwriting, drawing, reactions to pictures, participation in psychodrama, and the Rorschach test. Through projection, the patient gives the examiner many clues to the likes, dislikes, fears, hopes, and ambitions that go to make up his personality. Admitting the subjectivity of interpretation, which is an essential step in the use of these techniques, Hunt thinks that the emphasis is shifting, nevertheless, from more objective to more subjective methods of psychodiagnostics.

2. METHODS OF EXAMINATION

The Examiner's Use of the Special Senses.   The doctor, as one might expect, uses his sense of sight, feeling, hearing, and even smell in making medical judgments, though his natural powers of sight and hearing have been extended by instruments and he usually substitutes modern methods of laboratory analysis for judgments that might be based on the detection of odors. Terms used in medical parlance for these common universal functions are inspection, palpation, percussion, and auscultation.

Inspection means observing with the naked eye. The doctor notes the general size and body contour, posture, color of the skin, presence of rashes, swelling, scars, and any external visible pathology by simply looking at the patient.

Palpation is feeling with the hands. By palpation also the physician and nurse determine the rate or character of the pulse beat. Soft tissues are examined this way. The various organs of the abdomen and pelvis can be felt with the hands by applying pressure on the abdominal wall. Some of the organs are always palpable, and changes in size, shape, and location may be felt. Others are palpable only when enlarged or displaced. In either case palpation plays an important part in diagnosis.

Percussion is the tapping of an area of the body to determine the condition of the internal part by the sounds that are produced. The physician places the fingers of one hand flat on the area to be examined and taps those fingers with the tips of the fingers of the other hand. This method is of use particularly in examination of the chest and abdomen. It is by no means a new method, for it was discovered in 1761 by a physician named Auenbrugger. He, however, was the only one to use it; and so it had almost disappeared when, according to Howard W. Haggard in *The Doctor in History*,[13] a French physician, Corvisart, revived its use and wrote a book on the subject many years later. Since then it has become an indispensable part of every examination. Percussion is based on the fact that a hollow organ, such as the lung, if filled with air gives a characteristic sound when tapped, but if filled with fluid gives a duller sound. It is, therefore, possible to find out whether the lungs are well aerated or whether there is fluid or congestion present.

Auscultation is a term applied to the art of listening to sounds within the body. The ear may be placed directly against the body, but it is more common to use a stethoscope (*stethos*=breast or chest, and *skopein*=see, look). This instrument is of extremely simple construction and was designed by Laennec, a pupil of Corvisart. Laennec invented this instrument quite by accident. According to Haggard, Laennec had been unable to hear any sounds through the chest wall of an obese patient. One day he observed children tapping on a wooden beam and other children listening to the sounds produced at the other end. Seeing how that same principle could be used to solve his difficulty, he rolled a paper, placed one end on the patient's chest, and put his ear at the other. He could hear the sounds very well. The modern stethoscope is based on this same principle. It consists of two rubber tubes, one end of each being connected to a small ear piece. The other end of each tube is connected to a disk or cone-shaped device through which the sounds are transmitted to the listener's ears. Auscultation is used in examination of the heart, lungs, and arteries where variations in sounds are of extreme importance. The stethoscope is simply a device to facilitate listening to these sounds. Because the sounds are often faint and the differences between them slight, the room should be very quiet.

Examinations with Special Instruments. There are in current use many special instruments designed to test or examine specific body functions. The commonest is the thermometer used to determine the body temperature. Pulse and respiratory rates are usually counted while the body temperature is determined because they are so closely related. If one of the three varies, the other two usually show a corresponding change. The nurse is responsible for making these measurements and reporting the findings to the physician. The blood pressure, measured by means of the sphygmomanometer, is a part of every physical examination, and this is another measurement that the nurse must be able to make. (For a discussion of the techniques involved in determining body temperature, blood pressure, the respiratory and pulse rate, see Chapter 10.)

Accurate tests for visual acuity and hearing are of more recent origin but are now included in most examinations. It has recently been estimated that 50 per cent of the people in the United States have impaired hearing, which indicates the need for widespread efforts to prevent deafness. The audiometer is an instrument for testing persons individually or in groups.

Cavities and hollow organs that cannot be inspected with the naked eye may be seen by means of electrically lighted tubes through which, with a system of mirrors reflecting the light, the walls of the orifice, or the organ, are brought before the eye of the examiner. Intended to extend the range of sight (hearing in the case of the stethoscope) they are called "scopes" with prefixes to indicate their use; for example, ophthalmoscope for the eye, otoscope for the ear, cystoscope for the bladder, bronchoscope for the bronchi, and proctoscope for the rectum.

Tissues in any part of the body are made visible, in a sense, by x-rays. The outlines of dense tissues are most easily seen in roentgenograms, or hollow organs that can be filled with opaque substances. Certain deductions can be made about soft tissues by their displacement with air introduced into nearby cavities. Microscopic photographs extend the powers of sight to include objects invisible to the naked eye. When polarized light (light made to vibrate in a single plane) is thrown on an object under the microscope, internal structures within living and dead tissues are seen in a wide range of colors. This development in the microscopic examination of tissue makes it possible to learn far more than was learned from staining techniques used in the past for identification of cell and tissue structure.

Machines that make tracings of electrical charges within the heart and brain are commonly used in the medical examination. Special diagnostic tests are described in Chapter 19.

Laboratory Tests in the Physical Examination.   The role of the laboratory worker in making the diagnosis and in measuring the normal activities of the body is important. Innumerable tests are made on the urine and blood, the most common of which are described in Chapter 19. The contents of the body cavities, secretions from wounds, and pieces of living tissue are examined by a variety of methods.

3. EXAMINATION OF BODY AREAS, ORGANS, AND SENSES

In making a complete physical examination the physician adopts a more or less definite pattern or sequence of procedures. The following is the order most commonly used.

Examination of the Eyes.   The eyes are examined with the patient in a sitting position with the head resting against the back of the chair. Superficial eye examinations may be made when the patient is lying down. If the examination is made by daylight, the patient faces the light; if artificial light is used, the light is placed to the back and a little to one side of the patient. The examiner, facing the patient, frequently uses a head mirror that reflects the light to the patient's face. The first examination is one of inspection to determine such things as the movements of the eyes, reaction to light, accommodation to near and far objects, and the general appearance of the eyes. Pressure on the eyeball, which might be caused by a brain tumor, can be detected by palpation. For more detailed examination of the interior of the eye, an ophthalmoscope is used. With this instrument the examiner can see changes in the internal structures of the eye that occur in various systemic diseases, such as nephritis, diabetes, acute leukemia, and arteriosclerosis. The only place in the human body where blood vessels may actually be seen is the retina and then only by means of the ophthalmoscope. The tonometer is an instrument used for testing the tension, or pressure, within the eyeball, an extremely high pressure being characteristic of glaucoma.

For various examinations it is desirable that the eye be completely at rest. By instilling drops of certain drugs (mydriatics), it is possible to dilate the pupil and prevent its reaction to light. Two or three drops are placed in each eye every 10 minutes until the pupil is sufficiently dilated. The practice of dilating the pupil for examinations is not universal—in fact some authorities believe that the eye should be untreated in order to get a correct impression of visual acuity.

Examination of the Ears. For the examination of the ears, the patient may be either lying down or seated in a chair with the head supported. In either case the head should be in such a position that the ear to be examined is turned toward the examiner. The head must be held very still to permit a thorough examination and to prevent injury from the speculum, a funnel-shaped instrument that the physician places in the auditory canal. The nurse should stand behind the patient ready to support the head. The light should be placed behind the patient so that it may be reflected into the ear by means of the head mirror.

Articles required for the examination are a head mirror, ear specula of various sizes, cotton-tipped applicators, and an otoscope for observing the tympanic membrane.

By inspection and palpation the ears are examined for discharges and growths. The mastoid area is observed for soreness and swelling. By means of the otoscope, the tympanic membrane is observed. Glossiness, discoloration, and bulging of the membrane are symptoms of a diseased condition. Hardened secretions in the auditory canal that interfere with the examination may be removed by applicators or an irrigation. Hearing may be tested in a somewhat superficial way by the use of a tuning fork or by having the patient listen to the ticking of a watch. For more exact examinations an audiometer is used. This test is exact because the subject writes what he hears through earphones attached to a machine that plays a talking record with measured volume. Hallowell Davis[14] has constructed a "Social Adequacy Test for Hearing," designed to determine the person's need for a hearing aid. He also describes pressure tests, using water and mercury in the outer meatus, to differentiate between deafness caused by defects in conduction of sound by bone and defective nerve function. Since the test depends upon the subject's voluntary response, it is not as accurate as a recently developed technique that measures by means of electrodes placed on the skin electric charges, which represent an involuntary response to sound.[15]

Examination of the Nose, Throat, and Mouth. For the examination of the nose and throat the patient is usually seated with the head resting against the back of the chair. The examiner faces the patient. If the inspection of the throat is a part of the general examination, it is frequently made with the patient in the recumbent position. A light is placed behind the patient and reflected on his throat by means of the examiner's head mirror. A flashlight is also a convenient source of light for ear, nose, and throat examinations.

The instruments required for examination of the nose consist of nasal specula and possibly a probe. For examination of the throat, a tongue depressor and a good light are all that are needed.

The nasal passages are examined for discharges, growths, and the condition of the nasal septum. A deviated septum, though in itself a comparatively minor defect, often contributes to sinusitis and other infections of the upper respiratory tract. When there is inflammation of the mucous membrane sterile swabs may be passed over the surface, and cultures or smears made to be examined in the laboratory. The mouth and throat may show pathological conditions, such as anemia, syphilitic patches, or diseased tonsils. The number and condition of the teeth, the condition of the gums, and an odor of the breath are also noted. For satisfactory examinations of the eye, ear, nose, and throat in uncooperative children or adults, some sort of restraint may be necessary.

Examination of the Skin, Hair, and Nails.   Although the skin of the entire body is inspected, as the examination progresses the skin of the face and head are particularly observed. The color or texture of the skin may show the presence of jaundice, anemia, cyanosis, or rash. Conditions of the hair and scalp may show evidence of many diseases, classic examples of which are myxedema and syphilis. Cyanosis appears early in the lips, and nail beds; chronic pulmonary and cardiac conditions produce distorted nails in many cases, and jaundice is most easily noted in the eyes and the skin of the face.[16, 17]

Examination of the Neck.   The neck is palpated and inspected for evidences of growth or deformities with special attention to the size of the lymph nodes and thyroid gland. To test for stiffness the neck is gently flexed.

Examination of the Chest.   For the examination of the anterior chest, the patient is usually in a dorsal recumbent position with the head on one pillow. The chest is examined in several ways; it is percussed to determine the presence of fluid or congested areas, and the physician listens to sounds within the chest by means of the stethoscope. The posterior chest is examined in the same manner. The patient should be placed in a sitting position with a pillow close to the lower back to give support. The physician often prefers that the patient place each hand on the opposite shoulder and lean forward. He will, however, give these instructions if he desires that the patient assume this position. He may also ask the patient to cough or whisper at intervals while he listens to the sounds.

The *heart* is examined by percussion and auscultation by which means organic disorders and enlargement may be discovered. The area that the heart occupies is sometimes outlined with a skin pencil in order that the physician may visualize its size. The modern physician relies heavily upon an electrocardiogram and x-ray of the heart.

The *breasts* are examined by palpation for the presence of lumps or growths. Most physicians used the technique illustrated in Figure 121, and are encouraging women to examine the breasts monthly, just after the menstrual period and monthly after the menopause. (This practice is recommended by the American Cancer Society.)

The doctor should be protected against the spray from the nose and mouth during the chest examination when he must work close to the patient. A folded paper towel held between the patient's face and the doctor is an effective screen. The patient should be given a paper handkerchief to hold over his mouth when he is asked to cough. Exposure of the chest is reduced to a minimum when an examining cape, a chest blanket, or a towel is judiciously manipulated by the nurse.

Examination of the Abdomen. The abdomen is examined while the patient is in a horizontal recumbent position, with a pillow under the head and the knees flexed slightly to promote relaxation of the abdominal muscles. The abdomen is palpated to discover tender areas or hardness and the size and position of the organs in the abdominal cavity. The area is percussed to detect the presence of fluid and is observed for shape and size, scars, and growths.

Examination of the Spine. With the patient in a standing position, usually, the spine is examined for curvature. The patient should be provided either with paper slippers or with some other protection, such as disposable paper squares, for his feet. Unnecessary exposure should be avoided.

Examination of the Genitalia. For the examination of the genitalia of the male patient, the physician is left alone with him unless the nurse is a man; for the examination of the woman patient, the woman nurse is always present if the doctor is a man. The external genitalia are examined first by observation. The patient must be in a lithotomy position (see Fig. 122) when the vaginal canal or any part of the reproductive tract is examined. The vaginal canal may be dilated by a speculum and the wall of the canal and the cervix observed. A bimanual examination, in which the physician places one hand on the abdomen and one or more fingers of the other in the vaginal canal in order to feel the uterus and ovaries, is almost always made. For this examination clean rubber gloves are used. A vaginal speculum and lubricant also are required. All these articles must be sterile if the patient is pregnant and at term, if she is a post-partum patient, or a postoperative case. The draping for this position is discussed on page 567.

Examination of the Extremities. The extremities are observed for deformities and for limitation of motion. The fingers are observed for color, texture, and shape. Clubbed or spatulated fingers are typical of certain heart disorders. The legs are examined for varicose veins and enlarged joints. Inspection is the chief method of examination for these areas.

Neurological and Orthopedic Examination. In addition to the general physical examination, an examination of the nervous and motor systems may be made. This follows the other aspects of the physical examination and the history taking. It is never done as a single and complete examination. The physician tries to determine whether there are disease processes going on in the nervous and motor systems and

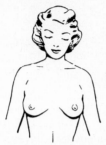

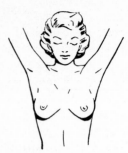

(1) Careful examination of the breasts before a mirror for symmetry in size and shape, noting any puckering or dimpling of the skin or retraction of the nipple.

(2) Arms raised over head, again studying the breasts in the mirror for the same signs.

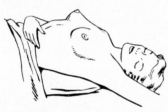

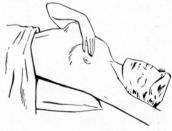

(3) Reclining on bed with flat pillow or folded bath towel under the shoulder on the same side as breast to be examined.

(4) To examine the inner half of the breast, the arm is raised over the head. Beginning at the breastbone and, in a series of steps, the inner half of the breast is palpated.

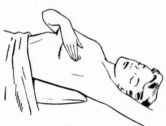

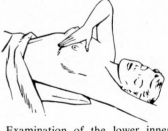

(5) The area over the nipple is carefully palpated with the flat part of the fingers.

(6) Examination of the lower inner half of the breast is completed.

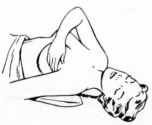

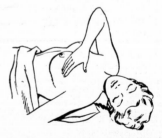

(7) With arm down at the side, self-examination of breasts continues by carefully feeling the tissues which extend to the armpit.

(8) The upper outer quadrant of the breast is examined with the flat part of the fingers.

562

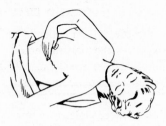

(9) The lower outer quadrant of the breast is examined in successive stages with the flat part of the fingers.

Figure 121. Breast self-examination. (*The Nurse and Breast Self-Examination*. American Cancer Society, Inc., New York City, 1952.)

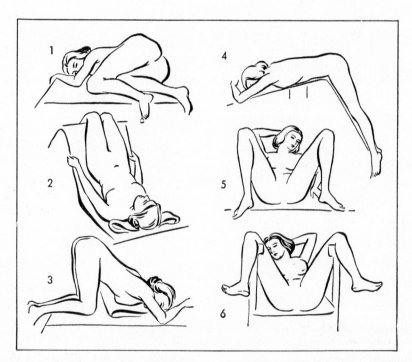

Figure 122. Positions used in examinations and treatments: (*1*) lateral or Sims' position (position may be right or left lateral); (*2*) Trendelenburg position; (*3*) knee-chest or genupectoral position; (*4*) jackknife position; (*5*) dorsal-recumbent position with knees flexed; (*6*) lithotomy, or dorsal-recumbent, position with knees supported.

the location and type if they are present. In order to make a thorough examination of the neuromuscular bony systems the person should wear trunks or a loin cloth and if the patient is a woman, a halter. Since the physician will ask the patient to move about his feet should be protected by slippers. The equipment includes that used for the physical examination and, in addition, substances of pronounced smell, taste, and texture: mints, coffee, violet perfume, tobacco, cloves, and vinegar to test the senses of smell and taste; stoppered vials of hot and cold water to test sense of heat and cold; and fabrics of various textures, objects such as buttons, coins, keys, screws, cotton sponges, and common pins to test the sensory powers of the skin. Most of this equipment is used in testing the cranial nerves whose functions are extremely important. The condition of the autonomic system is assessed by the behavior of superficial blood vessels of the skin, the sweat glands, and the appearance of the hair and nails; also, by the presence or absence of bladder and bowel control.

No less important is the locomotor system that is tested by observation of posture, gait, muscular development, symmetry, coordination and the reflex muscular response to muscle stretching, and cutaneous stimuli. Normally there may be wide variations in reflex responses, but any marked increase or decrease in the reaction is significant. Examples of reflex tests are those of the forearm, the abdomen, the leg, the toes (Babinski), and the fingers (Hoffmann).

If this briefly outlined examination suggests possible pathology, additional tests and measurements are made, as, for example, x-rays, electroencephalograms, pneumoencephalograms, and lumbar, cisternal, and ventricular punctures.[18, 19]

Proctoscopic Examination.   The proctoscopic examination is discussed here because it is probably the simplest example of the examination of an organ by means of a lighted tube. The principles underlying the use of the "scopes" are the same but when the instruments should be sterile, when anesthesia is required, or when x-ray photography is combined with the procedure it is more complicated. The proctoscopic examination is about the only one that is not made in a special examining, or operating, room. The equipment and hands of the operator should be clean, but sterility is not necessary since the intact rectum seems to be relatively immune to infections as indicated by the fact that normal feces always contains pathogenic organisms.

It is traumatic to make any examination against the wishes of the patient; therefore, the physician will explain what he intends to do and get the person's assent. Sometimes the physician leaves the explanation to the nurse. There should be a definite understanding about this; otherwise the person may be unprepared and, consequently, uncooperative during the procedure. Tension and attendant discomfort are reduced in most persons when the doctor and nurse explain and encourage throughout the examination. It also helps to have the room warm and to drape the area so that the anus only is exposed. Since the purpose is to observe the condition of its walls the rectum should be empty. This is usually ensured by enemas the day before, and morning of, the examination. The equipment includes the proctoscopes, the necessary connections to a battery or light socket, a rheostat for adjustment of the light, several long and well-covered cotton applicators, Celluwipes, paper bag for disposal of waste, and rubber gloves for the physician. Sterile swabs and glass slides should be available if laboratory tests are desired. The nurse places the patient in the prescribed position, usually knee-chest or Sims, and assists the physician throughout the examination. She should, of course, know the sequence of steps in this examination, so that she may give adequate assistance. This is at best a rather distressing examination, and the nurse can do much to reduce the person's discomfort. The patient should be adequately draped and sufficiently warm. Only a very small area need be exposed for this examination.

4. FUNCTIONS OF THE NURSE IN THE MEDICAL EXAMINATION

Preparation of the Patient. A physical examination is in many cases accompanied by a good deal of anxiety on the part of the patient. He may fear the news that he has a serious or fatal disease or he may dread hospitalization which would jeopardize his economic security. A young person may be afraid of losing time from school, or a mother may be unhappy over the prospect of separation from her family. Modesty is a common trait, and the person more often than not dislikes the thought of exposure of the body necessitated by the examination. The nurse's presence does much to relieve the woman patient who is being examined by a man physician. The nurse should try to adjust her assistance to the particular needs of each person. Explaining the procedures in the examination will somewhat overcome a natural fear of the unknown. The patient should be dressed in a loose garment and should lie on the back, with one pillow under the head and with the knees flexed and supported. Adequate covering for the patient should be provided both to ensure effective draping during the examination and to give sufficient warmth, as often a person is "cold with fear" and unable to relax. Cotton blankets are better than sheets except in very hot weather. The patient should be scrupulously clean and all discharges removed, unless the physician wants to see the nature and amount of the discharge.

Preparation of the Physical Environment and the Equipment. The examination is most easily made in a room designed for the purpose but may take place at the patient's bedside. Good light, preferably daylight, is one of the first requisites. The room should be warm, about 27° C or 80.6° F. An adjustable table equipped with a mattress and pillows is desirable, but an ordinary bed can be used.

The equipment needed for the examination is usually laid out in convenient order on a table if the examination is made in an examining room, or assembled on a tray or small portable table if it is made at the bedside. The equipment should include a stethoscope, sphygmomanometer, percussion hammer, flashlight or portable electric light, head mirror, tongue blades, applicators, otoscope with ear specula, ophthalmoscope, nasal specula, skin pencil, and, if a vaginal examination is included, sterile rubber gloves, vaginal specula, and forceps. Syringes and needles, culture tubes, and other specimen containers may be needed if specimens of blood, body secretions, and the like are to be collected for examination. Rectal examinations require rubber gloves and lubricant. The specific equipment for neurological and proctoscopic examinations is listed in the discussion of those examinations.

Admission departments and clinics should be so arranged that a person with a communicable disease may be examined without danger to others.

Assistance with the Examination. The nurse may often be asked by the physician to take his notes on the patient's condition. She must, therefore, be familiar with the purposes of the tests made and the medical terminology used. She eases the strain of the examination by seeing that every requisite is on hand to prevent delay and by being familiar with each step in the procedure. She assists the patient in assuming the desired positions, keeps the patient adequately draped, and at the same time exposes the part that is to be examined. The nurse protects the doctor from body discharges as, for example, the spray from the nose and throat, and supervises the care of used instruments and materials in such a way as to prevent contamination of other materials. In clinics or offices she is more or less the hostess who shows the patient where to undress and dress and who follows up the physician's directions with any further explanations that are needed. During the examination, if she is alert, the nurse can learn much about the patient that will serve as a basis for planning his nursing care, if, as is desirable, he is later assigned to her care. The nurse records any observations she may have made when the physician was not present, or she may discuss them with the physician.

5. POSITIONS AND DRAPING USED FOR PHYSICAL EXAMINATIONS

General Methods of Draping. Methods of draping vary with the position the patient is to assume, the examination to be done, and the temperature of the examining room; also different hospitals may require specific draping for certain examinations. There are, however, general considerations that apply to all draping. The draping should be arranged so as to avoid all unnecessary exposure, but at the same time not to interfere with a thorough examination. If the draping is loose enough not to outline the figure the patient feels less naked. While many persons are unembarrassed by exposure of the body, methods of draping should be designed with consideration for those who are. Loose draping has the additional advantage of allowing a quick change of position, but should be anchored so securely as not to be displaced by the patient's movements. The importance of warm covering during examinations has been emphasized. Draping should be arranged so that only the part to be examined is exposed. Special sheets or clothing, such as trunks, may be needed for special or neurological examinations. At times it is necessary to expose almost the entire body. Specific methods of draping are included with the following descriptions of positions.

Horizontal Recumbent Position. The patient lies on his back with the legs extended or slightly flexed to relax the abdominal muscles. One pillow is placed under the head, and two or more if the physician wants the abdomen relaxed. The arms may be crossed on the chest or lie loosely at the sides of the body. Lightweight blankets should be used unless the room is very warm. One or more blankets are spread over the patient but not tucked under the mattress.

Dorsal Recumbent Position. The dorsal recumbent position is like the one just described except that the legs are slightly separated, the thighs flexed on the body and the legs on the thighs, so that the soles of the feet rest on the bed. If the patient is on a table, the buttocks are brought to the extreme edge and the feet placed on extensions. This position may be used for a vaginal examination or a digital examination of the rectum. Slightly different draping is required for this position. Two blankets or two sheets are placed lengthwise over the body; they are then separated so that one covers the right leg, and one the left, leaving the genitalia exposed.

Dorsal Lithotomy Position. The dorsal lithotomy position is the same as the dorsal recumbent except that the legs are well separated and the thighs are acutely flexed on the abdomen and the legs on the thighs. The buttocks are brought to the extreme edge of the table or a little beyond. To maintain this position and further separate the legs, upright rods with stirrups attached are fastened to the sides of the table and the legs supported in the stirrups. The word lithotomy comes from two Greek words (*litho* = meaning stone, and *tome* = meaning incision). The position was so called because it was used in the operation for removing stones from the bladder. It is now used for cystoscopic examinations, examinations and operations on the perineum, vagina, cervix, bladder, and rectum. The draping is essentially the same as for the dorsal recumbent position.

Sims', or Left Lateral-prone, Position. In this position the patient lies on the left side obliquely across the bed or table. One small pillow is placed under the head with the left cheek resting on it. The left arm is drawn behind the body and the body inclined forward so that some of its weight is on the chest. The right arm may be in any position comfortable for the patient. The thighs are flexed, the right sharply against the abdomen and the left less sharply. This position is used for vaginal and rectal examinations and treatments; draping for this position is practically the same as for the horizontal recumbent. The anus or the vaginal orifice may be exposed by folding back a small portion of the sheet or blanket.

Knee-chest, or Genupectoral, Position. As the term implies, the patient rests on the knees and chest. The head is turned to one side with the cheek on a pillow. The arms should be extended on the bed, flexed at the elbows and resting so as partially to support the patient; they should not be under the patient. The weight should rest on the chest and knees, which are flexed so that the thighs are at right angles to the legs as they rest on the bed or table. A small pillow may be placed under the chest, but the abdomen remains unsupported. The position is used for examinations of the rectum and vagina and as an exercise for post-partum patients. The draping may be done with two sheets, one for the upper and one for the lower part of the body, or with a large sheet having an opening in the center.

Trendelenburg Position. The Trendelenburg position is used in the operating room during operations on the pelvic organs in order to displace the intestines from the pelvis into the upper abdomen. A special table is required, one that can be adjusted so that the patient's head is low, the body on an inclined plane, and the knees flexed over the adjustable lower section of the table, which is lowered. The patient is carefully supported to prevent slipping. Draping depends upon the kind of operation to be performed.

Standing, or Erect, Position.   In the standing position—that is, standing erect with both feet on the floor, the patient is examined for orthopedic conditions and for certain neurological abnormalities. The patient should wear slippers, or the floor should be covered to protect the feet. If this position is used for a vaginal examination, one foot should be placed on a low stool. The legs should be separated as far as is comfortable so that the examination is made as easy for the patient as possible. She should have some support, such as a chair to hold, as this is a difficult position to maintain.

Jackknife Position.   The jackknife position is one used for rectal surgery rather than for examination. The patient must be well supported on the table because this position is very uncomfortable. Draping should expose only the necessary area and should keep the patient warm.

REFERENCES

1. Brodman, Keeve, et al.: "The Cornell Medical Index-Health Questionnaire II: As a Diagnostic Instrument," *J.A.M.A.,* **145:**152, (Jan.) 1951.
2. Chapman, A. L.: "Multiple Screening for a Variety of Diseases," *Hospitals,* **24:**37, (May) 1950.
3. McDougall, J. B.: "Role and Responsibility of the General Hospital in the Diagnosis and Treatment of Tuberculosis," *Bull. World Health Organ.,* **3:**325, 1950.
4. Kline, Carl L.: "Should the General Hospital Provide Psychiatric Services?" *Wisconsin M. J.,* **49:**901, (Oct.) 1950.
5. MacBryde, Cyril M. (ed.): *Signs and Symptoms: Their Clinical Interpretation,* 2nd ed. J. B. Lippincott Co., Philadelphia, 1952.
6. Clark-Kennedy, A. E.: "The Patient and His Disease," *Lancet,* **2:**661, (Dec.) 1950.
7. Hunt, Howard F.: "Clinical Methods: Psychodiagnostics," *Ann. Rev. Psychol.,* **1:**207, 1950.
8. Kretschmer, Ernst: *Physique and Character: An Investigation of the Nature of Constitution and of the Theory of Temperament,* 2nd ed. rev., with an approval by E. Miller. Humanities Press, Inc., New York, 1951.
9. Sheldon, William H., and Stevens, S. S.: *The Varieties of Temperament: A Psychology of Constitutional Differences.* Harper & Brothers, New York, 1942.
10. Draper, George, et al.: *Human Constitution in Clinical Medicine.* Paul B. Hoeber, New York, 1944.
11. Strecker, Edward A.: *Fundamentals of Psychiatry,* 4th ed. J. B. Lippincott Co., Philadelphia, 1947.
12. Diethelm, Oscar: "The Evaluation of a Psychiatric Examination," *Am. J. Psychiat.,* **105:**606, (Feb.) 1949.
13. Haggard, Howard W.: *The Doctor in History.* Yale University Press, New Haven, 1934, p. 331.
14. Davis, Hallowell (ed.): *Hearing and Deafness.* Murray-Hill Books, New York, 1947.
15. Doefler, Leo G., and McClure, Catherine: "The Measurement of Hearing Loss in Adults by Galvanic Skin Response," *J. Speech & Hearing Disorders,* **19:**184, (Jan.) 1954.

16. Cecil, Russell L., and Loeb, Robert F. (eds.): *A Textbook of Medicine,* 8th ed. W. B. Saunders Co., Philadelphia, 1951, pp. 328, 1227, 1359.

17. Bereston, Eugene S.: "Examination of the Nails as a Diagnostic Aid," *J. Insur. Med.,* **6:**38 (Dec.–Feb.) 1951.

18. Holmes, Gordon: *Introduction to Clinical Neurology.* Williams & Wilkins Co., Baltimore, 1946, p. 10.

19. De Gutiérrez-Mahoney, Carlos G., and Carini, Esta: *Neurological and Neurosurgical Nursing.* C. V. Mosby Co., St. Louis, 1949, p. 65.

Additional Suggested Reading

Bryant, Zella: "Tuberculosis Case Finding in General Hospitals," *Pub. Health Rep.,* **65:**710, (June) 1950.

Dwyer, Sheila M., and Fish, George W.: *Modern Urology for Nurses,* 2nd ed. Lea & Febiger, Philadelphia, 1945.

Geldard, Frank A.: "Somesthesis and the Chemical Senses," *Ann. Rev. Psychol.,* **1:**71, 1950.

Hewson, Louise R.: "The Wechsler-Bellevue Scale and the Substitution Tests as Aids in Neuropsychiatric Diagnosis," *J. Nerv. & Ment. Dis.,* **109:**159, (Feb.) 1949, and **109:**246, (Mar.) 1949.

Kalkman, Marion E.: *Introduction to Psychiatric Nursing.* McGraw-Hill Book Co., New York, 1950.

Loewenberg, Samuel A.: *Medical and Physical Diagnosis,* 8th ed. F. A. Davis Co., Philadelphia, 1951.

Logie, Henry B. (ed.): *Standard Classified Nomenclature of Disease, Compiled by the National Conference on Nomenclature of Disease,* 2nd ed. American Medical Association, Chicago, 1937.

MacCarthy, D., et al.: "Discussion: Growth and Development Standards and Their Clinical Application," *Proc. Roy. Soc. Med.,* **43:**823, (Nov.) 1950.

Major, Ralph H.: *Physical Diagnosis,* 4th ed. W. B. Saunders Co., Philadelphia, 1951.

Miale, John B., and Gunn, James A.: "The Vaginal Smear: Its Value in General Practice," *Wisconsin M. J.,* **49:**918, (Oct.) 1950.

Newman, Edwin B.: "Hearing," *Ann. Rev. Psychol.,* **1:**49, 1950.

Osgood, Edwin E.: *A Textbook of Laboratory Diagnosis with Clinical Applications for Practitioners and Students,* 3rd ed. Blakiston Co., Philadelphia, 1948.

Pullen, Roscoe L. (ed.): *Medical Diagnosis,* 2nd ed. W. B. Saunders Co., Philadelphia, 1950.

Sigerist, Henry E.: *Man and Medicine: An Introduction to Medical Knowledge.* W. W. Norton & Co., New York, 1932.

Weiss, Edward, and English, O. S.: *Psychosomatic Medicine: The Clinical Application of Psychopathology to General Medical Problems,* 2nd ed. W. B. Saunders Co., Philadelphia, 1949.

CHAPTER 19. ASSISTING WITH DIAGNOSTIC TESTS

1. RESPONSIBILITY OF THE NURSE
2. URINE AND KIDNEY-FUNCTION TESTS
3. EXAMINATION OF SPUTUM
4. EXAMINATION OF FECES
5. TEST MEALS AND EXAMINATION OF THE GASTROIN-
   TESTINAL TRACT
6. GALLBLADDER TESTS
7. EXAMINATION OF THE BLOOD
8. EXAMINATION OF SPINAL FLUID
9. SMEARS AND CULTURES
10. BASAL METABOLISM
11. ELECTROCARDIOGRAPHY
12. ENDOSCOPY
13. DIAGNOSTIC X-RAY
14. PSYCHOMETRICS
15. NEUROLOGICAL DIAGNOSTIC TESTS

1. RESPONSIBILITY OF THE NURSE

While diagnosis is the function of the physician, many diagnostic tests are carried out entirely by the nurse. Her responsibility varies greatly according to the nature of the test and the particular situation. In almost every case, however, she is responsible for the preparation of the patient, preparation of equipment to be used by the physician, and frequently for the collection of specimens; in addition, it may be her function to label specimens and to supervise the transportation of materials to special laboratories where they are analyzed. The findings should be recorded by those who make the analysis, but the nurse usually notes on the patient's chart the fact that the test was made.

Labels for specimens should contain the following items of information: the patient's name, his address (in the hospital this means the room or nursing unit), the nature of the specimen, the date and sometimes the hour of collection, the type of analysis requested by the physician, and the name (sometimes the address) of the physician.

2. URINE AND KIDNEY-FUNCTION TESTS

Collection of the Single Urine Specimen. The examination of urine is one of the most common laboratory tests, and the collection of the specimen for examination is in many cases the responsibility of the nurse. The urine is usually examined at the outset of an illness and frequently during the progress of a disease. When the patient is in the hospital, a specimen of urine is ordinarily taken soon after admission, frequently the following morning, and at specified times thereafter. Since urine varies from time to time during the day, the physician may request that specimens be collected at different hours in order to get a more accurate picture of the

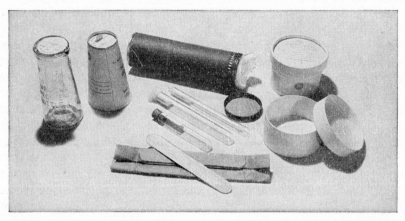

Figure 123. Specimen containers. (*Left to right*) A glass and a paper bottle for urine with space on the cap for writing patient's name, etc.; a carton in which a specimen may be mailed; two paper feces containers. Sterile spatulas are used to transfer feces from the bedpan to the paper cup for bacteriological tests. In the center are sterile test tubes for smears and blood samples. (Courtesy of Clay-Adams Co., New York City.)

condition. Such a specimen is known as a *single* or, less properly, a *routine* specimen. The latter term has been used to refer to the specimen that is almost always collected at the outset of the illness or on admission to the hospital. It is, however, a misleading term, as other types of specimens may be examined as often and as regularly. A single specimen is the urine passed in one voiding, all of which may or may not be sent to the laboratory for examination. From 100-120 cc of urine are sufficient for the usual tests.

To collect a single specimen, the patient is given a bedpan or urinal in which to void. A sufficient amount of urine (100-120 cc) is transferred to the specimen bottle, which is usually a 120-200 cc, wide-mouthed glass bottle. A pasteboard cover is used to close the container. Each specimen should be clearly labeled with the patient's name, hospital number, room, date, and the tests desired. Since urine should be examined while fresh, it should be taken to the laboratory as soon as possible. It goes without saying that all receptacles used should be scrupulously clean. A single specimen may be obtained also by catheterizing the patient (see Chapter 31). In this instance the specimen bottle is sterile. The reason for catheterization is usually because the physician desires a sterile specimen.

The nurse in the clinic or assisting a physician in his office will often find it necessary to instruct patients how to collect a specimen and bring it to the laboratory for examination. Such instruction should include directions as to the hour the specimen is to be collected, the amount necessary, and the kind of container to use. Generally speaking, a container with a screw cap is preferable to one having a cork. State and city departments of health often provide containers and cartons for mailing if the specimen is to be examined in their laboratories. This equipment may include a receptacle for collecting the specimen as well. Since this urine specimen cannot be examined while fresh, a preservative is provided in the container. (For illustrations of specimen containers, see Fig. 123.)

Collection of a urine specimen from infants is often a difficult problem, especially in the case of infant girls. A specimen may be collected from a boy baby in a specially constructed test tube held in place with a T-binder having an opening through which the tube is passed. Various appliances are used for collecting specimens of urine from girl babies. They are not entirely satisfactory. Glass vessels that fit over the vulva and can be held in place with a specially constructed T-binder are now available. A simple way of collecting a specimen from a girl baby is to place a small tray or shallow pan under the buttocks. The buttocks only rest on the tray. The gown may be turned back or otherwise arranged so that it will not rest on the tray. The edge of the tray, or pan, is padded, and the infant supported and placed in a comfortable position over the pan with pillows and soft restraining cloths until a sufficient amount of urine is collected.*

Common Tests Made on Single Urine Specimens. The tests made on the single urine specimens have come to be more or less standardized, and include the following:

1. *The reaction,* that is, whether it is acid or alkaline. Normal urine is acid because, on a mixed or average diet, more foods are eaten that yield acid waste products as a result of their metabolism than foods that yield alkaline. The reaction may vary somewhat, therefore, with the diet.

2. *The specific gravity,* which depends upon the amount of solids in the urine in proportion to the amount of water. It is based upon water as a standard—1 liter of water at a certain temperature weighs 1000 gm. Urine is heavier than water, because of the solids contained in it. The specific gravity of normal urine varies

---

* Since collection of urine specimens from babies is difficult, one nurse used the following method. At the time the rectal temperature was to be taken, the nurse placed in the unit an appropriate glass container. Then as she was holding the thermometer in the rectum, she placed the test tube or glass vessel over the penis or vulva. Frequently, the baby would void while the thermometer was in the rectum. Thus the nurse was able to collect the urine specimen *without* the restraining binder.

Another method is to apply a cellophane diaper so that there is a collecting portion between the legs. After the baby has voided, the diaper is removed carefully; the nurse then cuts the end of the cellophane diaper so that the urine will run into an appropriate container.

from 1.006 to 1.025.[1] The normal kidney adjusts the specific gravity according to the state of hydration of the patient. For example, with an increased fluid intake, more water will be excreted, and the urine will be "dilute," with a low specific gravity; whereas if water is withheld, the urine will become concentrated, with specific gravities up to 1.030. The ability of the kidney to concentrate in the face of water deprivation is a very simple but useful test of renal function. The glomerular filtrate has a specific gravity of 1.010, and the finding of a constant or "fixed" specific gravity in this range indicates poor renal function. Unusually high values for specific gravity, for example, above 1.030, suggests the presence of large amounts of solid constituents in the urine, such as glucose in a diabetic patient.

3. *The urinary sediment* is examined after centrifuging a specimen and pouring off the supernatant fluid. This examination should be done only on fresh urine. The sediment may include epithelial cells, red blood cells, leukocytes or white blood cells, casts, and inorganic crystals. The entire urinary tract is lined with epithelium, some cells of which are constantly being worn out and shed into the urine (just as cells of the outer skin), so that epithelial cells will be found in normal urine, as will very small numbers of blood cells and protein casts of the renal tubules. However, in the presence of disease, these constituents may increase in number; for example, in the presence of infection increased numbers of epithelial cells and leukocytes will be seen, and in nephritis increased numbers of red blood cells and casts.

4. *The Presence of Albumin.* Albumin is a body protein that circulates in the blood to supply the cells and forms a necessary constituent of all body cells. Normally in the urine there is a slight, or faint, trace of albumin, but too small an amount to be detected by the ordinary tests used. The products of inflammation— many epithelial cells, leukocytes, or pus—will cause an increased amount of albumin in the urine, so that in inflammation of any part of the urinary tract— kidneys, ureters, or bladder—albumin will be present in the urine. This inflammation may occur as a result of bacterial invasion, poisoning, or circulatory disturbances. Some people are said to have a functional disturbance of the kidneys, that is, the urine will contain albumin after a cold bath, excessive exercise, a high-protein diet, or a lordotic posture, without having inflammation of the kidneys. The presence of albumin in the urine, however, may be an indication of nephritis, which is a very serious disease, important to recognize in its early stages. So generally is this accepted that no life insurance policy is ever granted without testing the urine for albumin. If a large amount of albumin is found, the insurance policy is sometimes not granted.

5. *The Presence of Sugar or Glucose.* Normally there is a very faint trace of sugar in the urine. Eating a large amount of candy may temporarily cause a marked increase of sugar to appear in the urine in a perfectly healthy person. With no such cause, however, the presence of sugar indicates that the patient is suffering from a very serious disease—diabetes. In this disease the body cells are unable to burn the normal amount of sugar supplied them as fuel, and so are unable or have difficulty in producing the necessary heat and energy for the body processes. As the

sugar eaten cannot be used fully by the body, the level of sugar in the blood is abnormally high, and exceeds the renal threshold; sugar is then eliminated through the urine. In severe cases of diabetes the amount of sugar in the urine may rise as high as 10 per cent.

The presence of sugar in the urine does not indicate disease of the kidneys. Students frequently have the impression that because the presence of sugar in the urine is abnormal, the kidneys must be diseased. This is not the case. However, the presence of large amounts of sugar in the urine makes it a favorable medium for the growth of bacteria, so that urinary tract infections are a frequent complication of diabetes.

Tests for the Early Diagnosis of Pregnancy. Chorionic gonadotrophin is a hormone which is produced by the body shortly after the implantation of the fertilized ovum, and is excreted in the urine. It may readily be detected in the urine by its action on the gonads of various laboratory animals after injection of the patient's urine. Though not an infallible test, it is highly accurate, and of value when it is desirable to make an early diagnosis of pregnancy.

The principle of this test was first described by Aschheim and Zondek, but their original method has been modified by others, decreasing the time required, and increasing convenience and simplicity. A commonly used test today is the Friedman test. A morning urine specimen is collected, and 10 cc of the specimen are injected into the ear vein of a nongravid mature female rabbit. Twenty-four hours or more after injection the rabbit is anesthetized and the ovaries explored for the presence of hemorrhagic ruptured follicles, which indicate a positive reaction. Other methods are also used, varying primarily in the type of animal and anatomic changes indicating positive reactions.

Collection of the 24-Hour, or Fractional, Urine Specimen.   When it is desirable to make a quantitative rather than a qualitative analysis, all the urine voided in a 24-hour period is saved for examination. While the qualitative or single urine specimen will show the constituents of the urine, only the 24-hour specimen—the total amount secreted by the kidneys—will show what substances the kidneys are eliminating and the quantity of each. The diagnosis, diet, and general treatment for the patient may to a large extent be based on the findings in this examination; therefore, extreme care should be exercised in the collection of the specimen to ensure the inclusion of all urine voided during the specified period.

In beginning the 24-hour specimen the bladder is emptied and the urine discarded because the purpose of the test is to find how the kidneys are functioning, not merely the amount expelled or voided by the bladder, and the urine in the bladder may have been stored for a considerable length of time. The specimen is frequently started at 6:00 A.M. as this seems to be a convenient hour to begin and cease collection of the specimen. If this time period is adopted, the patient should void at six o'clock the first morning and the urine should be discarded. All urine voided up to and including 6:00 A.M. of the following morning must be included in the specimen sent to the laboratory. It is important that the patient void at exactly 6:00 A.M. of the following or second morning to complete the collection of all the urine secreted by the kidneys in the 24-hour period and so make possible an accurate estimate of the work performed by the organs concerned.

A 24-hour urine specimen is placed in a large container (usually a glass bottle) properly labeled and stoppered as was suggested in the case of the single specimen. Prevent, if possible, having the patient void at the same time as the defecation. Two bedpans may be used to make sure the urine specimen is not contaminated, collecting the urine specimen first. If by accident urine should be lost or mixed with fecal matter, a note should be made of this on the container and on the patient's chart.

It is common to have the urine voided in a 24-hour period collected in fractions of that period. The total amount of urine voided in 24 hours is saved, but instead of being placed in one container, the period is divided into three or four parts and the urine voided in each of these shorter periods placed in separate containers; for example, the prescribed periods may run from 6:00 A.M. to 12:00 noon; from 12:00 noon to 6:00 P.M.; from 6:00 P.M. to midnight, and from midnight to 6:00 A.M. In some instances the third period extends from 6:00 P.M. to 6 A.M.* All the urine voided in each period is placed in a container, stoppered, and labeled as before and the hours included are also indicated. This type of specimen is frequently used for the diabetic patient because it is a more accurate aid in determining the diet and the amount of insulin necessary than the other type of 24-hour specimen. Except for the several containers used, the specimen is collected in the same manner as described above.

Common Tests Made on 24-Hour Specimen. The examination of the 24-hour specimen may be for:

1. THE TOTAL NORMAL CONSTITUENTS or waste products of metabolism normally eliminated by the kidneys. The ability of the kidneys is tested by measuring the total volume of urine, on a known intake of fluids and diet. The volume may be greatly reduced in acute nephritis (water is retained in the body with resulting edema), or it may be greatly increased in some forms of chronic nephritis. When the patient is edematous, he is usually placed on "restricted fluids." In some forms of nephritis the patient may be encouraged to drink fluids. The nurse, however, should never give even a small amount of water without finding out whether it will invalidate the test.

The *specific gravity* (amount of solids in proportion to the amount of water) is always an important test. In chronic nephritis without edema, the volume may be greatly increased and the specific gravity may be very low, showing that the kidneys have difficulty in eliminating solids and are trying to dilute them with a large amount of water. In acute nephritis the volume is low and the specific gravity is high—the patient is edematous.

Ashes of Protein Metabolism. The intake of protein in the diet should be known. Tests may include the following: *total nitrogen.* The elimination of protein wastes is one of the chief functions of the kidneys. As all protein and protein wastes con-

---

* The times for collection will vary in different hospitals—usually the collection period ends one-half hour before mealtime.

tain nitrogen, and nitrogen is the essential element that distinguishes protein from all other foods, the efficiency of the kidneys to eliminate protein ashes can be tested by measuring the total nitrogen in the urine. Nitrogen forms 16 per cent of the weight of a protein molecule; if the amount of nitrogen in the urine is ascertained, then the amount of protein from which it was derived (the protein metabolism in the body) can easily be estimated and this result can be compared with the intake of protein in the diet; for instance, the normal daily output of nitrogen on a regular diet is about 15 gm; as nitrogen equals 16 per cent of the weight of a protein molecule, this daily output is the waste resulting from the metabolism of about 94 gm of protein. Part of the nitrogen in the urine comes from the breakdown of body tissues. Making allowances for this latter amount, the difference between the nitrogen in the urine and that given in the diet represents the amount retained in the body—retained either for growth and repair, or because the kidneys failed to eliminate it.

The rate of nitrogen excretion may also be measured by the *urea clearance test*, where the total urea excreted over a certain period, usually two hours, is measured, and the blood concentration of urea determined. Thus the amount of blood cleared of urea per hour may be computed. This may also be done by measuring the total urea in a 24-hour specimen; 85–90 per cent of all nitrogen excreted is in the form of urea, and thus a fairly accurate picture of protein metabolism and kidney efficiency may be obtained. Urea is an inert substance, relatively harmless to the body cells, which is formed primarily in the liver from the intermediate products of protein metabolism. A rise in its blood concentration is characteristic of uremia, the clinical syndrome of nitrogen retention. This is a serious condition, the real cause of which is unknown. It was once supposed that the accumulation of urea was the direct cause of uremic poisoning, but urea may be injected into the blood without causing any of the symptoms of uremic poisoning and it will quickly be eliminated in the urine.

Even if the results of these tests show that the kidneys are not eliminating the ashes as they should, reduction of the amount of dietary protein is of little if any therapeutic value.[2] This is chiefly because of the fact that, in the absence of dietary protein, the body tends to break down body cells to serve as a source of protein, resulting in the formation of the metabolic products. Other dietary restrictions, primarily salt, may be necessary if the patient is edematous.

Inorganic Salts. As chlorides in the urine comprise more than all the other salts combined, the efficiency of the kidneys in eliminating salts is tested by measuring the total chlorides eliminated on a known diet. The normal daily output of chlorides on a regular diet is from 10 to 15 gm. Only sufficient salt is normally retained to keep a percentage of salt (0.9 per cent) essential to the life activities of the tissues.

Hormonal Excretion Products. Twenty-four-hour urine specimens may also be examined for the total excretion of 17-ketosteroids and corticoids. These are the metabolic degredation products of certain of the adrenocortical and gonadal hormones. The level of these excretion products in the urine is often of great aid in the diagnosis of pituitary, adrenal, or gonadal diseases in which the function of one or more of these glands is altered.

2. TOTAL ABNORMAL CONSTITUENTS. In a 24-hour specimen of urine the total amount of albumin or of sugar may be accurately measured. Other abnormal constituents for which the specimens may be examined are the acetone bodies (acetone, diacetic acid, and β-oxybutyric acid), indican, ammonia, mucus, pus, blood, urobilin, bilirubin, casts, calculi, iron, iodine, sulfur, and bacteria.

Clinitest, Benedict's, and Fehling's Tests for Sugar. When nursing in the home (either in private duty nursing or as a visiting nurse from a public health association), or in a doctor's office, and in other occupational settings, a nurse is frequently required to examine single specimens of urine for abnormal constituents. The Clinitest reagent tablets are frequently used for testing urinary sugar in the office and home because of the simplicity, ease, and rapidity with which the test may be made. More elaborate are the Benedict's and Fehling's tests, used in hospitals, although the Clinitest method is frequently used there as well. The nurse may be called upon to teach the patient to make such tests in the home.

For the _Clinitest_ method, put 5 drops of urine and 10 drops of water in a test tube; add one reagent tablet. Do not shake the test tube during the reaction or for 15 seconds after boiling inside the test tube has stopped. Then shake the test tube gently and compare the color of the solution with the color scale to determine the presence and amount of sugar in the urine. (In this test external heat has been eliminated, since the reagent tablet generates heat.) The color scale of the Clinitest reaction is shown in Plate III.

For the _Benedict's_ test, put 5 cc of the reagent and 8 drops of urine in a test tube. Immerse the tube in a water bath of boiling water and keep the water boiling. At the end of exactly 5 minutes, remove the tube and allow it to cool. If the fluid is opaque, it indicates the presence of sugar. If no sugar is present, the fluid remains clear, or only a faint turbidity results which is due to urates. The color reactions are shown in Plate II.

To make _Fehling's_ test, put about 3 cc of urine in a test tube. Add about 5 cc of boiling Fehling's solution, then boil the mixture and place the tube in a rack. The formation of a typical red or golden-yellow precipitate indicates the presence of sugar.

These tests are based upon the fact that sugar is a reducing agent; that is, it will precipitate or separate heavy metals from their compounds. Fehling's solution, for instance, is a compound containing copper, which, when precipitated, gives the usual copper color to the solution. The Benedict test is a more sensitive one than Fehling's, because the reagent is not reduced by uric acid, creatinine, and other substances that are in the urine, as Fehling's solution may be. The Clinitest is based on the principles of copper-reduction methods.

Test for Acetone. Drop a crystal of sodium nitroprusside in 5 to 10 cc of water. Add 1 to 2 cc of this solution and a few drops of glacial acetic acid to 5 cc of urine and stratify strong ammonia over the mixture. A purple ring at the junction of the fluids indicates that acetone is present.

The Diacetic Acid Test. Add a few drops of 10 per cent ferric chloride to about 10 cc of urine, drop by drop. If a precipitate forms, filter and add a few more drops of ferric chloride. A "Burgundy" red indicates that diacetic acid may be present. If the tube is then boiled, the red color will fade if the reaction is due to diacetic acid. However, if the patient has been taking phenol, salicylates, aspirin, acetanilid, or antipyrine, a dark color will also be produced on the addition of ferric chloride to the urine, but this color will persist when the tube is boiled.

Tests for Albumin. The nurse is frequently expected to make tests for albumin; the following tests are suggested. To make the _heat and acetic acid test,_ fill a test tube two-thirds full of urine. Add about 5 drops of 2 per cent acetic acid (enough to make the reaction acid), and boil at the top, holding the tube at the bottom with a test-tube holder and directing the flame against the upper portion of fluid. Add a few more drops of acid; then examine the tube by transmitted light against a black background for a clouding in the top portion as compared with the portion just below it. If the precipitate is flocculent, take the tube in a holder and heat the entire contents to boiling and stand the tube in a rack. When the precipitate has settled, 15 minutes or more afterward, mark the percentage of albumin according to the estimated proportion of the column of urine occupied by the sediment. The result may be reported as 1 + to 4 + according to the amount of precipitate.

Coagulation of albumin by concentrated nitric acid is done by pouring about 2 cc (½ dram) of nitric acid into a test tube. Then an equal volume of urine is allowed to flow in slowly, so as to form a layer above the heavier acid. A white ring at the junction of the fluids indicates the presence of albumin.

These tests are based upon the fact that albumin is coagulated, either by heat or strong acids.

The _Esbach_ test also is frequently used. It is a quantitative test that indicates the total amount of albumin excreted in 24 hours.

The Guaiac Test for Blood. To about 4 cc of urine, add 1 cc of glacial acetic acid and 2 cc of ether; shake gently; pour off the ether, and add a few drops of freshly prepared guaiac tincture and 1 cc of hydrogen peroxide. (Never use a test tube with yellow copper oxide on its wall resulting from Fehling's or Benedict's sugar test.) A blue color indicates the presence of blood. Tests for blood have definite limitations, and the guaiac test, according to James C. Todd and associates,[3] can be relied upon only when the test is negative.

Phenolsulfonphthalein Test (P.S.P.). One of the most useful tests in determining the function of the kidneys is the phenolsulfonphthalein test. This test is indicative of the functional capacity of the kidneys, but does not, according to Todd,[4] necessarily represent permanent anatomic changes. No one test, however, should be relied upon as a total evaluation of renal function.

To administer this test, the phenolsulfonphthalein, which is a harmless dye excreted only by the kidneys, is given intravenously or intramuscularly, the urine collected for a stated period, and an instrument known as the colorimeter used to determine the amount of dye excreted in the urine. Before the dye is given, the patient drinks 300–400 cc (2 glasses) of water to make sure he can void

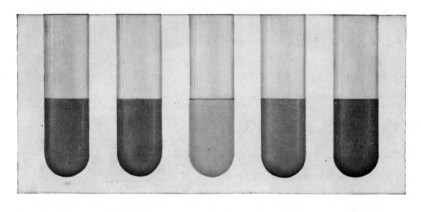

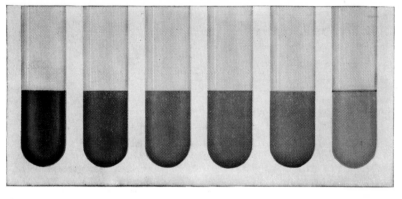

Reaction	Reaction	Reaction	Reaction	Reaction
Grade O	Grade 1	Grade 2	Grade 3	Grade 4

Plate II. (*Top*) The Benedict color scale for sugar in urine. (Courtesy of Eli Lilly and Co., Indianapolis, Ind.)

Negative	Trace	+	++	+++	++++
0%	¼%	½%	¾%	1%	2%

Plate III. (*Bottom*) The Clinitest color scale for sugar in urine. (Courtesy of Ames Co., Elkhart, Ind.)

at the specified times, and about 20 minutes or a half hour later the patient voids. As soon as possible after the voiding, 1 cc of phenolsulfonphthalein is injected intravenously or intramuscularly. Although the test may be carried on in different ways, the patient is usually ask to void in 1 hour and 10 minutes and again 2 hours and 10 minutes after the drug is given. All the urine collected at each voiding is saved in separate containers and sent to the laboratory for examination. Normally 40–50 per cent of the dye is eliminated in the first hour and 60–75 per cent at the completion of the test. Such a test is of use in the diagnosis of nephritis.

Dilution and Concentration Tests. The dilution and concentration tests are widely used tests of renal function; they are valuable in that they measure the functional capacity of the kidneys under extreme conditions, and may be the first tests to change in early renal disease.

The original *concentration test* was described by Mosenthal, but numerous modifications have since been made in the interests of simplicity and in saving time. One test used today is the Fishberg concentration test. In this test, the patient is allowed to eat supper, after which he is permitted nothing by mouth. Any urine specimens passed during the evening are discarded; then the first specimen of urine voided at 6 A.M. the next morning is saved, as are specimens voided at hourly intervals thereafter, and the specific gravity of each is measured. During this time the patient is allowed no food or fluid. Specimens are usually collected until noon, when the patient is again allowed to resume normal activity and diet. With good renal function, at least one specimen during the morning should show a concentration to 1.030 or nearly so.

The *dilution test* measures the opposite function of the kidneys; that is, its power to dilute urine. Again the methods vary, but in general the patient is given no breakfast and is required to drink from 1000 to 1500 cc of water. Specimens in this test are collected more frequently, usually at 8:30, 9:00, 9:30, 10:00, 10:30, 11:00, 11:30 A.M., and 12:00 noon. The rest of the urine voided, until the test ends at 8:00 A.M. the following morning, is put into one container. Again, as in the concentration test, the amount of urine voided and the specific gravity of each specimen are measured. According to Thomas H. Ham,[5] the normal kidneys will dilute the urine to a specific gravity of 1.002, and will excrete a volume equal to, or larger than, the amount of water ingested. He also states, however, that this test is a less reliable one than the concentration test.

3. EXAMINATION OF SPUTUM

Collection of the Specimen. Specimens of sputum for examination are collected by having the patient cough up the material from the bronchi or lungs and expectorate it into a container. The container most commonly used is a waterproof, waxed sputum cup, though in disorders such as bronchiectasis, a tall glass container*

---

* When this type of container is used, the nurse covers the outside of the container with a paper towel, fastened in place with Scotch tape, so that the contents are not visible to the patient and his visitors. A paper cover is affixed to the top of the container.

may be used to observe the characteristic layering of the sputum. If a sterile specimen is desired, the container used is generally a wide-mouthed glass bottle with a paper or screw cap, or a sterile Petri dish. Care should be taken in either instance to prevent the contamination of the inside of the container. Specimens are usually collected in the morning before food is taken. The mouth should be cleaned previous to the collection of the sputum because the presence of food particles in the material may be confusing in the examination. The patient must be instructed to raise material from the lungs by coughing and not simply expectorate saliva or the discharges of the nose and throat.

Occasionally the physician wishes to have the total sputum expectorated in the 24-hour period examined. The size of the container used will depend upon the quantity of sputum, but in most instances the waxed sputum cup is used. The waxed cup is desirable because it can be so easily destroyed after use. The most commonly collected specimen is the small quantity that is examined microscopically. State and city health departments have containers suitable for mailing specimens available for those who have no laboratory facilities at hand.

Gross Examination of Sputum.   Normally no sputum is expectorated, and in disease in which there is sputum produced, the amount may vary from a minute quantity to several hundred cubic centimeters. The measurement of the amount need only be approximated. A simple way to estimate the quantity of sputum is to fill a similar container with water to approximately the same level as the sputum reaches and then measure the water. Another method is to weigh the waxed sputum cup, subtracting the known weight of an empty container; in this way the number of grams of sputum that a patient has expectorated within a given period (usually 24 hours) can be easily determined. If the sputum is not to be saved for microscopic examination, the cup is filled with sawdust and placed right side up in a container lined with a paper bag, until such material can be disposed of by burning. Color is also observed and this, too, varies considerably. Blood may be detected in sputum by a red color; if a bright red, it is of recent origin; if dark, it has probably been in the lung for some time. In pneumonia the sputum has a rusty color, while in lung abscesses, bronchiectasis, and carcinoma, the sputum may be greenish. In gangrenous conditions of the lung, the color is usually brown. Sputum also may be colorless, gray, or yellow.

The consistency of sputum varies from a thin watery fluid to thick purulent material. Sputum may have no odor at all or it may have a most unpleasant odor, as, for example, in lung abscesses or gangrene.

Microscopic Examination of Sputum.   Sputum is examined microscopically for the purpose of determining the presence of certain specific bacilli, especially tubercle bacilli, and cells. If acid-fast bacilli with the morphologic characteristics of tubercle bacilli are found in the sputum, the diagnosis of tuberculosis is generally made. In pneumonia the organism causing the disease may be seen, and the type of pneumonia determined; this makes it possible to use the sera that are available for certain types of pneumonia. Bacilli causing other infections of the respiratory tract also may be seen in the sputum.

4. EXAMINATION OF FECES

Collection of the Specimen.   A stool for examination is collected in a clean bedpan and transferred by means of wooden spatulas into the container in which it is sent to the laboratory. The container is usually made of paper heavily waxed to make it waterproof. Care must be taken in transferring the specimen to avoid contaminating the outside of the container. The specimen should not be mixed with urine, and it is wise to have the patient void first into one bedpan and replace that with a clean one before the feces is passed. Stools should be sent to the laboratory when fresh; and when an examination for amebae is to be made, the stool should be sent to the laboratory while warm and kept warm during the examination, so that the movements of the amebae may be seen. Sometimes it is necessary to give a cleansing enema to collect the specimen. If this is done the solution used is preferably saline or tap water, because other solutions may affect the stool. Specimens of feces may be sent by mail in specially prepared containers for examination by state health department laboratories. A preservative of some kind is added to these stools; but when the patient is hospitalized and the specimen is examined in the hospital laboratory, no preservative is needed. The amount required is usually small, but occasionally the whole stool is saved for observation. Such an examination is usually a gross examination, observing that which can be seen with the naked eye, as for example, worms, or portions of worms.

Gross Examination of Feces.   The number, frequency, color, odor, and the presence of unusual matter in the stools are important in the total examination of the feces. These factors and the examination for intestinal parasites are discussed in some detail in Chapter 14. On close examination, gallstones may be observed.

Microscopic Examination of the Feces.   The microscopic examination serves often to verify the examination made by gross observation. Leukocytes and pus cells may appear if there are ulcers of the intestinal tract. Eggs of the various intestinal parasites also may be seen. Many very small worms cannot be seen except through the microscope. The stool may also be examined, after staining, for fat and starch, which may be present in abnormal amounts in certain diseases of the gastrointestinal tract characterized by absence of specific digestive enzymes; for example, fibro-cystic disease of the pancreas and sprue.

Chemical Examination of Feces.   One of the most important tests is the test for *blood*. Blood in large quantities can usually be noted, but traces of blood are harder to detect and often are much more important. The diagnoses of carcinoma of the stomach and colon and of gastric ulcers are often made as a result of finding traces of blood in the stool. The *guaiac* or *benzidine* tests are commonly used for this purpose. Tests for the presence of urobilin and urobiligen in the feces are also done, because these pigments are absent in obstructive jaundice. The chemical examinations may be extremely detailed, but the most common and probably the most important is that for blood. Others include the reaction of the feces, which is largely dependent on the diet of the individual, and tests for fermentation. The quantity required for chemical examination is very small.

Tests for Bacteria. Because such a large proportion of the feces in healthy individuals is made up of bacteria, special bacterial culture media have been devised which suppress the growth of the bacteria normally present, and selectively encourage the growth of those which may cause disease. The most important test of this type is the one for typhoid bacilli. It is often made in trying to determine whether an individual is a carrier of the disease. Other bacilli that may be found in feces and for which examinations are made are paratyphoid bacilli, *Shigella dysenteriae*, *Salmonella enteritidus*, and *Bacillus anthracis*.

5. TEST MEALS AND EXAMINATION OF THE GASTROINTESTINAL TRACT

Methods of Securing Specimens. The examination of the contents of the stomach is one of the most widely used means of determining pathology of the stomach. The specimen may be obtained for examination by various means. The simplest method (not always available) is saving vomitus. Gross examination of the material vomited and the observation of the manner in which it was vomited are of importance as well as the more detailed laboratory examination. Though this is the simplest method of securing stomach contents, it is by no means the most common. It is more often necessary to introduce a tube into the stomach and aspirate the contents.

A Rehfuss tube that has a metal tip with large openings is the type most often used. The aspiration of stomach contents is usually done in the morning before the patient has had any food. According to Charles H. Best and Norman B. Taylor,[6] the stomach normally contains at this time about 50 cc of gastric juice, because the stomach, if healthy, is continually secreting. For some purposes this amount of material is sufficient; but because the amount of gastric juice varies and because the secretion is influenced by the presence of food, test meals are often given.

Test Meals. The food given in different kinds of test meals varies, but the same purpose prompts the giving of the food in any case—the excitation of the glands to secrete gastric juice. The *Ewald test meal* is frequently chosen and consists of two slices of bread or toast (without crusts) and about 400 cc of water, or tea without cream or sugar. A slight variation of this is the *Dock test meal*, which uses shredded wheat instead of bread, because bread contains lactic acid and yeast cells. The *Riegel test meal*, which, according to Todd and associates,[7] consists of 400 cc of bouillon, 150–200 gm of broiled beefsteak, and 150 gm of mashed potato, is another example. Careful mastication is very important in this last meal, because if large particles of food are swallowed they may clog the tube and interfere with removal of the stomach contents.

Most of these meals are used in the so-called fractional method of analysis. In this method the patient has no breakfast, and the contents of the stomach are aspirated in the morning by means of a syringe attached to a Rehfuss tube.

When the stomach is completely empty, it is often washed out. This, however, may be omitted and the test meal administered immediately. Then for 2 hours after the ingestion of the test meal, about 5 cc of the stomach contents are aspirated every 15 minutes. Each individual specimen, collected in individual tubes or bottles and carefully labeled to make sure the course of the gastric secretions is correctly observed, is examined for free hydrochloric acid, lactic acid, and for

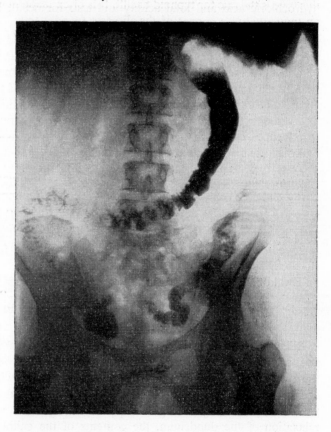

Figure 124. X-ray of intestines after the administration of a barium meal. This is one of a series in the x-ray examination of the alimentary tract. (Courtesy of Columbia-Presbyterian Medical Center, New York City.)

total acidity. During the progress of the test the samples as taken may be tested for acidity by Töpfer's reagent. A drop of Töpfer's reagent added to the gastric juice will cause it to turn bright red if there is free hydrochloric acid in the specimen. The test is usually discontinued when free hydrochloric acid is observed.

If, after the required number of aspirations, no free hydrochloric acid is present histamine hydrochloride, which acts rapidly to stimulate the secretion of gastric juice, may be given, and the aspirations continued after a period of about 15 minutes has elapsed. Should there still be no hydrochloric acid present, the test is discontinued. Because these tests are frequently done to ascertain either achlorhydria, the complete absence of hydrochloric acid, as in pernicious anemia, or the maximum acid response as in peptic ulcer, many clinics use only the most powerful stimulant, namely histamine, rather than first using one of the test meals. Sometimes alcohol, 50 cc of 7 per cent solution, is administered instead of the histamine, but only when the tests preceding the alcohol fail to show hydrochloric acid.

In addition to the tests for hydrochloric acid in the specimens aspirated, following the test meals, the specimens are usually sent to the laboratory for more detailed examination. Such tests include the quantitative tests for free and combined hydrochloric acid and total acidity and tests for occult blood, rennin, pepsin, and bile.

The reaction of the gastric contents is normally acid and after the Ewald meal, according to Todd and associates,[8] it may vary from 0.1–0.2 per cent or between 25 and 50 degrees of acidity. It is believed that no pathology of the stomach exists when the amount of acid is within the normal limits. If there is a marked increase, a peptic ulcer may be present, although neurotic conditions may affect the acidity. Decreased hydrochloric acid is noted in pellagra, early carcinoma, and gastritis. In advanced carcinoma, pernicious anemia, gastritis, and gallbladder disease, free hydrochloric acid is either entirely absent or markedly decreased in amounts.

Tests for Stomach Motility.   The motility of the stomach, or the speed with which the ingested food passes through the stomach, also is important. This may be tested by aspirating the contents of the stomach when it normally contains no food, for example, before breakfast in the morning. Sometimes easily recognized foods, such as rice pudding with currants, are given, and the contents of the stomach removed within 6–7 hours when normally all this food should have left the stomach. Todd[9] and others state that, if 100 cc of fluid can be aspirated 1 hour after an Ewald meal has been given, the motility of the stomach is deficient.

6. GALLBLADDER TESTS

Biliary Drainage.   To drain the contents of the gallbladder a Rehfuss tube is swallowed, as for aspiration of the stomach contents. After the tube has reached the stomach, the patient must be on the right side with the hips elevated. The end of the tube will gradually find its way into the duodenum. R. B. H. Gradwohl[10] states that, by adding a 25 per cent magnesium sulfate solution to promote relaxation of the duodenum, the contents of the gallbladder will drain. The use of this test is based on the belief, which at one time was quite general, that three different kinds of bile come from three different parts of the biliary tract. Gradwohl[11] states that this is a misconception and that the only value of this test lies in the collection of material for microscopic examination if that is desired.

Liver-function Tests.   These tests rest upon the fact that certain dyes are excreted solely by the bile. The dyes used are Bromsulphalein, phenoltetrachlorophthalein, and iodophthalein. If the latter drug is used, liver-function tests and gallbladder tests may be done simultaneously. These dyes are administered intravenously, and the liver removes the dye and excretes it. The rate of excretion is measured by drawing a blood sample shortly after the injection of the dye to measure its concentration, and then drawing repeated samples to measure the residual dye. Under normal functioning of the liver, about three quarters of the dye is excreted in about one-half hour. Correspondingly, if there is any abnormality present in the liver, the excretion of the dye is delayed in proportion to the amount of abnormality.

The *icteric index* is also an indication of the presence or absence of liver impairment. A sample of blood is taken by venipuncture and allowed to clot. The color of the serum is compared to a colorimeter. The normal icteric index is between 2.5 and 5. The *galactose-tolerance test* also is used to determine liver function. Galactose is given to the patient who has had no food for 12 hours. Since galactose is changed to glycogen by the liver, the excretion of sugar in the urine indicates the presence of liver damage.

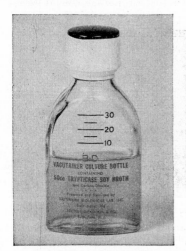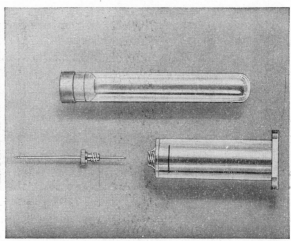

Figure 125. (*Left*) Commercially prepared media and container into which blood specimen is injected for culture. (*Right*) Sterile disposable syringe, prepared commercially, for collection of blood sample. (Courtesy of Becton, Dickinson and Co., Rutherford, N. J.)

7. EXAMINATION OF THE BLOOD

Methods of Securing Specimens. The method of obtaining blood for examination depends upon the type of test to be made. The blood normally remains very much the same, but disease conditions of various kinds produce changes in the blood that are of definite assistance in diagnosis. Certain tests, such as the Wassermann, require from 3–5 cc of blood, and therefore the blood is obtained by venipuncture. In this procedure the doctor or a laboratory technician aspirates the required amount of blood from a vein, commonly the median basilic. This may be done with a sterile syringe and needle, or a disposable unit of sterile syringe and needle may be used (see Fig. 125, *right*). (For the suggested technique for venipuncture, see Chapter 26.) With the exception of the Wassermann, the blood for tests is usually taken in the morning before the patient has had breakfast, since at this time the blood is most likely to give a correct picture.

For tests which require only a very small amount of blood, such as leukocyte, erythrocyte, and differential counts, a sufficient amount may be obtained by puncturing the edge of the lobe of the ear or the tip of a finger. In this method the skin is cleaned, and a quick stab is made with a sharp needle. The blood is collected in a pipette as it oozes from this puncture. (See Fig. 126.)

Blood Counts. The *erythrocyte, or red-cell, count* is one of the tests most commonly made in conjunction with the examination of the patient. The average healthy man has about 5,000,000 red cells per cubic millimeter of blood. The number for women is slightly less, being about 4,500,000. There may at times be an increase in the number of red cells, but this is rarely of clinical significance. Maxwell M. Wintrobe[12] states that individuals who live in the higher altitudes

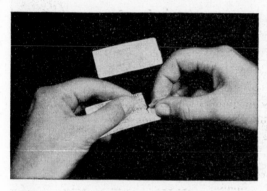 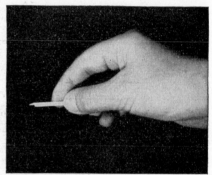

Figure 126. Sterile disposable instrument used to pierce the finger or ear lobe when collecting a small blood specimen. (Courtesy of Becton, Dickinson and Co., Rutherford, N. Y.)

habitually have a higher red-cell count. A decrease in the red-cell count is more common and also more significant. The change in the red-cell count is usually accompanied by a change in hemoglobin, but they need not necessarily correspond. Decreased red-cell count is present in almost all the anemias, and the count may drop to as low as 1,500,000. Leukemia also is characterized by a marked decrease in the red-cell count.

The *leukocyte, or white-cell, count* is of considerable importance clinically, because a change in the number of leukocytes occurs frequently. The normal leukocyte count varies from 5000 to 10,000 per cubic millimeter of blood. An increase in the white-cell count, or leukocytosis, may occur when the blood-forming organs produce an unusually large number of cells. This is noted when an unusually large number of leukocytes are produced to counteract an infection. Leukemia, while it is marked by a decrease in the red-cell count, also shows a definite increase in the white-cell count. The number may increase tremendously, sometimes to 1,000,000 per cubic millimeter of blood. In the case of infections it is generally believed that, if the leukocyte count is high, the individual is resisting the infection. The leukocyte count may not be increased if the individual is offering little or no resistance to the disease or if the infection is of little importance. Leukopenia, or a marked decrease in white cells, is a sign of overwhelming infection, or may be due to agranulocytosis, in which the blood-forming organs do not function properly.

The *differential count,* or the differentiation of the kinds of leukocytes, is fully as important as the simple leukocyte count, if not more so. It is made by staining the blood by one of several means. Ham[13] states that of the total leukocytes 25–33 per cent should normally be lymphocytes; 3–7 per cent monocytes; 54–62 per cent polymorphonuclears, 1–3 per cent eosinophils, and 0–1 per cent basophils. In certain diseases, such as pernicious anemia, lymphatic leukemia, pertussis, and exophthalmic goiter, the lymphocyte count is increased. In other diseases there is a change in the number of the other types of leukocytes as, for example, the monocyte count is high in malaria and typhoid fevers and the polymorphonuclear cells are increased in inflammatory conditions when the body seems to be successfully combating the inflammation. Eosinophilia, an increase in eosinophils, is characteristic particularly of parasitic and allergic diseases. Myelogenous leukemia may be characterized by a 500 per cent or more increase of polymorphonuclear leukocytes, with many immature forms, which constitute a definite diagnostic aid. Because the different kinds of leukocytes vary in number in certain diseases, a differential count is often of more value than simply a leukocyte count alone.

Platelet Count. The platelets are the smallest formed element in the blood, with a diameter of less than one half that of a red blood cell.* Their chief function is related to blood clotting, which is aided by the agglutination of platelets. Because of their small size and tendency to agglutinate, direct counting is difficult, and there is considerable variation in what are considered normal values. The number of platelets may also be estimated from the blood smear used for the differential count. Decreased numbers of platelets result in a tendency to bleed easily, particularly under the skin, producing a hemorrhagic rash, or purpura. The platelets may be decreased in diseases of the bone marrow, such as leukemia or extensive metastatic carcinoma, or may be depressed without obvious reason, as in idiopathic thrombocytopenic purpura.

Hemoglobin. Hemoglobin is a protein compound having a great affinity for oxygen. It is found in the red blood cells, and the amount of hemoglobin is usually proportional to the number of red cells. The amount normally present in the blood is 16 ± 2 gm per 100 cc of blood in the adult male, 14 ± 2 gm in the adult female.[14] In the past hemoglobin was frequently expressed as a per cent, but a wide range of standard or 100 per cent values were used, making the system a confusing and often inaccurate one. The use of the absolute value of hemoglobin is now preferred and is a much more satisfactory way of expressing the hemoglobin level. An increase—that is, above normal limits—is uncommon and may not be important. On the other hand, a decrease is both common and important as it is found

---

* The average diameter of a red blood cell is 7.2 microns or 7.2 one-thousandths of a millimeter. (Ham, Thomas H.: *A Syllabus of Laboratory Examinations in Clinical Diagnosis.* Harvard University Press, Cambridge, 1950, p. 109.)

in the anemias, leukemia, hemorrhage, and malignant diseases. It is estimated in various ways and is commonly used as a diagnostic aid.

Coagulation, Bleeding, and Prothrombin Times.   The *bleeding time* is the measure of the length of time required for a standard wound, usually a finger puncture, to stop bleeding. *Coagulation,* or *clotting time,* is the time necessary for the blood to clot after it has been removed from the vein and placed in a container. The normal values for these tests vary with the technique or method used. (See Appendix IV, p. 1194.) The bleeding or clotting time, or both, may be abnormally elevated in diseases of the blood-clotting mechanism, such as hemophilia. The danger of trauma or surgery without proper preparation to such patients is self-evident.

Another useful test in the clotting mechanism is the *prothrombin time*. This test is a measure of the level of prothrombin in the blood; prothrombin is a circulating protein which takes part in the process of clotting. Both the coagulation time and prothrombin time are valuable tests for following patients under anticoagulation therapy, so that desirable levels may be maintained, without decreasing the blood coagulability to dangerous levels. These tests are usually done once a day, but at times may be performed more frequently. The coagulation time is used to measure heparin dosage, whereas the prothrombin time is used when bishydroxycoumarin (Dicumarol) or other anti-prothrombin drugs are given.

Bone Marrow.   The direct microscopic examination of the bone marrow is a valuable method of diagnosis of many diseases of the blood and blood-forming organs. Bone marrow specimens are usually taken from the iliac crest, the spinous process of a vertebra, or the sternum. This is done by introducing, under local anesthesia, a needle directly into the marrow cavity of the bone. A small amount of marrow is then aspirated and smeared on glass slides, which are stained and studied microscopically. This technique is called bone marrow aspiration.

Another bone marrow study is that of biopsy. A biopsy is the removal of a small piece of tissue for fixation and microscopic study, and is also a widely used diagnostic method. A segment of marrow is obtained in a similar way to the aspiration, except that a special, large-bore needle is used which removes a small cylinder of tissue. The specimen is then fixed and sectioned, rather than being smeared. This method is generally used when repeated aspirations have proven unsatisfactory. These techniques are utilized in the diagnosis of many blood diseases, such as leukemia, pernicious anemia, and aplastic anemia. They may also aid in the diagnosis of metastatic neoplasm, but since the specimen is small, such lesions may not appear in it.

Sedimentation Rate.   It is a well-known fact that the red blood cells will settle down to the bottom of the container in which blood is allowed to stand. Blood is collected by means of a venipuncture and allowed to stand, and the speed with which the cells settle is measured. As yet there is no uniformity either in amount or the time they are observed, since different workers describe a variety of methods. Westergren's method is often used. Various factors, such as the number and size of red blood cells, the protein content of the blood, and the viscosity of the blood, play a part in the rate of sedimentation. In the Westergren test, blood is placed in fine glass tubes calibrated in millimeters. The rate at which sedimentation normally occurs with the Westergren method is usually stated as less than 15 millimeters in one hour. The sedimentation rate is a nonspecific test which may be altered by a large number of disease processes, much like the body temperature. It is of special value in following the activity of certain chronic diseases such as rheumatic fever, tuberculosis, and arthritis.

Serologic Tests for Syphilis. These tests are made on the blood serum to detect the presence of an antibody present in patients who have syphilis. The first test of this nature was described by Wassermann, and since then many variations in method have been developed; so that, besides the Wassermann test, there are many others, including the Kolmer test, the Kahn test, the Mazzini test, and the V.D.R.L. (Venereal Disease Research Laboratory). While these tests are usually accurate in the diagnosis of syphilis, they are not entirely specific, and certain other diseases may produce a small number of false positive reactions. The diagnosis may be accurately made, however, by combining the clinical findings with several of the different tests, including their repetition at various intervals.

One form of serologic test is usually done as part of every routine examination, requiring about 5 cc of clotted blood obtained by venipuncture. The widespread use of these tests has been one result of the increasing public health crusade against venereal disease, which has also reduced the number of complications of syphilis, such as abortion, in addition to neurologic, mental, and cardiac disease.

A new serologic test is the treponema immobilization test (T.P.I.), named after the spirochete *Treponema pallidum,* the etiologic agent of syphilis. This test is a measure of a specific antibody in a patient's blood, which is capable of inhibiting the normal motility of the spirochetes. This examination is an elaborate one, but valuable in confirming the diagnosis in borderline cases. It is probably not, however, of practical value for large numbers of screening examinations.

Blood Chemistry. A large number of chemical determinations may be made on the blood when indicated, each of which usually requires 5–10 cc of blood obtained by venipuncture. If whole blood or plasma is required, sodium oxalate or sodium citrate should be placed in the test tube to prevent the blood from clotting; whereas, if serum is desired, the blood is placed in a dry tube and allowed to clot. Blood specimens are usually drawn early in the morning, as many of the tests require that the patient be in a fasting state.

Blood Cultures. Cultures are made to determine the presence or absence of bacteria and therefore should be taken by venipuncture under careful aseptic conditions. The blood is added to culture media and incubated. It is observed over a period of time, frequently as long as two weeks. Some of the organisms that can be determined by means of blood cultures are the typhoid bacilli, pneumococci, staphylococci, and streptococci.

Blood Grouping. Because certain types of blood are incompatible, it is necessary to type the blood used in a transfusion so that the bloods of the donor and of the recipient are compatible. Untoward reactions and sometimes death of the patient will result if two types of blood not suited to each other are combined.

This problem is discussed more completely in the section on blood transfusion (see Chapter 26).

8. EXAMINATION OF SPINAL FLUID

Method of Obtaining Specimen.   The spinal fluid for examination is obtained by inserting a special needle into the subarachnoid space between the third and fourth lumbar vertebrae. This procedure is usually called a lumbar puncture because the needle is inserted in the lumbar region of the spinal column. (See Chapter 28 for a more complete discussion of this procedure.) When the stilette is removed from the needle that is in the spinal canal, the fluid will drop out of the needle. The fluid is collected in three sterile test tubes (or a sterile medicine glass may be used). Usually a total of from 6–10 cc is collected, the greatest amount being collected in the second tube. The fluid in the first tube may contain a few drops of blood as a result of a slight injury to the tissues as the needle passed through the tissues, and therefore is of little value for testing.

Characteristics of Normal Cerebrospinal Fluid.   Normal cerebrospinal fluid is clear and colorless. It is alkaline in reaction and has a specific gravity of from 1.001–1.010. Protein and sugar are present in small quantities and, with a few leukocytes, comprise the solid materials in the fluid. A cell count from 0–5 is considered normal. The fluid is normally under sufficient pressure to support 60–200 mm of water. This pressure causes the fluid to drop out of the needle at a rate slow enough to be counted, usually about 1 or 2 drops per second. Under high pressure the fluid may spurt out of the needle. Pressure on the jugular vein causes an increase in spinal fluid pressure. The amount of cerebrospinal fluid, according to Ham,[15] is thought to be 125–200 cc in a normal adult. The speed with which it is formed is unknown. The first fluid that drops from the needle may be blood-tinged, but after a few drops there should no longer be any trace of blood.

Abnormal Variations in the Cerebrospinal Fluid.   In inflammation of the meninges the cerebrospinal fluid may show an increase in pressure, in specific gravity, in the amount of protein, and in the number of leukocytes. In acute infections the fluid may also be cloudy or yellow in color, the specific organisms causing the infections may be found, and the cell count markedly increased (the cell count may reach several hundred). Pure pus may be present in the fluid, especially in acute meningitis, causing it to be very turbid. In tumors of the brain the fluid may be under increased pressure. Blood, usually dark in color, may be indicative of injury to the spinal cord above the site of the puncture or subarachnoid hemorrhage. Increased protein concentration may lead to clot or pellicular formation due to the increased amount of fibrinogen. W. R. Brain[16] states that in disorders characterized by a marked increase in protein, such as subarachnoid block and polyneuritis, the clot may solidify the whole specimen; whereas the clot of meningitis, particularly tuberculous, is a delicate pellicle which may take up to 24 hours to form, because the protein is less markedly elevated.

Tests on Cerebrospinal Fluid. In addition to the gross examination of the fluid the tests include those for specific bacteria, a test for syphilis, a test for protein, and a cell count. The bacteriological tests may include cultures and smears for meningococci, tubercle bacilli, influenza bacilli, and various other organisms. The presence of any of these organisms in the spinal fluid makes a specific diagnosis possible. The tests for syphilis of the spinal fluid are the same as those for the blood. The spinal fluid must, however, be free of blood. If positive, it further substantiates· the diagnosis of syphilis, especially of the central nervous system.

There are many different tests for measuring the spinal fluid protein, and also determining the levels of albumen and globulin. The protein concentration may be elevated in many diseases of the central nervous system such as inflammatory, neoplastic, and degenerative conditions.

The cell count usually includes a differential as well as a white-cell count. The few leukocytes which may normally be seen in the fluid are lymphocytes. An increase of leukocytes, chiefly lymphocytes, up to 500 cells per cubic millimeter is usually seen with poliomyelitis, tuberculous meningitis, viral meningitis, and syphilis. Acute purulent meningitis may have a cell count of from several hundred up to 20,000, almost all of which are neutrophils. The spinal fluid sugar is usually markedly decreased in both tuberculous and bacterial meningitis, which serves as another valuable diagnostic aid in the differential diagnosis of such conditions.

9. SMEARS AND CULTURES

Means of Securing Smears. A small quantity of the secretions of any body cavity or wound may be taken by means of a cotton applicator and transferred to a clean glass slide. After the applicator is saturated with the material to be examined it is rubbed across the surface of the slide until the middle part of the slide is covered. The material is allowed to dry on the slide before examination. Extreme care should be taken to prevent contaminating the whole slide, because very often these secretions are laden with virulent bacteria.

Types of Smears. Smears are taken from many different parts of the body, including eyes, ears, nose, throat, urethra, and vagina. Urethral smears are particularly valuable in the diagnosis of gonorrhea. Wounds and abscesses may also be studied in this manner. Smears should, however, generally be used in conjunction with cultures when facilities for the latter are available. Smears are stained by appropriate methods, and then examined microscopically for bacteria in an effort to make a specific diagnosis.

Making Cultures. In order to determine the nature of a bacterial infection in any person, secretion or material from a wound, skin, or mucous surface may be transferred to a medium that encourages the growth of microorganisms and the growth subsequently studied in the laboratory. The articles required for most cultures are sterile cotton applicators and a stoppered test tube or bottle (see Fig. 125, *left*) of sterile broth. The culture may be made on an agar plate instead of in a liquid medium. In securing the material to be cultured, it is essential that the applicator and tube of broth be protected from contamination from all other sources. The applicator is applied to the affected area and then inserted in the broth; the tube is carefully plugged with sterile cotton after flaming the mouth. The contents of the tube are subjected to conditions that favor the growth of the suspected organisms and then examined in the laboratory.

Blood, urine, and spinal fluid cultures are made by adding a small amount of these fluids to the media selected. Specimens must be collected under aseptic conditions.

Cultures of wounds, infected throats, eyes, and ears are common for diagnostic purposes. The procedure of collecting the specimen is usually carried out by the laboratory technician, but the nurse should be able to give this service.

Exfoliative Cytology. This is a relatively new technique for the diagnosis of malignant disease in which smears of body fluids or tissue scrapings are made and examined microscopically for the presence of tumor cells. The most valuable and extensively used test is the Papanicolaou cervical smear for the detection of carcinoma of the cervix. These smears are taken during a routine vaginal examination by the physician, who scrapes the external os of the cervix with a wooden applicator and places the obtained material on a glass slide. The attending nurse should then immediately place the slide in a fixative solution, taking care that the container is properly identified as to the patient from whom the specimen was taken. Other examinations, which concern the nurse less directly, are made on smears of the centrifuged sediment of sputum, bronchial washings, pleural or ascitic fluid, or urine. The interpretation of these smears is difficult, and is usually made by a physician particularly trained in these fields; with proper facilities, this technique is a useful diagnostic aid in the detection of malignancy.

10. BASAL METABOLISM

Definition. Metabolism may be defined as the sum total of all the chemical changes of the body. By means of these chemical processes, heat and energy are produced and growth results. It was Lavoisier who first discovered that the heat in an animal body was produced by burning foodstuffs in the body and was in no way different from the burning of carbon outside the body. He went further in his experimentation and found that in the oxidation of a given amount and kind of foodstuffs in the body the carbon dioxide eliminated is equal to that produced when oxidation of the same amount and kind of foodstuff occurs outside the body. This established the relationship between heat produced and carbon dioxide eliminated. Similar studies were made to show the relationship between the amount of oxygen required to burn the foodstuffs and the heat produced. It is therefore possible to measure the heat production and heat loss by measuring the amount of oxygen consumed and carbon dioxide eliminated. Furthermore, for each type of foodstuff the amount of oxygen needed for combustion and carbon dioxide expired have been ascertained, and the production of heat can be accurately determined by measuring the gases exchanged in the respirations.

It is a well-known physical law that energy can neither be created nor destroyed and that it can be changed from one form to another. Experimentation on dogs showed that this law applies to the living body as well as to all forms of matter. The heat produced in the oxidation of foodstuffs in the body, as measured by direct calorimetry, is equivalent (or nearly so) to the amount of heat it is estimated that the same foods produce if burned outside the body.

It has previously been stated that different foodstuffs require specific amounts of oxygen for burning and that they give off specific amounts of carbon dioxide. When referring to the oxidation of foodstuffs in the body, the ratio between the oxygen used and the carbon dioxide given off is called the *respiratory quotient*. A common method of showing this relationship is the following:

$$\text{the ratio} = \frac{\text{volume carbon dioxide expired}}{\text{volume oxygen inspired}}$$

Although the amount and kinds of food ingested play a very great part in determining the metabolism, other factors must, of course, be considered. The activity of the individual affects the metabolic rate. Best and Taylor[17] state that, if other things are equal, an individual who is sleeping has a metabolic rate that is from 10–13 per cent lower than if he were awake. The age and sex of the individual play some part, but most of the experimental work has been done on adults between the ages of twenty and fifty, and so less is known about the metabolism of children. It is well known, however, that the energy requirements of children per unit of body surface exceed those of the adult.

It is quite evident that size also would have an effect on the metabolism, and, at first, units of weight were used as a basis for measurement. That proved to be somewhat inaccurate, because although the total amount of heat produced by two bodies of different sizes varied, the amount per unit of body surface was the same; therefore the surface area of the body was substituted. The surface area is usually determined on the basis of height and weight of the individual rather than upon actual measurement. The activity of the individual affects his metabolism as does the temperature of the surrounding area. The body temperature also influences the metabolic rate.

Indirect calorimetry is the method now most commonly used to measure the metabolism in therapeutic practice. In this method the gases used in respiration are measured, and the heat and energy production estimated from that. For certain more specific experimental work on metabolism, the actual heat production is measured, and this method is known as *direct calorimetry*.

Because so many factors influence the metabolism, it is necessary to choose a time when the influencing factors are within the control of the patient and the technician. The usual time for making these measurements is early in the morning after a prolonged rest period.

The *basal metabolism* of an individual is the lowest energy requirement of the body (or the least amount of heat produced by the body) while it is at rest. The various body processes are going on at as low a rate as possible. Determination

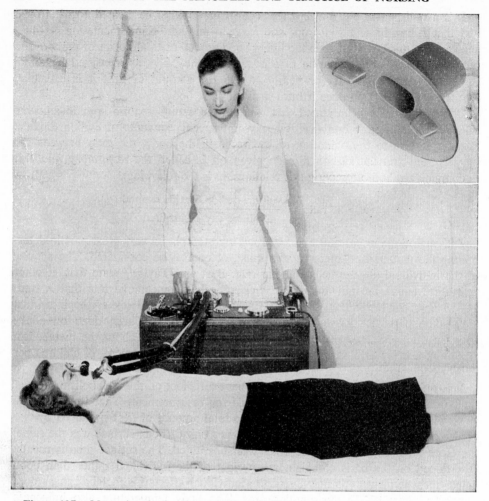

Figure 127. Measuring the basal metabolic rate. Note the clamp which prevents breathing through the nose. The patient breathes oxygen through the mouth piece; see inset: note the phalange that fits between the inside of the lips and the gums. The patient bites down on the small projections to hold mouth piece in place throughout the test. (Courtesy of Sanborn Co., Cambridge, Mass.)

of the basal metabolism rate is a useful diagnostic test in the evaluation of thyroid function.

Preparation of the Patient. The patient who is to have the basal metabolic rate estimated should have a very complete explanation as to what the test is for, how it is to be made, and how to prepare for it. If the patient is in the hospital, the nurse must direct the activities of the patient so that the measurement may be accurate. For the patient who is to go to the laboratory, detailed instructions must be given to ensure adequate preparation.

At least 10–12 hours of sleep are required preceding the test. A sedative may be given to ensure a good night's rest. No food should be taken after the evening meal on the day previous. Smoking should be restricted during the evening preceding also. The muscular activity of the individual in the morning after waking should be reduced to a minimum. For the bed patient, this means that no nursing care except the most necessary should be given. The person who is going to the laboratory from home should arise just before going for the test. He should ride and not walk to the laboratory. He should avoid walking up and down stairs. For about one-half hour before the test, the patient should lie quietly in the room in which the test is to be made. A slightly longer period might be required for the outpatient. The room temperature should be about 20° C (68° F), and the patient should lie comfortably and quietly on a bed. The height and weight and the body temperature are measured before the test. From the height and weight the surface area of the body is determined. All computations are made by the technician or the physician.

Conducting the Test. The test is usually carried out by an especially trained technician in a room designed for the purpose. (In some instances the instrument or equipment may be taken to the patient's bedside.) The nurse prepares the patient for the metabolism test and transports him to the room where it is to be made. The apparatus used may vary in type, but all pieces of such equipment are based on the same principles. The amount of oxygen that the patient breathes in and the amount of carbon dioxide expired are measured, and the calculations based on those measurements.

Interpretation of Test. The basal metabolic rate (B.M.R.) is recorded as normal or as being above or below normal. The basal metabolic rate has been found to be, according to Best and Taylor,[18] 35 to 40 calories per square meter of body surface per hour. They also say that the amount of heat produced per square meter of body surface is determined by dividing the amount of heat produced in one hour by the surface area of the individual. If this amount falls within the average normal limits (35–40 calories), the individual is said to have a normal basal metabolic rate. If it is more or less than normal, it is said to be a given percentage above or below normal. In stating the results of a test, the number is given, and the fact that it is a percentage is implied as, for example, a basal rate of − 10 really means 10 per cent below the normal level. The normal basal metabolic rate is usually considered as ranging from − 10 to + 10.

Radioactive Iodine. This is another useful diagnostic test in the evaluation of thyroid function. For this procedure a small dose of radioactive iodine or I^{131} is given to the patient either in a liquid or as a capsule, after which the uptake of radioactive iodine in the thyroid may be measured by placing a Geiger counter over the thyroid gland 24 hours later; or the radioactive iodine excretion may be measured by collecting a 24-hour urine specimen and measuring its radioactivity, also by means of a Geiger counter. Normal limits for these tests are not definitely established, most clinics evaluating the results on the basis of their own past experience. Radioactive iodine excretion indirectly also measures the uptake by the

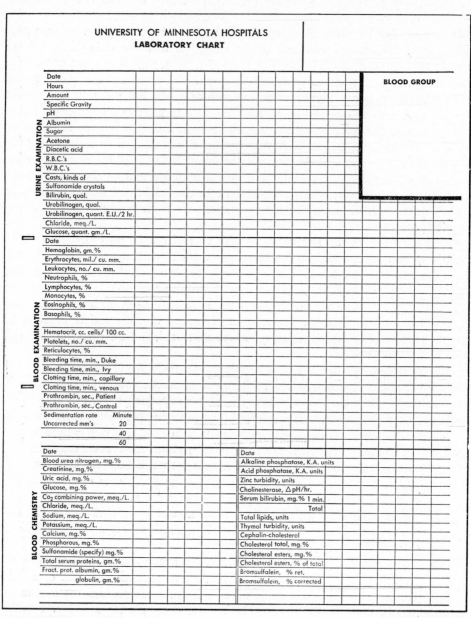

Figure 128A. Laboratory chart, showing face of form. (Courtesy of University of Minnesota Hospitals, Minneapolis, Minn.)

BACTERIOLOGY

Date	Specimen	Examination

SEROLOGY							STOOL EXAMINATION					
	U. of M. Lab.		State Board				Date					
Date	Wass.	Kahn	Wass.	Kline			Color					
							Blood:					
							Benzidine					

GASTRIC ANALYSIS Alcohol ☐ Histamine ☐

								Guaiac					
Date								Ova					
Time													
Amount													
Free acid°								Parasites					
Total acid°													
Lactic acid								Pus					
Blood:								Mucus					
Benzidine								Fat					
Guaiac								Urobilinogen, quant., E.U./100 gm.					

CEREBRO-SPINAL FLUID						BODY CAVITY FLUID					
Date						Date					
Erythrocytes, no./ cu. mm						Amount, cc.					
Leukocytes, no./ cu. mm.						Kind					
Neutrophils						Erythrocytes, no./ cu. mm.					
Mononuclears						Leukocytes, no./ cu. mm.					
Other cells						Neutrophils					
Protein, mg.%						Lymphocytes					
Chloride, meq./L.						Eosinophils					
Glucose, mg.%						Other cells					
Sulfonamide (specify) mg.%						Protein (Esbach) gm./l.					
Colloidal Gold Curve						Specific Gravity					
						Mucin					

MISCELLANEOUS REPORTS

Date	Specimen	Examination

Figure 128B. Back of laboratory chart, or reverse of form shown in Figure 128A. (Courtesy of University of Minnesota Hospitals, Minneapolis, Minn.)

thyroid gland, since, after 24 hours, virtually all the radioactive iodine still in the body is in the thyroid, so that the uptake is merely the total amount less the amount excreted. Values for both uptake and excretion are expressed as percentages.

[The physiologic basis of this test lies in the fact that the thyroid gland utilizes iodine in the production of thyroid hormone, and thus the greater the function of the gland, the higher the radioactive iodine uptake will be, and conversely in hypofunction of the gland, the uptake will be very low] This test is of no value if the patient has received radioactive iodine during the previous six to eight weeks, or if he has taken large amounts of iodine or iodine-containing substances; the first, because there may be retained radioactive iodine in the gland making the reading too high; the second, because the gland may be saturated with iodine, producing an incorrect low value. Because radioactive measurements are made so frequently within the hospital, many medical personnel do not recall that most patients are not familiar with the test. As many people tend to associate x-ray treatments and radioactivity only with cancer, a few reassuring words from the nurse about this safe and valuable test may prove most helpful to an anxious patient. (When such tests are made, it is important to discontinue the use of iodine solutions as skin disinfectants. Their use may invalidate these sensitive measurements.)

11. ELECTROCARDIOGRAPHY*

Nature of a Cardiogram.   The electrocardiogram is a photograph of the electrical currents produced by the activity of the heart muscle. It is an accepted fact that tissue in activity has a negative charge as compared with other tissues. These electrical currents are directed from the body by means of wires attached to the arms and legs and the apex region of the heart; the wires are attached to a string which vibrates with the heartbeat and the vibrations of the string are photographed. The vibrations of this string are the same as the currents given off from the heart; thus a photograph of heart activity is produced. This is recorded on a tape moving at a standard speed, and marked according to time (horizontal axis) and voltage (vertical axis). The advent of the electrocardiogram has made possible finer distinctions in the diagnosis of heart diseases and has increased tremendously the knowledge of abnormalities of the heart. Previously, diagnoses of heart disease were dependent on the interpretation of the history and physical examination. It must be remembered, however, that no matter how important a diagnostic aid the electrocardiograph is, it must be viewed as but a part of the total examination and should not be considered exclusive of other findings.

Conduction of the Test.   This examination is frequently carried out by a trained technician at the bedside, in a special department, or in the physician's office. Since

---

* Material on "Conduction of the Test" based on *Heart Disease,* 4th ed., by Paul D. White (The Macmillan Company, New York, 1951); material on "Interpretation," based on *PQRST, A Guide to Electrocardiogram Interpretation,* 3rd ed., by Joseph E. F. Riseman (The Macmillan Company, New York, 1952).

the nurse may often, in many situations, be called upon to make or participate in making this test, she should understand its basic mechanisms.

(1.) PLACING OF THE ELECTRODES. With the patient lying on a bed, strap electrodes are placed on both right and left arms just above the wrists, and another just above the left ankle. The area of skin over which the electrode will lie should be rubbed with conducting jelly before fastening the electrode in place, and the surface of the electrode should likewise be covered with a film of the jelly. The precordial or chest leads (Fig. 129) should then be located and similarly prepared with jelly, and the chest electrode then likewise coated, though not placed for

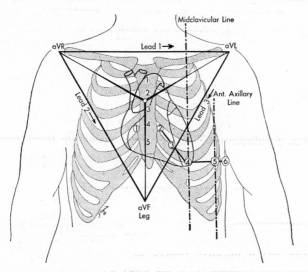

Figure 129. Diagram showing bipolar limb leads (1, 2, 3), unipolar limb leads (aVR, aVL, aVF), and precordial leads (V₁ to V₆ inclusive). The outline of the heart is shown under the sternum and ribs; the level of the first five interspaces is indicated. Einthoven's triangle is represented, as is also the spatial relationship of the remote electrode to the limb electrodes in the case of the unipolar limb leads. (White, Paul D.: *Heart Disease,* 4th ed. The Macmillan Company, New York, 1951.)

recording. The appropriate wires from the electrocardiograph are then connected with the limb electrodes, and the various leads are taken.

(2.) THE LEADS. The various leads are taken by controlling on the machine the electrode or combination of electrodes which are recording. This is usually done by merely setting a control dial.

Bipolar Limb Leads: In these leads, two electrodes are recording.

Lead 1: This is the recording of the right and left arms.

Lead 2: This is the recording of the right arm and left leg.

Lead 3: This is the recording of the left arm and left leg.

Unipolar Limb Leads: These leads are taken from the three limb electrodes, only one of which, however, is an active or exploring electrode, the other in this case being an indifferent one. These leads are designated aVR for the right arm, aVL for the left arm, and aVF for the left leg.

Precordial Leads: These chest leads, usually designated V_1 to V_6 according to their location in the chest wall, are taken with the exploring electrode held in the proper position by the patient. These leads are also unipolar, the other electrode being an indifferent one. Leads V_7 to V_9, continuing posteriorly around the chest, are less frequently used.

Interpretation. The electrocardiogram is most valuable and definitive in the diagnosis of the cardiac arrhythmias or abnormal rhythms of the heart. It is also valuable in evaluation of the state of the myocardium, especially the ventricular

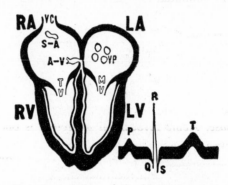

Figure 130. Diagrammatic representation of the heart at rest.

RA Right atrium	VC Vena cava
RV Right ventricle	VP Pulmonic veins
LA Left atrium	TV Tricuspid valve
LV Left ventricle	MV Mitral valve
S-A Sinoatrial node	

A-V Atrioventricular node, bundle of His and its branches

(Riseman, Joseph E. F.: *P-Q-R-S-T: A Guide to Electrocardiogram Interpretation,* 3rd ed. The Macmillan Company, New York, 1952.)

musculature, but aids little in the diagnosis of valvular lesions, and reveals nothing of the prognosis of the particular case.

The normal electrocardiograph wave is the PQRST complex as illustrated in Figure 130. The amplitude of the waves may vary with the lead taken, the anatomic position and physiologic state of the heart, and certain cardiac medications.

P WAVES represent the rhythmical impulses from the sinoatrial node or pacemaker, and contraction of the atria which each one initiates. Normal waves with irregular rate or rhythm indicate an arrhythmia of sinoatrial node origin. Abnormalities in size, form, duration, or direction indicate that either the stimulus has originated in the atrium, rather than the sinoatrial node, or that there are abnormalities of the atrial musculature.

PR INTERVAL is the segment from the beginning of the P wave to the beginning of the QRS complex. It is the measure of the time necessary for the spread of the impulse from the sinoatrial node to the intraventricular conducting system. Prolongation of the PR interval is the most common abnormality, and indicates delay or block in atrioventricular conduction, due usually to cardiac damage. Shortening of the interval is indicative of either premature ventricular beat or an abnormality of the atrium producing a shortened atrioventricular conduction time.

QRS COMPLEX represents the spread of the impulse through the ventricles; this complex is conducted from the atria by way of the A-V bundle or bundle of His. R is the first upward, or positive, deflection of the complex; Q the downward deflection which precedes it; and S the downward deflection following the R wave. Abnormalities in duration of QRS indicate disturbances in the conducting mechanism, while abnormal amplitude is indicative of abnormalities of the ventricular musculature.

RS-T SEGMENT AND T WAVES. The ventricular contraction, which begins before the QRS is completed, is represented by the RS-T segment and T waves, the terminal portion of the latter representing the recession of the stimulus and beginning of ventricular relaxation. Abnormalities represent changes of the ventricles, secondary to disease, anoxia, medication, or physiologic changes. For example, elevation or depression of the RS-T segment is usually due to myocardial anoxia, secondary to any cause. Acute myocardial infarction is one of the most frequent and most serious causes of these changes.

Leads. BIPOLAR LIMB LEADS are most valuable in the diagnosis of arrhythmias and in the preliminary search for myocardial changes.

UNIPOLAR LIMB LEADS permit recognition of cardiac position and diagnosis of posterior myocardial infarction.

PRECORDIAL LEADS are helpful in the diagnosis of myocardial infarction (except posterior), the differentiation of right and left bundle branch block, and the diagnosis of ventricular hypertrophy.

It should be remembered that electrocardiograph interpretation requires considerable skill and experience on the part of the physician. It is an immeasurably valuable adjunct in the diagnosis of cardiac disorders when interpretations are made by the expert.

12. ENDOSCOPY

Endoscopy is the technique of direct visual examination of certain body organs by means of hollow lighted instruments. This is obviously a valuable method in allowing pathology to be directly visualized and biopsied if so desired. These examinations are discussed in Chapter 18.

13. DIAGNOSTIC X-RAY

The use of x-ray as a diagnostic aid has become a very helpful and widespread technique. The applicability of x-ray lies in the fact that different tissues and substances vary in the resistance which they offer to the passage of x-ray or roentgen rays. Thus radiologists recognize four degrees of penetration, or x-ray densities; namely, air, fat, muscle, and bone, in order of increasing resistance to or absorption of x-rays. The film registers the amount of x-ray which penetrates the tissues; the greater the penetration, the darker the shadow on the film.

It should be remembered that the x-ray films are merely the two-dimensional projection of the varying densities of the tissues, rather than an actual "picture" of the various organs and tissues; correct interpretation of the shadows requires skill and experience. Fluoroscopy is a method of x-ray in which the image, instead of being recorded on a film, is focused on a radiosensitive plate, and the shadows may be directly studied by the radiologist. As a continuous stream of x-rays may be used with this technique, the dynamics of the body may be studied, for example, the action of the heart, the motion of the diaphragm, and the motility of the gastrointestinal tract. The technique of "plain" x-ray is adequate for the study of bones, their diseases, fractures, maturity, and size; and also for the study of the chest and to a lesser extent the abdomen. However, the use of either introduced gas or radiopaque substances to provide contrast has greatly increased the value of x-ray in the study of specific organs or organ systems.

Direct Introduction of Contrast Media.   This method allows the visualization of various body cavities and organs by the direct introduction of radiopaque material. For example, the upper gastrointestinal tract may be studied by having the patient ingest such a substance. The esophagus, stomach, and duodenum may then be viewed with both fluoroscopy and films as the material passes through the various organs (see Fig. 124). Likewise the large intestine may be outlined by the use of a radiopaque enema. In this fashion abnormalities of the entire gastrointestinal tract may be visualized radiologically—tumors, ulcerations, and scarring of the lining epithelium; abnormal anatomy, position, or motility; or pressure deformities secondary to extrinsic masses.

Other organs may likewise be visualized, at times requiring the use of special catheters or instruments to facilitate the introduction of the radiopaque dye. These examinations include study of the bladder, renal pelves, and ureters by the introduction of bladder and ureteral catheters, in order to demonstrate such lesions as tumors, tuberculous infections, strictures, and other structural abnormalities. The uterus and Fallopian tubes may be outlined by injecting dye into the uterus. This is particularly valuable in detecting uterine abnormalities and tubal patency in the study of sterility. The bronchi of a portion of the lung may likewise be defined, which is particularly useful in the diagnosis of bronchiectasis. The extent of sinus tracts and cutaneous fistulas are studied by the injection of dye directly into the opening after which films are taken. This procedure may be very valuable prior to surgical intervention.

The choice of the _radiopaque material_ to be used varies with the organ to be studied. Barium suspensions are used for the gastrointestinal tract, and various iodine-containing dyes for the other tests described. A slightly different technique is the introduction of a negative contrast medium, _air,_ which is used retroperitoneally. Formerly the air was injected perirenally through a lumbar needle, but now is usually injected through a needle placed anterior to the sacrum. This technique is of particular value in the localization of adrenal tumors.

Excretion of Contrast Media.   These tests utilize the ability of certain organs to excrete the radiopaque iodine-containing dyes. In this way the gallbladder and kidneys may be visualized. For the gallbladder, a dye such as sodium iodophthalein may be used. This dye is excreted selectively by the liver with the bile, and is then concentrated by the gallbladder, which may thus be visualized. The dye is usually given orally 12 or more hours prior to the time of actual x-ray; it may be also administered intravenously. Then, at the time of x-ray, a gallbladder stimulant, usually fatty food, is taken by the patient, and the motility may be seen fluoroscopically. In studying the kidneys, a radiopaque dye is administered intravenously shortly before the x-ray films are taken. The dye is rapidly excreted by the kidneys, and the kidneys, renal pelves, and ureters may be visualized. This method of intravenous pyelography is less difficult a procedure than the direct introduction of dye by catheter (retrograde pyelography) and demonstrates the outline of the kidney proper, which the latter method does less well. However, intravenous pyelography does not show the pelves and ureters with as great detail, and at times retrograde films must still be made.

It is obvious that for these x-ray tests to be useful, the organ under examination must have good function; for with poor function the dye will not be excreted in sufficient amount to be visualized radiologically.

Direct Injection for the Study of the Heart and Blood Vessels.   This method is merely that of direct injection of dye, which may then be studied as it flows in the circulation. It is important in these studies that the bolus of dye be injected rapidly so that it is not overly diluted with blood before films of the portion of the vascular tree under study may be taken. To demonstrate the heart, the dye is usually injected rapidly into an arm vein. Serial x-rays are then taken at short intervals to visualize the passage of the dye through the various heart chambers. This study of the heart is called *angiocardiography*, and is useful in the diagnosis of cardiac anomalies. The arterial system may be studied in a similar fashion, by the injection of the dye into an artery proximal to the part under study. Thus a needle may be introduced through the lumbar region of the patient's back into the descending aorta, or the injection may be made into the peripheral arteries. With this technique, termed *arteriography*, anomalies and diseases of the arteries may be demonstrated.

Most of these x-ray methods are utilized in neurological diagnosis, which is described on page 605.

Many of the procedures require special preparation, directions for which vary with the examination and preference of the individual physician; therefore, specific orders are written by the doctor prior to the examination. For example, the examination of the upper gastrointestinal tract is done on the fasting patient; catharsis and cleansing enemas are used prior to a barium enema. Often with other abdominal x-ray examinations, such as an intravenous pyelogram, the radiologist will order catharsis and enemas so that visualization is not hampered by retained gas or feces in the colon. X-ray examinations are usually not painful, unless special methods must be used to introduce contrast media. The responsibility for the explanation of these procedures to the patient, as well as the reason for the x-ray examinations, lies with the physician, but nurses or x-ray technicians usually amplify his explanations and directions by conference and written instructions.

14. PSYCHOMETRICS

The use of the psychometric examinations in the psychiatric evaluation of the patient has become a very useful adjunct to the clinical impression of the psychiatrist. These tests include the Wechsler-Bellevue, Rorschach, and Thematic Apperception tests; since they are usually administered individually by a trained clinical psychologist, they do not directly involve the nurse. However, their use is so widespread today that their significance and indications for use should also be understood by the nurse, for many patients react badly to first learning of such tests, feeling that they are being labeled "insane" or neurotic. The nurse can help to explain the true value of these tests to the patient. This duty is, however, primarily that of the physician, and the nurse should supplement his explanation or reassure the patient in general conversation until he is seen by the physician.

In a broad sense, all these tests measure the response of the patient to direct questions, to visual stimuli, and so on. They are designed to measure the mental processes of the individual—such as intelligence, imagination, emotions, and association. Since many parts of the examination require description or interpretation on the part of the patient as well as short answers, it is important that the tests be carried out in quiet privacy, free from interruption, so that valid results may be obtained.

The interpretation of each test is based on the results obtained by administering them to a large series of individuals, both normal and abnormal. The results of these series have been tabulated, and tables defining the range of normal and abnormal responses have been determined. The evaluation of the individual examination is made by the examining psychologist both on the basis of the responses of the patient, as compared with the normal scale, and also on his reactions during the period of examination.

Intelligence Testing.   There are many standard tests for this examination. Some are for adults, while others are designed for children, even on a preschool level, where the motor development and intellectual achievements of the child are determined by his ability to solve problems based on manual dexterity. One of the most frequently used adult examinations is the *Wechsler-Bellevue scale,* which measures different mental abilities, including comprehension, memorization, and problem solving. While it is obvious that native intelligence cannot be measured completely, free of the factor of education, such tests as the Wechsler-Bellevue have reduced the effect of education on test results to a minimum. In the testing of school children, this is less of a problem, as the degree of learning may be used as one measure of intelligence.

Rorschach test consists of a series of standard "ink-blot" patterns, each of which is presented to the patient who is asked to describe what he sees in the pattern. This test varies with both the normalcy of the mental and emotional processes and with intelligence, for the more intelligent individual may see things represented which would not occur to the mind of the less imaginative individual. Persons with disturbed thoughts or emotions may, on the other hand, describe the images in terms of their own subconscious fears or phobias.

Thematic Apperception Test. In this examination, a series of pictures is shown to the patient, who is then asked to first describe the picture and then to make up a brief story of the action which might be going on pertaining to the picture. In persons with markedly disturbed function, the actual descriptions of the pictures may be altered, while the less severe abnormalities may be indicated by the themes used in describing the dynamic action surrounding them.

These tests illustrate only three of the many forms of psychological tests available, all of which are designed to test the patient's reactions much as has been described.

The psychometric evaluation is useful not only in the diagnosis of mental disorders but has other values. Many organic diseases of the brain may first manifest themselves by personality changes, loss of reasoning ability, or disturbance in emotions; and serious illnesses may either produce mental changes in themselves or may precipitate latent mental disturbances. Thus the psychometric examination is a valuable diagnostic tool, when properly administered and interpreted, in helping the physician obtain a valid over-all view of the patient.

15. NEUROLOGICAL DIAGNOSTIC TESTS

The fields of neurology and neurosurgery utilize a number of special diagnostic tests; the principles of some of which have been outlined previously in the description of x-ray examinations. One of the most important is the examination of the spinal fluid which has been described on page 590. The others are complex examinations which require highly trained personnel and special equipment. The responsibility of explaining the procedures lies with the physician in charge, and in many instances written permission is necessary.

Electroencephalography. This examination may be likened to the electrocardiogram in that numerous electrodes are placed over the skull in specific areas, and then recordings of the electrical activity of the various segments of the cerebrum are made. Like the electrocardiogram, the recordings are usually made by a trained technician, and then read by a specially trained physician. The test is useful in helping to establish the diagnosis of conditions such as brain tumor, brain abscess, and epilepsy.

Electromyography is carried out by inserting needle electrodes directly into the bodies of different muscles in turn and then observing their electrical activity, both at rest and when active, by means of an electronic recording apparatus. It is a useful aid in the diagnosis of peripheral-nerve disorders and also certain spinal-cord and brain disorders.

Myelography is an x-ray examination of the spinal cord and its canal by means of an injection of a radiopaque substance into the spinal canal through a lumbar puncture needle. The spinal canal may then be visualized by means of fluoroscopy and x-ray films. It is a test of great value in localizing tumors and certain other disorders of the spinal cord, and also demonstrating external pressure on the cord from tumors, herniated disk, or bone fractures.

Pneumoencephalography consists of the withdrawal of spinal fluid and injection of gas, usually oxygen, into the subarachnoid space through a lumbar puncture needle. The gas rises in the spinal canal, and if it is not obstructed will usually fill the ventricles of the brain, so that x-rays may then be taken to visualize lesions of the brain itself. This test may demonstrate displacement and distortion of the ventricles caused by brain tumor, abscess, or other masses. (See Figs. 192 A and B.)

Ventriculography. This test is similar in principle to the pneumoencephalogram, and is done when a pneumoencephalogram is either felt to be unsafe or cannot be done satisfactorily. Ventriculography is the direct introduction of gas into the ventricles, and, except in infants (when the needle can be inserted through a fontanel), requires an operative procedure to make two small holes in the cranium through which the brain needles may be inserted. Oxygen is then injected directly into the ventricles, and x-ray films are taken and interpreted as with the pneumoencephalogram.

Arteriography is the method of injection of a bolus of radiopaque dye into the carotid, or, less frequently, the vertebral artery or arteries. By taking one or more x-ray films at short intervals after the injection, the arterial, capillary, or venous systems may be outlined. This is very useful in demonstrating abnormalities of the cerebral circulation and also the presence of other disease, such as the increased vascularity of certain tumors, or displacement in the normal position of the vessels.

REFERENCES

1. Ham, Thomas H.: *A Syllabus of Laboratory Examinations in Clinical Diagnosis.* Harvard University Press, Cambridge, 1950, p. 248.
2. Cecil, Russell L., and Loeb, Robert F. (eds.): *A Textbook of Medicine,* 8th ed. W. B. Saunders Co., Philadelphia, 1951, p. 958.
3. Todd, James C., et al.: *Clinical Diagnosis by Laboratory Methods,* 12th ed. W. B. Saunders Co., Philadelphia, 1953, p. 325.
4. Todd, James C., et al.: *op. cit.,* p. 145.
5. Ham, Thomas H.: *op. cit.,* p. 273.
6. Best, Charles H., and Taylor, Norman B.: *The Physiological Basis of Medical Practice,* 5th ed. Williams & Wilkins Co., Baltimore, 1950, p. 517.
7. Todd, James C., et al.: *op. cit.,* p. 474.
8. Todd, James C., et al.: *op. cit.,* p. 485.
9. Todd, James C., et al.: *op. cit.,* p. 493.
10. Gradwohl, R. B. H.: *Clinical Laboratory Methods and Diagnosis,* 4th ed. C. V. Mosby Co., St. Louis, 1948, p. 1050.
11. Gradwohl, R. B. H.: *op. cit.,* p. 1051.

12. Wintrobe, Maxwell M.: *Clinical Hematology*, 3rd ed. Lea & Febiger, Philadelphia, 1951, p. 710.
13. Ham, Thomas H.: *op. cit.*, p. 62.
14. Wintrobe, Maxwell M.: *op. cit.*, p. 95.
15. Ham, Thomas H.: *op. cit.*, p. 457.
16. Brain, W. R.: *Diseases of the Nervous System.* Oxford University Press, London, 1951, p. 128.
17. Best, Charles H., and Taylor, Norman B.: *op. cit.*, p. 622.
18. Best, Charles H., and Taylor, Norman B.: *op. cit.*, p. 620.

Additional Suggested Reading

Bodansky, Meyer, and Bodansky, Oscar: *Biochemistry of Disease,* 2nd ed. The Macmillan Company, New York, 1952.
Duffy, B. J., Jr., and Howland, J. W.: *Radioiodine* (I^{131}) *Principles of Diagnosis and Therapy of Thyroid Disease.* University of Rochester, Atomic Energy Project, Rochester, 1950.
Hodges, F. J., et al.: *Radiology for Medical Students.* Year Book Publishers, Chicago, 1947.
Markovits, Emerik: *Visceral Radiology.* The Macmillan Company, New York, 1951.
Rapaport, D.: *Diagnostic Psychological Testing.* Year Book Publishers, Chicago, 1945–1946.
Riseman, Joseph E. F.: *P-Q-R-S-T, A Guide to Electrocardiogram Interpretation,* 3rd ed. The Macmillan Company, New York, 1953.
Werner, S. C.: "Diagnostic Technique with Radioiodine," *M. Ann. District of Columbia,* **22:** 12-16, (Jan.) 1953.
White, Paul D.: *Heart Disease,* 4th ed. The Macmillan Company, New York, 1951.

CHAPTER 20. BASIS FOR THE SELECTION OF
METHOD IN THERAPEUTIC PROCEDURES

Basis for Methods Suggested in This Text. Part IV, to which this chapter is an introduction, is devoted to procedures. Before outlining the steps in any suggested method, an attempt is made to show why it is advocated. Sources of information on which conclusions are based are given insofar as time and space allow. In some cases experimental evidence is cited; in others expert opinion.

The methods themselves in no case duplicate those used in any one institution. Rather, an attempt has been made to set up a composite method, representing what the writer believes to be the best elements of many. Association with graduate nurses from all sections of the United States and from a number of foreign countries has resulted in a familiarity with many opinions and techniques. It is through the combined efforts of many students (graduate nurses) that an accumulation of information on so wide a range of subjects is possible. Even so, the material referred to represents only a part of the available sources.

No claim is made to presenting either the best or "perfect" procedure. Nursing, which is an applied science, is developing rapidly; with new discoveries its methods must change. A physiological concept of today is altered by discoveries of tomorrow; the most modern equipment of the present may seem clumsy or wasteful in comparison with that of next year. Any method should be regarded critically, and it is expected that nurses, like physicians, will be alert to possibilities of improvement.

Variability in Nursing Methods. A study of hospital manuals or "procedure books" shows that techniques vary widely in even the best hospitals in the United States, although they often seem to remain unchanged in a single institution over long periods. Differences existing in the country as a whole indicate unfamiliarity with many scientific discoveries, a lack of well-established standards, and very possibly a wide range of economic conditions, which directly influence selection of equipment. The fact that hospital methods tend to remain constant suggests a lack of the necessary interest, ability, time, or facilities for studying and revising techniques. As data in the physical and social sciences accumulate and are more widely known, techniques will inevitably change to conform to established laws, and less variation will exist in the technical aspects of medicine and nursing.

To what extent nursing procedures can or should be standardized is an ever-recurring question, a brief discussion of which seems appropriate here.

Standardization and Evaluation of Method.   Application of scientific techniques to the management of industry has resulted in a high degree of standardization in working conditions, processes, and products. Time, energy, and materials are wasted and products are unequal in quality when production methods, tools, and working conditions vary from those found to give optimal results. Where the process is a mechanical one, uniformity of the product desired is important. Impressed with the rapid advances in industry brought about by standardization, workers in other fields have adopted the same principles. The results, however, are often disastrous. Attempts to standardize education, religion, music, or any of the arts are generally believed to have an unwholesome effect. In the arts, standardization seems to destroy initiative and to produce a mediocre product. If these generalizations are true, the question resolves itself into one of deciding which, if any, nursing activities are like industrial processes that can be profitably standardized and which are characteristic of an art that when it is standardized ceases to be an art.

An analysis of nursing has led many authorities to refer to it as both an art and a science. Adapting nursing care and medical treatment to the individual patient is certainly an art. On the other hand, the nurse and the physician often have technical tasks to perform. For example, the nurse is in some situations responsible for sterilization of equipment for, let us say, a drug given intravenously; the physician is ordinarily responsible for preparation of the drug. Both of these tasks are technical and should be highly standardized.

In operating a hospital, as in managing a home, there are many processes, many technical problems, concerned with inanimate things: cleaning floors, laundering clothes, heating and lighting homes, washing dishes, and ordering and transporting supplies. An efficient way of doing any of these having been found, it is obviously economical to standardize the method. Time, energy, and materials are wasted if different tools are used each day, if they are stored in different places, and if the product is so varied in quality that the process has to be repeated.

In contrast to the mechanical aspects of operating a home or an institution, however, are the activities involving human relationships. For example, guests must be received and welcomed, meals must be modified according to age and the likes and dislikes of those concerned, and furnishings selected with reference to the size and age of those who are to use them. Suppose these activities become standardized; suppose the greeting is stereotyped, the Sunday dinner always the same, the clothing alike for everyone, the beds the same size, the blankets the same weight, and the chairs the same height. Under such circumstances there is far less comfort and pleasure in living than when individual needs and desires are considered.

Carrying this into the field of treatment and nursing care, suppose every patient is given bath water of the same temperature, the same quantity of infusion, and is catheterized with a tube of uniform size, no matter how the anatomical structure of individuals differs.

Anyone can see immediately the danger of standardization where human beings are concerned. The fact that no two persons are identical means that each responds differently and that he should be treated as an individual. Not only is the charm of human relationships destroyed by standardization, but there is also a possibility that irreparable injuries may be done to the person who deviates markedly from the average. These few examples may serve to illustrate the point that mechanical activities associated with nursing and medicine, as, for example, the marking and preparation of drugs, cleaning and sterilization of supplies, may be standardized, but aspects of all treatments concerned with the patient must vary with the needs of each person.

Directions for any medical or nursing procedure should state which factors are to remain constant and which must be modified by the patient's needs. Within nursing organizations it is highly desirable to have a committee or committees constantly studying and evaluating nursing procedures. In order to estimate their reliability, some common standards of measurement must be agreed upon. Isabel M. Stewart,[1] discussing the "Possibilities of Standardization in Nursing Technique" in 1919, emphasized the importance of using flexible standards. She said in effect that the reliability of each procedure should be judged on the following basis:

1. Does it provide maximal *safety* for the patient, the nurse, and other persons involved?

2. Is it *therapeutically effective?*

3. Does it provide the greatest degree of *comfort and happiness (or least amount of pain) for the patient* that is consistent with accomplishing the therapeutic aim?

4. Is it as *economical* of time, effort, and materials as it can be made without sacrificing the first three factors?

5. Does the equipment present a pleasing appearance and [does] the performance give an impression of finished workmanship?

6. Is the procedure as *simple* as it can be made without destroying its therapeutic effectiveness, safety, and comfort, and is it *adaptable* to hospital and home nursing?

The writer suggests that another criterion be added:

7. Does it provide for maximum patient independence, participation, and learning?

Miss Stewart might have intended that items 2 and 3 be interpreted to include 7.

Acceptance and application of these standards result in flexibility. If the comfort of the patient enters into the picture, methods must vary with the individual's physical and aesthetic reaction. There is great variation, for example, in reaction to temperature. What is comfortable for one person is unbearably hot or disagreeably cool to another; an injection of a liter of water into the colon may be painless to one patient but may cause agonizing pain to another who has a fresh abdominal wound.

Hospital nursing methods are often unnecessarily complex and wasteful. When an institutional nurse is introduced to visiting nursing, she is amazed to find that she can carry out any nursing procedure and most of the common therapeutic procedures with the equipment she carries in a small bag, supplemented by what is found in an ordinary home. She soon realizes that sterile towels are unnecessary in catheterization, that often soap and water may be effectively used in place of the many skin antiseptics employed in hospitals, and that a sterile solution may be poured on a compress from a pan or applied with a syringe to make a sterile hot wet dressing, instead of using forceps and other expensive equipment.

These are only a few instances; hundreds might be cited to show that, if the reliability of procedures is held up to these criteria, the result will be a method that will be consistent with certain principles but will vary with the particular needs of each patient and the available facilities.

Scientific Basis for Nursing Methods. To make a procedure safe, therapeutically

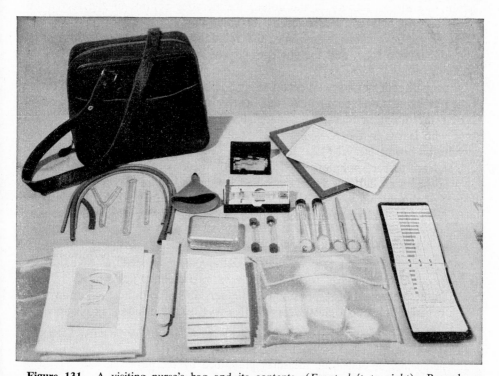

Figure 131. A visiting nurse's bag and its contents. (*Front, left to right*): Records as needed in plastic case (family folder, family health record, fee book, physician's instruction sheet, postcards, V.N.A. cards), apron, cord tie in coin envelope, tongue depressors in envelope, paper towels, plastic case (containing cord dressings, cotton balls, paper cups, Denco,* safety pins), nurse's handbook. (*Background, left to right*): Small catheter (#12 French), rectal tubes (medium, #18 French; large, #24 French), small piece of rubber tubing, glass connecting tubes (1 straight and 1 Y tube), test tube, rubber funnel, soap and soap dish, needles with stylettes (2 subcutaneous, #25, in hypodermic case; 2 intramuscular, #21 and #22, in glass needle holder; 2 intramuscular #19 and 1 #21, 1 in., in glass needle holder), hypodermic syringes (1 2-cc syringe in case, 1 5-cc syringe in box), file for ampoules, thermometers (oral, 2 in vial of 90% isopropyl alcohol; rectal, 2 in vial of 90% isopropyl alcohol), surgical scissors, forceps (or clamp). (Courtesy of Visiting Nurse Association of Brooklyn, Brooklyn, N. Y., and Clay-Adams Co., New York City.)

* Preparation used at the time this photograph was taken for making urinalysis.

effective, or even comfortable for the patient, it is necessary to know a good deal about physiology, chemistry, physics, bacteriology, and psychology. An ignorant person may learn a "model method" of giving an enema, memorizing the temperature to use, the amount of solution, the height of the can (pressure of the fluid), and the position of the patient. The model method may be satisfactory for the average person, but totally unsuitable for the postoperative case, the highly nervous individual, the person with hemorrhoids, or a paralyzed patient.

Intelligent adaptation of the procedure of giving an enema depends upon such scientific knowledge as the capacity of the colon, the structure of the anus and rectum, the motor activity of the colon, the nervous control of the rectum, the factors influencing pressure exerted by the solution and the rate of flow, the effect of chemicals on mucous membrane, the relationship between emotional excitement and muscle tone, and the susceptibility of mucous membrane to injury and infection.

In many directions we see an encouraging emphasis put upon principles. Teachers of the nursing arts are encouraging students to criticize, select, and modify methods, keeping the attention focused on fundamental principles rather than on rules. A nurse who learns in the physiological laboratory that the immersion of a muscle in water as hot as 50° C (122° F) stops the contraction of the muscle does not have to learn to keep solutions used for body irrigations below this point. The person who has seen cultures from unwashed hands and those cleaned with varying degrees of thoroughness does not have to learn by rule to wash his hands before going from one patient to another and to use sterile gloves if surgical asepsis is indicated.

Professional Responsibilities in Relation to Method. If nursing is a profession, its members must accept responsibility for studying its procedures and designing its methods. Overlapping of function in the various medical fields has led to confusion in the placement of responsibility. The nursing staff of a hospital or any other health organization might classify procedures used into the following groups:

1. Hygienic measures that may be prescribed and carried out by the nurse.
Examples: cleansing bath, cleaning the mouth.
2. Therapeutic or diagnostic measures prescribed by the physician and carried out by the nurse.
Examples: eye irrigation, hot wet dressing to a wound, or a subcutaneous injection of a drug.
3. Therapeutic or diagnostic measures prescribed by the physician and administered by him with the assistance of the nurse.
Examples: intravenous injection, lumbar puncture, irrigation of the ureter.
4. Therapeutic or diagnostic measures prescribed and administered by the physician without the assistance of the nurse.
Example: x-ray of some parts of the body, certain blood tests, or an encephalogram.

It would seem that a nursing committee should take full responsibility for the first group; this same committee should initiate and assume the major share of responsibility for the second group but work with medical representatives as consultants or as members of the committee. Physicians on the staff should assume responsibility for the third group and take the initiative in revising such procedures, but since the nursing staff also is vitally concerned, nursing representatives should work with the physicians as consultants or as members of the committee. Methods used for the fourth group of procedures are obviously the responsibility of the medical staff.

The work of procedure investigation and revision is unending, with unlimited possibilities and interest. Problems that arise carry the student into every field of science. A hospital or visiting nurse staff should be organized so as to utilize all available resources. Nurses and physicians will find that they need not only mutual assistance but also the cooperation of bacteriologists, chemists, physicists, nutritionists, psychologists, economists, special therapists, and social service workers. The most effective type of organization for the study of methods is one that facilitates cooperation among all these groups.

REFERENCE

1. Stewart, Isabel M.: "Possibilities of Standardization in Nursing Technique," *Mod. Hosp.,* **44:**46, (Oct.) 1919.

Additional Suggested Reading

American College of Surgeons: *Manual of Hospital Standardization.* The College, Chicago, 1946.
American Hospital Association, Committee on Simplification and Standardization of Hospital Furnishings, Supplies and Equipment . . .: *Manual of Specifications for the Purchase of Hospital Supplies and Equipment,* Bulletin 208. The Association, Chicago, 1940.
American Hospital Association: *Hospital Records Administration; Manual of Procedure.* The Association, Chicago, 1949.
Barnes, Ralph M.: *Motion and Time Study,* 3rd ed. John Wiley & Sons, New York, 1949.
Kitchell, Myrtle E.: "Analyzing and Developing Nursing Procedures," *Am. J. Nursing,* **51:**179, (Mar.) 1951.
Levitt, W. M.: "Liability of Manufacturers for Injuries to Patients from Defective Apparatus," *Brit. M. J.,* **2:**1122, (Nov.) 1950.
MacEachern, Malcolm T.: *Hospital Organization and Management,* rev. ed. Physicians Record Co., Chicago, 1940.
Smith, Martha R. (ed.): *An Introduction to the Principles of Nursing Care,* 2nd ed. J. B. Lippincott Co., Philadelphia, 1939, p. 395.
US Public Health Service, Division of Nursing Resources: *For Better Nursing in Michigan.* Cunningham Drug Co. Foundation, Detroit, Mich., 1954.

CHAPTER 21. BATHS AND PACKS

1. PRINCIPLES UNDERLYING THERAPEUTIC BATHS AND PACKS

Baths and packs are used in the treatment of inflammatory conditions of the joints and nerves, such as arthritis and neuritis, or conditions of the pelvic organs, such as painful menstruation or prostatitis; or they may be prescribed in skin diseases as, for example, scabies and urticaria, in which relief is afforded by chemicals in the baths. Baths at body temperature are used to relieve tension and induce sleep; cold packs are also sedative because they soon reach body temperature. Cool sponge and spray baths are prescribed for the relief of discomfort and the reduction of temperature in fevers, although none of these treatments is used now as frequently as in the past.

Heat is applied in the form of hot air, steam, or vapor, and water. Heliotherapy is the use of light rays in the treatment of disease; infrared rays have a heat effect.

General applications of heat are rarely used for seriously ill patients; they have a profound effect, beneficial or harmful, according to the intelligence and skill with which they are applied. Before attempting to give these treatments, the nurse should know the patient's condition, the disease from which he is suffering, the action of heat, the effects desired, and how the particular procedure should be carried out to achieve the desired effect. Rebekah Wright says:

Like our most potent drugs, hydrotherapy is a "two-edged sword." Good results depend not alone upon the prescribing physician's knowledge of the subject and the mental and physical condition of his patient but also upon the intelligence, training, tact, kindness, firmness and fidelity of the nurse who administers the treatment. The technique of hydrotherapy is one of the specialties of nursing. The treatments should be administered by a capable graduate nurse who is conscientious in reporting observation of effects.*

John S. Coulter and George M. Piersol, discussing the physiological reactions from general application of water, say:

The effect of immersing the entire body in water is to bring about changes in temperature. The stated mean skin temperature of the healthy adult is about 33.9° C (93° F). If the water is generally applied above body temperature, a rise in the patient's temperature will occur. If the temperature of the water is below that of the body, the opposite effect is produced.†

The results depend upon: (1) the difference between the patient's skin temperature and that of the bath or pack; (2) the suddenness of the application; (3) the method of applying the hot or cold medium; (4) the extent of the skin surface covered by the bath or pack; and (5) the duration of the treatment.

The effect of heat and the results of both local and general applications, but particularly the latter, depend upon the condition of the subject, the age, weight, vitality, and individual reaction, the basis for which is not understood. Victor R. Ott, discussing "the physiological basis of hydrotherapy and allied methods of physical medicine," in Francis Bach's text,[1] makes a point of these opposite effects of heat in different persons. He cites studies of the blood sugar levels and the heart action of subjects during and immediately following hot baths. Some of them showed the physiological response typical of stimulation of the sympathetic division of the autonomic nervous system; others, an opposing reaction characteristic of stimulation of the parasympathetic division of the autonomic system. This suggests to Ott the necessity of studying the specific effect of hydrotherapy on each patient.

A tabulation of the effects of hot and cold on the average person appears on page 616. The data are compiled from several sections of the American Medical Association's *Handbook of Physical Medicine and Rehabilitation,*[2] Frank H. Krusen's *Physical Medicine,*[3] Krusen's *Physical Medicine and Rehabilitation for the Clinician,*[4] William Bierman and Sidney Licht's *Physical Medicine in General Practice,*[5] and Richard Kovac's *A Manual of Physical Therapy.*[6]

Cold applications can be very injurious if they are prolonged, or if the patient hasn't sufficient vitality to carry the effects into the "reaction" phase. Elderly and

* Wright, Rebekah: *Hydrotherapy in Psychiatric Hospitals.* Tudor Press, Inc., Boston, 1940, p. 96.

† American Medical Association, Council on Physical Medicine and Rehabilitation: *Handbook of Physical Medicine and Rehabilitation.* Blakiston Co., Philadelphia, 1950, p. 175.

Comparative Effects of Cold and Hot Applications

EFFECT OF BRIEF APPLICATIONS OF COLD (TONIC EFFECT)	EFFECT OF BRIEF APPLICATIONS OF HEAT (ATONIC EFFECT)
1. Peripheral vasoconstriction (pale skin)	1. Peripheral vasodilatation (reddened skin)
2. Sensation of chilliness and tension	2. Sensation of warmth and general relaxation as bath progresses
3. Increase in output of blood with each heartbeat. Some authorities say the pulse rate is increased; others that it is decreased	3. Decrease in output of blood with each heartbeat is probable. The pulse rate tends to rise 10 beats with each degree Fahrenheit of body temperature
4. Increase in depth and rate of respiration	4. Increase in respiratory rate. One authority says the fall in alveolar carbon dioxide may produce an alkalosis. The pH is said to rise from 0.1 to 0.3 during the hot bath
5. Rise in blood pressure	5. Fall in blood pressure, although this effect varies
6. Shivering, leading to increased heat production and the "reaction" to cold that lasts from 20 to 30 minutes	6. Decrease in heat production and profuse sweating
Reaction effect	7. Increase in number and motility of leukocytes
Peripheral vasodilatation with reddened skin	
Sensation of warmth and relaxation	
Decreased pulse rate with increased cardiac output	
Decreased respiratory rate	
Fall in blood pressure	

debilitated subjects rarely "react" to general applications of cold; therefore, they are seldom prescribed for them or anyone with lowered vitality. Whenever cold treatments are used, temperatures should be modified to suit the condition of the patient; the more robust, the lower the temperature tolerated, as a rule.

Generalized hot applications can be so debilitating that the patient is prostrated. These treatments are rarely seen now. In the recent past, artificial fever produced with hot-water, vapor, and light baths has been used to combat infection. Other agents (the sulfonamides and antibiotics) have so nearly replaced this therapy that a discussion of it seems unnecessary.

Many hydrotherapeutic procedures include the contrasting effects of heat and cold. Hot-water or vapor baths are followed by cold showers, or extremities are immersed alternately in hot and cold water.

Hot baths are occasionally used in general nursing, but if they are prescribed they are more likely to be given in a hydrotherapy department under the direction of experts.

Temperatures to be used in hydrotherapy and heliotherapy should be prescribed by the physician. Temperature equivalents are given from two recognized sources:

ADJECTIVE USED TO DESCRIBE TEMPERATURES	A.M.A.: Handbook of Physical Medicine and Rehabilitation*		REBEKAH WRIGHT: Hydrotherapy in Psychiatric Hospitals†
	Centigrade	Fahrenheit	Fahrenheit
Very cold	Below 13°	Below 55°	32° to 60°
Cold	13° to 18°	55° to 65°	60° to 70°
Cool	18° to 27°	65° to 80°	70° to 80°
Tepid	27° to 34°	80° to 93°	80° to 90°
Neutral or warm	34° to 37°	93° to 98°	92° to 97° (neutral)
Hot	37° to 40.5°	98° to 105°	94° to 98° (warm) 98° to 104°
Very hot	40.5° to 46°	105° to 115°	104° to 120°

* American Medical Association, Council on Physical Medicine and Rehabilitation: *Handbook of Physical Medicine and Rehabilitation.* Blakiston Co., Philadelphia, 1950, p. 174.
† Wright, Rebekah: *Hydrotherapy in Psychiatric Hospitals.* Tudor Press, Inc., Boston, 1940, p. 94.

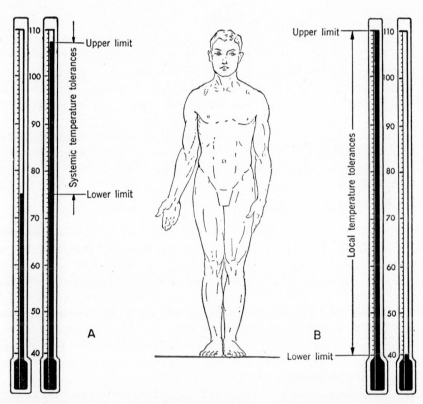

Figure 132. Temperature limits of the viable human body. Temperatures which can be tolerated for long periods of time without producing irreversible changes. (*A*) Systemic; (*B*) local. The indicated upper limit of systemic temperature is 107° F; the lower limit 75° F. The temperature tolerances of local tissues vary between 110° and 40° F. (Bierman, William: *Physical Medicine in General Practice.* Paul B. Hoeber, New York, 1944.)

617

Several authorities comment on the high degree of discrimination that some normal subjects have for temperature of immersion baths. The difference of 1 deg can often be recognized. On the other hand, particularly with local application of heat, the greatest care must be taken to protect the patient without a high degree of discrimination. He may be burned. Morris B. Bender[7] found that if stimuli are applied simultaneously to two points on the body, for example, the face and the leg, the person is aware of only one stimulus. The face sensation will, in this case, take precedence over, or obliterate, that of the leg. In like manner, severe pain in any body area, or a strong emotion, can obliterate the sense of discomfort from heat; therefore, the patient may be burned without his awareness. *Any form of heat applied to living tissue should be measured with a thermometer.*

Hydrotherapy and other means of lowering or raising the systemic or local body temperature have been used in the treatment of almost every known disease. Because water is the most universal solvent it is used in conjunction with drugs for their chemical or physical effects. It is needless for nurses to try to memorize *all the uses* of heat and cold. Rather, they should study the physiological action of different temperatures. This will enable them to understand why a cold, neutral, or hot application should be used; they will also be able to carry out procedures more critically. Figures 137 and 139 show the response of capillaries to heat and cold. Seeing a microscopic moving film in which the vasodilation from a hot application is shown to persist for several hours usually convinces the nurse that hot dressings can promote healing of wounds. Watching a film that depicts the vasoconstriction of capillaries with the application of cold should explain the reduction in swelling after a sprain, for example, when cold compresses are applied. Treatment by water and sunlight has been used throughout the ages and in all cultures. It is not possible to list all the hydrotherapeutic measures the nurse is likely to encounter. Tabular material on page 619 is an attempt to organize those most frequently mentioned in medical texts under general applications of heat and cold.

The *dangers* of excessive and prolonged cold and hot environments have been discussed in Chapter 5 and 10; they are also treated in Chapter 43. Immersion of the body in cold and hot water and in steam has an effect similar to, but more marked than, surrounding it with cold and hot air. Danger of prolonged local applications of intense cold and heat is similar in that both paralyze the discriminatory power of the skin and interfere with the circulation.

To avoid injury from local applications of heat and cold, the physician should prescribe (1) the method and area to be covered, (2) the temperature of the application, and (3) the duration of the treatment. In many cases alternating applications of heat and cold prevent local hemostasis. Nurses must be alert to skin discoloration and sensory changes.

In general applications of heat and cold there is a redistribution of the circulating fluids. Cerebral congestion can be controlled by cold applications to the forehead or back of the neck. Chilliness is mitigated by a hot application to the feet. These two practices are nearly always followed in giving sponge, spray, and hot-air baths as well as packs.

Types of General Cold, Neutral, and Hot
Hydrotherapeutic Applications

COLD	NEUTRAL	HOT
1. *Immersion* (water) *bath* for tonic effect	1. *Immersion* (water) *bath* for sedative effect; if prolonged, it is called "continuous bath"	1. *Immersion* (water) *bath* to induce sweating and relaxation
3. *Shower* or *douche* for tonic effect. Often alternated with hot shower or douche	2. *Shower* or *douche* for sedative effect	2. *Shower* or *douche* to induce relaxation. Often alternated with cold shower or douche
3. *Wet sheet pack* with blanket wrapping for sedative effect	3. *Wet sheet pack* with blanket wrapping for sedative effect (used when patient cannot tolerate cold packs)	3. *Wet sheet pack* with blanket wrapping usually to induce sweating; occasionally to induce sedation
4. *Wet sheet* or *towel application* ("pack") for temperature reduction	4. *Sponge bath* for temperature reduction—water, or water and alcohol	4. *Steam bath* to induce relaxation and sweating (prolonged use for production of artificial fever or fever therapy)
5. *Spray bath* or affusion for temperature reduction (patient recumbent)	5. *Spray bath* or affusion for temperature reduction (patient recumbent)	5. *Hot-air bath* or hot-air cabinet to induce relaxation and sweating (prolonged use for production of artificial fever or fever therapy)
6. *Cold wet hand rub* for tonic effect	6. *Medicated baths* for sedation or for soothing or antiseptic effect on skin (a) "Nauheim"—water baths charged with gas for sedation (b) Starch, bran, or other cereal, and sodium salts for soothing effect on skin (c) Sulfur for antiseptic effect on skin	6. *Medicated baths:* Mustard to induce relaxation in actual or threatened convulsions, especially in babies
7. *Medicated baths* for tonic effect (a) Saline (b) "Nauheim"—water baths charged with gas for tonic effect		

To guard against injurious effects, the pulse and respiration are taken before and after generalized hydrotherapy, and, if prolonged, they are checked at intervals. The bath or pack is terminated if the patient is reacting unfavorably according to these signs or to what he says.

The types of general cold, neutral, and hot hydrotherapeutic applications are shown above. For a full description of these methods the nurse should consult such standard texts on physical medicine as those in the list of references for this chapter. The following description of some selected methods is largely based on these sources.

2. HOT TUB BATH

Selection of Method. This bath is similar to the cleansing bath with which everyone is familiar; it needs no definition. It is sometimes prescribed to induce sweating or to relax muscles, tendons, and ligaments in the treatment of arthritis. It is ordered for its relaxing effect, but if the water is very hot and contact with it very brief, the result is excitement and muscular contraction rather than relaxation. The temperature should rarely exceed 41.1 C (106 F). The bath should not last more than 10 minutes. (N.B. A warm or neutral rather than a hot bath should be used for a sedative effect.)

Suggested Procedure. Underlying principles and precautions to be observed in giving the hot tub bath are the same as in all general applications of heat. Note the pulse, the patient's breathing, color, and expression for symptoms of excitement or signs of cerebral congestion, such as headache, nausea, and vertigo. To avert such reactions, apply cold compresses or an icecap to the head and raise the temperature of the bath slowly until perspiration begins.

Normal rate of perspiration is 1 or 1½ oz per hour or 2 pt in 24 hours, but by hot applications this may be increased to more than an ounce a minute. Remember that the loss of so much fluid has a very depressing effect on the heart, similar to that of hemorrhage. Except in edematous or dropsical conditions, encourage copious drinking of water before and during the bath.

Take every precaution to avoid burning the patient. The *temperature* of the water varies from 36.7° to 40° C (98° to 104° F), although sometimes, depending on the patient's condition and the effect desired, it may be increased, but never above 43.3° C (110° F). The *duration* varies from 2 to 30 minutes. After the bath the patient should lie down for at least 1 hour.

3. SEDATIVE BATH

Definition. A bath surrounding the skin with an environment free from irritation or stimuli is called a sedative bath because it favors relaxation and sleep. It is also called a neutral bath because the water is kept at about the same temperature as that of the skin, or around 33.3° C (92° F).

Therapeutic Uses. The sedative bath is used principally in insomnia to induce sleep and muscular relaxation, whenever indicated. A neutral bath is used also in diseases of the heart and blood vessels, when hot or cold applications must be avoided because they tax the circulation.

Selection of Method. A bath at body temperature produces no marked change, either thermal or circulatory, but surrounds the body with a medium that shields it from all external stimuli or irritation of nerve endings from air, clothing, pressure, and changes in temperature. The bath is therefore soothing and quieting. If the body is supported, the patient often sleeps in a neutral bath. Until recently sedative baths were widely used in the treatment of psychiatric patients, but some current texts on therapy barely mention them or omit any reference whatever.[8]

Hydrotherapeutic measures are at best palliative, and with the development of shock therapy and various forms of psychotherapy less emphasis is placed on them. Moreover, hydrotherapy demands more personnel and equipment than many of our overcrowded, understaffed psychiatric hospitals can boast. Insomnia and tension in many patients, even in general hospitals and homes, could, however, be relieved with sedative baths.

Suggested Procedure. The sedative bath is given in a full tub at a *temperature* from 33.3° to 36.1° C (92° to 97° F). Its good effects depend upon maintenance of the proper temperature. Its *duration* varies from 15 minutes to 1 hour, and the best time for it is just before bedtime. The subject then has the necessary rest following the bath with no danger from chilling.

In homes a sedative bath can be taken with ordinary bathroom facilities by simply regulating the temperature of the water. Physiotherapy departments and certain bathrooms in psychiatric divisions of general hospitals are provided with special tubs for prolonged or "continuous" sedative baths.

4. CONTINUOUS BATH

Definition. When the sedative bath is continued for hours or days, it is called a continuous bath. The effect on the nervous system is the same as that of the sedative bath.

Therapeutic Uses. Continuous baths are used (1) to quiet motor and psychic activity in diseases of the nervous system when the patient is hyperactive, excited, and unable to sleep; (2) in certain skin diseases; (3) in badly infected wounds; and (4) in extensive burns and bedsores. Some physicians believe the healing process is stimulated by continuous baths; others think that it is hard for the body to form granulations and scar tissue when macerated with water. A great disadvantage of the bath lies in the fact that it cannot be made aseptic.

Suggested Procedure. Support the patient on a hammock or other device with the body immersed, the head resting comfortably on a rubber pillow. Apply cold compresses or an icecap to the brow or nape of the neck. Watch the patient very closely and take special care to see that the neutral temperature of the water is maintained. It should be changed at least every 12 hours and the tub thoroughly cleaned. In a hydrotherapeutic department there are special tubs with provision for a constant removal of water and a fresh supply at the desired temperature. In many hospitals the water is thermostatically controlled, so that when the mechanism is set, no further adjustment is necessary. In any case, however, the thermometer should be suspended in the water so that the nurse can check the temperature.

Rub the patient's skin with petroleum jelly or oil to prevent maceration. Cover the tub with a sheet during the treatment so that there is no exposure of the patient. (Restraining devices that are buckled to the sides of the tub have been used for irrational patients.) Take care to prevent chilling the patient by wrapping him warmly at the termination of the treatment or if he has to leave the tub temporarily to empty the bladder or bowel, and by having him rest in bed afterward for several hours.

5. COLD OR TEPID SPONGE BATHS

Therapeutic Uses.   General cold baths are given in febrile conditions to relieve discomfort, to stimulate the circulation, and, where high temperatures exist, as in heatstroke, to reduce temperature. If used for temperature reduction, the treatment must be continued for some time to make it effective.

In the hydrotherapy department, cold spray and slush baths and cold douches are used for their tonic effect.

In the cold wet hand rub and the cold sponge bath, the *temperature* varies from 4.4° to 24° C (40° to 75.2° F) or from 18.3° to 32.2° C (65° to 90° F), according to the age of the patient and his ability to react. The *duration* is usually about 10 minutes.

Suggested Procedure.   Before starting the treatment bring everything required to the bedside. See that the room is warm. Cover the patient with a large sheet, while fanfolding the bedclothes to the foot of the bed; remove the pillows and gown. Adjust a loin cloth and place a large waterproof rectangle covered with a sheet under the patient to protect the bed. See that the body is warm before the treatment is given. Apply brief friction first to stimulate the skin, prevent chilling, and hasten the reaction. Place a hot-water bottle at the feet for comfort and to encourage the desired vascular reaction. Apply cold compresses to the head.

During the treatment the upper sheet may be removed, or it may be manipulated so that the parts under treatment are exposed in succession, then covered as reaction sets in. Vasodilatation should be induced by rubbing. Two nurses may give the treatment, one applying water with her hands or with washcloths to the face, anterior surface of the trunk, and upper extremities, while the second nurse treats the lower extremities; this should last 3 minutes. The patient is then turned and the posterior surfaces treated, beginning with the neck, shoulders, chest, and so on, with special attention to the spine; this might take 7 minutes.

Watch the patient's color and pulse; if there is any indication that he is reacting unfavorably, discontinue the treatment immediately and report his condition to the physician.

When the bath is completed, pat the skin dry and cover the patient with the sheet. Remove the waterproof protector and sheet under the patient and put a warm gown on him. Arrange the pillows and bedding to make the patient comfortable. A tonic reaction to cold is promoted by hot drinks.

6. ALCOHOL SPONGE BATH

Definition.   The alcohol sponge bath is a tepid or cold bath given with a 25 to 50 per cent solution of alcohol.

Therapeutic Uses.   The alcohol sponge bath is prescribed for the same purposes as the tepid- or cold-water sponge—when the patient is to be disturbed as little as possible with turning or moving. Since alcohol evaporates at a lower temperature than water, the sponged parts dry more quickly, the patient's reaction is less violent, and the bedding is not so likely to be wet by the bath.

Suggested Procedure. Give the bath in the same manner as the cold sponge just described. Since, however, the alcohol solution evaporates so quickly, no rubber protectors are necessary for the bed, and, therefore, it is not necessary to turn the patient so often. Bath towels are placed at either side of the patient and under the legs. The sponge or washcloth should be only slightly wet. The back may be rubbed with the hand, moistened with alcohol, instead of with the sponge and, if advisable, without turning the patient.

7. SALINE BATH

Definition. This is an artificial sea-water bath, in which 8 lb of sea salt to 30 gal of water are used. By using 5 to 8 lb of ordinary table salt, practically the same effects may be produced. For partial baths, use 4 oz of salt to 1 qt of water.

Therapeutic Uses. Cold saline baths are used for their tonic effect. Health claims of the spas are based, rightly or wrongly, on the effect of the salts in their local waters.

Selection of Method. Sea water feels much warmer than fresh because the salt irritates or stimulates the nerves in the skin and so hastens vasodilatation. The *temperature* of the bath is usually 21.1° C (70° F). The *duration* is usually 10 minutes, with friction during and after the bath. The usual precautions are taken to prevent chilling or exhaustion.

8. ALKALINE BATHS

Definition. An alkaline bath is one of natural alkaline waters or a bath prepared by the addition of an alkaline salt such as sodium bicarbonate to water.

Therapeutic Uses. Alkaline baths are most commonly used in skin diseases, to relieve itching.

Suggested Procedure. Add 4 to 12 oz of sodium bicarbonate to 30 gal of water. For local applications ½ oz of sodium bicarbonate to 1 qt, or up to 8 oz of sodium bicarbonate to 1 gal, of water may be used. The *temperature* of the water should be about 36.7° C (98° F).

Encourage the patient to lie quietly in the bath for the prescribed duration. Do not apply friction during or after the bath. At its termination, wrap the patient in a sheet that has been warmed and dry by gently patting over it.

9. SULFUR BATH

Definition. A sulfur bath is a water bath (usually warm) to which potassium sulfate is added.

Therapeutic Uses. Sulfur is very toxic to lower forms of vegetable life. It is used extensively in the form of an ointment and occasionally in the form of a bath in acne and in other skin diseases such as scabies, where it is lethal to the itch mite lying within the burrows it has made in the skin. (A mixture of benzyl benzoate, DDT, benzocaine, and an emulsifier is perhaps more often used now for scabies.)

Suggested Procedure. Dissolve from ½ to 2 oz of potassium sulfate in a small amount of hot water and add this to the bath water (15 gal). The *temperature* of the bath usually varies from 32.2° to 35.6° C (90° to 96° F); the *duration,* from 10 to 30 minutes.

Metal bath tubs should be protected, as sulfur corrodes them. When the bath is given to relieve infectious skin diseases the tub must be decontaminated after use. (The writer believes this treatment is now rare.)

10. MUSTARD BATH

Definition. A mustard bath is a warm- or hot-water bath to which powdered mustard is added.

Therapeutic Uses. Mustard is an irritant, inducing vasodilatation. It is sometimes used to relieve the spasm or convulsions of infants and young children.

Suggested Procedure. Add 1 tbsp of mustard to 1 gal of water for a child of 10 years; half this much, for infants. The mustard must be mixed into a paste with tepid water in the usual way, then further dissolved and thoroughly stirred into the bath water.

Suit the *temperature* to the patient's condition, but it may be lower than when water alone is used. It is usually 26.7° to 32.2° C (80° to 90° F), if the full effect of the mustard is desired. When the temperature is from 40.6° to 43.3° C (105° to 110° F), the mustard helps at first by hastening the desired reaction, but its effect is soon destroyed by the heat. The *duration* of the bath is prescribed by the physician, but the patient must be removed from the tub when the skin is a rosy pink.

11. EMOLLIENT OR SOOTHING BATHS

Definition. An emollient bath is a neutral tub bath to which some substance such as starch or a cereal has been added.

Therapeutic Uses. The bath is used to relieve skin irritation.

Suggested Procedure. Add 1 lb of corn starch or 4 to 6 lb of bran to 30 gal of water. The starch is boiled into a smooth paste, or the bran is boiled in a bag for 20 minutes. Either must be strained to remove large particles that would clog the plumbing. The thick liquid is then added to, and mixed thoroughly with, the bath water. The *temperature* is usually from 33.9° to 35.6° C (93° to 96° F).*

12. HOT PACK

Definition. A general hot pack is the application of blankets wrung out of water as hot as the patient can endure without pain or injury. A second wrapping of dry blankets is used to delay cooling of the hot wet pack.

---

* Aveeno is a patented colloid fraction of oatmeal prepared for baths and made by the Musher Foundation, Inc., New York. Its chief advantage is that it requires no boiling or straining.

Therapeutic Uses. A hot pack was at one time prescribed in diseases accompanied by suppression of urine; for example, nephritis, uremic poisoning, bichloride of mercury poisoning, and eclampsia.

Results desired are sweating, relief of edema, elimination of waste products not eliminated by the kidneys, and lowering of arterial tension. A review of medical literature shows, however, that the therapeutic value of the hot wet pack is questioned, and there is considerable doubt whether it produces any such results as was once believed. There is great question about the ability of the skin, during packs or at any other time, to eliminate in appreciable quantities wastes ordinarily eliminated by the kidneys. Granted that the skin might help to do the work of the kidneys, many physicians believe that any benefit derived from stimulation of perspiration is overbalanced by water loss and exhaustion produced by the pack. Hot local packs used in poliomyelitis are described in Chapter 22, but the enveloping general hot pack is so rarely used that a description here is scarcely justified. Dana W. Atchley, who advocated their use in the past, says repeatedly in the 1951 revision of Russell L. Cecil and Robert F. Loeb's *Textbook of Medicine* that purges and sweatings are useless and often harmful in the condition for which hot packs were used.[9, 10]

13. COLD AND TEPID PACKS FOR THE REDUCTION OF TEMPERATURE

Definition. A temperature-reducing pack is one in which the body is enveloped in wet sheets or towels applied at a temperature lower than that of the body.

Therapeutic Uses. So-called antipyretic packs are used to reduce dangerously high fever. They are also used as sponge baths are to make patients more comfortable and to stimulate the circulation when the body temperature goes above 39.4° C (103° F).

Selection of Method. When cold is applied to the body for the reduction of temperature, care must be taken to prevent the sensation of chilliness and the consequent muscular reaction of shivering. It has already been pointed out that shivering raises the body temperature, and if the treatment is given to make the patient more comfortable, this purpose is also defeated when the treatment is associated with the disagreeable sensation of being cold. This reaction is avoided by the use of friction accompanying the pack, which increases the blood supply in the skin. According to C. Lovatt Evans[11] and other physiologists, people feel warm when the cutaneous vessels are dilated and vice versa. Bringing blood to the skin with friction not only keeps the patient from being chilly but also hastens the reduction of temperature by increasing the volume of blood exposed to the cooling action of the pack.

It is obvious that, when a cold pack is used for the reduction of temperature, the patient, wrapped in the cold sheet or pack, must be exposed to the air. The cooling effect of the pack is largely due to the process of evaporation. When water is changed into vapor, heat is required for the physical process, and this heat is taken from the body.

The *temperature* of the water prescribed for an antipyretic pack varies from 15.6° to 36.1° C (60° to 97° F), the higher temperatures being more commonly used than very cold ones at the present because it is believed that very low temperatures are more likely to elicit the shivering reflex and the general tonic reaction of the body to intense cold.

The *duration* of the pack varies from 15 to 30 minutes, but the treatment is discontinued at any time if any unfavorable reaction occurs.

Suggested Procedure. Prepare the patient by removing the gown and applying a protector over the pubic area, covering the lower bedding with a large waterproof rectangle, and replacing the top covers with a bath blanket. Apply a hot-water bottle to the feet, and an icecap or cold compress to the forehead.

The pack can be given with 2 or 3 small cotton sheets or 6 bath towels; the object in both methods is to keep the body covered with cool wet cloths. Encase the body with the exception of the head, feet, and hands in wet sheets or wet bath towels. Keep sheets or towels cool by having an extra sheet or towel kept in a basin of water the prescribed temperature and used as a replacement when the heat of the skin warms the covering. When sheets are used, change them about every 5 minutes; when towels are used, keep them rotating almost constantly. Apply light friction over sheets or towels. At the termination of the treatment, which usually lasts 20 minutes, dry the patient, remove the rubber and wet sheets or towels, put a dry gown on the patient and leave him to rest with an icecap on his head and a hot-water bottle at his feet. If there is any tendency to chilliness during the treatment, the pack is removed and external warmth applied.

To see whether the treatment has reduced the fever, the temperature is taken and recorded just before and an hour after the pack. Record the pulse at these times and at intervals during the treatment as indicated by the patient's condition.

During febrile states the physician ordinarily prescribes a high fluid intake because of the excessive water loss. While the nurse is giving an antipyretic bath or pack, she has an excellent opportunity to urge the patient to drink such fluids as are included in his diet.

Recording the Treatment. Record the treatment, the time it was given, the duration, the temperature of the water used for the pack, the patient's temperature and pulse just before and an hour after the pack, and any marked reaction to the pack, favorable or unfavorable.

14. SEDATIVE PACK

Definition. Sedative packs are prolonged applications of wet sheets to the body. Evaporation and cooling of the sheets, and also motor activity, are controlled by wrapping the body tightly in blankets.

Therapeutic Uses. Sleeplessness, hyperactivity, and excitement are indications for the use of a sedative pack. These symptoms occur in organic and functional diseases of the nervous system and in abnormal mental states associated with many kinds of pathology. The action of a sedative pack is similar to that of the continuous sedative tub. The chief reason why it is more popular is probably because facilities for its use are more generally available, and it is a form of protective restraint for the hyperactive person.

Selection of Method. Sedation, or quieting the patient and inducing sleep, is the purpose of the pack. This result is chiefly accomplished by having the sheets wet with water at the proper temperature, by insulating the wet sheets with snug wrappings, by seeing that the body is in a comfortable position, by the removal of stimuli from the environment, by continuing the treatment until the subject is relieved, and possibly by preventing cerebral vasodilatation.

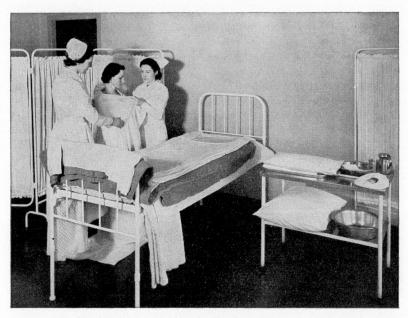

Figure 133. Patient and bed prepared for sedative pack. Patient draped with a sheet, dry blankets and wet sheets arranged on bed ready to be wrapped around the body; all other necessary articles assembled in the unit. (Courtesy of New York State Psychiatric Institute and Hospital, New York City.)

Attention was called in Chapter 15 to the various theories on sleep. The most generally favored are that sleep is induced by muscular relaxation, by reducing the blood volume in the brain, and by chemicals that inhibit the activity of brain cells. Treatments used to induce sleep are designed to bring about one or more of these conditions, depending on the theory or theories accepted by the physician prescribing them.

Of the various factors affecting the success of a sedative pack, the *temperature* of the sheets is possibly the most important. A study made by Marguerite Kennedy et al.[12] in 1936 showed that water ranging from 8.9° to 100° C (48° to 212° F) for wetting sheets in packs was being used at that time in 24 mental hospitals.

These workers experimented with temperatures of from 10° C to 100° C
(50° F to 212° F), using 15 young women in good health as subjects. The results of the investigation showed more complete relaxation and longer periods of
sleep with cold sheets than with hot. Wright recommends temperatures of 8.9° C
(48° F) for "the active robust" patient, 15.6° to 21.1°C (60° to 70° F) for patients of "average vitality," and 33.3° to 36.1° C (92° to 97° F) for less active patients. The less vigorous the person, the less able he is to stand low temperatures;
several authorities say that the temperature of the pack should be determined in

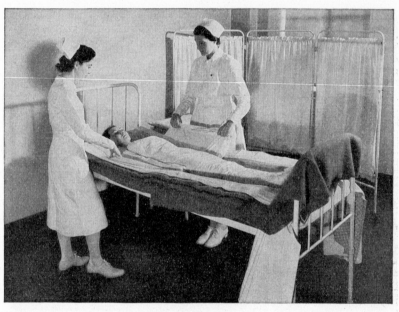

Figure 134. First sheet has been wrapped around the body so that skin surfaces are
separated. The second sheet is drawn around the arm and under the back, thereby limiting
motion. (Courtesy of New York State Psychiatric Institute and Hospital, New York City.)

each case by the condition of the individual and the room temperature. Age is an
important factor; elderly patients rarely respond favorably to cold. In some cases
temperatures of 42.2° C (108° F) are used for them. Wright recommends hot
foot baths as preparation for the sedative pack.

The *duration* of the treatment, as shown in the study of Kennedy and others,
varied from 20 minutes to 6 hours; the average period was 2 hours. It is questionable whether any appreciable relaxation is effected when the duration of the pack
is less than 1 hour, and longer periods seem desirable for the maximal benefit. If
the pack lasts more than 3 or 4 hours, it is usually necessary to remove the blankets
to enable the patient to void or defecate. When this necessity arises and it interrupts
the prescribed time period, the pack is replaced. In cases of involuntary micturition

or defecation, the patient must be removed from the pack, bathed, and re-enveloped in fresh sheets and blankets.

One of the most important points in the application of a pack is the proper adjustment of the sheets and blankets. It is important that the pack be snug, especially around the neck, so that there are no air pockets around the body; the covering must be smooth and the sheets so arranged that no skin surfaces touch. During the pack the patient perspires freely, and before sedation is accomplished, there may be friction from restless movements. In such cases excoriation is almost

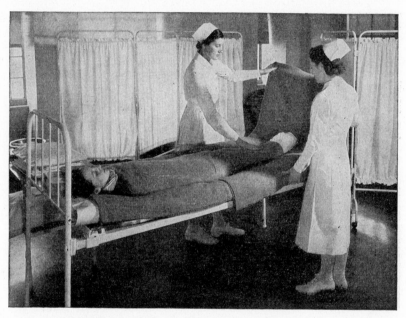

Figure 135. First blanket has been arranged mummy fashion, the second used to cover the feet, and the third applied like the first. Note sheet drawn over blanket at the neck. (Courtesy of New York State Psychiatric Institute and Hospital, New York City.)

certain to result if skin surfaces are not separated. It is also important to make sure that the arms are beside the body and not caught under it. There is a difference of opinion as to whether the feet should be wrapped in the wet sheets and blankets or only in the dry blankets. It probably makes little difference in the final result, but it may be easier to keep the feet warm if they are not first encased in cold sheets. The feet should be warmed by a hot-water bottle throughout the treatment.

In all cases it is desirable to have the body firmly encased in the sheets and blankets, but this is essential if the person is resisting the treatment. Excited, irrational patients will work themselves out of this covering or, wrapped like a cocoon, will bounce themselves off the bed. For this reason protection sheets are placed over the chest, and sometimes over the knees as well, in order to prevent such accidents.

Special restraining devices are used in a few institutions, but ordinarily the patient is held in bed with folded sheets that are fixed tightly around the rods that run lengthwise of the bedframe. The element of restraint is psychologically traumatic, and uncooperative patients are not forced to have this treatment if there are better sedative measures available.

Relaxation, which is such an important factor in promoting sleep, is not induced by the dorsal recumbent position unless the knees are flexed and supported. A pillow under the knees relaxes the leg, thigh, and abdomen. Lateral and supine

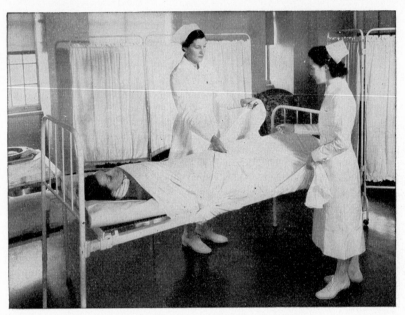

Figure 136. Diagonally folded sheets are tied over an uncooperative patient to prevent her from falling out of bed. (Courtesy of New York State Psychiatric Institute and Hospital, New York City.)

positions are impractical for the patient in a pack because the arms are bound to the body.

Appreciable amounts of fluid are lost during the pack in perspiration. It is therefore important to have this made up either before, during, or after the pack. The practice of forcing fluids just before and during the treatment is questionable, both because of the inconvenience of voiding and the objection to arousing a drowsy patient to drink. A more reasonable practice is to make certain that the fluid intake is increased a few hours before and after the pack.

It is customary to apply an icecap to the forehead or the back of the neck; the latter practice seems more logical if its purpose is to constrict the vessels carrying blood to the cerebrum. In some hospitals an icecap is applied to the nape of the neck and cold wet compresses to the forehead. Changing the compresses disturbs the sleeping patient; therefore, this is discontinued as soon as he is quiet and shows a favorable reaction to the treatment. Some authorities suggest that the ice-cap be removed after the first reaction to the pack has subsided, if there is no headache, marked flushing of the face, or other indication for its use.

Sedative packs are generally said to be contraindicated in organic heart disease, in exophthalmic goiter, in advanced arteriosclerosis, certain atrophic muscular diseases, paralysis, old age, and during pregnancy and menstruation.

It is very desirable to gain the cooperation of the patient in this treatment since struggling against the pack delays its sedative effects and is psychologically traumatic. An explanation should precede the application of the pack. The nature of the explanation, as in all similar cases, is determined by the patient's powers of comprehension, his vocabulary, and his condition.

Suggested Procedure. Fanfold the top covers to the foot of the bed; protect the foundation bed, as suggested for other packs; place a blanket crosswise on the bed so that there is an excess on one side; place a second blanket, folded crosswise, on the bed in such a way as to cover the feet on the lower third of the mattress; place a third blanket crosswise on the bed with an excess at the opposite side. The wet sheets are laid on top of the blankets. Three sheets are used, two large ones and a draw sheet in between, the latter placed crosswise on the bed approximately 10 in. below the top edge of the blankets.

While one worker is arranging the bed, another prepares the patient. She explains the treatment and determines the pulse and respiratory rates. The patient is undressed, is usually draped in a sheet, and care is taken to see that he empties the bladder. The nurses then draw the wet sheets quickly over the body, the left side of the pack sheet over the patient's left leg, under the right leg and across the body, leaving the arms free. The end of the draw sheet is brought up between the arms and the body, over the arms, fixing them to the side with the palms against the thighs. The third sheet goes over the body, covering the right leg and the feet. The blankets are wrapped around the body in mummy fashion; the neck and chin are protected from contact with the blankets by a cuff made of the sheets. If protection sheets are used, place them over the chest, and if the patient is uncooperative, place these sheets also over the knees; adjust rubber-covered pillows under the head and knees; draw the top covers up and tuck a towel under the patient's chin to protect it from contact with the blankets.

Although the natural tonic reaction to the pack is a chilly sensation, this must not be prolonged. Provide a hot-water bottle for the feet and extra blankets if the patient feels cold. Apply an icecap to the back of the neck and cold compresses to the forehead. Ventilate and darken the room, and disturb the patient as little as possible during the treatment. Take the femoral pulse and respiratory rates every 30 minutes until relaxation occurs; and if there is any abnormality noted in the heart action or the respiration, as indicated by a weak, rapid pulse or cyanosis, terminate the treatment. As soon as the patient shows signs of drowsiness, remove the icecap, and adjust the top covering so that he is comfortable and warm.

On removal of the pack, rub the body with alcohol, rearrange the bed, put on night clothes and encourage the patient to rest for at least a half hour. The duration of the pack is prescribed by the physician. The treatment is not considered successful unless the person is relaxed or, better still, actually sleeps.

Recording the Treatment. Chart the time the treatment was given, when begun and terminated. Indicate the nature of the patient's reaction, the pulse and respiratory rates before and during the pack, and the sedative effects of the pack.

REFERENCES

1. Bach, Francis (ed.): *Recent Advances in Physical Medicine.* Blakiston Co., Philadelphia, 1950.
2. American Medical Association, Council on Physical Medicine and Rehabilitation: *Handbook of Physical Medicine and Rehabilitation.* Blakiston Co., Philadelphia, 1950, p. 175.
3. Krusen, Frank H.: *Physical Medicine.* W. B. Saunders Co., Philadelphia, 1941.
4. Krusen, Frank H.: *Physical Medicine and Rehabilitation for the Clinician.* W. B. Saunders Co., Philadelphia, 1951.
5. Bierman, William, and Licht, Sidney (eds.): *Physical Medicine in General Practice,* 3rd ed. Paul B. Hoeber, New York, 1952.
6. Kovacs, Richard: *A Manual of Physical Therapy,* 4th ed. Lea & Febiger, Philadelphia, 1949.
7. Bender, Morris B.: *Disorders in Perception.* Charles C Thomas, Publisher, Springfield, Ill, 1952, p. 16.
8. Alexander, Leo: *Treatment of Mental Disorders.* W. B. Saunders Co., Philadelphia, 1953.
9. Atchley, Dana W.: "The Treatment of Chronic Nephritis," *M. Clin. North America,* **9:**427, (Sept.) 1925.
10. Cecil, Russell L., and Loeb, Robert F. (eds.): *Textbook of Medicine,* 8th ed. W. B. Saunders Co., Philadelphia, 1951, pp. 954, 958.
11. Evans, C. Lovatt (ed.): *Starling's Principles of Human Physiology,* 10th ed. Lea & Febiger, Philadelphia, 1949.
12. Kennedy, Marguerite, et al.: "The Sedative Wet Pack," *Am. J. Nursing,* **36:**53, (Jan.) 1936.

Additional Suggested Reading

Buettner, K.: "Effects of Extreme Heat on Man: Protection of Man Against Conflagration Heat," *J.A.M.A.,* **144:**732, (Oct.) 1950.
Cooksey, F. S.: "Advances in Physical Medicine," *Practitioner,* **165:**417, (Oct.) 1950.
Ebaugh, F. G., and Thauer, R.: "Influence of Various Environmental Temperatures on the Cold and Warmth Thresholds," *J. Appl. Physiol.,* **3:**173, (Oct.) 1950.
Grayson, J.: "The Sensitivity of the Cold and Warmth Vaso-Constrictor Responses," *J. Physiol.,* **3:**39, (Oct.) 1950.
Hines, H. M., and Randall, B. F.: "The Effect of Temperature and Various Methods Used in Physical Medicine to Increase Temperature or Local Circulation," *Physiotherapy Rev.,* **30:**504, (Dec.) 1950.
Kersley, George D.: *Outlines of Physical Methods in Medicine.* W. Heinemann, London, 1945.
LeQuesne, Ruth M., and Granville, Mary: *Hydrotherapy; A Textbook for Students,* 2nd ed. Cassell and Co., London, 1946.
Watkins, Arthur L. (ed.): *Physical Medicine in General Practice.* J. B. Lippincott Co., Philadelphia, 1946.
Wright, Rebekah B.: *Hydrotherapy in Psychiatric Hospitals,* 2nd ed. Tudor Press, Inc., Boston, 1940.

CHAPTER 22. LOCAL APPLICATIONS OF HEAT, COLD, AND CHEMICALS FOR CIRCULATORY EFFECTS

1. USES AND EFFECTS OF LOCAL APPLICATIONS OF HEAT

Uses. Heat is applied locally for comfort to warm a cold skin area; for this purpose it may be instigated by the nurse, unless heat is contraindicated by the patient's condition. When heat is used as therapy the physician prescribes the size and mode of application, the intensity, and duration. Applications to a circumscribed part of the skin or mucous membrane are most often applied in acute or chronic inflammation of the superficial tissues lying underneath or in reflexly related, deeper tissues. Another and more reliable means of getting the effect of heat in the deeper tissues and viscera is the passage of an electric current through them. The resistance offered to the current by tissues raises their temperature.* Diathermy and other electrotherapeutic procedures are discussed in Chapter 24.

Effect of Local Applications of Heat. The effect of heat applied locally is the same as that discussed under general hot applications except that it is more, but not entirely, circumscribed. John H. Gibbon and Eugene M. Landis[1] showed that immersion of the forearm in water of 43.3° C (110° F) raised the skin temperature of the big toe from 21.1° to 32.2° C (70° to 90° F) in about 40 minutes. This shows that local application of heat induces a general vasodilatation, but the effect of a hot arm bath on the pulse and respiration cannot be compared with the systemic

* We can see "hot dogs" cooked by this method at many roadside stands.

633

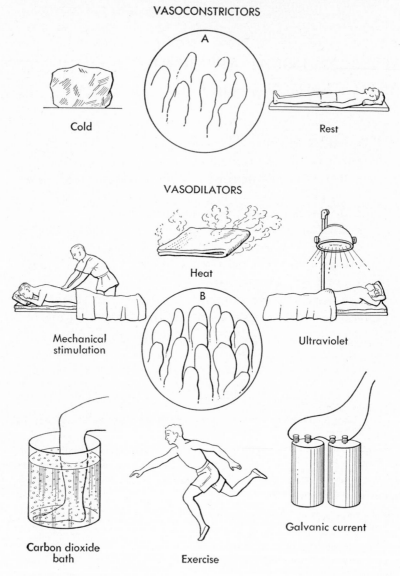

VASOCONSTRICTORS

A

Cold

Rest

VASODILATORS

Heat

B

Mechanical
stimulation

Ultraviolet

Carbon dioxide
bath

Exercise

Galvanic current

Figure 137. Physical agencies causing vasoconstriction and vasodilatation. (*A*) Constricted capillaries; (*B*) dilated capillaries (schematic). (Bierman, William: *Physical Medicine in General Practice.* Paul B. Hoeber, New York, 1944.)

effect of a general hot bath. For this reason heat of greater intensity and duration is used for applications to a circumscribed body area than to the entire body. This difference of temperature tolerance in systemic and local applications is shown in Figure 132. For local applications William Bierman and Sidney Licht give 43.3° C (110° F) as the upper limit to which the skin temperature should be brought. Temperatures hotter than this, they believe, cause irreversible tissue changes.

Bierman and Licht give the temperature changes in the superficial and deeper tissues with local applications of heat and cold to the leg, arm, abdomen, forehead, urethra (male), and vagina. Basing their judgments on their own studies and those of H. C. Bazett and L. Scribyatta,[2] Albert Kuntz,[3] Selling Brill,[4] Norman C. Lake,[5] and others, they show that local hot and cold applications respectively raise and lower the temperature of the skin, subcutaneous tissue, and muscle lying under the hot or cold object; however, the effect is less intense in the deeper tissues, and there is a lag in its appearance. Bierman and Licht had an opportunity to observe that a cold application to the forehead reduced the temperature of the brain 1.5° F,

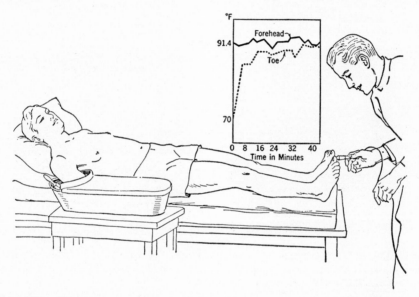

Figure 138. Changes in temperature of the skin surfaces of the forehead and toe when the forearm is immersed in hot water (Landis-Gibbon test). The test is useful in the diagnosis of cardiovascular disease. (Bierman, William, and Licht, Sidney [eds.]: *Physical Medicine in General Practice,* 3rd ed. Paul B. Hoeber, New York, 1952.)

but the evidence of temperature changes within the stomach from applications of heat to the abdominal wall are conflicting. To quote from their text:

Typical temperature changes produced by a hot-water bag placed on the calf of the leg were as follows:

Interior of hot-water bag			133°	F
Outside of towel covering hot-water bag			122°	F
Cutaneous temperature rose from	90°	F to	110°	F
Subcutaneous temperature rose from	91.2°	F to	105.5°	F
Intramuscular temperature rose from	94.2°	F to	99.6°	F

It required about thirty minutes for the skin surface temperature to reach maximum height; about forty minutes for the subcutaneous temperature; and about fifty minutes for the intramuscular temperature.*

* Bierman, William, and Licht, Sidney (eds.): *Physical Medicine in General Practice,* **3rd** ed. Paul B. Hoeber, New York, 1952, p. 5.

Results of recent studies by Harry M. Hines and Barbara F. Randall[6] are more or less consistent with these finding and opinions.

There is much controversy about the distant or reflex thermal response to local hot and cold applications. The fact that the skin temperature in the toe rises in response to a hot immersion of the arm proves that there is a general vasodilatation with an accompanying rise in the temperature of the circulating blood. Some authorities believe that there is an even more marked circulatory effect in a specific related viscus or skin area. Theoretically, the nerves carrying outgoing, or efferent, impulses to this specific viscus or skin area come from a center in the central nervous

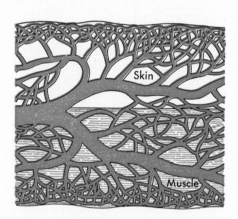 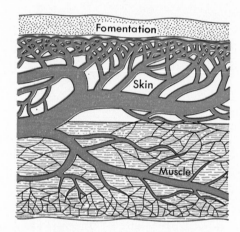

Figure 139. (*Left*) Diagram showing collaterally related vascular areas. (*Right*) Hyperemia of skin with collateral anemia of underlying muscle produced by a hot application. (Kellogg, J H.: *Rational Hydrotherapy.* Modern Medicine Publishing Co., Battle Creek, Mich., 1928.)

system receiving the incoming, or afferent, impulses, from the skin area where heat is applied. Some doctors depend upon the application of heat to a related skin area to improve the circulation in a related deep-lying viscus, such as the uterus; others doubt the efficacy of such treatment and would substitute the deep-heating action of an electric current in the form of diathermy.

Vasodilatation is the only action of heat that has been mentioned, chiefly because this is more easily measured. Other changes accompanying vasodilatation—increased metabolism and relaxation of muscle and connective tissue—are discussed in Chapter 21. Heat applied to a local infection hastens the physical and chemical process of suppuration. Moist hot applications, especially, promote drainage from wounds and skin lesions.

The effect of temperature depends upon the size of the area covered, whether it is intense or moderate, whether it is dry or moist, and the duration of the treatment (Chapter 21). It also depends upon the part of the body to which it is applied, the age and condition of the patient, and particularly the difference between the temperature of the hot application and the skin area involved.

Contraindications to Local Hot Applications and Their Dangers. Nurses see hot applications ordered by one physician and cold applications ordered by another in what appears to her to be similar situations. Depending upon the way in which they are used both may increase the local blood supply; used alternately they are very effective in doing this. Heat is usually contraindicated when vasodilatation would increase pain, as in a swollen sprained ankle or when expansion of fluids or gases would intensify discomfort as in an infected tooth. In the first case cold applications are indicated, or contrasting temperatures; in the second case hot applications should be avoided. The pain in an infected tooth is caused by the pressure of gas formed by the bacteria infecting the tooth. There is less avenue for its escape in the untreated tooth, and the only relief comes from the contraction of the gas and blood vessels in the infected area. Heat is rarely applied to the head because vasodilatation of cerebral vessels makes pressure on the rigid cranium with resulting pain or discomfort.

Heat is believed to hasten a suppurative process; it is therefore contraindicated when this should be avoided, as in appendicitis. Patients with this condition who are awaiting operation, or trying to avoid one, have ice applied intermittently to the area for hours or days. Few patients other than the comatose will tolerate general applications of heat without considerable complaint; local applications at injuriously high temperatures may go unnoticed if the person's attention has been diverted by pain or absorbing thoughts. Those who apply heat must see that the skin temperature is never raised above 43.3° C (110° F). This is the maximum temperature for wet applications since water is a good conductor of heat. Air is a poor conductor, and the skin therefore tolerates higher temperatures in air baths. Hot objects, however, and even air baths, soon induce sweating, and this may convert a dry application, for example, an electric pad, into a wet one. Some tissues, notably the mucous membrane of the mouth and pharynx, tolerate brief contact with food and drink at temperatures of 49° C (120.2° F) which could not safely be used on the skin. This should not influence the nurse to be less cautious in applications of hot treatments.

Methods. Table 8 shows most of the common and some of the less common means of modifying local temperatures. Cold, neutral, and hot applications are combined to offset the disadvantages of prolonged cold and heat. For example, the vasodilatation that accompanies prolonged applications of heat results in edema, and this can be avoided by alternating applications of heat and cold.

If light is used that gives off rays having chemical as well as thermal effects, there will of course be a difference between its action and that of a hot-water bottle. Many electric-light bulbs, however, produce only a heat effect. For convenience, the therapeutic use of light, both for its thermal and chemical effect, is discussed in Chapter 24, although, as a means of applying heat, it more properly belongs here.

If applying heat over a painful area, weight is to be avoided. In such cases an electric pad is preferable to a hot-water bottle, or lights suspended from a cradle placed over the area are even more desirable. When accurate regulation of temperature is important, a hot-water bottle is preferable to an electric pad, because these devices have not yet been perfected so that danger of overheating is completely eliminated.

If the physician wants to promote drainage, moist heat in the form of a bath or compresses is usually indicated. Poultices used over open wounds must be separated from the wound by a sterile waterproof fabric, paper, or cellulose film. Since the heat from them is very penetrating, some physicians prefer them to hot-water bottles and electric pads. Compresses, kept at the same temperature by changing them frequently or by applying hot-water bottles or an electric pad over them, have the same effect as a poultice.

The following suggested procedures include the more common methods of applying heat locally, with the exception of the heated-air bath, which is discussed in Chapter 24.

2. LOCAL HOT-WATER BATHS

Selection of Method.   Local baths used in the treatment of wounds and some skin eruptions should be *sterile*; if the skin is intact and the bath is prescribed for its thermal effect only, it need be nothing more than *clean*. The *temperature* of the bath depends upon the effect desired, the sensitivity of the area, and the temperature tolerance of the patient. For therapeutic baths the physician usually stipulates the temperature he wishes to have used. The average adult tolerates water at temperatures as high as 43.3° C (110° F); a child's skin is more sensitive and more easily injured. Generally speaking, the ventral body surface is more sensitive than the dorsal surface, and the foot and leg more sensitive than the hand and arm. Temperatures that are not bearable at first are tolerated if the bath is gradually brought to that point by adding hot water. *A thermometer should always be used to test the temperature as the skin may tolerate water hot enough to burn it.*

No matter whether the treatment is an arm bath, a foot bath, or a sitz bath (immersion of the buttocks and pubic region with the patient in a sitting position), the *posture* should be a comfortable one. The body must be supported, and the legs or arms protected from the rim of the tub with a pad of some kind. The skin must be protected from chilling during and after the bath. A foot bath or sitz bath is commonly ordered to last for 20 minutes, but may last for a much shorter or longer period.

Water is used for hot local baths ordinarily, but drugs are sometimes added and are especially likely to be used in baths for the treatment of wounds. *Solutions* commonly used for wounds are sodium chloride, sodium bicarbonate, boric acid, and magnesium sulfate, and tannic acid for burns. Mustard is sometimes added to a hot foot bath in the proportions of 1 tbsp to 1 gal of water when the bath is used to induce hyperemia of the intact skin. The mustard should be well dissolved in tepid water before it is added to the bath water to ensure its even distribution. If this is not done, particles of mustard may burn or blister the skin. When mustard is used, the temperature of the bath may not be more than 37.8° to 40.6° C (100° to 105° F), because the irritating quality of the mustard makes the bath seem hot to the patient.

Suggested Procedure for a Clean Foot Bath. Give the bath with the patient sitting comfortably in a chair, or in bed. When in a chair, wrap the upper part of the body in a blanket, cover the legs with a second blanket, and enclose the bath. When the patient is in bed, turn back the bedclothes, protect the bed with a rubber sheet, and cover the legs and enclose the bath with a blanket. Before immersing the feet, apply cold to the head. Place the bathtub so that the feet and legs are in a comfortable position. Support the knees with a knee rest or pillow, and pad the rim of the tub with a towel. Immerse the feet gradually to accustom the patient to the high temperature.

In removing the legs at the termination of the bath, which may last from 5 to 30 minutes, avoid exposure and chilling. Dry the legs and feet thoroughly and leave them wrapped in the blanket for 20 to 30 minutes.

Record the time at which the treatment was given, the duration of the treatment, and the patient's reaction.

Suggested Procedure for a Sterile Foot or Arm Bath. Scrub the foot or arm as in preparation for surgery and leave the extremity wrapped in sterile towels until it is immersed in the bath, using a sterilized tub. Cover the tub with a lid made of the same material as the tub, an opening being left at the top and to one side for the arm or leg (Fig. 138). The solution used for the bath should be sterile. A sterile thermometer must be available for testing the temperature of the water. At the termination of the bath a sterile dressing is applied to the wound, and the remainder of the area is dried with a clean towel, protecting the wound from contact with anything that is not sterile.

The nature of the solution, its temperature, and the duration of the bath are prescribed by the physician. Physicians often prescribe such a bath as a more or less continuous treatment, and in such cases it is necessary to keep adding hot water to maintain the desired temperature. A thermostatically controlled electric heating device, such as that described by R. Fortescue Fox,[7] is ideal for the solution but is rarely available.

Record the time the bath was given, its duration, the nature and temperature of the solution. If a wound or skin lesions are present, describe their appearance before the bath, their appearance afterward, and the amount and kind of discharge observed in the bath water.

Suggested Procedure for a Sitz Bath. This bath derives its name from the German word meaning *seat* because it is taken in a sitting position. If a special tub is available the patient may sit in the water with his feet outside. A nearly similar effect can be secured by having the patient sit in an ordinary bathtub full of water. This is the method commonly used.

When the patient is in the bath, apply cold compresses to the head. An ice collar on the back of the neck is also very effective. A bed jacket or blanket is placed around the shoulders of the patient, and a blanket over the thighs and legs and drawn around to enclose the tub if one is used.

The prescribed temperature is usually as hot as the patient can bear it. If the heat is gradually increased, a temperature of 43.3 C (110° F) may be tolerated, but it must never exceed this. The duration of the bath is from 5 to 60 minutes according to

Frank H. Krusen.[8] Should the patient show signs of exhaustion before the termination of the prescribed period, he is of course removed from the bath.

Record the time the bath was given, its duration, the nature and temperature of the solution, and the patient's reaction.

3. HOT WET COMPRESSES AND FOMENTATIONS (OR STUPES)

Selection of Method. Flannel and pieces of old woolen blankets are satisfactory materials for hot compresses, because a woolen fabric is light and holds a propor-

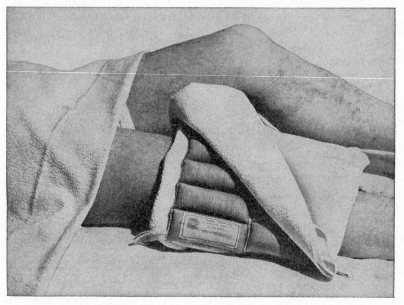

Figure 140. Moist heat applications with a Hydrocollator steam pack that can be applied for periods up to 30 minutes. The pack is designed so that it can be rolled along one dimension; it can also be hinged into a "V" along the other dimension. Thus, it can be adapted to practically any body contour. (Courtesy of Chattanooga Pharmacal Co., Chattanooga, Tenn.)

tionately large amount of water. The pieces may be laundered afterward and used many times, but very hot water soon makes them hard, scratchy, and unsuitable for this purpose, so that they must be replaced with new compresses at frequent intervals. In many hospitals thick gauze pads are used instead of woolen squares; expendable cellucotton and gauze pads also may be used with excellent results. The last-mentioned type of compress is the most economical and probably the most satisfactory. Whatever type of material has been selected, see that it is cut or folded to cover the area that the physician wishes to have covered. This depends upon the objective. When it is to cause an increased volume of blood in the skin and relieve congestion in the adjoining parts or internal organs, make the fomentations very large, so as to withdraw a large volume of blood; for instance, applications to relieve congestion in the kidneys must cover the whole central and lower part of the back and come well around to the sides; to relieve inflammation of joints, the application should be closely wrapped completely around the joint and extend several inches above and below it; to relieve pain in the stomach, the application must extend from the fourth rib to the umbilicus and between the two axillary lines; to relieve pain or congestion in pelvic organs, the application must extend over the whole lower abdomen and well down over the hips and thighs; to relieve pain in abdominal organs, the application must extend from above the waistline and well down over the hips; to relieve inflammation or congestion of the breasts, the application should be applied closely around the breasts, but the nipples must never be covered.

When applied for a purely local effect, as in the relief of an infected finger or boil, the application should be no larger than necessary, in order to avoid dilating the artery supplying the part and thus increasing the congestion; for instance, when the object is to relieve the inflammation of the eyeball, the application should cover the eye and extend over the brow (but not over the cheek); when applied to relieve toothache or earache, the application should be made to the face only, and should never extend below the jaw as this would dilate the carotid artery and its branches supplying the face, thus increasing congestion and pain.

Suggested Procedure for Clean Compresses. Protect the patient from chilling, both during and after the treatment, by exposing no more of the body than is necessary and by covering the area of hyperemia, produced by the treatment, with a dry piece of flannel after the wet compresses are removed.

Before applying the compresses, wring from them the prescribed solution. Test the temperature of the water or the liquid solution with a thermometer. Keep a thermometer in the liquid, so that it can be maintained at the desired temperature; this should not exceed 55° C (131° F), for compresses wrung out of water hotter than this are likely to burn the patient unless very carefully cooled before they are applied.

Wring the compress as dry as possible. A saturated compress is heavy, and water trickles from it over the patient. If the area is not tender, a single compress may be applied and kept at the desired temperature with a hot-water bottle or an electric pad; but if the weight of either of these causes discomfort, electric-light bulbs suspended from a cradle may be used. In case the physician wants the effect of heat moderated by periodic removal of the compress, the method employed is to use two cloths and as the application cools renew it with a fresh hot one.

To protect the bedding and clothing, cover the wet compress with a moistureproof material, such as cellophane, a processed paper, oiled silk, or rubber tissue. This also acts as insulation and helps to maintain the application at the desired temperature. A dry piece of flannel over the waterproof material also helps to provide insulation. When an electric pad is used, take special care to prevent wetting the pad as this is likely to cause a short circuit. Special pads are designed to avoid this danger. It is desirable to hold the compress in place with a loosely applied binder, so that the patient is not obliged to stay in one position throughout the treatment.

If turpentine stupes are ordered, paint the skin with a carefully blended mixture of 1 part turpentine and 3 parts sweet oil. For children the proportions should be 1:6 instead of 1:3. Since turpentine is a very irritating substance, observe the area closely. The physician usually orders the treatment to extend over a period of 15 to 20 minutes. If the skin is deeply flushed before the prescribed period has expired, the treatment should be discontinued. The application of the turpentine-and-oil mixture is made three or four times during the 20-minute period, or oftener if the skin does not show the desired reaction of flushing. The greatest care must be taken to prevent burning the skin. Wring the flannel as dry as possible. Apply it gradually and, if it causes pain, lift it up for a second and then replace it, so that the patient may accustom himself to the extreme temperature. Oil the skin if tender or if applications are made frequently.

Avoid chilling the part before, during, or after the treatment. It is first covered with a soft, dry, warm piece of flannel, large enough to extend well beyond the area on all sides. All applications are made beneath this flannel. Avoid currents of air or exposure during the applications, as this will cause loss of heat and chilling. Avoid any evaporation of heat or cooling of the part by using two hot fomentations in succession, applying one as soon as the other is removed.

Maintain the desired temperature by changing the compress every 2 or 3 minutes. The treatment is repeated every 2, 3, or 4 hours, as the case demands, and may last each time from 10 to 20 minutes. In some cases one application is left on for 15 to 20 minutes, then removed, a fresh application being made each hour.

After removal of the last hot compress, dry the part and leave it covered with the soft, dry, warm flannel to prevent chilling. Oil the skin if very red or tender.

When fomentations are applied to the abdomen for the relief of distention, an order is usually given to insert a rectal tube into the rectum before beginning the treatment and to allow it to remain during and for some time after. The free end of the tube must be in a receptacle in the bed because fecal matter is frequently expelled with gas.

Chart the treatment as given and its effect on the patient.

Suggested Procedure for Sterile Hot Wet Compresses. If wet dressings are applied directly over a wound, they should be sterile. Sterilize the compress itself and the insulating material; the solution used should be sterilized by steam under pressure. Provide a sterile thermometer to ensure the application of the compress at the right temperature. To keep the compress sterile while being moistened, wring it with sterile forceps, steam it in a sterile sieve over a sterile pan of boiling water, or, best of all, place the dry pad on the wound and wet the pad with the prescribed solution, using a sterile Asepto syringe to apply the liquid. Cover the wet compress with a waterproof material and insulate it further with a clean dry compress or a piece of flannel. (Other methods of maintaining the desired temperature are those described for clean compresses.)

Hot compresses to the eye are generally sterile because they are used in conditions that make the conjunctiva very susceptible to infection. Several gauze sponges, 2 by 2 in., or a pad made of cellucotton covered with gauze may be used.* Moisten compresses by immersion in a bowl of sterile solution, then wringing them with sterile forceps; by steaming them in a sieve; or by wetting the pad with a solution applied with an Asepto syringe. Change the compresses as soon as they cool, and use a fresh compress each time. (A special forceps should be provided for handling the contaminated dress-

---

* Specially prepared eye cotton and eye gauze pads are frequently used to prevent pieces of lint or ravelings from falling on the eyeball.

ings.) The duration of the treatment is usually 20 minutes, changing the compresses every minute (because of the thickness of the compress, sufficient heat is retained for this period). If only one eye is affected, protect the other eye with a clean dry dressing or shield. In addition, keep the patient's head turned slightly toward the affected side so that the solution cannot run into the unaffected eye. If both eyes are under treatment, avoid contaminating one eye with material from the other; use a separate tray for each eye.

Since the eye is very sensitive, regulate the temperature of the compress accurately, so that it will be comfortable (it should never exceed 50° C [122° F]), and avoid putting any pressure on the eye. Place the patient in a recumbent position, the head on a pillow protected with moistureproof material, and over this an absorbent cover.

Small pads are available that will keep eye compresses hot for hours. They have waterproof covers and are filled with chemicals that, when moistened, generate heat. When available and their weight tolerated, they simplify the procedure.

4. HOT MOIST PACKS IN POLIOMYELITIS

Selection of Method. The value of heat in relieving the muscle spasm of anterior poliomyelitis and in relaxing muscles in preparation for reduction of a fracture is generally recognized. It has been popularized by Sister Kenny's methods of application. While the patient might be immersed in a tub, during the acute phase of the disease he is in great discomfort or pain, and the application of hot packs, cut to fit the extremities and the trunk, is more satisfactory. Warm baths in pools, tanks, and tubs are used in the later stages. The warmth relaxes muscles and softens tendons and ligaments, making exercise less painful. A body supported in water is moved with a fraction of the effort required when it is not. Until recently "polio packs" were pinned on but this required considerable movement. To reduce the patient's activity to a minimum, "lay-on" in contrast to "pin-on" packs are more often advocated now, especially during the stage of painful spasm. Sometimes pin-on and lay-on pack treatments are alternated.

"Kenny packs" are made of three layers: (1) inner moist, hot woolen (or woolen and cotton) fabric in double layers; (2) dry waterproof cover; and (3) dry outer woolen (or woolen and cotton) layer. Pin-on packs are cut in rectangles to envelop the foot, leg, back, abdomen, chest, neck, forearm and hand; triangles to envelop the thigh and shoulder. For lay-on packs the inner moist woolen layer alone is used. The larger rectangles cut for pin-on packs are suitable for this purpose. Waterproof covers may be made from cellulose film, waxed paper, oiled silk and rayon, or pliofilm. The covers should be light and flexible.

Since the packs are applied as hot as can be tolerated without fear of burning, a means of heating the packs must be provided. Special portable steamers are economical of time and effort. Portable electric washing machines and wringers are the next choice. Since these treatments may be prescribed at 2-hour intervals, "polio packs" are a major economic problem in understaffed hospitals. It is important that efficient portable equipment be provided. Instrument sterilizers, tubs, stoves, and wringers of all sorts have been used, and improvisation in homes is necessary, except in centers where special electric steamers may be rented. Heating units must decontaminate packs as well as heat them unless they can be isolated.

A loin cloth should be provided for all patients, and a breast protector for older girls and women; breast and abdominal binders and pins are also needed. Thick moist cloths favor the growth of microorganisms, particularly yeasts and molds; so they must be sterilized after each use and, if possible, dried in sunlight or ultraviolet light. Washing in detergents and boiling for 20 minutes are recommended. The patient's skin must be watched closely for signs of infection, and a rash is a contraindication for "packing." Certain patients are intolerant of contact with wool, some physically, others psychologically. Turkish-toweling packs can be substituted, but they are heavier and will not hold heat as long as wool. A layer of gauze next to the skin makes the wool pack bearable in some cases.

Sponge baths may be indicated between packs to reduce fever and remove lint left by packing. The skin must be dried gently, for it is subject to irritation and maceration from repeated applications of packs. Oils and ointments are not recommended. There is great difficulty in preventing discoloration and odor in pack materials; heat quickly hardens woolen fibers, and this makes it necessary to replace packs frequently.

The procedure should be described to the patient, and his cooperation enlisted before any equipment is brought to the bedside. A warm environment for packing is essential, for subsequent chilling would more than counteract the benefit of the packs. Speed is also important to prevent cooling the packs before they can be adjusted. At least two workers should give the treatment; more can be used with benefit in turning the patient and applying the packs, especially if the equipment necessitates wringing water from the cloths.

Suggested Procedure.* Gain the patient's understanding of and cooperation in the treatment if possible. See that the room is warm. Replace the patient's gown or pajamas with a pubic binder or loin cloth and protect the breasts of adolescent girls and women. Leave the patient in the desired position and bring the pack materials to the bedside.

For lay-on packs have the patient supine if pads are to be applied to the chest; prone if to the back. Apply a rectangle of moist (not wet) woolen (or woolen and cotton) blanketing large enough to cover the prescribed area. Lay it on gently, having shaken out all wrinkles, and make sure that it is not too hot. A patient's first packs should be only moderately hot to accustom him to the treatment. Fear must be avoided as it induces muscular contraction. Do not insulate the pack, but replace the cooling rectangle with a hot one every 5 minutes for the prescribed period, or until the spasm is relieved. After treating the chest, and in some cases the anterior surface of the arms and legs, put the patient in the prone position and pack the posterior surface. If packs are to be applied to the legs as well as the back, use one large rectangle over the neck, shoulders, arms, back, and buttocks and another over the thighs and legs. Tuck the pack at the sides to prevent air currents. Maintain good body alignment throughout

* This technique is based on that described in the booklet *Nursing for the Polio Patient,* prepared by the Joint Orthopedic Nursing Advisory Service of the National Organization for Public Health Nursing and the National League of Nursing Education, New York, 1948. N. B. It is hoped that the effective use of vaccine to prevent poliomyelitis and sera to treat it will soon make this cumbersome treatment obsolete.

the pack and promote relaxation with the use of pillows, pads, and sandbags as discussed in Chapter 15.

For pin-on packs the patient and his environment are prepared as described for lay-on packs except that abdominal and chest binders in addition to the three pack layers are placed under him ready to be drawn up over the packs after they are adjusted. Apply the inner packs, the insulating layers next, and the dry woolen layers, folding them firmly but not tightly over the inner and middle layers. Pin the binders over the packs. (In some methods binders are omitted, and the outer layer of wool is pinned over the wet and insulating layers.) Move the patient gently and support the extremities when necessary by placing the hands under the joints. Leave the packs on the patient for the prescribed period and repeat them according to the doctor's directions. Remove the packs if signs of prostration (rapid pulse and increased respiration, pallor or cyanosis, or excessive sweating) indicate an unfavorable reaction.

Record the time the pack was applied, its duration, and any systemic or local reactions.

5. POULTICES

Nature of a Poultice. A poultice is an application of moist heat in the form of a soft spongy mass that retains its heat for a varying length of time, according to the ingredient used. The effects of poultices depend upon the heat they supply. Few physicians order them, for other simpler methods of applying heat are usually available.

Flaxseed or linseed is commonly used. Bread, oatmeal, and other edible cereals were formerly used in home nursing, but this unesthetic practice is seldom seen now. Flaxseed has mucilaginous and oily ingredients; it is soothing to the skin and may be used at high temperature without burning, and air can be readily incorporated in it, making it light in weight.

Suggested Procedure for a Flaxseed Poultice. Make the poultice large enough to cover the desired area completely. When the application is prescribed for the treatment of one lung, the patient should lie on the unaffected side, and the application should extend from the neck to the base of the lung and from beyond the midline in front to beyond the midline in the back. The poultice, flannel cover, and binder used to hold it in place should each be shaped so as to fit under the arms and at the neck.

Before beginning to make the poultice, see that everything needed is at hand to avoid unnecessary delay in applying it. Add the flaxseed to the boiling water gradually, at the same time stirring constantly with a spatula. (The water should not stop boiling.) When the mixture will drop clean from the spatula, it is of the right consistency. Beat the mixture thoroughly, so as to introduce air and make it as light as possible. The addition of 1 tsp of sodium bicarbonate increases this effect. Spread it evenly on muslin and protect it with another piece of muslin, in each case leaving sufficient margin to turn in neatly, so that there can be no possible escape of the flaxseed mixture. Then wrap it in a warm towel or piece of flannel and take it to the bedside on a hot-water bottle. This flannel may be left on the part after the poultice is removed, to prevent chilling.

Unnecessary weight is particularly to be avoided when a poultice is to be applied to the chest if breathing is already an effort, as in pneumonia. The flaxseed mixture should not be more than ¼ in. thick. Also, when applied to the abdomen for distention or to other tender areas, the poultice should be as light as possible. To other areas, such as the extremities, where lack of weight is not such an important factor, the poultice may be ½ in. thick or more.

The care of the skin and protection of the part is much the same as in the application of fomentations. Oil the skin if the applications are frequent, or if the skin is tender; apply the poultice gradually; keep raising part of it until the patient is accustomed to the heat. Avoid exposure of the part before, during, or after the treatment. Cover the poultice with flannel or oiled muslin, so as to retain the heat. Fasten it in place with the binder or bandage the part may demand. A patient who is restless, or who is in pain, should not be obliged to stay in one position or to worry about keeping a poultice in place. Fasten binders on the trunk only tightly enough to hold the poultice in place, not enough to restrict breathing.

When applying a poultice over an abdominal dressing to relieve distention in postoperative cases, a gauze dressing and a sterilized piece of moistureproof material may be placed between the poultice and the dressing to protect the latter. The dressing next to the wound must never be interfered with.

The duration of the application in all cases should be only as long as the heat is retained (never longer than 1 hour).

After the removal of the poultice, dry the part and inspect the skin. It should have a pink glow. Oil it if tender or red, and cover with soft flannel to prevent chilling.

When a poultice is applied to relieve distention, a rectal tube is usually inserted into the rectum (by order) to aid in the expulsion of gas.

Record giving the treatment and the patient's reaction.

6. HOT-WATER BOTTLE AND ELECTRIC PAD

Suggested Procedure. Test the temperature of the water with a thermometer. It may vary from 49° to 65° C (120.2° to 149° F), depending upon the thickness of the cover used, the area to which the application is made, and the condition of the patient and the skin. The solution should not be hot enough to burn the patient should the bag leak or the rubber burst, and the bag should be completely and suitably covered.

The avoidance of unnecessary weight is important. If the patient must support the weight of the bag, as when applied to the abdomen, it should be one-third full and all the air carefully expelled. If even this weight is unbearable, suspending it from a cradle or by some other means make it unnecessary for the patient to support it.

If the application is to be continued, see that the bag is regularly refilled and kept hot. Notice the position of the bag. The patient may be restless (particularly if in pain), displace the bag, roll over on it, and get burned.

Earthenware and glass bottles, if they can be tightly stoppered, are very good substitutes for rubber bags. Here the application is used to warm the feet, the chest, abdomen, or other body area. In home nursing it is often necessary to find a substitute for a rubber bag.

It is usually important to record that a hot-water bottle has been given to a patient whether for therapy or comfort and also to note the area to which it is applied.

An electric pad is an efficient substitute for a hot-water bottle, but there is always danger of its overheating. Observe the patient frequently while it is in use. The heating unit should be encased in a waterproof jacket to prevent short circuits.

7. USES AND EFFECTS OF LOCAL APPLICATIONS OF COLD

Uses. Cold is prescribed therapeutically to contract the blood vessels, thereby reducing the circulating fluids in an area and relieving pain caused by pressure. It is also used to control hemorrhage, check inflammation, and prevent suppuration. A cold application may be used to affect the skin and the tissues immediately under the skin or to effect internal circulatory changes by reflex action. The latter was discussed with relation to the effect of heat (p. 636).

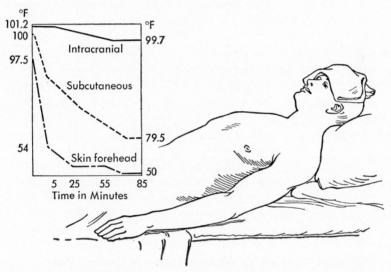

Figure 141. Temperature changes produced by application of ice bags to head. (Bierman, William, and Licht, Sidney [eds.]: *Physical Medicine in General Practice,* 3rd ed. Paul B. Hoeber, New York, 1952.)

It is essential that those who use it understand the action of cold, because, if used improperly, it may be harmful.

Action and Effects. The physiological action of cold applications and the effects produced depend upon: (1) the mode of application—whether in the form of moist or dry cold, for this affects the intensity; (2) the temperature; (3) the duration; (4) the surface of the body covered by the application; and (5) the condition of the tissues and the general condition of the patient.

Moist cold, like moist heat, is more penetrating in its action, because water is a better conductor of cold than air. A patient can tolerate an ice bag (a form of dry cold) for a much longer period than a local ice-cold bath.

Bierman and Licht give the following changes in skin, subcutaneous, and muscle temperature with the application of an ice bag:

With the application of cold, heat is transferred from the body to the colder substance. An ice bag placed on the calf of the leg caused the following temperature changes:

Interior of ice bag	32° F
Outside of towel covering ice bag	40° F
Cutaneous temperature declined from 84° to 43° F	
Subcutaneous temperature declined from 94° to 70° F	
Intramuscular temperature declined from 98° to 79° F	

The time required for the fall in skin temperature was fifteen minutes; for the subcutaneous temperature, about one hour; for the intramuscular, about two hours.*

The effect of cold on mucous membrane is the same as that on the skin except that it is less sensitive to either heat or cold. The effect may be seen by holding ice in the mouth: the lining pales; bleeding, if present, is checked; nerves are numbed so that sensations are dulled. Ice held in the mouth before taking an obnoxious drug will make it much less distasteful. Surgeons and dentists anesthetize with a volatile liquid which, in evaporating, markedly lowers the temperature locally.

Cold, if too prolonged, not only threatens destruction of tissue by retarding the circulation, but it lessens the activities of cells to such a degree that their function and even life may be destroyed. This effect of prolonged chilling can be seen when cold weather makes the fingers blue, numb, stiff, and clumsy.

The interference of prolonged cold applications with the blood supply, temperature, and function of the part, as well as the danger of lowered resistance, delayed healing, death, and sloughing of tissues, should always be remembered by the nurse. The *first symptoms*—a blue, purplish, mottled appearance of the skin, with numbness or stiffness of the part—*should be reported at once and the applications removed*.

Reflex Action of Cold on an Internal Organ or Distant Part. "The distant thermal changes," as Bierman and Licht describe them, are as well established in cold as in hot applications. It is generally accepted that the supply of blood to internal organs is modified in response to changes in the blood volume of the skin. In appendicitis, for example, cold is applied to the area of the abdomen lying over the appendix, and experience indicates that this allays inflammation internally. While this might result from conduction of cold through the abdominal wall, it is generally believed that cold affecting blood vessels in the skin is the first link in a chain of nerve reflexes carried through the central nervous system that result in vasoconstriction of related internal organs.

Contraindications to Local Cold Applications. If signs of circulatory stasis are present, cold is contraindicated. Cold is rarely applied to injured tissue or any condition that suggests poor nutrition in the part. Some authorities think that a local application of cold increases the blood supply in the surrounding area, and they

* Bierman, William, and Licht, Sidney (eds.): *op. cit.*, pp. 5-6.

therefore hesitate to use cold applications when pain might be caused by congestion in the surrounding tissues.

Because warmth is associated in most minds with comfort, hot applications rather than cold are likely to be used for the relief of pain. Actually, the choice should depend upon the ultimate relief that results from correct treatment, and this is to be determined in each case by taking into consideration the cause of the pain or discomfort. It is a misconception to think that heat relieves pain and cold does not. Either can relieve pain, according to whether pain is produced by muscular contraction, a collection of pus, or dilated blood vessels causing pressure on sensory nerve endings.

In some cases, to avoid the injurious effects of too prolonged application of heat or cold, they are made alternately, as has been noted.

8. COLD WET COMPRESSES

Suggested Procedure. Cut or fold layers of gauze or turkish toweling so that they make a compress about ½ to 1 cm (⅙ to ⅓ in.) thick and shaped to fit the part. A chest compress, for example, should be made the shape of a binder with armholes; a compress for the eye should be approximately the shape of the eye socket.

If this treatment is used repeatedly and the compress is a large one, it is wise to make it so that it will withstand laundering. Small towels are suitable for compresses to some body areas. An eye compress is discarded after one use if the eye is infected; but, if there is no infection present, an entire treatment may be given with two compresses applied alternately.

Protect the bedding and clothing from wetting by using impervious paper, cellulose film, oiled silk, or rubber tissue. See that the patient is in a comfortable posture before starting the treatment.

Cold compresses are usually wrung from water containing ice, which means that the water is only slightly above the freezing point. In a warm room the temperature of the compress changes before it can be applied; therefore, wring the compress with the hands and apply it as quickly as possible. There must be sufficient ice to maintain a very low temperature; use large pieces rather than chips, which might cling to the compress and irritate the area. Cold compresses are never sterile, because ice is not sterile, strictly speaking. If they are applied over an area that should be kept sterile, the technique of application can be made fairly safe by the use of sterile equipment, and forceps for handling the compresses.

Do not cover the compress. A cold compress that is covered soon reaches body temperature, and the effect is then that of a neutral or warm application. The physician should stipulate the effect he wishes, the desired temperature, and the duration of the treatment. If cold compresses are applied to a large area, place a hot-water bottle at the feet and take all necessary steps to prevent the sensation of chilliness.

The prescribed duration of cold compresses is usually 15 to 20 minutes, repeated every few hours. During the 15-minute period the compress is changed as it is warmed by the body; ordinarily this is every minute. In some cases, as, for example, when the patient has a bruised eye or an infected tooth, he may be well enough to change the compress himself and will prefer to do so, because he knows best when it loses its coldness.

If the area is infected, as in a gonorrheal conjunctivitis (which is usually treated with cold compresses), care must be taken to protect the unaffected eye of the patient, the worker's eyes, and other persons who may come in direct contact with the infectious material. The patient's unaffected eye should be covered with a clean dressing or shield, the nurse should wear glasses to protect her eyes from the contaminated liquid that might be splashed into them, and the strictest medical asepsis practiced in all other respects. Used compresses should be handled with forceps, discarded into a paper bag, and burned. The gonococcus is readily killed by soap and hot water, so that it is unnecessary for the nurse to wear gloves. Because mucous membrane is peculiarly susceptible to infection by the gonococcus, however, every effort is made to protect the nurse's eyes. If by accident her eyes or the unaffected eye of the patient is contaminated, the conjunctival sac should be freely irrigated with sublimate lotion and penicillin solution instilled every few minutes for half an hour and then some half dozen times at half-hour intervals. The eye is carefully observed for a conjunctivitis.[9]

Record the time the treatment was given and the patient's reaction.

9. ICECAP AND ICE COLLAR

Suggested Procedure. Select an icecap or ice collar to fit the part to which the application is to be made. Fill the cap or collar approximately one-half full of pieces of ice about the size of a walnut. Expel the air before closing the cap. (Air decreases the flexibility of the bag and increases the rapidity with which the ice melts.) Test the cap for leakage. If there is leakage, a new washer may be all that is needed. Cover the cap with a soft absorbent bag or case made of a fabric such as Canton flannel. Water condenses on the outside of the bag; if the cap is used without a cover, bedding and clothing are likely to be wet, and the cold may be too intense.

If the application is made over a tender area, or if it is applied over the chest and likely to restrict breathing, the bag should be suspended from a cradle, so that it is in contact with the skin but its weight is not borne by the body.

Icecaps are ordinarily filled with ice, but various freezing mixtures are now used with more or less success. The cap is filled with a water solution of alcohol or glycerin and then placed in an electric refrigerator until the liquid is frozen to a mushy consistency. Since the freezing point is lowered by increasing the specific gravity of the water with alcohol or glycerin, this type of ice bag is colder than one filled with ice, and it is therefore particularly important to cover it with a thick cover. The advantage of this method is that the solution may be left in the icecap, and after the outer surface has been properly cleaned and decontaminated it can be put back in the refrigerator and refrozen. In this way the nurse's time and effort are conserved.

Observe the skin carefully every hour or so. Report blueness, or mottling immediately, for the physician will probably want to stop the treatment. If an ice bag is applied over a period of days, it is usual to remove it every few hours for a short period to allow the circulation in the area to return to normal. (Gangrene may result from too prolonged applications of icecaps.)

An icecap used for its therapeutic effect must be kept cold. The rate at which the ice melts depends upon the size of the pieces of ice, the type of freezing mixture, the size of the icecap, and the temperatures of the room and the patient's body. Note the approximate length of time the bag stays cold and then establish regular hours for refilling it.

Record the application of the ice collar and any visible reaction of the patient or that which the patient describes.

10. USES AND EFFECTS OF CHEMICAL COUNTERIRRITANTS

Uses.   Chemical skin irritants are used as are hot applications to induce vasodila·· tation in the superficial tissues, or to affect the circulation or muscle tone in an underlying area or distant part by reflex action. Chemical counterirritants have been prescribed in bronchitis, pleurisy, pneumonia, joint pain, headache, abdominal dis-· tention, and many other conditions but are now seldom prescribed. Commercially prepared analgesic plasters are used by the public for "backache" and various types of rheumatic pain. In some cases their use is justified; however, the cause of the pain should be determined, and, except in emergency, nurses should discourage treatment not prescribed by the physician.

Action and Effects.   Mustard and turpentine, camphor, menthol, and other aromatic substances found in linaments are the chemical counterirritants most often seen. (Older texts mentioned a plaster made of the powdered bodies of a fly named *Cantharis vesicatora*.) Their action is similar. When absorbed by the skin they irritate the sensory nerve endings and produce a vasodilatation. Most of them blister the skin if they are left in contact with it long enough. Absorption of any drug is hastened if the drug is carried in an oil; counterirritants, called linaments, are therefore oily.

Choice of Method.   Application of linaments is not described here because it presents no problem other than the protection of bedding and clothing and the control of an odor which may be offensive to some persons. Their use should be avoided in nursing units for this reason.

Addition of turpentine to hot compresses is described on page 642, but this treatment is rarely prescribed. Almost as unusual is the application of mustard, but nurses may find local mustard baths and mustard plasters prescribed in some situations.

In the dry form, mustard has no irritant quality; but when combined with water, a ferment or enzyme (myosin) breaks up a glucoside in powdered mustard into dextrose and volatile oil. The enzymes in the mustard flour are destroyed by a temperature of 60° C (140° F). Therefore, when the irritant effect of the volatile oil is desired, tepid water only should be added to the dry mustard.

In former years the effect of counterirritants on the skin was sometimes carried far enough to produce a blister. This practice is no longer believed beneficial; it is, on the other hand, considered dangerous, because infection of the blistered area is unavoidable. The only reason to produce a blister purposely is when the serum formed in a blister is needed in the production of an autogenous vaccine. A blister is occasionally made over a rheumatic joint, the fluid aspirated under aseptic conditions, and a vaccine prepared and administered to the same patient.

Suggested Method of Procedure.   To prepare a *mustard paste* or *mustard plaster,* mix mustard and flour in the prescribed proportions and make into a smooth paste with tepid water. The proportions of mustard and flour are usually 1:4 for an adult, 1:8 for a child, and 1:12 for an infant. If the individual has a very sensitive skin, the mustard may be diluted even more with flour. The greater proportion of mustard, the less time is required for the plaster to have the desired effect and the more often the color of the skin must be checked to prevent a burn or blister. It is better to use less mustard and avoid burning the skin. The nurse must remember, however, that a weak mixture can also burn if left on the skin long enough. The application of any mustard preparation makes it essential to look at the area frequently to prevent too intense a reaction.

Make a paste that can be spread easily but is not runny. The plaster should feel moist but not wet to the touch. A clammy plaster is uncomfortable, and the patient will shrink from it. Spread the plaster on a piece of muslin large enough to cover the area, and turn up over the edges and back of the plaster. Take the plaster to the patient on a hot-water bottle, so that the application will feel warm. Turn the bed-clothes down to expose the area of application, and protect the upper part of the

**Table 8. Types of Local (Cold, Neutral, and Hot)
Hydrotherapeutic Applications**

COLD	NEUTRAL	HOT
1. *Compresses, wet dressings,* or *packs* to induce vaso-constriction, reduce swelling, and retard the suppurative process. Alternated with hot applications to improve the tone of mucle tissue, particularly the blood vessels. Sometimes applied for reflex effect on deeper tissues	1. *Compresses, wet dressings,* or *packs* to soften exudates and induce drainage	1. *Compresses, wet dressings,* or *packs* to induce vasodilatation and leukocytosis, to increase the metabolic rate locally, to relax muscles and connective tissue, to hasten suppuration and promote drainage. Alternated with cold applications to improve the tone of muscle tissue, particularly the blood vessels. Sometimes applied for reflex effect on deeper tissue
2. *Immersion baths* to induce vasoconstriction, etc., as above; whirlpool baths—water kept in motion giving the effect of massage to some extent (cold sitz bath for immersion of pelvic area rarely used)	2. *Immersion baths* to induce drainage and relieve pain and irritation in burns and other skin lesions. Whirlpool baths—water kept in motion giving the effect of massage to some extent	2. *Immersion baths* to induce vasodilatation, etc., as above. Sitz baths for immersion of pelvic area. This is not alternated with cold bath and is used chiefly for reflex action on pelvic organs. Whirlpool baths—water kept in motion giving the effect of massage to some extent
3. *Spray baths, douches, or irrigations to body surface and communicating cavities.* Same effects as item 2.	3. *Spray baths, douches, or irrigations to body surface and communicating cavities.* Same effect as item 2.	3. *Spray baths, douches, or irrigations to body surface and communicating cavities.* Same effect as item 2.
4. *Air baths or cabinets* to induce vasoconstriction and improve the tone of all muscle tissue in the local area	4. *Air baths or cabinets* to relieve pain and irritation and promote healing of skin lesions	4. *Air baths or cabinets* to induce vasodilatation and promote healing of skin lesions

5. *Cold objects*—collars, caps, and bags of various sizes filled with ice or frozen glycerin mixtures; coils and Elliot applicators containing circulating ice water have about the same effect as described under item 1

5. *Hot objects*—collars and bags of various sizes filled with hot water or chemicals that react and produce heat when water is added; electrically heated pads and bricks or stone heated in a stove produce same effect as item 1, except that it does not promote drainage to the same extent

6. *Poultices* have same effect as item 1

7. *Semisolids*—paraffin and mud, same effect as item 4

8. *Counterirritant chemicals*, liniments, and plasters induce vasodilatation and relaxation of muscle and connective tissues. Sometimes applied for reflex effect on deeper tissues

9. *Diathermy* (the passage of an electric current through the tissues) heats the deeper tissues, producing in them effects similar to those listed under items 1 and 2 (it is described in Chapter 24)

body with a blanket if the room is cool. Arrange a binder in position, then apply the plaster and over it a piece of waterproof material the same size to prevent wetting or soiling the clothing. Fix the plaster in position by pinning the binder; arrange it so that observations of the skin under the plaster can be made every few minutes.

Leave the plaster in place until the skin is a deep pink. There is no stated time required for this reaction; it depends upon the individual's skin. It may redden in a few minutes, or it may be 20 minutes before a flush appears. After the removal of the plaster, wash the area gently with soap and water and leave it well covered. If the skin shows signs of irritation, apply sweet oil, petroleum jelly, or cold cream. A thin coating of oil to the skin before the plaster is applied delays and decreases the intensity of the action. Ordinarily this is not necessary, but for patients who have a very tender skin it is a desirable precaution. Apply a dressing if oil is left on the skin, to avoid soiling the clothing.

A mustard leaf or paper (which consists of a preparation of mustard on muslin or paper) is cut to the required size, dipped in tepid water, allowed to drip for a moment or two, and applied directly to the skin. The application is then covered with a towel or with the flannel or blanket. It must be watched closely, as the skin reddens in from 4 to 8 minutes.

Record the time at which the plaster was applied and removed, the area of application, and the reaction of the patient.

REFERENCES

1. Gibbon, John H., and Landis, Eugene M.: "Vasodilation in the Lower Extremities in Response to Immersing the Forearms in Warm Water," *J. Clin. Investigation,* **11:**1019, (Sept.) 1932.
2. Bazett, H. C., and Scribyatta, L.: "Effect of Local Changes in Temperature on Gas Tensions in the Tissues," *Am. J. Physiol.,* **86:**565, (Oct.) 1928.
3. Kuntz, Albert: "Relation of Autonomic Nervous System to Physical Therapy," *Arch. Phys. Therap.,* **19:**24, (Jan.) 1938.
4. Brill, Selling: "Effect of Abdominal Thermal Applications on the Intraperitoneal Temperature," *Ann. Surg.,* **89:**857, (June) 1929.
5. Lake, Norman C.: "An Investigation into the Effects of Cold Upon the Body," *Lancet,* **2:**557, (Oct.) 1917.
6. Hines, Harry M., and Randall, Barbara F.: "The Effect of Temperature and Various Methods Used in Physical Medicine to Increase Temperature on Local Circulation," *Physiotherapy Rev.,* **30:**504, (Dec.) 1950.
7. Fox, R. Fortescue: "An Arm-Bath at Rising Temperature; for Relief of Vascular Hypertension," *Lancet,* **1:**984, (Apr.) 1935.
8. Krusen, Frank H.: *Physical Medicine.* W. B. Saunders Co., Philadelphia, 1941, p. 502.
9. Duke-Elder, Sir Stewart: *Parsons' Diseases of the Eye,* 12th ed. The Macmillan Company, New York, 1954, p. 136.

Additional Suggested Reading

See "Additional Suggested Reading" for Chapter 21, page 632.

CHAPTER 23. MASSAGE, THERAPEUTIC EXERCISE, AND PRESSURE

1. MASSAGE
2. THERAPEUTIC EXERCISE
3. PRESSURE AS THERAPY
4. ULTRASOUND

1. MASSAGE

Definition. Massage is scientifically designed and rhythmic manipulation of the tissues, although animals use a form of massage instinctively. Kneading, stroking, or friction may characterize the motions used.

Physiological Effect and Therapeutic Uses. Donald B. Erickson, reviewing research on massage in Frank H. Krusen's *Physical Medicine and Rehabilitation for the Clinician,*[1] says that there is little accurate data on its physiologic effect. It has been shown to raise *skin* temperature from 2° to 3° C (4° to 6° F), and it helps to remove debris from the skin. Controlled animal experimentation has failed to show that it reduces *fatty tissue,* and according to the source just cited there is no proof that massage strengthens *muscles.* However, according to the movements used, it can be a stimulant or a sedative to motor activity. General massage causes *peripheral vasodilatation,* with a visible reddening of the area manipulated. With the dilation of the capillaries there is increased permeability so that the interchange of fluids and solids between the blood stream and the tissue cells is accelerated. It is doubtful whether there is an appreciable effect on the metabolism although vasodilatation may have a local effect of this nature.

Massage has been considered a *sedative to nervous activity* for many years. It is difficult to find the scientific explanation. Mothers and nurses know from experience that they can induce sleep with rhythmic stroking motions. How much of this results from the comfort of their presence and the sympathy conveyed by their touch, how much to the monotonous motion, or how much to the local vasodilatation and muscle sedation is a question. Certainly an unsympathetic and rough operator can have the very opposite effect and so irritate the subject that relaxation and sleep will be delayed rather than induced.

Whether or not the effect can be shown to rest on a scientific foundation, massage is prescribed by the physician in abnormal conditions of muscles and nerves associated with disease or injury. It is also prescribed by the doctor or used at the nurse's discretion as a nerve sedative.

The physician should indicate when he wants massage used as a stimulant and when as a sedative. If a physical therapist is to carry out the prescription, he or she will know what motions to use. Since, in many cases, this type of worker is not available, both the physician and the nurse should be familiar with the effect and nature of the common movements in massage so that he can prescribe them and she can use them. If a physical therapist is a member of the medical team serving the patient, he or she may give a weekly or daily treatment and direct or guide the nurse in supplementary massage. In conditions that need long-term

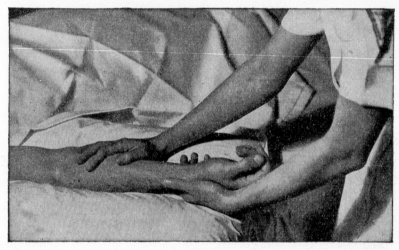

Figure 142A. Stroking or effleurage, one of the common movements in massage. (Krusen, Frank H. [ed.]: *Physical Medicine and Rehabilitation for the Clinician.* W. B. Saunders Co., Philadelphia, 1951.)

home care either or both the physical therapist and the nurse are called on to teach the family to give simple massage. Massage of the back is taught in home nursing courses and is as common as any comforting nursing procedure. It is, in the last analysis, a substitute for active exercise when the patient's condition prohibits this.

William Bierman and Sidney Licht[2] say that vigorous massage results in significant increase in the average blood flow of an extremity. They agree on almost every point made by Erickson on the effect of massage.

Massage is contraindicated when there are skin lesions and where lesions in underlying tissues are known or suspected. It is particularly dangerous to massage an extremity when the patient complains of pain in it since the pain may be caused by a clot. Massage may loosen the clot, and send it out into the blood stream where it may occlude a blood vessel supplying a vital organ or produce a hemorrhage.

Common Movements in Massage. Figures 142 A, B, and C show the three most common movements in massage: (1) *stroking* or effleurage, (2) *kneading* or petrissage, and (3) *friction*. Percussion or tapotement, which is rarely used, is not illustrated.

Suggested Procedure. See that the subject is in a relaxed (usually recumbent) position, in good alignment, and supported by pads or pillows as described in Chapter 15. Expose the area to be massaged, but make sure that the room temperature and covering are adequate to prevent chilling. (Relaxation is difficult under such circumstances.) Stand in a relaxed position facing the direction which the massage movements will take. Separate the feet sufficiently to give a firm base on which the operator's weight may be shifted from the front to the back foot when long stroking movements are used. Lubricate the hands with powder, cocoa butter, mineral oil, or lanolin. Using the prescribed motions start with moderate force and rhythm; increase the force and then decrease it. Do not use the same motion on the same area more than three times but

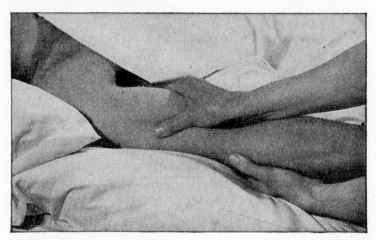

Figure 142B. Kneading or petrissage, another common movement in massage. (Krusen, Frank H. [ed.]: *Physical Medicine and Rehabilitation for the Clinician.* W. B. Saunders Co., Philadelphia, 1951.)

move on to another area before the subject begins to tire of the pressure or friction. Watch the patient's response and moderate the force used if he does not seem to enjoy the treatment.* Discourage talking by being quiet since both subject and operator should be relaxed. The following are more specific suggestions for each movement.

STROKING. Use long, slow, rhythmic movements, upward from the hand, foot, or buttocks, according to the part under treatment, and very lightly downward to begin the next stroke. Keep the entire hand or hands in contact with the patient's skin throughout and use firmer pressure on the upward than on the downward movement, or the return to the starting point. The force used depends upon the effect desired and the tone and bulk of the muscles. It should be graduated so that the movement begins and ends gently. When stroking the back use both hands; when stroking an extremity support it under the joint with one hand while massaging with the other.

KNEADING. Use a series of rhythmic, short, squeezing, wringing, or compression movements in the direction taken by the muscle kneaded. Keep as much of the hand

---

* The interest, sympathy, or compassion of the operator is literally felt by the subject. It is impossible to massage effectively while thinking of something else.

as possible in contact with the subject's skin, but in this movement pressure is exerted with the thumb and the distal phalanges. Both hands are used in kneading back muscles, but in treating extremities it is necessary to support and steady the part with one hand. Pressure varies with the purpose of the massage and the patient's reaction.

FRICTION. With the thumb and distal phalanges exert pressure with a deep rolling or circular movement around (never over) joints or scars when the purpose of the massage is to break up adhesions.

PERCUSSION. The nurse is rarely expected to use this type of massage, but it may be of interest to know that rapid, light, cutting, loose-wrist motions are made with the little-finger side of the operator's hand.

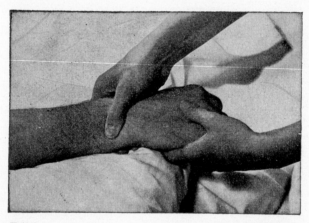

Figure 142C. Friction, a third type of movement commonly used in massage. (Krusen, Frank H. [ed.]: *Physical Medicine and Rehabilitation for the Clinician.* W. B. Saunders Co., Philadelphia, 1951.)

Aftercare. Excess lubricant may be removed with alcohol or soap and water if desired. This is refreshing in some cases but may tend to rouse the patient when massage is used for sedation.

2. THERAPEUTIC EXERCISE [3]

The effect of exercise and its lack were discussed in relation to health in Chapter 15. If some one else will feed a human being, life can be maintained by movement of the involuntary, or visceral, muscles and those voluntary or skeletal muscles used in respiration that function reflexly and of whose action the individual is unconscious until it is interrupted. Exercise means to most people those body movements not associated with, or essential to, visceral activity. When these movements are prescribed by a physician they are termed therapeutic. Specialists in body mechanics are often more highly trained in this branch of therapy than the general medical practitioner but they rarely practice independently of the doctor who should initiate, or prescribe, the treatment.

Since the services of the physical therapist are not available to the majority of persons who need, or would benefit from, therapeutic exercise, physicians and nurses who are trained in this special branch of medicine have an opportunity to hasten the rehabilitation of many patients. In fact, there are few cases of illness lasting more than a week or two where some form of exercise should not be used just to keep the patient from losing muscle tone. This principle has been recognized by many surgeons who make exercise a regular part of pre- and postoperative care (see p. 991; p. 1028). The same principle applies to the medical condition as has been thoroughly demonstrated by Joel E. Goldthwait and his associates.

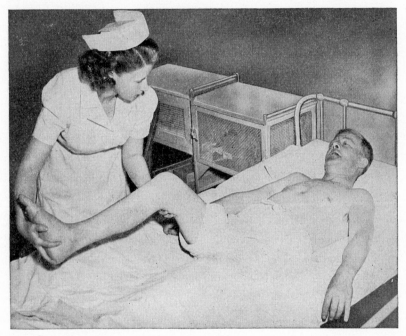

Figure 143. Daily passive motion of involved parts is important in the prevention of contractures. (Courtesy of Veterans Administration, Washington, D.C.)

Nurses who expect to take a very effective part in kinesthesiology should make a special study of the neuromotor system in its relationship to the underlying bony structure. When exercises are prescribed for their effect on a particular muscle, it is important to know its origin and insertion and its action or function. Texts devoted to this subject describe such exercises, and anatomical monographs are available on the locomotor system that describe and illustrate every voluntary muscle that has been identified. It is not possible, however, in this text to give anything more than a bare introduction to the subject of therapeutic exercise. The student should pursue the matter in some of the references listed at the end of the chapter.

As stated earlier, therapeutic exercises are prescribed by the physician to help a patient regain and/or maintain normal function of a part. Such exercises may be directed toward correction of abnormalities (structural, functional) as well as toward rehabilitation (social, mental).

The doctor considers the type of exercise, duration, frequency, and anticipated result; he also evaluates the patient's general condition, physical abilities, and particular needs. After all these points have been carefully weighed, the physician orders the exercise or exercises to be carried out.

The exercises may be *passive* and carried out by the operator or physical therapist without any assistance from the patient. Passive movement is frequently

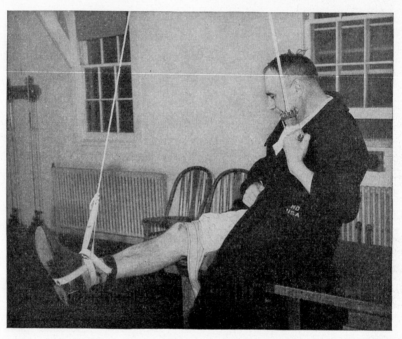

Figure 144. Pulley therapy requires the patient to actively participate in his exercise program. (Courtesy of Veterans Administration, Washington, D.C.)

used following the removal of a leg or arm cast since it helps to restore normal muscle tonus and to prevent or overcome atrophic muscle changes.

When the patient carries out the exercise, the movement is termed *active*. There are three grades, or levels, of active exercise: (1) When the patient is assisted by the operator or by other means such as weights and pulleys to achieve the desired result, the exercise is termed *assistive*. (2) When the exercise is made more difficult by resistance of the operator or by other means such as gravity, it is termed *resistive*. (3) However, when the exercise is carried out by the patient himself, it is termed *free*.

These local corrective exercises are selected and graduated according to the patient's immediate needs. They require careful supervision by the operator and the physician. Any adjustments to be made in the scope and duration of the exercises are prescribed by the physician.

In addition, the physician may utilize facilities for immersion of a part in water. The arms or legs can be placed in a whirlpool tank, or the patient can carry out the prescribed exercise in a swimming pool. Water reduces the influence of gravity, and free movements can be carried out more easily, without tiring the patient, when resistance to gravity is so minimized. Water therapy is frequently used for patients who have had poliomyelitis.

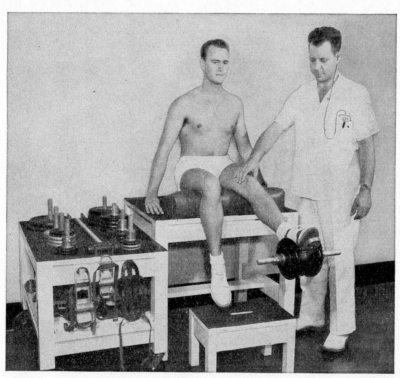

Figure 145. Heavy resistive exercises are applied by progressively increasing the weight of the bar-bell which is attached to the shoe. (Courtesy of Veterans Administration, Washington, D.C.)

Occupational activities are also useful. The patient may be instructed in a craft such as weaving where a number of muscle groups will be used and strengthened, or crafts such as knitting or blockprinting, where movements are finer, may be selected.

Although the nurse does not usually carry out or supervise local corrective exercises, she must be familiar with them and the desired results. It is important that the nurse know the time the patient was served his meal so that he will not go to the physical therapy department for exercises until one hour after he has eaten.

She should observe the patient's pulse and respiration, note, and report to the physician any marked, sustained increase (prior to and following the exercises). After the treatment the patient may complain of stiffness of the muscle groups exercised; the nurse must report such muscle stiffness to the physician since it may indicate that the exercises are too severe. It is also the nurse's responsibility to make certain that the temperature and humidity in the patient's environment are suitable; such exercises produce peripheral vasodilatation, and the patient must not be exposed to too cold an environment following such activity.

The nurse charts the subjective as well as objective symptoms of the treatment.

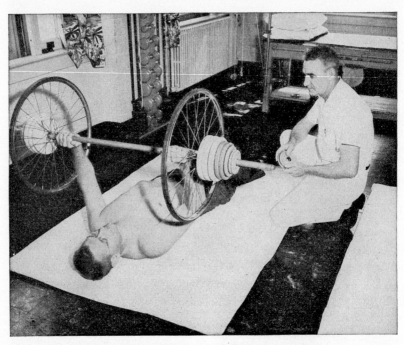

Figure 146.   The strengthening of the upper extremities is necessary, preparatory to ambulation, for the paraplegic. (Courtesy of Veterans Administration, Washington, D.C.)

In recent years, Thomas L. DeLorme, who has contributed the section dealing with therapeutic exercise in Bierman and Licht's text,[4] and other kinesthesiologists have studied the effect of exercise on the size and power, or strength, of muscles. There seems to be considerable evidence that *exercise against resistance* is essential for maximum muscular development. Thus the physical therapist may initiate a series of exercises, prescribed by the doctor, which combine passive and active motions and include those in which the patient pushes with his hand or foot against the operator's hand, or against a weight or some other object that offers resistance. Unless the nurse has special preparation she cannot implement the physician's prescription without the supervision of an expert; she can, however, encourage all patients except the most seriously ill or incapacitated to use simple forms of exercise that will keep their joints free-moving and prevent loss of muscle tone.

3. PRESSURE AS THERAPY

Uses. It has been found that circulation in an area can be stimulated by the alternate applications of pressure that is first more, then less, than atmospheric

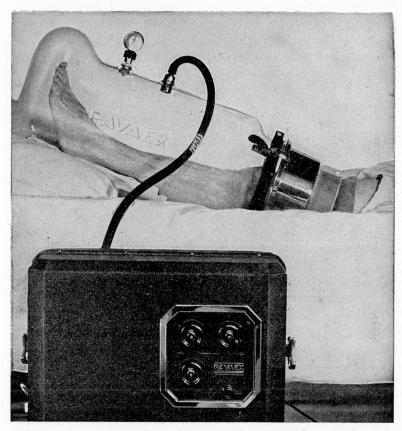

Figure 147. Pavaex suction pressure boot. A similar apparatus is available for the arm and hand. (Courtesy of Taylor Instrument Co., Rochester, N. Y.)

pressure; in other words, by alternate applications of positive and negative pressure. Some of the conditions in which this treatment is prescribed are thromboangiitis obliterans, acute peripheral stasis, as in chilblains or frozen extremities, arteriosclerosis (certain types, not all), varicose ulcers, and to re-establish the circulation following the healing of a fracture.

It is interesting to note that "cupping," used in the past to produce hyperemia of the skin, was based on the same principle as the Pavaex chamber. It was, however, used for treatment of inflammatory rather than circulatory conditions. A negative pressure was created in glass cups by burning alcohol in the cup and clapping the cup over the skin just as the flame was extinguished. Since this practice is no longer followed, it is unnecessary to give details of the method.

Effects of the Pavaex Chamber.   In peripheral vascular disease some of the vessels of the extremities may be obliterated or partially occluded. This interference may lead to areas of ulcerations and gangrene. Great benefit is derived

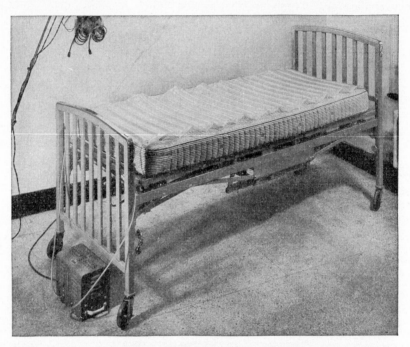

Figure 148.   Alternating pressure point pad unit. The pad, a pneumatic massaging mattress, is placed on the bed mattress; in order not to lessen its effect, it is covered by only a single bed sheet. Parallel rows of air cells are contained within the unit, and alternate series of these air cells are filled and emptied approximately every three minutes by means of a small electric pump that operates quietly 24 hours a day. The patient's skin blanches and flushes as the air cells inflate and deflate every three minutes. Use of the pad helps to prevent the development of decubiti as well as making possible more rapid healing if a decubitus has developed. (See also Fig. 185, in Chapter 27, which illustrates a rocking bed.) (Courtesy of Air Mass, Inc., Cleveland, Ohio.)

from the action of a pressure chamber that alternately draws blood into the leg or arm and forces it out. Patency of vessels may be re-established or a nearly normal circulation established by increasing the capacity of collateral vessels. Changes in the environmental pressure are thought to stimulate the arterial circulation more successfully than either heat or massage.

The extremity is placed in a suction-pressure chamber like that shown in Figure 147, which is made airtight by the use of a rubber cuff around the arm or leg at the point at which it is introduced into the chamber. The inner aspect of the chamber is connected with a motor that forces air in and sucks it out. A manometer indicates the amount of negative or positive pressure inside the chamber. *Pavaex* is a coined word from the initial syllables of the words in the phrase, *passive vascular exerciser*. The apparatus is portable, and the treatment is given to the patient in his own bed. The time cycle and the pressures are ordered by the physician. Controls enable the operator to set the machine for the prescribed amount of negative and positive pressures and to time the phases.

As the pressure inside the chamber is reduced below that of the atmosphere, the atmospheric pressure on the remainder of the body forces an excess amount of blood into the vessels of the extremity to fill the vacuum in the chamber. During this period, the skin flushes, the rapidity and the intensity of the reaction depending upon the extent of damage that disease has produced in the vascular system. The more intense the reaction, the less suction is needed and the shorter the time cycle indicated. After the application of suction, air is forced into the chamber until the pressure is greater than that of the atmosphere. This phase is shorter than the suction phase, but should last long enough to force the excess blood back into the circulation. A typical cycle is one in which the period of negative pressure lasts 12 seconds and that of positive pressure lasts 3 seconds. L. Hobson[5] suggests bringing the negative pressure to 80 mm of mercury gradually and following this with a positive pressure that reaches 20 mm of mercury in the average. It is important that this change from negative to positive pressure be gradual.

In many hospitals the apparatus used for Pavaex treatment is operated by a physical therapist; in others, by a nurse. In either case it is desirable for the nurse to undertand the method, and if not responsible for the treatment to cooperate intelligently with the person who is.

Suggested Procedure.   Before starting the treatment, explain it thoroughly to the patient, giving him some idea of the sensations he will have. If he sees the apparatus before he has had this explanation, the sight of it may frighten him; the nature of the explanation should vary, as in all such cases, with the patient's physical condition and his powers of comprehension.

Place the patient in a comfortable position. Since the treatment may last for as long as a period of 5 or 6 hours, it is important that this position be one that the patient can maintain without strain. Elevate the extremity so that the foot or hand is slightly higher than the heart; this facilitates the return of the venous blood to the large veins.

If the leg or arm is ulcerated, remove the dressings so that the vascular changes around the ulcerated area may be observed. Protect open lesions by placing one or more sterile towels under the part in the chamber. The leg or arm should rest on a soft pad. Since the extremity moves up and down in the chamber with the alteration of pressure, friction must be reduced to a minimum. The opening of the chamber for the admission of the leg or arm is made airtight by the use of a cuff. Powder the part where the cuff is adjusted to facilitate application and removal. Adjust and remove the chamber carefully to avoid injury to the skin. (The condition for which this treatment is used are ones which interfere with the healing process; therefore, any break in the skin may have serious consequences.)

Set the apparatus for the time cycle and pressure phases prescribed by the physician. Observe the skin and if satisfactory color changes are not produced, report it immediately for the physician will undoubtedly wish to change the prescription. (An effective cycle is one in which the extremity is flushed during the period of negative pressure and the flush disappears during the period of positive pressure. The desired intensity of these changes must be determined by the physician prescribing the treatment.) Having once established a satisfactory cycle, the apparatus may be left to run automatically.

The treatment causes no discomfort if properly given, and the patient often experiences great relief if the condition is one that responds to this type of therapy. An exaggeration of the former discomfort is an indication that the treatment should be discontinued; it is, therefore, very important to report the sensations experienced by the patient. While constant attendance is not necessary, the patient should have careful supervision throughout the treatment for some part of the machinery may get out of order or other untoward incidents occur.

Record the time at which the treatment was begun and ended, skin color changes, and the subjective reaction. Also record the amount of negative and positive pressures used and the time relationship of the two phases.

The Rocking Bed.* Changes in blood volume in dependent parts may be accomplished by alternately elevating and lowering the parts. This treatment, combined with hot applications, is advocated in a circulatory disease described by Buerger and named after him. The exercises are also called *Buerger's exercises.* The same effect is produced by placing the patient on a bed that oscillates (see Fig. 185). This motorized bed which lowers first the head and then the feet at a very slow rate may also be used for patients who have spent some time in a respirator; it is, therefore, a valuable adjunct in the transition period when a patient is learning that he can breathe without such mechanical assistance.

4. ULTRASOUND †

An ultrasound generator bears some resemblance to a short-wave diathermy generator. The ultrasound head is applied to the body or to the surface of a pan of water in which the hand or foot rests; it is a form of energy, and when waves are applied to the skin, changes have been observed by numerous scientists. Fritz Frieland, discussing ultrasound as a therapeutic agent in the text edited by Bierman and Licht,[6] says we should not accept the claims that have been made for ultrasound therapy uncritically but neither should we reject them. There are reports of the use of ultrasound in the treatment of several thousand patients with tumors and inflammatory conditions. Reduction in the size of growths and relief from pain have been reported. It is suggested that the effect may be the result of reflex

* Also called an oscillating bed.
† "Sound waves are periodic density oscillations of a medium; their speed of propagation will vary with the medium through which they travel. In air it is 1083 ft per second; in water, about 4920 ft per second; in steel, about 19,700. Speeds which are greater than that of sound are called supersonic, whereas the word 'ultrasound' is reserved for sound waves of a frequency above the level heard by human ears. . . ." (Bierman, William, and Licht, Sidney [eds.]: *Physical Medicine in General Practice,* 3rd ed. Paul B. Hoeber, New York, 1952, p. 277.)

action on the autonomic nervous system. One authority claims that ultrasound is an aid in mapping out pathological areas in the brain. This recent addition to the list of physical agents is in its experimental stage. It is mentioned here as a matter of interest rather than a treatment in which the nurse plays an active part.

REFERENCES

1. Krusen, Frank H. (ed.): *Physical Medicine and Rehabilitation for the Clinician.* W. B. Saunders Co., Philadelphia, 1951.
2. Bierman, William, and Licht, Sidney (eds.): *Physical Medicine in General Practice,* 3rd ed. Paul B. Hoeber, New York, 1952, p. 299.
3. Bierman, William, and Licht, Sidney (eds.): *op. cit.,* pp. 385-96.
4. Bierman, William, and Licht, Sidney (eds.): *op. cit.,* p. 398.
5. Hobson, L.: "Suction Pressure Treatment," *Am. J. Nursing,* **37**:1091, **(Oct.) 1937.**
6. Bierman, William, and Licht, Sidney (eds.): *op. cit.,* p. 293.

Additional Suggested Reading

Fash, Bernice: *Kinesiology in Nursing.* McGraw-Hill Book Co., New York, 1952.
Gardiner, M. Dena: *The Principles and Practice of Exercise Therapy,* 2nd ed. The Macmillan Company, New York, 1957.
Goldthwait, Joel E., et al.: *Essentials of Body Mechanics—In Health and Disease,* 5th ed. J. B. Lippincott Co., Philadelphia, 1952.
Kraus, Hans: *Principles and Practice of Therapeutic Exercises.* Charles C Thomas, Publisher, Springfield, Ill., 1949.
Prosser, Edith M.: *Manual of Massage and Movements,* 3rd ed. J. B. Lippincott Co., Philadelphia, 1952.
Wakim, K. G., et al.: "The Effects of Massage on the Circulation in Normal and Paralyzed Extremities," *Arch. Phys. Med.,* **30**:135, (Mar.) 1949.

CHAPTER 24. RADIATION THERAPY
AND ELECTROTHERAPY

1. GENERAL PRINCIPLES UNDERLYING THE SELECTION
OF METHOD IN RADIATION THERAPY

Definition.   The term radiation therapy refers to methods of therapeutic treatments: (1) radiations, such as clinical applications of sun rays, infrared rays, ultraviolet rays, and short-wave diathermy; (2) radiations, during medical applications of x-rays, and radioactive substances.

The term *radiotherapy* refers only to the therapeutic applications of ionizing radiations, mostly derived from x-ray apparatus and radioactive materials.

Sources of Therapeutic Rays.   Radiation therapy in itself is not new, but new forms have been developed, and the whole subject has acquired added interest. *Sunlight is a natural source of visible rays, ultraviolet rays, and infrared rays*; therefore, the sun is an effective source of near infrared and near ultraviolet rays.[1] The effectiveness of the sun varies with the latitude, the season, the time of day, and weather conditions. The intensity of the ultraviolet rays is greatest in the middle of the day and in the summer months. Artificial sources of radiation include heated solids, liquids, and gases. *Any object hotter than its surroundings gives off infrared rays.* Heat may be transmitted by convection, conduction, or radiation. In the case of a hot-water bottle or an electric pad, much more heat is transmitted by conduction than by radiation; therefore, we seldom think of such objects as sources of infrared rays, because their radiant value is relatively slight. If a stove, radiator, or lamp is heated so that it is unbearable to the touch, it cannot be used as a form of conductive heat, but it becomes an effective source of radiant heat; there is a proportionate increase in the infrared rays given off as the temperature is raised.

To further increase the efficiency of a source of infrared rays, a reflector may be placed behind a flame, a heated metal rod, or a heated wire to bring the rays given off from the source to a focus on a small area. Therapeutic infrared lamps usually consist of a heating unit surrounded by a concave metal reflector. The heaing unit may be a metal rod or wire wound around a refractory nonconducting material, such as porcelain. In some cases the heating unit, such as a carbon filament, is encased in glass; the chamber may also contain a gas. It is not possible in a text of this general nature to mention the many types of therapeutic radiation units. The public should be alert to both their possible dangers and ineffectiveness. Another type of heating unit is an incandescent lamp or ordinary electric-light bulb. Therapeutic infrared lamps contain a unit heated electrically to approximately 800° C (1472° F).[2]

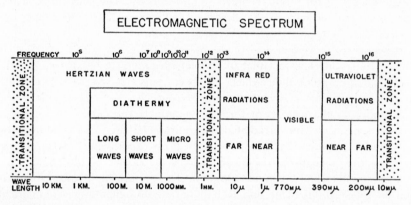

Figure 149. Electromagnetic spectrum. (Bierman, William, and Licht, Sidney [eds.]: *Physical Medicine in General Practice,* 3rd ed. Paul B. Hoeber, New York, 1952.)

The electromagnetic spectrum, or light spectrum, may be divided into different regions according to ranges of wave lengths, and hence according to the physiological effects of the rays on the body. The penetration of the ultraviolet rays is superficial as compared to the penetration of the near infrared rays. The visible rays lie in between the ultraviolet and infrared rays. The more penetrating infrared rays are in the visible spectrum. Rays further away from the visible spectrum are less penetrating and less heat producing. Far infrared rays are produced by units heated to 213° C (415.4° F). Figure 149 shows the spectral regions and their wave lengths.

A source of heat may give off heterogeneous rays (ultraviolet, light, and infrared rays), or only certain ones. Lamps and heaters made to use as sources of infrared rays give off ultraviolet rays but in negligible amounts. According to the American Medical Association, Council on Physical Medicine and Rehabilitation, it is necessary to raise the temperature of the radiating substance to 3000° C (5432° F) or higher to get a sufficient amount of ultraviolet radiation to be therapeutically effective.[3] Such high temperatures destroy metals; therefore, *electric arcs* made with electrodes of carbon, of metals, and of mercury vapor enclosed in a tube of quartz glass are used as *sources of ultraviolet rays*. Reflectors are placed around the arc to focus the rays on the area under treatment; though they alter the direction of the rays, they do not alter their nature. If heating units give off many kinds of rays, as they usually do, screens or filters may be introduced between the source and the patient, which allow only rays of certain wave lengths to pass through. In this way the infrared rays from a therapeutic lamp may be partially excluded, and the luminous and ultraviolet rays reduced to a fairly narrow range of wave lengths. White and colored glass, water cells, and other materials that are known to absorb rays of certain wave lengths are employed as filters.

Therapeutic Effects for Which Radiation Is Prescribed.   Radiation is used for its heat effect, for its power to produce chemical changes (actinic action) in the tissues, and for its inhibiting effect on bacteria; it may be prescribed for its immediate effects or for ultimate effects upon the body. The heat effect of infrared radiation is exactly the same as that described in Chapter 22 for other types of heating devices.

There seems to be a good deal of doubt as to the exact nature of the chemical reaction to radiation. The fact that ultraviolet rays seem to be specific in arresting rickets led to the assumption, which has been substantiated by experimentation, that they stimulate certain metabolic processes in the cells. This action is sometimes described as the process of forming vitamin D from the fats present in the subcutaneous tissues.[4] Milk, irradiated with ultraviolet rays, can be shown to have a high vitamin D content by its arresting effect on experimental rickets in rachitic animals. Another recognized chemical effect is the power of ultraviolet rays and x-rays to precipitate and coagulate albumin. The American Medical Association's Council on Physical Medicine and Rehabilitation says that some commercial sun lamps emitting ultraviolet radiation of short wave lengths, less than 2900 Angstrom, can with excessive exposure coagulate the lens and cause cataract.[5]

Light stimulates the formation of histamine-like substances that dilate blood vessels; in addition, protective bodies (immune bodies) appear in the skin in great numbers, if pathogenic microorganisms are present, and the process of their destruction is therefore hastened. It is believed that this reaction occurring in the reticuloendothelium affects the composition of the blood, increasing the body's capacity to overcome bacterial invasions of superficial and deep tissues.

The type of radiation chosen depends primarily upon the effect desired. If the purpose of the treatment is to produce an increased temperature in the superficial or underlying tissues, infrared rays are used. This type of radiation also may be prescribed with the hope that by reflex action circulatory changes will be produced in related internal organs or distal parts. According to William Bierman and Sidney Licht, there are three general indications for the use of infrared radiation: (1) relief of pain, (2) relief of spasm in painful conditions, and (3) promotion of healing through an increased blood supply to a part. Infrared radiation is utilized in some forms of arthritis and some of the neuralgias, as well as for strains, sprains, and bursitis. Irradiation with infrared rays may also be used prior to massage (passive or active) since relaxation of tissues, especially skin and muscles, occurs after such treatment, making the massage more effective. However, when the skin has been damaged and replaced by scar tissue, caution in the use of infrared radiation is indicated because the thermal sensitivity of the skin may not be normal and overexposure could cause a burn.

Infrared radiation has the advantage of being free from weight when administered to the patient; it penetrates more deeply and can be used with more ease and comfort to the patient than hot-water bottles, electric pads, and hot baths.

Certain pathological conditions occur in which the physician hopes to produce changes within the tissues other than those ordinarily produced by tolerable forms of heat. Such changes are generally classified as chemical changes. Ultraviolet radiation, for example, is used sometimes to speed up metabolic processes in the treatment of a metabolic condition such as rickets, although an adequate vitamin intake usually makes this unnecessary. Ultraviolet radiation is used for its direct effect upon microorganisms in skin lesions and on the operative field.[6] There is some evidence that when wounds are exposed to carefully regulated ultraviolet irradiation in the operating room, they heal more rapidly and with a lower percentage of infections. Erysipelas, tubercular skin lesions, ringworm, psoriasis, and other skin conditions respond favorably to this treatment. The fluorescence produced in skin lesions by the filtered rays from a quartz-mercury arc burner is a diagnostic aid in certain skin diseases.[7] When ultraviolet rays are used to kill bacteria in air and water the far, or short, wave lengths are used, *not* the near ultraviolet energy that is made use of therapeutically.[8]

In cases in which an effect is desired in tissues so far below the skin that external applications of infrared and ultraviolet rays do not penetrate to them, x-rays, radium, and other forms of electrotherapy are employed. Both normal and pathological cells in the interior of the body can be treated by electric currents passing through them and may be coagulated and destroyed if the action is sufficiently intense. Fortunately, diseased tissues are more sensitive to the ionizing action of these radiations and electric currents, and thus tumor cells may be inhibited or destroyed by x-ray and radium whereas normal body tissues are left unaffected or unharmed. Electric currents are used to produce heat and chemical changes of sufficient intensity in the interior of the body to discourage the growth of bacteria.

Sensitivity. Care must be used in regulating the dosage of radiation from any of the sources discussed. Individual differences, the body area, and the amount of moisture in the atmosphere, or on the skin, are some of the factors that influence sensitivity and determine the period of exposure and intensity of administration. Methods of determining sensitivity, and preventing overdosage, are fairly well established; they will be discussed in relation to the use of infrared and ultraviolet radiation. Regulation of dosages in x-ray, radium, and electrotherapy is entirely outside the province of nursing, but the intelligent observation of expected or untoward effects on the patient must be reported immediately by the nurse.

Other Forms of Therapy Used for the Patient. It is well known that chemical reactions are accelerated by heat. It is not surprising, therefore, that drugs may be activated by concurrent radiation. When ultraviolet rays, x-rays, or radium is used,

the physician may discontinue all external medication, although in some cases radiation is used purposely to intensify the effect of the drug.

2. HELIOTHERAPY

Definition. Heliotherapy is the exposure of the body to the rays of the sun,
helios being the Greek word for sun.

Therapeutic Uses. The stimulating effect of the sun's rays on the growth of
plants is well known. Plants show their need by turning toward the sun and by
their sickly appearance if deprived of sunlight. Radiations of different lengths are
given off by the sun and include the near ultraviolet rays (shorter waves), luminous
rays of the visible spectrum, and the near infrared rays (longest rays). Therefore,
sunlight has both the chemical effect of light and ultraviolet rays and the heat
effect of infrared radiation. An overdose of sunlight produces the same toxic symptoms that result from excessive exposure to ultraviolet and infrared rays, although
what we call sunburn is produced by the ultraviolet irradiation. Ultraviolet
rays are thought to stimulate the production of a histamine-like substance that dilates
the skin capillaries. Ultimately it thickens the superficial layer of the skin. From
ancient times both the healing and destructive effects of the sun's rays have been
recognized. Exposure to intense heat and light from the sun withers plants and burns
and prostrates animals and human beings. To avoid this, the toleration of the
organism must be carefully developed. The minimal erythemal dose (M.E.D.) for
the sun is variable with the time of day, time of year, latitude, and the condition
of the atmosphere. The amount of pigmentation in the skin of the patient will also
influence the length of exposure. Exposure should be gradual; a period of 15
minutes has been suggested when the treatment is instituted, with an increase in
length of exposure of about 5 minutes each day.[9] The rate of increase will vary
with each patient, depending on the skin reaction. In the past, heliotherapy was
used for erysipelas, furunculosis, and extrapulmonary tuberculosis; however, such
conditions are now being treated with other types of therapy such as chemical
and antibiotic preparations. In general, heliotherapy is still utilized in a number
of types of skin pathology as well as for its beneficial effect on the convalescent.

Ultraviolet rays are believed to be completely absorbed by the skin, and their
effect is thought to be due to chemical changes effected there. Likewise, injuries to
the eye from sunlight are the result of its effect on the conjunctiva and cornea.
Extreme exposure may ulcerate the cornea, causing permanent impairment of
vision.[10] Medical scientists admit the generally wholesome effect of sunlight and the
dependence upon it of most living organisms; recent animal experimentation has,
however, cast doubt upon its specific action in the treatment of disease.[11]

One of the more common types of skin cancer is the basal cell carcinoma (rodent
ulcer), occurring mainly on the face, and in some patients it seems to be associated
with too prolonged exposure to the sun since its highest incidence is in outdoor
workers such as farmers and seamen.

The action of sunlight and its effect on health is discussed in more detail in Chapter 5.

Regulation of Dosage.   Care must be taken to prevent overexposure to sunlight as to other types of radiation. The physician prescribes a short exposure at first, increasing the period from a few minutes daily to an hour or more if tolerance is developed and if the treatment seems beneficial. Reddening of the skin is an indication of the patient's tolerance. Nature's protective device is apparently the production of the dark pigment, melanin. Some persons, for example, redheads, often lack this capacity and never get a "suntan" but continue to redden and blister. The eyes may be protected with dark glasses, if the sunlight is intense or exposure prolonged, or the head shaded. A method of zoning is ordinarily used; that is, the area of exposure is increased from day to day until the whole body is exposed. A covering is provided for the genitalia.

Symptoms of overexposure, other than erythema, are headache, elevation of temperature, nausea, and vomiting, and in severe cases collapse. Heliotherapy is rarely ordered if the patient is febrile or has a gastrointestinal disorder.

The skin should be protected against the rays of the sun, when conditions necessitate prolonged exposure and especially when the skin lacks protective pigments. Ointments and suntan preparations are temporarily effective because they prevent or reduce the passage of the ultraviolet rays to the skin area on which the suntan preparation has been applied; however, if the preparation is to provide effective protection against sunburn, it is advisable to reapply the preparation after each swim as well as every two or three hours of exposure.[12] Therefore, it seems apparent that protection against sunburn by special preparations is only partial.

Suggested Procedure.   Remove the patient's clothing and adjust a loin cloth or a pair of very short trunks. Protect the patient adequately while conveying him to a porch, roof, or yard—wherever the treatment is to be given. His condition and the facilities available determine whether he should walk or be conveyed by chair, stretcher, or bed. Shade the head (if necessary protect the eyes with dark glasses), and shield the patient from drafts. If there is any indication of overexposure, terminate the treatment and report the symptoms to the physician. Daily exposure is usually prescribed and it should fall between the hours of 10 A.M. and 2 P.M. When the radiation (the difference between the temperature in the shade and the sun) is over $-6.67°$ C ($20°$ F) the time of exposure is usually cut to two thirds the prescribed period.

In very cold climates exposure to the sun in front of a window made of special glass (fused quartz), which does not screen out all the ultraviolet rays, is of some value but is not as effective as outdoor exposure.

Specific directions should be given to patients for the use of ultraviolet energy from the sun if heliotherapy is to be carried out in the home.

Recording the Treatment.   Note the patient's condition, especially any symptoms that indicate an unfavorable reaction to the treatment; indicate the time, duration, intensity, radiation, and zones exposed. In some hospitals a special form is used for recording such treatments.

3. ELECTRIC-LIGHT BATHS (HEATED-AIR BATHS)

Definition. An electric-light bath is the exposure of the body to light from ordinary incandescent lamps or electric-light bulbs inserted in a cabinet that has a reflecting metal lining. This may be constructed so that the patient can lie or sit. From 20 to 50 lights are provided; a few or all of them may be used in the treatment. A partial electric-light bath is administered by exposing any portion of the body to ordinary artificial light. Bulbs are inserted in the roof and sides of a cradle or box. (See Fig. 150.) There are many kinds of such devices. Bulbs suspended from an ordinary cradle make an effective substitute for the commercial type illustrated. The bulbs must be 30 cm (11½ in.) or more from the skin area.

Therapeutic Uses. There is great similarity between the action of an artificial light bath, using ordinary incandescent bulbs, and a natural sun bath except that the ultraviolet radiation effect is lacking. An ultraviolet unit can, of course, be added to any cabinet or baker, but such a device should be considered under the heading of ultraviolet therapy. As compared to ultraviolet lamps, the action of these ordinary light bulbs is mild. However, if sufficiently powerful bulbs are used and placed close to the skin, burns can result. Actually this treatment is an application of infrared radiation. The effect is similar to that of a hot pack, the result of surrounding the body with a blanket of still hot air. Sweating is profuse, and the blood vessels of the skin are dilated.

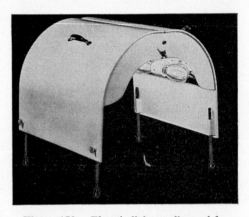

Figure 150. Electric-light cradle used for a partial light bath. (Courtesy of Burdick Corp., Milton, Wisc.)

There is a difference of opinion on the value of hot-air baths, particularly systemic baths. The water loss from excessive sweating is admittedly dangerous unless the fluid loss is replaced by that ingested. Some of the values of hot-air baths are said to be that they lower blood pressure, increase blood alkalinity, relax muscles, and put the patient in a condition to benefit from massage and passive exercise. General hot-air baths have been most frequently prescribed in nervous and mental disorders. They are so rarely used now that the method is not described in this text. Local hot-air baths are used in arthritis, rheumatism, gout, lumbago, and neuritis; to promote healing of wounds, burns, excoriation, and skin eruptions; to stimulate circulation in the extremities; and postoperatively in the treatment of fractures after a cast has been bivalved or while the patient is in traction. In such cases a moderate temperature, not higher than 80° C (176° F), is used.

Suggested Procedure for a Partial Electric-light Bath. Give a suitable explanation of the treatment. Adjust the patient's posture so that it is a comfortable one, because he may be obliged to stay in this position for some time. Support a painful extremity on pillows or pads; place a blanket directly under the part. Protect the part to be treated from contact with metal. (If the head is to be treated, the patient must wear dark glasses.) Place the baker in position over the part to be treated. Draw the blanket that is under the part over the box or cradle and snugly around the opening, to prevent admission of air. An additional blanket over the top of the cradle may be needed, according to the size and nature of the apparatus.

Maintain the prescribed temperature of the air inside the cradle for a designated period. (All bakers and heated cradles must be provided with a thermometer.) Observe the color of the skin at frequent intervals and reduce the dosage of heat and light if there is excessive reaction. If the cradle used is equipped with ordinary electric-light bulbs, several of the bulbs can be loosened to reduce the temperature. Following this, check the thermometer recording to be sure that the temperature has not been too drastically reduced.

The duration of the treatment varies. It may be resorted to daily or several times a week, and each treatment may last from a few minutes to several hours (usually one hour), depending upon the temperature used, the sensations of the patient, and the nature of the case under treatment. In the treatment of wounds and burns, it may be necessary to maintain a temperature slightly above that of the body for periods of days or weeks.

If a high temperature has been maintained inside the baker, chilling should be prevented afterward. After removing the baker, keep the part wrapped in blankets until the circulation has returned to normal and sweating has ceased.

Some cradles are equipped with a heating unit that is thermostatically controlled. Such a device may be used over long periods of time since the air inside the cradle never goes below the prescribed temperature. Such a gentle heat is believed to be particularly valuable in the treatment of peripheral vascular disease.

Recording the Treatment. Note the time the treatment was given, the area exposed, the duration, the temperature employed, and the patient's reaction.

4. INFRARED RADIATION

Definition. Infrared radiation is the exposure of the body to an electrically heated unit capable of emitting therapeutic doses of infrared rays.

Therapeutic Uses. The application of infrared radiation has the effect produced by any form of heat; it is therefore used in the same conditions as those for which conductive types of heat are prescribed (see Chapter 22). Infrared radiation dilates blood vessels, and relaxes connective tissue and muscles. In some conditions it relieves pain. Its advantages over hot applications that transmit heat by conduction are that dosage can be regulated easily, the application has no weight, and the patient can be made more comfortable throughout the treatment. This is the type of home treatment prescribed for some skin diseases, and patients can easily be taught to use it safely. As more specific methods of treatment are developed, use of infrared radiation therapy decreases.

Regulation of Dosage.   In order to prevent burning the skin with infrared radiation, the intensity of the heat at the source, the distance of the heating unit from the skin, the sensitivity of the patient, and the duration of the treatment must be considered.

Infrared lamps are usually placed from 30 to 60 cm (1 to 2 ft) above the skin area, depending on the size and intensity of the heating unit. A sensation of pleasant warmth should be produced, and with the responsible patient the subjective reaction serves as a guide; with infants and irrational adults, the operator cannot rely upon this. The color of the skin must be closely observed; burns may result

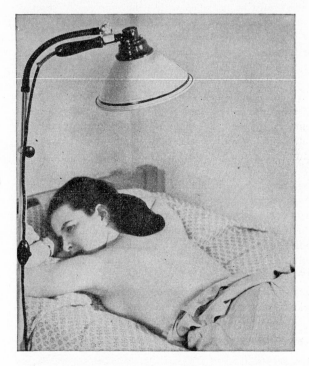

Figure 151. Infrared treatment in the home. Note the failure to use a pillow under the abdomen and thereby to preserve good alignment of the vertebral segments. (Courtesy of Burdick Corp., Milton, Wisc.)

through a failure to do so. It is dangerous to allow the skin to become too reddened. It is a fair guide to place the bulb of a bath thermometer within the heated area at the same distance from the heating unit as the skin. A temperature of 46° C (114.8° F) is a safe one and will not burn the patient. The treatment ordinarily ranges in duration from 20 to 40 minutes and may be given once or twice daily, or, if mild enough, may be extended to several hours. Excessive reddening of the skin, pain, and/or discomfort are indications for discontinuing the treatment or reducing the dosage.[13]

Suggested Procedure.   Place the patient in a position that he can maintain comfortably for the duration of the treatment. Expose the area to be irradiated and protect the rest of the body with suitable covering. Adjust the heating unit at a distance from the skin area that gives the patient a pleasant sensation of warmth. (If the distance is correctly estimated, it is not necessary to keep the heating unit in motion to avoid burning; but if lamps are used that throw their rays on a small area, it may be necessary to move the lamp several times during the treatment in order to cover the prescribed area.) Increase the distance between the heating unit and the skin if there is marked flushing or if the patient complains. Some patients think if a little is good more is better; in their desire to get relief they may ask for more intense heat; therefore, the operator must not rely entirely on the patient's reaction at first. Ultimately the patient and the family should be taught to use an infrared lamp if the patient is ambulatory and the treatment drawn out.

Cover the area with warm clothing or bedding after the baker is removed, and protect the part treated from exposure to cold air until normal circulation is reestablished.

Recording the Treatment. Note the area treated, the hour and duration, the distance of the unit from the skin, and the patient's reaction.

5. ULTRAVIOLET RADIATION

Definition. Ultraviolet radiation is understood to mean exposure of the body to an electrically heated unit that gives off ultraviolet rays in therapeutic doses. Less powerful, but nevertheless therapeutically effective, ultraviolet radiation may be accomplished by exposure to the sun.

Therapeutic Uses. Ultraviolet rays have little power of penetration and therefore affect the superficial, rather than the deeper, tissues. Its probable therapeutic value and its uses have been pointed out in the discussion of heliotherapy (p. 672).

Regulation of Dosage. Serious injury may be done the patient if the dosage of ultraviolet rays is not carefully regulated. In many hospitals radiation therapy (with the exception of heliotherapy) is entirely in the hands of experts; in some institutions nurses are expected to perform this service and therefore they should understand the underlying principles and the techniques involved. Some authorities say the use of ultraviolet lamps in the home should be discouraged.[14]

Ultraviolet radiation produces an erythema that does not appear until several hours after the treatment is administered. The reaction may be so intense as to burn and blister the skin. This effect is seldom desired except in a skin disease, such as erysipelas, when the physician may actually want to kill bacteria and destroy infected tissue. The degree of erythema produced by artificial means depends upon the source, the distance between the lamp and the patient's skin, the duration of exposure, the area of the body treated, and the sensitivity of the individual. The lamps vary greatly; each one should indicate the M.E.D. (minimal erythemal dose) in terms of seconds of exposure. The physician prescribes in terms of so many M.E.D.'s, using a specific piece of equipment. The size of the dose may be increased from 1 to 10 or more minutes daily according to the lamp. The physician alone must decide whether ultraviolet radiation is to be used, what source is best, what area is to be treated, what dose should be used initially, how often he wishes the treatment given, and how to increase the exposure.

The following is a method of testing the patient's sensitivity: Cut a series of holes 2 cm in diameter in a large piece of white paper. Place this paper over the medial surface of the forearm or thigh. (The area must be untanned.) Cover all but the lowest opening and expose the underlying skin to the action of the lamp for a period of 15 seconds; at the end of this time uncover the next opening and expose the underlying skin to 15 seconds of exposure; uncover the next and the last openings in the same manner so that the first area radiated will have been exposed for one minute. At the end of 18 to 24 hours, note the erythema produced on these four spots, and in giving the treatment use the length of exposure that produces

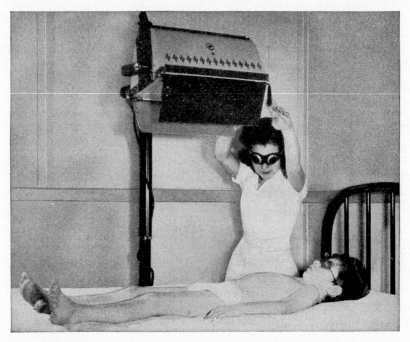

Figure 152.   Ultraviolet treatment in the hospital. Note that both the patient and physical therapist are wearing protective goggles. (Courtesy of National Society for Crippled Children & Adults, Inc., Chicago, Ill.)

the desired skin reaction; or increase the exposure if one minute is not long enough. Generally speaking, men tolerate larger doses than women, brunettes are less sensitive than blonds, and a tanned skin tolerates far larger doses than an untanned skin. (Blondness as used here refers to a fair skin, not to the color of the hair.) As the skin becomes pigmented, the dosage is increased. *Both the patient and the operator must wear dark glasses* (see Fig. 152) to avoid irritation of the conjunctiva and cornea.

Suggested Procedure.   Except for the protection of the eyes with goggles, the preparation of the patient is the same as for infrared radiation. However, because there is no sensation of heat, as with infrared radiation, the patient's reaction does not protect him, and ultraviolet radiation must therefore be even more carefully applied.

Neither is there immediate reddening of the skin with ultraviolet radiation to guide the operator; the erythema appears several hours later. If the test for sensitivity has been properly carried out and the results considered in administering the treatment, there need be no fear of burning the patient.

If it should be deemed advisable to prescribe treatment with an ultraviolet lamp at home, the patient must be thoroughly instructed in its use. He should be warned of the danger of being burned if he falls asleep while under the lamp, as well as being injured should the lamp be broken by a movement while he is asleep.

6. X-RAY, RADIUM, AND RADIO-ISOTOPE THERAPY

The *value* of radiation—whether applied with x-ray, radium, or radio-isotopes —is due to its destructive effect on living cells, especially rapidly growing cells such as those found in most tumors. The cells of malignant tumors are more sensitive than those of normal tissue from which the tumor arises. A major problem facing radiotherapists is how to produce a maximal effect upon abnormal cells and a minimal one upon normal cells. Agents of radiotherapy are dangerous only if they are mishandled; therefore, nurses who regularly care for patients undergoing radiation should study the action of the therapeutic agents and should learn to handle them expertly, which includes working rapidly to reduce the duration of their exposure to the medium. A more specific discussion of this subject follows (p. 684).

The amount of radiation from any source is directly proportional to the time of exposure. In most institutions the skilled nurse and trained technician, under the direction of the medical specialist, work closely in its safe management.

Medical personnel who work with patients undergoing treatment with x-ray, radium, or radio-isotopes should bear in mind the public's dread of cancer. Most patients, regardless of their various ways of cloaking it, are in a state of stress, anxiety, or sometimes terror. There is no easy way to dispel this fear because cancer does threaten the patient's life, and love of it is inherent in normal human beings. Those associated with such patients must gradually build up the hope that with treatment he may live out his normal life span if this is justified or help him develop a philosophy that enables him to accept a briefer expectancy. Since tumor cells proliferate at such different rates of speed according to the type of cell and tissue environment, there is always an element of uncertainty that justifies hopefulness. The possibility of developing better methods of treatment and the conviction of some medical authorities that we are on the threshold of solving the riddle of cancer result in an optimistic attitude which medical personnel unconsciously transmit to their patients.

Just listening to an expression of a patient's anxiety relieves him if he senses a sympathetic attitude. Ivan Stevenson, a psychiatrist, points out, however, that the value of "ventilation" has its limits.[15] Yet, sooner or later all doctors and nurses will have to develop some personal convictions as to whether they are going to be entirely honest, evasive, or deceptive in answering patients' questions. This is a philosophical, moral, and therapeutic issue on which there is great range of opinion. Two monographs on this subject are *Morals and Medicine; . . .* by Joseph Fletcher and *Psychiatry and Catholicism* by James H. VanderVelt and Robert P. Odenwald.

In general, Fletcher takes the position that an untruth is a moral and a thera-peutic mistake, but since the doctor's opinion is often only an opinion and not the *truth,* he can and should withhold it in some cases. He and others point out that as soon as the patient discovers that the truth is being withheld, or that he is being deceived, his faith is destroyed in the very persons on whom he should be able to depend for support. A practical difficulty in successfully using deception is that the medical personnel can rarely "get together on the deception." Dana Atchley, reviewing Fletcher's monograph,* presents the point of view of a physician who believes that the truth should be avoided and that the family, rather than the patient, should be honestly dealt with.

Since diagnosis and prognosis are the doctor's prerogative the nurse is relieved of the ultimate responsibility in answering patients' questions on these matters. She should, however, know the doctor's approach with each patient, for by what-ever she says, by her manner of referring a question to the doctor, or by her silence, she may convey an impression that is more disquieting to the patient than the stark truth might be.

Patients undergoing the type of radiation therapy under discussion fear the agent as well as the condition treated. The fact that medical personnel must protect themselves from overexposure to x-ray, radium, and radio-isotopes isolates the patient during treatment. He feels as if he is in the presence of a mysterious and powerful force. Someone should explain why it is dangerous for medical personnel to remain with him but not dangerous for him to have this carefully regulated exposure to the therapeutic agent. In many cases a detailed teaching program is essential for the protection of others and for the complete reassurance of the patient.

X-ray Therapy.   Roentgen rays (x-rays) are produced by the passage of a high-voltage electric current through a glass-walled vacuum tube; with the exception in wave length, they are similar in character to the gamma rays of radium producing similar results. Even though a nurse is not occupied in this special field, she can promote public understanding and break down misconceptions about the value, uses, and dangers in x-ray, radium, and radio-isotope therapy. So often the patient's emotional reaction to this kind of therapy depends upon what he knows or thinks he knows, misconceptions from neighbors' stories, or misunderstandings from what the physician has told him. On the other hand there can be tragic results when these agents are employed by the inexpert who may permanently injure the skin by overexposure, and who may treat conditions with these agents when surgery might be more effective. The public should realize that the physician can show evidence of preparation in this field of therapy.

The size of the x-ray machine and the idea of being left in the room alone are likely to be a source of concern to the patient. Knowing that there is an inter-communication system over which he may talk with the technician or that the technician is always able to see him will help to allay his fears.

* *Saturday Review of Literature,* Oct. 2, 1954.

The physician is responsible for determining the dosage of x-ray therapy and for observing and controlling systemic and skin reactions that may occur. A systemic effect varies with the dosage applied, the size of the area irradiated, and the emotional state and general condition of the patient. However, the nurse must know that the administration of radiation sometimes results in a systemic reaction known as *radiation sickness*. Walter M. Levitt says that the term radiation sickness "embraces every degree of postradiation alimentary disturbance from simple nausea to quite severe and prolonged vomiting."* Such a reaction may develop after the treatment; however, the degree of reaction and time of appearance vary greatly because of individual, patient tolerance. When the area of irradiation is small, milder symptoms such as headache, some mental depression, and general lassitude may develop. The symptoms generally clear up in a matter of days after the treatment has been terminated.

Neither the physician nor the nurse should suggest or imply that such symptoms are to be expected, but whether an in- or outpatient, he should be led to report at each visit on his appetite or any discomfort.

If a systemic reaction occurs, medications such as pyridoxine and dimenhydrinate (Dramamine), prescribed for "motion sickness," may prove helpful by preventing nausea and loss of appetite. However, J. Walter and H. Miller[16] say that no particular drug can be depended upon to control the symptoms of radiation sickness. They have found that sedative drugs may be useful and that several of the vitamins, especially B and C, have been of value. Loss of fluids by vomiting must be replaced by intravenous fluids; otherwise the dehydration may prolong the nausea and vomiting.

With large doses of radiation, there may be a *skin reaction*. The appearance and intensity of the symptoms usually depend on the site and volume of irradiated tissue, rate of administration, and the patient's skin sensitivity. The nurse may reassure the patient by reaffirming what the doctor has already told him, which is usually that the dose of radiation needed to treat the illness often cannot be delivered without affecting the skin in some degree and that the reaction will fade in time. Such an area should be referred to as a reaction, *not* as a burn.

Several factors influence the degree of skin reaction. (1) Since people vary in their sensitivity to radiation as in the case of ultraviolet rays producing sunburn, fair-skinned persons may be expected to experience a skin reaction more quickly and in greater degree than darker-skinned persons. (2) In addition, different parts of the body, such as the face, are more sensitive to radiation. (3) Because friction in areas such as the axillae and inguinal region may irritate the skin, these portions of the skin are to be observed carefully.

Walter and Miller[17] recommend that the patient be warned at the start of the treatment that a skin reaction will probably occur during or soon after the course of treatment. In addition, the patient should be told that all forms of irritation (mechanical, thermal, or chemical) which will increase the severity of the reaction

* Levitt, Walter M.: *A Handbook of Radiotherapy for Senior and Post-Graduate Students.* Harvey and Blythe, Ltd., London, 1952, p. 68.

are to be avoided. The patient should be cautioned not to wash the part under treatment. When the jaw area of a man's face is being treated, he should be told not to shave until the reaction has disappeared.

In *first- and second-degree reactions* the chief complaint is usually itching. Early application of a simple starch powder* will relieve the itching and help control the reaction since the patient will not be inclined to touch and further irritate the part under treatment. In *third- and fourth-degree reactions,* dressings may be needed to prevent infection; in addition, if vesication should occur, the area may be treated with bland ointments such as boric acid ointment or vitamin A and D ointment; this will facilitate the removal of the dressing, which is apt to adhere to the skin when there is serous oozing. Too thick an application of an ointment such as petroleum jelly is to be discouraged according to Walter and Miller since it hinders the natural discharges and thus might promote infection. Discharges may be removed gently with mineral oil and cotton applicators. Fourth-degree reactions are treated in the same manner as third-degree reactions, but respond more slowly to treatment.

When the course of radiation therapy has been completed and the skin reaction has subsided, the treated skin will remain more sensitive and therefore more liable to damage. The patient must be cautioned against further irritation from sunburn, hot-water bottles, strong winds, excessive cold, and the like. In addition, exposed parts such as the hands or parts subject to friction such as the feet need constant attention.

When the patient is followed as an outpatient, the tiny tattoo mark or colored lines ordinarily used for showing the center of the skin ports† must not be removed. Most doctors ask that no water or aqueous solution come in contact with the skin ports until the treatment has been terminated. The nurse explains this to the patient and helps him to understand that his cooperation is essential. The patient should be encouraged to drink more liquids than usual, one to two quarts over his customary intake. This can be taken in the form of fruit drinks, soda water, milk, tea, coffee, or water. Loss of appetite may be a temporary symptom. A nourishing diet, with frequent small meals, may be better tolerated than three large meals. In any event the daily diet should be a complete one including fresh fruits and vegetables and meat, fish, eggs, or cheese.

Radium Therapy.   Radium is one of the most important of the earth's radioactive elements. Radioactivity results from the emission of penetrating rays during the slow disintegration of an element, in this case radium (see Fig. 153). For therapeutic purposes, radiation is obtained from the element itself (radium) and from radium emanation (radon), the gas which results from the continuous disintegration of radium. Radium is commonly applied in needles, small glass tubes,

---

* Walter and Miller say that the ordinary dusting powders should not be used since many of them contain the metal zinc; the presence of zinc in the powder will give rise to secondary radiation which will only irritate the skin further.

† Skin ports are those areas of skin designated by indelible markings made by the doctor to indicate the path of entry of x-rays when an internal organ is being treated.

and plaques, and occasionally as a large "pack." Radon* is usually applied in the form of small gold tubes or "seeds," also called implants.

In radium therapy, the nurse usually carries more responsibility than in x-ray therapy, since she often helps with the insertion and removal of the radium appliance and cares for the patient while it is in place. The dose and time required

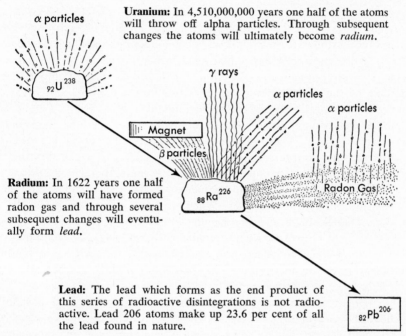

Uranium: In 4,510,000,000 years one half of the atoms will throw off alpha particles. Through subsequent changes the atoms will ultimately become *radium*.

Radium: In 1622 years one half of the atoms will have formed radon gas and through several subsequent changes will eventually form *lead*.

Lead: The lead which forms as the end product of this series of radioactive disintegrations is not radioactive. Lead 206 atoms make up 23.6 per cent of all the lead found in nature.

Figure 153. Radioactive atoms are transformed into stable atoms. (Goostray, Stella, and Schwenck, J. Rae: *A Textbook of Chemistry,* 7th ed. The Macmillan Company, New York, 1954.)

to give the necessary amount of exposure are calculated by the doctor, and specific information as to location of the radium and exact time at which it is to be removed by the doctor must be noted in the chart when the nurse assumes responsibility for the observation of the patient. Any shifting of the position of the radium

* According to Walter and Miller, it is not difficult to separate radon from its parent element, radium. Because radon does not readily escape from a solid radium compound such as radium sulfate, it is necessary to start the procedure with a soluble compound such as radium chloride. Radon escapes from the solution readily and is then collected. However, the radon contains other gases which must be removed. The mixture will contain oxygen and hydrogen which were produced by the chemical decomposition of water under the influence of emitted radiations. A minute trace of helium is present as well as carbon dioxide because of the action of the radiations on any inorganic matter that may be present. After gases other than radon have been removed by a series of steps, radon is pumped into suitable containers and sealed off. The complete purification of radon is difficult to attain; however, for therapeutic uses this is not essential. (Walter, J., and Miller, H.: *A Short Textbook of Radiotherapy.* Blakiston Co., Philadelphia, 1950, pp. 125-27.)

applicator, whether suspected or seen, should be reported immediately to the doctor for it may decrease the dosage to the affected area and irradiate normal tissues. In treatments of, or near, pelvic organs the patient is asked first to empty the bladder and colon since, if distended, they may be subjected to unnecessary irradiation and because distention adds to the patient's discomfort.

Radon seeds are placed within a lesion and are allowed to remain there because they contain the gas and not the element, radium; they, therefore, become harmless "foreign bodies" after their radioactivity has for all practical purposes ceased.[18] The nurse's responsibility for the applicators containing radium which the doctor will insert is to assist the doctor with their placement as well as to prevent loss of the element or the radon seeds. Prevention of loss is of utmost importance, not only because of the cost (radium, $20,000–$23,000 per gram) but because unknowing persons may be exposed to the emanations.

Radium applicators and radon seeds should be kept in thick lead-lined containers until they are to be used. These items are then transferred to portable lead carriers; radon seeds are later transferred to a small lead chamber in which they are boiled in a water sterilizer for 10 minutes. Whenever the nurse handles a radium applicator, she holds it at arm's length by means of the long handle and places it promptly in the portable lead carrier. When working with radon seeds, the nurse should always handle them at arm's length with long forceps, preferably working behind a lead shield (Fig. 154, *right*). Appliances soiled with dry blood and mucus are often difficult to clean. They are washed immediately after use by placing them in a basin containing a 5 per cent soap solution; they are not taken apart. *Any loss must be reported at once.**

Possible dangers of unwarranted radiation to bed patients and hospital personnel should be ascertained routinely by the physics department. A Geiger-Müller counter† is used whenever there is a question of contamination and especially after the discharge of a patient before personnel clean the room and dispose of linen, dressings, and excreta.

Nurses who regularly care for patients being treated should perform their duties as quickly as possible; however, there is no need for undue haste if this work is done within the time limits set up by the doctor or physicist.

Because keeping up the patient's morale is so important, the nurse must be able to work quickly and effectively without giving the patient a feeling of being hurried. Adequate reading materials and a radio or television may be provided to keep the patient occupied. In some instances, visitors may be permitted within 5 ft of the patient and limited to less than one-half hour a day. It is not necessary to alternate visitors each day because the amount of exposure to any one visitor is so much less than it is to the nurse who returns to care for the patient at intervals. Nursing supervision of visitors may be done through the glass panel in the door. Patients

---

* To help prevent loss, all sinks in areas where radium appliances and radon seeds are used should be equipped with special traps; this will prevent the introduction of radioactive material into the sewerage system.

† A Geiger-Müller counter is a sensitive detection instrument primarily used for qualitative estimate of contamination. This device is especially effective in the detection of beta and gamma rays.

on discharge may be considered nonhazardous in any contact with other members of their families and visitors unless specific precautions are given in writing to the contrary by the doctor (for example, urine, stool, and vomitus precautions may be continued).

Patients receiving radium treatment should not be allowed bathroom privileges because of the increased danger of loss of radium. Some of the following items may

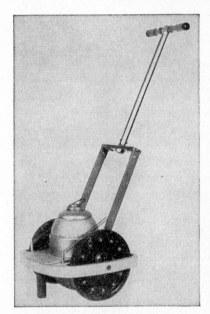 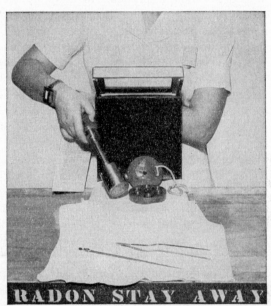

Figure 154. (*Left*) Movable lead carrier for transportation of vaginal and rectal radium applicators from permanent storage container to treatment room. (*Right*) Transfer of radon (gold) seeds from lead hand-carrier to circular lead chamber for sterilization. In background is lead shield, 2 in. thick, with lead glass. Nurse is wearing both a wrist monitor (badge) and a monitor over left breast pocket. In the foreground are a gold-seed needle and long forceps. (Courtesy of Memorial Center, New York City.)

be indicated; their use will be determined by the length of time the radium applicators remain in place, and by the physician's specific instructions:

1. A hamper frame with a laundry bag so that linen used during the treatment may be discarded into it

2. A waste can lined with a heavy paper bag and operated by a foot pedal for discarded dressings and other similar waste

3. A large dark bottle so that urine may be discarded into it through a funnel placed in the neck of the bottle

4. A galvanized pail with a tight-fitting cover for the disposal of feces (a second pail may be provided for the disposal of vomitus)

These containers are placed in a bathroom which adjoins the patient's room where they will be conveniently at hand and yet not conspicuous to the patient and his visitors. All soiled linen, dressings, waste, and excreta should be kept until the radium has been removed from the patient and accounted for. If the waste containers need to be emptied before the radium is removed, the nurse notifies the physicist who will see that the contents are monitored for possible loss of radium and who will supervise the disposal of the material.

A placard hung on the foot of the bed while the patient is being treated may state: "No linen changed without supervision—no bedpans to be emptied or pads discarded without inspection." In addition there should be a sign on the door which reads: "Radium"; such a door sign should alert all personnel. The competent nurse makes accurate note of the reaction of the patient and gives him emotional support throughout the treatment, as was discussed on page 679.

The exposure of medical personnel to radium and radon (applicators, needles, and seeds) can be reduced and controlled by intelligent application of principles and by using suitable equipment and accessories. Containers for the transportation of applicators, etc., are designed to protect personnel during transit time only (see Fig. 154) and should not be considered adequate for permanent storage. All workers who are exposed to radiation should be monitored or tested for the presence of accidental, accumulative, radioactive contamination by means of *film badges*. A film badge is an effective device and contains a photographic film which, when the worker has been exposed to radiation, measures both the beta and gamma radiation since the degree of exposure of the photographic film is directly proportional to the number of disintegration rays that have passed through the film badge.[19] Film badges are worn by x-ray technicians and by nurses who prepare radon seeds and who assist the doctor with the implantation. The badge is pinned to the uniform over the left breast pocket. When nurses are sterilizing radon seeds, a second badge is worn on the wrist (Fig. 154, *right*). (Right-handed persons wear the badge on the right wrist, and left-handed persons, on the left wrist.)

Differential and total white-cell counts are often required for personnel having close contact with sources of radiation; these counts are made at regular intervals such as once a month, or more often at the discretion of the doctor in charge. Walter and Miller[20] recommend that each worker's normal count should be determined when he starts to work with radioactive substances so that it will serve as a basis of comparison. They regard a white-cell count of 6000 or more as satisfactory; however, they stress the importance of watching the *relative* effect (e.g., increase and/or decrease of the various kinds of white blood cells—not just the total count) for each individual as compared with the normal differential and total count established earlier. To ensure a uniform and comparable technique, they also recommend that white-cell counts be done by the same person, if possible.

Radio-isotope Therapy. These substances* are calculated and administered by the physician with the assistance of a trained physicist. Because these isotopes

---

* A radio-isotope or radioactive isotope is one exhibiting the property of spontaneous decomposition, usually referring to an element rendered radioactive by artificial means. The isotope has the same atomic number as the element but a different atomic weight. Some examples of radio-isotopes include: (1) radioactive sodium (Na^{24}), injected intravenously to determine the rate of circulation of the blood; (2) treatment of hypothyroidism and cancer

are radioactive, all precautionary measures should be taken to forestall accidents that could cause exposure of personnel to contamination and radiation. Nurses caring for patients so treated must be adequately instructed. The treatment of patients with radio-isotopes is usually not dangerous to nurses and other hospital personnel if the precautions and regulations, as set up by experts, are understood and observed.

The nurse must know the isotope used and the dose; the time and date of administration should also appear on the patient's chart, on the "bed tag," and on the "door tag." Since the patient is often in a room or area isolated from other patients, the nurse must be prepared to give a simplified explanation and emotional support to the patient who is apt to become alarmed over this "new" treatment. An intercommunication system enabling the patient to talk with the nurses at any time reassures him. A small glass panel in the door will permit the nurse to observe the patient frequently without entering the room.

Detailed instructions must be given the patient concerning the handling of his own vomitus, urine, and stool; the nature of the instruction depends upon the radio-isotope used. He must know whether he has bathroom privileges or whether he should collect his excreta and add it to special containers in the bathroom (see p. 685). The procedure to be carried out is determined by the physician and physicist.

In some instances, a bath should not be given within the first 48 hours following administration of the radio-isotope unless specifically ordered, as it may be when patients are very ill. Clothing and bed linen require special handling by workers wearing rubber gloves. Since the use of rubber gloves may frighten the patient, the nurse must explain that the gloves are to prevent contamination of her hands in case of spillage, that this is done for each patient and for the general welfare of all patients and personnel. Occasionally, rubber aprons, protective goggles, and waterproofed, lined containers for dressings are necessary. If a treatment, such as a paracentesis or thorocentesis, is done following the administration of a radioactive substance, the equipment should be monitored with a Geiger-Müller counter for contamination soon after use.

The main hazard when caring for patients treated with radio-isotopes is the deposition of radioactive material in the body (resulting from ingestion, inhalation, or absorption through the body surfaces) rather than external radiation that is practically small to begin with and easy to control. This source of contamination is a greater hazard because it involves the radioactive substance coming in direct contact with the nurse either on hands, feet, or clothing, from the end of a cigarette, or in food (such as the patient's candy which may be offered to the nurse). Therefore, the nurse's fingernails must be kept short and cleaned frequently; eating in patients' rooms is restricted, and smoking by nurses prohibited (radio-isotopes burned on a cigarette may be drawn into the lungs).

Rehabilitation. Rehabilitation really begins before the treatment is started.

---

of the thyroid with radioactive iodine (I^{131}), since iodine is selectively absorbed by the thyroid gland.

In clinical units where patients are treated with radioactive iodine, the use of iodine preparations as disinfectants should be suspended. Their use may upset the calculation of the dosage.

Pleasant surroundings, attractive trays, friendliness, and understanding on the part of the nurse and all personnel are important. By eliciting the help of visitors and family, the nurse can often suggest recreational and/or occupational activities that the patient can begin in the hospital and that will prove of interest and value when he returns home. By including the family in the doctor-nurse-patient discussions, the family will more fully realize the important role they may play in helping the patient maintain a continuing interest in everyday activities. In communities where a community nursing service is available, an important contribution both to the patient and family may be made by the community nurse who acts as a liaison in promoting a more rapid recovery from, or better adjustment to, a disability.

Conclusion. Regardless of the type of therapy used, there are the following factors which must be considered in giving nursing care to patients receiving radiation therapy: (1) the accuracy of the dose and intelligent understanding of the agent, (2) proper care of the treatment area to prevent irritation and infection, (3) building up the patient's physical condition, (4) giving him emotional support or building up his morale, and (5) protecting the self and others from radioactive substances.

7. ELECTROTHERAPY

Definition. The passage of any electric current through living tissue for chemical, physical, or heat effects falls under the general classification of *electrotherapy*. If an electric current is used to cauterize or destroy tissue cells, the process is referred to as *electrosurgery*. The usual classifications of electrotherapy include:

I. High-frequency currents (heat action)
   A. Surgical
      1. Electrocoagulation
      2. Desiccation
      3. Fulguration
      4. Radiocutting knife
   B. Medical
      1. Conventional (long-wave) diathermy
      2. Short waves (90–30 meters)
      3. Ultrashort waves (6 meters and below)
II. Low-frequency currents (mechanical or chemical action)
      1. Galvanic current
      2. Faradic current
      3. Sinusoidal current
      4. Static current

Infrared and ultraviolet radiation from artificial sources also belong in a classification of electrotherapy, but they have been discussed at length and are not referred to in this section (see p. 675; p. 677). The forms of electrotherapy may be used alone or in combination.

At the present time the nurse, unless she is also a physical therapy technician, is rarely responsible for the operation of electrotherapy apparatus, other than that used for infrared radiation. She often prepares the patient for the treatment and takes care of him during the treatment and afterward; she should, therefore, have some knowledge of the principles and methods involved.

Diathermy. If alternating high-frequency currents are passed from one electrode to another through living tissue, the process is called *medical diathermy*. The resistance offered by the tissues to the passage of the current produces heat. With an alternating current of high frequency, the ions in the body fluids move to and

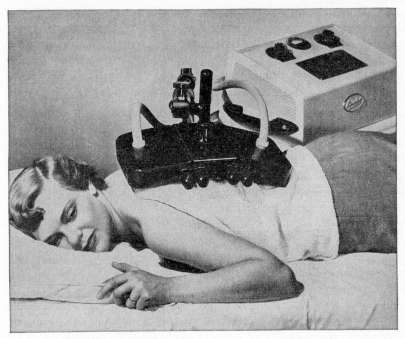

Figure 155. Diathermy treatment being carried out in the physician's office. Note the failure to use a pillow under the abdomen and thereby to preserve good alignment of the vertebral segments. (Courtesy of Burdick Corp., Milton, Wisc.)

from the electrodes so rapidly that there is no appreciable chemical change in the tissues. The only therapeutic result is believed to be the heat effect. This may be mild and produce a moderate hyperemia or may be so intense as to coagulate or "cook" the tissues. In medical diathermy the strength of the current is regulated in such a way that the temperature changes within the tissues fall within a therapeutically effective range. Its advantage over other forms of hot applications is that it affects all the tissues of the body lying between the electrodes. Internal organs can therefore be treated as easily as superficial tissues. Because different types of tissue offer varying amounts of resistance to electric currents, the effect is not uniform throughout the body, and some tissues respond more favorably to treatment with diathermy than others.

Diathermy may be used for any condition in which heat is indicated. Many physicians claim to have seen excellent results in a number of inflammatory diseases—namely, bronchitis, bronchial asthma, pleurisy, arthritis, and neuritis, to mention a partial list. It is also used in joint injuries such as bursitis.[21]

Diathermy is employed in fever therapy, often in combination with infrared radiation. The operation of the apparatus is always in the hands of a physician or special technician. Nursing care of the patient is the same, regardless of the medium employed to produce artificial fever therapy. Because it is so seldom used, the procedure is not described in the text.

When diathermy is employed by the physician to treat a "frozen" shoulder or other joint with limited motion, he may prescribe exercises for the patient. The nurse assists the patient with such exercises; if there are untoward effects, such as increased severe pain, the nurse reports the reaction to the physician immediately.

Electrosurgery might be termed *surgical diathermy,* for high-frequency alternating currents also are used for this purpose. The chief difference between this and medical diathermy is the strength of the current. To limit the area of desiccation, coagulation, or cutting with electricity, the electrodes used must be of various shapes and sizes, and there must be a nice adjustment of the strength of the current.

Surgical diathermy is used for the destruction or removal of warts, moles, and papillomas. It is rarely used in removing large growths or for major surgery.

Low-voltage Currents.   Alternating (sine wave), galvanic, and pulsating direct currents are low-voltage currents used in electrotherapy. Their effects may be mechanical or chemical or a combination of the two. Sine wave, or sinusoidal, currents stimulate involuntary muscle movements and in this way produce the mechanical action of passive exercise or massage. The nonsurging galvanic current produces chemical changes or ionization within the tissues as it passes from one electrode to the other; an astringent effect is produced at the positive pole (anode) and a relaxing effect at the negative pole (cathode). The astringent effect is anti-hemorrhagic. Ionization of metallic salts in human tissue is another effect aimed at in electrosurgery.

Electric currents are commonly used to test the function of muscles and nerves when those structures have been injured or an injury is suspected.

Nurses, unless trained as technicians in physical therapy, are not expected to operate apparatus used in electrotherapy. (More detailed discussions of this subject are found in texts on therapeutics and monographs on this aspect of physical therapy.)

REFERENCES

1. American Medical Association, Council on Physical Medicine and Rehabilitation: *Handbook of Physical Medicine and Rehabilitation.* Blakiston Co., Philadelphia, 1950, p. 75.
2. American Medical Association, Council on Physical Medicine and Rehabilitation: *op. cit.,* p. 80.
3. American Medical Association, Council on Physical Medicine and Rehabilitation: *op. cit.,* p. 78.

4. Bierman, William, and Licht, Sidney (eds.): *Physical Medicine in General Practice,* 3rd ed. Paul B. Hoeber, New York, 1952, p. 266.
5. American Medical Association, Council on Physical Medicine and Rehabilitation: *op. cit.,* p. 102.
6. Walter, Carl W.: *Aseptic Treatment of Wounds.* The Macmillan Company, New York, 1948, pp. 193-99.
7. Bierman, William, and Licht, Sidney (eds.): *op. cit.,* p. 746.
8. Krusen, Frank H. (ed.): *Physical Medicine and Rehabilitation for the Clinician.* W. B. Saunders Co., Philadelphia, 1951, p. 61.
9. Bierman, William, and Licht, Sidney (eds.): *op. cit.,* p. 238.
10. Maxcy, Kenneth F. (ed.): *Rosenau's Preventive Medicine and Hygiene,* 7th ed. Appleton-Century-Crofts, Inc., New York, 1951, p. 797.
11. Maxcy, Kenneth F. (ed.): *op. cit.,* p. 980.
12. Bierman, William, and Licht, Sidney (eds.): *op. cit.,* pp. 748-50.
13. Krusen, Frank H. (ed.): *op. cit.,* p. 240.
14. Maxcy, Kenneth F. (ed.): *op. cit.,* p. 981.
15. Stevenson, Ian: "The Nurse and Her Patient in Long Term Cases," *Am. J. Nursing,* **54:** 1462, (Dec.) 1954.
16. Walter, J., and Miller, H.: *A Short Textbook of Radiotherapy.* Blakiston Co., Philadelphia, 1950, p. 187.
17. Walter, J., and Miller, H.: *op. cit.,* pp. 175-76.
18. Walter, J., and Miller, H.: *op. cit.,* p. 196.
19. Goostray, Stella, and Schwenck, J. Rae: *A Textbook of Chemistry,* 7th ed. The Macmillan Company, New York, 1954, p. 58.
20. Walter, J., and Miller, H.: *op. cit.,* pp. 181, 406.
21. Bierman, William, and Licht, Sidney (eds.): *op. cit.,* pp. 140-41.

Additional Suggested Reading

Ashbrook, James B.: "Not by Bread Alone," *Am. J. Nursing,* **55:**164, (Feb.) 1955.
Best, Nelliana: "Radiotherapy and the Nurse," *Am. J. Nursing,* **50:**140-43, (Mar.) 1950.
Cancer Nursing, A Manual for Public Health Nurses. A joint project of the National Cancer Institute and the New York State Department of Health, 1950.
Cromwell, Helen: "Religion in Nursing Practice," *Am. J. Nursing,* **49:**768, (Dec.) 1949.
Duffy, Benedict J., Jr.: "Atomic Energy in the Diagnosis and Treatment of Malignant Diseases," *Am. J. Nursing,* **55:**434, (Apr.) 1955.
"Emotional Relief for Cancer Patients" (Medical Highlights), *Am. J. Nursing,* **55**:14, (Jan.) 1955.
Fletcher, Joseph: *Morals and Medicine; The Moral Problems of: the Patient's Right to Know the Truth, Contraception, Artificial Insemination, Sterilization, Euthanasia.* Princeton University Press, Princeton, 1954.
Glasser, Otto, et al.: *Physical Foundations of Radiology,* 2nd ed. Paul B. Hoeber, New York, 1952.
Handbooks of the National Bureau of Standards (available from the Superintendent of Documents, Government Printing Office, Washington 25, D.C.):
No. 38. "Protection of Radium During Air Raids."
No. 41. "Medical X-ray Protection up to Two Million Volts."
No. 42. "Safe Handling of Radioactive Isotopes."
No. 51. "Radiological Monitoring Methods and Instruments."
No. 52. "Maximum Permissible Amounts of Radioisotopes in the Human Body and Maximum Permissible Concentrations in Air and Water."
Levitt, Walter M.: *A Handbook of Radiotherapy for Senior and Post-Graduate Students* Harvey and Blythe, Ltd., London, 1952.

Johnson, Dallas: *Facing the Facts About Cancer.* Public Affairs Committee, New York, 1951.

Kiernander, B.: *Physical Medicine and Rehabilitation.* Charles C Thomas, Publisher, Springfield, Ill., 1953.

Kovács, R.: *Electrotherapy and Light Therapy,* 6th ed. Lea & Febiger, Philadelphia, 1949.

————: *Light Therapy.* Charles C Thomas, Publisher, Springfield, Ill., 1950.

Osborne, S. L.: *Diathermy: The Use of High Frequency Currents.* Charles C Thomas, Publisher, Springfield, Ill., 1950.

Quimby, Edith H.: "Safety in the Use of Radioactive Isotopes," *Am. J. Nursing,* **51**:240, (Apr.) 1951.

Schorr, H. A.; Nagle, R. A.; and Priest, B. R.: "The Patient's Spiritual Needs," *Am. J. Nursing,* **50**:64, (Feb.) 1950.

VanderVelt, James H., and Odenwald, Robert P.: *Psychiatry and Catholicism.* McGraw-Hill Book Co., New York, 1952.

Wolff, Ilse S.: "Should the Patient Know the Truth?" *Am. J. Nursing,* **55**:546, (May) 1955.

CHAPTER 25. ADMINISTRATION OF MEDICINES

1. **PREVENTION OF DISEASE BY ADMINISTRATION OF DRUGS**
2. **DRUG THERAPY**
3. **FACTORS MODIFYING DOSAGE AND EFFECTS OF DRUGS**
4. **ROUTES OF ADMINISTRATION**

1. PREVENTION OF DISEASE BY ADMINISTRATION OF DRUGS

"Medicines" are sometimes used to promote health and prevent disease. Vaccines and sera, for example, are given to protect people and animals from communicable diseases; quinacrine (Atabrine) is taken regularly as a preventive by susceptible persons living where malaria is rife; drinking water is reinforced with iodine in certain regions to prevent goiter, and in some places with fluorine to control dental caries; insulin is occasionally used to promote the appetite; and vitamins are given in the form of a medication when the diet is substandard in quantity or quality. Ordinarily, however, drugs are given to cure or control a disease or to allay the accompanying pain and discomfort.

2. DRUG THERAPY

Responsibilities of the Nurse. Giving drugs is one of the nurse's most serious duties. A person who is under treatment but who does not need nursing care may prepare and take his own medication. He can, in many cases, learn enough about the drug and his condition to do this with safety and he should be helped to gain this independence. The nurse, in contrast, has a more difficult task because she must know about *many* drugs and in giving these must be able to follow many physicians' plan of therapy for many patients. To get the best results, drugs should be given exactly as the doctor prescribes them in relation to route and time of administration, preparation, and dosage. At the same time the person who is giving, or taking, the drug must know enough to carry out the doctor's directions and to recognize and report reactions that would make the physician want to change his prescription. It is desirable, therefore, that the nurse (as an administrator of drugs) know the nature of the drug; its local and systemic action and something of the physiological explanation; why the drug is ordered in each case and the result the physician hopes to get; the signs of the intended effect; and the signs of an overdose or of a cumulative toxic effect, or indications that the patient has an idiosyncrasy to the drug. The nurse must know how to use the apothecaries' and metric systems of measurement and how to convert one to the other since both systems are used in this country (see Appendix II for tables of equivalents). All those who take part in drug therapy should know the minimum and maximum dosage of any drug they use. Nurses should know how age, sex, body weight, and time of administration affect the dose. She should know how drugs are excreted, for the excretory organ is the first to show signs of poisoning. For example, the kidneys are irritated by mercury, arsenic, and the sulfa drugs. The nurse should understand that drugs cannot change the functions of body cells but they can stimulate or depress these functions and eventually destroy the cells if either of these effects is carried beyond physiological limits. A knowledge of the selectivity of drugs will help her to understand the wide variety of reactions to medication. The person giving or taking the drug should know when it is to be pushed to its physiologic limit—that is, until the first symptoms of poisoning occurs. A classic example is digitalis which is often given until the pulse is slowed to 60 beats per minute.

While the physician is primarily responsible for ordering the medication in the correct dosage he, being human and often overworked, is subject to error. Lives have been saved by nurses who have recognized mistakes in written orders for drugs, and lives have been lost because similar mistakes were not detected. Moreover, a nurse can be successfully prosecuted for carrying out a doctor's order for the wrong drug, or a toxic dose, if the court is persuaded that the preparation of the nurse qualified her to recognize the danger of the drug or the dosage. Emanuel Hayt and Lillian R. Hayt in discussing the duty of the nurse to execute the physician's orders say:

Duty of Nurse to Execute Physician's Orders. Nurses and internes at a general hospital are charged with the duty of carrying out the instructions of the attending physician, except in cases of emergency. A patient entering the hospital has the right to expect that the instructions of his physician will be complied with. While he relies on the skill of his own physician, he knows nothing of the ability of the internes and nurses. In an emergency it is, of course, incumbent on the nurses and internes to exercise their own judgment until [a] report can be made to and instruction received from the attending physician.

In the discharge of duty, nurse and interne must obey the orders of the physician or surgeon in charge of the patient, unless such orders are so obviously negligent as to lead any reasonable person to anticipate that substantial injury would result to the patient. The law contemplates that the physician is solely responsible for the diagnosis and treatment of his patient; nurses are not supposed to be experts in the technique of diagnosis or the mechanics of treatment. However, nurses are expected to exercise their judgment: if a physician "should order a nurse to stick fire to a patient," no nurse would be protected from liability for damages for undertaking to carry out the orders of the physician. The law does not expect blind obedience from a nurse.*

* Hayt, Emanuel, and Hayt, Lillian R.: Legal Guide for American Hospitals. Hospital Textbook Co., New York, 1940, p. 353.

It is obvious that in order to protect the patient and herself the nurse should know the therapeutic and maximum doses of the drugs she gives and she should be informed on her legal status in drug therapy. It is a protection to know the laws and regulations restricting the use of drugs, the most important law being the Federal Food, Drug and Cosmetic Act that in 1940 replaced the Pure Food Law of 1906 and the (federal) Harrison Anti-Narcotic Act of 1914 (revised many times since) with the related (state) Uniform Narcotic Drug Acts.[1, 2, 3]

This competence is not acquired in any "course" but it is built up gradually through a study of each patient and the medication used for him. The nurse must know some chemistry and physiology and some general principles of therapy in order to read medical reports with understanding. She should be familiar with the indexes to current medical periodicals; she should know that "U.S.P." indicates that a drug is made according to the standards published in the *United States Pharmacopoeia,*[4] that the *National Formulary*[5] ("N.F.") supplements that publication, and that a digest of these two is available in the form of the *Epitome of the Pharmacopoeia of the United States and the National Formulary.*[6] To get information about new drugs not included in official publications students must use *New and Nonofficial Remedies*[7] published annually by the American Medical Association, recent texts on pharmacology, and reports in current medical journals. A nurse should develop the habit of looking up every unfamiliar drug she gives. Drugs should be thought of as potentially dangerous, and no nurse should dare to be ignorant, uninterested, or mechanical in the administration of them. There are, in some institutions, regulations permitting graduate nurses to give on their own judgment a few mild drugs like sodium bicarbonate. Such regulation should be written, and nurses should avoid responsibility for the most harmless medication except in a situation where doctors are not available.

Patients ask nurses many questions about drugs prescribed for them and patent preparations they use on their own. The nurse should have a clear understanding of what the physician wants the patient to know about the medication used in his treatment. Increasingly, doctors like their patients to be partners in the therapeutic plan and usually they are very frank about the nature and purpose of the drugs they prescribe. (Exceptions to this rule are generally made in the case of habit-forming drugs.) In the treatment of diabetes, pernicious anemia, hypothyroidism, and many long-term diseases, control is only possible if the patient and his family understand the use of therapeutic agents. Nurses should listen with interest to anything the patient may ask or tell her about medication, his mental attitude toward the treatment, the experiences he has had with drugs, and particularly any idiosyncrasies to drugs. The latter should be reported at once, but at all times the nurse should take every opportunity to learn from the patient himself and she should report what she knows promptly and accurately. On the basis of the nurse's observations drugs are often discontinued and dosage changed.

In general the nurse should reinforce the doctor's information to patients by teaching them how to prepare and take drugs, by explaining that certain results, as, for example, a dry mouth from belladonna, or dark stools from bismuth, or diarrhea from oxytetracycline (Terramycin), are to be expected, while warning them to watch closely for toxic signs such as a reduction in urine with sulfa drugs or headache and skin eruptions from bromides. Nurses should impress patients with the danger of self-medication. They should also teach them to look for evidence of high standards of quality in drugs. Instruction must often include demonstrations and supervised practice in the measurement and administration of drugs. It is as much the nurses's function to teach the patient how to take medications as to give them to him.

Accuracy, Punctuality, and Efficiency. To ensure that the right patient is given the right medicine at the right time, each hospital has developed or adopted a system for the administration of medicines, which usually includes the following steps.

On each ward there is a *doctor's order book* in which the doctor's orders are written. Except in extreme emergencies, no medicine should be given a patient unless the doctor writes the order and signs it. When an emergency prevents this, the order should be dictated and signed later. All orders must be clearly written. (A nurse should never give a medicine if in doubt as to the drug or dosage.) Sometimes there is a separate order book for day and night, but, in any case, the date and hour should be clearly indicated. Nurses should look at this book frequently, because a doctor may write an order without calling the attention of a nurse to it and the patient may be suffering from want of the medication. In some hospitals the doctor puts a red tag on the front of the patient's chart to show that an order has just been written. When the medicine ordered is not to be repeated, the order should be marked off with red ink as soon as the drug is given and the time of administration indicated. The order and the time are copied on the chart. If such an order is not marked off, the drug may be given a second time and endanger the life of the patient. Those orders for drugs that are to be repeated are marked off when transferred to the medication tickets, or cards. Colored "tickets" (2 in. square) are commonly used, each color indicating the time of administration as in the following:

COLOR OF TICKET	TIME OF ADMINISTRATION
Plain yellow	Every 4 hours
Yellow with corners cut	Four times a day
Plain pink	Three time a day
Pink with corners cut	Every 3 hours
Orange	Before meals
Orange, ½ ticket	Every night
Blue	After meals
Pale orange	Twice a day
Red	Every 6 hours
Red, ½ ticket	Every morning
White	Every 2 hours
Green	When required

These tickets can be protected by dipping them in an ether solution of paraffin or by rubbing with a piece of paraffin.* So treated they will stay clean and the writing

* The medicine cards can also be coated with shellac, but this method is not as convenient since sufficient time must be allowed to permit the shellac to dry thoroughly.

clear and distinct. Commercial cardboard covers for medicine glasses are available that have space for writing all the information given on the ticket. If they have different colored borders they serve the same purpose as medicine tickets and also provide covers for the glasses. (See Fig. 157.) Some workers prefer to have all cards the same color, depending entirely on what is written on the card.

It is necessary to give the following information on each card: ① the patient's full name, ② the drug, ③ the dosage, and ④ the hour and frequency. It is convenient to give the room or the bed number, the date the drug was ordered, and the date on which it is to be discontinued, if this is known. In most places it is assumed that drugs are to be given by mouth unless otherwise indicated on the card.

When the ticket system is used, the doctors' orders are transferred from the order book to tickets, usually by one person, such as the head nurse. In any event it must be clearly understood who is responsible for this. The tickets should be kept near the medicine closet in a convenient holder that assorts them according to the time of administration. There should be a record by which the number of medications to be given at different hours can be checked daily. This should be tallied with the medication cards and the patients' charts. When an order for a drug is altered or discontinued the ticket is often put on the desk and destroyed by the head nurse, or by the person assigned the responsibility for seeing that drugs are accurately given.

When the nurse administers the medications she places the tickets of the drugs to be given at that hour in a row. As she prepares each dose she attaches the corresponding ticket to the glass and does not remove the ticket until she gives the medication to the patient. In some institutions tickets are placed on the head nurse's desk to indicate that the medicines have been given.

The following rules, or precautions, in giving drugs make for accuracy.

1. Arrange, if possible, to be free from interruption while preparing a medication. Avoid conversation or anything that prevents concentration on the task in hand.

2. Check the doctor's order and make certain that it is signed. Read the medicine ticket and be sure that it tallies with the doctor's order; keep the ticket in sight while preparing the medication.

3. Check the order (medicine ticket) with the label on the bottle. Read the label three times—before taking the bottle from the shelf, before pouring the medication, and before returning the bottle to the shelf.

4. Measure the dose exactly, using standard weights and measures: use graduated glasses for measuring cubic centimeters (milliliters), ounces, and drams; a minim glass for minims, and a pipette or medicine dropper for drops. Never give minims for drops, or vice versa. (Some pipettes are calibrated for minims and drops.)

5. When measuring fluids hold the graduate so that the eye is on a level with the line indicating the desired quantity.

6. Shake fluid medications. Don't use a fluid if there is a change of color, or if there is a sediment in a preparation that does not have "shake well" on the label.

7. Give each liquid drug in a separate glass, or cup.

8. If an excess of the drug is poured do not return it to the bottle; in general this is dangerous, even with pills, tablets, and capsules.

9. Take the drug to the patient with the identifying ticket on it. (The nurse who measures the drug should give it; drugs should not be sent to a patient by another patient.) Use the person's name in handing him the drug to give him a chance to correct mistaken identity.

10. Stay with the patient while he takes the drug but try to avoid the impression of compulsion and haste. If circumstances make it impossible or undesirable for the person to take the medication at the time ordered, consultation with the doctor may be indicated. The drug should not be left with the patient, but a fresh dose taken to him if the medication is given later.

11. Be sure that the person is able to take the medication as it is prescribed. Semi-conscious and irrational patients should not be given drugs in liquid form. Pills, capsules, and tablets may be held in the mouth or they may be inhaled and lodge in the trachea, occluding the air passages. (Patients whose swallowing reflex is absent should not be given anything by mouth.)

Medications should be given to each patient by the nurse assigned to care for him. In this way the patient is most likely to have the maximum help from the nurse, and she is likely to learn most about the clinical uses of the drug and its relationship to the patient's progress. The graduate nurse should require no supervision of this function; for the welfare of all concerned medications given by student nurses should be checked by the graduate staff. Many hospitals assign the giving of drugs to one nurse even though most of the nursing care of patients is individualized.

Recording Medications. A part of every medical record is the sheet on which the doctor's orders for the patient are written. This gives the date, the drugs prescribed, their dosage and route of administration, and the date of cancellation. Another part of the record is the sheet on which nursing care is reported. On this is a record of the medications—the day, the hour, the dosage, and route of administration. Practice in charting medications varies in several respects. In certain hospitals the nurse is asked to record every drug she gives; in other hospitals she is expected to record giving only selected drugs, a list of which is posted. In some agencies the nurse is required to sign her initials or her name after every medication she gives but in most places after potent drugs only. Nomenclature used in all records should be official, and abbreviations, when used in records, should be taken from a standard source. (See Appendix III for a list of abbreviations with which nurses should be familiar.)

The Medicine Cupboard and Care of Drugs. If possible, medicines should be kept in a separate room near the head nurse's station, or office. A sink with running water should be a part of the unit. It is necessary to prevent some patients, occasionally with suicidal intent, from taking hospital supplies. For this reason particularly the medicine cupboard is always locked; the keys are tagged and given to qualified personnel only. Solutions, ointments, and liniments for external use should be in a compartment which separates them from substances for internal use. Solids and liquids are separated; poisons should be in a special part of the cupboard in bottles clearly marked *poison,* differentiated by color, roughened surface, and shape. All potent drugs such as morphine and strychnine, usually given hypodermically, should be in a separate compartment. The alphabetical arrangement of drugs within the groups just mentioned saves time in finding the desired substance. Organic oils should be kept in a cool place—they are decomposed by heat and made rancid by exposure to air. Sera, vaccines, and antibiotics,

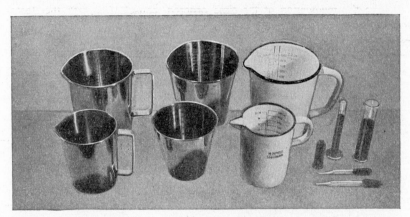

Figure 156. Calibrated measures used in preparing solutions and medications. (Glass measures are available in large sizes also.) (Courtesy of Clay-Adams Co., New York City.)

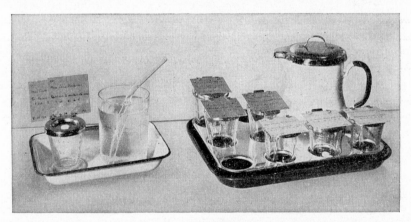

Figure 157. Equipment for administering medicines by mouth. (*Left*) Tray to be used when medications are given individually; (*right*) convenient setup for group technique in giving medicines.

such as penicillin and oxytetracycline, are kept in a refrigerator. The medicine cupboard should be well supplied with all drugs likely to be required, but it should not be overstocked. Its contents should be checked frequently. Day nurses should see that there is sufficient for the needs of the day and should be particularly watchful to see that the necessary supply is on hand for the night. Drugs should be ordered in small amounts since many deteriorate or lose their effectiveness if not fresh. Any change in color, odor, or consistency should be reported. Bottles should be tightly covered and labeled. Labels should be indestructible and clean. No nurse, however, should alter or change labels—this should be done by the pharmacist. In some hospitals the personnel of the pharmacy check drugs in the clinical divisions and assume responsibility for providing, storing, and maintaining supplies of drugs.

To avoid soiling the label when pouring the solution from the bottle, the label should be held uppermost. The rim of the bottle should always be cleaned afterward. Medicine should never be left in an unmarked glass or bottle. If a drug has two commonly used names it is wise to have both names on the label. The dosage

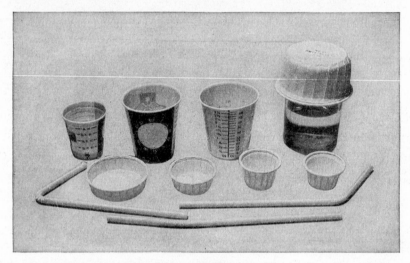

Figure 158. Calibrated paper medicine cups, fluted soufflé cups for pills, and paper drinking tubes. Note use of larger soufflé cup to cover drinking glass. (Courtesy of Field Research Division, Paper Cup and Container Institute, New York City, and Clay-Adams Co., New York City.)

of potent medicines is sometimes printed on labels. Shelves, bottles, and labels should be clean and orderly. Bottles for drugs of the same group should be of a uniform size and shape, and arranged so that each label is visible. To avoid overcrowding, discontinued prescriptions should be returned to the drug room. There are desirable types of bottles for powders, liquids, and tablets. When a screw cap is used, it covers the mouth of the bottle and protects it from contamination. Glass-stoppered bottles, while very attractive looking, are expensive and impractical, the stoppers not being interchangeable and affording no protection to the bottle lip.

3. FACTORS MODIFYING DOSAGE AND EFFECTS OF DRUGS

As has been said, a nurse is not responsible for the dose ordered but it is often her function to see that the patient gets the drug in the amount intended by the physician. To help prevent errors in medication she must know, or be able to find information on, the minimum and maximum dosage and she should have some appreciation of the way in which the following factors modify dosage.

Age. Since it is impossible to memorize doses for all ages, rules have been set up for computing the child's dose from the adult therapeutic dose. The rules are usually based on age and weight. Of these Louis S. Goodman and Alfred Gilman[8] think Clark's rule the most serviceable. (Child's dose $= \dfrac{weight\ of\ child\ in\ pounds}{150}$ × adult dose.) John D. Crawford et al.,[9] however, think that the child's dose should be based on the area of body surface.

No formulas can be applied mechanically because children respond differently to different kinds of drugs. For instance, children require small doses of narcotics, while, on the contrary, the child's dose of a cathartic approaches that of an adult. In old age the dose of weakening or depressing drugs, such as irritant cathartics or narcotics, is smaller than the usual therapeutic dose.

Sex. The adult dose is based upon the average weight of a man. As women weigh less than men, the dose ordered is often smaller. Women are more susceptible to the action of certain drugs, and, during pregnancy, drugs acting on the uterus are avoided.

Previous Habits or Toleration. When a patient has been in the habit of taking drugs, such as morphine or alcohol, it is often dangerous to stop the drug suddenly. For instance, following an accident or in pneumonia, when the patient has been in the habit of drinking heavily, whisky is administered to prevent delirium tremens. In such cases large doses are necessary to produce any effect. If the patient has been in the habit of taking morphine only a large dose will relieve pain or induce sleep. Patients quickly develop a tolerance for all sedatives.

Idiosyncrasy and Susceptibility. Certain foods and drugs that may be given to most people with safety produce in others very unusual and poisonous effects; for instance, some people have a decided intolerance for cocaine or derivatives of opium, so that even small doses cause nausea or other toxic symptoms.

Condition of the Patient. Rate of Excretion and Cumulative Action. When pain is great, large doses of morphine may be ordered. When the patient's breathing is already difficult, smaller doses of morphine are given, and the patient is watched closely for further depression of the respiratory center. In shock or collapse, the dosage of stimulants ordered may be larger than usual. When drugs are given as antidotes for poisoning, large doses are ordered. On the other hand, in diseases of the kidneys or in any disease with edema, smaller doses of drugs eliminated by the kidney may be ordered, and at greater intervals. Failure of the kidneys to eliminate the drug makes it accumulate in the body. In edema, the drug may accumulate and be dissolved in the excess fluid. In conditions that prevent the elimination of a drug through the normal avenue of excretion the nurse should be on the alert for symptoms of cumulative poisoning.

Nature and Form of Medication. Some drugs are eliminated very rapidly, as, for example, ammonia and epinephrine (Adrenalin). The effect of such drugs is fleeting, therefore, and they can be repeated in therapeutic doses without fear of toxicity; other drugs, such as digitalis and iron, are eliminated slowly and for this reason they are effective when given less frequently, but the patient must be watched for signs of cumulative poisoning.

Liquid medications, particularly drugs dissolved in water, act more rapidly than pills and powders. Powders should be dissolved or given in capsules. Absorption of powders and capsules is hastened, and swallowing made easier, if they are taken with a large quantity of liquid.

Some drugs have a *biphasic action;* that is, doses on different levels have different effects. Small doses of atropine slow the heart rate by stimulating the vagus nerve; large doses increase the cardiac rate by freeing the heart from vagal inhibition.[10]

Time of Administration.   The effect of drugs given by mouth is more marked if the stomach and upper part of the intestinal tracts are empty. For instance, the same amount of alcohol is much more intoxicating taken before than after a meal. If given after meals, larger doses of drugs are usually necessary to produce the effect desired.

Drug Combinations.   When two drugs that have similar actions are given at the same time the dosage of each is smaller than if it were given alone. Drugs that act in this way are called *synergistic;* drugs whose actions oppose each other are termed *antagonistic.*

The Route of Administration.   The dose varies with the rapidity with which it is absorbed; for instance, when given intravenously, the dose is small because the full effect of the drug is felt immediately. When given by rectum the dose ordered may be larger than when given by mouth because the rate and amount of absorption are generally less rapid and certain.

Route of Excretion.   Drugs are selective in their avenues of excretion. They may be eliminated by one or all of the following routes: the kidneys, the alimentary tract, the lungs, the skin, and mucous membranes of the nose and throat. When the patient's disease cripples the excretory function of any of these routes the physician avoids, or gives in small dosage, drugs that must be eliminated by them.

4. ROUTES OF ADMINISTRATION

Medicines may be given by any of the following routes depending upon the effect desired (a direct local effect, a systemic effect, or a remote local effect), the rapidity of action needed, the nature and amount of drug to be given, and the condition of the patient: (1) by needle injections—intra-arterial, intravenous, intramuscular, subcutaneous, intracardial, intraperitoneal, intraspinous, intraosseous, and intradermal; (2) by mouth—swallowed and sublingual; (3) by inhalation; (4) by the mucous membranes of the rectum, vagina, urethra and bladder, the eye, ear, nose and throat; and (5) the skin. The speed of action according to route is more or less in the order given, from the most rapid to the least rapid. (The introduction of drugs through the skin by means of a jet of liquid under high pressure gives results comparable to needle injections. This procedure is in the process of development and is discussed on page 731.)

Since the techniques of giving drugs with needles and through tubes into body cavities require detailed directions they are described in the section of the text devoted to therapeutic procedures; other methods of medication are described here.

By Mouth. Drugs are given by mouth in the following *forms:* (1) liquids—oils, water solutions as infusions, decoctions, or suspensions, and alcoholic solutions as extracts or tinctures; (2) solids—tablets, powders (often put in capsules), pills, and lozenges.

The person preparing an oral medication should consider the effect desired and how to get it, the nature of the drug, how to protect the mouth and teeth if the drug has an injurious action on them, and how to make the dose acceptable to the patient.

It is important to know why a medication is given in order to decide whether it should be well diluted or given in a more concentrated form. If, for example, a systemic or a remote local effect is desired, drugs should be well diluted to aid absorption. (As water is usually the best solvent, all drugs, except oily preparations, are given with water unless otherwise ordered.) Water is given freely with all diaphoretics, diuretics, and narcotics. A hot drink following administration of such drugs is thought to hasten their action. When sweating is induced by drugs such as the salicylates, care should be taken to keep the patient from getting chilled.

Some drugs, such as aromatic spirits of ammonia, although given for a systemic effect, owe their action to a reflex response following irritation of nerve endings in the mucous lining of the mouth or throat. Such drugs must be diluted sufficiently to prevent irritation to the tissues, but not to the extent of preventing irritation of nerve endings.

Drugs, such as syrup cough mixtures, prescribed for a local soothing or sedative effect on the mucous lining of the respiratory tract, are usually given undiluted. Drugs given for a local effect on the stomach are only slightly diluted. They may be given before meals, when the stomach is empty and at rest, to soften mucus or to stimulate the flow of gastric juice. They may be given *during* or *after* meals to supply a deficiency of hydrochloric acid or enzymes, or to counteract abnormal conditions present.

Time of administration is chosen with reference to the desired effect. Drugs given by mouth for a systemic effect usually depend upon absorption from the intestines rather than the stomach. They act most rapidly when the stomach and upper intestines are empty (as has been noted); they are therefore prescribed between meals. Sodium bicarbonate, when given in acidosis, to neutralize an acid tendency in body fluids, is usually given between meals. If given after meals, more of the alkaline salt is combined with hydrochloric acid, and absorbed as sodium chloride. It should rarely be given in a capsule but should be dissolved in a glass of water and followed by more water.

In order to give a sedative or narcotic intelligently a nurse must know the effect desired, and also the time required for the drug to act. The *hour* of administration is often left to her judgment. Before giving the drug the nurse should see that the patient's surroundings and his mental and physical condition are all conducive to rest. Because of the depressing effect of all sedatives and narcotics the character of the patient's sleep should be noted.)

The effect desired sometimes determines the _amount of drug_ given. For instance, when ipecac is used to cause vomiting by a direct local effect on the stomach, a large dose is given well diluted; but when used as an expectorant, through its remote control effect on the bronchial tubes, a small dose is given undiluted in a cough mixture.

Cold water is commonly used to dilute drugs; but when a drug, such as peppermint, is given for a carminative effect, hot water should be used, as heat promotes the expulsion of gas from the stomach or intestines.

The _nature of the drug and its possibly injurious effects_ should be fully considered by the nurse. Many drugs, such as dilute acids, iron, arsenic, salicylates, iodides, bromides, digitalis, and mercury, are irritating to the mucous lining of the stomach and may cause pain, nausea, and vomiting. All such drugs should be well diluted. They are usually given after meals so that they may be mixed with the stomach contents which reduces the effect on its walls. Dilute acids such as hydrochloric acid and liquid preparations of iron are also destructive to the teeth. They should be given through a glass tube or a straw. Dilute hydrochloric acid is frequently added to a drinking glass of water, and the patient is asked to sip it during the meal, in this way approximating the normal secretion in the stomach. The mouth should receive careful attention when such drugs are given. Some doctors prescribe bicarbonate of soda with aspirin and other preparations of the salicylates to lessen the irritation in the stomach and to prevent acidosis.

Every nurse should know how to make medicine as acceptable as possible to a patient. There are a few drugs, such as the bitter stomachics, quinine, gentian, and nux vomica, that owe their stimulating effect on the appetite to their bitter taste. These drugs are therefore given undiluted with no attempt to disguise the taste. In all other cases the taste should be made as unobjectionable as possible. Unpalatable drugs should be diluted, and cold water should be given immediately afterward from a clean glass. Ice may be held in the mouth before and after the medication in order to numb the nerve endings which include the taste buds. It is unwise to try to disguise the taste with food because this is likely to turn the person against the food.

Although a nurse's manner should not be hurried when giving a medication she should encourage the patient to take it promptly. Delay only prolongs the period of dread and intensifies dislike of the drug. Mouthwash should be offered persons who must take unpalatable concoctions or who are getting drugs which, like the iodides, are excreted in the saliva.

Castor oil is a heavy oil with a taste universally disliked in this country. A tasteless preparation is on the market but the consistency is still unpleasant, and memory supplies the taste to those who know it. To make this drug acceptable to most persons it should be disguised. It may be bought flavored with peppermint or its cloying consistency may be changed by mixing it thoroughly with a carbonated drink such as root beer. The following method is simple and satisfactory.

(The medicine glass is first rinsed with lemon juice. About a teaspoonful of lemon juice is poured into the glass, then the oil, and on top of that more lemon juice. The glass is then placed in a small saucer and surrounded with small pieces of chipped ice. The taste of the chilled oil is much less disagreeable. The patient is given ice to hold in his mouth before and after taking the oil. Taking orange juice, Vichy or Seltzer water, or an olive afterward will often prevent the feeling of nausea that sometimes follows a dose of castor oil.)

Pills or tablets should be broken up, powdered, and dissolved when it is difficult for patients to swallow them. Powders that will not dissolve readily or that have a disagreeable taste may be given in capsules. Because compound licorice powder is not easily dissolved, it should be mixed into a paste with a small amount of water. Sufficient water should be added to enable the patient to swallow it; adding too much water is likely to cause nausea.

Attractive looking equipment helps to make medicines less distasteful to patients. The articles shown in Figure 157 were chosen for their neat appearance, durability, and convenience. Disposable paper medicine cups and drinking tubes save labor. Medicine glasses and glass tubes must be "sanitized" as described for dishes in Chapter 7. A short drinking tube has an advantage over a long one because it is better balanced. When drugs are given to a group of patients an extra water supply is carried on the tray, but the nurse giving the medicines should see that each patient who is to receive medicine is provided with a drinking glass and fresh water on the bedside table.

By Inhalation. Drugs may be given by inhalation for either a *systemic* or a *local* effect. The systemic effect is produced immediately because of the large surface area of the lungs and the rich supply of blood vessels. Drugs used for *local effect* may be in the form of medicated steam and fumes, although the latter method is rarely used. Fumes from stramonium leaves (or stramonium with belladonna) may be inhaled to relax spasms of the involuntary muscles. Stramonium leaves may be made into cigarettes, or they may be burned in a fireproof vessel and the fumes inhaled through a cone fitted over the vessel.

Some drugs that are used for their *systemic effect* are: Ammonia gas (from ammonia water or smelling salts) is inhaled as an emergency heart and respiratory stimulant in fainting or mild collapse. Amyl nitrate is inhaled to relax the coronary arteries and relieve an attack of angina pectoris or to relax spasms of the muscles of the bronchial tubes in asthma. This drug comes in small glass capsules, or pearls, which are broken in a paper or gauze handkerchief and held a short distance above the nose for a few minutes.

The inhalation of fumes from volatile drugs, or burning drugs, is *dry inhalation*; the inhalation of plain steam or steam impregnated with a drug is *moist inhalation*.

Moist or *steam inhalations* are used chiefly for the following purposes: (1) to relieve inflammation of the mucous membrane in acute colds and in sinusitis; (2) to relieve inflammation of the larynx; (3) to soften thick, tenacious mucus and relieve coughing from many causes; and (4) to warm and moisten the air when, following operations such as a tracheotomy, room air is drawn into the trachea without being warmed and moistened by the nose and upper respiratory passages as it is in normal breathing.

Steam for moist inhalations is generated, most often, in an electrically heated unit as shown in Figure 159. Antiseptics, such as tincture of benzoin, turpentine, menthol, creosote, and eucalyptol, are sometimes vaporized in the steam. Most authorities, however, believe that the virtue of an inhalation lies chiefly in the action of moist heat. Some physicians believe that the patient should stay in a very humid

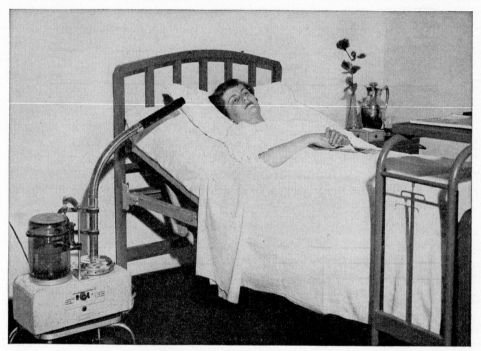

Figure 159. A steam inhalator with an automatically controlled electric heating unit. (If indicated, a canopy may be draped over a frame that fits on the bed.) (Courtesy of New York Hospital, New York City.)

room rather than inhale steam intermittently. Windows and doors are kept closed, and steam is released from a special outlet on a steam radiator, from an electrically heated humidifier, or from a kettle of water boiling in the room over any source of heat. Usually, the treatment is given intermittently for a period of one-half hour every three or four hours during the day. The method depends upon the equipment available. Inhalations with incorporated electrical heating units are most convenient and safest.

A croup tent arranged around and over the head of the bed is advisable, particularly for a child with croup, and in all cases in which it is desirable to have a patient breathe warm moist air continuously or for a prolonged period. This prevents the discomfort, strain, and exhausting effect of keeping the face turned con-

stantly toward the steam and overcomes this difficulty during sleep. In this, and
in all other methods used, the greatest precaution must be taken to protect the
patient from burns or scalds. The outer covering of the tent may be a cotton sheet,
but the inner layers must be a blanket or a large piece of turkish toweling to absorb
the moisture; otherwise, the hot condensed steam would fall on the patient or bed.
The head of the bed must be securely enclosed to prevent the escape of steam. There
should be ample ventilation however, and, although there must be no drafts, the

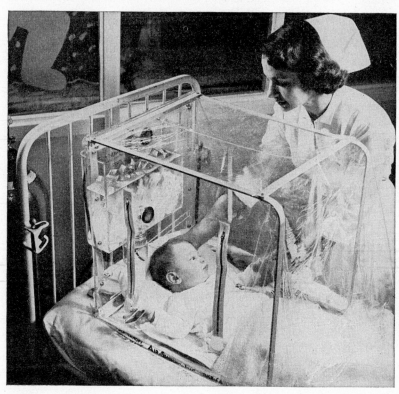

Figure 160A. "Croupette," a humidity and oxygen tent unit. (Courtesy of Air-Shields, Inc.,
Hatboro, Pa.)

tent should not be kept so warm that both patient and nurse get a steam bath.
The humidifier or kettle should be on the floor, a low table, or chair, according to
the design, with the spout extending into the tent at the side or back. The spout
must not extend far enough for the patient to touch it or for condensed steam to
fall from it on the patient. When electric inhalators are not available other methods
of generating steam may be used. Boiling water or the boiling medicated solution
may be poured into a narrow-necked pitcher, and a towel, or a cone of cardboard
or oiled paper, placed over it to direct the steam toward the mouth and nose of the
patient. (To avoid burning the patient the pitcher must be filled only two thirds

full.) An ordinary teakettle may be used in the same way. The earthenware Maw's inhaler is sometimes used as it retains heat for a long time. The croup kettle—a tin kettle with a long spout—is occasionally used in the hospital. An electric stove is the best and safest means of keeping the contents of the kettle steaming hot. In all methods, the patient must be in a comfortable position for inhaling the vapor.

Inhalations involve a risk of scalding the person or of scorching his bedding. Every precaution should be taken to prevent such accidents, and the patient should be closely watched. During this treatment blood vessels of the skin and mucous mem-

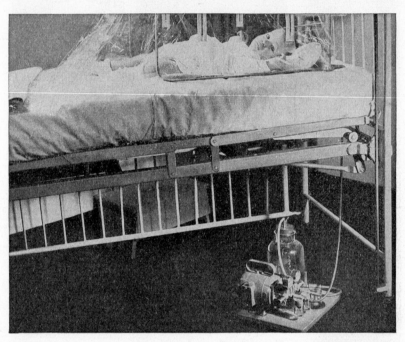

Figure 160B. Motor compressor-aspirator unit for "Croupette," illustrated in Figure 160A. (Courtesy of Air-Shields, Inc., Hatboro, Pa.)

brane of the head are dilated. For this reason the patient is easily chilled; therefore, he should not go into a cold atmosphere for several hours.

Many persons suffering from chronic upper respiratory disease get considerable relief from inhaling steam. Very often the doctor prescribes this treatment to be used by the patient in his home. The nurse should, in such cases, devise and teach the patient a method that is adapted to the circumstances in which he lives.

Another way of medicating the respiratory passages is to *spray* the nose or throat with very finely divided liquids. If the particles are extremely small the liquid is said to be *nebulized*. Devices for mechanically dividing medications are called atomizers and nebulizers. Both operate on the principle that a column of gas forced through a liquid will collect and carry with it particles of the liquid. Air is forced through the atomizer with the hand bulb, or a stream of oxygen may be passed through the nebulizer. The latter is one way of giving antibiotics, such as penicillin, when the patient has a lung infection. Because the lungs have such an abundant blood supply inhaled nebulized drugs, such as epinephrine, may be rapidly absorbed and show immediate systemic action.[11]

When nebulizers are used the physician wants the drugs to reach the lungs. (The finer the particles the more likely they are to penetrate the lungs.) Patients must be taught to inhale as the bulb collapses in order to draw the vapor into the lungs and to avoid swallowing the drug. If swallowed it may be inactivated and wasted, or it may cause discomfort. The exact dose is put in the nebulizer; the mask is fitted to the patient, and oxygen allowed to flow through the nebulizer at the rate of 5 or 6 liters a minute until all the drug has been vaporized.

Gases—oxygen, helium, and carbon dioxide—are given by inhalation as therapeutic agents. Because there is so much detail to be discussed in connection with their administration, Chapter 27 is devoted to this subject.

By Mucous Membranes. There are numerous blood vessels in the mucous membrane under the tongue (sublingual vessels). Tablets and lozenges held under the tongue in the front of the mouth are rapidly dissolved and absorbed. Goodman and Gilman[12] say that nitroglycerin is absorbed more efficiently by the sublingual than by the intestinal route. While drugs to be absorbed are most often given by mouth they can reach the circulation from the mucous lining of the oropharynx, nose, eyes, rectum, vagina, urethra, and bladder. Ordinarily those regions are medicated for a local effect, but sometimes it is convenient to give systemic medications by these routes, as, for example, general anesthesia by rectum. Topical medications and irrigations of these areas and the introduction of suppositories into these various body cavities are described in Chapters 30, 31, 32, and 33.

By the Skin. In the simplest forms of life the surface of the organism is very sensitive to its environment, chemicals penetrate the outer cells, and the organism dies if it is not in a fairly stable medium. The higher forms of life, in contrast, are able to exist in more unstable surroundings because most chemicals in their (outer) environment do not penetrate their skins, or hides. Drugs, therefore, are rarely applied to the skin for anything but a local effect. If the skin is clear and the drug is carried in an oil, or fat, it can penetrate the hair follicles and sebaceous glands and through them the subcutaneous tissue according to Goodman and Gilman.[13] They say also that drugs that ionize can be made to migrate through the epidermis by means of a galvanic current, a procedure called *iontophoresis.* Discussing the danger of industrial exposure to chemicals Anna M. Baetjer,[14] in Kenneth F. Maxcy's text, says all oil-soluble substances can penetrate the skin to some degree. With an instrument called the *Hypospray,* described in Chapter 26, a jet of liquid drug can be directed at the skin with such force that it will penetrate the unbroken skin and will give a systemic effect similar to that of a hypodermic.

Drugs carried in fats or oils and applied to the skin for their systemic effects are called *inunctions.* Mercurial ointment was formerly used this way in the treatment of syphilis. A drug is absorbed most readily in regions where the skin is thin, such as the axilla, the inner surface of the arm, the thigh, and groin. The skin should be clean and the blood vessels dilated by a warm bath. The ointment or oil should be warm also. To prevent irritation the ointment is never applied to the same area on successive days. The areas just listed may be used in rotation on successive days; this is called a "course" of applications. The treatment is then omitted for a day and the parts are washed to remove any of the ointment which may remain in the pores of the skin. The "course" is then begun again in the same order. A record of the treatment should be indicated on the chart each day. If a nurse is rubbing an irritating drug on a patient's skin she should wear gloves, otherwise her hands may be affected or the drug may be absorbed and act on her systemically. Most applications to the skin are made for the purpose of cleaning, soothing, or disinfecting the skin. The concept of "feeding the skin" with fats, vitamins, and proteins has in the past had little credence in medical circles. The effectiveness of local applications to the skin of fat-soluble vitamin ointment in conditions associated with constant removal with soap and water of skin oils is evidence that the skin can, in a sense, be "fed" certain food elements.

REFERENCES

1. United States Government: *Organization Manual 1951–52.* Federal Register Division, National Archives and Record Service, General Service Administration, Washington, D.C., 1952, p. 364.
2. Lesnik, Milton J., and Anderson, Bernice E.: *Legal Aspects of Nursing.* J. B. Lippincott Co., Philadelphia, 1947, p. 245.
3. Hayt, Emanuel, and Hayt, Lillian R.: *Legal Guide for American Hospitals.* Hospital Textbook Co., New York, 1940, p. 298.
4. *Pharmacopoeia of the United States of America,* 15th revision, by Authority of the United States Pharmacopoeial Convention. Mack Publishing Co., Easton, Pa., 1955.
5. American Pharmaceutical Association (ed.): *The National Formulary,* 9th ed. The Association, Washington, 1950.
6. American Medical Association, Council on Pharmacy and Chemistry: *Epitome of the Pharmacopoeia of the United States and the National Formulary,* with comments, 9th ed. J. B. Lippincott Co., Philadelphia, 1951.
7. American Medical Association, Council on Pharmacy and Chemistry: *New and Nonofficial Remedies,* rev. J. B. Lippincott Co., Philadelphia, 1952.
8. Goodman, Louis S., and Gilman, Alfred: *The Pharmacological Basis of Therapeutics.,* 2nd ed. The Macmillan Company, New York, 1955, pp. 10-11.
9. Crawford, John D., et al.: "Simplification of the Drug Dosage Calculation by Application of the Surface Area Principle," *Pediatrics,* **5:**783, (May) 1950.
10. Goodman, Louis S., and Gilman, Alfred: *op. cit.,* pp. 546-47.
11. Smith, Austin: *Techniques of Medication.* J. B. Lippincott Co., Philadelphia, 1948, p. 216.
12. Goodman, Louis S., and Gilman, Alfred: *op. cit.,* p. 736.
13. Goodman, Louis S., and Gilman, Alfred, *op. cit.,* p. 8.
14. Maxcy, Kenneth F. (ed.): *Rosenau's Preventive Medicine and Hygiene,* 7th ed. Appleton-Century-Crofts, Inc., New York, 1951, p. 1038.

Additional Suggested Reading

Barach, Alvan L.: *Physiologic Therapy in Respiratory Diseases,* 2nd ed. J. B. Lippincott Co., Philadelphia, 1948.

Bastedo, Walter A.: *Pharmacology, Therapeutics and Prescription Writing for Students and Practitioners,* 5th ed. W. B. Saunders Co., Philadelphia, 1947.

Blumgarten, A. S.: *Textbook of Materia Medica, Pharmacology, and Therapeutics,* 7th ed. The Macmillan Company, New York, 1937.

Byrne, Anne K.: "Errors in Giving Medications," *Am. J. Nursing,* **53:**829, (July) 1953.

Cramp, Arthur J.: *Nostrums and Quackery and Pseudo-Medicine,* Vol. III. American Medical Association, Chicago, 1936.

Cushny, Arthur R.: *Pharmacology and Therapeutics,* 13th ed. (thoroughly revised by Arthur Grollman and Donald Slaughter). Lea & Febiger, Philadelphia, 1947.

Cutting, Windsor C.: "Drug Reactions: What to Watch For and What to Avoid," *Am. J. Nursing,* **48:**166, (Mar.) 1948.

————: *A Manual of Clinical Therapeutics: A Guide for Students and Practitioners,* 2nd ed. W. B. Saunders Co., Philadelphia, 1948.

Faddis, Margene O., and Hayman, Joseph M., Jr.: *A Textbook of Pharmacology for Nurses,* 4th ed. J. B. Lippincott Co., Philadelphia, 1953.

Muse, Maude B.: *Pharmacology and Therapeutics,* 4th ed. W. B. Saunders Co., Philadelphia, 1944.

Sister Mary Carl Re: "Narcotics in Vials," *Hosp. Progr.,* **31:**356, (Dec.) 1950.

Sollmann, Torald H.: *A Manual of Pharmacology and Its Applications to Therapeutics and Toxicology,* 7th ed. W. B. Saunders Co., Philadelphia, 1948.

World Health Organization: *International Pharmacopoeia,* Vol. 1. Columbia University Press, New York, 1951.

Wright, Harold N., and Montag, Mildred: *Materia Medica, Pharmacology and Therapeutics.* W. B. Saunders Co., Philadelphia, 1951.

CHAPTER 26. ADMINISTRATION OF MEDICINE, FOOD, AND FLUIDS BY NEEDLE INJECTION (PARENTERAL THERAPY)

1. GENERAL CONSIDERATIONS IN PARENTERAL THERAPY

Definition. Parenteral therapy is a term for the giving of therapeutic agents, including foods, outside the alimentary tract (*para* = beside; *enteron* = intestine). By definition, inhalation and insufflation of drugs might fall under parenteral therapy, but the conventional use of the term is confined to the administration of drugs by the routes with the corresponding procedures given in the table on page 713.

Parenteral fluids might conceivably be given in any but the most unyielding tissues. Those tissues (and areas) enumerated are injected in current practice although some procedures are rarely used.

Choice of route depends upon whether a local or systemic action is desired, how rapid an effect is needed, the amount of fluid to be injected, the nature of the fluid, whether blood vessels are accessible and suitable for injection, the wishes of the patient and his family, and the skills and preferences of the physician or operator.

Materials Injected. Water, salts, vitamins, sugars, digested proteins, whole

TISSUES AND CAVITIES INJECTED	NAME COMMONLY GIVEN THE PROCEDURE
*1. Skin	Intradermal injection
2. Subcutaneous or areolar tissue	"Hypodermic," if a small amount is given ("Hypospray," a substitute for a hypodermic) Hypodermoclysis or subcutaneous infusion if a large amount is given
3. Muscles	Intramuscular injection
4. Bone marrow	Intraosseous injection
5. The peritoneal cavity	Intraperitoneal infusion or injection (and intraperitoneal irrigation)
6. The spinal cavity	Intraspinal infusion or injection
7. Blood vessels	Intravenous infusion Intra-arterial infusion Tranfusion if blood is given

* Arranged in order from the least rapid to the most rapid rate of absorption.

blood and its component parts, so-called "blood substitutes," vaccines and protective sera, and many drugs used for diagnosis and therapy are all given parenterally.* Some of the fluids most often given by each route are discussed under each procedure heading.

Dangers Common to All Injections.   Whenever the skin is punctured or incised there is risk of *infection*. (This risk is reduced to a minimum when the equipment is prepared as for a surgical operation.) Many of the substances injected are foreign and often toxic so that the patient may have an *allergic* or *toxic reaction* to the treatment. This is likely to be most severe with intravenous and intra-arterial injections because they are most rapidly absorbed.

Tissue trauma is the inevitable accompaniment of an injection. If the treatment is given skillfully, tissue destruction is negligible and the wound heals readily, but it is possible to inflict a lasting, or fatal, injury with a needle. For example, a nerve can be severed with a needle or in striking a bone the bone may be injured, or the needle broken off and left embedded in the tissues. The injection into blood vessels of irritating drugs that should have been injected into the muscles or subcutaneous tissues has injured the vessels and produced toxic symptoms.

Needles range in size from 27 gauge (the finest) to 13 gauge (the largest). The finest gauge that can be used effectively should be chosen in each case. All injections elicit some degree of fear in persons not accustomed to them. *Psychic trauma* is a factor to be considered in parenteral therapy. *When food and drugs can be taken orally they should not be given by less natural routes.*

Choice of Equipment.   Skin-cleansing equipment is needed for all injections; in some cases this includes articles for shaving the area. It is most convenient if the skin-cleansing equipment is sterilized separately in units such as those shown in Figure 30. Waterproof disposable containers can be substituted to bring **to**

* Fat solutions are still in an experimental stage and are not available commercially.

the patient sponges, or applicators, already wet with the cleansing and disinfectant solutions.

Any preparation for parenteral use (including drugs) should be put up in a sealed plastic or glass ampoule, vial, flask, or bottle from which the contents can

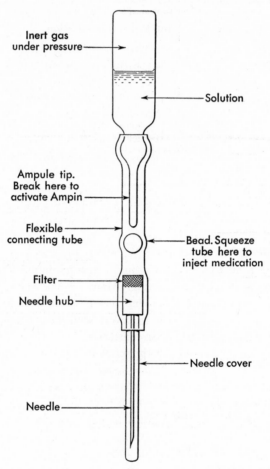

Inert gas
under pressure

Solution

Ampule tip.
Break here to
activate Ampin

Flexible
connecting tube

Bead. Squeeze
tube here to
inject medication

Filter

Needle hub

Needle cover

Needle

Figure 161. Disposable subcutaneous injection unit—"Bead" Ampin. Syringe, needle, medication in one unit, sterile and ready for instant use. (Courtesy of Strong Cobb & Co., Inc., Cleveland, Ohio.)

be removed without contaminating it. (The solute and solvent are put in separate containers when the drug in solution is unstable.) Commercially prepared parenteral fluids in plastic or glass containers from which they are dispensed are one of the most important developments in modern asepsis and medical economy. Sterile disposable syringes, needles, and tubing have been brought within a possible cost range for most sections of the country, and, in many cases, their purchase represents a saving. When commercially prepared sets are not used a reservoir for the solution must be provided. For small quantities (up to 60 cc or 2 oz) a syringe is used; for larger quantities a burette or flask. The burette (a glass cylinder from which the solution flows by gravity in an open system) is going into the discard for it necessitates transferring solutions from one container to another with the inherent danger of contamination. The Fenwal flask is a satisfactory reservoir because the solution can be both sterilized in it and dispensed from it. Varieties of flasks, tubing, and syringes are illustrated and discussed in Chapter 8. The importance of selecting equipment that will not react with the water, food, and drugs given parenterally was emphasized. When needles are sterilized in the hospital it is convenient to have them in glass vials or transparent envelopes so that they may be seen when selected and extra needles kept sterile if not used. Choice of needle, as to length, gauge, and bevel, is discussed with each procedure.

Tubing, sufficient in length to reach without tension from the reservoir to the needle, is needed. The transparent or semitransparent type is desirable. A heavy-walled pure gum rubber is often used, and plastic tubing that withstands autoclaving is available and rapidly replacing other varieties. Whatever the kind, it must be fitted with clamps to regulate the flow. The drip bulb is usually placed just below the reservoir so that the rate at which the solution is flowing can be timed and regulated with exactness. The end of the tubing to be attached to the needle is fitted with an "adapter."

Some operators feel more secure if the site of injection is surrounded with sterile towels and if they wear sterile rubber gloves when injecting veins, giving transfusions, or injecting the spinal canal. In most cases the operator works without gloves or from any sterile area, other than that made by the inside of the covering of the sterile equipment. The patient's clothing and bedding should be protected by paper or cotton squares backed by waterproof paper, plastic, or rubber, if, during the procedure, they are likely to be wet or soiled.

Preparation of Equipment. Sterilization of needles, syringes, tubing, and solutions was discussed in Chapter 8. It was emphasized that such materials used for surgery should be sterilized with steam under pressure, or hot air at very high temperatures, to destroy spore forms of microorganisms. Tetanus and the gas-forming bacilli, common in nature, are particularly dangerous if they are injected into the tissues with a puncture wound. While there are comparatively few reported cases of tetanus and gas gangrene following injections, it is well known that the reported cases represent a small percentage of accidents that have occurred.[1, 2] Epidemics of infectious hepatitis have been attributed to improperly disinfected syringes, needles, and surgical implements.[3, 4] A pressure cooker may be used when an autoclave is not available. Boiling-water sterilization should not be used, even in homes, when steam under pressure is available. Sterilization with chemicals is uncertain and risky. Equipment for injections should be prepared in central supply services by technicians. The use of sterile, assembled, disposable equipment prepared by reliable commercial firms gives maximum protection and is economical where labor costs are high. It is widely used in military medicine and in disasters. When assembled sterile disposable units are not available and it is necessary to protect a community by vaccinating thousands of persons in a short time, platinum needles that can be sterilized with a flame are used, and many injections are made with the same syringe. The necessity for immediate immunization may outweigh the risk of poor aseptic technique.

Psychological Preparation of the Patient.   Medical personnel, accustomed to seeing very painful treatments accepted by many patients with little visible protest, tend to forget man's natural fear of the unknown and the unwillingness of most persons to acknowledge this fear. The writer has seen strong men faint in anticipation of "a hypodermic." It is routine to give an infusion to any persons undergoing major surgery, but to the patient or his family it may be an indication that he is very ill. Except in emergencies, when time is of the essence, the purpose and nature of the treatment should be explained to the patient. The physician may prefer to do this himself, but, if not, the nurse should assume the responsibility after consultation with the physician. The explanation should be given before the patient is faced with the syringe or infusion or transfusion set. The patient should understand the treatment and be willing and ready to submit to it. He should know how much discomfort he can expect. (When feasible, pain should be minimized with local anesthetics and substances, like *hyaluronidase,* that speed absorption.) Restraint seldom is needed when this approach is used. For any treatment involving fear, discomfort, or pain, tension is reduced by keeping the patient warm and relaxed in a sitting or recumbent position.

Preparation of the Skin at the Site of Injection.   Skin disinfection was discussed at length in Chapter 7 and will not be treated in detail here. An injection of a needle is a minor surgical procedure, and the area should be prepared as for surgery. A cleaning agent, such as alcohol 70 per cent, ether, or water and a detergent, should be followed by a skin disinfectant, such as tincture of iodine or benzalkonium (Zephiran). Disinfectants that stain clothing, such as iodine, should be removed when the treatment is over. Many operators rely solely on alcohol, but this is especially questionable when the needle is injected into the deeper tissues. Applicators or sponges and forceps, with which the disinfectant is applied, should be sterile.

Restraint of the Patient.   It is obviously desirable to immobilize a joint, such as the elbow, if a needle is inserted into this part of the arm. Ordinarily, adult patients are not restrained for injections unless they are irrational. Infants and very small children may require restraint, but it should be avoided whenever possible.

Technique for Injecting the Needle.   Whenever a needle is injected the object is to get the needle into the intended locale with minimum discomfort for the patient and injury to body tissues. Almost everyone, brave or cowardly, is tense as he waits for an injection. A sharp needle injected skillfully *into relaxed tissue* is so unexpectedly painless, however, that the patient is often waiting for the prick when the treatment is over. There are various ways of evoking the desired relaxation. A diverting thought, a deep breath, or a light blow or pinch near the site of injection will usually relax the patient. For subcutaneous and intramuscular injections a successful technique is that of striking the patient sharply with the hand, then immediately inserting the needle. A similar effect results from grasping the area to be injected between the thumb and forefinger, or pinching the area, as in Figure 162. The tissues grasped in this fashion make a firm cushion, which the needle punctures easily. The second method is safer with thin patients, for it draws the muscle away from the bone and makes striking the bone less likely. Injecting the needle quickly, as one throws a dart, minimizes the discomfort.

Injecting needles between the layers of the skin, into veins, serous-lined cavities, and bones present special problems. While the nurse does not ordinarily make these injections, the techniques are discussed briefly under the procedures involved.

The angle of the needle and the depth to which it should be inserted depend upon what lies between the skin at the site of injection and the spot in the tissues that the needle point should reach when the needle is in place. Knowledge of anatomy, judgment as to the amount of fat lying in the subcutaneous tissue, and experience all contribute to making successful injections. Figure 162 shows the angle at which needles are ordinarily inserted for subcutaneous medication.

Factors That Favor Absorption. It is obvious that fluids injected into the blood stream will most rapidly find their way to all parts of the body. Likewise substances injected into the muscles or into red bone marrow are quickly distributed by the abundant blood supply in these tissues. When fluids are deposited in the subcutaneous tissues, they are taken up less readily because there are relatively fewer blood vessels. Fluids may accumulate in subcutaneous tissues to a dangerous degree. By any route, however, liquids may be given more rapidly than they can be absorbed.

Application of heat over the site of the injection or the use of warm solutions has been recommended. Microfilms have proven that heat dilates blood vessels and that the effect on the capillaries lasts for hours. August K. Krogh[5] has shown that dilated capillaries are more permeable, and it follows that their capacity for absorption is increased. Raising the temperature of the solution, therefore, within the limits of physiological tolerance, should theoretically increase the rate of absorption. Many devices for maintaining the temperature of the solution at the desired point have been described. In some methods heat is applied around the reservoir; in others, around the tubing. Hot-water bottles, heating pads, and other devices have been used as the source of heat. Walton Dutton and George B. Lake[6] (1936) recommend solutions at body temperature for parenteral therapy unless heating affects the chemical composition of the fluid. Austin Smith[7] (1948) says subcutaneous infusions should be heated to a temperature slightly above that of the body. While solutions flowing into the veins slowly (2 to 3 cc per minute) need not be above room temperature, Smith thinks blood temperature most desirable. Elmer L. De Gowin[8] et al. report that blood given at 10° C (50° F) caused no untoward reaction. Accidents have been reported from overheated solutions. Dutton and Lake recommend inserting in the tubing near the needle a long glass-connecting tube containing a thermometer (an "infusion thermometer") so that the temperature of the solution as it enters the body can be checked. Temperatures above 42° C (107.6° F) can cause tissue burns or necrosis.

In spite of the probability of hastening the absorption by warmth the practice of heating parenteral fluids is disappearing. With all known methods it is time consuming and with most methods uncertain. A solution that is heated in a reservoir drops from 2.3° to 9° C (5° to 20° F) according to room temperature and other conditions, as it flows through the tubing. Heating the tubing may result in dangerously hot injections. It is now customary to store parenteral solutions in warmed closets; no other attempt is made to keep the solution above room temperature.

Massage is believed to increase the local blood supply and increase the rate of absorption. It is usual to follow a hypodermic or an intramuscular injection with gentle massage.

The rate of absorption differs with the *composition of the fluid* injected. In parenteral therapy, especially intravenous and intra-arterial therapy, it is well to bear in mind Claude Bernard's thesis that all vital mechanisms of the body have but one object—to preserve constant conditions of life in the internal environment.[9] In sections of this text dealing with nutrition, fluid balance, and emotional stability, it was pointed out that the aim of therapy is "to keep the lymph constant around the cells." Whatever interferes too greatly with the equilibrium of body fluids endangers life. When liquids, too foreign in nature or too large in quantity, are injected into the body, the processes that ordinarily maintain equilibrium of the lymph cannot prevent a mild or serious reaction. When a solution with a lower content of solids than is present in blood or lymph is injected into the tissues, the tissue cells take in some of the water solvent and give off some of their solids to equalize the hydrostatic pressure inside the cells and in the fluids surrounding them. Likewise when a liquid with a higher content of solids than is found in the blood and lymph is injected, the cells give off some of their water content and take in some of the solids to equalize the pressure inside the cells and in the fluids surrounding them. This process of osmosis (the passage of water molecules through a membrane) and dialysis (the passage of solid molecules through a membrane) if carried far enough can destroy cells by shrinking them as they give off water, or by bursting them as they take in more water than the cell membrane can support. A liquid is spoken of as isotonic when it exerts the same osmotic pressure as the blood; hypertonic when it exerts a greater osmotic pressure, and hypotonic when it exerts a lesser osmotic pressure. Hypertonic solutions can shrink, or crenate, cells and sclerose tissues; hypotonic solutions can hemolyze cells ("lake" the blood) and cause generalized edema. Fortunately, a cell's membrane has a selective action and will allow some molecules to pass through and not others. The exchange of solids and water that goes on between the cell and its environment is constant and, within limits, physiological. If given time, a cell can adjust itself to many changes in its fluid environment. Generally speaking, however, fluids that are isotonic, with the blood and lymph, or nearly so, are most easily absorbed.

Absorption can be markedly increased by the addition of a substance that tends to break down the natural resistance of the tissues to the injected fluid. Research of the past twenty years has established the fact that extracts of certain mammalian organs, leeches, some bacteria, and snake venom contain a "spreading factor." Hyaluronidase is the name given this enzyme because it breaks down, or depolymerizes, hyaluronic acid, a mucopolysaccharide which is the main component of the intercellular ground substance, or cement substance, of tissues. Karl Meyer[10] says hyaluronic acid "holds cells together in a jelly-like matrix and serves as a lubricant and shock absorber in joints." Because hyaluronidase breaks down this matrix, injections of it have proved useful as an accompaniment of hypodermoclysis solutions and irritating drugs (such as heparin), in speeding the action of topical and injected local anesthetics in joint hematomas, in dispersing subcutaneous hematomas and unabsorbed drugs, and in some forms of arthritis. Occasionally it is used to hasten the dispersion of a dye in studies of living tissue. Actually, hyaluronidase is such a relatively new drug that its full usefulness is unknown. Current and future experiments may show that it has a much greater therapeutic application than is indicated here.

Hyaluronidase is available for clinical use as a pyrogen-free extract of bovine testes. It is put up in crystalline form in "turbidity-reducing units." After the addition of the solvent (sterile physiological saline) the solution is stable for two weeks, if refrigerated. The dry powder is stable at room temperatures indefinitely but is destroyed by heating. It is best to prepare the solution just before using it. Dosage varies according to the area involved. The dose is most often measured in turbidity-reducing units. One unit is defined as: the amount of hyaluronidase required to reduce the viscosity (of hyaluronic acid) 50 per cent in thirty minutes.[11] David V. Habif[12] recommends the use of 300 turbidity-reducing units in 1000 cc of clysis solution. One unit per cubic centimeter of procaine as a local anesthetic is advocated by J. N. Thorpe.[13] Dosage is always prescribed by the physician, and the nurse's responsibility is the same here as in other medication. Fortunately hyaluronidase seems to be nontoxic. Improvement in its preparation is said to have eliminated occasional allergic reactions. When *hyaluronidase* is given with small quantities of another drug it may be drawn into the same syringe or injected first into the selected site; when given in hypodermoclysis it may be introduced into the tubing with a needle immediately after the fluid starts flowing into the tissues, or it may be incorporated with the solution in the reservoir. Habif recommends injection of the drug into the tubing. The bulk of fluid entering the tissues in hypodermoclysis exerts enough pressure to stimulate absorption; when hyaluronidase is injected into a hematoma a pressure bandage should be applied over the area.

More specific discussion of the major types of injections follows. The sequence chosen has nothing to do with the rate of absorption by the different types. It seems more reasonable to discuss first the procedures most commonly used, "the hypodermic," and the intramuscular injection. The chapter should be read as a whole because in each section there is an assumption that the reader is familiar with the preceding sections.

2. SUBCUTANEOUS MEDICATION OR HYPODERMIC INJECTION
(INCLUDING INSULIN ADMINISTRATION)

Definition. *Hypodermic* is derived from *hypo* (under) and *derma* (skin). In common parlance and medical practice the term "hypodermic" is used for the introduction of a small quantity of fluid into the subcutaneous tissues with a needle.

Therapeutic Uses. A drug is given by "hypodermic" when (1) the patient cannot or will not swallow a drug or when it is dangerous for him to attempt it; (2) the person is vomiting or having gastric suction; (3) the action of the drug is destroyed by secretions of the gastrointestinal tract or is irritating to the tract; and (4) the drugs act more quickly or effectively if absorbed from the subcutaneous tissues.

Selection of Method. The importance of sterility for all injection equipment has already been stressed, and the best method of *sterilization* discussed. Maximum safety probably lies in the commercially prepared ready-to-use disposable unit, such as the *Ampin** or the *Syrette†* (see Fig. 161). Developed for military uses, disposable injection units are equally suitable for civil medicine.[14] Robert R. Cadmus [15] reports a substantial saving when Ampins were substituted for a common method of hypodermic injection in one of Cleveland's large hospitals. The Ampin containing the drug is so designed that the solution flows into the tissues when the tip of the ampoule is broken and light pressure made on the rubber tubing connecting it with the needle. Since this type of unit is a relatively new development, and since only a limited number of drugs are available in the disposable units, nurses must be familiar with other methods of giving hypodermic injections.

The sterilization in the central supply service of an assembled syringe and needle put up in a glass or metal tube is probably, next to the disposable unit, the method of choice. A rack to hold them and vials of drugs to be used with them has been described by Thelma Dodds et al.[16] Drugs in multiple dosage in rubber-stoppered vials are prepared commercially and in hospital pharmacies. The difficulty of sterilizing the rubber stoppers, through which the drug is drawn with the needle and syringe, makes this type of container less safe than the single-dosage sealed glass ampoule. The latter method is thought by many to be too expensive for general use, but in some European countries all drugs given by injection are prepared in ampoules.

When vials or ampoules are not used, *preparation of the solution* is a problem because the drug is in tablet form. Lack of moisture in the bottle discourages the growth of bacteria, but it can hardly be claimed that the contents of a bottle that is opened repeatedly remain sterile. Tablets must be mixed with a solvent, but the solution should not be boiled afterward because heating might alter its chemical composition. While tablets can be handled in such a way as to reduce contamination of the solution to a minimum, hypodermic injections prepared with tablets are

* Strong, Cobb and Co., Inc., Professional Products Division, Cleveland, Ohio.
† E. R. Squibb and Sons, New York.

never free from microorganisms. Sterile physiological saline and sterile distilled water are commonly used as solvents. Walter A. Bastedo,[17] Torald H. Sollmann,[18] and Arthur Grollman and Donald Slaughter[19] recommend the former. When neither is available, as in homes, boiled tap water must be substituted. There is some question as to whether minerals in natural waters combine with the drug to make it less active or irritating. About 2 cc (30 m) of the solvent is ordinarily used.

The site of injection may be almost any of the less sensitive areas of the body where no bones or large blood vessels are near the surface. The outer aspect of the arms and thighs fulfill the requirements and are convenient sites, but muscular areas of the body wall may be used also. When a patient is getting hypodermics frequently, the sites of the injection should be rotated and an attempt made to avoid puncturing the same spot twice.

Preparation of the skin was discussed in Chapter 7 and again on page 716.

Insertion of the needle is described in general terms on page 716. For subcutaneous injections the needle should be held at an angle of about 60 deg and inserted quickly, as a dart is thrown, to the depth of 1½ cm (½ in.). If the individual is obese the needle can be inserted as much as 2 cm or more; if he is emaciated an injection 1 cm in depth will take the drug into the areolar tissue.

Factors affecting the rate of absorption are numerous. There is general agreement on some points but not on all. Drugs given in aqueous solution are absorbed more rapidly than those given in oil or wax suspensions. When the physician wants to slow the rate of absorption so that the drug will be available to the body over a period of hours (as with penicillin or insulin), he prescribes it in an oil or wax suspension. Carl J. Wiggers[20] cites experiments demonstrating the presence of drugs in the thoracic duct two minutes after they (in aqueous solution) were injected subcutaneously. John J. R. MacLeod[21] says that methylene blue injected in the thigh appears in the urine before it is seen in the thoracic duct. Smith says that because absorption is so rapid the common practice of massaging the site gently after the removal of the needle is unimportant. While it is evident that the drug gains access immediately to the blood and lymph circulations, it is probably true that massage and heat, both of which dilate blood vessels, hasten absorption. When irritating drugs are given, gentle massage and the application of heat may reduce discomfort caused by the continued presence of the drug in the tissues.

Equipment. Because hypodermic injections are often given in an emergency, with an immediate response the prime object, it is particularly important that the equipment be ready for use. Obviously, a presterilized assembled unit, such as the Ampin, is most satisfactory. When this is not available, the syringe with needle attached that has been sterilized by steam under pressure is the best substitute. Any containers or wrapping for a needle should protect the point. Extra needles in glass tubes should be available. Ampoules, files, and sterile paper or gauze squares, to protect the hands in breaking ampoules, should be stored nearby. If tablets are used they, too, should be kept with the other articles used in giving hypodermics. Solvents should be sterilized in small flasks with a rubber cover through which the liquid can be drawn, or a cap that can be replaced without contaminating the lip of the flask. Sterile sponges, handling forceps, and a skin disinfectant complete the essential equipment unless tablets are used; then it is necessary to have a small flat-bottomed receptacle in which the tablet can be dissolved, such as tiny waxed paper cups, a birdseed dish, or a saltcellar. Small packages may be made for individual injections containing a dish, the sponges needed, and a small square of waxed paper on which the prepared "hypodermic" may be carried to the bedside. Very large cotton applicators in a waterproof paper envelope, in which they may be carried wet with the skin disinfectant, are a convenience in keeping the applicators uncontaminated and the bedside table clean and dry. The practice of embedding the needle in an alcohol sponge is undesirable because the discomfort of the injection is increased.

In some hospitals and in home nursing it is necessary to boil the syringe and needle and even the solvent. In a very few places chemical disinfection of syringes and needles is practiced, but this should be considered the last resort. When boiling a hypodermic syringe and needle or when sterilizing them in a pressure cooker it is convenient to support them in a sieve. The point of the needle in the sieve swings free and so is protected from blunting. Attempts to sterilize a needle in a spoon over the flame from a lamp should be discouraged.

Syringes should be made of heat-resistant alkaline-free glass. A small gauge needle should be used whenever possible because it punctures the skin more easily than a large needle and causes less pain and tissue damage. Most subcutaneous needles have a moderately long bevel or cutting edge. Some operators believe that the needle with a lateral bore causes least discomfort. The length of the needle for ordinary subcutaneous injections should be about 2 cm (¾ in.) and the gauge 25 or 24. A larger gauge is necessary when oily drugs that do not readily pass through a fine needle are administered; longer needles are used when it is desirable to inject the drugs deep in the tissues. *Safety or security* needles have a beadlike construction just below the juncture of the shaft and the hub. The needle is most likely to break at this point, and the bead keeps the broken-off shaft from getting lost in the tissues.

Suggested Procedure. If a sterilized assembled disposable unit is available, take this from the cabinet in which it is stored, observing the usual precautions to see that the drug and its dosage are correct. Carry the unit on a small tray to the bedside with a waterproof paper or envelope containing sponges or applicators, one or more wet with the skin antiseptic. After cleaning the skin remove the guard over the needle, release the solution according to the directions of the manufacturer of the unit, and after striking, or grasping, the area insert the needle as a dart at an angle of about 60 deg. (The patient is less likely to feel the prick if he is diverted, and if he is not watching the process.) Inject the solution slowly. Remove the needle quickly while exerting pressure over the area with a dry sponge; maintain the pressure for a few seconds and rub the area gently.

When a sterile assembled needle and syringe are used with the drug in an ampoule, collect these articles and the skin-cleaning equipment. Warm, but do not heat, the drug if it is a thick oil or suspension that cannot be drawn readily through the needle. Twirling the vial or ampoule between the palms of the hands both warms and mixes

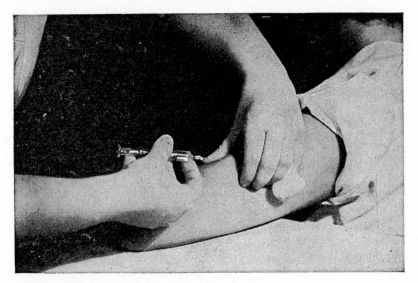

Figure 162. Subcutaneous medication; *first step*. Note arm grasped firmly to make a cushion and the needle held at an angle of approximately 60 deg.

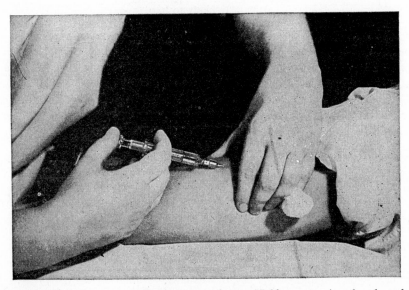

Figure 163. Subcutaneous medication; *second step*. Hold on arm is relaxed, and needle has been inserted 1½ cm (approximately ½ in.).

a suspension. (Work quickly and give the injection immediately; otherwise, the drug will stiffen and "lock" the syringe.) Clean the neck of the ampoule with alcohol. Collect all the drug in the bottom of the ampoule by tapping the tip until the liquid leaves it. File the neck of the ampoule and break it, protecting the fingers with a sterile gauze or paper square; then withdraw the contents, or part of the contents of the ampoule, as prescribed, through the needle into the syringe. If the drug is in a rubber-stoppered vial, clean the rubber stopper. Draw into the syringe as much air as drug to be withdrawn from the vial. Insert the needle into the vial cap and force the air into the liquid; the pressure of this air makes it easy to withdraw the drug from the vial. Before giving the medication see that all but a small bubble of air is expelled from the syringe. This air bubble will rise to the surface of the liquid as the hypodermic is given and, being injected last, tends to fill the channel left by the needle as it is removed. Theoretically, this prevents leakage of drugs through the skin opening, and the air is soon absorbed. In carrying the equipment to the patient protect the needle with a sterile, dry gauze or cotton sponge.

When a tablet is to be used, the solution is prepared in the following manner: Pour a small amount of saline solution into the mixing receptacle; draw up 2 cc (30 m), or the desired amount, into the syringe and discard what remains. Drop the tablet into the vessel and discharge the saline solution from the syringe upon it; draw the solution back and forth in the syringe until the tablet is dissolved; fill the syringe and attach the needle. The remainder of the procedure is carried out in the same way as when an ampoule is used.

Clean the syringe and needle at once with a fat solvent, such as ether, alcohol, or benzine. Wax suspensions are particularly likely to harden, or "freeze" in the needle and syringe.

Insulin Administration. A very important procedure in the care of the diabetic is the administration of insulin. Insulin lowers the blood sugar, promotes combustion of carbohydrates, and prevents acidosis. It is not a cure, or a substitute for strict regulation of the diet, but it is an aid of immeasurable value in arresting the disease, in prolonging life, and in restoring the patient to health more quickly. It is given when the patient's own insulin production is so deficient that regulation of the diet alone is not enough to keep the urine sugar-free and the blood sugar normal. It is always given in diabetic coma, and it is used in the pre- and postoperative treatment of diabetic patients.

No set rules can be given for the dosage, time, or frequency of administration as they vary with the diet and with the individual and also at different times for the same individual. Louis S. Goodman and Alfred Gilman[22] say that when diet alone does not control glycosuria, insulin is generally given before breakfast since the blood sugar is usually at its highest level then. When moderate amounts of insulin have been ordered by the doctor (usually 40 units or less daily), it is given before the morning and evening meals or in a single dose in the morning should a modified insulin be used. They feel that individuals receiving more than 40 units of insulin a day may require an injection of insulin before each meal. Because doctors differ in their method of prescribing insulin, it is important for the nurse to see that the treatment is carried out exactly as ordered.

There are five types of insulin in use today, and experimental work is being done to develop other types.[23] See Table 9 where these five types are listed and where the time of onset, period of maximum action, and duration of action are given.

Insulin injection (or regular insulin) is absorbed rapidly and therefore acts quickly upon the metabolic processes. Protamine zinc insulin acts much more slowly, and its effect is more lasting. With protamine zinc insulin it is possible to provide the daily requirement in one injection; however, its onset is slow (see Table 9), and frequently regular insulin must also be given, alone or in combination, with the protamine zinc insulin. When given in combination, the two types

Table 9. Properties of Various Insulins*†

TYPE OF INSULIN	TIME OF ONSET	PERIOD OF MAXIMUM ACTION	DURATION OF ACTION
	Hours	Hours	Hours
Insulin injection (regular insulin)	1	3	6
Crystalline zinc insulin injection	1	3	8
Globin zinc insulin injection	2–4	8–16	16–24
Protamine zinc insulin injection	6–8	12–24	48–72
Isophane insulin injection	2	10–20	28–30

* A 2:1 mixture of regular insulin and protamine zinc insulin behaves essentially like isophane insulin; a 3:1 mixture, like globin zinc insulin.
† Goodman, Louis S., and Gilman, Alfred: *The Pharmacological Basis of Therapeutics*, 2nd ed. The Macmillan Company, New York, 1955, p. 1629.

of insulin are mixed immediately prior to the injection. Since regular insulin has its time of onset in 1 hour, it is usually given one-half hour before meals so that the body will be prepared to take care of the ingested food. Protamine zinc insulin is broken down more slowly over a period of hours, and therefore produces a gradual fall in the blood sugar throughout this longer period (see Table 9).

The method of administering insulin is by hypodermic injection, although it may be given intravenously in cases of coma. All the usual precautions in giving hypodermic injections are to be carefully observed; they include: (1) a suitable syringe (see Fig. 164) and a sharp, tightly fitting needle to avoid trauma; (2) introduction of insulin into loose subcutaneous tissue and not into skin, muscle, or over pressure points; (3) rotation of doses in different areas; and (4) maintenance of asepsis. The patient, or a relative, should learn all the details of giving hypodermic injections of insulin in the home.

The procedure taught the patient by the doctor or the nurse should utilize equipment that is readily available, and the method employed should be simply and fully explained and demonstrated. The procedure of preparing a hypodermic in the home that is described on page 722 applies to the administration of insulin.

Figure 116 shows a nurse teaching a diabetic child and her mother how to prepare and administer insulin. The method is being taught in a hospital with equipment, some items of which can be found in or bought for the home. Children as well as adults should be taught and encouraged to practice self-administration of insulin. The nurse should not consider that she has taught thoroughly until the patient can demonstrate with competence. Alcohol is usually advocated to clean the skin and the rubber stopper of the insulin vial. Medicated rubbing alcohol, 70 per cent, can be obtained in any drugstore and is a satisfactory preparation to use. A device for holding the insulin syringe for automatically injecting the needle is available for persons who find it difficult to inject the needle into their tissues (see Fig. 164).

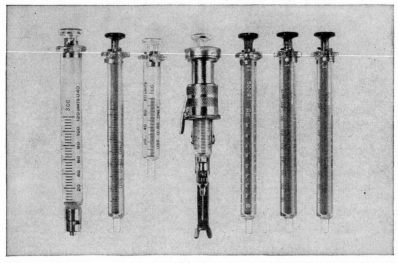

Figure 164. Different types of insulin syringes. In the center is a device for holding insulin syringe that will automatically inject needle when pressed. (Courtesy of Becton, Dickinson and Co., Rutherford, N. J., and Clay-Adams Co., New York City.)

Because protamine zinc insulin is a suspension, the vial must be rotated gently or rolled between the hands before use to ensure an even distribution of the insulin particles and thus to ensure accurate dosage. Formation of foam on the surface should be avoided and, if present, should not be drawn into the syringe and considered part of the dose. Although protamine zinc insulin is said to be a stable compound if kept at room temperature, authorities recommend storing all insulin preparations in a cool place such as a refrigerator. However, if a diabetic is traveling and it is not possible to keep the vial of insulin in a refrigerator, there should be no anxiety, especially when the insulin is self-administered by the patient at least once daily. (This would result in emptying the vial within a matter of days.)

Goodman and Gilman say there is a low incidence of serious untoward reactions to insulin. Local reactions may occur, but these are frequently the result of poor injection technique. Allergic reactions may prove troublesome, and are indicated

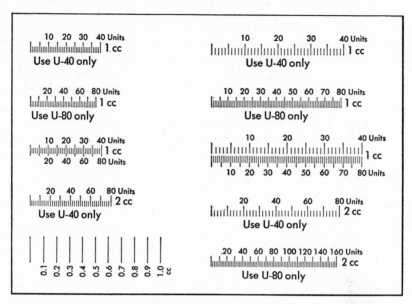

Figure 165. Scales for measuring insulin. (Courtesy of Becton, Dickinson & Co., Rutherford, N. J.)

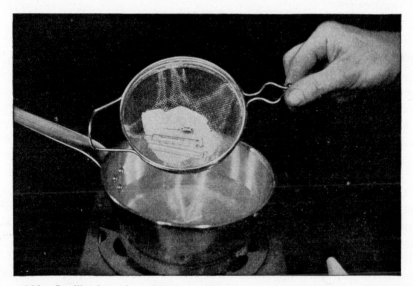

Figure 166. Sterilization of an insulin syringe and needle in the home. The syringe is taken apart and placed with the needle in a strainer lined with a gauze square. The strainer is then put into a pan of water. Add water to cover syringe and needle. This is heated and then boiled for 10 minutes. After boiling, the strainer is lifted out, the water poured from the pan, and the strainer returned to the pan until the syringe and needle have cooled. (Courtesy of Dr. Henry Dolger and New York Diabetic Association, New York City, and Clay-Adams Co., New York City.)

by swelling, erythema, and itching at the site of injection. Generalized urticaria and a severe constitutional reaction are seen occasionally. The following are other symptoms that may appear: swelling of the lips, reddening of the eyes, puffiness of the face, weakness, epigastric pain, nausea, and vomiting. If the reaction cannot be traced to poor technique, hypersensitivity in some cases can be controlled by changing the brand of insulin.

Insulin is a very potent substance and must be used with caution and exactitude. An error in dosage, time, and frequency of administration or in the diet to which it bears a direct relationship may prove serious. The following are other factors that affect the insulin requirement: interferences with the absorption of the diet such as vomiting and diarrhea; or anything that makes great demands on the patient's energy such as unusual exercise, overexertion, exposure to cold, or emotional disturbances.

If the amount of insulin given is not sufficient to balance the diet, or if a dose is omitted without regulating the diet, the result will be glycosuria, hyperglycemia, acidosis, and, eventually, coma. Patients should be warned of these dangers. They should be urged to carry a card stating that they have diabetes so that, if one of these untoward complications develops, they will receive prompt treatment. In addition, it is important for each diabetic to keep an adequate supply of insulin as well as an extra syringe and needle on hand.

3. INTRAMUSCULAR INJECTION

Definition.   The meaning of the term is self-evident. The term is applied to the injection of drugs in quantities that usually range from 2 to 10 cc. Much larger doses of sera or blood are occasionally introduced into the muscles.

Therapeutic Uses.   Fluids are injected into muscles for the same reasons that they are given subcutaneously. The intramuscular route is chosen in preference to the subcutaneous route when (1) the substance is irritating, (2) more rapid absorption is desired than is thought possible with the subcutaneous route, and (3) when there is a larger quantity of the fluid (as with injection of blood and some sera) than the subcutaneous tissues can absorb easily. Some writers think there is confusion in the uses of subcutaneous and intramuscular injections. Smith says, for example, that while irritating drugs are more rapidly absorbed by muscle than areolar tissue, certain drugs (he specifies emetine) are more painful if given intramuscularly.

Selection of Method.   Intramuscular injections involve more risk than subcutaneous injections because there is a greater likelihood of striking nerves and large blood vessels. Intramuscular injections were formerly done by physicians, but now nurses in this country regularly carry out this procedure, and, with the more widespread use of agents injected into the muscles, the patients and their families must be taught the techniques in some cases.

Any muscular area of the body may be used for the *site of injection.* The buttock is most often injected if bulky doses are given because the gluteal muscles are so thick. The area in which the operator is least likely to hit bones, large nerves, and blood vessels is above and to the outer side of the intersection of two lines dividing the buttock into four equal parts. (See Fig. 167.) Intramuscular injections of small bulk are often given in the outer aspect of the arm and the front of the thigh. For the person who is sitting or lying down constantly the thigh and arm muscles may be better sites for small intramuscular injections.

Sterilization of equipment, preparation of the drug, and preparation of the skin are the same as for a subcutaneous injection. The *technique for injecting the needle* is similar except that the needle is injected at right angles to the skin since it must penetrate the muscles. When the injection is given into the buttock, the skin is stretched and held taut with the palm of the hand. The thighs and arms can be grasped, or pinched, as shown in Figure 162. When the drug is injected the patient should be in a relaxed position. For injections in the buttocks Dutton and Lake suggest the prone position with the head turned on one side, the arms hanging over the edge of the treatment table or bed and the knees bent, with a pillow under the shins to support the legs.

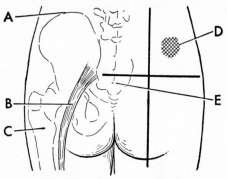

Figure 167. Gluteal intramuscular injection. *A,* crest of ilium; *B,* sciatic nerve; *C,* femur; *D,* injection sites; *E,* sacrum. The site of injection is varied by using not only alternate buttocks but also a number of points within the safety zone, *D.* (Musser, Ruth D., and Bird, Joseph G.: *Modern Pharmacology and Therapeutics.* The Macmillan Company, New York, 1958.)

Equipment. The articles required are practically the same as those needed in giving a subcutaneous injection, the size of the syringe varying with the amount to be given and the gauge and length of the needle with the type of drug it is intended to carry and the condition of the tissues. Sizes commonly used range from 19 to 22 gauge and from 3½ to 6 cm (1½ to 2½ in.) in length. Fine needles may be used for thin liquids, heavier ones for suspensions; short needles are satisfactory when the person is thin and flabby; longer needles are necessary when the patient is obese. For injections into the arms or thighs, needles range from 2.5 to 3½ cm (1 to 1½ in.) in length. The size of the syringe depends upon the amount of liquid to be injected.

Suggested Procedure. Prepare the drug and carry the equipment to the bedside in the same way as for a subcutaneous injection, first being sure that the patient is willing to have the treatment. If the injection is to be made into the buttock, place him in the prone position with head turned on one side, arms hanging over the side of the treatment table or the bed, knees bent and legs supported by a pillow; the buttock and hip should be exposed, but the remainder of the body should be covered with sufficiently warm bedding to keep the patient from feeling chilly. Clean and disinfect an area about 7½ cm (3 in.) in diameter near the inner angle of the upper outer quadrant of the buttock.

The following technique for the administration of the injection and the treatment of complications is taken from Dutton and Lake's text, *Parenteral Therapy:*[*]

". . . . Before injection of the solution the syringe should be inverted and the piston withdrawn sufficiently to allow 0.2 cc of air to enter the barrel, and then reverted for injection. The air aids the diffusion of the drug, minimizes the pain and prevents the leakage of the solution along the puncture canal into the subcutaneous tissue. . . . The syringe should be held in the right hand (if the operator is right-handed), between the index and middle fingers, and thumb, with the point downward and the weight of the hand resting on the tip of the little finger, which rests upon the skin.

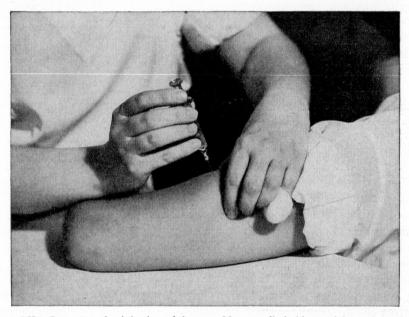

Figure 168.   Intramuscular injection of the arm. Note needle held at a right angle to the skin.

The left hand is placed flat on the buttock, the thumb and index finger approximating the angle of the upper-outer quadrant, and with moderate pressure moved firmly downward toward the patient's thigh, flattening and fixing the tissues. When ready to insert the needle, the weight is shifted from the little finger to the thumb, index and middle fingers; then the needle is thrust to one-half the desired depth with a firm bold pressure. A second light pressure is made, pushing the needle to the proper depth. The left hand is then removed from the buttock. This causes the syringe to slant slightly upward. . . . When the needle has been introduced to the desired depth, the syringe is held by the left hand while the piston is pulled gently upward with the right hand. The attempt to aspirate should be continued for a few seconds with a thin soluble solution, or emulsion, and ten seconds for a thick emulsion. If blood should appear, the needle should be withdrawn and introduced again 2 cm. from the original point. Then, if blood is not aspirated, the contents of the syringe may be *slowly* in-

[*] Dutton, Walton, and Lake, George B.: *Parenteral Therapy.* Charles C Thomas, Publisher, Springfield, Ill., 1936, pp. 29-30.

jected. . . . The injections should be alternated in the two buttocks. The areas of injection should be two centimeters apart each way. No two injections should be given in the same area during a course of treatment."

[If the needle breaks, the operator is urged to keep his head and while holding the left hand in the same position try to remove the needle with the right hand. If this attempt is unsuccessful and the needle is lost, a surgical operation will have to be performed. The importance of using needles with sharp points and otherwise in perfect condition is given great emphasis.]

"Treatment of Complications. . . . Insoluble preparations and irritating materials frequently cause superficial indurations or nodules. They may be treated by applications of iodine ointment and rubbed between the thumb and forefinger.

"Painful, deep indurations may be alleviated by hot, moist applications of magnesium sulphate and massage. The patient is much relieved by moving about after the injection. If discomfort continues more than two hours after a soluble, or twenty-four hours after an insoluble, salt is injected, a technical error or idiosyncrasy is the probable cause. In some cases, however, indurations are unavoidable.

"Persistent local reactions are usually traceable, either to a highly irritating material or to some technical fault. Indurations and nodules represent a certain amount of encapsulated drug and may be suddenly released for absorption by a slight trauma, such as sitting down heavily on an uncushioned chair. This sudden release of a large amount of a drug, such as insoluble mercury salts, may cause salivation or other constitutional symptoms. . . . Abscess formation is rare, but resolves promptly on evacuation. Sciatica is evidence of technical error in injecting too deep and too near the sacral plexus and the great sciatic nerve."

4. THE "HYPOSPRAY"

Definition. The administration of a drug through the skin, without a needle, in the form of a jet of fluid under high pressure is called the *Hypospray*.* The jet of fluid is discharged from an instrument that looks like a metal syringe.

Therapeutic Uses. The Hypospray is in the process of development. Theoretically, it may be substituted for the subcutaneous and intramuscular administration of an unlimited number of therapeutic agents. It may therefore have the same uses as the "hypodermic" and intramuscular injections.

Method. The Hypospray is a metal barrel with a very small opening at the end from which the drug is discharged. It contains a plunger operated by a spring, and the drug is in a metal cartridge. Release of the spring forces the plunger against the cartridge, and as it breaks the drug is forced out in a fine stream, or spray, under high pressure. Robert Hingson et al.[24] and W. Royce Hodges[25] report two similar studies on the Hypospray in venereal disease clinics. Approximately 150 patients were treated with penicillin given by the Hypospray and approximately 50 with penicillin by needle injection. Hingson et al. report 97.5 per cent cures using the Hypospray and 97.9 per cent cures using needle injection. Hodges' results with

---

* R. P. Sherer Corp., Dayton, Ohio.

virtually the same number of patients in the experimental and control groups were identical.

The obvious advantage of the Hypospray is that the skin is not broken in the administration of the drug. Release of the spring makes a rather loud report that may frighten the patient at first, but in these studies the child patients were unafraid of the treatment after the first dose. Hingson et al. found that the concentrated preparation of penicillin administered by the Hypospray caused pain and irritation; this could be corrected with a more dilute solution. Mild erythemas at the site of administration disappeared after 24 hours. If the patient moves against the instrument when the spring is released he will be scratched or bruised. Skins differ in their ease of penetration. It is possible that this instrument will be made with springs of varying power. A limited number of drugs are available in the cartridges. Smith says of this instrument that it offers interesting possibilities.

No procedure is suggested for the Hypospray. The mechanism is in a developmental stage, and the operator should be guided at present by the directions furnished by the designers.

5. INTRADERMIC OR INTRACUTANEOUS INJECTION

Definition.   *Intradermal injection* is the term used to describe an injection into the corium or the upper layers of the skin.

Therapeutic Uses.   When the physician wants to see the local reaction of tissue to bacteria, their toxins, or foreign proteins, he introduces them under the superficial layer of the skin. Because absorption from the skin takes place more slowly than from the areolar tissue or muscle, it may be desirable to inject intradermally therapeutic doses of very potent substances that produce severe generalized body reactions. Dutton and Lake say that intradermal injection may be used to induce reactions in skin cells and embryologically related tissues in the treatment of infectious conditions of the skin, and mucous and synovial membranes.

Selection of Method.   Because intradermal injections are used for diagnostic purposes and sometimes dangerous or delicate therapy, the physician generally prefers to prepare the drug, inject it, and watch the reaction. The nurse may, in some situations, prepare the equipment or she may carry out the entire procedure.

The *sterilization of equipment* and *preparation of the drug* are the same as for subcutaneous and intramuscular injections. Drugs given intradermally are nearly always put up in ampoules because, if used for diagnostic purposes, it is essential that they be pure.

The *site of injection* is usually the inner aspect of the forearm. Local reactions, if they occur, are most easily recognized if the skin is relatively free from hair and pigment and if the skin is thin. Disinfectants that discolor or irritate are avoided in the *preparation of the skin* because the physician does not want the reaction of the skin to the injected agent to be obscured. Alcohol 70 per cent is commonly used.

Injecting the needle so that the point goes no deeper than the first layer of the skin is very important; in order to do this the needle is held at a very slight angle to the skin with the opening of the needle up and the point of the bevel lying on the skin. The needle is injected about 2 mm or ⅛ in., and when in position for the injection the opening of the needle should be visible through the skin.

Equipment. Materials for cleaning the skin are required as in any injections. A slender syringe that enables the operator to hold the needle at a slight angle and to measure very small doses in the syringe should be provided. The most desirable type of needle is one with a rounded sloping hub that allows the shaft to lie close to the skin. It should be about 1 cm (⅜ in.) in length and from 26 to 27 gauge. When injections are made for diagnostic purposes, at least two syringes and needles are necessary since a control wheal is usually made.

Suggested Procedure. Give the patient a suitable explanation of the treatment if there is any doubt about his understanding it. See that the patient is in a comfortable position with the forearm supported on a firm surface. He may be sitting or lying, but if there is any tendency on the part of the patient to be nervous about the treatment, he is less likely to become faint or nauseated if he is in a recumbent position. Clean an area about 7½ cm (3 in.) in diameter on the inner surface of the forearm midway between the wrist and the elbow; allow the skin to dry. Holding the needle and syringe almost parallel with the arm, introduce the needle about 2 mm (⅛ in.) with the opening upward. The bevel of the needle should be visible under the skin. When the needle is in place, introduce the drug, making a wheal, or circumscribed elevation of the skin. The area is not cleaned or massaged following the removal of the needle.

When foreign proteins are administered, a very minute amount is usually given and the patient observed for symptoms of allergic shock before proceeding with the administration of the total dose. In serum therapy, in which an anaphylactic reaction is likely, a preparation of epinephrine should be available for immediate subcutaneous administration.

If injections are made for diagnostic purposes, a control injection of sterile saline solution is given on the other arm and a careful record kept to avoid possible errors in reading the tissue reaction.

6. SUBCUTANEOUS INFUSION OR HYPODERMOCLYSIS

Definition. The word *hypodermoclysis* is derived from *hypo,* meaning under, *derma,* the skin, and *clysis,* to cleanse. In medical practice the term is used to designate an injection of a large amount of fluid into the subcutaneous tissues by means of a needle, for the purpose of supplying the body with fluids, and not, as the name implies, for the purpose of cleansing the area into which the solution is injected.

Therapeutic Uses. Subcutaneous injections are given (1) to supply the body with fluids when the patient is unable to take adequate amounts by mouth and by rectum and when administration of fluids into the veins is contraindicated or impractical; and (2) to supply the body with the salts of the tissue fluids, chiefly sodium chloride, and occasionally to furnish food in the form of glucose, amino acids or protein hydrolysates, and vitamins. Smith says that glucose has marked limitations because it is irritating to the tissues, its absorption uncertain, and the caloric yield low for the amount tolerated. Charles S. White and Jacob J. Weinstein say that protein hydrolysate is absorbed as readily as saline and causes no greater discomfort and no local reactions.[26] Intravenous injections have largely replaced hypodermoclysis, but the latter is still used when the venous route is impractical or contraindicated.

Selection of Method.   In some hospitals every step of this procedure is carried out by the nursing staff; in others, the physician injects the needles and starts the flow of solution; in both cases the nurse may prepare the equipment, regulate the flow of solution, and take care of the patient before, during, and after the treatment. Since the physician and the nurse share the responsibility for this procedure, the basis on which the selection of method is made is a matter of concern to both. The chief objectives in any method are the promotion of rapid absorption and the prevention of undue distention, irritation, infection, and unnecessary pain or discomfort to the patient.

The *solution* is prescribed by the physician. An isotonic solution of sodium chloride (0.9 per cent) was most commonly used in the past; Ringer's and Locke's solutions that contain the chief salts of the blood in physiological concentrations are also used. Dutton and Lake recommend Hartmann's solution, a hypotonic preparation of buffer substances (sodium, potassium, and calcium chloride, and lactic acid), designed especially for the treatment of alkalosis or acidosis. While Bastedo says that if a solution is not almost isotonic with the blood it may cause gangrene, Smith advocates a 0.45 per cent solution of sodium chloride because it is more "thirst quenching" and "less irritative." Glucose may be used in 5 per cent or less concentrated solutions. White and Weinstein report favorably on the parenteral administration of a 5 per cent solution of digested protein (*protein hydrolysate solution**).

The preparation of parenteral fluids and the dangers of pyrogens were discussed in Chapter 8; their composition as nutrients in Chapter 13.

Maintaining the *temperature of the solution* at, or near, body heat was discussed on page 717. Unless the physician requests that the fluid be warmed, subcutaneous infusions are, in most places, given at room temperature. The flask of solution, if stored in a warmed closet, is near body heat at the start of the treatment.

The *amount of solution* to be given depends on the size and condition of the patient. Dutton and Lake say that amounts from 50 to 500 cc (1⅔ to 16 oz) are used; seldom as much as 1000 cc (1 qt). Bastedo gives 1500 cc (1½ qt) as the outside estimate and says that clinical experience has shown the danger of giving large amounts. White and Weinstein report the daily administration of 1000 cc of *protein hydrolysate solution* subcutaneuosly in the thighs to postoperative patients. In Chapter 13 the importance of adjusting the amount to the individual's need was stressed.

The *rate of administration* is determined by the individual's rate of absorption and by his needs. A large quantity may be given more rapidly if the solution is

* Baxter Laboratories, Inc., Glenview, Ill.

injected into two areas of the body simultaneously. Fluids are absorbed more rapidly by thin than by fat persons because the areolar tissue is not so packed with fat cells. Tissue that is dehydrated absorbs fluid more rapidly than edematous tissue. Hobart Hare[27] believed that it is not safe to inject more than 4 cc (1 dram) to each pound of body weight in a 15-minute period. This means that 600 cc (20

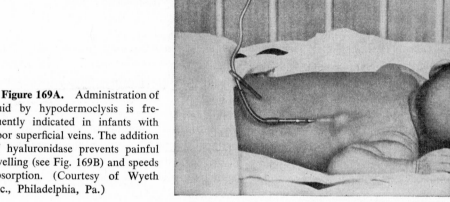

Figure 169A. Administration of fluid by hypodermoclysis is frequently indicated in infants with poor superficial veins. The addition of hyaluronidase prevents painful swelling (see Fig. 169B) and speeds absorption. (Courtesy of Wyeth Inc., Philadelphia, Pa.)

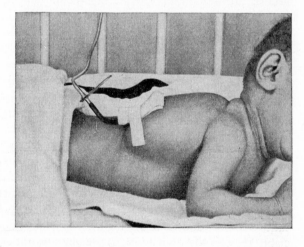

Figure 169B. Note swelling of tissues following a hypodermoclysis to which hyaluronidase has not been added. (Courtesy of Wyeth Inc., Philadelphia, Pa.)

oz) is the most that should be given in a 15-minute period to a man weighing 150 lb. Dutton and Lake stress the importance of giving the solution slowly, stating that it should take from 30 minutes to 1 hour to give 500 cc (1 pt). Smith says the administration of 500 cc (1 pt) should consume from 15 to 30 minutes. These time estimates would be reduced if *hyaluronidase* were added to the solution.

A nurse should make every effort to give the fluid at the prescribed rate, but she should exercise judgment to prevent engorgement of the area injected. Discomfort and pain are caused by pressure of the fluid, and Bastedo says gangrene may result from marked interference with the circulation when fluid is given too rapidly.

Areas most commonly used for the *site of subcutaneous injection* are (1) under and near the outer margin of the breast, (2) the abdominal wall above the crest of the ileum, and (3) the front of the thighs midway between the knee and the hip. Bastedo includes the buttocks and the back below the scapula. James Morrison[28] urges that an area be used postoperatively that does not limit chest movement, although he thinks because the tissues under the breast are loose the area favors absorption. He recommends directing the needle toward the axillary line when this site is chosen. Smith suggests the outer border of the pectoral muscle and says that the needle should be inserted midway between the nipple and the head of the humerus. In choosing the area the objects are to select loose tissue; to avoid large blood vessels, nerves, and glands; and also to limit the patient's movements as little as possible.

Preparation of the skin and *sterilization of the equipment* are based on the principles discussed in Chapters 7 and 8 and in the beginning of this chapter.

The *position of the patient* should be one in which he is relaxed and comfortable. If the fluid is given under the breast, the patient is probably most comfortable lying on his back; if it is given in the abdominal wall above the crest of the ileum, he should be turned on the opposite side and supported with pillows. When the needles are introduced into the thighs, the patient is placed in the dorsal recumbent position with the knees slightly flexed and supported in this position.

The *technique of injecting the needles* varies according to the area into which the solution is given. When injecting the needles under the breast, it is important to lift the breast away from the body and insert the needle into the space between the chest wall and the mammary gland. The needle should be held almost parallel with the body wall to avoid the possibility of striking a rib, passing the needle through the intercostal muscles, or injuring the glands of the breast. When inserting the needle into the thigh, the tissue should be grasped firmly in the left hand and the needle introduced quickly, at a slight angle, for a length of approximately 3 cm (1¼ in.). If the needle is sharp and the injection made with a quick movement, it is only slightly more painful than a hypodermic injection. The fluid entering the tissues and the resulting pressure produce a burning, tingling sensation that is very uncomfortable and nerve-racking even to a well person. Some physicians inject the area first with a local anesthetic, such as procaine (Novocaine), and this appreciably reduces the discomfort. Hastening absorption with hyaluronidase eliminates most of the sensations induced by pressure of the fluid.

There is some question as to whether *massage* should be used during and following hypodermoclysis to hasten absorption. Although a very representative group of therapists favor gentle manipulation because it stimulates the circulation of body fluids, there would seem to be no justification for massaging the part while the needle is injected; the movement of the point of the needle is obliged to destroy the surrounding tissue cells and to cause a good deal of pain. Robert T. Gants[29] and O. P. Humpstone,[30] reported fatalities following the administrations of hypodermoclysis under the breast and in the thigh, and each concludes that one of the injurious factors was the massage that accompanied the administration of the fluid.

Equipment. If small amounts of solution are administered, it may be convenient to give the treatment with a Luer or Record syringe, but in most cases a reservoir of some type is used. It is desirable that this reservoir is the flask or bottle in which the solution is sterilized in order to prevent the possibility of bacterial contamination in transferring the solution. An Erlenmeyer, a Fenwal, or a Florence flask may be used. Commercially prepared solutions are used in most hospitals and almost universally in home, office, industrial, and military medicine. A 180-cm (6-ft) length of plastic or rubber tubing about 1 cm (⅜ in.) in diameter is needed to deliver the solution; if two needles are used, a glass Y tube should be introduced into the tubing with about 35 cm (14 in.) of tubing attached to each arm of the Y tube. The end or ends of the tubing to be connected with the needle, or needles, must be provided with suitable adapters. The tubing should be equipped with a drip bulb, so that the solution may be regulated to drops per minute, if so ordered. A screw clamp is necessary above the drip bulb to control the rate of flow.

Needles used range from 22 to 19 gauge and from 3.7 cm (1½ in.) to 5 cm (2 in.) in length and have a moderately long bevel. Small needles cause less discomfort and less tissue damage. Some physicians use a very small-gauged needle as a means of slowing the rate of flow; if a sufficiently fine needle is employed, the drip bulb and screw clamp can be dispensed with. An irrigating pole or standard is necessary to support the reservoir. If a siphonage system is used, a syringe to start the flow of solution from the reservoir should be provided.

Materials for cleaning the skin include the disinfectant and either sponges and forceps or cotton applicators. Four or five gauze squares to be used as dressing and strips of adhesive on crinoline may be sterilized in the package with the tubing. A small basin for waste solution and a paper bag for soiled sponges are needed. A moistureproof bed protector with a soft cover to place under the puncture area is desirable; sterile towels are not necessary, but one may be used for convenience to supply a sterile field on which to handle the tubing and needles. Sterile rubber gloves are also unnecessary because it is possible to manipulate the equipment with sterile forceps and clean hands without contaminating any surfaces that should be kept sterile. The drip bulb, the glass Y tube, and the adapters should be inserted into the tubing before they are sterilized. If the solution is to be kept warm throughout the treatment, an infusion thermometer should be introduced into the tubing about 5 cm (2 in.) from the needle, and a heating device, such as a rubberized electric pad or two hot-water bottles provided. The writer has found it difficult to maintain a stable and correct temperature with an electric pad around the tubing. Hot-water bottles at 44.4° C (112° F), refilled every 15 or 20 minutes, will keep the solution at the needle between 35° C (95° F) if it is flowing at the rate of 1000 cc in 40 minutes.

One or more treatment blankets should be available for draping the patient.

A cart on which the equipment can be wheeled to the bedside saves time and effort. (See Fig. 29.)

Preparation of the Patient.   Hypodermoclysis is often used after operations when patients are unconscious or too ill to want an explanation of the procedure. The importance of gaining the rational patient's understanding and cooperation has been discussed.

The room should be comfortably warm; the patient placed in a suitable position and well supported to avoid strain; the bed covers turned down to expose the area in which the needles are to be injected; patient's clothing and his bedding arranged to avoid soiling; and treatment blankets properly adjusted to protect uncovered parts of the body. Only the necessary skin area should be exposed. The skin is prepared as for any surgical operation. The fold of upper bedclothes just below the site of injection may be covered with a sterile towel or a square of soft crepe paper. If the equipment is not brought into the room on a treatment wagon, a table must be cleared and placed at the bedside.

Suggested Procedure.   If the puncture is made on a hairy part of the body, shave the area before starting the treatment. Clean and disinfect the skin as described and inject the local anesthetic if it is to be used. Attach the tubing and its connections to the reservoir; hang the reservoir about 90 cm (3 ft) above the level of the bed and allow the solution to fill the tubing, and, at the same time, expel the air from the tubing. Pierce the center of a square gauze dressing with the needle; then, holding the needle at a slight angle, inject it quickly into the subcutaneous tissue at the specified site. Attach the tubing to the needle by the adapter. Fix the needle (or needles) in position with a strip of adhesive brought around the needle hub and carried over the gauze square to the skin on either side. When the needles are in position draw the bedding or treatment blanket over the patient. Adjust the flow of solution to the prescribed rate. When hyaluronidase is used it is injected with a fine needle into the tubing as the solution starts to flow. In all cases the rate at which the fluid is given should be such that the tissues around the needle stay nearly normal in tension and appearance. If the rate of absorption is very low, the physician may want the treatment discontinued before the prescribed amount is given. The injection may last from 30 minutes to 6 hours or more according to the rate of flow and the amount of fluid needed by the patient. If the temperature of the solution is to be maintained near that of the body, hot-water bottles or an electric pad may be placed around the tubing on the bed beside the patient. The position of this heating device may be fixed by pinning the four corners of the covering of the electric pad or hot-water bottles to the bedding. The temperature of the solution is checked at frequent intervals by the infusion thermometer. (This is now thought unnecessary.)

At the end of the treatment withdraw the needles quickly, making pressure over the puncture wound with a sterile gauze dressing. Fix a dry, sterile gauze square over the wound with adhesive. Arrange the patient's clothing and bedding.

It is important that the nurse stay nearby while the solution is flowing to prevent the occurrence of accidents and to reassure the patient. The screw clamp may loosen and allow the solution to flow in too quickly; a sudden movement of the patient may disconnect the tubing from a glass connection; or the patient may turn and displace a needle.

Recording the Treatment. Indicate the nature, amount, and temperature of the solution given; state the rate of flow and the total amount of time over which the treatment extended; report briefly the patient's reaction to the treatment.

7. INTRAVENOUS INFUSION OR INJECTION

Definition. *Infusion* comes from *infundere,* to pour into. *Intravenous infusion* is used to designate the giving of fairly large amounts of fluids into the veins. *Intravenous injection* is the term more often used if the quantity is small and if it is a drug. If blood (and sometimes its component parts) is given, the infusion is called a *transfusion.*

Therapeutic Uses. Intravenous infusions are given (1) to supply the body with fluids, salts, and foods when the patient is unable to take an adequate supply orally; (2) to supply the body with food in the form of glucose, amino acids, protein hydrolysates, or whole blood when there is a hypoproteinemia from burns or other causes, or when there is a metabolic crisis, such as acidosis, with an immediate need for a food like glucose in the tissue fluids; (3) to bring about alterations on vascular pressure by introducing hypertonic saline and/or glucose solutions, acacia, dextran, or albumin solutions; and (4) to supply one or more of the blood's components by injections of whole blood, cell suspensions, plasma, "plasma substitutes," or elements of plasma. Some of the indications for infusing blood, blood components, and their substitutes are discussed under *transfusion* on page 747.

Drugs are injected into the veins when (1) a very rapid effect is needed, (2) when the drug is given for its action on the blood stream or the vessels, and (3) when the drug would be irritating or ineffective given by other routes.

Selection of Method. Because so many risks are inherent in the procedure physicians, in the past, have preferred to give intravenous medications, or to train special technicians for this task. With the increased demand for hospital care and for intravenous therapy, and the disproportionate increase in physicians and medical technicians, there is a movement on foot in some quarters to include nurses in the personnel prepared to give intravenous medications.* In World War II each soldier was taught to give blood and blood substitutes in emergencies, and the whole world is attuned to first aid by civilians in disasters. It is possible that police and other civil servants will be taught to give intravenous solutions to injured persons with symptoms of shock when medical personnel are not available. In general, doctors

* In the *American Journal of Nursing* for October, 1951 (**51**:603), there was an editorial report of expert opinion on the question "Should Nurses Do Venipunctures?" Those who commented were: George F. Lull, M.D., secretary and general manager of the American Medical Association; Malcolm T. MacEachern, M.D., director of professional relations, American Hospital Association; Peter B. Terenzio, assistant director, Roosevelt Hospital, New York, N. Y.; Emanuel Hayt, legal counsel for the New York State Hospital Association and the American Association of Nurse Anesthetists; and Charles U. Letourneau, M.D., secretary, Council on Professional Practice, American Hospital Association.

Only one of these authorities is unequivocally opposed to nurses doing venipunctures. There is recognition by the majority that in some situations they are being forced to accept this function.

are shifting much of what has been considered medical procedure into other hands. It is unlikely that this tide will turn until there is an increase in the ratio of physicians to population.

Those who give intravenous injections, and this applies to nurses in some situations even now, should know how to locate blood vessels suitable for injection; they should have sufficient knowledge of anatomy to avoid injury to nerves, bones, and glands; they should understand the nature and action of the substances they inject and know enough to check the dosage; they should be keenly aware of the dangers involved and, obviously, they should be skilled in the procedure itself. In the writer's opinion the average nurse who carries out this treatment at the present time, except as the agent of the physician and under his direction, subjects the patient to a medical risk and herself to the charge of malpractice. Few nurses are prepared to carry out this procedure skillfully or to deal with the serious reactions to intravenous medication that are all too common. Until there are enough nurses to give nursing care it is wasteful of nursing potential to convert nurses into medical technicians.

Whether or not the nurse actually finds and injects the vein she has an important role in intravenous therapy. She should participate in designing the method used for infusions since she is the person who most often regulates the flow of solution and who watches and records the patient's reaction throughout the treatment. Physicians rarely stay with the patient if a large volume of fluid is given. Nurses frequently prepare and assemble the equipment (although this is most economically done by technicians in a central supply service). Throughout the procedure the nurse should work with the physician; the more thoroughly she understands the treatment, the better her service to the patient.

The method selected should be as simple as possible to reduce hazards to a minimum, introduce the fluid at the desired rate in each case, and eliminate unnecessary pain or discomfort for the patient.

The *solution* is prescribed by the physician. He may be giving it to supply any one or several of the following: water, salts (electrolytes), or drugs; or food in the form of glucose, amino acids, protein hydrolysates, or vitamins. If the blood volume is diminished, or if there is a lessening of the cell or plasma content, the physician will order whole blood, plasma, or plasma substitutes. Infusion of blood, plasma, or the so-called substitutes is discussed in detail under the heading of *transfusion* on page 746.

Effects of introducing *hypotonic, isotonic,* and *hypertonic* solutions were treated on page 718. The reader is referred to that discussion, since the dangers of intravenous therapy cannot be understood without some knowledge of the reaction of the blood to solutions of varying osmotic pressures.

Sodium chloride solution at approximately 0.9 per cent is considered isotonic with the human blood, and is the strength commonly used. Other saline preparations, such as Ringer's, Locke's, Fisher's, and Hartmann's solutions, containing a number of the plasma salts beside sodium chloride, are also used. Frederick A. Coller and Walter G. Maddock, discussing water and electrolyte balance in Frederick Christopher's *Textbook of Surgery*,[31] say there are individuals incapable of tolerating even small amounts of salt (sodium chloride) in the immediate post-operative and postanesthetic period. Quantities in excess of 4–5 gm daily may be held in the body and upset the fluid balance. Many of the untoward effects of infusions can be avoided when their prescription is based on blood analysis. When the blood tends toward an acid reaction (acidemia), sodium lactate from 1.5 to 5 per cent solutions may be administered Smith believes that the giving of 5 per cent solutions of sodium salts a heroic measure and says that a safe dose is ordinarily 0.5 gm per kilogram of body weight. Sodium bicarbonate solutions should never be heated because heat converts this salt to the very toxic sodium carbonate solution. For this reason sodium lactate is preferred, and commercial solutions prepared under special conditions should be used if possible. Alkalemia is rarely severe enough to require treatment. When it is, acid sodium phosphate 2 per cent may be given. Hartmann's solution is designed to correct both *acidemia and alkalemia.*

Glucose is administered in 5, 10, 25, and even 50 per cent solutions, although concentrations over 5 per cent are hypertonic. According to Smith, hypertonic solutions may be given without sclerosing the vessel if they are injected slowly. Although some blood cells may be destroyed by hypertonic solutions, this effect does not appear to be sufficiently extensive to be dangerous. Smith says that concentrations below 3½ per cent should not be used. Hypertonic saline and glucose solutions have been given to draw fluid from the tissues into the blood vessels for the relief of such conditions as generalized and local edema and increased intercranial pressure. Glucose in 50 per cent solution has been used to sclerose varicose veins; but in such cases it is injected with a special technique, more rapidly than in an infusion for a systemic effect. Glucose is most often given in saline solutions, but if there is no object in administering sodium chloride, the solution may be prepared with distilled water. Glucose is administered with insulin in diabetic coma.

Amino acids prepared from enzymatic digests of complete protein are given in saline and glucose. Amino acids and protein hydrolysate solutions supply the body with the same end products of protein digestion that are found in normal blood plasma. *Parenamine,** an acid hydrolysate of casein, is available in a 15 per cent solution, and *Amigen,*† an enzymatic hydrolysate, is available in a 5 per cent solution with or without glucose. These and similar preparations are said to be capable of bringing the person with hypoproteinemia into nitrogen balance. (Protein preparations should be given with glucose. As in the metabolism of a complete diet, the body uses the glucose for energy and the protein is left for tissue growth and repair.) Dextran,‡ a polydipseroid polymer of glucose with a molecular weight similar to albumin and a specific gravity between blood and plasma, like albumin, gelatin, acacia, and pectin, is given to increase the volume of circulating fluids rather than to serve as food.[32] The molecules of all these solutions are sufficiently

* Winthrop-Sterns, Inc., New York.
†Mead Johnson Co., Evansville, Ind.
‡ Dextran is made by Pharmacia, Stockholm, Sweden. (Intradex, a form of dextran, is made by Crookes Laboratories, Ltd., New York.)

large to keep them from passing through the capillary walls readily and so they hold water in the blood system. These preparations are given chiefly because whole blood and blood plasma are not available in sufficient quantity to serve the public need. Most blood substitutes have limited value and are in a developmental stage.[33]

Whether the *temperature of the solution* affects the efficacy of the treatment is still a question. There is a growing tendency, as has been noted, to give parenteral fluids at room temperatures. Lee Rademaker[34] claims that nonpyrogenic solutions may be given at 20° to 44° C (68° to 111.2° F) without causing unfavorable reactions. Samuel Hirschfeld et al.[35] think the temperature unimportant, and Samuel A. Thompson,[36] reporting 300 infusions, makes about the same statement as does Rademaker. Thompson reports favorable results from the use of cool solutions to lower fever. Paul Titus,[37] on the other hand, advocates maintaining the temperature of the solution between 38° and 43° C (100.4° and 109.4° F). Several authorities express the opinion that the vein is more likely to stay patent if the solution is given at body temperature. The dangers of overheating parenteral solutions and the precautions to be preserved in preventing this were discussed on page 717.

The *amount of solution* and the *rate of flow,* as in hypodermoclysis, varies with the size and condition of the patient, the nature of the solution used, and the purpose of the treatment. Dutton and Lake say:

> The tolerance on the part of the organism to large intravenous doses of many substances and great quantities of fluids, provided the rate of flow is not more than 4 cc. per minute (intravenous drip) for amounts over 250 cc. and 5 to 15 cc. a minute for smaller amounts, has been firmly established, except in surgical shock and hemorrhage when large amounts are administered in a few minutes, to bring the blood pressure up to a normal level.*

Hirschfeld and his associates call attention to unfavorable reactions which they attribute to solutions introduced too rapidly. Because some solutions given intravenously can pass quickly from the capillaries into the tissues, it is obviously possible to produce an edematous condition. (The much dreaded pulmonary edema has resulted from an infusion.) W. Kenneth Jennings says in Christopher's *Textbook of Surgery* that a person can absorb 0.8 gm of glucose per kilogram of body weight per hour. When glucose is given more rapidly it acts as a diuretic and dehydrates the individual. (Using hyaluronidase with infusions speeds up the dispersion of the fluid in the tissues.) Too rapid administration of protein preparations may cause nausea, vomiting, flushing, abdominal pain, mild fever, and phlebitis. Makers of Amigen recommend administration at 2.7 to 3.3 cc (40–50 gtt) per minute.† White and Weinstein say that a 5 per cent solution of Amigen with 5 per cent glucose can be given to a child weighing 5 kg (11 lb) at the rate of 1 cc per minute. They think it safe to give it to adults at the rate of 5 to 10 cc per minute. They report a series of postoperative cases in which they gave daily: 1000 cc (1 qt)

* Dutton, Walter F., and Lake, George B.: *Parenteral Therapy.* Charles C Thomas, Publisher, Springfield, Ill., 1936, p. 51.
† Mead Johnson, Evansville, Ind. Personal communication.

of 5 per cent *protein hydrolysate solution* in the thighs subcutaneously in the afternoon, and 1000 cc (1 qt) of 5 per cent *protein hydrolysate solution,* with 500 cc
(1 pt) of 25 per cent glucose solution, intravenously both morning and evening. In
this way they provided the patient with 18.78 gm of nitrogen (the equivalent of
117.37 gm of protein), 250 gm of dextrose, and 4000 cc (4 qt) of fluid.

While the physician prescribes the amount and rate of flow for infusions, the
nurse usually keeps the apparatus adjusted to maintain the desired rate. As with
other such treatments she should know the purpose of the treatment, understand the
method, and be able to recognize unfavorable reactions and report them correctly.

The *site of the injection* is most often the median basilic or cephalic vein at
the inner aspect of the elbow (see Fig. 175). Some operators prefer to inject one of

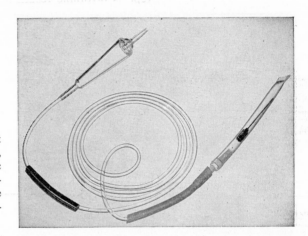

Figure 170. An intravenous set
including a tapered drip chamber,
tubing, and a needle in a plastic
shield that can be attached aseptically to the adapter with a simple
twist. (Courtesy of Cutter Laboratories, Berkeley, Calif.)

the veins of the lower forearm above the inner aspect of the wrist when a continuous
drip is used, because inserting the needle in the vein at the bend of the elbow necessitates splinting the arm, and prolonged immobilization is uncomfortable. The
saphenous vein above the ankle is another point at which the injection may be made.
With infants and small children, the jugular, femoral, and popliteal veins are used,
and in some cases, when the anterior fontanel is not closed, the fluid is given into the
longitudinal sinus. In each case the physician selects a vein accessible to the exterior
of the body, and if possible in an area where limited motion does not cause the
patient unnecessary discomfort.

Patients who cannot eat and drink are kept alive during a protracted illness with
parenteral fluids. Repeated injections of veins tend to sclerose the walls, and
ultimately it is difficult to find an accessible vein that is patent. Some patients
have poor veins, and under certain conditions it is hard to enter anyone's veins.
These facts have led to the use of *intravenous catheters* that are "indwelling" or
fixed in the vein. Catheters are believed by some persons to be less irritating than
a needle.[38] Some operators get excellent results with the indwelling Lindemann
needle, which is blunt at the end and has a sharp cannula and trochar, which are

removed after the needle is in place. Michael Ladd and George E. Schreiner[39] and Lawrence Meyers[40] describe the successful use of plastic intravenous catheters. They come in sizes equal to needles of 27 to 19 gauge. A catheter is passed into the vein for 4 to 5 in. through a needle, which is then removed. The free end of the catheter is attached to the reservoir of solution by tubing, or to a syringe. In both cases appropriate adapters are needed. Ladd and Schreiner say that the tip of the catheter should be in a large vein. They recommend the femoral, rather than the axillary "route." Meyers says the catheter should be rotated to keep the solution injected from hitting the same spot as it enters the vein. There has been some difficulty in the use of these catheters, and it is doubtful whether their advantages outweigh their disadvantages.

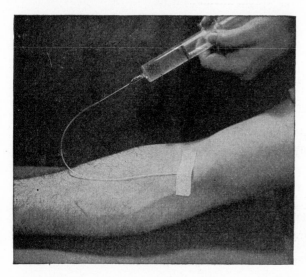

Figure 171. Polyethylene tubing for intravenous therapy; sometimes used instead of a needle when treatment extends over a period of hours. (Courtesy of Clay-Adams Co., New York City.)

Solutions are very occasionally injected into arteries. The procedure is difficult and hazardous. The skin preparation and the preparation of the equipment is the same as for intravenous injections.

Whether to *immobilize the area* in which the needle (or catheter) is inserted depends in each case on the site of injection, condition of the patient, and duration of the treatment. If a nurse is in constant attendance, immobilization is usually unnecessary.

The *preparation of the skin* is the same as for any skin puncture or incision. What has been said about the importance of complete *sterilization of equipment* for other injections applies to infusions.

Unfavorable reactions to intravenous injections have been all too common in the past. The most frequent cause is said to be the presence of *pyrogens* (the products of bacteria) in the solutions. (See p. 759.) A. H. Perkins[41] lists, as other possible causes, improperly treated rubber tubing, too rapid administration, solutions injected at unsuitable temperatures, too large amounts, the presence of alkaline impurities from glassware, or other factors responsible for too high or too low a hydrogen ion concentration in the solution. Particles of glass, a mechanical hazard, and individual susceptibility to the solutions used may explain some reactions. Preparation of the solutions and tubing requires intelligent direction, well-trained technicians, and good equipment. The use of tubing and solutions prepared and tested for purity by reliable firms is more and more widespread and eliminates many risks.

The *technique of injecting the needle* concerns all those who participate in the treatment. The vein should be dilated with a tourniquet or digital pressure between the site of injection and the heart, and the pressure released as soon as a flow of blood from the needle indicates that the vein has been entered. If the attempt to enter the vein is unsuccessful and the process long drawn out, the circulation is allowed to return to normal before the next attempt. In some cases it is necessary to make an incision and expose the vein. When an incision is made a local anesthetic is always used; some physicians anesthetize the area in preparation for a needle puncture.

Equipment. Small amounts of solution may be given with a Luer or Record syringe, but when the quantity is sufficient to necessitate refilling the syringe, a reservoir is more convenient. The reservoir, tubing, regulating clamps, and adapters are similar to those used for subcutaneous infusions. Intravenous needles range in length from 4 to 5 cm (1½ to 2 in.) and from 20 to 18 gauge. They should have a medium bevel. The Lindemann needle is often used when the infusion is to last for days. It is less likely to injure the lining of the blood vessel and to become clogged. An irrigating pole or standard is necessary when a reservoir is used. Materials are needed for skin disinfection as in all injections. Gauze dressings and strips of adhesive on crinoline may be sterilized with the tubing or in a separate package. Sterile towels enable the operator to handle the area surrounding the point of injection without contaminating his hands. Like sterile gloves they are a convenience rather than a necessity. If the physician prescribes the administration of a solution above room temperature a heating device must be provided and the safeguard of an infusion thermometer. (See p. 717 for suggested method.) A tourniquet is required for dilating the vein to be injected. A moistureproof pillow is often needed to support the part of the body in which the injection is made. A small blanket may be needed to cover the shoulders or exposed areas of the body according to the room temperature. Containers for liquid and dry waste should be provided. As in all such treatments it is convenient to bring the equipment to the bedside on a moving table or cart. Splints and restraints are selected according to the requirements of each patient. A small hair pillow strapped to the arm makes a less uncomfortable elbow restraint than the rigid type.

Preparation of the Patient. Because the area of injection is different, the patient's position and the arrangement of his clothing and bedding are different; in other respects the preparation of the patient is the same as for a subcutaneous infusion. The operator needs a good light on the area where the vein is to be injected, and the patient's eyes must be shielded in some cases.

Suggested Procedure. Attach the tubing with its connection to the reservoir. (If a syringe is used, attach the needle and fill the syringe with the solution.) Expel the air inside the tubing with solution from the reservoir before attaching the needle to it. Hang the reservoir about 90 cm (3 ft) above the bed. (If a local anesthetic is used, it is given at this point.) Apply the tourniquet above the site of the puncture; as soon as the vein is sufficiently distended inject the needle into the vein, and when the flow of blood from the needle shows that the vein has been entered, release the tourniquet.

If the syringe method is used, the operator remains with the patient and himself injects the total amount; but if the solution is delivered from a reservoir, the nurse caring for the patient keeps the apparatus adjusted so that the solution flows at the prescribed rate. Fix the needle in the vein by passing a strip of adhesive around the needle hub and applying the ends to the skin.

When the puncture is made in the bend of the elbow a padded splint is attached to the arm. Other necessary restraints, as determined by the condition of the patient, the site of injection, and the amount of nursing attendance available are applied by, or under the direction of, the physician. The patient should be under constant observation as long as the solution is flowing and the needle is in the vein, in order to prevent the occurrence of accidents and to reassure the patient. There is always the possibility that the clamps on the tubing may loosen and allow the solution to flow into the vein too rapidly, a sudden movement of the patient may disconnect the tubing from one of its connections, or he may displace the needle and injure the surrounding tissues.

(If the temperature of the solution is to be maintained near that of the body, place hot-water bottles or an electric pad around the tubing on the bed near the site of injection, and fix this heating arrangement in place by pinning the four corners of the covering of the bottles or pad to the bedclothes. When a heating device is used, check the temperature of the solution at the infusion thermometer frequently. The electric pad at low heat or hot-water bottles filled with water at 44° C [111.2° F] will keep the infusion solution in the tubing at 35° to 38° C [95° to 100.4° F] if it is flowing at the rate of 1000 cc in 40 minutes. It is now usual to allow the solution to flow into the vein at room temperature.)

Throughout the treatment watch the patient for signs of unfavorable reaction, particularly when the solution is given rapidly and in large quantity. The nurse should note and report immediately to the physician any marked changes in the pulse, respiration, or color; also nausea, headache, nervousness, excitement, restlessness, or any unfavorable signs in the patient's condition.

When the prescribed amount of solution has been administered, remove the needle, making pressure over the wound with a sterile gauze dressing. It is usual to apply a dry dressing over the site of injection, held in position by a bandage or adhesive. The physician may or may not want to apply an antiseptic to the area.

Recording the Treatment. Indicate the nature, amount, and temperature of the solution given; the rate of flow and the total amount of time over which the treatment extended; report briefly the patient's reaction.

8. TRANSFUSION

Definition. *Transfusion* is the transfer of blood from the veins of one person (the donor) to the veins of another (the recipient). Blood may also be infused into the arteries, the muscles, the marrow cavities, and the peritoneal cavity. While transfusion primarily refers to the transfer of whole blood, any discussion of it must include the infusion of the component parts—cells, plasma, and plasma derivatives.

Therapeutic Uses. Blood or its constituents are infused when (1) the circulating blood volume is suddenly reduced, as in acute hemorrhage or shock; (2) the red cell volume or hemoglobin content of the blood is reduced, as in anemias; (3) the leukocyte content of blood is reduced as in agranulocytosis and neutropenia; (4) there are defects in the factors controlling hemostasis as in hemophilia or erythroblastosis foetalis; (5) the quantity of the protein is reduced as in malnutrition, excessive loss of protein from burns, or vesicular skin diseases; and (6) when there is an infection with lowered immunity that might be raised by giving the ill person some blood or plasma from a person who has just recovered from the same disease.[42]

In case this listing gives the impression that blood transfusion is used extensively, it may be well to state that all authorities consulted say that even with the most up-to-date methods and skillful operators transfusion still involves serious risks. Ronald B. Scott, in Geoffrey Keynes' text, estimates that untoward reactions occur once in every 20 transfusions or oftener. Robert C. Hardin in De Gowin's text[43] says that blood transfusion has proved fatal in 0.14 per cent of cases and should be used only when the "inherent dangers are overshadowed by the expected benefits."

Selection of Method. There are two distinct problems in blood transfusion: the first is the collection of blood from the donor; the second, the administration of blood to the patient or recipient. *Since the blood of one individual may be incompatible with the blood of another individual and may contain disease-producing microorganisms the donor must be selected with great care.* When it is decided that the person is to have a transfusion, his blood is tested in order to determine its inherited or acquired characteristics according to "group" or "type." ("Group" is often used to refer to the O, A, B, AB characteristics only and "type" to the Rh factor. In the following discussion "group" will be used to refer to either characteristic.) Blood from a donor is then found that is free from disease and is *compatible* with the patient's blood—meaning that it does not agglutinate (clump) or hemolyze the patient's red blood cells.

Knowledge of blood compatibility and the relationship of heredity to blood groups, both from the standpoint of medicine and genetics, is expanding so rapidly that it is difficult to make an up-to-date statement on the subject. The following outline of developments in the clinical use of blood is taken largely from *Blood Groups in Man* by Robert R. Race and Ruth Sanger[44] and *Blood Transfusion* by De Gowin and associates.[43]

There are records of attempts to transfuse blood from animals and well human beings to sick persons as far back as the seventeenth century. These attempts were rare because the methods were crude; there was little understanding of blood compatibility, and the chance of surviving the treatment was about fifty-fifty.

In 1900 Landsteiner reported that red cells from one human being were agglutinated, or clumped, when mixed with the blood serum of some human beings but not others. Within two years he and his associates were able to announce that people can be divided into four groups according to the behavior of their blood cells and sera. This led to wide experimentation by scientists in various parts of the world. A conflicting nomenclature sprang up for these blood groups and the mysterious qualities or factors that make some bloods compatible, others not.

The following table shows three systems of naming the Landsteiner groups although the O, A, B, AB system, recommended by the Division of Hygiene of the League of Nations, has almost replaced numbering.

Table 10. Landsteiner Blood Groups as Defined by Anti-A and Anti-B Factors

PERCENTAGE OF THE POPULATION IN UNITED STATES AND EUROPE	INTERNATIONAL NOMENCLATURE	JANSKY NUMBER-ING	MOSS NUMBER-ING	AGGLUTINOGENS OR ANTIGENS IN RED BLOOD CELLS	AGGLUTININS OR ANTIBODIES IN SERUM
45	O	I	IV	O	Anti-A (alpha factor) Anti-B (beta factor)
42	A	II	II	A factor	Anti-B (beta factor)
10	B	III	III	B factor	Anti-A (alpha factor)
3	AB	IV	I	A and B factors	None

As can be seen when one studies the table, a person who has group O blood has red blood cells that are not agglutinated by the blood serum from any of the other groups. He is often (with undue confidence) called a *universal donor*. A person with group AB blood has serum with no anti-A and anti-B agglutinins to clump the cells from the A and B groups, so he is termed the *universal recipient*.

Table 11. Interactions of the Four Blood Groups

CELLS	AB SERUM NO AGGLUTININS	B SERUM (ANTI-A)	A SERUM (ANTI-B)	O SERUM (ANTI-A, ANTI-B)
AB	−	+	+	+
A	−	+	−	+
B	−	−	+	+
O	−	−	−	−

(+ means agglutination, or clumping; − means no agglutination.)

Actually, these statements are oversimplifications. Since the discovery of these four blood groups, O, A, B, and AB, subgroups have been recognized in A and AB groups. These are designated as subgroups A_1 and A_2, A_1B and A_2B. (Differences in the behavior of bloods of two persons belonging in the A group or the AB group are clinically significant and point to the necessity of proving the blood of the donor compatible with the blood of the recipient before each transfusion.)

De Gowin says that perhaps next in importance to the discovery of the original blood groups was the introduction in 1914 of sodium citrate as an anticoagulant by Lewinsohn in the United States, Hustin in Belgium, and Agote in Argentina. This made "delayed transfusion," with a simple aseptic procedure, possible. The discovery of *pyrogens* by Seibert in 1923, and the development of blood banks and blood preservation from 1933 to the present have all contributed toward safer transfusions.

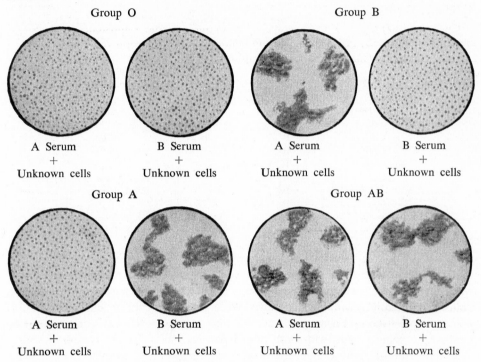

Figure 172. Diagrams showing the behavior of blood when compatible or incompatible blood serums are added. *Upper left:* The corpuscles of *group O* are not agglutinated by serum from groups A and B. *Lower left:* The corpuscles of *group A* are agglutinated by group B serum. *Upper right:* The corpuscles of *group B* are agglutinated by serum from group A. *Lower right:* The corpuscles of *group AB* are agglutinated by serums of groups A and B. (Courtesy of LaVerne Ruth Thompson and Clay-Adams Co., New York City.)

In 1927 Landsteiner and Levine reported that human beings could again be divided into three groups according to the way their blood cells reacted to two sera, one of which they named anti-M and the other anti-N. Bloods agglutinated by anti-M serum they designated *type M,* those agglutinated by anti-N they termed *type N;* those agglutinated by both sera, *type MN.* In 1947 Race reported an *S group* which he classifies with the MN category. Another category of blood groups Landsteiner and Levine have reported as *type P+* and *type P—.*

A much more important discovery, from the clinical standpoint, is the *Rh factor* (antigen or agglutinogen) reported by Landsteiner and Weiner in 1940. They described studies in which rabbits were injected with red cells of the Rhesus monkey, the rabbits developing an antiserum that was found to agglutinate the red cells of human beings in about 85 per cent of those tested, regardless of the absence, or presence, of the agglutinogens AB, MN, or P. They called the agglutinogen or antigen in the cell the *Rh factor* after the Rhesus monkey. Persons whose erythrocytes are agglutinated by the antiserum are termed *Rh positive;* those whose cells

Table 12.   The Frequency of the Rh Chromosomes in England*
(From Race, Mourant, Lawler, and Sanger, 1948)

Fisher	*Short notations much used*	*Wiener,* 1949	
CDe	R_1	R^1	0.4076
cde	r	r	0.3886
cDE	R_2	R^2	0.1411
cDe	R_0	R^0	0.0257
C^wDe	R_1^w	R^{1w}	0.0129
cdE	R''	r''	0.0119
Cde	R'	r'	0.0098
CDE	R_z	R^z	0.0024
C^wde	R'^w	r'^w	
CdE	R_y	r^y	of very low
C^wDE	R_z^w		frequency
C^wdE	R_y^w		

* Race, Robert R., and Sanger, Ruth: *Blood Groups in Man,* 2nd ed.   Charles C Thomas, Publisher, Springfield, Ill., 1954.

were not agglutinated are termed *Rh negative.* About 85 per cent of the Caucasians are estimated to be *Rh positive,* 15 per cent *Rh negative.* At first the *Rh factor* was thought to be a single antigen; now it is known to be what De Gowin calls a "mosaic" of antigens. Table 12 shows Weiner's nomenclature and the C, D, E nomenclature used by Fisher and Race for this "mosaic." Medical workers must be familiar, to some extent, with both nomenclatures until a single system is widely accepted. International organizations are working on the problem of standard terminology.[45]

Since the *Rh factor* was recognized and publicized as the cause of severe transfusion reactions and erythroblastosis foetalis (hemolytic anemia of the newborn characterized by jaundice with an increased number of nucleated red blood cells), the *Rh factor* has come to be a familiar term in this country. Many nonmedical persons know the danger in transfusing an *Rh negative* individual with *Rh positive* blood; they even know the precautions that must be taken to protect the *Rh negative* woman and her offspring if she marries an *Rh positive* man, or if she gets transfusions of *Rh positive* blood. It will be a good thing when everyone knows that *Rh positive blood should never be given to any person who is Rh negative.* This has often been done in the past, and, as a result, many *Rh negative* persons who have received repeated transfusions of *Rh positive* blood have developed antibodies against the *Rh positive* cells, or they have been "sensitized" to *Rh positive* blood. The *Rh negative* mother carrying a fetus who has (inherited) *Rh positive* blood cells may develop antibodies against the *Rh positive* cells of the fetus, and these antibodies in the mother's blood cause erythroblastosis foetalis. This reaction, or sensitization, is more marked with each *Rh positive* fetus the mother carries. This explains why the third or fourth child is more likely to develop erythroblastosis than the first born. If the sensitized *Rh negative* mother is given a transfusion of *Rh positive* blood she is likely to have a very serious reaction, which can be fatal. Victor C. Vaughan[46] says that erythroblastosis can be predicted by testing maternal serum for antibodies at 35 to 36 weeks' gestation. If the test is positive and there is a likelihood of disease in the offspring, plans should be made for an "exchange transfusion" as soon as the baby is born. The erythroblastotic blood of the infant is replaced with *Rh negative* blood from a female donor. The exchange transfusion is often made through the umbilical vein. (*Rh negative* persons should be urged to donate blood to blood banks so that their blood will be available in such eventualities. *Rh negative* blood should never be used for *Rh positive* recipients.) Fortunately, only a small percentage of *Rh negative* mothers are sensitized to *Rh positive* blood either by transfusion or by *Rh positive* fetuses. Therefore, erythroblastosis foetalis is a comparatively rare condition. Other blood groups not yet thought to be very significant from the clinical standpoint are the *Lutheran,* reported by Callender and Race in 1946, the *Kell* and *Lewis* groups, reported in 1946 by Coombs, Mourant, and Race, and the *Duffy* groups by Cutbush, Mollison, and Parkin in 1950. The names of these groups have been taken from the patients in whom the antigens were first found. It must be obvious from even so brief an account of blood groups that medical workers must be alert to new progress in the study of blood physiology.

The fact has been established that blood groups are inherited through the Mendelian law of inheritance. Given the blood group characteristics of a baby, the experts in genetics can say whether it is possible or impossible for a man, on the basis of his blood characteristics, to be the father of the child. Blood grouping has therefore a very important role in *forensic* (pertaining to a law court), or legal, medicine. Blood tests may help an accused man to prove that he is not the father of a child, or they may help a man suspected of a crime by proving that the blood stains on him were not made by the blood of the victim. It has been suggested that

Rh Positive*	Rh Negative (type Rh)*
Group A_1	Group A_1
Group A_2	Group A_2
Group B	Group B
Group O	Group O
Group A_1B	Group A_1B
Group A_2B	Group A_2B
Group O M	Group O M
Group O N	Group O N
Group O MN	Group O MN
Group O Rh_0	
Group O Rh_1	
Group O Rh_2	
Group O Rh_1Rh_2	
Group O rh′	
Group O rh″	

* Certified Blood Donor Service (ed.): *Save Time,* 1952. Jamaica, N. Y., p. 15.

newborn infants have their blood tested and records kept. This means of identification would be a protection for hospitals in lawsuits over the ownership of babies.

A commercial blood donor service has on hand a number of cells to be used by laboratories in checking blood types, but it is only occasionally that some of these cells are needed. (See table on p. 751.)

Minimum Requirements: Citrated Whole Blood (Human), set up by the National Institute of Health,*[47] gives very specific recommendations for *the selection of donors and typing their blood.* Donors must have a normal temperature and blood pressure, be free from syphilis, malaria, and upper respiratory disease and give no history of viral hepatitis. They must not have been pregnant within the last six months, and their hemoglobin must not fall below 12.5 gm per 100 cc of blood. When the blood is collected from the donor a sample is taken, and from this sample a serological test for syphilis is made and the blood is "typed" or "grouped." (Blood from a syphilitic patient is either rejected or used in such a way that transmission of the disease is impossible. Actually, the spirochete causing syphilis is easily killed and, according to the N.I.H. will not survive in blood that is stored for 96 hours.) All blood is typed for *O, A, B, and AB* groups and for the *Rh factor,* using an anti-Rh_0 (anti-D) typing serum. Because *group O* blood is sometimes used for *groups A and B,* it may be "titered" (strength measured) for *isoagglutinins.* (The prefix *iso* comes from the Greek word, *isos* = equal or same. Here this refers to the same group.) If *group O* blood has a high titer of isoagglutinins, "group specific substances" may be added to reduce the titer so that the blood is more compatible with other groups. The National Institute of Health says this practice is not universally recommended by immunologists and suggests that *group O* blood be marked "low titer" to indicate that it might be used safely for other groups. "High titer" *group O* blood should not be used for other groups. Some writers say that the terms "immune sera" and "universal donors" should be discarded because they give a false impression. They point out that transfusions of *group O* blood, or plasma, to other groups may have cumulative effects that are at first unnoticeable but build up to marked blood changes.

The donor's blood may be used as citrated whole blood or the cells and platelets and the plasma may be used separately. Until recently it has been thought safe to give *pooled plasma*—that is, a mixture of the plasma from eight or more donors. It was assumed that the titer of agglutinins was lowered sufficiently by mixing (and to some extent by storing) to prevent reactions. White and Weinstein say that while the pendulum is swinging back and forth they have never advised pooling plasma; De Gowin says it multiplies the danger of transmission of infectious hepatitis; and Max M. Strumia and John J. McGraw[48] say that the use of "group-specific plasma" transfusion is "theoretically ideal."

In summary, the serological test is made for syphilis on the donor's blood. It is typed for *O, A, B groups* and the *Rh (CDE) factor.* It is titered and subtyped in special cases. Before the whole blood (blood cells) from any donor is given to any recipient it must be crossmatched. The donor's cells are mixed with the re-

* Referred to hereafter as N.I.H.

cipient's serum (plasma), and the recipient's cells are mixed with the donor's serum. All these tests must be negative for agglutination before the blood can be safely given. Ordinarily, plasma or its proteins (albumin and globulin) are given without crossmatching; some physicians, in some cases, insist on group-specific plasma. All containers of blood and plasma must be clearly marked with the information as indicated above.

The technique of collecting blood from the donor and giving it to the patient has been revolutionized in recent years. Textbooks continue to list *direct* and *indirect* methods. De Gowin thinks more descriptive terms are *immediate transfusion* [(1) vessel anastomosis, (2) cannula anastomosis, (3) vein-to-vein connection by tubing and valve or pump, (4) paraffined tube method, and (5) multiple syringe method] and *delayed transfusion* [(1) two reservoir method, with collection of blood in open or closed container, and (2) one reservoir procedure with temporarily open systems or completely closed systems].

In the *immediate* or *direct* methods the donor and recipient are placed side by side, and blood taken from one person is given directly to the other so that, theoretically, the blood has no time to clot. Actually all direct techniques are difficult and hazardous compared with indirect methods. Direct transfusion, now rarely used, is a procedure for the operating room and will not be discussed in this text.

With *delayed* or *indirect* transfusions, blood is taken from the donor and given to the recipient days or weeks later in, perhaps, another hemisphere. *Clotting is prevented* by the addition of an anticoagulant solution and the blood preserved by refrigeration. The N.I.H. has set up the following standards: (1) Citrated whole blood must not be used after three weeks, (2) the anticoagulant must be chemically clean, pyrogen-free, and sterile. The following formulas are specified for the anticoagulant solution.

Table 13. Formulas for Anticoagulant Solution

	SOLUTION A	SOLUTION B
Trisodium citrate	22.0 gm	13.2 gm
Citric acid	8.0 gm	4.8 gm
Dextrose	24.5 gm	14.7 gm
Water to make	1000 $\begin{cases} cc\ or \\ ml \end{cases}$	1000 $\begin{cases} cc\ or \\ ml \end{cases}$

For each 100 cc of blood to be drawn, 15 cc of solution A, or 25 cc of solution B, is put into the reservoir, or receiving unit. The anticoagulant should be sterilized in the receiving unit, or reservoir, in such a way that the dextrose is not damaged. (See Chapter 7.)

The equipment for the collection of blood from the donor and the administration of blood to the recipient is very similar. Materials for disinfecting the skin are identical. The container in which the blood is collected from the donor serves as the reservoir in which it is stored and from which blood is given to the recipient. Commercially prepared, disposable units that include reservoirs, tubing, needles, filter, and clamps offer by far the best protection and are, in the long run, most economical in this country. In the donor set the reservoir is connected with the donor's vein by a 60-cm (2-ft) length of plastic or rubber tubing that has a needle on each end. One needle is inserted into the top of the reservoir and one into the vein of the donor. (All sterile areas of the equipment are well guarded.) Blood is drawn from the donor by gravity, or with suction created by a vacuum in the reservoir. De Gowin calls attention to the dangers of collapsing the donor's veins with too powerful suction and, conversely, forcing air into the veins. A small amount of air is not thought to be dangerous, but a large air embolus can interfere with the circulation. The gravity method is probably safer. A motorized holder for the reservoir to keep it in motion during the collection of blood is laborsaving. Blood and anticoagulant solution must be mixed with a swirling movement as the donor is bled. (*The mixture must be gently agitated.*) A means of regulating the flow in collecting and giving blood should be provided. Some operators believe that in both instances the flow can be automatically controlled by using a 16-gauge needle as the inlet or outlet to the reservoir. In any event it is desirable to have the tubing fitted with a disposable clamp.

For administering the blood, a longer tube is used, 120 to 180 cm (4 to 6 ft). The tubing is fitted at the reservoir end with a needle, or a tube, that is inserted into the reservoir. Incorporated in the tubing is a filter. *Filtration of the blood going to the patient is essential.* The N.I.H. says the filter must be one that removes "particulate matter of a size potentially dangerous to the patient" but must not reduce the rate of blood flow unnecessarily. A drip bulb may be placed in the

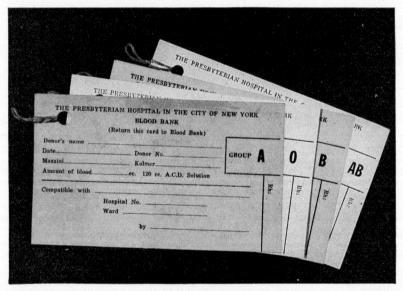

Figure 173A. Tags for flasks to safeguard the administration of blood. The tag for each group has an identifying color as an added precaution. (Courtesy of Columbia-Presbyterian Medical Center, New York City, and Clay-Adams Co., New York City.)

tubing a few inches below the reservoir. A dressing to cover the puncture wound is needed for the donor and recipient. Splints and restraints may be required for the recipient. Blood and plasma are given at room temperatures, or lower. *Blood must never be heated.* The reservoir in which it is collected should be chilled and the blood is refrigerated at 4° to 6° C (39.2° to 42.8° F). While blood is often given in tandem with saline, or saline and glucose, the practice of mixing nutrients or drugs with blood is frowned on.

Disinfection of the skin at site of puncture is the same as for the other procedures described in this chapter. The donor and the patient should both be prepared to cooperate through suitable explanations of what is to happen. *The sites for transfusion* are virtually the same as those for infusion. Blood is ordinarily collected from the median basilic or cephalic vein of the donor after an application of a tourniquet, but any good-sized patent vein may be used. Blood is given to the recipient in veins of the arm, leg, hand, foot, or neck. When for any reason the veins cannot be used, blood is injected into the peritoneal cavity, into muscles, and bone marrow. Occasionally when a patient is in a critical condition, blood may be given into an artery, especially if an artery is exposed as during an operation. Transfusions for infants are difficult because their veins are small. Sometimes, while the fontanel is still open, blood is given into the longitudinal superior sinus. Because, however, the danger of a hematoma in the cranium is so serious, this site seems to be unanimously condemned.

The amount of blood taken from the donor is usually 500 cc (1 pt) and it may be collected rapidly in less than 10 minutes. The amount given the patient depends upon his condition and the purpose of the transfusion. In the treatment of shock De Gowin suggests that as much as 1000 cc (1 qt) of blood may be given in 30 minutes if the systolic blood pressure is below 85 mm of mercury. (The blood pressure should rise from 10 to 20 mm of mercury for every 500 cc of blood.) It is

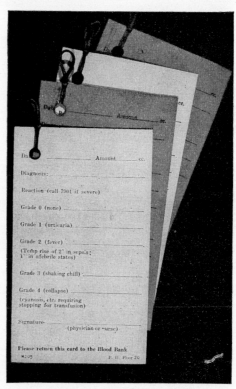

Figure 173B. Back of tag illustrated in Figure 173A. Following the transfusion the physician or nurse fills in the card and returns it to the blood bank. (Courtesy of Columbia-Presbyterian Medical Center, New York City, and Clay-Adams Co., New York City.)

suggested that *the rate of flow* be reduced to 3 to 5 cc (45-75 gtt) per minute when the blood pressure reaches 90 mm mercury and be continued "until the circulation

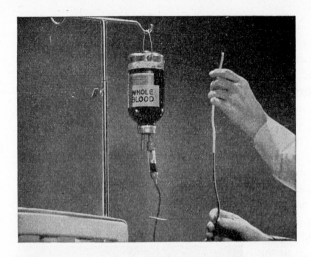

Figure 174A. Preliminary step in the administration of blood. Displacing air from tubing.

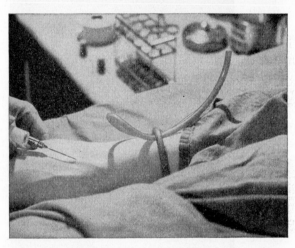

Figure 174B. Tourniquet in place; needle about to be inserted into the vein.

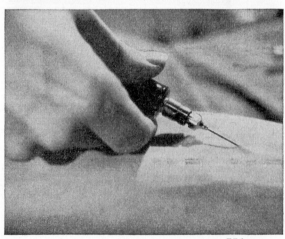

Figure 174C. Needle in vein.

is stabilized." Blood has been introduced very slowly, as a continuous infusion, over a period of as long as 24 hours when there is a hemorrhagic condition that cannot be controlled. Blood introduced slowly and continuously helps to make up the constant loss of blood without raising the intravascular pressure which, if raised, tends to increase bleeding. To keep the citrated blood agitated and further reduce the danger of clotting, a tank of oxygen may be connected with the cylinder of blood and bubbles of gas allowed to pass through it.

In anemia the object of transfusion is to increase the red blood cell count until a given hemoglobin concentration is reached. This can be calculated by established formulas. Roughly, 500 cc of blood should raise the hemoglobin concentration in an adult 10 per cent. Slow (drip) administration of blood gives best results. Even at

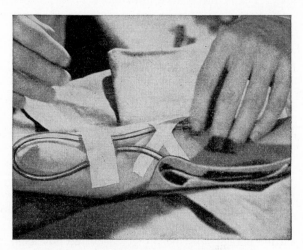

Figure 174D. Needle in vein is fastened securely in place with tape, and tubing looped and taped to prevent tension on needle.

(Figs. 174 A-D from "Guide for Venipuncture and Intravenous Therapy in Emergency Medical Services," prepared by the New York State Department of Health, Albany, New York, 1952.)

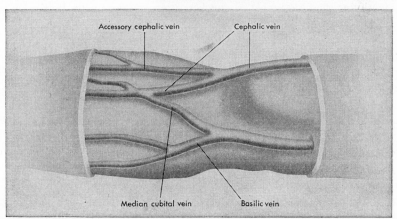

Figure 175. Diagram to show veins used for collection of blood from the donor and administration of blood to the recipient. ("Guide for Venipuncture and Intravenous Therapy in Emergency Medical Services," prepared by the New York State Department of Health, Albany, New York, 1952.)

this slow rate, blood is rarely given continuously, so it may take almost four days to raise the hemoglobin concentration 30 per cent. To keep from "overloading the circulation" anemic and cardiac patients are sometimes given concentrated suspensions of erythrocytes (whole citrated blood from which some of the plasma has been removed.)

I. S. Ravdin and William T. Fitts[49] say there are *no substitutes for whole blood* (the writer's italics). When the oxygen-carrying red blood cells are needed, citrated whole blood should be used. In some conditions the blood count is normal, but the volume of circulating fluids is low. In such cases blood plasma (fresh, frozen, or dried) is used. Albumin solutions prepared from human blood are also given. Substitutes for plasma are discussed briefly on page 741 under *infusion.* Even with blood banks, the collection of blood from persons who have met accidental death, and the improved methods of preserving whole blood, blood cells, plasma, and albumin, there is still an insufficient supply. Medical workers should take every opportunity to make the public mindful of this need. Considerate, appreciative treatment of donors and skillful collection of blood are most effective in promoting both voluntary and paid donations.

Accidents, Reactions, and Complications. Scott, writing in Keynes' text, lists the following "dangers and complications": (1) hemolytic reactions, (2) simple febrile reactions, (3) allergic and anaphylactoid reactions, (4) reactions from bacterial contamination of transfused materials, (5) potassium intoxication, (6) citrate intoxication, (7) circulatory overloading, (8) transmission of infections and infective agents, and (9) miscellaneous local and remote sequellae.

Many of these dangers are eliminated by the blood bank, or the blood collecting service, if the department furnishes the patient with compatible pyrogen-free and sterile plasma or blood, properly treated with an anticoagulant. From this point on the patient must be protected by the physician and by all who work with him. Labels identifying the blood must be checked and rechecked with the patient's name by several persons who understand the danger involved. (The writer has recently seen the administration of the wrong blood to a sick man prevented by the vigilance of a student nurse in her preliminary study period.) Forms shown in Figures 173 A and B illustrate a method of requesting and marking blood designed to prevent the use of incompatible blood.

No matter what precautions are taken, the patient must be watched closely during and after a transfusion. Symptoms of hemolytic *reactions* caused by blood incompatibility vary. Some reactions are severe and may result in death; others are so mild that they may be unnoticed. A severe reaction is described by Alexander S. Wiener[50] more or less as follows. During the injection, even after as little as 10 cc of blood, the patient begins to complain of fullness in the head, oppression in the chest, generalized tingling sensations, and later a *sudden sharp pain in the lumbar region.* Wiener and Keynes both stress the last symptom as indicative of blood incompatibility. Those observing the patient can see that his face is flushed; the veins of the neck are distended; he is dyspneic and coughing, and is restless and anxious. A severe reaction may terminate very rapidly in collapse, coma, and death. If the patient survives the initial phase he will have a chill with a rise of temperature, and this is followed by an "interval phase" in which he seems to improve, but he soon goes into uremia and may die from kidney damage. Milder reactions due to blood incompatibility are evidenced by chills and rise in temperature with blood changes that may be detected by laboratory studies. Pyrogens also are often responsible for chills and fever. Epinephrine is usually given at once for any severe reaction. Compatible blood transfusions may be indicated. Treatment for the uremic stage is too complex to be discussed here.

Another type of reaction is the allergic reaction that, if severe, resembles anaphylactic shock. An allergic reaction may occur immediately or it may be delayed. Urticaria is a characteristic sign of an allergic reaction. Edema of the respiratory mucous membrane and other allergic symptoms are relieved by epinephrine (the recognized antidote for allergic poisoning) if not too severe and if treated immediately.

Reactions believed by some persons to be caused by the sodium citrate in modified blood are said by Wiener to resemble mild reactions (chills, anxiety, and a rise in temperature) produced by incompatibilities of bloods. They are treated in the same way and are usually harmless except for the discomfort of the patient.

Suggested Procedure. *For the removal of blood from the donor's vein* place the patient in a comfortable recumbent position, the arm or leg to be injected supported and the table or bed on which it rests protected. (The individual should have a thorough understanding of what is to be done, and the attendants should try in every way to relieve him of any anxiety he may feel. Keeping the person engaged in conversation helps to prevent fainting which is thought to have a psychic origin.) Disinfect the skin; apply a tourniquet but release it as soon as the needle enters the vein. Allow 500 cc (1 pt) of blood to flow into the receiving unit unless the donor is faint or nauseated, in which case it may be necessary to terminate the procedure. Keep the blood and anticoagulant in a gentle swirling motion throughout the collection of blood. Fill a small test tube with blood to be used for laboratory tests and attach it to the receiving unit at the end of the procedure. When the needle is withdrawn cover the wound with a dressing. Provide a half hour's rest and quiet for the donor. Give him a palatable drink to replace some of the body fluid he has just lost.

For the administration of blood to the recipient prepare him as for an infusion. Check and recheck the blood or plasma to be given. Prepare the patient as for any infusion and give the blood or plasma with the usual technique for infusions with the following exceptions: Be sure that a filter is incorporated in the tubing; give the blood very slowly at first and watch the patient carefully for an adverse reaction. If a physician is not present and the patient is extremely nervous and complains of any of the symptoms listed on page 758, stop the blood flow and report the condition at once. (Epinephrine should be available for immediate injection.)

Recording the Treatment. Different institutions have different regulations for recording transfusions. Whether the physician or the nurse records the treatment, it is important to indicate the time and manner in which the blood was administered, by whom the treatment was performed, the amount of blood injected, and the patient's reaction to the treatment. This report is normally made on the patient's chart, and a second report is often sent to the blood bank supplying the blood.

9. INTRAPERITONEAL INFUSION OR INJECTION
(AND INTRAPERITONEAL IRRIGATION)

Definition.   The injection of fluid into the peritoneal cavity by means of a needle is an intraperitoneal infusion or injection. (If the fluid is aspirated after it is injected, the treatment is termed an irrigation.)

Therapeutic Uses.   When it is difficult to give fluids by vein, as with infants and small children, the peritoneal route is used. Smith says that the peritoneal cavity is sometimes *"irrigated"* for several days in acute uremia or anuria, this procedure theoretically removing some of the metabolic products that are not eliminated by normal processes.

Selection of Method.   An intraperitoneal infusion or injection is like a subcutaneous and an intravenous infusion except that the needle is injected into the abdominal, or peritoneal, cavity. *The equipment* is the same except that a short needle with a short bevel is used. Smith recommends a 20-gauge needle, 3¾ cm (1½ in.) in length. Obviously the length of the needle should be chosen with relation to the thickness of the abdominal wall. A short bevel makes puncturing the intestine less likely. The needle is inserted in the midline halfway between the umbilicus and the symphysis pubis with the needle pointing upward. It is important that the bladder be emptied in preparation for the treatment. A full bladder can rise to the point of the injection and the thin wall of the distended bladder is easily penetrated with the needle. To avoid the danger of puncturing the abdominal or pelvic organs some operators make a small incision and introduce a blunt needle, or trochar. If the peritoneal cavity is to be irrigated, a glass Y tube must be inserted in the tubing from the reservoir of solution. One arm of the Y tube is attached to the tubing with the needle on its distal end; another is attached to a length of tubing connected with a drainage bottle. Smith says the irrigating fluid can be adjusted to the electrolytic balance of the patient. He thinks there is great danger of infection with the treatment and gives this as one reason why the peritoneal cavity is rarely irrigated.

Preparation of the equipment and preparation of the skin at the site of injection are the same as for infusions. As is the case of any injection where a large needle must be used, a local anesthetic lessens discomfort. It is important with this, as with all treatments, to gain the understanding and cooperation of the patient. Intraperitoneal injections for the administration of blood or nutrient fluids are more often given to infants and small children than to adults; for these patients restraints are usually necessary. The *solutions* are approximately the same as those given by vein. Smith says that some drugs are absorbed more slowly from the abdominal cavity than from the vein but that the effect may be more lasting. He thinks that not more than 100 cc (3⅓ oz) of fluid should be given a child at one time. White and Weinstein report the successful use of plasma given intraperitoneally for dehydrated infants. They think that intraperitoneal injection is a simple procedure applicable to home and hospital practice when it is impossible to infuse (or transfuse) intravenously.

10. INTRACARDIAC INJECTION

Definition. As currently used, an *intracardiac injection* refers to the introduction of a drug into the atrium or ventricle of the heart by means of a needle.

Therapeutic Uses. Charles S. Beck in Christopher's *Textbook of Surgery* lists, in effect, the following uses: When the heart stops beating suddenly as a result of anesthesia, hemorrhage, respiratory paralysis, status lymphaticus, electrocution from cautery, vagus inhibition, pneumothorax, asphyxia, or cardiac trauma. The patient can often be saved in these cases if given an intracardiac injection, with aeration of the lungs with 100 per cent oxygen through a tracheal catheter, heart massage, and parenteral fluids. Smith says that there are proposals to make atrial puncture routine in deaths from an "asystolic heart."

Selection of Method. It is obvious that only the physician is qualified to give a cardiac injection. In cases such as those listed, the ventricle of the heart is injected through the chest wall with 1 cc (15 m) of epinephrine, 1:1000 in 2 to 3 cc of sterile normal saline solution. At the same time the lungs are aerated through an intracheal tube. If a coordinated heartbeat does not result, the chest is opened, the heart massaged, or stimulated electrically, and epinephrine (the same quantity as above) dripped over the heart. Beck says that too much epinephrine throws the ventricles into fibrillation. Smith recommends a needle of 20 gauge, 10 cm (4 in.) in length, for ventricular puncture; a slightly curved 20-gauge (4 to 4½ in.) needle for atrial puncture through the chest wall. Any hypodermic syringe will serve the purpose. The skin should be disinfected as for a surgical operation, but the entire procedure must be carried out with the utmost speed. The area just to the left of the sternum in the fourth or fifth intercostal space is used for ventricular puncture and just to the right of the sternum in the third intercostal space for atrial puncture. (The latter is said to be the more difficult operation.) In some emergencies the surgeon may think it wiser to risk infection than to take time for aseptic precautions.

11. INTRAOSSEOUS INFUSION OR INJECTION

Definition. The introduction of fluid into the marrow cavities of bones is called an interosseous infusion.

Therapeutic Uses. This procedure is carried out when it is difficult or impossible to give fluids intravenously, as, for example, when there are extensive burns.

Selection of Method. First described in 1941, intraosseous infusions have been used for adults and children, but chiefly for the latter. Smith says that the action of an intraosseous injection is almost as rapid as that of an intravenous injection. The puncture is always made by the physician. As in all procedures the patient's understanding and cooperation are sought. If the patient is a child the parents should have the treatment explained carefully since this is a relatively new procedure.

A thorough *preparation* of the skin is of particular importance for the treatment

is very traumatic and the injured bone is especially susceptible to infection. *The equipment* is similar to that used for any infusion (or transfusion) except that a local anesthetic, such as procaine, is always provided and the needles used in entering the bone are quite different.[51, 52] The outer guiding needle is 14 gauge, the inner trephine needle 17 gauge. The outer needle is 2 cm (¾ in.) in length and has a cutting tip and a stylet. This outer needle is left in the bone and is the tube through which the fluid flows into the bone marrow. The inner needle is a trephine. It is passed through the outer needle and used to saw and remove a plug of bone to make a pathway for the introduction of the larger outer needle. When the outer needle is in place the inner needle is removed. The outer needle is equipped with an adapter that will fit a syringe or tubing. Besides its stylet the needle has a cap that can be fitted over the hub. If repeated infusions are given through the needle, the opening or hub may be protected from gross contamination by the cap. The right-angle "observation tube" is said to make it easy to tape the tubing to the skin. (An advantage in this method of giving parenteral fluids over the intravenous method is said to be the ease with which the needle can be kept in position.) The most common *site of insertion* of the needle is the midline of the sternum just above the junction of the manubrium with the body, or about 4 cm (1⅝ in.) below. In children up to 3 years (or 5 years, if they are not robust) the upper third of the shaft of the tibia and lower third of the shaft of the femur are used because the sternum is said to be insufficiently developed. After 14 years the tibia and femur should not be used because the character of the bone marrow changes and it is not so well supplied with blood vessels. When the long bones are used the needle is, of course, inserted into the shaft rather than the head of the bone. In the tibia the site is 2 to 3 cm (¾ to 1¼ in.) below the tibial tuberosity.

Solutions should not be irritating although bacteriostatic drugs (sulfonamides and penicillin) have been successfully given by this route. Saline, glucose, and plasma are said to be readily absorbed by bone marrow, but blood is not successfully given by this method. Advocates of this technique report that adults can tolerate a *rate of flow* of 50 cc (1⅔ oz) per minute in some cases, while admitting that too rapid flow causes discomfort and pain. H. I. Arbeiter and J. J. Greengard[53] report that infants were given plasma in the tibia with an average rate of flow 1.44 cc (22 gtt) per minute. Small quantities of fluid can be given with a syringe, but the administration of the fluid from a container, in which it has been sterilized, offers better protection from infection.

It is generally conceded that the administration of fluids by the intraosseous route presents difficulties and hazards. Osteomyelitis, mediastinitis, subcutaneous abscess, and arterial thrombosis have been reported in the literature as results of this procedure.[54]

REFERENCES

1. "Tetanus Following Subcutaneous Injections of Saline Solution" (editorial), *J.A.M.A.*, **81:** 2210, (Dec.) 1923.
2. "Gas Gangrene from Injections" (editorial), *J.A.M.A.*, **87:**453, (Aug.) 1926.

3. Howells, Leonard, and Kerr, J. D. Olav: "Hepatitis after Pencillin Injections," *Lancet,* 1: 51, (Jan.) 1946.

4. Capps, Richard B.: "A Syringe-Transmitted Epidemic of Infectious Hepatitis," *J.A.M.A.,* 136:12, (Mar.) 1948.

5. Krogh, August K.: *The Anatomy and Physiology of Capillaries.* Yale University Press, New Haven, 1922, pp. 96-103.

6. Dutton, Walton, and Lake, George B.: *Parenteral Therapy.* Charles C Thomas, Publisher, Springfield, Ill., 1936, pp. 32, 47.

7. Smith, Austin: *Techniques of Medication.* J. B. Lippincott Co., Philadelphia, 1948, pp. 94, 103.

\. De Gowin, Elmer L., et al.: "Studies on Preserved Blood: Transfusion of Cold Blood into Man," *J.A.M.A.,* 114:859, (Mar.) 1940.

9. Bernard, Claude: *Introduction to the Study of Experimental Medicine* (translated by Henry C. Greene). The Macmillan Company, New York, 1927.

10. Meyer, Karl: *Conference on the Ground Substance of the Mesenchyma and Hyaluronidase.* New York Academy of Science, Dec. 3-4, 1948.

11. Schwartzman, Joseph, and Levbarg, Morrison: "Hyaluronidase: Further Evaluation in Pediatrics," *J. Pediat.,* 50:79, (Jan.) 1950.

12. Habif, David V.: Department of Surgery, College of Physicians and Surgeons, Columbia University, New York. Personal communication.

13. Thorpe, J. N.: "Procaine with Hyaluronidase as a Local Anesthetic," *Lancet,* 1:210, (Jan.) 1951.

14. Rovenstine, Emery A., and Baterman, Robert C.: "The Use of Ampin, an Automatic Ampule Injector for Routine and Emergency Hypodermic Medications," *J. Lab. & Clin. Med.,* 35:795, (May) 1950.

15. Cadmus, Robert R.: "Medication Cost Study," *Mod. Hosp.,* 75:68, (Sept.) 1950.

16. Dodds, Thelma, et al.: "Simplifying Hypodermic Injections," *Am. J. Nursing,* 40:1345, (Dec.) 1940.

17. Bastedo, Walter A.: *Pharmacology, Therapeutics and Prescription Writing for Students and Practitioners,* 5th ed. W. B. Saunders Co., Philadelphia, 1947, p. 33.

18. Sollmann, Torald H.: *A Manual of Pharmacology and Its Application to Therapy and Toxicology,* 7th ed. W. B. Saunders Co., Philadelphia, 1948, p. 71.

19. Grollman, Arthur, and Slaughter, Donald: *Pharmacology and Therapeutics,* 13th ed. Lea & Febiger, Philadelphia, 1947, p. 32.

20. Wiggers, Carl J.: *Physiology in Health and Disease,* 5th ed. Lea & Febiger, Philadelphia, 1949, p. 1089.

21. MacLeod, John J. R.: *Physiology and Biochemistry,* 6th ed. C. V. Mosby Co., St. Louis, 1930, p. 112.

22. Goodman, Louis S., and Gilmen, Alfred: *The Pharmacological Basis of Therapeutics,* 2nd ed. The Macmillan Company, New York, 1955, p. 1631.

23. Goodman, Louis S., and Gilman, Alfred: *op. cit.,* pp. 1628-29.

24. Hingson, Robert, et al.: "Hypospray Administration of Penicillin in the Treatment of Gonorrhea," *J. Ven. Dis. Inform.,* 29:61, (Mar.) 1948.

25. Hodges, W. Royce: "Continued Use of Hypospray in Treatment of Syphilis and Gonor-rhea," *Anesth. & Analg.,* 28:231, (July-Aug.) 1949.

26. White, Charles S., and Weinstein, Jacob J.: *Blood Derivatives and Substitutes.* Williams & Wilkins Co., Baltimore, 1947, p. 281.

27. Hare, Hobart: *A Textbook of Practical Therapeutics,* 19th ed. Lea & Febiger, Philadel-phia, 1925, p. 608.

28. Morrison, James: "A Study of Postoperative Hypodermoclysis," *Anesth. & Analg.,* 8:75, (Mar.-Apr.) 1929.

29. Gants, Robert T.: "Fatal Thrombosis Following Hypodermoclysis," *J. Kansas M. Soc.,* 33:13, (Jan.) 1932.

30. Humpstone, O. P.: "Unusual Sequelae of a Submammary Hypodermoclysis," *M. Rec.,* **65:**216, (Feb.) 1904.
31. Christopher, Frederick (ed).: *A Textbook of Surgery,* 5th ed. W. B. Saunders Co., Philadelphia, 1949.
32. Thorsen, Gunnar: "Dextran as a Plasma Substitute." *Lancet,* **1:**132, (Jan.) 1949.
33. White, Charles S., and Weinstein, Jacob J.: *op. cit.,* p. 263.
34. Rademaker, Lee: "The Cause and Elimination of Reactions after Intravenous Infusions," *Ann. Surg.,* **92:**195, (Aug.) 1930.
35. Hirschfeld, Samuel, et al.: "Influence of Velocity on the Response to Intravenous Injections," *Arch. Int. Med.,* **47:**259, (Feb.) 1931.
36. Thompson, Samuel A.: "Preparation of Dextrose and Saline Solutions and Apparatus for Intravenous and Subcutaneous Use," *Am. J. Surg.,* **22:**127, (Oct.) 1933.
37. Titus, Paul: "Combined Needle Adapter and Thermometer for Intravenous Infusions," *J.A.M.A.,* **102:**1676, (May) 1934.
38. Anderson, L. H.: "Venous Catheterization for Fluid Therapy: A Technique and Results," *J. Lab. & Clin. Med.,* **36:**645, (Oct.) 1950.
39. Ladd, Michael, and Schreiner, George E.: "Plastic Tubing for Intravenous Alimentation," *J.A.M.A.,* **145:**642, (Mar.) 1951.
40. Meyers, Lawrence: "Intravenous Catheterization," *Am. J. Nursing,* **45:**930, (Nov.) 1945.
41. Perkins, A. H.: "Preventing Dangerous Reactions in Intravenous Therapy," *Mod. Hosp.,* **38:**69, (Feb.) 1932.
42. Keynes, Geoffrey (ed.): *Blood Transfusion.* Williams & Wilkins Co., Baltimore, 1949, pp. 44-109.
43. De Gowin, Elmer L., et al.: *Blood Transfusion.* W. B. Saunders Co., Philadelphia, 1949, p. 250.
44. Race, Robert R., and Sanger, Ruth: *Blood Groups in Man,* 2nd ed. Charles C Thomas, Publisher, Springfield, Ill., 1954, pp. 16-268.
45. Wiener, Alexander S.: "Heredity and Nomenclature of the Rh-Hr Blood Types," *Bull. World Health Organ.,* **3:**265, 1950.
46. Vaughan, Victor C., III: "The Rh Factor: Practical Considerations," *Connecticut M. J.,* **14:** 1089, (Dec.) 1950.
47. National Institute of Health: *Minimum Requirements: Citrated Whole Blood (Human),* 2nd ed. Public Health Service, Federal Security Agency, Bethesda, Md., (Aug.) 1951, p. 8.
48. Strumia, Max M., and McGraw, John J.: *Blood and Plasma Transfusions.* F. A. Davis Co., Philadelphia, 1949, p. 223.
49. Ravdin, I. S., and Fitts, William T.: "The So-Called Blood Substitute," *Am. J. Surg.,* **80:** 744, (Nov.) 1950.
50. Wiener, Alexander S.: *Blood Groups and Blood Transfusion,* 3rd ed. Charles C Thomas, Publisher, Springfield, Ill., 1943, pp. 119-28.
51. Strumia, Max M., and McGraw, John J.: *op. cit.,* 176-97.
52. De Gowin, Elmer L., et al.: *op. cit.,* pp. 254-55.
53. Arbeiter, H. I., and Greengard, J. J.: "Tibial Bone Marrow Infusions in Children," *J. Pediat.,* 25:1, (July) 1944.
54. Quilligan, J. J., Jr., and Turkel, H.: "Bone Marrow Infusion and Its Complications," *Am. J. Dis. Child.,* **71:**457, (May) 1946.

Additional Suggested Reading

Barnett, Roy N., et al.: "Hepatitis Following the Use of Irradiated Human Plasma," *J.A.M.A.,* **144:**226, (Sept.) 1950.
Best, Charles H., and Taylor, Norman B.: *The Physiological Basis of Medical Practice,* 5th ed. Williams & Wilkins Co., Baltimore, 1950.
Ciliberti, Benjamin J., and Dickler, Donald J.: "Intra-Arterial Transfusion in Hemorrhagic Emergencies," *J.A.M.A.,* **144:**382, (Sept.) 1950.

French, L. Edward: "Intra-Arterial Transfusion," *Mississippi Doctor,* **28:**196, (Nov.) 1950.

Hecter, Oscar, et al.: "The Clinical Use of Hyaluronidase in Hypodermoclysis," *J. Pediat.,* **30:** 645, (June) 1947.

Howat, H. T., and Schofield, B.: "An Intravenous Apparatus with Automatic Warning Devices," *J. Physiol.,* **3:**29, (Oct.) 1950.

Koucky, R. W.: "Transfusion Problems," *Minnesota Med.,* **33:**1015, (Oct.) 1950.

Mason, Robert L., and Zintel, Harold A. (eds).: *Preoperative and Postoperative Treatment,* 2nd ed. W. B. Saunders Co., Philadelphia, 1946.

Meyer, Karl: "The Biological Significance of Hyaluronic Acid and Hyaluronidase," *Physiol. Rev.,* **27:**335, (July) 1947.

Rosenthal, Helen, and Rosenthal, Joseph: *Diabetic Care in Pictures,* 2nd ed. J. B. Lippincott Co., Philadelphia, 1953.

Varney, J. Howard, et al.: "Successful Treatment of Mismatched Blood Transfusion," *J.A.M.A.,* **145:**978, (Mar.) 1951.

Wyeth, Inc: *Lyophilized Wydase (Hyaluronidase): A Review of the Nature, Actions and Clinical Application of the Spreading Factor.* The Company, Philadelphia, 1951.

CHAPTER 27. ADMINISTRATION OF OXYGEN AND OTHER GASES, AND THE USE OF RESPIRATORS

1. ADMINISTRATION OF OXYGEN
2. ADMINISTRATION OF HELIUM
3. ADMINISTRATION OF CARBON DIOXIDE
4. USE OF RESPIRATORS

Oxygen in excess of that in the atmosphere is administered in a number of conditions, and under these circumstances the gas that is normally inhaled is considered a therapeutic agent. Oxygen therapy is used in conditions in which there is a direct or indirect interference with normal oxygenation of tissues. Some of these conditions include: respiratory diseases, heart disease, shock, infections with fever, industrial asphyxia,* to mention only a partial list. Oxygen may be used instead of air in diagnostic treatments such as a pneumoencephalogram (see p. 810). Since oxygen is absorbed more rapidly than air, the excruciating headache which is a frequent sequela of the treatment disappears more rapidly and the patient's discomfort is greatly eased; occasionally oxygen may be prescribed by the physician and is then administered by means of a face mask following the treatment and its subsequent x-rays.†

Besides oxygen, other gases are used in inhalation therapy. These gases and vapors have little in common except that they are absorbed chiefly by the respiratory tract; on a pharmacological basis, they have been classified into three main groups (e.g., therapeutic, noxious, and inert). In the therapeutic group are the anesthetic gases and vapors, oxygen and carbon dioxide, as well as helium. Helium, even

---

* Several simple industrial asphyxiants include nitrogen, hydrogen, and acetylene. When such gases are used, there may be insufficient oxygen present; thus they can act as asphyxiants. Examples of chemical asphyxiants include carbon monoxide and cyanide. Because carbon monoxide has the property of combining with the hemoglobin of the blood, thus excluding oxygen, it is called a chemical asphyxiant. Cyanide may be a chemical asphyxiant since it acts upon the tissues and temporarily deprives them of the capacity to use the oxygen in the blood.

† This therapy supplements other more general measures such as urging the patient to lie flat in bed, keeping the room darkened and adequately ventilated, and offering the patient fluids at frequent intervals and in small amounts—all of which will help the patient obtain needed rest and sleep until the headache has subsided.

though it is an inert gas, is included among the therapeutic gases since it has valu-able therapeutic actions because of its physical properties (see p. 784).[1] Of the therapeutic gases, only oxygen, helium, and carbon dioxide are discussed in this chapter.

1. ADMINISTRATION OF OXYGEN

Nature of the Gas and Definition of Oxygen Therapy. Oxygen, which com-prises 20.93 per cent of normal air, is a colorless, odorless, and tasteless gas that is heavier than air. It is a constituent of air, water, crust of the globe, and all plant and animal life. It supports combustion and must be kept away from inflammable materials.

Tissue cells must be constantly supplied with oxygen by the circulation since they have no reserve store; oxygen inhalation in humans is therefore essential for life. However, there is a wide difference in the critical need of oxygen by the various body cells. Cells in the cerebrum must have oxygen constantly; if the supply of oxygen to the cerebral cells is cut off for from five to seven minutes, irreversible changes occur in the cells. In the heart, however, the myocardial cells would have to be completely deprived of blood (and the oxygen the blood contains) for from 30 to 40 minutes before irreversible changes occur.[2]

Oxygen may be administered by tent, face mask, and oropharyngeal or intranasal catheter. Since World War I the therapeutic value of oxygen has been scientifically investigated, and oxygen is now recognized as a valuable therapeutic agent.[3]

Physiological Basis of Therapeutic Use. Oxygen is used principally to relieve *anoxia,* or oxygen want, which occurs in diseases of the respiratory and cardio-vascular systems, as well as in conditions secondarily affecting these systems. (The older term *anoxemia* is now generally restricted to mean *anoxic anoxia.*)

It is not a function of this text to give in detail the physiological phenomena of respiration; however, to understand oxygen therapy it is essential to know that the lungs and the circulatory system supply oxygen to the tissues and remove carbon dioxide in a continuous cycle which consists of four phases: (1) *ventilation,* or the movement of air into and out of the lungs, (2) *absorption,* or passage of oxygen from the alveoli of the lungs into the blood hemoglobin, (3) *transportation,* or movement of the oxygenated blood through the cardiovascular system from the lungs to the tissues, and (4) *tissue absorption,* or passage of the oxygen into the cells of the body from the blood. A failure of any one phase of the respiratory cycle will cause a deficiency in the oxygen supply available to the cells of the body (in part or completely). The anoxia which results may be classified according to the type of disturbance of the oxygen-supplying mechanism by which it is caused.[4]

(1) *Anoxic Anoxia.* Disturbance of the *phase of ventilation* may produce anoxic anoxia. This type of anoxia is characterized by a low arterial oxygen tension with the result that the exchange of oxygen in the lungs is interfered with. When such conditions as pulmonary edema, atelectasis, or bronchospasm are present, they act as a mechanical hindrance in the lungs and prevent the free diffusion of gases from

the alveoli into the lungs. There is sufficient concentration of oxygen in the lungs, but the amount in the arterial blood is below normal because it does not diffuse readily.

2. *Anemic Anoxia*. Disturbance of the *phase of absorption* may result in anemic anoxia. This condition occurs when the hemoglobin in the blood is reduced in quantity with a consequent reduction in the capacity of the blood to carry oxygen. Causes of this condition include hemorrhage and anemia. The tissues, therefore, fail to receive an adequate supply of oxygen.

3. *Stagnant Anoxia*. Disturbance of the *phase of transportation* of the oxygenated blood from the lungs to the tissues may result in stagnant anoxia. The tissues receive insufficient oxygen because their circulation is inadequate in conditions such as the following: reduction of blood volume (dehydration), lowered arterial blood pressure (shock, hemorrhage), and local circulatory insufficiency from constricted or diseased blood vessels.

4. *Histotoxic Anoxia*. Disturbance of the *phase of tissue absorption* may result in histotoxic anoxia, which is caused by an interference in the ability of the cells to utilize oxygen. Alcohol, narcotics, and certain other poisons can cause such interference.

Because several varieties of anoxia can exist at the same time, there is a fifth type, referred to as the *combined form*. For example, the patient with shock from hemorrhage has both the anemic and stagnant forms of anoxia.

When an oxygen want exists, the basic cause or type of anoxia must be determined so that effective therapy can be instituted. Thus, in anemic anoxia, the basic condition—anemia—must be treated; in histotoxic anoxia, the cause of the diminished ability of the cells to utilize oxygen must be determined. In general it may be stated that oxygen therapy is most effective in anoxic conditions when the anoxia arises from inadequate oxygenation of the blood passing through the lungs (e.g., *anoxic anoxia*). Unless shock is preceded by or accompanied by hemorrhage, oxygen therapy does little to relieve stagnant anoxia because the blood, even though its circulation time has been greatly slowed down, is being saturated with oxygen to a normal degree.

Indications for Oxygen Therapy. The first essential in oxygen therapy is early recognition of the developing anoxia. The nurse is the person most often in a position to observe the signs of oxygen want, and she should be alert to observe and report them promptly. The signs of anoxia include one or more of the following: an increase in pulse rate, rapid and shallow breathing, occasionally cyanosis, and an increasing restlessness. Sometimes symptoms such as headache, cardiac pain, and muscle twitching develop.[5]

Arthur E. Guedel[6] says that cyanosis may be a useful index in evaluating anoxia but that the presence and observation of cyanosis are determined by four factors. These include: color of the skin, thickness of the epidermis, density of the capillary network, and lighting and color effects in the patient's unit or in the operating room. (1) In fair-skinned persons the threshold value for the appearance of cynosis is lower than in persons with a darker skin. (2) Because there are no blood vessels in the epidermis, it acts as a screen through which the cyanosis must be observed; cyanosis in areas of thick epidermis is not as readily apparent as when the epidermis is thin. (3) When capillaries are abundant and the epidermis thin (as in an ear lobe), cyanosis can be observed more quickly and accurately. (4) The evaluation of cyanosis is influenced by the character of the light in which it is observed; cyanosis can be observed more accurately and promptly in bright daylight than in artificial light.

Therapeutic Uses. The factors upon which a normal supply of oxygen to the tissues depends are: (1) an adequate oxygen pressure in the atmosphere; (2) an unobstructed passageway from the nose or mouth to the lungs; (3) an adequate lung capacity; (4) an adequate supply of blood to the lungs; and (5) blood characterized by a red blood cell count, a hemoglobin content, and a buffer salt content all within physiological limits. Any atmospheric condition or disease that interferes with these requirements produces a state of oxygen want or anoxia. The administration of air rich in oxygen is of at least temporary benefit whenever the body tissues are receiving an inadequate supply no matter what the cause, but only in marked oxygen want and under certain conditions is it prescribed.

Fliers and mountain climbers who expect to reach great altitudes carry tanks of oxygen with them. During a gradual ascent, the normal body can adjust to marked changes in oxygen pressure; but in flying, and often in climbing, there is not enough time for the body to alter the composition of the blood or to compensate in other possible ways. Harry G. Armstrong in 1952 stated that in Army aviation oxygen is used by the pilot during the day when an altitude of 10,000 ft has been reached; and at night at an altitude of 5000 ft in order to retain normal vision for night flying.[7]

Any obstruction in the respiratory passageways or any diseases that limit the capacity of the lungs mean that the body must make a conscious effort to draw in a sufficient amount of air to get the necessary oxygen requirement from it. If the person breathes air in which the oxygen content is increased above the 20.93 per cent in the atmosphere, a smaller volume of inspired air is required to meet the body needs. Oxygen is therefore administered to those who have any sort of growth, such as a tumor or a thyroid enlargement, obstructing the respiratory passageways; to those who have asthma and emphysema; and to patients with pneumonia or any disease of the lungs that markedly decreases the vital capacity.

Oxygen therapy is of marked benefit to patients with cardiac insufficiency that decreases the supply of arterial blood to the lungs or incompletely empties the pulmonary veins resulting in pulmonary edema. Pulmonary edema occurring in postanesthesia patients is likewise treated with oxygen. Convalescence from major surgical operations, such as thoracoplasty and pneumonectomy, is believed by many surgeons to be hastened by oxygen therapy postoperatively. The dyspnea and other signs of anoxia seen in such patients soon disappear when they are placed in an environment in which the oxygen content is high.

Whenever the red blood cells and their hemoglobin content are markedly reduced, there is necessarily a condition of oxygen want, for hemoglobin is the carrier of oxygen in the blood. Oxygen and hemoglobin form oxyhemoglobin, a compound that dissociates to give off oxygen as needed by the tissue cells. The chemical processes involved in the production and dissociation of oxyhemoglobin are affected by the acid balance of the circulating fluids. This is a physiological pheomenon that is difficult to describe accurately in any simple statement; however, it is safe to say that anything that increases the hydrogen ion content of the blood (decreases its alkalinity) produces an oxygen want. Acute alcoholism and the acidosis occurring in diseases such as diabetes are striking examples of conditions in which there is oxygen want due to chemical changes within the blood. The reduction of red blood cells as a result of hemorrhage produces a marked anoxia. "Air hunger" is often cited as a characteristic symptom of hemorrhage. All these conditions are relieved, although not cured or permanently corrected, by oxygen administration.

To summarize, any person who shows signs of oxygen want, such as increase in pulse rate or labored breathing, is benefited, or at least made more comfortable, by increasing the oxygen content of the inspired air.

The administration of oxygen in anoxia produces marked physiological changes. Cyanosis, if present, decreases or disappears altogether, and the respiratory rate and the character of the respiration more nearly approach the normal or may return to normal. The pulse rate usually decreases, and there may be a temperature reduction in a febrile patient with relief of the accompanying physical distress and anxiety. Until the cause of the oxygen want is corrected, however, anoxia will reappear as soon as the patient is returned to normal atmospheric conditions; since the body is unable to store oxygen, the treatment therefore must be continuous to be of value.

Dosage and Means of Controlling It.   Atmospheric air contains 20.93 per cent oxygen, 0.03 per cent carbon dioxide, and 79.04 per cent nitrogen. To be effective therapeutically, the inspired mixture of gases must contain considerably more oxygen than ordinary air.

Oxygen therapy alleviates anoxia because it raises the amount (often expressed as concentration or percentage) of oxygen in the lungs; with increased oxygen tension in the lungs, additional oxygen is passed over into the blood. Albert H. Andrews, Jr., has said that "it is not the amount of oxygen flowing into the administrative device that is important, but the concentration or percentage of oxygen in the lungs."* In generalized conditions (many conditions of the respiratory and cardiovascular systems), a 50 per cent concentration or higher is indicated; when the condition is local as in coronary occlusion, high oxygen concentrations up to 100 per cent are used.[8] In local conditions in which a high concentration of oxygen is utilized, the partial pressure is raised as well as the volume of oxygen in the blood; therefore, more oxygen passes from the blood into the anoxic tissues. When an oxygen concentration of 50 per cent is not clinically satisfactory, the percentage of oxygen is increased.

Premature infants are frequently placed in an individual unit which controls

* Andrews, Albert H., Jr.: *Manual of Oxygen Therapy Techniques,* 2nd ed. Year Book Publishers, Chicago, 1947, p. 17.

humidity and temperature, and permits the administration of oxygen. The concentration of oxygen must be carefully determined since very high concentrations over a long period of time have resulted in lesions developing in the retina. Arnall Patz and associates[9] have shown that oxygen produces microscopic lesions in animal retinas that closely resemble the lesions in the human retina seen in retrolental fibroplasia. Causative mechanism and other factors that may be involved require further study.

When patients have had oxygen therapy over a period of time, it must be discontinued gradually. The higher the concentration of the oxygen therapy, the more gradual should be its termination and concentration reduction. At such times a careful watch is maintained, and the pulse and respiratory rate observed closely. If there is no increase in pulse and respiratory rate following the decreased concentration, it may be assumed that the patient's general condition is satisfactory, and additional decreases can be carried out over a period of hours. Throughout the gradual discontinuance of the oxygen therapy, pulse and respiratory rate serve as guides to the patient's condition.

Oxygen should be ordered and administered in specific dosages as is any other medication, and accurate recordings are made by the nurse of the duration of the therapy, including the patient's physical and mental reactions.

Andrews has compared oxygen administration by tent, catheter, and mask, and he thinks that the effectiveness of the therapy is unrelated to the device used.[10] He considers the maintenance of the desired oxygen concentration more important than the device and says the selection of the device is determined by other factors such as the preference of the patient. Some patients will be more comfortable and relaxed in an oxygen tent, whereas others may benefit more when a mask or catheter is used.

Dosage in oxygen inhalation therapy is expressed in percentage of the total inspired atmosphere. Because the *liter flow per minute is not an accurate guide,* the only way to determine accurately the percentage of oxygen in the inspired air is to make a chemical analysis of a sample of the air that the patient is breathing. In oxygen therapy this should be done every few hours and following any treatment that has necessitated a loss of oxygen from a tent or room. The technique of making this analysis is discussed on page 784.

Regulation of Carbon Dioxide Content in the Inspired Air.   Atmospheric air contains 0.03 per cent carbon dioxide; expired air, 4 per cent. The concentration of this gas in the air we breathe can be increased markedly without any appreciable effect; however, the effect of too great concentrations is injurious since carbon dioxide in the blood stream stimulates the respiratory center in the medulla. According to Louis S. Goodman and Alfred Gilman, as little as 2.0 volumes per cent of carbon dioxide in the inspired air increases its alveolar concentration.[11] Concentrations above 2.0 volumes per cent for patients receiving oxygen therapy are undesirable, because the deep respirations produced may be exhausting.

Since the expired air contains such a high concentration of carbon dioxide, there is some danger of the air inside an oxygen tent or chamber containing too large a proportion of this gas. Trays of soda lime may be used inside oxygen tents and oxygen chambers to absorb the carbon dioxide; however, in many types of oxygen apparatus this is considered unnecessary. Canopies and rubberized fabric sides of collapsible oxygen tents have been found to be permeable to carbon dioxide, so that the concentration of this gas tends to remain within desirable limits even though no absorbing material, such as soda lime, is used. It has been found also that with a fairly high dosage of oxygen (around 50 per cent concentration) the circulation of air produced in a tent by the inrush of oxygen (maintenance flow, 8–10 liters per minute) is sufficient to blow the carbon dioxide out and keep its concentration down below 2.0 volumes per cent.

If soda lime is employed, it must be changed as soon as it loses its effectiveness, the length of time depending upon the amount of carbon dioxide exhaled by the patient and the amount eliminated from the tent in other ways than by absorption with the soda lime. Some types of soda lime change color when the carbon dioxide absorbing power has been exhausted. If used, soda lime should be removed and replaced at least once in 24 hours. However, the only certain method of maintaining the desired carbon dioxide concentration in the oxygen tent, or chamber, is to make chemical analyses at regular intervals. A different solution is used in making the test, but the principles underlying the analyses for oxygen and carbon dioxide are similar. A carbon dioxide analyzer requires greater accuracy than an oxygen analyzer because the concentrations are usually below 2.0 volumes per cent, whereas the oxygen concentrations in a tent are generally 50 per cent or higher.

Control of Humidity. It is very important in both health and disease to provide a sufficient amount of moisture in the inspired air. A discussion of this subject may be found in Chapter 5. For patients receiving oxygen therapy, the regulation of the humidity is especially important.

If oxygen is administered by a nasal or oropharyngeal catheter, the common practice is to pass the gas through a water bottle or humidifier because such catheters, depending upon the depth of insertion, bypass (in part or completely) the mucous membranes by which the inspired air is moistened. The use of oxygen without a humidifier dries and irritates the lining of the nose and throat.

In oxygen mask therapy, a humidifier is not necessary. Usually sufficient water vapor from the expired air collects in the face piece of the mask and the rebreathing bag. However, moderate humidification may be of value at the higher concentrations approaching 100 per cent since the patient's mucous membrane system cannot vaporize the higher concentration.

Oxygen tents and chambers are so constructed that the atmosphere is air-conditioned. Ice chambers and refrigerating coils are used to cool the oxygen and by condensation of water vapor in the expired air to remove excess moisture from the environment. A 50 per cent relative humidity is generally considered desirable.

Methods of Administering Oxygen. Oxygen may be administered in the following ways: (1) by introducing a catheter into the oro- or nasopharynx, (2) through hollow tubes that fit into the nose (nasal inhaler), (3) by a face mask, and (4) by an oxygen tent or chamber. Whatever method is selected, the means of administering oxygen is connected with a supply of oxygen (either individual tank or an outlet from the oxygen piping system) to which an oxygen regulator has been attached.

The *choice of method* depends upon the patient's condition, concentration desired, the facilities available, and the patient's and the doctor's preference. Should a patient be more comfortable wearing a face mask than with an oropharyngeal catheter in place, the former method would then be the preferred one if the prescribed concentration can be maintained. Less oxygen is usually required to maintain therapeutic concentrations using a catheter, nasal inhaler, and mask than to operate a tent, and the administration of oxygen in the oxygen chamber is even more costly. Nursing care is given with the greatest ease if the patient is in an oxygen chamber (although a special nurse is required), and probably with most difficulty if he is in a tent. Catheters and inhalers irritate the mucous membranes if a humidifier is not used, and irrational patients are likely to pull them out of the nose or to jerk off a face mask. Pliofilm canopies used in tent therapy overcome to a great extent the patient's feeling of claustrophobia.

Responsibility for the operation of oxygen-therapy apparatus varies from one institution to another, as well as in homes. In large hospitals there are usually oxygen-therapy technicians who make the initial adjustment of the apparatus, inspect it at frequent intervals, test the inspired air for oxygen and carbon dioxide concentrations, and repair the equipment as necessary. Some of this work may be done by physicians when such technicians are not available, but in most institutions and homes, the nurse gives this service and should be competent in maintaining prescribed conditions. Even if technicians are available, their presence is not sufficiently constant to prevent errors of dosage and other untoward incidents. The nurse should understand the manipulation of cylinders, regulators, humidifiers, catheters, inhalers, face masks, and tents; how to replenish ice and soda lime; and how to adjust canopies. She should be able to make analyses of the air for concentrations of oxygen and carbon dioxide, know how to clean all this equipment and to store it so that deterioration is reduced to a minimum. It is her particular responsibility to study and devise ways of giving nursing care so that there is no interruption in the administration of oxygen and no waste of gas.

An important factor in successful oxygen therapy is the cooperation of the patient. Unless the treatment has been adequately explained, he will be fearful, anxious, and tense. Explanation is also given to members of the patient's family who will otherwise be apprehensive; they must also be told of the great danger of smoking in the patient's room—signs on the tent and the door are not sufficient warnings.

No matter what technique is used, an *adequate supply of oxygen* must be maintained. This gas is most economically purchased in large cylinders that contain 220 cu ft of U.S.P. oxygen. The tanks may be taken directly to the patient's bedside or the oxygen delivered to the clinical division through an outlet from a manifold, or group of oxygen tanks, kept in a special oxygen-supply room. On account of the danger of fire and explosion, installation of an oxygen manifold in a hospital is very desirable since the weight of tanks makes transportation difficult and since there is a possibility of errors in marking tanks "full" and "empty." Oxygen cylinders (or tanks) should be stored in a cool temperature away from inflammable material and where they are not likely to be knocked over. High temperatures cause expansion of the gas with consequent loss through the safety valve. While in use, an oxygen cylinder should be strapped to the tent, bed, or wall. In some types of oxygen tents there is space for the tank in which it is secured by a metal door.

The supply of oxygen must always be equipped with a regulator. A regulator changes the pressure at which the oxygen escapes from the tank to that needed for oxygen administration and keeps it flowing evenly. The flow gauge is usually calibrated in liters of oxygen per minute. The operator sets the gauge for the prescribed flow, and the regulator automatically controls it.

Before attaching a cylinder to a regulator it is important to do what is known as "cracking the valve." This means opening the valve at the top of the cylinder slightly until a hissing sound is heard and then closing the valve quickly. Dust particles that may have lodged in the opening are thus removed. A failure to take this precaution may result in an injury to the regulator and possibly to the person operating the apparatus. The person cracking the valve should stand at the side, rather than the front, of the outlet.

A general rule in using any oxygen regulator is to avoid the use of oils. In the presence of high oxygen concentrations, oils are likely to ignite and explosions have occurred as a result. A set of directions is supplied with each piece of oxygen equipment, and every operator should study and follow them carefully.

No rule can be given for regulating oxygen flow. To maintain a concentration of 50 per cent oxygen in the inspired air, Andrews says a minimum flow of from 6 to 10 liters per minute is required according to the method of administration and the construction of the equipment; if no oxygen analyzer is available, flows of 10 to 14 liters per minute are indicated. As previously stated, the only sure method of maintaining the prescribed dosage is to make frequent analyses of samples of air available to the patient.

A cylinder should not be replaced until it is entirely empty. A special gauge on the regulator shows the amount of oxygen in the tank at any given time.

When the amount of oxygen is low (about 300 lb) as indicated on the regulator, another cylinder is ordered from the oxygen-therapy unit so that it can be connected when the tank in use registers "empty." This will ensure continuous treatment. (At 8 liters per minute, the 300 lb remaining in the cylinder should last nearly 2 hours.*)

Every doctor, nurse, technician, patient, and his visitors should be aware of the *danger of fire and explosion* in oxygen therapy. Warning signs should be placed outside and inside oxygen tents and chambers. With the catheter and mask, the signs should be placed where anyone near the bed can see them. As far as the writer has been able to discover, all fires that have been reported in connection with oxygen therapy have been caused by the lighting of a cigarette or pipe in a tent or in the vicinity of the oxygen supply.

* Andrews' formula to determine duration of flow from oxygen cylinders is useful. He says: (1) multiply the pressure by 3, and (2) divide by flow in liters per minute. E.g.: $300 \times 3 = 900 \div 8 = 112\frac{1}{2}$ minutes (or about 1 hour and 50 minutes). (Andrews, Albert H., Jr.: *op. cit.*, p. 23.)

The hazard in using oil or grease on oxygen apparatus has been mentioned. Andrews says that the patient should not be rubbed with alcohol or oil because of the danger of fire. Oil may be dangerous if left on the nurse's hands while she manipulates the regulator. Electrical devices and open flames should be banned. The patient is supplied with a hand bell instead of the usual electric signal light, hot-water bags should be used instead of electric pads, and so on. While the danger of accidents must be stressed in order to avoid them, there is no reason to be afraid of using oxygen apparatus if proper precautions are taken. Fires are always the result of carelessness or ignorance and they need never occur. The same is true of explosions.

Oropharyngeal Catheter Technique.   Administration of oxygen by oropharyngeal catheter makes it less difficult to examine the body, give nursing care, or any sort of treatment. One of the great advantages of this method is that the patient is able to move about freely in bed; on the other hand, administration of oxygen by catheter is likely to produce some irritation of the mucous membrane. It is the combined responsibility of the physician and the nurse to get the patient to accept the treatment willingly and then to reduce the irritation of the nose and throat by the use of a humidifier and by changing the catheter when indicated.

Suggested Procedure.   Attach a rubber catheter (size #8 to #10 French for children and size #12 or #14 French for adults, perforated with fine holes in its terminal 2½ cm [1 in.]) by a metal adapter to a 150-cm (5-ft) length of rubber tubing. Connect this tubing at its other end to a humidifier that in turn is screwed on the oxygen regulator. Attach the regulator to a cylinder of oxygen or an outlet from the oxygen manifold. To insert the catheter:[12]

1. Measure the distance from the tip of the nose (external nares) to the lobe of the ear (tragus), and mark this point on the catheter with a small piece of tape (to indicate the approximate distance the catheter is to be inserted).

2. After the humidifier,* tubing, connector, and catheter have been assembled, set the regulator to deliver 3 or 4 liters of oxygen per minute.

3. Lubricate the catheter sparingly while the oxygen is flowing; then hold the tip of the catheter in a glass of water to make sure the terminal holes are not plugged with the lubricant.†

4. Determine the direction of the natural "droop" of the catheter: (a) hold the taped part with the thumb and forefinger, and (b) slowly rotate the catheter until its tip hangs at the lowest level.

5. Elevate the tip of the nose, and pass the end of the catheter (in the position of its greatest "droop") gently along the floor of the nasal cavity into the oropharynx, *with the oxygen flowing*. Observe the position of the catheter through the patient's open mouth.

6. To make certain the catheter is in the correct position, insert it slowly beyond the measured depth until the patient has swallowed a bolus of oxygen; then withdraw it back to a point where no swallowing is observed (about ⅔ cm or ¼ in.). (This part

---

* The humidifier is filled with distilled water to the indicated water level. If there is no level mark, fill the bottle *only half full*. When indicated by the manufacturer, tap water may be used, but it is preferable to use distilled water.

† A lubricant that is not soluble in water (e.g., petroleum jelly) is satisfactory.

of the procedure can be followed only when the patient is conscious.) The tip of the catheter will now rest approximately opposite the uvula. (See Fig. 176.)

7. Tape the catheter in position over the end of the nose and brow with strips of adhesive. If the patient prefers, the tube may be fastened to the cheek and brought over toward the ear where it is taped to the side of the face. (See Fig. 177.)

8. With the catheter in correct position in the oropharynx and firmly fastened to the patient's face, increase the oxygen flow up to 4 to 6 liters per minute or to the concentration prescribed by the physician.

9. Pin the tubing—attached to the catheter and leading to the humidifier—to the pillow or back of the mattress. (See Fig. 177.) See that there are no kinks in the tubing.

10. Before leaving the patient, make sure he is as comfortable as possible and that his call bell is within reach since he may be apprehensive about the treatment.

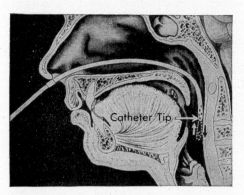
Catheter Tip

Figure 176. Sagittal section of the head to show depth to which oropharyngeal catheter is inserted. (Courtesy of Linde Air Products Co., New York City.)

At stated intervals check the humidifier and add water as indicated.* Also check the catheter to be sure it does not adhere to the inside of the nose. Depending upon the amount of mucous secretion, the catheter is changed every 12 hours or as ordered by the doctor. It is then replaced in the other nostril by a freshly lubricated catheter. The soiled catheter is washed and sterilized before it is inserted again.

In giving oxygen by this method, there is some difficulty in accurately determining the concentration of oxygen in the inspired atmosphere, because it is not possible, as it is with the tent method, to test a representative sample of the air the patient is breathing.

Nasopharyngeal Catheter Technique.   Some physicians prefer to insert a catheter in the nasopharynx rather than the oropharynx. The equipment needed and the procedure of administration are the same as in oropharyngeal technique, except that the tip of the catheter is inserted to within 1.2 cm (½ in.) of the nasopharynx. The catheter is taped, and the tubing fastened with a safety pin as mentioned earlier. The catheter is changed when indicated.

A double catheter can be used, but this does not add materially to the efficiency of this method. Also, a catheter in each nostril will be discomforting to the patient. If a double catheter is indicated, a metal nasal inhaler may then be selected as the method of choice.

Metal Nasal Inhaler.   Metal nasal inhalers, also called cannulas, are metal tubes of various sizes with tips that fit into the nostrils. The prongs are made of malleable metal and can be bent to fit the facial contour; the ends of the prongs are lubricated

* When water is to be added to the humidifier, turn off the oxygen before adding water and fill quickly so that the patient is without oxygen for a minimal period.

and then inserted into the nostrils about ¼ to ½ in. Occasionally short pieces of rubber tubing are placed on the ends of the prongs. The prongs must not occlude the nostrils since the patient would then be forced to breathe through the mouth, negating the beneficial effects of the treatment by diluting the concentration of oxygen. Because the vapor collects in drops of water in the nosepiece, a humidifier is not used unless the patient complains of dryness of the nasal mucous membrane. The inhaler is held in position with a head band.

This method may be valuable in tapering off oxygen therapy; also it is easily adapted for self-administration.

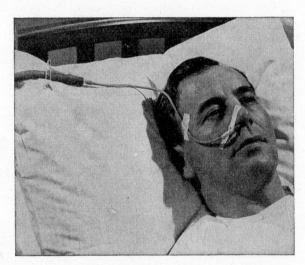

Figure 177. Oropharyngeal catheter in place and fastened to the patient's face with adhesive tape. Note how tubing is securely fastened to pillow with safety pin. There must be sufficient slack to permit free movement of the patient's head. (Courtesy of Linde Air Products Co., New York City.)

Oxygen Face Mask. Face masks are used to administer oxygen in varying concentrations, as prescribed by the physician. They are available in two types: the nasal type which covers only the nose, and the oronasal which covers both the mouth and the nose. With the nasal type the patient may take medication and food without removing the mask; however, his cooperation is essential for the success of the treatment depends upon his keeping his mouth closed and breathing through his nose. Only with such cooperation can dilution of the oxygen be prevented. If the patient cannot carry out such instructions easily, the oronasal mask must be substituted.

It is important to remember that face masks may have to be worn for days and even weeks. Therefore, the mask must fit the patient's face, and careful adjustment of the head band is essential. The conscious patient can tell the nurse whether the head band should be placed above or below the ears for greater comfort. The nurse must be meticulous in the placement of the band so that there is no pressure on the top of the ear. A piece of gauze or sponge rubber over the bridge of the nose prevents irritation when a rubber face mask must be in position for a long time.

When oxygen therapy by means of a face mask is instituted, the nurse must spend sufficient time with the patient to be certain that he understands and will tolerate this treatment. When she leaves him, she makes sure the call bell is close at hand.

*The B.L.B. mask** is a partial rebreathing face mask in which part of the exhaled air is trapped in the reservoir bag and rebreathed. It comes in two sizes. After the appropriate size has been determined by the patient's facial contour, the tubing from the mask is connected by an adapter to a 150-cm (5-ft) length of rubber tubing that, in turn, is attached to the outlet of the oxygen regulator. The flow of oxygen is usually set at 6 to 8 liters per minute. The mask is applied to the patient's face as he exhales into the mask. Oxygen enters the mask through perforated rubber tubing that opens directly under the external nares. Most patients breathe more deeply or more rapidly when a mask is first applied. For this reason, it is advisable to increase the flow up to from 10 to 12 liters per minute. As soon as

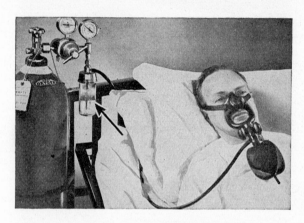

Figure 178. Oxygen therapy with a nasal face mask. Note placement of water bottle between oxygen tank and the mask to ensure adequate humidification of the gas. (Courtesy of Linde Air Products Co., New York City.)

the initial abnormal breathing has subsided, the flow is reduced to from 6 to 8 liters per minute; the breathing bag should almost, but not quite, collapse during inspiration.

Usually the mask is removed at stated intervals (every 2 hours) so that the patient's face may be washed, dried, and powdered lightly before the mask is reapplied.

A disadvantage of the oronasal face mask is that oxygen administration must be discontinued when the patient eats and drinks. It is used, however, because the equipment is inexpensive, because it simplifies nursing care, and because some patients with a tendency to claustrophobia prefer a mask to a tent. It does not have the disadvantage of irritating the oronasal mucous membranes as does the catheter technique.

With *the O.E.M., meter, or Barach mask* the oxygen flow is regulated by an attached concentration meter, and *not* by the liter flow per minute as with the B.L.B. face mask. With the meter mask, the flow of oxygen, to prevent the reservoir bag from collapsing completely, will vary with each patient's pulmonary ventilation.

* The name, B.L.B. mask, is taken from the first letters of the surnames of the men who devised it: W. M. Boothby, W. R. Lovelace, and A. H. Bulbulian.

When the bag rises and falls sharply as the patient breathes, the mask is in the correct position and the liter flow accurate. An occasional deep breath may cause the bag to collapse completely; however, this is not an indication that the liter flow should be increased. The appropriate rhythm of rise and fall of the bag will occur when the patient assumes his more normal rate of respiration. Should the action of the bag seem sluggish, it usually indicates that there is leakage or that the liter flow requires adjustment.

When the oxygen concentration is changed by resetting the meter disk, the liter flow must be either raised or lowered. Close observation of the reservoir bag at this time is particularly important. During regular normal breathing, the bag must never completely collapse. The plug in the meter mask can be removed if suction is indicated. If removed inadvertently and not replaced, there will be a loss of oxygen by leakage.

The meter mask comes equipped with specially designed large-diameter tubing. It is important to use this tubing; if a smaller diameter tubing is substituted, the percentage of oxygen actually administered will vary from that shown on the meter. There must be no kinks in the tubing.

The meter mask is available in both nasal and oronasal styles. The meter which mixes air with oxygen and on which the required concentration of oxygen is indicated is attached to the outlet of the oxygen regulator after the hose nipple and nut have been removed. (It is important to store these two items carefully to prevent loss.) The large-diameter tubing from the mask is attached to the outlet at the back of the meter.

Suggested Procedure. Check the inlet connection of the mask to make sure the large-diameter tubing has been attaached so that the inlet connection is pointing downward at a slight angle. Then turn the meter disk to the prescribed oxygen percentage by rotating the disk so that the number corresponding to the desired percentage is at the top. Have the meter disk set at approximately 10 liters when applying the mask. After the patient has been breathing normally for several minutes, turn the flow of oxygen down to from 6 to 8 liters per minute. The patient is to exhale as the mask is being applied. Adjust the head band so that it fits snugly; be sure that there is no pressure on the top of the ears. The breathing bag which must not collapse completely during inhalation indicates correct application and flow of oxygen.

Should the patient complain of dryness of the mouth, nose, and throat, increase the moisture of the inhaled oxygen by injecting 15 to 20 cc of water into the meter, either through the large hole in the meter disk or through the hose connection on the back of the meter.

Remove the meter mask at stated intervals (usually every 2 hours) so that the patient's face can be washed, dried, and powdered lightly.

Oxygen Tent. An oxygen tent consists of a cabinet that may be connected to a supply of oxygen and a canopy to cover the patient and the whole or part of his bed. There are various oxygen tents on the market. They may be grouped under the classification of motor-driven and motorless tents. In the first type, oxygen is forced into the tent by a motor-driven rotary blower. The oxygen is air-conditioned

motorless

in the cabinet before it enters the canopy. In the second type, oxygen is forced into an air-conditioning chamber by pressure from the oxygen cylinder only. Because cold air is heavier than warm air, currents form inside the canopy and cabinet, cold air falling as hot air rises. If the outlets in the cabinet are properly placed and the whole mechanism well constructed, therapeutic concentrations of oxygen can be maintained in a motorless tent with a very much lower oxygen consumption than in the motor-driven tents. Motor-driven tents require a flow of from 6 to 12 liters to maintain oxygen concentrations around 50 per cent while some motorless tents maintain the same concentrations with a flow of from 6 to 10 liters. When an oxygen analyzer is not available, Andrews recommends an oxygen flow of from 10

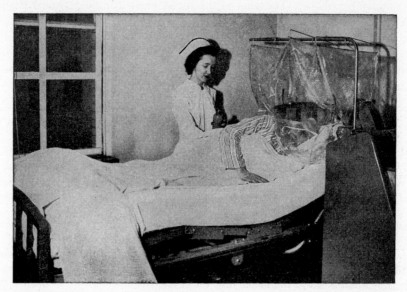

Figure 179. Patient being cared for in an oxygen tent. The canopy is tucked under the pillow, above the shoulders, so that he receives continuous oxygen. (Courtesy of New York Hospital, New York City. West, John P.; Keller, Manelva W.; and Harmon, Elizabeth: *Nursing Care of the Surgical Patient,* 6th ed. The Macmillan Company, New York, 1957.)

to 14 liters per minute to maintain a 50 per cent concentration; in addition, after the tent has been opened, it should be generously flooded.

The temperature of the air can be satisfactorily regulated with either type. A desirable temperature is thought to range around 21° C (69.8° F) although higher temperatures may be indicated for infants and the aged. The ice chamber cools the incoming air and removes excess moisture from the exhaled air. The vapor condenses on the ice and runs off with the melted ice. A relative humidity of 40 to 60 per cent should be maintained.

Canopies are made of rubberized fabrics and transparent plastic film. The larger the transparent area, the better the patient likes it and the more easily the nurse can observe the patient. From the occupant's standpoint, canopies that cover the entire bed are preferable, but they require a higher oxygen consumption than the smaller canopies and make nursing care more difficult.

While taking care of a patient in an oxygen tent, a nurse is often responsible for maintaining the prescribed oxygen concentration, a desirable temperature and humidity, and for renewing ice and, if used, soda lime. She should feel that it is her responsibility to give nursing care in such a way that the patient's needs are adequately fulfilled with the minimum loss of oxygen from the tent.

It is essential that each institution set up its own nursing procedure for oxygen tent therapy in accordance with the type of tent in current use at that institution, even though the basic principles in effective tent therapy are applicable to any type of tent. The following method summarizes the steps in starting tent therapy:

Suggested Procedure

1. Check the tent and its accessories outside the patient's room to make sure the unit is complete; then fill the cabinet with chunks of ice about the size of a grapefruit.

2. With the canopy over the top of the frame, wheel the tent into the patient's room, having first talked with him and explained the advantages of the treatment and tried to discover and minimize his anxieties. Place a shoulder wrap around the patient.

3. Turn on the oxygen flow. Adjust the tent canopy over the patient, being careful that the edges of the canopy do not touch the patient's face. Then tuck the canopy under the mattress as far as it will go at the head and sides of the bed. With a sheet or cotton flannel bath blanket, fasten the front of the canopy by making a wide double cuff; tuck the ends firmly under the mattress.

4. Flood the tent with oxygen either with the flush valve for at least two minutes or by raising the oxygen flow to 15 liters per minute and maintaining this flow for approximately 15 minutes. At the end of this period, analyze the atmosphere within the tent to make certain the patient is receiving the prescribed oxygen concentration (usually 50 per cent).

5. Place the drain bucket in position and open the water drain.

6. Check the thermometer within the tent to make sure the temperature is not too low for the patient's comfort. If he feels cold, give him an extra shoulder wrap and/or raise the temperature control to medium or warm. *No electrical appliances* (such as an electric heating pad, signal cord, or device of any kind) *are to be used within the tent.*

7. After the oxygen content within the tent has been analyzed and found to be the prescribed concentration, reduce the rate of flow, usually to between 6 to 10 liters per minute.

8. Before leaving the room make sure the patient has a hand bell.

If the patient has accepted the tent therapy without undue apprehension and seems relaxed and comfortable, it is wise for the nurse to explain again briefly and calmly why no electrical appliances are to be used within the tent as well as emphasizing that visitors are not to smoke in the room while the treatment is in progress. The nurse must check to make sure there are no matches and cigarettes in the patient's bedside stand. It is also the nurse's responsibility to give the family adequate and frequent reminders of these hazards. Signs on the tent canopy and door of the patient's room need reinforcement through repeated verbal warnings to the patient and his visitors, just as the warning has been repeated within this chapter.

To conserve oxygen, the following precautions should be taken: (1) examine the canopy frequently for cracks and tears; (2) keep the canopy well tucked under the mattress, sealing the free edge with a folded sheet or cotton bath blanket if the canopy does not entirely cover the bed; (3) when using the sleeve or zippered opening to hand the patient food or drink, bathe the face, or clean the mouth, draw the sleeve tightly around the arm; (4) in bathing the patient's body or making the bed, slide the canopy up around the neck of the patient and tuck it under the pillow (see Fig. 179). In some hospitals, patients are removed from the tent and given oxygen by catheter or mask while they are bathed.

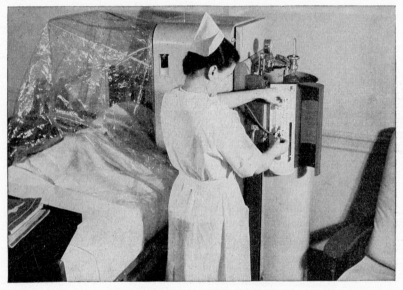

Figure 180A. Nurse making an analysis of the oxygen concentration in the tent. (Hawthorne, M.; Henderson, V.; Montag, M.; and Warfield, M.: "A Study in Some Nursing Aspects of the Operation of the Oxygen Tent," *Am. J. Nursing,* **38**:1203, [Nov.] 1938.)

The value of a rubber sheet over the upper third of the mattress to conserve oxygen is controversial. If it is used, a quilted pad is placed over the rubber sheet to make the bed more comfortable for the patient.

For the febrile patient, low temperatures inside an oxygen tent are usually comfortable. It is wise, however, to provide a head and shoulder wrap, for the air entering the tent on the side with the cabinet is very cool and the unprotected neck and shoulders are likely to be chilled. If the tent has louvers, they are adjusted so that the incoming atmosphere is not blown directly on the patient.

Analyses of the air inside the canopy should be made at regular intervals (every 3 or 4 hours) and whenever examinations or treatments necessitate opening the canopy. Either the liter flow per minute is increased to 15 for a 15-minute period, or if the tent is equipped with a flush valve, the tent may be flooded rapidly with extra oxygen for 2 minutes. However, when the latter method is used, the patient must be warned of the rushing sound this makes. Even though the flow of oxygen is always increased following treatments, there is no certainty that the prescribed concentration has been re-established until an oxygen analysis of the atmosphere in the tent has been made. (See Figs. 180 A and B.)

When oxygen therapy is to be discontinued, it may be advisable to taper off the treatment. This may be done by loosening the canopy to create leakage; however, this is an expensive method. As an alternative, the patient may be removed from the tent for short intervals of 15 to 20 minutes. If the pulse rate does not increase,

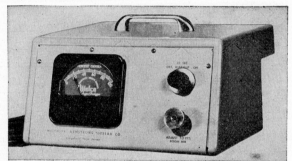

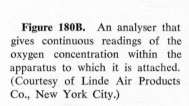

Figure 180B. An analyser that gives continuous readings of the oxygen concentration within the apparatus to which it is attached. (Courtesy of Linde Air Products Co., New York City.)

such intervals can be lengthened. A third method would be to give the patient oxygen either by catheter or face mask, with a slower rate of liter flow per minute. A very slow rate of oxygen flow cannot be utilized in a tent because of the possibility of carbon dioxide build-up within the tent should the flow of oxygen be so reduced that there is insufficient force to blow out the excess carbon dioxide.

At the termination of the treatment the tent should be thoroughly washed with soap and water and aired before it is stored. Washing with alcohol is advocated by some authorities, but it is doubtful whether it is effective in such brief contact. Alcohol clouds Plastoceal windows and must never be used on this material. Great care should be taken in storage to prevent tearing or cracking tents. If space is available, it is best not to fold them at all. Transparent canopies made of Pliofilm are very fragile and can rarely be used a second time. Tears in this material can be mended with Scotch tape, whereas adhesive tape should be used to mend rubberized canopies.

A modification of the ordinary oxygen tent is the *open-top tent*. This is an open box that fits over the head and leaves the body free. Therapeutic concentrations of oxygen can be maintained in such tents, because oxygen is heavier than air and tends to collect around the patient's nose and mouth. The great disadvantage of this apparatus is that the sitting position, which is the most comfortable for many patients, disturbs the concentration of oxygen around the head. This apparatus is ideal for infants and young children and can be rapidly improvised in an emergency.

The procedure for the open-top tent is similar to the adult canopy tent. For example, assembling the tent and filling the ice container are the same. However, when the open-top tent canopy is adjusted, there are some different steps to be carried out: With a child the front opening is closed by securing the canopy around the child's waist; for infants the front opening can be closed by folding the sleeve into itself. The tent must be tilted in such a manner that the patient's face does not touch the front of the canopy, and the tent's supports are then tightened to keep the canopy in the desired position. After the oxygen has been flowing for a 15-minute period, the oxygen atmosphere is analyzed to determine the concentration.

It is important that an open-top tent not be used in a drafty room. Any movement of air over the canopy will increase the rate of diffusion of oxygen from the top of the tent, and it will be impossible to maintain adequate concentrations of oxygen within the tent.

Oxygen Chambers. The ideal but most expensive method of administering oxygen is the oxygen chamber. This is an airtight room into which a sufficient quantity of oxygen is introduced to maintain a therapeutic concentration. Many hospitals have special rooms built for this purpose. It is obvious that this method of oxygen therapy allows the patient more freedom than any other, with the additional advantage of making it possible to give medical and nursing care without interruption of the administration of oxygen.

In an oxygen room or chamber, more than one patient may be treated at the same time. Such therapy has been used for children with acute rheumatic carditis.[13]

Analysis of Air for Oxygen Content. Oxygen and carbon dioxide analyzers may vary in construction but they all depend upon the fact that either of these gases can be bubbled through a liquid that absorbs it. A measured sample of air is removed from the tent or chamber in a syringe or other collecting device and immediately injected into a measured quantity of the testing solution. The amount of oxygen (or carbon dioxide) in the sample is equal to the decrease in the volume of the sample of gas introduced into the testing solution. Figure 180A shows a nurse making an analysis of the concentration of oxygen in a tent, and Figure 180B illustrates a typical oxygen analyzer. All such equipment is provided with detailed instructions for operation. The process of making the analysis is a very simple one, but *most important* to ensure adequate oxygen therapy.

2. ADMINISTRATION OF HELIUM

Nature of the Gas. In 1866, J. Norman Lockyer observed the chromosphere of the sun through a special telescope that he had designed, and saw a yellow line in the solar spectrum that could not be identified as sodium. This bright yellow line was later identified as the gas, helium (*helios* = sun). However, it was not until 1895 that its existence on earth was determined and confirmed by Sir William Ramsey, a London professor. Its therapeutic use was reported by Alvan L. Barach in 1934. "Helium is an inert gas which owes its pharmacological actions exclusively to its physical properties."*

* Goodman, Louis S., and Gilman, Alfred: *The Pharmacological Basis of Therapeutics*, 2nd ed. The Macmillan Company, New York, 1955. p. 922.

Helium is an odorless, colorless, and tasteless gas. It is found in the atmosphere, in minerals, and in natural gases, the latter being the commercial source. Helium is an extremely light gas, and a mixture of 80 per cent helium and 20 per cent oxygen is only one third as heavy as air. Other physical properties include its low coefficient of solubility and high rate of diffusion.

Therapeutic Uses. The act of inspiration requires an energy expenditure which, as Barach has pointed out, is influenced by the weight of the volume of air that is moved in the respiratory act. Normal respiration is effortless and unconscious. However, if the respiratory passage is obstructed by a growth, or by a narrowing of the bronchioles, inspiration is labored. When obstruction of the respiratory tract of an acute nature occurs, great relief is experienced by the patient if helium is substituted for the nitrogen in the inspired air. In status asthmaticus, the patient is often refractory to drug therapy and in great need of oxygen since only a limited amount of air can reach the alveoli of the lungs through the constricted bronchioles; Goodman and Gilman also state that the administration of helium-oxygen mixture leads to partial relief at once and that helium is valuable in the treatment of inflammatory obstructions in the air passages.[14] Such obstructions may have been caused by infection or mechanical irritation following instrumentation (e.g., bronchoscopy). Other indications for the use of helium may occur in anesthesia should a patient's trachea be partially compressed by an adjacent growth. Helium mixtures have been used successfully for patients with emphysema, bronchiectasis, and pulmonary fibrosis. Barach and P. Swenson based their recommendation of the use of helium and oxygen therapy under positive pressure on roentgenographic studies. Such studies showed that the smaller bronchi are further enlarged at the end of expiration when positive pressure is used.[15]

Because of its physical properties helium is effective in shortening the decompression period of divers and other persons who have breathed compressed air under high pressure. Since nitrogen has a high solubility and relatively low rate of diffusion, a long period of time is required to rid the body of excess nitrogen. When a helium-oxygen mixture is used, the period of decompression is much shorter. This is due to the low solubility of helium and its poor affinity for lipids which limit the amount of helium dissolved in body fluids. The rapid escape of helium is further increased by its high rate of diffusion.

Knowledge of the physical properties of helium is essential in determining its effective use in untoward respiratory conditions.

Method of Administration. Because of its low molecular weight and density, helium-oxygen escapes more easily than nitrogen-oxygen (air). A face mask (B.L.B. or meter) is a better method than the tent or oropharyngeal catheter. However, if a tent is used, it should be made of a special fabric that is helium proof.

Administration of helium is started by the physician or a specially trained technician, and the nurse may continue the treatment after its successful initiation. It is much more important to prevent the access of air into the mask or canopy in helium administration than in oxygen therapy. As in oxygen administration with the tent method, the mixture is passed through an air-conditioning cabinet before it enters the canopy (see pp. 779-80).

Helium mixed with oxygen in the desired proportions is available in large cylinders. Special regulators calculated for helium should be used. A regulator that has been used for helium, or for carbon dioxide, or for mixtures of either gas with oxygen, must not be used on an oxygen cylinder. Some helium and carbon dioxide cylinders are compressed with oil-lubricated compressors, and may contain very fine particles of oil. If any of these particles lodge in the regulator, it is hazardous to use the regulator on a cylinder of oxygen. Oil coming in contact with oxygen under high pressure can ignite violently.

3. ADMINISTRATION OF CARBON DIOXIDE

Nature of the Gas.   Carbon dioxide was discovered by J. B. van Helmont (1577-1644) in the products of combustion and fermentation. It is a colorless gas, with a faint pungent odor and a slightly acid taste. It occurs in the atmosphere, is a product of metabolism in animal life, and can be made commercially in various ways. In pure form it is highly toxic and can cause death. According to A. S. Blumgarten, carbon dioxide snow ("dry ice") is a strong caustic that destroys living tissue.[16] For medicinal purposes, carbon dioxide is usually administered in combination with oxygen, and cylinders (both large and small tanks) containing the two gases in varying proportions (carbon dioxide 3 to 10 per cent and oxygen 90 to 97 per cent[17]) are available. The pressure and volume during carbon dioxide administration are regulated by a gauge.

Therapeutic Uses.   In normal physiology, carbon dioxide is a gas of paramount importance in the control of both the respiration and circulation.[18] It stimulates the respiratory center located in the medulla oblongata, increasing the rate and depth of respiration. The intensity of this action is affected by: (1) concentration of carbon dioxide in the blood, which is determined by the composition of the alveolar air inhaled; and (2) the responsiveness of the respiratory center. If the center has been depressed by morphine, the response to carbon dioxide is minimal.[19] Carbon dioxide also contracts the involuntary muscles of the blood vessels, thereby raising the blood pressure.[20]

Carbon dioxide is used therapeutically as a respiratory stimulant and in the resuscitation of the newborn, the drowned, and persons with drug poisoning. Carbon dioxide inhalations have been widely used to increase the depth of respiration in the postoperative patient. Because this treatment increases the volume of tidal air, excretion of anesthetics eliminated by the lungs is hastened, and the period of recovery from anesthesia is reduced. The fact that it increases the depth of respiration and thus lung expansion prevents pulmonary congestion and atelectasis, both of which predispose the lungs to infection. Carbon dioxide has proved of value in hiccup, the possible explanation lying in the stimulation of the respiratory center which leads to more rhythmical contractions of the diaphragm.

Carbon dioxide is of value in the treatment of asphyxiation of all kinds because it stimulates spontaneous respiration, and the increased oxygen intake helps to overcome the symptoms of anoxia or oxygen want. In carbon monoxide poisoning, administration of carbon dioxide has a special advantage in that the increased carbon dioxide content in the blood hastens the dissociation of carboxyhemoglobin.

Some physicians have recommended the administration of carbon dioxide with oxygen in the treatment of pneumonia; others have stated that increase in the depth of respiration is exhausting and therefore harmful. Some favorable results have been reported with the explanation that carbon dioxide causes expansion of the lungs to a maximum and so promotes drainage and prevents atelectasis.[21]

Contraindications. According to Goodman and Gilman the contraindications are relative rather than absolute. Whenever concentrations of 5 per cent carbon dioxide are administered for a period of 30 minutes or more, the patient should be observed carefully for signs of toxicity. These include the following: unbearable dyspnea, vomiting, disorientation, and a markedly elevated systolic blood pressure.[22] When such symptoms appear, administration of the gas must be discontinued at once. In general, it seems best to discontinue its use as soon as the desired effect on respiration is observed.

Whenever respiratory obstruction is present, caution in the use of carbon dioxide is definitely indicated. The gas which stimulates the respiratory center results in an increased respiratory rate which, in turn, may cause pulmonary edema. "For the same reason pulmonary edema enjoins caution in the use of carbon dioxide and only low concentrations (below 5 per cent) should be employed in the presence of this complication."*

Methods of Administration. Carbon dioxide may be administered with the type of mask used in anesthesia that delivers a mixture of oxygen and carbon dioxide in prescribed percentages (3 to 10 per cent carbon dioxide in oxygen, but usually 5 per cent); it may also be given with a B.L.B. or meter mask (oronasal type). Andrews recommends that the physician give the first treatment; the doctor adjusts the mask for 100 per cent administration and turns on sufficient flow to keep the bag from collapsing completely. If the patient does not respond by increased breathing after six inhalations, the treatment is stopped to prevent a dangerously high carbon dioxide blood level. Other indications to terminate the treatment include: dyspnea and a change in the quality and rate of the patient's pulse (pulse weaker and more irregular and/or an increase of 15 pulsations per minute—that is, from 80 to 95 beats or higher per minute).

During the administration of carbon dioxide it is important that the doctor or the well-prepared nurse stay with the patient. He requires constant attention to prevent overstimulation of the respiratory center in the medulla with subsequent hyperventilation. The effectiveness of the treatment is determined by a *satisfactory* increase in the rate and/or depth of respiration.

Carbon dioxide is sometimes ordered postoperatively to stimulate respirations in order to prevent pulmonary complications or to control hiccup (see p. 1038; p. 1041). In such cases the procedure is usually carried out by the nurse.

* Goodman, Louis S., and Gilman, Alfred: *op. cit.,* p. 921.

Suggested Procedure

1. Before the treatment is started, explain to the patient that the gas which is about to be used is *not* an anesthetic and that he is to breathe normally.

2. Collect and bring to the bedside the following equipment which includes: (a) small cylinder of carbon dioxide and oxygen in the percentage prescribed by the physician; (b) a face mask, with an inhaling bag, connected to the cylinder by rubber tubing.

3. Turn down the upper bed linen so that the chest movements may be observed.

4. Inflate rubber face cushion moderately so that it conforms to the patient's facial contour.

5. Close exhaling valve on mask; then open tank valve to fill bag with the carbon dioxide and oxygen mixture; close tank valve. Do not fill the bag too full.

6. Place the mask over the patient's face so that it is airtight; open exhaling valve and instruct the patient to breathe in and out for several minutes, until the rate and depth of respirations have been increased.

7. Close the exhaling valve just after the patient has completed an expiration. The bag is thus left inflated.

8. As deeper respirations subside, repeat the procedure, refilling the bag as necessary. The length of the treatment is determined by the physician.

(Carbon dioxide and oxygen inhalations may be ordered every four hours or three times a day for a period of 24 to 48 hours postoperatively.)

Charting.   Note and record the rate and depth of respiration before, during, and at the end of the treatment; the general appearance and reaction of the patient (e.g., color of the patient's face and lips, presence or absence of chest pain, etc.). Record the duration of the treatment and the number of bags of carbon dioxide and oxygen mixture administered as well as the percentage of gases used.

A simple means of increasing the carbon dioxide content in the inspired air is to place a paper bag over the face. This necessitates rebreathing the expired air which contains approximately 4 per cent carbon dioxide. This method can easily be applied and is useful in terminating hiccup.

Forms of carbon dioxide therapy are essentially hazardous, and should be administered only under the direction of experts.

4. USE OF RESPIRATORS

Definition and Principles of Action.   The cylinder respirator is one means of providing artificial respiration.* The patient's body with the exception of the head is inserted into a hollow cylinder. The pressure within the cylinder is decreased below the atmospheric pressure and returned to atmospheric pressure by the movements of a diaphragm on the cylinder which is attached to an electric motor.

Because the electric motor operating the apparatus may, like any other mechanism, get out of order, respirators are provided with a handle (see Fig. 181) that allows the diaphragm to be moved rhythmically by hand while the motor is being repaired.

* Other mechanical aids to respiration include: chest-abdomen respirator, chest respirator, and rocking bed; all designed to provide the patient with adequate pulmonary ventilation.

Placement of the Patient in the Respirator.   The physician and the nurse who will care for the patient in the respirator, while telling the patient about the treatment, can reassure him by emphasizing that the machine will give him needed rest and that it is a temporary measure. He must be assured that he will never be left alone. At the same time a second nurse is preparing the respirator cot and checking the respirator to make certain that all equipment is at hand.* The cot may be made up with two sheets, one over the upper half and the other over the lower half, or the cot mattress may be covered with one sheet, and a second small sheet used as a drawsheet under the buttocks. Either method will facilitate change of linen after the patient has been placed in the respirator.

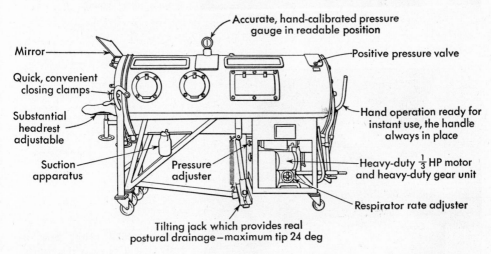

Figure 181.   Diagram of a tank respirator. (Courtesy of Emerson Co., Cambridge, Mass.)

A team of at least four persons is needed to move the patient in a supine position to the respirator either by the hand-carry method or the use of a lifting sheet. After the patient has been placed on the respirator cot, his neck is protected with soft material such as cotton flannel, a strip of sponge rubber in stockinette, or several layers of sheet wadding, and then his head is passed through the collar. One nurse stands at the head of the respirator and protects the patient's nose and mouth with her hand as she guides his head through the collar,† unless it is the type shown in Figure 183 which can be opened wide. The collar is immediately adjusted, and the body of the respirator moved into place and locked. All locks should be fastened securely, and all armports inspected to make sure there is no leakage which would decrease the efficiency of the apparatus. The degree of negative pressure and rate of respiration are determined by the physician who adjusts the pressure dial. He informs the nurse whether the patient is to have negative pressure

* In many hospitals, the engineer is also present when a patient is to be placed in a respirator.

† This is particularly important when a sponge rubber collar is used.

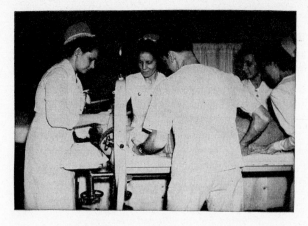

Figure 182A. A patient being placed in a respirator. His body is *lifted,* not pulled up. It requires at least four people to assist in getting the patient's head through a sponge-rubber collar.

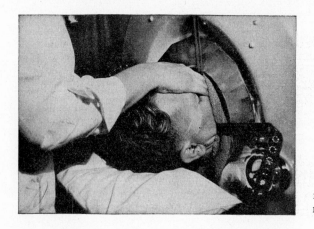

Figure 182B. Note how the nurse's hand protects the patient's nose.

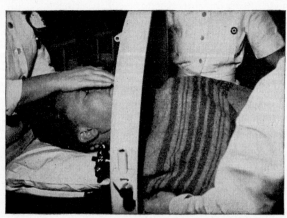

Figure 182C. The headrest is adjusted so that the patient's head is in a good position (parallel). The patient is covered with a light-weight blanket.

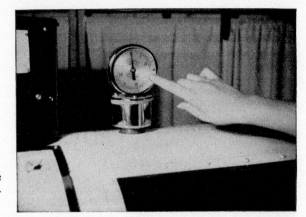

Figure 182D. Pressure gauge on a respirator is checked frequently.

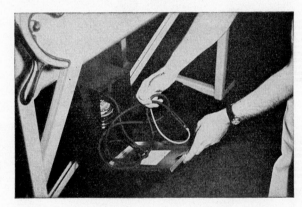

Figure 182E. Suction apparatus is an essential part of a respirator's equipment. Patients in respirators may need to be suctioned frequently. Such aspiration is done only when the patient exhales.

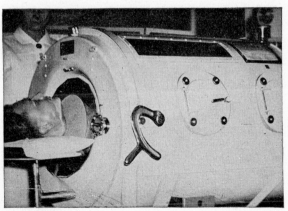

Figure 182F. Patient in a respirator that has been properly adjusted.

(Figs. 182 A-F, courtesy of Bellevue Hospital, New York City, and Clay-Adams Co., New York City.)

only or a combination of negative and positive pressure (see p. 794). In the meantime the nurse at the head of the respirator adjusts the headrest and teaches the patient to breathe with the machine. When the collar moves in, the nurse says the word "inhale," and when the collar moves out, "exhale." The patient must be taught to speak and swallow sips of liquid on expiration only. Throughout this early period as well as later on, the patient's color and rate of respiration are carefully observed.

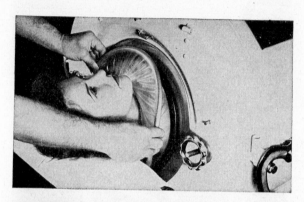
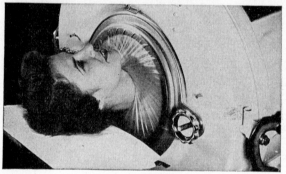

Figure 183. A plastic collar for a respirator. (*Top*) Collar being closed by rotation of the outer ring. (*Bottom*) A properly adjusted collar that remains taut and resists in-and-out motion. Collar is nonirritating to skin of patient's neck; therefore, no stockinette or sheet wadding indicated. (Courtesy of Emerson Co., Cambridge, Mass.)

Figure 184 illustrates an adult model respirator with a positive-pressure dome; Figure 181, the structure of a respirator. The metal chamber opens at one end to admit the patient and the cot. A support outside the respirator is provided for the head. To prevent entrance of air into the chamber during the low-pressure (e.g., negative) phase of the cycle, the patient's neck is encircled with a collar that fits snugly. Observation windows in the sides enable the physician and nurse to see the body of the patient within the chamber. Openings of several sizes along the sides make it possible for attendants to reach any part of the body to give treatments and nursing care. Round openings provided with doors are equipped with sponge-rubber cuffs that fit closely to the arm to keep air from rushing in around the nurse's or doctor's arm during the periods of reduced (e.g., negative) pressure within the chamber; the larger opening for the bedpan has a door but no cuff.

The action of a respirator is based on the physical principle that air pressure within the body tends to equalize with the pressure of the external air around it. Pressure within the normal human body is approximately the same as the atmospheric pressure surrounding it. When the person is in a respirator, the body is subjected to periods when it is surrounded by an atmosphere of reduced (e.g., negative) pressure at regular intervals. Equalization of pressures can only occur if air is drawn into the body or into the chamber. When a tank respirator's diaphragm moves out, pressure within the cylinder becomes less than the atmospheric pressure

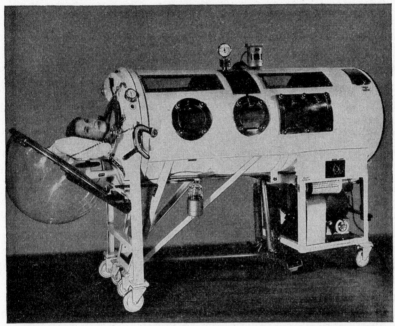

Figure 184. Body respirator equipped with a positive-pressure dome. (Courtesy of Emerson Co., Cambridge, Mass.)

outside.* Since the head is outside, and subjected to atmospheric pressure, this pressure, being greater than that inside the chamber, forces air into the lungs through the nose and mouth (or tracheotomy tube), simulating the physiological act of inspiration. When the diaphragm moves outward (ascends), air pressure within the cylinder then returns to atmospheric pressure, and air is forced out of the lungs because there is an elastic recoil of the lungs. If the patient needs more assistance in the act of expiration, the respirator may be adjusted to provide a positive pressure which is greater than that of the atmosphere and which follows the period of reduced (e.g., negative) pressure. Usually in the early stages the rate is set to correspond with the patient's respiratory rate. Later, when the patient is less toxic and less apprehensive, the respiratory rate per minute may be reduced.

To summarize the action of the respirator: The phase of lowered (e.g., negative)

* This is true of an Emerson tank respirator. Outward motion of its diaphragm, however, corresponds in its effect to downward motion of the bellows on a Collins respirator, for example.

pressure expands the lungs somewhat as subatmospheric pressure in the pleural cavity expands them in normal respiration, and the following period of atmospheric pressure allows the recoil of the lungs to occur as in normal expiration.

Recently, however, experimental evidence indicates that under some circumstances a combination of negative and positive pressure is more beneficial than negative pressure alone. James V. Maloney, Jr., and James L. Whittenberger in 1951 wrote as follows:

> . . . evidence . . . to demonstrate that respiration produced by decreasing the pressure around the body (as in the body respirator), is physiologically and mechanically the same as respiration produced by increasing the pressure in the upper airway (as by a pressure dome over the head). The circulatory depression produced by the body respirator in the presence of a failing circulation may be profound; this effect can be minimized or averted by addition of a positive phase within the respirator.*

They suggest that when such circulatory depression is present, a pressure range of -10 cm to $+10$ cm of water may be indicated instead of a pressure range of -20 cm to 0 cm of water because the former pressure range is considered to have a less deleterious effect on a failing circulation.

Therapeutic Uses.   A condition that is characterized by a temporary paralysis, or exhaustion, of the respiratory muscles is an indication for the use of a respirator. Poliomyelitis (infantile paralysis) is the most common cause of this condition and is the disease in which respirators are most often used. If available, they are occasionally used in resuscitation of the newborn and in the treatment of persons poisoned by morphine, carbon monoxide, or any drug causing respiratory failure.

The early signs of a developing anoxia include headache, increased pulse rate, restlessness, and anxiety. It is important to see that the patient is placed in a respirator without delay. Subsequently an effort is made to maintain a free airway and remove mucus by suction if indicated. The nurse must watch the rate of the respirator, for while adequate ventilation is important and must be maintained, hyperventilation is to be avoided. To aid in drainage, the respirator chamber that is mounted on a frame can be tilted; this enables the physician to employ postural drainage and artificial respiration at the same time. The Trendelenburg position must not be maintained for too long a period, however. When a patient has poliomyelitis, constant use of this position should be avoided as the weight of the abdominal viscera against the diaphragm might further embarrass respiration and reduce cardiac output.

Operation of a Respirator.   Of special importance in the successful operation of a respirator are the determination and maintenance of a respiratory rate that permits adequate ventilation of the lungs. In short-term artificial respiration, oxygenation of the patient's arterial blood is of primary concern. However, when artificial respiration must be carried out over longer periods, removal of carbon dioxide from the blood becomes as important as arterial oxygenation. Since arterial carbon dioxide pressure (pCO_2) is sensitive to slight changes in lung ventilation, the

* Maloney, James V., Jr., and Whittenberger, James L.: "Clinical Implications of Pressures Used in the Body Respirator," *Am. J. M. Sc.*, **221**:425, (Apr.) 1951.

amount of carbon dioxide to be removed will be a determining factor in establishing adequate ventilation by means of the respiratory rate for which the mechanism is set.[23]

It is obvious that the respiratory movements of the patient (feeble though they may be) should be synchronous with the chest movement induced by pressure changes within the chamber. Earlier respirators had only two or three respiratory rates at which the mechanism could be set; later models can be operated at any rate. E. Smith[24] has said that the normal respiratory rate of the patient should be used. When this is done, it does not take very long to synchronize the action of the respirator and the respirations of the patient. The rate used for infants is around 45 per minute; that for adults, 15 to 20 per minute.

According to the authority just quoted, the amount of negative pressure within the chamber must be adjusted to the patient. It is recommended that a negative pressure of not more than 10 cm of water pressure be used at the beginning of the treatment for children under 10 years of age. The pressure may be increased 1 cm every three or four days until a maximum pressure of 15 cm is reached. A pressure of 15 cm of water pressure is usually employed for adults.

Air passages should be free from mucus when the patient is placed in the respirator. Aspiration of the nose and mouth may be indicated preceding and sometimes immediately after starting the treatment. Talking or swallowing during the reduced (e.g., negative) pressure phase of artificial respiration (inspiration) is likely to cause insufflation of the material in the mouth. For this reason it may be necessary to feed the patient by infusion until he learns to swallow during expiration. In addition to suction apparatus, oxygen equipment and a tracheotomy set should also be near at hand, for immediate use.

Should the motor of the respirator stop, the nurse pushes down on the emergency handle (at the foot of the respirator) and operates the diaphragm by means of this handle. At the same time, the nurse in charge is notified of the emergency, and she calls the physician and hospital engineer at once.

Nursing care must, of course, be adapted to the particular needs of the patient. The initial fear of the machine, the restriction of motion, and later the anxiety over removal from the respirator all present psychological problems. The chief physical and mechanical problems are care of the skin to prevent pressure sores, special care of the neck, feeding in such a manner as to avoid insufflation of food, the necessity of frequent change of position to avoid hypostatic pneumonia, and the mastery of the operation of the respirator. The nurse must be able to regulate the rate of respiration, the pressure and temperature within the chamber, and to give necessary nursing care without interruption of respiration. As mentioned earlier, facilities for the administration of oxygen should be in readiness throughout the duration of the treatment. A mouth gag, a tongue clamp, and an airway should be part of the bedside equipment as well as suction apparatus and a tracheotomy set.

While the patient is in the respirator, and this period may extend over months (in rare cases over years), his attention should be diverted to minimize the depressing effect of enforced inactivity. Placement of a mirror above the patient's head enables him to see persons entering the room and to see the nurse should she not be in direct line of vision. The confidence of the nurse and doctor, who should always be present when the patient is taken from the respirator for the first time, will do a great deal toward reassuring him. The patient is never removed from the cabinet until he realizes that he can breathe without mechanical assistance. Even so, he should be told that he will be returned to the cabinet if he experiences any difficulty.

Throughout the treatment frequent change of position is encouraged. This necessitates rearranging pillows and pads, and it is extremely desirable that two nurses do this to prevent unnecessary interruption of the desired air-pressure changes within the cabinet. Covering the upper half of the mattress with one sheet and the lower half with another makes it easier to change the bedding as it is soiled. These sheets should lap in the center of the bed, and quilted pads or cotton and rubber draw-sheets used to protect the bedding under the buttocks. The entire mattress is first covered with a waterproof fabric.

To prevent pressure sores, small gauze-covered cotton pads are used between all skin surfaces that are likely to rub together. Small cotton or sponge rubber rings (doughnuts) are used under the elbows and heels and occasionally a rubber ring under the hips. The patient is bathed daily and oftener if indicated. Frequent rubbing with lanolin or alcohol is helpful. Special back care is needed for incontinent patients.

Because the fluctuating collar tends to irritate the skin, special neck care is necessary. The area is washed gently with soap and water and dried thoroughly. To do the job quickly, two persons are needed; one holds the head and retracts the collar while the other washes. Powder or ointment is not used because they might cake and cause the protective neckband to rumple. When the neckband is not smooth, the patient is uncomfortable; in addition there is the possibility that air might leak into the chamber.

Lights within the cabinet provide warmth if needed, but a cotton bath blanket is usually kept over the patient. Care must be taken to prevent the air inside the cabinet from becoming uncomfortably warm.

It is necessary for the nurse to feed the patient. She must teach him how to eat easily and safely. The nature and spacing of the feedings depend upon the patient's condition. The attention given to elimination, oral hygiene, and other bodily needs is that demanded in the care of any sick and helpless patient.

The relief experienced by the person who is having respiratory difficulty when he is placed in the respirator makes him more than willing to accept the treatment; his improvement often seems miraculous. It must not be assumed, however, that the critical state is passed until the cause of abnormal respiration is removed.

Since each respirator is equipped with detailed directions for its operation, it seems unnecessary to give the procedure in detail here. Respirators operate on the same principles but differ slightly in their construction. The directions of the manufacturer must be followed carefully to get satisfactory results.

A recent development is the *plastic dome*[25] which can be attached to the head of the respirator (see Fig. 184). The dome is a positive-pressure attachment of transparent material shaped in a hemisphere. When it has been locked onto the head of the respirator, the respirator may be kept open for short periods. A valve on the inside of the respirator controls the amount of positive pressure within the dome. Patients vary in their tolerance of the positive-pressure dome. The first time it is used should be a demonstration period only so that the patient will be assured that he can breathe as easily in the dome as in the respirator. After the patient's

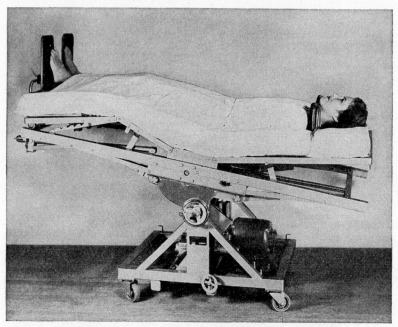

Figure 185. An oscillating bed. Note supports for shoulders and feet. (Courtesy of Emerson Co., Cambridge, Mass.)

confidence in the equipment has been built up, he will then be able to stay out of the respirator for periods of varying length. When the patient is in the dome and the respirator open, baths, physical therapy, and treatments such as catheterization can be carried out more quickly, with better technique, and with less discomfort to the patient.

When not in use, the dome may be suspended upon the frame of the respirator where it will be readily available but out of the way.

Charting. When a patient is in a respirator, charting is especially important. The nurse observes respiratory rate and temporal pulse carefully and keeps a record of the vital signs as ordered by the physician. Any deviation from normal is reported immediately. She observes and charts the attitude and mental outlook of the patient, as well as his ability to speak without effort, ability to take liquids by mouth, time at which treatments and medications were given and any untoward reaction, whether he breathes easily with the respirator or tries to "fight" it, presence of mucus and frequency of suctioning, and whether he gets sufficient rest and sleep.

The physician decides the proper time for the *termination* of the treatment. Because many patients usually become psychologically dependent on the respirator,

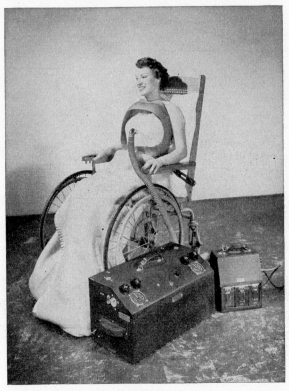

Figure 186A. A chest-type portable respirator. (Courtesy of J. J. Monaghan Co., Denver, Colo.)

the transition period requires careful supervision. The nurse can instill confidence in the patient and help him believe that he can breathe easily and adequately without mechanical help. A beginning step might be the opening of portholes regularly a few times a day. Later on, after the patient has shown his tolerance of this step, he may be wheeled out of the respirator for a period of 15 to 20 minutes; however, the respirator motor should not be shut off. Knowing that he can be returned to the respirator immediately, the patient may make a greater effort to stay out for a longer period. The patient's head is not removed from the collar until he can breathe without the respirator for approximately one hour. By the time the patient can remain out of the respirator for a period of at least two hours, it is usually safe to transfer him to a bed for gradually lengthening periods. This last step will do much to increase the patient's confidence and improve his morale. *However, the patient should not be left alone until the physician feels he has acquired sufficient self-confidence in his ability to breathe normally.*[26]

As the condition of the patient improves, one of several mechanical aids to respiration may be utilized. These include : (1) the *chest-abdomen respirator* which

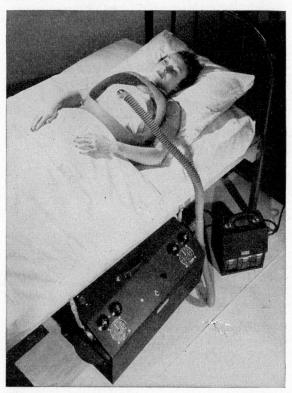

Figure 186B. A chest respirator is also used for a bed patient. (Courtesy of J. J. Monaghan Co., Denver, Colo.)

facilitates care of the patient and permits treatments to be carried out more easily, (2) the *chest respirator* which is useful for the patient in a chair, and (3) the *rocking bed*. Any of the above pieces of equipment can be used during the transition period; the physician will indicate which method is best suited for an individual patient. Selection will be determined by the patient's general condition and by the degree of impairment of accessory respiratory muscles.

The chest-abdomen and chest respirators operate on the same principles as a cylinder respirator.

The Respir-aid rocking bed[27] can be adjusted to rock 12 to 40 times a minute, and the degree of movement can be increased as indicated up to 45 degrees.

During operation when the head of the bed moves upward, the abdominal viscera shift downward, thus encouraging movement of the diaphragm and drawing air into the lungs, favoring inhalation. When the head of the bed moves downward, the viscera shift up toward the diaphragm, helping expiration. The nurse must instruct

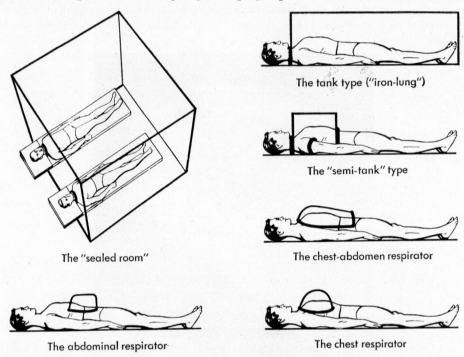

The tank type ("iron-lung")

The "semi-tank" type

The chest-abdomen respirator

The "sealed room"

The abdominal respirator

The chest respirator

Figure 187. Some external-pressure respiratory devices. (*Left, top*) The "*sealed room.*" The patient's head extends through an opening in the wall, sealed off by a collar at his neck. The atmosphere within the room is evacuated at a normal breathing rhythm. (*Left, bottom*) The *abdominal respirator.* A shell whose coverage is restricted to the abdominal area of the body. Air seal is maintained by flexible sheeting wrapped around the patient, or by straps.

(*Right, top to bottom*) The *tank type* ("*iron lung*"). Here a mobile tank is substituted for the sealed room. The principle is identical. The "*semi-tank*" type. The chest is sealed off from the rest of the body by airtight sleeves. The *chest-abdomen respirator.* A cuirass which covers not only the chest but the abdomen as well. The seal is maintained by a soft sponge-rubber cushion which conforms to the body contours. The *chest respirator.* A domed shell covering the anterior rib cage of the patient. It is rimmed with a continuous rubber gasket which becomes an air seal when the shell is strapped to the patient. (Courtesy of Conitech, Ltd., New York City.)

the patient to inhale as the head of the bed rises, and to exhale when the head of the bed has been lowered. The circulation is also benefited.

Rocking beds and partial body respirators are very useful in helping the patient become acclimated to being outside a cylinder respirator. Such special equipment not only gives the patient the feeling of security he needs, but also makes him feel less restricted.

REFERENCES

1. Goodman, Louis S., and Gilman, Alfred: *The Pharmacological Basis of Therapeutics,* 2nd ed. The Macmillan Company, New York, 1955, p. 905.
2. Ivy, Andrew C.: "The Physiology of Respiratory Diseases," *West Virginia M. J.,* **43:**71, (Feb.) 1947.
3. Barach, Alvan L., et al.: *Physiology of Anoxia.* Linde Air Products Co., New York, 1943, p. 24.
4. Goodman, Louis S., and Gilman, Alfred: *op. cit.,* pp. 906-7.
5. Livingstone, Huberta M.: "Oxygen as Therapy," *Am. J. Nursing,* **48:**17, (Jan.) 1948.
6. Guedel, Arthur E.: *Inhalation Anesthesia,* 2nd ed. The Macmillan Company, New York, 1951, pp. 113-14.
7. Armstrong, Harry G.: *Principles and Practice of Aviation Medicine.* Williams & Wilkins Co., Baltimore, 1952, p. 228.
8. Andrews, Albert H., Jr.: *Manual of Oxygen Therapy Techniques,* 2nd ed. Year Book Publishers, Chicago, 1947, p. 17.
9. Patz, A.; Hoeck, L. E.; and de la Cruz, E.: "Studies on the Effect of High Oxygen Administered in Retrolental Fibroplasia. I. Nursery Observations," *Am. J. Ophthal.,* **35:**1248, (Sept.) 1952. Patz, A.; Eastham, Ann; Higgenbotham, D. H.; and Kleh, Thomas: "Oxygen Studies in Retrolental Fibroplasia. II. The Production of Microscopic Changes in Retrolental Fibroplasia in Experimental Animals," *Am. J. Ophthal.,* **36:**1511, (Nov.) 1953.
10. Andrews, Albert H., Jr.: *op. cit.,* p. 51.
11. Goodman, Louis S., and Gilman, Alfred: *op. cit.,* p. 918.
12. *Oxygen Therapy Handbook,* 3rd ed. Linde Air Products Co., New York, 1953, pp. 29–33.
13. Taran, Leo M., and Szilagyi, Nelly: "Oxygen Therapy in Acute Rheumatic Carditis in Children," *Am. J. Med.,* **5:**379-91, 1948; and "Effect of Oxygen Therapy on the Electrical Sequence of Events in the Cardiac Cycle in Children with Acute Rheumatic Carditis," *Am. J. Med.,* **5:**392-401, 1948.
14. Goodman, Louis S., and Gilman, Alfred: *op cit.,* p. 923.
15. Barach, Alvan L., and Swenson, P.: "Effect of Breathing Gases under Positive Pressure on Lumens of Small and Medium Sized Bronchi," *Arch. Int. Med.,* **63:**946, (May) 1939.
16. Blumgarten, A. S.: *Textbook of Materia Medica, Pharmacology and Therapeutics,* 7th ed. The Macmillan Company, New York, 1937, p. 297.
17. Blumgarten, A. S.: *op. cit.,* p. 297.
18. Goodman, Louis S., and Gilman, Alfred: *op. cit.,* p. 917.
19. Goodman, Louis S., and Gilman, Alfred: *op. cit.,* p. 224.
20. Blumgarten, A. S.: *op. cit.,* p. 297.
21. Goodman, Louis S., and Gilman, Alfred: *op. cit.,* p. 921.
22. Goodman, Louis S., and Gilman, Alfred: *op. cit.,* p. 921.
23. Radford, Edward P.; Ferris, Benjamin G., Jr.; and Kriete, Bertrand C.: "Clinical Use of a Nomogram to Estimate Proper Ventilation during Artificial Respiration," *New England J. Med.,* **251:**877, (Nov. 25) 1954.
24. Smith, E.: "Respiratory Failure and the Drinker Respirator in Poliomyelitis," *J.A.M.A.,* **100:**1666, (May) 1933.
25. Steigman, Alex J., and Rumph, Pauline H.: "The Positive-Pressure Respirator Dome," *Am. J. Nursing,* **52:**311, (Mar.) 1952.
26. Parisi, Carmela Di Piano: "The Patient in a Respirator," *Am. J. Nursing,* **51:**360, (June) 1950.
27. Wright, Jesse: "The Respir-aid Rocking Bed in Poliomyelitis," *Am. J. Nursing,* **47:**454, (July) 1947.

Additional Suggested Reading

Barach, Alvan L.: *Physiologic Therapy in Respiratory Diseases,* 2nd ed. J. B. Lippincott Co., Philadelphia, 1948.

Comroe, Julius H., and Dripps, R. D.: *The Physiological Basis for Oxygen Therapy.* Charles C Thomas, Publisher, Springfield, Ill., 1950.

Dillon, John B.: "Oxygen Therapy," *California Med.,* **76:**264, (Apr.) 1952.

Galloway, Thomas C.: *Treatment of Respiratory Emergencies including Bulbar Poliomyelitis.* Charles C Thomas, Publisher, Springfield, Ill., 1953.

Gray, John S.: *Pulmonary Ventilation and Its Physiological Regulation.* Charles C Thomas, Publisher, Springfield, Ill., 1950.

Livingstone, Huberta M.: "Safety Measures in Oxygen Therapy," *Hosp. Management,* **70:**46-48, (Sept.) 1950.

Moon, V. H.: "Symposium on Inhalation Therapy, The Origins and Effects of Anoxia," *Bull. New York Acad. Med.,* **26:**361-70, (June) 1950.

Nale, Thomas W.: "The Therapeutic Use of Oxygen in Industrial Medicine," *Indust. Med.,* **21:** 179-82, (Apr.) 1952.

Russek, H. I., et al.: "One Hundred Per Cent Oxygen in the Treatment of Acute Myocardial Infarction and Severe Angina Pectoris," *J.A.M.A.,* **144:**373-75, (Sept.) 1950.

Trovell, R. M., and Hellijas, C. S.: "Pipelines: Aid to Oxygen Therapy," *Anesth. & Analg.,* **31:**19, (Jan.) 1952.

West, Harold E.: "Treatment of Poliomyelitis with Involvement of the Respiratory System," *California Med.,* **73:**397, (Nov.) 1950.

CHAPTER 28. ASPIRATIONS AND INCISIONS OF BODY CAVITIES

1. GENERAL PRINCIPLES UNDERLYING SELECTION OF METHOD

Conditions Requiring Aspiration and Incision: General Purpose. In certain diseases, fluid collects in body cavities and tissues. This excess fluid may result from local inflammation or from an abnormal condition of a remote organ or organs. When a serous membrane, such as that covering the brain or the lungs or lining the abdominal cavity, is inflamed it secrets an abnormal amount. This fluid is nature's means of bathing and separating the affected tissues. It also protects the affected organs with a water cushion. When excessive fluid forms in the cranial, chest, or abdominal cavities, it exerts pressure on vital organs. This always causes discomfort or pain and menaces the function of the affected parts.

Fluid may collect in body cavities and tissues as a result of disease of the circulatory or excretory systems. In these cases drugs, such as meralluride sodium solution (Mercuhydrin), may be given intramuscularly to speed up elimination by the kidneys, although aspiration (removal of the fluid through a hollow needle or other instrument) may be used in conjunction with the diuretic. Aspirations not only relieve pressure caused by the fluid accumulation but also enable the physician to examine the fluid and make a more accurate diagnosis.

Classification and Character of Fluid Collected in Body Cavities. For clinical purposes the fluid is classified as an *exudate* (a fluid produced by the lining of the cavity) or a *transudate* (a fluid that escapes from the blood and lymph vessels and collects in the cavity). An exudate, occurring as a result of inflammation, may be serous (watery) or it may be purulent if suppuration has developed. It usually has a high specific gravity, contains white blood cells, and, in many cases, microorganisms. The meningococcus, streptococcus, pneumococcus, staphylococcus, and tubercle bacillus are among those infecting serous cavities. An exudate may also contain fibrin or blood. In malignancies, necrotic tissue may be present. A transudate has much the same character as blood serum; it is pale yellow or greenish yellow, is alkaline in reaction, and has a low specific gravity. The amount of protein is low, and blood cells are few in comparison with those in an exudate; there are no bacteria in the fluid. Salts, glucose, and urea are found as in plasma.[1]

Methods of Drainage or Suction Employed. Fluid may be drained through an incision if pressure on the organ or tissue is sufficient to cause drainage, or if gravity favors it. If an incision is likely to prove either ineffective or dangerous, a hollow needle, or cannula, is introduced, and suction applied by means of a syringe, vacuum bottle, or motor-driven suction pump. There are various ways of producing subatmospheric pressure (suction), but the underlying principle is the same. Air may be sucked out of a bottle or a tube, in order to create a partial vacuum, with a hand pump, a pump operated by an electric motor, or with running water.

Regulation and Measurement of Suction. As explained in Chapter 29, a vacuum is a void—theoretically, a space in which there is nothing. That "nature abhors a vacuum" is a well-known axiom of physics, and the consequence is that a complete vacuum does not exist, because an airtight chamber is difficult to construct and atmospheric pressure forces air through the smallest opening. A partial vacuum is, however, easily created and occurs whenever part of the air is forced out of a bottle or cavity so that the remaining air is rarefied, expanded, or under less than atmospheric pressure. In any vacuum system it is essential that connections between tubing and needles, manometers, bottles, and syringes are tight. Admission of air at the wrong time and place destroys the vacuum. Operation of the apparatus must be mastered before the treatment is started.[2]

In order to measure the power of a vacuum, a water, mercury, or spring manometer may be attached to the vacuum chamber. Some physicians believe that whenever suction is applied to a body cavity, its force, or pull, should be estimated. At present, this practice is uncommon except in the case of an instrument used to collapse the lung; such apparatus is equipped with a manometer that registers positive and negative pressures. Thus the physician is able to measure the pressure within the pleural cavity and that applied to produce a pneumothorax (collapse of the lung).[3]

In aspirating fluid from any body cavity, it is possible to measure the positive pressure the fluid is under in this cavity by attaching to the needle a perpendicular glass tube with a special adapter. The height to which the fluid rises indicates the pressure—the higher the fluid, the greater the pressure.

Importance of Asepsis. Cavities or tissues that require aspiration or incision are obviously those having no opening to the outside air. (Such cavities as open on the surface of the body may be drained through tubes inserted into these openings.) Nature has not provided closed cavities with the immunity to infection that exists in the mucous-lined cavities, and a more rigid asepsis is therefore required. Preparation of the skin area to be punctured or incised and preparation of equipment must follow the rules laid down in Chapter 7 for all surgical procedures. The skin is prepared by cleaning and by the application of an antiseptic; dressings and instruments should be sterilized by steam under pressure. It is desirable to sterilize the skin-cleaning equipment in a separate covered tray so that the nurse may handle these articles without contaminating instruments prepared for the surgeon. The nurse is often asked to prepare the skin while the doctor is scrubbing or preparing the local anesthetic.

Reducing the Danger of Trauma. A puncture or incision inevitably injures the tissues. A wound is made that nature must heal. The physician and nurse should try to reduce the amount of trauma to a minimum. Voluntary and involuntary movements of the patient during the procedure usually may be prevented by a thorough and appropriate explanation; he should be supported in a comfortable position; the possibility of striking a bone should be reduced by selecting the proper site of injection; and, above all, needles and scalpels should be sharp and of the right size.

Preparing the Patient. To patients and their families, aspirations are minor operations, and it is not unusual to see marked anxiety or even terror expressed in word or manner. An explanation from the physician is most reassuring, but the nurse should supplement this as she senses the need. Terms should be used that the patient can understand, and diagrams may be helpful.* Only in rare cases should treatments such as this be given without the patient's understanding. His cooperation is often essential to the success of an aspiration if he is conscious, and psychologically it is traumatic to have such an experience under duress. In some hospitals, patients are asked to sign permits; parents and guardians sign such forms for children and mental incompetents. A sedative given at the proper time may help the patient to stand the treatment much more easily. One authority recommends amobarbital (sodium Amytal) by mouth.

2. THORACIC, OR CHEST, ASPIRATION

Definition. A chest aspiration or thoracentesis is the withdrawal of fluid from the pleural cavity.

Therapeutic Uses. Aspiration is indicated if an accumulation of fluid causes pain, dyspnea, and other symptoms of pressure. A transudate may form as a result

---

* There was a case in which a patient sued a highly reputable hospital for damages. In court he testified that the nurse came in with a tray of instruments and told him he was going to have something done to him (he didn't know exactly what she said); then she turned him to the wall, tied his hands and feet, the doctor came in and hit him in the back, and he, the patient, hadn't been the same since. Any of us can recognize in this account a **failure** on the part of the medical worker to interpret a lumbar puncture in the patient's terms.

of heart, kidney, or vascular disease; an exudate is nearly always caused by tubercular pleurisy. Pleural infections, however, can be associated with infections of the lung, or secondary infections in other parts of the body, for example, the meninges. In such cases the microorganisms found in the fluid may be the pneumococcus, streptococcus, or meningococcus. If the effusion is purulent in nature, the patient is said to have empyema, and it becomes impossible to drain the cavity adequately through a needle. Fluid may collect in the pleural cavity as a result of malignant growths in the chest that press on blood vessels.

Pleural fluid is often removed for diagnostic purposes; that is, to discover the causative organism in pleurisy. For this purpose it is not necessary to collect a large quantity, and no attempt is made to do so unless the fluid is causing discomfort.

Equipment. The articles required are a rubber sheet to protect the bedding, towels or soft paper to cover the rubber, sterile draping materials (convenient, but not necessary); sterile cotton and skin disinfectants; a sterile hypodermic needle and syringe with ½ or 1 per cent procaine (Novocaine) for local anesthesia; sterile gloves and powder for the doctor; sterile dressings; and the aspirating set. When a motor-driven suctioning device is not available, a hand-operated apparatus is substituted. The later consists of a calibrated glass bottle having a rubber stopper in which there is a metal tube with two branches, each provided with stopcocks. To each branch is fitted rubber tubing with metal ends or adapters. The sterile aspirating needle fits the metal end of one piece of tubing, and through the other end air may be exhausted from the bottle with an exhaust pump, leaving a vacuum in the bottle into which the chest fluid will readily flow. Such equipment is known as a *Potain aspirating set.* Commercial sets are most satisfactory because the connections are usually airtight. If a Potain set is not available, adequate negative pressure may be created in a syringe. This is troublesome to use, however, because the amount of fluid removed is often larger than the capacity of the syringe, and air may enter the pleural cavity while detaching, emptying, and readjusting it. A suction apparatus must be used to collect fluid from the pleural cavity, because a subatmospheric pressure exists there and the fluid will not flow out by gravity. This low pressure is caused by the elasticity of the lung tissue and the resistance it offers to the elevated ribs and lung expansion. The downward pull of the elastic lung makes the atmospheric pressure greater than the pressure in the thoracic cavity, and fluid cannot run out by gravity until the external pressure in the bottle or syringe is less than the internal thoracic pressure.

When the air is exhausted from the bottle, both stopcocks must be closed; the apparatus having been tested on starting to ensure that the chest fluid will flow into the bottle. To test the apparatus place the tubing to be attached to the aspirating needle in a glass of water and open the stopcock of that branch only; if the water runs into the bottle readily, the chest fluid also will run into it when the needle is inserted into the pleural cavity and attached to the tubing.

Needles of different sizes should be provided. The bevels in all cases should be short to avoid pricking the lung, but the bores should vary so that a small needle is ready in case the exudate is of a serous nature or a large one for a purulent exudate. A 5-cm (2-in.) 20-gauge needle is recommended by A. J. Cohen[4] for a pneumothorax where only air is carried.

Preparation of the Patient. As in all treatments, the patient's mental and physical welfare should be considered throughout. To lessen the danger of shock, fainting, or fatigue it is wise to have him lie on his side in a semirecumbent position, and on the side of the bed most convenient for the doctor. Morris Braverman[5] urges that the recumbent be substituted for the sitting position. A small pillow or pad under the thorax arches the vertebrae laterally and widens the intercostal spaces; this helps to avoid the ribs in making the puncture. The arm of the

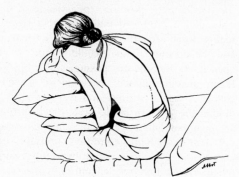

Figure 188. Sitting position for a patient about to have a thoracentesis. Note pillows used to support patient during treatment and covering provided.

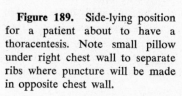
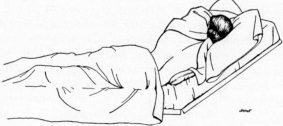

Figure 189. Side-lying position for a patient about to have a thoracentesis. Note small pillow under right chest wall to separate ribs where puncture will be made in opposite chest wall.

affected side may be held above the head or forward with the hand on the opposite shoulder. The position should be comfortable. The treatment may be given with the paient sitting on the side of the bed, his feet resting on a stool, and his arms on a pillow laid over the back of a chair. Sometimes the patient leans forward on a bed tray or table. He should be warmly clad to prevent chilling and to lessen the danger of shock. There should be no more than the necessary exposure.

The lungs do not completely fill the pleural sac, so that at the anterior and inferior borders sinuses are formed. Pathological fluids first collect in the interior or costophrenic sinus, but may collect also in the interlobular spaces. The physician always selects the site of insertion of the needle. He may clean and disinfect the skin, or the nurse may do it. In either case forceps are used to handle the sponges. If sterile drapery is used, the physician usually adjusts it after he has scrubbed his hands or put on sterile rubber gloves.

Suggested Procedure. The physician first anesthetizes the site of injection with ½ to 1 per cent procaine or similar drug and then inserts the needle in the skin area under which he believes the fluid to have collected. The site of puncture is determined by the chest sounds on examination that indicate the location of excess serum or pus.[6] The needle is injected midway between the ribs to avoid the intercostal blood vessels and during inspiration when the spaces are wider. Either the doctor or the nurse must instruct the patient not to move or cough while the needle is in the chest wall. If coughing is unavoidable, the physician may withdraw the needle temporarily. An adapter (a three-way stopcock) must be attached to the needle, so that entrance of air through the needle into the pleural cavity can be prevented by closing the stopcock. As soon as the needle is in position, the syringe or tubing from the vacuum bottle is attached. The suction produced pulls the fluid from the cavity. The stopcock to the pump remains closed after the treatment is started (unless it is necessary to renew the vacuum), and the opening to the needle should be closed until the physician asks the nurse to open it. As soon as this passageway is opened, fluid should flow into the vacuum bottle. If an uncontaminated specimen is needed for laboratory study, the physician may collect it with a syringe and transfer it to a small, wide-mouthed, covered bottle. Although the vacuum bottle is sterilized in preparation for the treatment, it is hard to get an uncontaminated specimen from this large container.

Watch the patient's condition carefully; throughout the treatment note his color, pulse, and breathing. Sudden withdrawal of pressure on the chest organs may cause fainting, or a hemorrhage may result from puncture of a blood vessel, or the lung may collapse as a result of being pricked.

On the withdrawal of the needle the physician applies a sterile dressing. After the treatment the patient rests for a prescribed period according to his condition. The sputum should be watched for the presence of blood, suggesting injury to lung tissue.

The bottle containing the fluid must be labeled with the date, patient's name, clinical division, nature of the fluid, and the purpose for which it is to be examined. If so desired by the physician, it should be sent immediately to the laboratory to be examined for specific gravity, differential white cell count, the Esbach test, and the specific organisms present. The Esbach test is a quantitative test for albumin, the amount of which indicates the degree of inflammation present.

Recording the Treatment. The amount, color, and type of fluid withdrawn, the time of treatment, coughing, any fatigue, syncope, or untoward symptoms either accompanying or following the procedure, as well as any beneficial effects observed, should be recorded. Note the collection of specimens and the purpose for which they were sent to the laboratory.

3. ARTIFICIAL PNEUMOTHORAX

Definition. _Pneumothorax_ means air in the pleural cavity. An artificial pneumothorax is the introduction of nitrogen gas, or air, into this cavity for the purpose of creating sufficient pressure to collapse and rest the lung. Some authorities believe that nitrogen gas maintains the pressure better than oxygen or air because it is less readily absorbed; others find air equally satisfactory.

Therapeutic Uses. Pneumothorax is used in tuberculosis involving one lung only. It is indicated when an x-ray shows a cavity or a progressive lesion. Complete rest gives the tissues a chance to heal and to check the disease process. There is no discomfort or dyspnea when the uninvolved lung is able to compensate. In some cases the phrenic nerve to one side of the diaphragm is cut (phrenicotomy) instead of performing a pneumothorax. This allows the diaphragm to rise on that side and act as a sort of splint for the lung.

Artificial pneumothorax is contraindicated if the untreated lung cannot take up the work of the collapsed lung and if pleural adhesions prevent the collapse of the lung. With the development of more effective drug therapy this treatment will be less common.

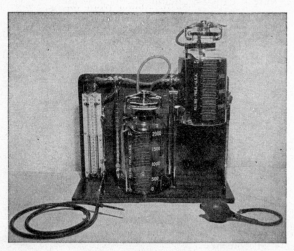

Figure 190. Pneumothorax apparatus. When the bottle with solution (*right*) is lowered, solution flows into the second bottle that contains air; this in turn forces air from the second bottle into the tubing that leads to the sterile needle placed earlier in the patient's chest wall. (After the needle has been inserted, the stylette is removed, and the tip of the needle is in the pleural cavity.) The manometer (*left*) records the pressure. (Courtesy Clay-Adams Co., New York City.)

Suggested Procedure. Strict aseptic measures must be observed. The patient lies on the unaffected side, and the skin—usually in the midaxillary line in the fifth or sixth intercostal space—is disinfected. The aspirating needle is then inserted, moved up and down to be sure it is free and not in lung tissue, and pure nitrogen or air is introduced from a special machine (Robinson or Zavod machines are commonly used) up to a positive pressure of from 40 to 50 mm of mercury. (A water manometer is preferred by some operators because it is more sensitive.) Cohen recommends a 5-cm (2-in.) 20-gauge needle attached to a three-way adapter and a 2-cc glass syringe. The treatment is repeated weekly or biweekly until the lung is gradually and completely collapsed. In most cases the pressure must be maintained over a period of months to enable the tissues to heal. Periods between treatments range from a few days to weeks, depending upon the condition of the lung.

This treatment is usually given in a special clinic, and in each institution the technique is highly developed. To some extent the method depends upon the apparatus

available. For a more detailed description of the procedure, the nurse should refer
to a textbook on chest surgery or the treatment of tuberculosis.

4. LUMBAR PUNCTURE WITH MYELOGRAM OR ENCEPHALOGRAM

Definition. A lumbar puncture is the introduction of a hollow needle into the
subarachnoid space of the spinal canal, usually in the lumbar region, for the purpose
of draining the canal or injecting substances into it. When opaque substances are
injected and x-ray pictures taken, the result is a myelogram; when air or oxygen is
injected, the procedure is called a pneumoencephalogram.

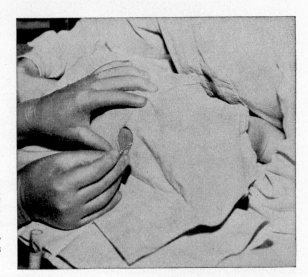

Figure 191. Spinal tap showing
infant draped and held in position
by the nurse. (Courtesy of Bellevue Hospital School of Nursing,
New York City, and Clay-Adams
Co., New York City.)

Therapeutic Uses. The cerebral and spinal subarachnoid spaces and the fluid
contained in them communicate freely with each other through the foramen magnum and with the cavity of the cerebral ventricles through the foramen of
Magendie in the lower part of the roof of the fourth ventricle. The cord is suspended
in cerebrospinal fluid. If the circulation of fluid is unobstructed, pressure of the
fluid varies with breathing, coughing, or abdominal straining. Manual compression on
large veins (jugular pressure usually) produces a rise in the pressure. A stationary
pressure indicates a block. In a relaxed recumbent position the spinal fluid is under
a pressure of 10 to 15 cm of water; 20 to 25 in a sitting position.[7] In disease
the pressure during relaxation may rise markedly. A lumbar puncture as a diagnostic or therapeutic measure depends upon this intercommunication and interchange of fluid and the responses to varying pressures within the body, referred to
as "spinal dynamics."

The subarachnoid space is entered in order to (1) withdraw cerebrospinal fluid
to relieve pressure, (2) secure a specimen of fluid for diagnostic purposes, (3)
inject sera or drugs in the treatment of disease, (4) inject a spinal anesthetic, (5)

introduce an opaque liquid before taking an x-ray for diagnosis of cord and brain lesions, and (6) measure the pressure of the spinal fluid under varying conditions. This last is referred to as the manometric test. The normal rise in spinal-fluid pressure on compression of the internal jugular veins is called "Queckenstedt's sign," because he first described it, hence "Queckenstedt's test."

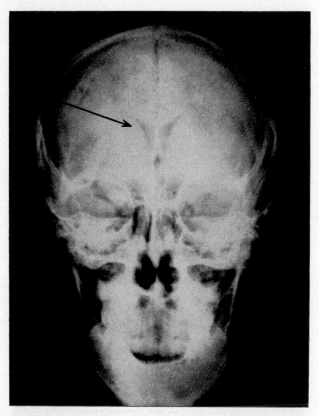

Figure 192A. Anteroposterior encephalogram showing normal size lateral and third ventricles. (Courtesy of Columbia-Presbyterian Medical Center, New York City.)

Removal of excess cerebrospinal fluid is often indicated in hydrocephalus and meningitis. Meningitis caused by the meningococcus and the pneumococcus was once treated by the introduction of sera into the spinal canal. The antibotics are occasionally given in this way. Israel S. Wechsler says that the chemotherapeutic agents are irritants when injected into the spinal canal. He implies that even antibiotics are more satisfactorily given in other ways. Antisyphilitic substances are injected into the meningeal spaces in some forms of neural syphilis, and spinal anesthesia is administered when other types of anesthesia are contraindicated. If a tumor of the brain or spinal cord is suspected, for diagnostic purposes an opaque substance* is injected into the subarachnoid space of the spinal cord, the enlargement of this space at the base of the brain, or into one of the lateral ventricles. A cavity filled with this substance shows up as a dark area on a film. A misplaced or distorted ventricle or an occluded area of the subarachnoid space indicates pressure made by a nearby tumor or lesion. Air is opaque to x-rays and is sometimes used instead of a drug.

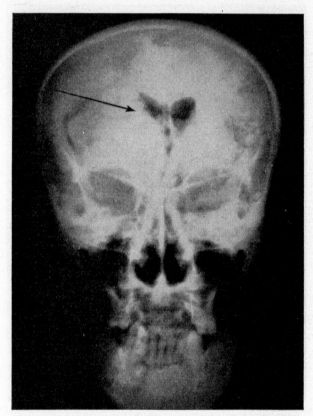

Figure 192B. Anteroposterior encephalogram showing moderate displacement of lateral and third ventricles to left due to a low posterior right frontal tumor. (Courtesy of Columbia-Presbyterian Medical Center, New York City.)

Equipment. Articles required are materials for cleaning and disinfecting the skin; sterile towels or a sterile fenestrated sheet for draping the patient; sterile rubber gloves, a mask, and gown (not universally considered essential) for the doctor; procaine (Novocaine) ½ to 1 per cent, a hypodermic syringe and two needles for administration of the anesthesia; 2 lumbar puncture needles; a water manometer for measuring the pressure of the cerebrospinal fluid; 3 small, sterile,

* Ethyl iodophenylundecylate (Pantopaque) or iodized poppy seed oil (Lipiodol) are drugs commonly used for this purpose.

capped bottles marked 1, 2, and 3 to receive specimens of the fluid; and a sterile dressing to apply to the wound after the removal of the needle. In addition to these items, a rubber square and cotton or paper cover should be provided to protect the lower bedding and a treatment blanket to cover the upper part of the body, unless the room is very warm. If the bed sags, it may be necessary to place a board under the mattress. Any lateral curvature of the spine distorts the intervertebral spaces in such a way as to preclude the introduction of the needle. A pad and pencil are needed to record pressure readings. Sterile handling forceps are a convenience. An alcohol lamp is used by some operators for flaming the mouths of specimen bottles. Drugs to be injected must be added to the equipment as ordered by the doctor.

In selecting needles for the introduction of the local anesthesia, choose one for the superficial tissues about 1¾ cm (¾ in.) and 25 gauge; for a deeper injection of the anesthetic, the surgeon will want a slightly longer and heavier needle. To reach the subarachnoid space, lumbar puncture needles of various sizes are used. Walter F. Dutton and George B. Lake recommend one 7½ cm (3 in.) long, 18 to 20 gauge, with a short bevel and a close-fitting stylet. For babies Wechsler advocates a 5-cm (2-in.) needle. It is desirable in most cases to have the needle equipped with a three-way stopcock. The needle may be attached directly to a syringe or to a manometer by an adapter, but with many types of apparatus it is connected to either of these with rubber tubing about 14 cm (5½ in.) long. This tubing should be the noncollapsible type; unless it is transparent, it should have a glass connecting tube within its length and adapters at each end to make it fit tightly to the needle and the syringe or to the needle and manometer, as the case may be.

Intraspinal medications usually come prepared in ampoules. A water bath at 40° C (104° F) is desirable to warm the liquid in the vial. The temperature of the bath must be carefully controlled because high temperatures may coagulate or change the chemical nature of a drug.

Preparation of the Patient. Explanation to the patient and his family should be made as discussed on page 805. As the patient must remain motionless during the treatment, it is essential to have his cooperation (if he is an older child or an adult). Successful restraint of an infant or small child is possible, but it is extremely difficult to keep an adult quiet by force. If manometric readings are to be made, the procedure must be thoroughly explained. The patient will be asked to strain (as if at stool) and to submit to manual pressure on the jugular veins or to pressure with a blood pressure cuff around the neck. Since the local anesthetic rarely reaches the meninges, pain is almost inevitable as the admission of the needle stretches the dura and pulls on the connective tissues surrounding the vertebrae. It is wise to tell the patient that a certain amount of unavoidable pain is involved; otherwise he may not be braced for it and will move involuntarily as the needle is introduced. His move may injure the spinal nerves or cord.

While the physician is scrubbing his hands, draw the patient to the right side of the bed or table if the operator is right-handed; otherwise to the left. See that a stool is provided for the operator. Have the patient arch his back so that his head is almost touching his knees. (The patient also moves his knees up toward the chest.) If the bed sags, place a board under the mattress to correct the resulting spinal curvature. Cover the body as far as the waist with a treatment blanket, fold the upper bedding down to the separation of the buttocks, and protect the bedclothes under the lumbar region. The skin area to be cleaned and disinfected lies in a line drawn between the crests of the two ilia if a puncture is to be made in the lumbar region. Dutton and Lake suggest painting these points and the skin over the spinous processes of the vertebrae with a disinfectant such as iodine to make it easy for the physician to find the intervertebral space that he wishes to puncture. The fourth lumbar interspace is the one most commonly used, but the spinal canal can be entered at other levels.

After the skin is prepared, it is usual to surround the area with sterile towels or a fenestrated sheet. This simplifies the maintenance of surgical asepsis but is not essential. It is wise for the nurse to ask the physician whether he wishes her to prepare the skin area or whether he prefers to do it himself. If the skin is hairy, it should be shaved; in any case shaving is a desirable precaution.

Wechsler says that the patient may be in a sitting position for this treatment, but in any position the back must be arched to separate the vertebrae; therefore, if a sitting posture is used, a table or chair must be provided for the patient to lean on. Any physical ordeal is more easily borne in the recumbent position; this should be used unless the physician prescribes otherwise.

Suggested Procedure. See that all sterile equipment is available and ready for the physician's use. If the patient is an infant or a child that the nurse must restrain, she will not be able to give the physician any other assistance during the treatment; therefore, everything must be ready for him, or a third member must be added to the team. After scrubbing his hands and putting on gloves, gown, and mask (the gown and mask are often omitted), the doctor introduces the needle. The resistance offered by the ligaments, and lastly by the dura, guides the doctor in making this puncture, which toward the last is made slowly and carefully. As soon as serum starts to drop from the needle, its position in the subarachnoid space is established. If the physician wishes to know the pressure the fluid is under, he attaches the manometer to the needle. He then expels the air by tilting it horizontally. While the patient is in a relaxed horizontal position, the initial reading is made. Then the pressure is read during and after straining and jugular compression. Any specimens desired for laboratory analysis are collected in small, open-mouthed bottles under aseptic conditions. In case a drug or serum is to be administered, an equal amount of spinal fluid is withdrawn before the therapeutic agent is introduced. Dutton and Lake say that a larger amount of spinal fluid should always be removed than is replaced by the drug. This is especially important if the pressure is abnormally high. The amount of serum commonly injected is from 20 to 30 cc (⅔ to 1 oz).

If a pneumoencephalogram or myelogram is to be made, the air or opaque liquid (about 3 cc) is injected, the needle removed, a dressing applied, and the patient with his head elevated on two pillows taken at once to the x-ray department. After the x-ray picture and fluoroscopic examination the opaque material is removed with a second lumbar puncture.

After the removal of fluid and possibly the introduction of some therapeutic substance, the stopcock is closed, the needle withdrawn, and a sterile dressing applied over the wound.

Throughout the procedure the nurse should note very critically the condition of the patient. Withdrawal of fluid from around the brain may cause pressure on vital centers in the medulla. Removal of spinal fluid takes away the water cushion on which the medulla rests and allows it to fall upon the uneven surface of the cranial bones. The introduction of a drug in too large amount may cause respiratory failure and other symptoms of intercranial pressure. If this occurs during the treatment, fluid is allowed to flow back through the needle. Note and call the doctor's attention to any changes in color, pulse, or respiration, and any complaint the patient makes of headache or nausea.

At the termination of the treatment keep the patient in a recumbent position for the time prescribed by the physician. He usually orders an elevation of the foot of the bed, particularly if a drug has been administered, and requires the patient to stay in bed for at least 24 hours in order to re-establish the circulation of the spinal fluid. It is usual for the patient to suffer from headache and backache for several days following a lumbar puncture. Quiet and good care are likely to reduce this discomfort (see also page. 766).

Recording the Treatment.   Note the amount and character of the fluid withdrawn—its color, whether cloudy or bloody—and whether withdrawn by gravity or suction. If blood is present, note whether it is in all three tubes or, as occasionally happens from trauma, merely in the first. Record the kind and amount of any drug injected and whether it was removed in whole or in part. X-rays, if taken, should be recorded. Any discomfort and any signs of the desired beneficial effects should be carefully noted. State whether specimens of fluid were sent to the laboratory for analysis. It is usual to indicate the exact time at which the treatment was given and the name of the physician who administered it.

5. CISTERNAL PUNCTURE

Definition.   A cisternal puncture is the injection of a needle into the cistern magna (an enlargement of the subarachnoid space just below the cerebellum) and is similar in nature to a lumbar puncture except for the area of injection. The lateral ventricle may be aspirated or injected, in which case the procedure is called a *ventricular puncture*; the x-ray picture following the injection of air, a *pneumoventriculogram;* or following the injection of an opaque drug, a *ventriculogram*. All these diagnostic measures are more thoroughly discussed in neurological texts such as Wechsler's or neurological nursing texts such as that by C. G. deGutierrez-Mahoney and Esta Carini.[8]

Therapeutic Uses.   It is desirable to enter the subarachnoid space at the cistern magna instead of the lumbar region (1) in cases of meningitis, as a means of diagnosing spinal block, and to introduce serum if inflammation of the meninges has blocked off areas of the spinal subarachnoid space; (2) as a means of getting a drug into contact with the meningeal spaces around the brain (a lumbar injection, according to some authorities, being rarely successful in so doing); and (3) to inject air or an opaque drug before making an encephalogram to discover the presence and location of brain lesions. (Air also may be injected directly into the lateral ventricles through the cranium. The needle can be introduced through the anterior fontanel of an infant or by way of a trephined opening through the skull of a child or an adult.)

Equipment.   The only difference between the equipment for a lumbar and a cisternal puncture is the use of a slightly different needle. It has a guard about 1 cm (⅜ in.) from the hub, is about 19 gauge, and approximately 7½ cm (3 in.) long, although it can be secured in several lengths. Since the area of insertion is always hairy, a razor is necessary to shave the site of injection. A lumbar puncture may be made at the same time, in which case it is necessary to include equipment for the two injections.

Preparation of the Patient.   With exception of the position, preparation is in general the same as that for lumbar puncture. It is important that the spinous processes of the vertebrae and the occipital protuberance should be in line; therefore the head must rest on a small hard pillow or a sand bag. The patient is told to tilt his head forward, to draw his legs up, and to fold his arms over his chest. The physician inserts the needle between the first and second cervical vertebrae, entering the cranium through the foramen magnum.

Suggested Procedure.   From the standpoint of the nurse there is no difference, after the preparation of the patient and the equipment, between this procedure and that for the lumbar puncture. In preparation for an encephalogram the physician alternately removes fluid and injects air, the amount of air depending upon the size of the ventricles. According to Dutton and Lake, the amount of air required to fill the ventricles varies from 15 cc (½ oz) to 300 cc in cases of hydrocephalus.

6. ASPIRATION OF THE PERICARDIUM

Definition.   The term defines itself; it is the removal of fluid from the pericardial sac surrounding the heart.

Therapeutic Uses.   Fluid is removed from the serous sac surrounding the heart (1) for diagnostic purposes or (2) to relieve intrapericardial pressure.

Normally, only a few cubic centimeters of clear citron-colored fluid are seen in the pericardium on post-mortem examination. In acute pericardial effusion, the parietal layer may be stretched so as to allow 360 cc (12 oz) or more of fluid to accumulate, while in chronic cases where the accumulation has been gradual and the parietal layer has had time to adapt itself, Johnson McGuire in Russell L. Cecil and Robert F. Loeb's text[9] says that 1½ to 2 liters (3 to 4 pt) may collect in the pericardium. A transudate also may collect in the pericardium in heart and kidney disease.

The pericardium is pear-shaped, the base in contact with the diaphragm, the apex above. If the sac is only partly filled, the fluid may shift its position with that of the body, so that when the patient is in the recumbent position, the fluid may extend into the apex, press on the bronchi, and interfere with breathing. If the patient is sitting up, the fluid gravitates to the base of the sac.

If the fluid is excessive, there is pressure on the heart, lungs, bronchi, trachea, and esophagus. This causes dyspnea; a dusky, anxious countenance; a rapid weak pulse; a cough; and dysphagia. The diaphragm, liver, and stomach may be displaced downward. Removal of the fluid in such cases relieves symptoms due to pressure. Successful antibiotic therapy has, however, reduced the necessity for pericardial aspiration.

Equipment.   Articles required for the procedure are the same as in aspiration of the pleural sac except that as the amount of fluid withdrawn is small, the aspirating set and large receptacle for the fluid are rarely required. A large, sterile syringe equipped with a three-way stopcock is ordinarily used to withdraw the fluid and a sterile bottle to receive it.

Preparation of the Patient.   As the patient's condition is critical and he is usually in great distress, he must always remain in the position in which he can breathe most easily and in which he is as free from strain as possible.

The area where the incision or puncture is usually made is the fourth, fifth, or sixth left intercostal space close to the left edge of the sternum or the fourth or fifth right intercostal space close to the sternum. McGuire says that recently some operators recommend inserting the needle just below the ensiform cartilage. The skin is cleaned and disinfected as for any surgical procedure. As in all such punctures, the greatest precaution is taken to prevent the entrance of infection or of air.

Suggested Procedure.   From the nurse's standpoint, there is little difference between this procedure and a thoracic aspiration. She should observe the patient critically and report immediately any unfavorable symptoms. Not only is this in itself a dangerous procedure, but the patient is nearly always very ill before the treatment is begun. The nurse should keep in mind the dangers. Any change in the rate or quality of the pulse, pallor, sighing, yawning, or coughing should be noted and reported immediately. A stimulant is usually kept at hand ready for instant use.

Recording the Treatment.   Follow the suggestions for recording similar procedures.

7. ABDOMINAL PARACENTESIS

Definition.   An abdominal paracentesis is removal of fluid from the peritoneal cavity. The condition in which a large amount of fluid has collected in the peritoneal cavity is called *ascites* from the Greek work *askos,* a bag.

Therapeutic Uses.   Fluid may be removed from the peritoneal cavity (1) for diagnostic purposes or (2) for drainage of an exudate in peritonitis and (3) to relieve pressure on other abdominal and chest organs if a transudate collects as a result of tumors of the kidney or heart and circulatory disturbances.

The peritoneal sac, like the pericardium, contains just enough fluid to lubricate its surface and to prevent friction between contiguous parts. The surface of the peritoneum is enormous, almost equal to that of the skin, and contains many lymph vessels. Its power of absorption is therefore great; but when irritated, the flow of lymph is reversed and an equal transudation or exudation may occur. This explains the rapid and repeated accumulation of fluid in the peritoneal cavity. A patient known to the writer received 200 treatments in a period of 4 to 5 years, about 13,000 cc (13 qt) being removed at each tapping. This patient was obliged to sit up constantly and had great difficulty in breathing. In another patient, 18,000 cc (18 qt) accumulated without causing any difficulty in breathing, and the patient slept comfortably in the recumbent position. This fluid was removed at one tapping or paracentesis. Where abdominal taps must be repeated often, some surgeons have advocated the introduction of a Murphy button into the abdominal wall. Offering a communicating channel between the peritoneal cavity and the tissues of the abdominal wall, it is supposed to drain the peritoneal fluid into these tissues. Thomas C. Chalmers et al.[10] report a highly unsuccessful trial of this procedure with 17 patients.

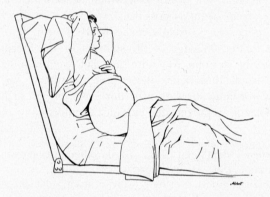

Figure 193. Sitting position of a patient in bed, about to have a paracentesis.

Equipment. Articles required are similar to those needed for pleural and pericardial aspirations, except that a trocar and cannula may be substituted for a needle. (See Fig. 35.) Fluid may be collected through tubing attached to the cannula and reaching to a bottle or pail. A slight preliminary incision is usually made; for this a scalpel will be needed. Sometimes one or two sutures may be necessary after the treatment is finished. If so, dressing forceps, needle holder, suture needles, and sutures will be required. No aspirating appartus is needed as the fluid flows out, impelled by gravity, the pressure of the viscera, and contraction of the abdominal walls. Since this is a slow process, a seat should be provided for the doctor.

Preparation of the Patient. As in all such treatments, the patient's cooperation and understanding should be assured before the treatment is begun. He should empty the bladder, because, if full, it is easily punctured during a paracentesis. Catheterization is indicated if he cannot micturate. Bring the patient close to that side of the bed from which the physician finds it easier to operate. The patient should be in a sitting position, well supported. Cover the chest with the gown or treatment blanket. Be sure that the patient is warm—nervousness is likely to produce a chilly sensation. Fold the upper bedding down to the pubic area. Protect upper and lower bedclothes with rubber or moistureproof paper, and cover such materials with cotton or soft paper squares. (The patient may find it more comfortable to be seated in an armchair.)

The incision is usually made in the midline of the abdomen, 2.5 to 5 cm (1 to 2 in.) below the umbilicus. The midline is chosen because an incision at the side might puncture the colon as it is fixed in position. Clean and disinfect this area as for any surgical procedure. Shave the skin if the site of injection is hairy.

Suggested Procedure.   After the usual preparation for a surgical procedure (scrubbing, adjusting gloves, gown, and possibly a mask), the surgeon incises the skin and introduces the trocar and cannula. The trocar is removed to allow the fluid to flow through the cannula. After the collection of specimens of fluid for laboratory analysis, the cannula is attached to tubing that reaches from the instrument to the drainage bottle. This bottle is usually placed on the floor or on a low stool. The greater the vertical distance between the incision and the end of the tubing in the drainage bottle, the greater the pull on the fluid in the cavity and the more quickly the cavity is drained. Too rapid withdrawal of fluid reduces the intra-abdominal pressure and so causes a distention of the deep abdominal veins, thus robbing the heart of its normal blood supply. A fatal syncope may result, or there may be a rapid outflow of fresh transudate from the lymph stream. Such results may be prevented by a gradual withdrawal of fluid and by external pressure made with an abdominal binder. Usually from one half to three quarters of the estimated amount of fluid is removed.

The patient should be reassured, and the treatment throughout made as simple as possible. (He is less likely to be nervous if he has had previous treatments, as he welcomes the relief that follows.) Avoid any unnecessary display of instruments, and divert the patient's attention if possible. The nurse must, however, remember the dangers involved; she observes the patient's color, pulse, and breathing, and notes immediately any signs of syncope. A glass of ice water and a stimulant should be at hand. A scultetus binder is placed behind the patient to be adjusted when required.

The thickness of the dressing depends upon the expected amount of drainage. It should be examined for drainage, and the patient's condition checked frequently after the treatment.

Recording the Treatment.   Follow the suggestions for recording similar procedures.

8. ASPIRATION OF EDEMATOUS TISSUES

When there is a transudate in the body cavities, the tissues are usually edematous. Eugene A. Stead, Jr., says that the tissues may be drained "if massive subcutaneous edema cannot be controlled. The patient sits in a chair; after the injection of a local anesthetic, number 14 needles are inserted through the skin of the legs and left in place for a few minutes."* After their removal alcohol sponges are lightly applied to the wounds, which are allowed to drain through the usual "tracts" left by the needles. Penicillin is given to control any infection that might result from such a procedure.

9. MYRINGOTOMY

Definition.   This minor operation consists of an incision, or paracentesis of the eardrum. It is performed with a special knife called a *myringotome*.

* Cecil, Russell L., and Loeb, Robert F. (eds.): *Textbook of Medicine,* 8th ed. W. B. Saunders Co., Philadelphia, 1951, p. 1066.

Therapeutic Uses. A myringotomy is made to provide a channel for drainage of pus or other fluid from the middle to the external ear. It is performed in otitis media when the drum is red and bulging with an accumulation of fluid or pus in the middle ear, when pain is severe, or when other symptoms, such as tenderness over the mastoid process, indicate the spread of the inflammation. Opinion among authorities consulted on the subject varies greatly as to indications for this operation. At present the tendency is to postpone the incision until there is reason to believe that the drum if not incised will burst from the pressure within the middle ear. It is thought that the incision made by the surgeon heals with less distortion of the drum than occurs after a rupture of the membrane. Most infections can be controlled by chemotherapy or the antibiotics; so this treatment is now very rare.[11, 12]

Equipment. Articles required are a myringotome, ear speculum, ear forceps, an applicator, sterile cotton, sterile cotton applicators, alcohol, and possibly hydrogen peroxide. Glass slides will be needed if smears are to be made from the discharge. A culture also may be desired. The surgeon may require sterile rubber gloves. The myringotomy knife is usually sterilized by immersion in a chemical disinfectant or by hot air. It should be protected against any hard surface, because it is most important that its sharp edge be preserved.

Preparation and Aftercare of the Patient. Have the patient on the edge of the bed or on an operating table. He should lie on the unaffected ear.

The surgeon performs the operation. The nurse prepares the patient, the required articles, and assists the surgeon, carries out the aftercare, observes and reports any results of the treatments, and any symptoms of complications that may develop.

A general anesthetic is nearly always given, as the incision causes agonizing pain, and local anesthetics do not desensitize the drum sufficiently. Moreover, the ear is very sensitive, and even the slightest involuntary movement might cause a serious accident. Nitrous oxide gas is commonly used. (Frequently in the case of very young babies, however, no anesthetic is given; they are wrapped firmly in a sheet.) In all cases, even when a general anesthetic is used, the head should be held to prevent voluntary or involuntary motion.

As in all operations, every precaution is taken to prevent secondary infection. If possible, a short time before the operation the auricle and surrounding area are cleaned. The canal is syringed with an antiseptic solution and packed with antiseptic gauze. When the surgeon is ready, sterile towels are placed across the shoulder and around the head covering the hair. A bright light should be placed so that it will be reflected by the doctor's head mirror into the patient's ear.

The treatment following the incision varies—the necessary articles should always be in readiness. Sometimes the canal is irrigated directly after the incision in order to wash out any blood clots that might block the incision if allowed to remain. Sometimes fluid is removed by suction. Some surgeons apply a moist dressing to absorb the discharge, or a sterile gauze wick may be inserted and a dressing and bandage applied. Dressings are usually impregnated with an antibiotic. They are changed as often as necessary, depending upon the amount of discharge.

After a myringotomy the canal is sometimes irrigated until the discharge has ceased; at first every 2 or 3 hours, then as often as the amount of discharge indicates. Sterile cotton or a gauze wick may be kept in the canal between treatments. Some surgeons keep the aural canal free from all dressings, believing that anything in the canal tends to block it. In such cases a sterile cellucotton pad with an impervious paper base or a rubber sheet is placed under the draining ear as the patient lies on this side. Irrigations of an ear with an open drum are dangerous because of the possibility of forcing infectious material back into the middle ear and possibly into the mastoid cells and Eustachian tubes.

10. PHLEBOTOMY OR VENESECTION

Removal of blood from a vein is a quick way to reduce blood pressure and for this purpose is occasionally used. Most often blood is withdrawn for diagnostic tests. (The technique is discussed under transfusion in Chapter 26.)

Bleeding and "leeching" were common in the past, so common that barbers did both. The striped pole in front of the barber shop represents the blood that was drawn and the white, the bandage applied to the wound. A leech (sucking worm) is said to withdraw 15 cc (½ oz) of blood before he is satiated. Another outmoded and unwarranted method of reducing blood volume is to place vacuum cups over incisions made in the tissues. These procedures are mentioned for their historical interest only.

REFERENCES

1. Todd, James C., and Sanford, Arthur H.: *Clinical Diagnosis by Laboratory Methods,* 11th ed. W. B. Saunders Co., Philadelphia, 1948, p. 607.
2. Flitter, Hessel H.: *An Introduction to Physics in Nursing.* C. V. Mosby Co., St. Louis, 1948, p. 90.
3. Dutton, Walter F., and Lake, George B.: *Parenteral Therapy.* Charles C Thomas, Publisher, Springfield, Ill., 1936, p. 88.
4. Cohen, A. J.: "Forty Years Experience with Artificial Pneumothorax," *Dis. Chest,* **17**:74, (Jan.) 1950.
5. Braverman, Morris: "Aspiration of Pleural Fluid," *Dis. Chest,* **18**:450, (Nov.) 1950.
6. Christopher, Frederick (ed.): *A Textbook of Surgery,* 5th ed. W. B. Saunders Co., Philadelphia, 1949, p. 855.
7. Wechsler, Israel S.: *A Textbook of Clinical Neurology,* 7th ed. W. B. Saunders Co., Philadelphia, 1952, p. 75.
8. DeGutierrez-Mahoney, C. G., and Carini, Esta: *Neurological and Neurosurgical Nursing.* C. V. Mosby Co., St. Louis, 1949, p. 65.
9. Cecil, Russell L., and Loeb, Robert F. (eds.): *Textbook of Medicine,* 8th ed. W. B. Saunders Co., Philadelphia, 1951, p. 1083.
10. Chalmers, Thomas C., et al.: "Evaluation of the Peritoneal-Button Operation for Ascites," *New England J. Med.,* **243**:857, (Nov.) 1950.
11. Boies, Lawrence R., and associates: *Fundamentals of Otolaryngology.* W. B. Saunders Co., Philadelphia, 1951, p. 66.
12. Rutherford, Miriam: "Proper Use of Antibiotics in Treatment of Acute Otitis Media," *California Med.,* **75**:98, (Aug.) 1951.

Suggested Additional Reading

Birch, C. A.: "Hazards of Medical Procedure; Lumbar and Cisternal Punctures," *Nursing Mirror and Midwives J.,* **91:**163, (May) 1950.

Stewart, J. B.: "Peritoneal Drainage," *J. M. A. Georgia,* **39:**399, (Oct.) 1950.

Wanamaker, G. T.: "The Dynamics of Lumbar Puncture," *U.S. Armed Forces M. J.,* **2:**67, (Jan.) 1951.

CHAPTER 29. INTUBATION—TO DRAIN, IRRIGATE, AND INTRODUCE FOOD INTO THE ALIMENTARY TRACT

1. INTUBATION OF THE STOMACH AND INTESTINES
2. GASTRIC LAVAGE

1. INTUBATION OF THE STOMACH AND INTESTINES

Definition. Intubation, decompression, suction-siphonage, and nasal suction are some of the terms used to indicate the introduction of a tube through the nose into the alimentary tract for removal of its contents by suction applied to the end of the tube outside the body. Any organ or cavity having an opening to the surface of the body may be decompressed in this way. Suction, or negative pressure, is exerted whenever a vacuum exists. "Nature abhors a vacuum," and atmospheric pressure forces into a vacuum any gas or fluid at the opening of the chamber in which the vacuum exists. Suction-siphonage, or decompression of the alimentary tract, occurs when a vacuum large enough (a negative pressure strong enough) to remove its contained fluids and gases is applied.

Therapeutic Uses. Intubation of the alimentary tract is used for four general purposes: (1) to remove gas and fluids in the prevention or treatment of distention following abdominal operations, (2) occasionally to study with x-rays the response of the alimentary tract to opaque liquids introduced through the tube, and (3) to remove the contents of the alimentary tract when its distension is caused by an obstruction. In the latter case when obstruction is the result of a mechanical condition, such as kinking, intubation alone may correct it; more often, suction-siphonage precedes surgical treatment.[1] (4) A fourth use of intubation is the removal of the stomach contents as preparation for, and during, general anesthesia. This is particularly important in surgery for which the patient is unprepared by fasting. Henry K. Beecher says:

Ideally, all wounded patients should have their stomachs emptied before being anesthetized in order to avoid the chance of aspiration of gastric contents. A further reason for this practice is found in the observation that distension of the stomach is great enough in some wounded men to interfere with the circulation, decided circulatory improvement occurring on evacuation of the stomach contents.*

* Beecher, Henry K.: *Resuscitation and Anesthesia for Wounded Men; The Management of Traumatic Shock.* Charles C Thomas, Publisher, Springfield, Ill., 1949, p. 104.

Aspiration of gastric contents is said by George Culver and his associates to be "a common and serious complication of anesthesia and surgery."* (To determine its frequency these physicians used dyes opaque to x-rays.) In a study of 300 unselected surgical cases at the Massachusetts General Hospital they found that 79 regurgitated and 49 aspirated gastric contents before the completion of the operation and there was "frank vomiting" in 24 instances with 16 of these aspirating gastric contents. Another 25 patients aspirated "silently"; thus it is apparent that the operative patient is in constant danger of infecting the lung with the stomach contents.

When the head is lowered during anesthesia and operation or when the side-lying position is used, the hazards are increased. Special care should be taken to keep the mouth free from aspirated material when the patient is in these positions. Gastric tubes during the operation are said to exert a protective effect. John W. Devine, Jr., and Robert L. Morrison recommend a tube inside a tube for this purpose. Occlusion, which often occurs with ordinary tubes when the mucosa is sucked into the holes on the side of the tube, is not possible with Devine's and Morrison's instrument according to their report.†

Selection of Equipment and Method.   Methods of intubation vary considerably, and Meyer O. Cantor believes these differences indicate that the procedure still presents difficulties to most, if not all, operators. He urges that the physician, usually a surgeon, himself participate actively. He thinks each patient presents a unique problem and says: "Intubation should not be relegated to the junior interne or the nurse on the floor. The attending surgeon must either supervise or pass the tube himself and must see the patient at frequent intervals during the first twenty-four hour period."‡ He thinks the operator requires "common sense above all" and says most of the errors are "the result of thoughtlessness on the part of the intubator." Nevertheless, his monograph shows very clearly that the operator should understand the anatomy and physiology of the alimentary tract, and should be familiar with the available instruments and the physical principles governing their use. In practice, nurses are often expected to carry a large share of the responsibility for intubation and until this situation is modified, they should study the procedure just as physicians must.

The choice of equipment is the physician's responsibility. He must decide how he wants negative pressure, or suction, created and what kind of tube to use. Five *types of suction* are described by Cantor: (1) simple suction; (2) continuous hydraulic, or water-displacement, suction; (3) electric, motorless pump exerting intermittent suction through expansion and contraction of air (Gomco thermotic

* Culver, George, et al: "Frequency of Aspiration of Gastric Contents by the Lungs During Anesthesia and Surgery," *Ann. Surg.,* **133:**289, (Mar.) 1951.

† Devine, John W., Jr., and Morrison, Robert L.: "New Tube for Rapid Evacuation of Stomach Contents Before Anesthesia in Emergency Procedures," *Am. J. Surg.,* **83:**396, (Mar.) 1952.

‡ Cantor, Meyer O.: *Intestinal Intubation.* Charles C Thomas, Publisher, Springfield, Ill., 1949, p. 178.

pump); (4) a pump "activated by electromagnetic coils on the same principle as the electric meter" (Stedman pump); and (5) motor-driven pumps.

Emptying the stomach with simple suction has been practiced for more than a century. Devices to induce vomiting were used in ancient times, but Philip Syng Physick (1800) is believed to be the first to wash out a stomach with a tube and syringe.[2] From this time on, stomach tubes have been improved, and in 1909 duodenal intubation was developed. It was found that when a tube was passed into the stomach or intestine their contents flowed out forcibly, since the liquids and gases in the alimentary tract, because of its muscular walls, are under greater pressure than the atmosphere. The longer the tube and the greater the drop from the patient to the container into which the contents flow, the greater the suction. When the flow ceases, it can be reestablished with a syringe or a vacuum bottle. With this method bubbles of gas are likely to block the tubing, and it is necessary to re-establish siphonage by their removal at frequent intervals. D. J. Leithauser[3] describes a method of doing this, or "priming" the siphon with a syringe when necessary in "A Simplified Suction Unit for Intestinal Decompression." Leithauser advocates this method because the patient can carry around all the equipment attached to his person, and this promotes ambulation which Leithauser believes so important.

Decompression with water displacement is commonly used where means of creating suction with electric power are unavailable. Hydraulic suction is based on the fact that negative pressure is created by the flow of water from a higher to a lower level. In this method a bottle, usually of 4-liter capacity, is suspended from an irrigating standard at any convenient height, but higher than the patients' bed. This bottle is connected by rubber tubing to one of similar size placed on the floor; water flowing from the upper to the lower bottle creates a vacuum in the upper that is transmitted through a tube to the patient's stomach or intestine. An airtight system is, of course, essential for the creation of a vacuum. The fluid or gas that may be in the alimentary tract is drawn into the upper bottle, causing the water in it to flow to the bottom bottle. According to James R. Paine and Elizabeth C. Phillips,[4] the average effective negative pressure is about 75 cm of water; Barnard Davis[5] says that while a pressure of 70 to 150 cm of water is usually adequate, a negative pressure of 1000

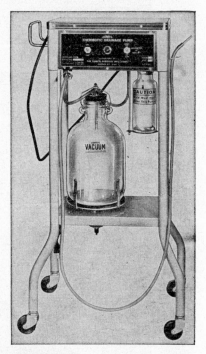

Figure 194. Electrically driven drainage pump; unit creates a negative pressure that can be regulated within the recommended range. (Courtesy of Gomco Surgical Manufacturing Co., Buffalo, N. Y.)

cm will not injure the alimentary tube. Commercial firms claim that the automatic evacuators exert a maximum negative pressure of approximately 2½ lb per square inch.*

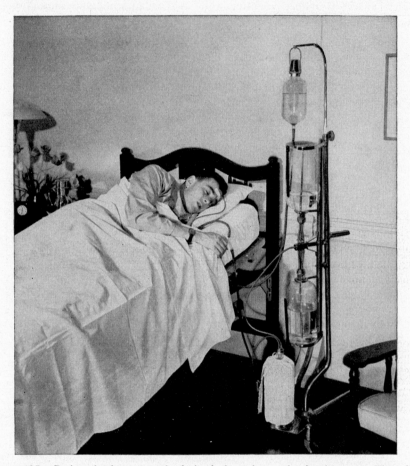

Figure 195. Patient having stomach drained through a tube in the nose. Three-bottle method is illustrated. Bottles that create suction are on a pivot. The upper bottle, which has no part in the suction-siphonage system, is attached to the nasal tube by a glass Y tube and contains saline solution that is used to wash out the tubing and to provide the patient with fluid as needed; the stomach contents are drawn into the lower bottle as a vacuum is formed there.

The greater the perpendicular distance between the level of the stomach and the drainage bottle, the greater the pull on the stomach, or the greater the negative pressure.

* If an apparatus is used that gives a subatmospheric pressure of 75 cm of water, this means that there is a, so-called, negative pressure exerted on the stomach of approximately 1 lb per square inch.

A third bottle may be added to the apparatus. Then the vacuum created by the flow of water from the upper to the lower bottle is transmitted to the third bottle and in turn to the tube inserted into the stomach or duodenum. The chief advantage of this modification is that the material aspirated from the stomach or the duodenum is kept in the third bottle. The material may be observed for color and consistency and may be more easily measured if kept separate from the water in the other two bottles. In this method only one of the three bottles is contaminated

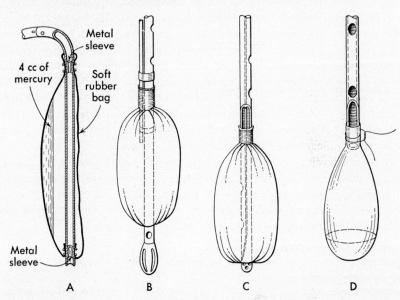

Figure 196. Tube heads of the most commonly used intestinal decompression tubes. (*A*) Harris tube, (*B*) Johnston tube, (*C*) Miller-Abbott tube, and (*D*) Cantor tube. The Johnston tube and Miller-Abbott tube are double-lumen tubes. Note position of balloon along the shaft of the tube. These tubes were designed for inflation of the balloon with air to propel the tube. Note the construction of the Harris tube head. It is exactly the same as the Miller-Abbott and Johnston tubes. It is a single-lumen tube and uses mercury as a weight. Note that in the Cantor tube the loose balloon at the tip of the tube permits an unrestricted free-flow of the mercury. (A later model of the Cantor tube is made with the balloon fixed to the tubing. See Fig. 197.) (Cantor, Meyer O.: *Intestinal Intubation.* Charles C Thomas, Publisher, Springfield, Ill., 1949.)

by the contents of the stomach, and the cleaning of the equipment is simplified. In the three-bottle method, it is a convenience to color the water in the two bottles used to produce the vacuum, because this enables the nurse to see the level of the liquid from a greater distance. A hospital-made water-displacement suction set can be assembled; its commercial counterpart is shown in Figure 195.

While effective decompression can be accomplished with the suction devices just described, electrically operated units are coming into general use. Of these the most desirable are the motorless ones because they are noiseless. Small portable units are more convenient than the large cumbersome variety. It is also important that pumps be made so that the operator can regulate and limit the negative pressure or suction. Cantor mentions that with one mechanism it varies from a minimum of 9 mm of mercury (126 mm of water) to a maximum of 12 mm of mercury (168 mm of water). This is of course a safeguard. He does, however, mention that experimentation with varying negative pressures has never been shown to injure the mucosa of human or animal subjects. Too great negative pressures will collapse the tube and for this reason make the treatment ineffective.

No matter how the suctioning device is constructed, it cannot be made "foolproof." The medical worker must understand the principles on which it operates. Since the nurse is most constantly with the patient during the days and nights when the tube is in place, successful decompression depends to a large extent on the faithfulness with which she checks the mechanism and her ability to use it effectively.

Four decompression tubes are in common use in this country. These are (1) the Harris, (2) the Johnston, (3) the Miller-Abbott, and (4) the Cantor tubes. A tube designed by Devine is so recently described and marketed that it is not yet generally known.* Also, there is the Aquiar tube used in South America, and there may be other modifications of these tubes in use elsewhere.

A very recent development is the use of a magnet-tipped tube. A. H. James uses a magnet so that he can determine the position of the tube in the alimentary tract with a compass; Devine and others claim that with their tubes the head can be drawn through the intestinal tract with a magnet (a 20-lb piece of alnico-5 metal) held against the abdomen. James says that with a compass:

. . . magnets of a size which can be used are detectable at a range of about 3½ in., and a compass pressed on the abdomen can be brought within the distance of most parts of the stomach and duodenum.

In practice there was never a convincing instance of a tube having entered the duodenum more rapidly with the magnet's help than without. . . . Magnet-tipped tubes are of value only for use in conjunction with a compass.†

Devine claims success in the manipulation of the head of the tube through the alimentary canal with a magnet, if the abdomen is not obese. The magnet he uses is heavy and relatively costly, and these features may discourage general use of his method.

Leon A. Frankel describes a "suction feeding tube employed in gastrointestinal surgery" that is different in construction from those just described but not used in exactly the same way. The Frankel instrument is two tubes, one longer than the other, joined by a collar. They are put in place during the operation. The shorter tube drains the stomach and duodenum; the longer is passed into the jejunum and the patient is fed through this tube. This instrument is passed through the incision and not through the nose. Frankel says, "The two tubes may be used as a single unit or independently."‡ While the nurse may not encounter this tube very often,

* Devine, John W., Jr., Lynchburg, Virginia. Personal communication.
† James, A. H: "Duodenal Intubation with Magnet-Tipped Tubes," *Lancet*, 1:209, (Jan.) 1951.
‡ Frankel, Leon A.: "A Suction Feeding Tube Employed in Gastrointestinal Surgery," *J. Internat. Coll. Surgeons*, 1:568, (Nov.) 1950.

the existence of an instrument whose two parts can be passed to different parts of the intestinal tract seems worth mentioning.

Cantor says the Levin tube is usually discussed in connection with decompression, but it is not in the same category with the four tubes mentioned because it will decompress only the stomach and duodenum. Nevertheless, these newer tubes are modifications of the Levin tube in use since 1921. The Levin tube is a #16 French rubber tube with a closed weighted tip and opening along the side. Because this tube would often fail to pass the pylorus and because it was not long enough to drain the length of the alimentary tract, as is sometimes necessary, variations have been designed. The Levin tube is rarely used except for decompression of the stomach if the distention is believed to be from gas.

In order to make the decompression tube pass beyond the pylorus, a number of modifications of the tip have been devised, and the decompression tubes have been lengthened and the number of holes in them increased so that negative pressure could be applied to any part of the intestinal tract. To combat the difficulty of obstruction of the tubes, their caliber has been increased.

The four decompression tubes in current use, shown in Figure 196, have balloons fixed to their tips, or just above them. The Miller-Abbott tube was the first. This is a single double-lumen tube with a weighted tip. The tube is passed with the balloon deflated, and it is not inflated until the tip of the tube has been carried through the pyloric valve of the stomach. The double lumen enables the operator to introduce air into, or deflate, the balloon at any point in the procedure. Because many operators had difficulty in getting the Miller-Abbott tube to go through the pyloric sphincter, this instrument has been modified.[6] Franklin I. Harris[7] found that if the balloon was weighted with 4 cc (1 dram) of mercury and if the patient's position favored it, the tube would be carried by gravity through the alimentary tract and the inflation of the balloon with air was unnecessary. The Harris tube is a single lumen tube, because it is not necessary to inflate the balloon. The Johnston tube is based on the same principle as the Miller-Abbott tube—that a balloon will be propelled onward by persistalsis of the alimentary tract. Charles G. Johnston[8] improved the Miller-Abbott tube by increasing the diameter of the decompression portion. The Miller-Abbott tube is a double-lumen tube enclosed in one sheath; Johnston's instrument is composed of two tubes attached to one tip and enclosed in one balloon a short distance above the tip which is an elongated fenestrated metal bulb. With Walter B. Cannon's findings in mind, that the pylorus would not open to the stimulus of a hard object, Cantor eliminated the hard tip and put the balloon containing mercury on the end of the tube. Because Cantor and Harris tubes depend upon the free flow of mercury to carry them by gravity through the intestinal tract, and because the balloon, with mercury in it, is passed through the nose, these are single lumen tubes. The Cantor tube is #18 French with a sufficient series of large holes to provide for decompression of the intestinal tract all along its course. There is least likelihood of stoppage in a tube of this type.

The decompression tubes described here are made of soft radiopaque rubber. In modern practice the surgeon depends upon the help of the x-ray in determining the position of the tube (unless like James he uses a magnetized tip and a compass). At certain stages in the passage of the tube he may work with the patient under the fluoroscope.

The *amount of mercury* used in the Harris tube is usually 4 cc (1 dram); Cantor varies the amount from 5 to 10 cc according to the age, size, and condition of the patient. If he anticipates sphincteric spasm, he uses 7 to 9 cc; in most cases he thinks the tube passes easily with 5 cc. When intestinal movement is normal, or nearly so, peristalsis will propel the tube onward; when the small intestine is atonic, as often happens if infection follows surgery, the weight of the tube rather than intestinal movement carries it onward.

Lubricants used in passing decompression tubes include water, glycerin, and vegetable and mineral oils. Cantor recommends the latter, but the danger of insufflation of mineral oil (see page 918) should be kept in mind.[9] A vegetable oil is a safer choice. The lubricant should be applied to the tube with a cotton sponge. If the tube is dipped in the lubricant, the excess is most likely to drop into the air passages. As long as the tube is in the nose the part just outside the nares must be kept lubricated; otherwise, a crust forms which is irritating to the mucous membrane and slows the passage of the tube.

The *temperature* of the tube as it is passed has been thought important. Many texts advocate icing the tube to stiffen it; with tubes in current use this is not generally thought necessary.

Successful intubation is dependent upon getting the tip of the tube through the pylorus. *Many methods of passing the tube through the pyloric sphincter* have been advocated. Stylets to stiffen the tube have been used. Under the fluoroscope the operator can then maneuver the tube to the pylorus. (He sometimes does this through the abdominal wall without a stylet.) This is uncomfortable for the patient and admittedly dangerous in any but the most skilled hands.[10] Henry T. Mayer, Jr.,[11] and Devine have recommended a magnetized head on the tube with a magnet used outside the body to pull the head through the pylorus. Amyl nitrate has been recommended to relax the pyloric sphincter. Cantor claims that if the patient's position favors it, the tube containing free-flowing mercury will, by gravity, pass through the pylorus and a paralyzed ileum with ease. The Cantor tube with the "mushy" balloon on the end most nearly approximates the consistency of the stomach contents, to which the pylorus normally opens. If, however, the operator cannot visualize the tortuous course of the alimentary canal, it is difficult for him to put the patient in postures that favor a passage of the tube through the canal by gravity. If he has opaque x-rays of the patient's stomach and intestines, made previous to the intubation, to which he can refer, his problem is somewhat simplified. Because the head of the tube may not reach the point in the intestinal tract intended by the surgeon within 24 or even 48 hours, the nurse must of necessity participate in promoting its progress in many situations. She should, in such cases, insist upon written and specific directions for changing the patient's position, for elevating the bed, and for getting the patient on his feet. She must also know whether the tube outside the nares should at any time be free or fixed to the face; and if the latter, how it should be fastened on the face. The nurse needs equally specific directions as to when and how much of the tube is to be fed into the nose. The point is made repeatedly that the tube should not be pushed forcibly. Intestinal movement and/or the weight of the tube will carry it toward the anus with almost no help if it is not held back. Cantor thinks 4 in. of tubing the maximum that should be fed at one time. If too much is pushed in at once, it tends to coil in the tract.

Gases in the alimentary tract have been known to permeate, distend, and stop the progress of the balloon. Cantor and associated physicists discuss this problem in his text. They say:

It has been well established that practically all the gas found in the gastro-intestinal tract in early post-operative intestinal distension is due to swallowed air, after the anesthetic agent has been dissipated if general anesthesia was used. . . . In cases of small bowel obstruction, however, . . . the composition of intestinal gases . . . is seen to consist of the following:

Nitrogen—70 to 80%. . . .
Oxygen—1 to 10%. . . .
Carbon dioxide—4 to 18%. . . .
Hydrogen—1 to 6%. . . .
Hydrogen sulphide—2 to 12%. . . .*

In such cases unless precautions are taken, the balloon could be dangerously distended, for natural rubber found in many of these instruments is highly permeable to carbon dioxide; and balloons of latex are permeable to hydrogen sulfide, as are Neoprene balloons to a lesser extent. Cantor says:

In a very small percentage of cases in which the intestinal tube is permitted to remain in the gastro-intestinal tract for longer than five days, it may be found that the balloon-tipped intestinal tubes take up gas into the balloon from the bowel. Because of this, check-up roentgen studies may show that the balloon is more inflated than the amount of air inserted, or the presence of air may be noted in the balloon of the Cantor tube where no air was supposed to be.†

When such accidents occur their correction is the surgeon's problem, but the nurse can help to prevent them. The Cantor tube provides an air vent by injecting the mercury into the balloon with a hypodermic needle. The tiny hole that is left permits the escape of gas. The nurse usually participates in the preparation of equipment and can see that this precaution is taken. The air-filled balloons of the Johnston and Miller-Abbott tubes can be deflated at any time by opening the communicating lumen of the tube. While intestinal tubes are used chiefly to remove gas and fluids from the intestinal tract, they are a means of washing it out and giving food, as tolerated. Intubated patients are usually very ill and for the first few days are ordinarily fed intravenously. Fluids are introduced during this time to keep the tube patent, to distend the tract ahead of the tube and make its passage easier, or to wash out

* Cantor, Meyer O.: *op. cit.*, p. 247.
† Cantor, Meyer O.: *op. cit.*, p. 184.

the tract. As the distention subsides, increasing amounts of food are given as tolerated by the patient. When food is taken without nausea or distention, and the bowels move normally, the tube can be safely withdrawn. Sodium chloride solutions are commonly used for cleansing the tract, although sodium bicarbonate solution may more successfully dissolve mucous plugs. Provision must be made for returning to the patient, intravenously or by mouth, the water and salts removed by suction- siphonage; otherwise the fluid-electrolyte, acid-base balance is dangerously upset (see pp. 392 ff.). Jonathan E. Rhoads mentions the upset in this balance as one of the abuses of the Miller-Abbott tube. He summarizes these abuses in the following terms:

Abuse has occurred mainly in cases of mechanical obstruction where it has some-times led to delay in operation in patients who have gangrene of the bowel. . . .

Abuse consists in leaving balloon inflated and fastening tube at the anterior nares. Peristaltic action of bowel makes persistent drag on tube, resulting in skin necrosis at the nares and mucosal ulceration at the cardia. When tube has advanced far enough, balloon should be deflated when tube is fastened. Since mercury can seldom be with-drawn completely, a tube with mercury in the balloon is best avoided when it is desired to fix tube at a particular level.

Passing tube requires skill and judgment must be exercised as to how much time, how much of patient's strength, and how much x-ray exposure can be justifiably ex-pended for this purpose.

To employ tube for suction without adequate negative pressure (usually about 5 ft of water), or without frequent irrigation, is an *abuse* in that it generally fails to function effectively.

Another abuse occurs when suction drainage is instituted without adequate re-placement of water and electrolytes, including sodium, potassium, chloride and bi-carbonate.*

The Psychological and Physical Preparation of the Patient.   More than in most procedures the preparation of the patient is of utmost importance. Fear and anger make successful decompression much more difficult. Before starting the procedure, the patient, if not too ill, should be shown the tube, pictures, and diagrams that help him to understand its function. Surgeon and nurse and roentgenologist need the patient's cooperation, and they are more likely to gain it if he understands the pro-cedure. An explanation from the physician in charge means most to the patient usually, but this may be left to the nurse. The patient with obstruction is so sick that he often welcomes something that promises relief. In all cases Cantor recommends the administration of morphine sulfate to allay nervousness and relax the stomach sphincters. (This is contraindicated for patients who are nauseated by morphine or have some other negative reaction to the drug.) It is, of course, essential that the subject be willing to swallow the tube when it passes into the oral pharynx. Figure 197 shows the *position of the patient's head* for intubation. This is one of the chief factors in successful passage of the tube through the nose, and the subject is most likely to maintain it if he visualizes the course the tube should take.[12]

* Rhoads, Jonathan E.: "The Use and Abuse of the Miller-Abbott Tube," *Surg., Gynec. and Obst.,* **92:**244, (Feb) 1951. By permission of *Surgery, Gynecology, and Obstetrics.*

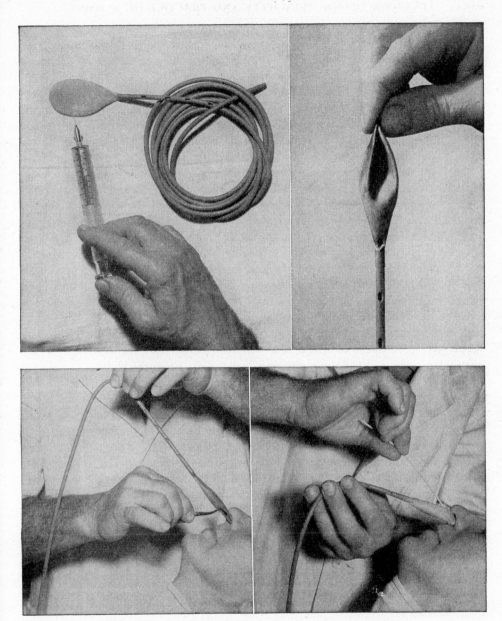

Figure 197. (*Top, left*) Mercury being injected into balloon of Cantor tube; (*top, right*) end of tube held by balloon so that mercury will flow to tip by gravity. (*Bottom, left*) Insertion of Cantor tube started with metal forceps, and (*bottom, right*) continued with a long cotton-tipped applicator. (After Cantor, Meyer O.: *Intestinal Intubation.* Charles C Thomas, Publisher, Springfield, Ill., 1949. Courtesy of Clay-Adams Co., New York City.)

Most physicians writing on this subject recommend painting or spraying the nostril to be intubated with a local anesthetic such as tetracaine (Pontocaine) 2 per cent. Shrinking the area with ephedrine 2 per cent is indicated when the passage is narrow.

Passing the tube into the stomach through the nose is the physician's responsibility, but the nurse can help him and the patient more effectively if she understands the technique. The patient's head should be in the hyperextended position shown in Figure 197. He may be sitting or recumbent. Hyperextension of the head is the position in which the weighted end of the tube can be made to fall most readily into the nasopharynx. The tube should be directed downward and backward as it is passed. It should never be pushed up into the nose. The deflated balloon, with or without mercury, is folded so that the tip of the tube is pointed or small; a Levin tube, of course, requires no special manipulation. Thorough lubrication facilitates passage of the tube, and for this reason an oily lubricant is preferred to water or glycerin by most operators.

The patient's discomfort during intubation should be minimized as much as possible, for at best this is a traumatic experience. The tube is a foreign body, and the mucous membrane secretes excessively in order to protect itself. The patient is conscious of what feels like a noxious mass lying in his throat, and, already nauseated, he must constantly swallow or spit out the excess and tenacious mucus. The throat soon gets sore and if the tube falls constantly over the openings of the Eustachian tubes a middle ear infection may result. Frequent change of position helps to prevent this. The best possible oral hygiene should be practiced before and after insertion of the tube. The teeth should be brushed three or four times daily, and a mouthwash kept in the unit for the patient. Some patients find very dilute cool lemon juice refreshing; others have used ginger ale because the bubbles of gas seem to break up the thick mucus that is so hard to spit out. Cracked ice to suck, chewing gum (sometimes Aspergum), and oil sprays are variously advocated to combat throat irritations and the parotitis (inflammation of the parotid gland) that sometimes accompany intubation.[13] Change of position and ambulation minimizes and equalizes the pressure of the tube on pharyngeal surfaces.

The patient's bedding and clothing should be protected. Nausea is often present, and intubation may precipitate vomiting. Several emesis basins and a box of paper wipes should be available. The nauseated patient usually prefers to be flat in bed, and the treatment may be started in this position with the head hyperextended over a pillow. Some operators think it easier to pass the tube through the nose when he is sitting.

Suggested Procedure. Having prepared the patient and gained his cooperation, bring the necessary equipment to the bedside. Check the suctioning device to be sure it is functioning properly. With an electrical device, or pump, see that it will draw water from a bowl into the attached bottle which will later receive the contents of the stomach and intestine. Establish suction in a hydraulic system by allowing water to run from the upper to the lower bottle. As soon as suction can be felt, or otherwise demonstrated at the opening of the tube from the source of the vacuum (to be connected with the intubation tube) it is clamped off. Protect the patient and his bedding with waterproof and absorbent covers and give him some paper handkerchiefs. See that the patient is sitting or lying with the head back, the neck hyperextended. The physician checks the condition of the tube and balloon, if one is used. He attaches the latter to the tube and inserts the mercury into the balloon with a syringe and 18-gauge needle. After aspirating the air he ties it off as described by the designer of the particular instrument. (Cantor suggests that a nasal speculum to stretch the mouth of the balloon facilitates its fixation on the tube. He also advocates a "25 pound pull fishline of braided silk" for the tie.) The physician next swabs or sprays the nostril with a local anesthetic (tetracaine 2 per cent), lubricates the tube, and passes it through the nostril into the nasopharynx. When the tip falls into the nasopharynx, the neck is straightened, the patient, preferably, sits up, and the nurse immediately gives him water through a drinking tube. This swallowing carries the tube into the stomach. With the Cantor tube an "S" (stomach) appears at the nares when the tube is in the stomach. With other tubes, measures in centimeters or inches, the points at which the tube would be in different parts of the alimentary tract, are predetermined by the operator. The nature of the fluid aspirated indicates the position of the tube to some extent. From the time the tube is in the stomach Cantor advocates the following program.*

1. For the first 2 hours keep the patient turned on his right side with the face inclined downward and raise the foot of the bed.

2. For the next 2 hours have the patient in Fowler's position (a position with the back rest elevated 18 to 20 in.) and gently feed another segment of the tube until the letter "D" (duodenum) appears at the nares. If the Johnston or Miller-Abbott tube is used, the doctor will inflate the balloon. The presence of bile in the aspirated fluid is some indication that the tube is in the duodenum unless there is reverse peristalsis. This side of the tube should be marked "Balloon—doctor only" and must stay clamped firmly.

3. For the third 2-hour period turn the patient on his left side and pass another 4 in. of tubing.

At this point check the position of the tube with the x-ray, and if it is satisfactory, encourage ambulation which increases peristalsis and helps by gravity to speed the passage of the tube through the tract to the desired point.[14]

Do not fix the tube to the face unless ample slack is allowed, for this will obviously stop its progress. This is a common mistake made by both doctors and nurses. Rhoads says the tube must not be fixed to the nose until the tube has advanced as far as desired and until the balloon is deflated.[15]

There are several methods of determining whether or not it has passed from the stomach into the intestine. One is to have the patient drink (or inject through the tube) a colored solution; then immediately aspirate the fluid or observe the liquid that comes back into the drainage bottle. A quick return of colored fluid obviously indicates that the tube is still in the stomach. Another test, with the Johnston or Miller-Abbott tube, is to inject the amount of air required to inflate the balloon. Attach a loose-fitting empty syringe to the tube and retract it slightly. If the balloon is in the duodenum, the rhythmical movements of the intestine produce changes in pressure on the balloon

---

* If gastric suction alone is desired, the tube (usually a Levin or a Devine rather than the Cantor, Miller-Abbott, or Johnston tube) is attached to a suction device and left to drain the stomach as long as indicated.

that will make the plunger move back and forth in the barrel. The latter test is always made by the physician.

Proceed with intermittent or continuous suction as prescribed by the physician. It may be necessary to irrigate the tube, or flush it with a syringe at intervals. When a double lumen tube is used, take every precaution to avoid injecting the irrigating solution into the lumen communicating with the balloon. This mistake can have very serious results. To irrigate the tube, stop the suction by shutting off the clamp on the tube leading to the vacuum. Attach a syringe to the tubing on one arm of the glass Y tube and gently force the irrigating solution through the tube. It may be aspirated with the syringe, or the suction may be turned on to remove the fluid. If a reservoir is attached to the Y tube, allow the desired amount of solution to run into the stomach and turn on the suction to aspirate the fluid.

The patient may assume different positions during the progress of this treatment, but care must be taken not to dislodge the tube. Give fluids by mouth up to 2000 cc daily as ordered by the physician. The patient is considerably more comfortable when able to drink fluids. Any clear strained fluid food or drink may be given. Paine recommends the administration of 2000 cc of normal saline parenterally each day. He considers that this amount and kind of fluid will help to prevent alkalosis by keeping a positive chloride balance in the body. Administered orally, sodium chloride is of little value, because the fluid is aspirated from the stomach almost immediately after it is taken, but if salt is given by mouth, it is better given in broth or in some other palatable form. To prevent irritation of the nasopharynx, use Albolene cream in the nostrils daily. This is destructive to the tubing, but the relief of the patient's discomfort is the first consideration.

The bottle into which the drainage is aspirated may be emptied as necessary. If the treatment is continued for a long period, it may be necessary to remove the tube, to give the nose and throat a rest for a few hours and introduce a clean tube. This has obvious disadvantages and is rarely considered essential.

When the treatment is to be discontinued, the physician slowly withdraws the tube through the nose. (If by accident the end has been passed through the anus it is withdrawn through the rectum.) Cantor says the removal of a tube should be gradual enough to consume 20 minutes or more.

Decontaminate all equipment by suitable methods. Do not soak intubation tubes in disinfectants, such as carbolics, that might leave an odor. Balloons are discarded. Disposable tubing has been designed for intubation, but plastic tubes are too easily collapsed to be satisfactory.

Recording the Treatment. Note the hour at which the treatment is begun, and record the patient's reaction. Record the amount of fluid the patient has received by mouth or parenterally daily. It is likewise important for the physician to know the amount of fluid and gas aspirated from the gastrointestinal tract. If a three-bottle method is used, the fluid in the third bottle may be easily measured and recorded. If the two-bottle apparatus, with hydraulic suction is used, the siphonage is begun with a known amount of water (4000 cc) in the upper bottle and in the lower bottle (400 cc). As gas and fluid are aspirated into the top bottle, fluid will flow into the bottom bottle. The difference between the amount originally in the lower bottle (400 cc) and the amount present at the time of the reading is the amount of gas and fluid aspirated from the stomach. The gas remains in the top bottle; it may be measured by means of the calibrations on the bottle. The total amount of fluid in the lower bottle minus the original amount of water in that bottle, minus the amount of gas aspirated will give the amount of fluid aspirated. Such readings should be taken and recorded at prescribed intervals and always when changing the apparatus.[16]

2. GASTRIC LAVAGE

Definition. Lavage is a French word derived from the Latin *lavare*, to wash out, and as used here it means the washing out of the stomach.

Therapeutic Uses. A gastric lavage is used (1) to remove undigested food and toxic substances in persistent vomiting, when the stomach may be enlarged or atrophied with lessened secretions; (2) in acute dilation of the stomach and to prepare the patient for gastric surgery; or (3) for emergency surgery as discussed on pages 823-24. More often in the latter case the gastric contents are removed by suction, but the stomach is not washed out.

Selection of Method. The gastric lavage is usually accomplished by means of the siphon. It is a well-known physical law that the atmosphere exerts a pressure equal to a column of water 34 feet high. If the two ends of a tube are each placed in a container of water, the fluid will run from the container that is on the higher level to the container on a lower level, because the atmospheric pressure plus the weight of the column of water in the tube forces the water into the lower container. In the lavage, one end of the stomach tube is resting under the level of the fluid in the stomach and when the funnel end of the tube is inverted and extended below the level of the distal end of the tube, the contents of the stomach will drain out. Slight suction may be used to begin the siphonage, but that is usually unnecessary. As long as the distal tip of the tube is below the level of fluid in the stomach and the funnel end of the tube inverted, the fluid will drain from the stomach. When continuous gastric drainage is indicated during an operation, a Levin tube is passed through the nose and attached to a suctioning device, such as those described on pages 824-25.

The most commonly used solution is soda bicarbonate. Tap water would suffice almost as well, but it is believed that soda bicarbonate is of some value in liquefying mucus. Other solutions are of little value because they remain in contact with the mucous membrane lining of the stomach too short a time to exert any action; however, in the removal of poison from the stomach a neutralizing solution may be used. The temperature of the solution may be from 37.8° C to 41.1° C (100° to 106° F). The quantity varies from 4000 cc to 12,000 cc (1 to 3 gal). When prescribed for cleansing purposes, the treatment may be continued until the return flow is clear.

The time and frequency of treatments vary, but a lavage is usually an emergency treatment in gastric dilatation or in poisoning. If repeated lavage is indicated, the intubation just described is more satisfactory. Some persons who habitually swallow more than the normal amount of air have learned to pass a stomach tube to relieve distention. This self-treatment should, of course, be discouraged, and the source of this neurosis corrected if possible.

Equipment.   Articles necessary for a gastric lavage include a stomach tube, a large pitcher for the irrigating solution, and a container for the return flow. A waste basin and paper handkerchiefs and a paper bag that may be discarded are also needed. The patient's bedding and clothing should be protected. A bib of rubberized silk or cellulose film and an absorbent cover provide satisfactory protection. Lubricants are likely to be unpleasant in taste and consistency and increase the tendency to nausea, but they reduce the irritation caused by passage of the tube.

Some operators ask that the stomach tube—a medium-sized, smooth, flexible tube about 4½ to 5 ft long—be placed on ice to prepare it for use. A stiff, cold tube is thought to be more easily passed. A funnel is attached to one end of the tube to receive the solution. Ordinarily no suction is needed to remove the stomach contents, but some stomach tubes are equipped with a small bulb about midway that can be used to produce mild suction. The tube is usually marked about 45 cm (18 in.) from the gastric end. If the tube is inserted this distance, it indicates, in the average adult, that the end of the tube is in the stomach. A tube is passed through the mouth to lavage a cooperative patient, but a smaller tube must be passed through the nose if an uncooperative patient bites the tube to prevent its passage.

Preparation of the Patient.   The first essential in the preparation of the patient is the explanation of the treatment. The physician usually makes this explanation, but the nurse may amplify it or in some instances be entirely responsible for it. If the patient cooperates by swallowing as the tube is passed, the passage will cause much less discomfort. He should be instructed to breathe through the mouth.

The patient should preferably be in a sitting or horizontal recumbent position. If the head is held slightly forward, swallowing is easier and the tube is passed more easily. The bedding and clothing should be well protected. The patient should either hold paper wipes in his hand or have easy access to them.

Suggested Procedure.   The doctor passes the stomach tube, the nurse giving whatever assistance is necessary. Passage of the tube is never forced. As soon as the tube is in place, permit the stomach contents, if present, to drain into the receptacle for the return flow. Fill the funnel with the irrigating solution, allowing the fluid to run in slowly. The solution should be poured so that the funnel never completely empties because this introduces air. When 2 or 3 funnelfuls have flowed into the stomach, and before the funnel is completely empty, pinch the tube, invert the funnel over the waste receptacle, and allow the solution to siphon back. If the tube is completely empty it may be difficult, if not impossible, to obtain any siphonage. About 500 cc of solution should be allowed to run in before it is siphoned back. Continue the treatment by alternately introducing fluid into the stomach and permitting it to run back until the return flow is clear or until the prescribed amount of solution has been used.

To discontinue the lavage, pinch off or clamp the tube and withdraw it quickly. The patient may appreciate the use of some pleasantly flavored mouthwash after the tube is removed. Wipe the mouth dry and remove the rubber protector. Remove the equipment from the bedside and clean and disinfect it appropriately.

Recording the Treatment.   Note the time of the lavage, the kind and amount of solution used, and the character of the return flow. In addition, record the reaction of the patient during and his condition following the treatment.

REFERENCES

1. Cantor, Meyer O.: *Intestinal Intubation.* Charles C Thomas, Publisher, Springfield, Ill., 1949, p. 154.
2. Cantor, Meyer O.: *op. cit.,* p. 20.
3. Leithauser, D. J.: "A Simplified Suction Unit for Intestinal Decompression," *J.A.M.A.,* **127**:157, (Jan.) 1945.
4. Paine, James R., and Phillips, Elizabeth C.: "Nasal Catheter Suction-Siphonage, *Am. J. Nursing,* **33**:525, (June) 1933.
5. Davis, Barnard: "Managament of Postoperative Distension: An Evaluation of the Nasal Catheter Suction-Siphon Drainage," *Northwest Med.,* **37**:234, (July) 1937.
6. Abbott, William E.: "Indications for the Use of the Miller-Abbott Tube," *New England J. Med.,* **225**:641, (Oct.) 1941.
7. Harris, Franklin I.: "A New Rapid Method of Intubation with the Miller-Abbott Tube," *J.A.M.A.,* **125**:784, (July) 1944.
8. Johnston, Charles G.: "Decompression in the Treatment of Intestinal Obstruction," *Surg., Gynec. & Obst.,* **70**:365, (Feb.) 1940.
9. Schneider, Louis: "Subclinical Mineral Oil Pneumonitis," *New York State J. Med.,* **51**:245, (Jan.) 1951.
10. Cantor, Meyer O.: *op. cit.,* p. 120.
11. Mayer, Henry T., Jr.: "Improved Miller-Abbott Tube Technic," *Modern Med.,* **13**:89, (Feb.) 1945.
12. Cantor, Meyer O.: *op. cit.,* p. 124.
13. Cleveland, Marion: *Relief of Throat Irritation During Intubation.* Unpublished Study, Nursing Education Division, Teachers College, Columbia University, New York, 1940.
14. Cantor, Meyer O.: *op. cit.,* p. 133.
15. Rhoads, Jonathan E.: "The Use and Abuse of the Miller-Abbott Tube," *Surg., Gynec. & Obst.,* **92**:244, (Feb.) 1951.
16. Kehoe, Rosemary; "Recording Suction Siphonage," *Am. J. Nursing,* **39**:126, (Feb.) 1939.

CHAPTER 30. DRAINAGE, IRRIGATION, AND MEDICATION OF THE COLON

1. SELECTION OF METHOD IN COLONIC TREATMENTS
2. CLEANSING, OR EVACUATING, ENEMAS
3. COLONIC IRRIGATION, OR ENTEROCLYSIS
4. PROCTOCLYSIS, MURPHY DRIP, RECTAL INFUSION, OR RECTAL SEEPAGE
5. HARRIS DRIP, OR PROCTOCLYSIS BY A TIDAL-STAND METHOD
6. RECTAL FEEDING, OR NUTRITIVE ENEMAS
7. MEDICATED RETENTION ENEMAS
8. RECTAL SUPPOSITORIES
9. IRRIGATION OF A COLOSTOMY

1. SELECTION OF METHOD IN COLONIC TREATMENTS

Anatomical, Physiological, and Physical Facts Influencing Colonic Treatments.
The large intestine begins at the ileocecal valve and extends to the anus. The colon surrounds or frames the small intestine; the transverse colon is closely associated with the liver and gallbladder, the stomach and spleen; the ascending and descending colons are in front of the kidneys. A hot or cold solution in the colon, therefore, acts as a local application of heat or cold to these organs. Hobart H. Hare says: "An injection of this kind goes into the very heat-citadel of the body, and if too cold, as it often is, produces dangerous chilling of organs which are ordinarily especially protected from cold by the omental apron and intestine."* Walter C. Alvarez[1] thinks the average adult's colon is around 2.4 to 3.0 meters (8 to 10 ft) long. Walter A. Bastedo[2] says that roentgen studies demonstrate that the average tonic colon is filled by the injection of 750 cc (1½ pt), while an atonic colon may hold as much as 4000 cc (8 pt).

There is some uncertainty as to the exact nature of the *movements* in the large intestine. (See also Chapter 14.) Thomas W. Todd[3] has shown that parts of the colon go through a lengthening and shortening process of an accordion-like nature

---

* Hare, Hobart H.: *A Textbook of Practical Therapeutics.* Lea and Febiger, Philadelphia, 1930, p. 611.

that tends to hold the contents in the ascending and transverse colon. Some writers refer to an "antiperistalsis" that would have the same effect; a number of physiologists say there is no such thing as antiperistaltic movements in the human being. There is general agreement among Alvarez, Arthur F. Hertz,[4] and other investigators that infrequent periodic "mass movements," most likely to occur after eating, carry the contents rapidly forward. Alvarez speaks of the "rounded masses" being "pushed into the rectum like cars on a track."* The presence of these fecal masses in the rectum arouses the defecation impulse, the sensitivity of the rectum varying with the individual. While some persons' defecating habits seem to keep the rectum

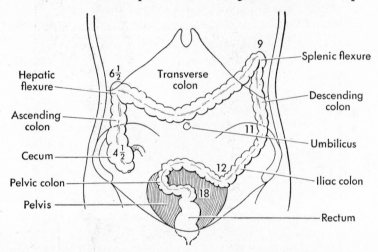

Figure 198. "Semidiagrammatic view of the large intestine; the figures give in hours the average times after taking a meal that its debris reaches the various parts. (Hurst.) This diagram shows the transverse colon in a higher position than it occupies when man is erect, and rather higher than the average even in the horizontal position." (Halliburton, W. D., and McDowell, R. J. S.: *Handbook of Physiology,* Blakiston's Sons and Co., Philadelphia, 1934.)

empty, Alvarez comments on the experience of physicians on finding feces in the rectums of many patients when making examinations in the office. If an opaque enema is injected into the rectum under moderate pressure with the rectal tube inserted 7½ to 10 cm (3 to 4 in.), Louis J. Hirschman,[5] Bastedo, and others claim that the liquid will reach the cecum in 5 minutes or less. Whether this is due simply to dilation of the colon by the liquid, or whether an antiperistaltic movement carries it toward the proximal portion, has not been determined. Frederick H. Morse[6] believes that in colonic irrigations there is some danger of forcing putrefactive bacteria present in the cecum and colon up into the small intestine; in other words, he thinks that the liquid may not only be carried throughout the full length of the large intestine but past the iliocecal valve into the small intestine. He advocates determining the competency of the valve by a radiograph before giving this treat-

* Alvarez, Walter C.: *An Introduction to Gastro-Enterology,* 4th ed. Paul B. Hoeber, New York, 1948, p. 574.

ment, and stresses the importance of gradual dilation of the colon in enemas and irrigations.

In medical practice, food, drink, and drugs are administered by rectum; therefore, a consideration of *absorption* in the large intestine is important in the study of colonic treatments. This is also discussed in Chapter 14. Complete digestion of a carnivorous animal's diet takes place before it reaches the large intestine, and the

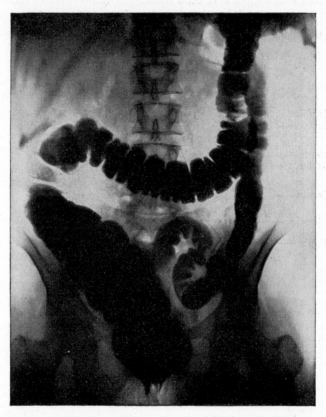

Figure 199. X-ray of colon immediately after the injection of a barium enema, showing that the whole length of the colon is completely filled by the liquid. (Courtesy of Columbia-Presbyterian Medical Center, New York City.)

absorption of most of the end products of digestion is believed to have been accomplished by the small intestine. Alvarez says that man's alimentary tract is similar to that of carnivorous types. Charles A. L. Evans[7] also says that the colon's role in the absorption of food is insignificant. Others imply, however, that a good deal of digestion started in the small intestine may continue in the colon and that a fair amount of absorption takes place, particularly if the diet contains a large amount of vegetable food.[8] Foods broken down into forms that are readily taken up and utilized by the cells *may* be absorbed in the large intestine. Evans says that the colon will absorb about 6 gm of glucose an hour. Reginald A. Cutting[9] found that dogs could absorb 30 gm an hour, whereas W. W. Ebeling[10] and A. B. Corkill[11] think that the amount absorbed is too small to make rectal feedings of much value.

Although the capacity of the colon to absorb foods is probably very limited, water passes from it into the blood stream in fairly large quantities. Evans estimates that an isolated large intestine of man absorbs about 80 cc an hour; Cutting found that the colons of dogs absorbed 240 cc an hour, and he believed that the same amount would find its way into other tissues from the human colon. The contents of the alimentary tract, as it enters the cecum, is about 90 per cent water, whereas a normal stool is a semisolid mass; this shows how much water passes from the large intestine into the tissues during its normal activity.

The amount and rate of absorption of drugs depend upon the drug and how it is injected. According to Bastedo, some drugs are absorbed from the rectum as rapidly as, or more rapidly than, from the stomach, though other medications are not absorbed at all. Besides the physical processes of osmosis and diffusion, by which water and solid particles pass through animal membranes, there appears to be a selective activity of the cells lining the large intestine, enabling them to accept certain materials and reject others. A great deal of experimental work has been done on absorption, but the findings and opinions vary. Importance has been attached to absorption from the large intestine of putrefactive or toxic products in constipation. Alvarez and others have cast doubt on this theory. However, there is evidence that glucose, certain salts, ether, and other drugs are absorbed. Injecting the solutions in hypotonic concentrations, under low pressure and near body temperature, favors absorption in the colon.

A number of writers comment on how little is known about the formation and absorption of gases in the intestine. In connection with a discussion of feeding and elimination in typhoid fever, William R. Houston says:

> Gas is constantly being formed in the intestines in large amounts . . . nearly all is absorbed into the blood and passes out with the breath . . . an excess may be expelled. An equable distribution of gas throughout the small and large intestines is essential to the proper functioning of the bowel. Some distention is a physiological necessity. . . . Gas pains following operations are due to the exposure and handling of the intestine which brings about spasmodic contractions . . . spasm and not gas causes the pain.*

A different conception of gas absorption in the intestine is found in Alvarez' text, for he believes that much of the gas is swallowed air and he differentiates between what happens to oxygen, hydrogen, carbon dioxide, and gases formed in the intestine. He says that nitrogen gas is being eliminated into and formed in the alimentary canal constantly and that since the process is irreversible (that is, since it is not absorbed from this tract into the blood stream), it must seek an outlet. Alvarez cites the work of Fries as showing that a normal man passes about a liter of gas in 24 hours and that a single discharge of the gas may vary from 50 to 500 cc.

* Houston, William R.: *The Art of Treatment*. The Macmillan Company, New York, 1936, pp. 106-7.

If it must be expelled, sickness, or any condition that lessens muscle tone, would tend to make the expulsion of gas more difficult. On the other hand, if absorption of gas does occur, disease and handling of the intestines might retard this process.

It is certainly true that the passage of gas along the intestinal tract requires a greater muscular effort than the passage of food. The writer has seen the violent contractions produced by the injection of air into a rabbit's alimentary canal whose motor function was preserved by suspending it in a tank of warm saline solution. Such contractions in the living animal may cause a pull on sensitive areas of the peritoneal attachments and so cause considerable pain. No matter what the mechanism, there is no doubt that discomfort and pain are associated with a distended abdomen, a condition known as *tympanites* or *meteorism*. Treatments, such as colonic irrigation, enemas, and proctoclysis, should be given in such a manner as to facilitate the escape of gas.

Experiments with dogs have shown that enemas of physiological salt solution, tap water, soap solution, and mixtures of ox gall, glycerin, and water did not have any effect on mobility of the small intestine but that injections of hypertonic salt solution do increase peristalsis of the small intestine and should therefore be more effective in relieving abdominal distention.

Austin Smith[12] gives the following formulas for "purgative enemas": Glycerin 30 cc, magnesium sulfate 60 gm, and water 120 cc; another larger preparation consists of warm soapsuds 0.5 liter, magnesium sulfate 60 gm, glycerin 60 cc, and oil of turpentine 15 cc emulsified in the yolk of an egg. Smith says that fecal impaction sometimes requires the donning of a finger cot or rubber glove and gentle manipulation with the finger in the rectum to break up the mass.

Physical principles *regulating* (positive) *pressure* when dilating the colon and suction (negative pressure) when draining it are of great importance. Persons administering such treatments must bear in mind the greater the height of the column of liquid, the greater the pressure, the more rapid the dilation, and the greater the stimulation of the intestinal musculature; also, the larger the caliber of the outlet of the column of liquid, the more rapid the flow. Likewise, the greater the drop, or length of the drainage column below the level of the anus, the greater the suction and the more rapidly the colon empties. If sufficient suction were exerted on the bowel, the mucosa might be sucked into the opening of the tube, occlude it, and possibly injure the mucosa. Nice regulation of the pressure and rate of flow in filling and draining the colon is for this reason important. Although the colon can probably stand a good deal of pressure without injury to the organ, Adolph Walkling[13] has reported several cases of rupture of the rectum resulting from distention during proctoscopic examinations. The nurse must not lose sight of this danger.

Physiological response to the *insertion* of a rectal tube or any foreign body into the anal canal is a contraction of the anal sphincter. This protective reflex makes the introduction of the tube difficult and possibly painful if the tube is forced into the canal while the body is trying to prevent its entrance. The following method should reduce the discomfort of the patient and the difficulty of the worker: Expose the anal region, keeping the patient as well covered otherwise as possible; a good light on the area is required; if he is able to cooperate, ask the patient to bear down as if he were having a stool (this opens the orifice) and to inhale deeply in order to relax the abdominal wall; then insert the tube slowly and gently. The tube should be well lubricated. Vegetable and mineral oils make effective lubricants, but the heavy hydrocarbons, such as petroleum jelly, are most effective. Since oils, and particularly hydrocarbons, are destructive to rubber, vegetable jellies, which have little if any effect on the life of rubber and are nearly as satisfactory as lubricants, are extensively used. If a small amount of solution is injected as the tube is inserted, the fluid will distend the rectum and leave a free passage for the introduction of the tube.

When introduction of the tube is painful or difficult, the nurse should remove the tube and report the condition. The patient may have hemorrhoids, a stricture of the rectum, an abscess, or some condition that would make the usual introduction of a rectal tube dangerous. The ability to determine whether an unnatural amount of discomfort is experienced by the patient is acquired through experience. Student nurses should err in being too careful rather than incautious in such cases.

2. CLEANSING, OR EVACUATING, ENEMAS

Definition. An enema given to remove fecal material from the colon is often called a *clyster*. This comes from the Greek *klysis,* meaning a washing out of stagnant or waste materials by means of injection of fluid. An enema for this purpose is given in such a way as to stimulate the defecation impulse.

Therapeutic Uses. A cleansing, or evacuating, enema may be ordered if the number or character of the stools indicates that waste products are not being properly eliminated or when the intestines are abnormally distended by gas. An enema given to stimulate the expulsion of gas is called a *carminative enema.* The purpose of the treatment is to soften hardened fecal matter and to stimulate the contraction of the colon by distending the walls or by irritating them with high or low temperatures or with chemicals. William Lieberman in "Some Historical Notes on the Enema"* says: ". . . the use of the enema recedes far into the past beyond the earliest recorded times." People are likely to resort to enemas without any medical advice whatever.

Some physicians warn against the continued use of cleansing enemas saying that they interfere with normal bowel movements, cause gradual dilation of the colon, and wash out the mucus which is the natural lubricant of the colon as well as the bacteria that function in cellulose digestion. Russell B. Grant and Murray S. Douglas[14] report a perforation of the rectum following a self-administered enema. This is not uncommon in the literature.

Selection of Method. The *kind* and *amount of fluid* depend upon the age and condition of the patient, the purpose of the treatment, and the judgment of the physician. Solutions most commonly given are sodium chloride, sodium bicarbonate,

* *Rev. Gastroenterol.,* **13:**215, (May-June) 1946.

and a weak solution of a neutral soap; plain water also is used. Medicated carminative enemas include solutions and mixtures containing purgative salts, glycerin, turpentine, oil, alum, ox gall, milk, molasses, asafetida, and other substances in various combinations and proportions. (Most texts list these substances but the writer thinks they are rarely used. Formulas for these various enemas are given in Appendix I.) There is good deal of variation in the nomenclature and in the proportions of the drugs used for enemas. Most hospitals give directions in their procedure manuals for preparing special enemas.

When the physician orders a cleansing enema and fails to prescribe *the solution,* the nurse is probably safe in using physiological saline solution. Attention has been called to the fact that physiological solutions are nonirritating. Although dilute soap solutions are used, they are irritating; this is dramatically demonstrated every time that soap gets into the eyes during a shampoo. In experiments with animals, soap-solution enemas have produced hemorrhages and ulcerations of the colon. Distention and irritation of the bowels by temperatures above or below that of the body are sufficient to stimulate peristalsis. Ordinarily, the physician prescribes the solution; he may indicate the strength of the drug and the proportions to be used in compounded enemas; or, if in a hospital, he may use the customary name which in that institution designates the particular solution or mixture.

Medical opinion and custom vary with respect to the *temperature* of solutions given. The practice of making the fluid about 41.7° C (107° F) so that it enters the rectum around 40.6° C (105° F) is probably most general. Temperatures above 43.3° C (110° F) should not be used, as they may injure the tissues. Recently, cool water has been advocated on the basis that it stimulates peristalsis, thereby avoiding the necessity of distending the bowel with large quantities of fluid. Houston[15] says that in some cases patients find cold-water enemas comforting and refreshing. Since this difference of opinion does exist, the nurse should be familiar with the preference of the physician in charge of the patient.

Apparently no rule can be laid down for the *amount* of solution, as quantities varying from 500 cc (1 pt) to 2000 cc (2 qt) are advocated. For infants and children, proportionately smaller amounts are injected. More recent reports indicate a growing disapproval of large quantities because abnormal distention of the bowel, especially if it occurs frequently, decreases muscle tone. Bastedo says that the amount of solution necessary depends upon the condition of the colon, in some cases a few ounces serving to stimulate bowel movements. In abdominal and pelvic surgery, if the abdomen is distended with gas and the pressure on the operative site from this distention is causing discomfort or actual pain, especial care should be exercised to avoid increasing distention any more than is necessary. If the patient is an adult, it is desirable to introduce about 240 cc (8 oz) and insert a rectal tube or allow the patient to use the bedpan before continuing to give the total amount prescribed. Usually the physician orders the enema as a means of emptying the lower bowel and is willing to have as little or as much solution used as is necessary to stimulate evacuation.

Much of the discomfort patients suffer during admininstration of enemas is caused by rapid dilation of the colon. Attention has been called to the importance of giving fluids under low *pressure*. This precaution is repeated here for emphasis. Mention has been made also of the fact that solutions injected into the rectum with a tube inserted 7½ to 10 cm (3 to 4 in.) have been shown to reach the cecum in 5 minutes or less. Higher insertions of the tube seem to be not only unnecessary but also to involve the possibility of injuring the rectum. Velvet-eyed catheters or rectal tubes (tubes with side rather than end openings) are preferred for all rectal injections. It is now generally agreed that the *position of the patient* makes little if any difference in the results of an enema. Abdominal relaxation decreases pressure and consequent discomfort; this is favored by having the patient in the lateral position with the knees flexed. In some cases, especially those in which there is loss of control over the anal sphincter, it is necessary to give the enema with the patient on the bedpan. As the patient may get very tired in this position a rubber-covered pillow should be placed under the small of the back so that he will feel supported, and unless he can keep his knees flexed without tiring, another rubber-covered pillow should be placed under them for support. When giving an enema to infants who are unable to retain the solution, provision must be made for its immediate return. In hospitals, regular treatment tables are provided for this purpose; in homes the infant may be supported over a douche pan or a waste container of any kind. Care must be taken to protect the infant from the edges of the pan.

Equipment.   The solution may be administered from a reservoir (an irrigating can or rubber douche bag) or it may be poured from a pitcher into a funnel attached to a length of tubing. Because it is more convenient for the worker and there is less likelihood of introducing air with the solution, the reservoir method is preferable. The funnel-and-pitcher method is frequently used by nurses in homes because it is easy for them to carry this equipment in their bags. If an irrigating can is used, a standard should be provided for its support. It is necessary to have a clamp on the tubing to stop or regulate the flow of solution. Tubing attached to the can and connected to the rectal tube by a glass connecting tube, should be approximately 90 cm (3 ft) in length. The rectal tube should be a #22 or #24 French, with a velvet eye; the smaller sized catheters are used in giving enemas to infants. (Hard-rubber rectal tubes are likely to irritate or injure the rectum, and their use should be discouraged.) A lubricant for the tube, such as a vegetable or petroleum jelly, is essential. Usually a small portion of the lubricant is brought to the bedside in a folded piece of toilet tissue by which means it is applied to the tube. A waste basin is needed for the used rectal tube. The bed should be protected by some means; this may be a piece of rubber sheeting with a cotton or paper cover, or a pad of cellucotton with a piece of impervious paper as a base. A pad made of newspapers and covered with old sheeting is an excellent protector to use in the home if rubber sheeting is not available. A treatment blanket covers the upper part of the body, and toilet articles must be at hand for cleaning and drying the patient after the treatment.

In order that it may enter the rectum at the proper temperature, the solution is prepared at a temperature a few degrees higher than that prescribed. If a soap-solution enema is ordered, the suds should be removed from the surface of the liquid, since, for reasons already pointed out, the injection of air into the rectum should be avoided. A tray or treatment wagon is used to convey the equipment to the bedside.

Recently placed on the market is a disposable unit for giving enemas. It is a plastic bag containing the solution with an attached rectal tip. The solution is forced into the rectum by pressure on the flexible bag. It is suitable for home and office use, and many hospitals are adopting this laborsaving device. Disposable units also are aesthetically appealing to patients. The solution can be warmed by immersing the plastic bag in a water bath.

Suggested Procedure.   Before taking the equipment to the bedside, explain the treatment to the patient and gain his cooperation. As in all such cases the explanation must be suited to the patient. Discomfort is reduced and the effectiveness of the treatment increased if fear and resistance are eliminated. Preparation of the patient includes protection of the bottom sheet, replacing the top bedclothes with one or more treatment blankets, screening the patient, and putting a sign on the door of a private room to ensure privacy.

If an irrigating can is used, hang it so that the level of the solution is never more than 45 cm (18 in.) above the anus. Ordinarily, half this height will result in a steady, slow injection, which is desirable. Expel air in the tubing by allowing a small amount of solution to run through it into a waste basin. With the patient in the proper position and the blanket adjusted in such a way that only the anal region is exposed, insert the lubricated rectal tube slowly and gently for a distance of approximately 10 cm (4 in.). *Let the solution flow into the rectum slowly.* Do not allow the can or the funnel to empty as this draws air into the rectum. If the patient complains of discomfort, the solution is probably flowing too rapidly and should be stopped to allow persistalsis to quiet down. In some cases it is desirable to remove the tube and ask the patient to use the bedpan. If a good bowel movement results, it may not be necessary to give the remainder of the solution. Irritation of the rectum is reduced to a minimum during the removal of the tube if this is done gently and quickly. Manual pressure over the rectum with a cellucotton pad inhibits defecation temporarily. In some instances it may be desirable to have the patient retain the solution for a few minutes before using the bedpan, but if a large amount of solution has been injected, he is seldom able to do this. The bedpan should be warm, and the diagonally folded protection sheet drawn up between the legs like a diaper to form a shield that prevents the upper bedclothes from being soiled and helps to control the odor. If the patient is weak or ill, he should not be left alone, since an enema is tiring and he may faint from the effort made to expel the solution. Ordinarily, the patient prefers privacy, but the nurse must be near and a means of summoning her within his reach. If she is not called within a reasonable length of time, the nurse should make certain that the patient is all right.

Sometimes a patient is unable to expel the enema. Retention of a cleansing enema is likely to occur if the patient is dehydrated. The solution injected is then absorbed to supply fluid of which the tissues are in need. In cases of this kind, reinsert the rectal tube, place the end in a bed pan, and if the nurse is a student she should report the condition to the head nurse. Further measures will probably be prescribed.

After the enema is expelled, the pan is removed, the patient turned on his side, and the buttocks cleaned with toilet tissue and bathed with soap and water. The bed protector is removed and the clothing readjusted.

Recording the Treatment. Consider the purpose of the treatment and chart the results—whether retained or expelled, whether the return was satisfactory in amount, whether it was fluid or contained small, hard masses, the amount of flatus, and the presence of any abnormality. Also note the effect on the patient—whether the treatment was accompanied by pain or discomfort, or followed by signs of weakness or exhaustion.

3. COLONIC IRRIGATION, OR ENTEROCLYSIS

Definition. *Enteroclysis* is derived from two Greek words: *enteron,* meaning intestine, and *klysis,* a washing out of stagnant or waste material. Bastedo says:

Between enemas and irrigations there would seem to be no sharp dividing line yet they are distinct in their purpose. In medicine the term *irrigation* conveys the idea of washing; therefore, while the ordinary enema is given with the purpose of inducing defecation, the irrigation is administered not to induce defecation but to wash out material situated above the defecation area and to lavage the wall of the bowel as high as the water can be made to reach. To accomplish its purpose an irrigation requires (1) that the fecal mass in the lower colon shall have been expelled, and (2) that the liquid shall be passed into the colon so gently that it does not arouse the defecation reflexes. Otherwise it is not a properly given irrigation.*

Therapeutic Uses. Colon irrigations are given for the following purposes: (1) To clean the colon of feces, gas, and excess mucus, bacteria and their products, in preparation for diagnostic examination or surgery or when the rectum is impacted with feces or when it is coated with a barium preparation, and in cases of poisoning to dilute and remove any of the toxic agent that may be present in the large intestine. (2) To supply heat to the colon, or to the pelvic and abdominal organs surrounding the large intestine, for the relief of pain and to bring about circulatory changes. Cold as well as hot irrigations may be used for the thermal effect on the colon and nearby organs. Arthur A. Stevens[16] suggests ice-water enemas in the treatment of sunstroke. (Houston in discussing the treatment of typhoid fever says, "A large cold-water enema will reduce temperature as much as a sponge."†) (3) As a means of applying local remedies to the colon in the treatment of infections and other pathological conditions. (4) To supply the body with the fluid that may be absorbed during the administration of the irrigation.

With the development of the sulfa drugs and the antibiotics, colonic irrigations are less often used in the treatment of infections.

C. O. Molander gives the following contraindications for colonic irrigations: "(1) loose sphincter, (2) painful hemorrhoids or fistula, (3) debilitation, (4) numerous polyps, (5) tuberculosis, (6) rectal infections, (7) painful skin

---

* Bastedo, Walter A.: "Colon Irrigations; Their Administration, Therapeutic Application and Dangers," *J.A.M.A.,* **98:**734, (Feb.) 1932.

† Houston, William R.: *op. cit.,* p. 107.

lesions around the anal opening, (8) syphilis, (9) massive carcinoma or other malignant tumors making it impossible to insert a rectal tube, and (10) severe diverticulitis."*

Selection of Method.   The equipment and method depends upon the purpose for which the treatment is ordered, the condition of the patient, and the facilities available. The physician may prescribe the method or simply order a colonic irrigation and leave it to the judgment of the nurse to decide the details of the procedure. In either case the nurse should have a thorough understanding of the basis on which the choice of method is made. She should determine whether the treatment is prescribed for its cleansing, thermal, or chemical action, or as a means of supplying fluid to the body; and whether the physician intends that the solution reach the entire length of the colon or only the distal portion. Having this information, the nurse administers the treatment, keeping in mind its purpose and the condition of the patient.

Variations in method most often mentioned are the use of one or two tubes. There is probably little difference in the results or in the ease with which the two methods are used. In the one-tube method, the rectal tube is attached to one prong of a glass Y tube, a drainage tube is attached to the other prong, and the tubing from the reservoir is attached to the base of the Y tube. Stopcocks on the inlet and drainage tubes enable the operator to introduce a given quantity of solution and then drain the bowel by closing the inflow tube and opening the drainage tube. In the second method an inflow and a drainage tube are inserted into the rectum at once, and the bowel may be drained constantly while the solution is being administered; or, with the use of the stopcocks on the tubing, the treatment may consist of periods of injection of the solution with the outflow tube closed and periods of drainage while the inflow is cut off.

A number of colon tubes have been designed by physicians and nurses making a special study of colonic irrigation. Bastedo[17] condemns the very heavy colon tube (#38 to #50 French) that some operators recommend. A tube the length of the colon is used by some workers, but its successful introduction requires special skill to prevent its coiling or injuring the mucosa. Its general use has been discredited by a number of writers; and, since a tube inserted into the rectum 4 in. results in the passage of the solution to all parts of the colon if a sufficient quantity is administered, such a difficult and hazardous procedure seems unjustified.

Regarding the methods of irrigation, Molander says:

The one we have used since 1933 is a pressure and vacuum gauge apparatus with a single metal piece which is inserted into the rectum. This apparatus has a reversible pressure inflow and outflow, producing first a positive pressure with inflow and then, by reversing the levers, a negative pressure on the outflow. A mercury manometer measures accurately both the inflow and the outflow. Such an apparatus can be controlled accurately; first, with the amount of fluid introduced and the amount of fluid expelled. The mercury gauge indicates the pressure, which is important and valuable in keeping the danger of pressure to a minimum. Thus by watching the gauge one can

* Molander, C. O.: "Colonic Irrigation," *Arch. Phys. Med.,* **30:**523 (Aug.) 1949.

control the treatment throughout, and by so doing potential dangers will be minimized. The apparatus has a metal tube which is easily inserted into the rectum and through which the fluid passes in and out of the rectum. These metal tubes are made in different sizes to fit most all patients. Therefore, because of the safety and ease with which a colonic irrigation can be given, we use the pressure and vacuum gauge apparatus.*

The value of a negative and positive pressure gauge is indisputable whenever hollow organs are filled and drained. If used consistently the danger and discomfort of such treatments would be minimized. Molander recommends draining the colon when the positive pressure begins to rise. This prevents overdistention with the cramps that accompany the intestine's reaction. Many will question the use of a metal rectal tube. An unyielding instrument is obviously more hazardous, and its manipulation by a person who does not know the anatomy of the rectum thoroughly should be condemned.

Equipment.   In any method the following equipment is necessary: a reservoir (an irrigating can, a large pail with a spigot at the base to which tubing may be attached, or a large glass cylinder, any of which must be calibrated so that the worker can determine the amount of solution injected into the patient), tubing for the solution, rectal tubes, and connecting tubes of suitable size. If the one-tube method is used, a #30 to #32 French with a closed end and velvet eye is generally satisfactory for an adult; if two tubes are employed, this size may be used for the outflow or drainage and a smaller size (#22 to #24 French) for the inflow. It is desirable to select tubes that are calibrated in centimeters or inches, with some indelible marking (silver nitrate may be used on rubber tubes). Clamps must be provided for both inflow and outflow tubes; a lubricant, such as a vegetable or petroleum jelly, is essential; a calibrated pail or jar for the return, which should be covered; an Asepto syringe that can be used to wash out the drainage tube if it clogs; pitchers or other containers for the total amount of solution to be used; a waterproof bed protector; an irrigating pole; and a suitable tray or treatment wagon for conveying this equipment to the patient. A bedpan should be available and toilet articles for cleaning and drying the patient after the treatment.

The *solution* used, its *temperature,* and the *amount* depend upon the purpose of the treatment, the condition of the patient, and the preference of the physician. For cleansing irrigations, Bastedo,[18] R. G. Snyder and S. Fineman,[19] Mark S. Shaine,[20] and other writers advocate the use of water; Hare[21] says that physiological saline solution is preferable to plain water because the latter irritates the mucosa. Sodium bicarbonate 1 to 2 per cent is frequently recommended. If the nurse must make the choice, physiological saline would be safe as this is the more normal habitat of body cells and it is reasonable to suppose that it could have little if any harmful effect.

Bastedo, Snyder and Fineman, and John H. Kellogg[22] recommend a temperature near that of the body; Eugene F. DuBois[23] gives the temperature of the internal organs as 37.2° C (99° F) or higher. If the treatment is to extend over a period of about 40 minutes and 8000 cc of solution (2 gal) are to be used, the writer suggests that the first gallon be prepared at approximately 40° C (104° F) and the

* Molander, C. O.: *op. cit.*

remaining half of the solution at 42° C (107.6° F) to allow for cooling as the solution runs through the tubing and stands in the containers. (This approximate drop takes place at a room temperature of 25° C [77° F]).

The amount of solution advocated for cleansing varies from ½ gal to 10 gal although the latter represents an extreme. Hare recommends using an amount sufficient to get a return of clear fluid from the intestine; in fact, he implies that this is the only way to determine the amount to be used for a cleansing irrigation. Molander thinks not more than 2 to 3 gal should be used and suggests that the patient will be unduly tired if the treatment lasts more than 30 to 45 minutes. Since the solution must be given under gentle pressure (slowly) to avoid stimulating peristalsis, the administration of large amounts consumes more than an hour's time and is likely to exhaust the patient. The nurse must stop the procedure before this happens, for no matter how much solution the physician orders, he does not want the patient unduly tired. If it is necessary for the nurse to determine the amount of solution, she probably should not use more than 4000 cc.

When the treatment is ordered chiefly for its thermal effect, the solutions are usually those mentioned. The temperature of the solution will be prescribed by the physician, and while Kellogg says that the mucous membrane endures a temperature 5.5° to 8.3° C (10° to 15° F) higher than can be borne by the skin, no references have been found to temperatures above 46° C (114.8° F). The use of a cold irrigation is uncommon, because it is seldom desirable to reduce the temperature of the abdominal and pelvic viscera, except in sunstroke.

Hirschman advocates the use of sodium bicarbonate in colonic irrigations for the removal of mucus; A. S. Blumgarten[24] mentions tannic-acid irrigation; Harry E. Bacon[25] advocates the use of silver nitrate 1:5000 to 1:1000, potassium permanganate 1:5000, tannic acid 1:100, thymol 1:500, and alum 1:100 for various conditions. The object in selecting an antiseptic solution, in any infection, is to find a drug that is specifically destructive to the causative organism in such a strength as will not be injurious to the tissues.

If the treatment is ordered for the purpose of supplying the body with fluids, the solution used should be hypotonic in order to encourage the passage of water from the intestine into the tissues. Plain water, or a sodium chloride solution of 1:200 or of lower concentration, may be used.

Position and Preparation of the Patient.   The room should be comfortably warm, and the bed table, floor, and furniture that might be injured by wetting suitably protected. Protection and privacy of the patient should be assured by draping, screening, and a sign on the door. Since the patient's cooperation is essential, the nurse should give an explanation, suited to his intelligence, experience, and condition. The position of the patient is usually prescribed by the physician; the dorsal recumbent, the right and left lateral, and the knee-chest positions are variously advocated. James T. Case,[26] reporting x-ray studies of the colon, found that it filled easily with the patient in the supine position unless there was "some gross obstruction." Molander uses first the lateral and then the dorsal recumbent position.

If the abdominal muscles are relaxed the patient has less sensation of pressure as the intestine is distended; therefore, regardless of whether he is on his side or back, the knees should be flexed. Bastedo[27] and others recommend giving the first gallon with the patient on the left side and the remainder with the patient on his back; this helps to prevent tiring the patient. He should be supported with pillows and made as comfortable as possible in whatever position he is placed. His clothing should be folded up above the waist and he should be covered with one or more treatment blankets, according to the room temperature and his condition. A cellu-cotten pad with a nonabsorbent base placed directly under the anus absorbs any seepage there may be around the tube and keeps the bed dry.

An important point in preparing a patient for a colonic irrigation is determining whether the rectum is empty or filled with fecal matter. If fecal matter is present, it may be hardened from having remained in the rectum where absorption of water takes place. This hardened mass is difficult to break up or soften and drain from the rectum with the drainage tube; it is likely to clog the tubing and should therefore be evacuated before giving the irrigation. Bastedo advocates a cleansing enema before the irrigation, but if the patient has had a normal stool a few hours earlier or is having daily colonic irrigations, this should not be necessary. If an enema is given, the irrigation should not be started for 20 to 30 minutes after the enema has been expelled, because the enema will have stimulated the defecation impulse, and stimulation of this reflex interferes with successful irrigation. Molander advocates giving mineral oil by mouth the day before the treatment. Before inserting the rectal tube he examines the rectum with a gloved or cotted finger. If there is fecal matter in the rectum he gives a cleansing enema to remove it. In order to reduce pressure within the abdominal and pelvic cavities, the bladder should be emptied before a colonic irrigation.

Suggested Procedure. Hang or support the reservoir so that the surface of the liquid is not more than 45 cm (18 in.) above the level of the anus; attach the large catheter (or small rectal tube) to the glass connecting tube; allow the solution to run to the tip of the tube to expel the air, and clamp off the tubing. Place the pail or jar for the return on a stool, chair, or stand, so that the top of the container is not more than 15 to 20 cm (6 to 8 in.) below the anus. To avoid splashing, see that the drainage tube reaches well into the container. Insert the tip of the smaller inflow tube into the eye of the larger drainage tube; lubricate the tubes and insert them together. When they are well in the rectum, about 5 to 7½ cm (2 to 3 in.), make traction on the smaller tube in order that the tip will be drawn out of the eye of the larger tube. Continue the insertion of the two tubes separately until the inflow tube is inserted 12½ to 15 cm (5 to 6 in.), and the outflow, or drainage tube 7½ to 10 cm (3 to 4 in.). If calibrated tubes are not available, mark with narrow strips of adhesive or on rubber tubing with a silver nitrate solution. As soon as the tubes are in place, start the inflow with the outflow tube closed. Allow the solution to run into the bowel at the rate of approximately 100 to 150 cc a minute under gentle pressure. When about 500 cc have been injected, open the drainage tube and adjust the height of the outflow column so that the bowel drains at the same rate of speed while the fluid is being injected; this keeps the bowel distended with approximately 500 cc of fluid until the end of the irrigation. Then the inflow tube is clamped off and the drainage tube is left open and in the rectum as long as there is any return flow. The outflow tube may be left in position for 10 minutes or more after the treatment, or the patient may be allowed to use the bedpan if he wishes.

In case the patient complains of abdominal pain during the treatment, clamp off the inflow and increase the rate of flow through the drainage tube by lowering the waste container, thereby lengthening the drop in the tubing. If the solution is given under sufficiently low pressure and not allowed to accumulate in or distend the colon too much, the patient should have no pain and very little sensation of any kind.

Should the drainage tube clog, pinch it or move it gently back and forth in the rectum to open it; if this is not effective, force some fluid through the tube with a bulb syringe or, if necessary, remove, clean, and reinsert. Note the nature of the return flow throughout the treatment and whether gas is expelled; this is indicated by bubbles seen through the plastic tubing or the glass connection in the drainage tube. As soon as the treatment is completed, clamp and remove the tubes gently and quickly; clean and dry the patient; remove the bed protection; readjust the clothing; and leave the patient in a comfortable position with his surroundings in order.

Recording the Treatment. Indicate the nature, amount, and temperature of the solution used; make a report of the fecal matter, the odor, and the presence of mucus, gas, and food particles if noted in the return. Describe briefly the patient's reaction to the treatment.

Modifications and Adaptions. A satisfactory irrigation may be given with the one-tube method, partially described under another heading.

One rectal tube is attached to a glass Y tube, to the other arm the drainage tube is attached, and the base of the Y to the tubing from the reservoir. The irrigation consists of a series of injections of approximately 500 cc each, with intervening periods of drainage through the outflow tube.

If a reservoir is not available, the colon may be lavaged just as the stomach is lavaged, with a tube and funnel. This method requires more care and skill in order to prevent the introduction of air and soiling the bedding and surroundings.

4. PROCTOCLYSIS, MURPHY DRIP, RECTAL INFUSION, OR RECTAL SEEPAGE

Definition. Proctoclysis comes from the Greek: *proktos,* meaning anus or rectum, and *klysis.* The treatment is sometimes called *Murphy drip,* after the noted surgeon who first used and described it. It is a form of rectal injection in which the solution is introduced drop by drop, with a device on the inflow tubing that provides for the escape of gas from the rectum. The treatment is designed to extend over a period of hours or days.

Therapeutic Uses. Rectal infusions are given in order (1) to supply fluid and sometimes food in the form of glucose during postoperative periods and acute stages of illness when the patient is unable to get sufficient water and nourishment by mouth, and intravenous and subcutaneous injections are not available or practicable; (2) to dilute toxins that may be in the intestines; and (3) to provide an outlet for the escape of gas from the colon and rectum. Because chemicals, antibiotics, and intravenous therapy are now so effective in combating most of the conditions for which proctoclysis was used, this procedure is now rarely seen in the United States. Some physicians are currently advocating, however, that the intestinal contents suctioned off with the Miller-Abbot tube be returned to the alimentary tract by proctoclysis. In this way the fluid-electrolyte balance may be more nearly maintained. Meyer O. Cantor[28] thinks, however, that the replacement of chloride, potassium, and other electrolytes should be made with infusions and/or feedings by mouth.

Guy W. Daugherty et al., reporting improvement in a patient with renal insufficiency, which they attribute to continuous lavage of the colon, say: "We feel that this experience demonstrates the value of the mucosal surface of the bowel as an avenue for the absorption of sodium chloride and that it re-emphasizes the value of proctoclysis when indicated. . . . Technically, the procedure seems to be entirely feasible. . . ."*

Equipment. The following articles are needed: an irrigating pole and a reservoir with attached tubing to deliver the solution (the reservoir may be a calibrated irrigating can or glass cylinder); and a drip bulb, which enables the worker to regulate the flow in drops per minute, introduced into the tubing about 30 cm (12 in.) below the reservoir. A glass Y tube is attached by one prong to the delivery tube a few centimeters below the bulb. The base of the Y is attached to the tubing inserted into the rectum; the other prong is attached to a piece of tubing long enough to reach up into the reservoir; this latter piece of tubing provides a means of escape for gas from the intestinal tract. A catheter, #20 to #22 French, is used to deliver fluid to the rectum, since a small tube is less irritating. Tubing should be supplied with sufficient clamps to enable the nurse to regulate the flow and to detach and clean parts of the equipment.

The *solutions* used should be hypotonic to favor their passage from the intestines into the tissues. Those commonly used are water, sodium chloride 0.5 per cent or lower concentration, and glucose 2 to 5 per cent in water or in hypotonic sodium chloride. The *amount* required depends upon the length of time over which the treatment is extended and the ability of the patient to absorb the fluid. Daugherty and associates used a solution containing sodium, potassium, magnesium, and calcium chloride with sodium bicarbonate, sodium acid phosphate (anhydrous), and glucose.

As it enters the rectum, the *temperature* of the solution should be near body temperature, or slightly higher, to promote absorption. Heating devices applied in and around the reservoir have proved ineffective because water passing through the tubing drop by drop cools to room temperature no matter how hot it is in the reservoir. When heating devices are used around the tubing, especially electrical appliances, an infusion thermometer should be inserted into the tubing to check the temperature of the solution as it enters the rectum. It has been found that by using an electric pad with the heat control turned to low around the tubing, the fluid may easily be raised as high as 50° C (122° F) or higher, which is sufficient

* Daugherty, Guy W., et al.: "Continuous Lavage of the Colon as a Means of Treating Renal Insufficiency; Report of a Case," *Proc. Staff Meet., Mayo Clin.*, **23**:209, (Apr.) 1948.

to irritate, if not injure, the mucous membrane. Sandwiching the tubing between two hot-water bottles at 43.3° to 44.4° (110° to 112° F) placed on the bed near the buttocks keeps the solution in the catheter at approximately 38° to 40° C (100.4° to 104° F). The hot-water bottles may be kept at a fairly constant temperature by refilling every 30 minutes. A thermostatically controlled electric heating unit would be ideal if a suitable one were available.

A lubricant, preferably a vegetable jelly, is necessary. Adhesive or Scotch tape is needed to strap the catheter to the buttock so that it will not be displaced when the patient moves. A perineal T binder and an especially designed tube that can be attached to the binder may be used for persons with very sensitive skin.

Waterproof protection for the bed should be provided. Since a rectal infusion is a protracted treatment, especial care should be taken to make the patient comfortable.

In order to keep accurate record of the amount of absorption, it is desirable to have paper and pencil at the bedside to chart the amount of solution added to the reservoir and the estimated absorption taking place.

The room and bed should be prepared and the treatment explained as described under colonic irrigation.

Since this treatment may be continued over a long period of time, no one position should be maintained; on the contrary, the nurse should encourage or help the patient to change his position frequently and so arrange the tubing, heating devices, and reservoir that this is possible. Relaxation of the abdominal wall is desirable and encourages retention of the solution. The bladder should be emptied frequently in order to reduce abdominal pressure. At the beginning of the treatment, the bedding may be folded to the anal region and the top of the body covered with a bath blanket; the patient's clothing should be folded up above the waist to avoid soiling.

It is important before starting this treatment, as it is before irrigating the colon, to make sure that the rectum is empty. Fecal matter in the rectum interferes with the introduction of the solution and its absorption, and particles of fecal material may occlude the tube. The physician may order a cleansing enema or a colonic lavage as preparation for the proctoclysis. Since an enema stimulates the defecation reflex, the proctoclysis should not be given for 20 to 30 minutes after the enema is expelled.

Suggested Procedure. Hang or support the reservoir high enough to keep the drip bulb in an upright position well above the level of the bed. Attach the catheter to the glass connecting tube and allow the solution to flow through it until it warms the catheter and eliminates the air in the tubing. Lubricate and introduce the catheter 10 to 12½ cm (4 to 5 in.); when in position, attach it to the side of the buttock with adhesive or Scotch tape; care must be taken not to apply it over the pubic hair. It may be necessary to shave the area. As soon as the catheter is in place, arrange two hot-water bottles or other type of heating unit near the anal region but not in contact with the patient; sandwich the tubing between the two bottles, arranging a cover around them so that the tubing will be held in place. The temperature of the water is regulated by noting the temperaure of the solution as it runs through the infusion thermometer, which is used in place of a glass connection between the tubing from the reservoir and the catheter; this catheter should be not more than 25 cm (10. in) in length, which brings the thermometer between the anal orifice and the hot-water bottles. As soon as the apparatus is adjusted and the patient comfortable, start the solution flowing at the rate prescribed by the physician; this may vary from 10 to 60 drops per minute, according to the patient's ability to absorb it. No matter what rate the physician specifies, however, he will expect the nurse to regulate the flow to prevent dilating the rectum and filling the tubing as far as the drip bulb. The nurse should note and report the rate at which the patient appears to be absorbing the solution. If all factors are favorable for absorption—that is, an empty rectum, a comfortable position, unoccluded tubing, a slow rate of injection, a nonirritating and hypotonic solution, and the temperature of the solution around that of the body—and yet there is little if any absorption taking place, the nurse should report the condition to the physician, who will probably stop the treatment. This treatment requires a good deal of skill on the part of the attendant, and a nurse can justifiably feel a fair measure of satisfaction if she is able to administer as much as 1000 to 2000 cc in 24 hours by this method. If the drainage tube becomes clogged, move it back and forth in the rectum; or pinching the tube may dislodge a particle of fecal material in the eye of the catheter. If the tube is still occluded, force solution through the catheter with a bulb syringe or remove and clean the tubing.

Recording the Treatment.   Throughout the treatment, note the amount of solution absorbed, the gas bubbling through the outlet tube, soiling of the solution by fecal matter, and the patient's reaction to the treatment. Make written reports at regular and frequent intervals so that the physician may be able to judge whether the treatment is effective or whether other means must be adopted to accomplish its purpose.

5. HARRIS DRIP, OR PROCTOCLYSIS BY A TIDAL-STAND METHOD

Definition.   This treatment is a modification of the Murphy drip, and is likewise named after the physician who designed it. The distinctive feature of this method of proctoclysis is that the reservoir for the solution is hung about the level of the rectum, so that there tends to be a flow of solution into the rectum from the reservoir and a return of the solution, with an expulsion of gas and fecal material from the rectum into the reservoir, according to changes in pressure within this area; such movement of the solution and the contents of the rectum is encouraged by periodically raising and lowering the reservoir.[29]

Therapeutic Uses.   The purposes of the Harris drip are the same as those listed under the Murphy drip. Paul Titus[30] thinks that this method of protoclysis is preferable to the Murphy drip.

Equipment.   The reservoir should be a calibrated irrigating can, not a transparent vessel, since the solution is soon mixed with fecal matter and gases. It should be covered with a sheet of cellulose film or other transparent material held firmly in place with a rubber band to help control odor in the room and at the same time enable the nurse or physician to see the contents of the can. A glass Y tube should be introduced into the drainage tube to facilitate emptying the rectum, flushing the rectal tube if it is occluded, and emptying the reservoir during the treatment. When the drainage tube is opened, a covered and calibrated container for the collection of the return from the rectum is needed; also when the reservoir is emptied, cleaned, and refilled with fresh solution. A closed-end velvet-eye catheter, about #28 French, is used as a rectal tube. The opening and diameter of the tube should be large enough to facilitate the escape of fecal particles from the rectum. In order to bring the infusion thermometer for checking the temperature of the solution near the anus, the tube should be about 25 cm (10 in.) in length. Tubing should be supplied with clamps to facilitate inserting and removing the catheter and detaching parts of the equipment when it is necessary to clean them.

Solutions used are similar to those listed under the Murphy drip. Several hospitals mention sodium bicarbonate 1 to 2 per cent or this solution combined with glucose. Titus expresses a preference for tap water and says that sodium bicarbonate is no longer used for the Harris drip. The *amount* depends upon the length of time over which the treatment is extended and the ability of the patient to absorb the solution. The amount in the reservoir should not be allowed to fall below 500 cc.

As it enters the rectum, the *temperature* of the solution should be near that of the body or slightly higher, and maintained at this point as suggested under Murphy drip. Lubrication of the tubing and protection of the bed are also similar.

As the fluid flows in and out of the reservoir and rectum, it soon acquires a fecal odor. Frequent change of solution, covering the reservoir, and cleaning the can and tubing constitute the most satisfactory way to reduce odor, but air conditioning, as discussed in Chapter 5, helps.

Preparation of the Patient.   The same steps should be taken that are described under the Murphy-drip method of proctoclysis.

Suggested Procedure.   Support the reservoir so that the surface of the liquid is not more than 10 cm (4 in.) above the anus. See that the tubing is connected to the glass Y tube, the infusion thermometer, and the catheter or rectal tube. Allow the liquid to flow through the tubing to warm it and expel the air. Lubricate and introduce the catheter 10 to 12½ cm (4 to 5 in.); when in position, attach it to the buttock with adhesive or Scotch tape avoiding the pubic hair. Sandwich the tubing between the two hot-water bottles placed near the anal region but not in contact with the patient. (The arrangemen is the same as that described under the Murphy drip.) Make sure that the drainage arm of the tubing is closed and open the clamp regulating the flow from the reservoir.

At the beginning of the treatment and periodically thereafter, especially if the patient complains of pain from distention, lower the can 20 to 25 cm (8 to 10 in.) to drain the rectum, then lift it to the original height of 10 to 12½ cm. (4 to 5 in.) above the anus. This should be done at half-hour intervals. With the reservoir adjusted so that the surface of the liquid is about 10 cm (4 in.) above the anus, the solution flows very slowly into the rectum, and as soon as the rectum is sufficiently distended there appears to be sufficient pressure to force the contents back into the reservoir. This back-and-forth movement of the liquid is referred to as a *tidal flow.*

It is very important to prevent complete emptying of the can, for when the liquid falls below the level of the outlet, air is drawn into the tubing and then into the rectum.

This procedure, like the Murphy drip, may extend over a week; therefore, it is essential for the success of the treatment that the patient be kept comfortable. He should be moved frequently, and the legs, abdomen, and back properly supported with waterproof pillows and pads. The catheter should be removed once daily, cleaned, lubricated, and reinserted.

Before discontinuing the treatment, drain the rectum by lowering the can, or leave the rectal tube in place with the end in a urinal for 15 or 20 minutes.

Recording the Treatment. The same type of report and record should be made for this treatment as that described under the Murphy drip.

6. RECTAL FEEDING, OR NUTRITIVE ENEMAS

Definition. A nutritive enema is the injection into the rectum of a liquid food selected on the basis of the supposed ability of the colon to absorb it. Since opinions differ on absorption in the colon, practice will differ in the use of nutritive enemas. It is conceded that liquid foods must be used that are broken down to such a simple state as to be ready for absorption.

Therapeutic Uses. Nutritive enemas are resorted to as a means of feeding the patient if oral feeding is contraindicated (for example, following operations on the mouth or upper alimentary tract) and in case nutritive infusions are unavailable; also when some condition, such as hemophilia, makes injection of a vein an undesirable proceeding. Nutritive enemas are now seldom used.

Equipment. Articles used in giving an enema that is to be retained differ in the following respects from those required for giving a cleansing enema: A catheter is substituted for a rectal tube in order to reduce to a minimum the irritation likely to stimulate defecation; a funnel and pitcher may be used instead of an irrigating can, because the amount of solution employed is so small that a proportionately large amount is lost adhering to the sides of the can and tubing, and it is cooled in passing through the can and tubing. A bedpan should be within reach, but since the object of the treatment is defeated if the patient expels the solution, it should not be within sight of the patient because it suggests defecation.

The food most commonly used is a glucose solution; whisky and brandy and predigested proteins were prescribed in the past. It has been noted that some physicians recommended that the intestinal contents recovered by intubation be reintroduced by rectum to maintain the electrolyte (salt) balance.

Although no fixed rule can be given for the *amount* of solution to be administered, 500 cc (1 pt) is probably the maximum prescribed for an adult and 240 cc (8 oz) is about the average amount given; proportionately smaller amounts are prescribed for infants and children. The *temperature* of the solution as it reaches the rectum should be near that of the body to avoid stimulating its contraction. The solution should be prepared at approximately 42°C (107.6° F) to allow for cooling while the patient is prepared, and for the drop in temperature as the solution passes through the funnel, or the reservoir and tubing.

Preparation of the Patient. The directions for preparing a patient for the administration of proctoclysis may be followed here. His cooperation is even more essential, and every effort should be made to gain it. Protection of the bedding is of course important. The position advocated is usually the left lateral, but the right lateral or dorsal-recumbent position, with the knees flexed, may be substituted. To reduce pressure within the abdominal cavity, the bladder and rectum should be empty. When rectal feedings are prescribed, the physician ordinarily directs that a cleansing enema or colon lavage be given once or twice daily and the feedings four or five times during the 24-hour period. To quiet the patient the physician may prescribe a sedative, sometimes an opium suppository, to be inserted before the feeding; or he may direct that a sedative be added to the enema. If the patient has hemorrhoids, or for other reasons the anal canal or rectum is very sensitive, it may be necessary to apply a local anesthetic.

Suggested Procedure. A nutritive enema is given in the same general manner as any other rectal injection to be retained. The following encourage retention and absorption: A small tube, well lubricated, inserted gently and slowly and removed gently but quickly, the height of the insertion probably not exceeding 12½ cm (5 in.); regulation of the temperature so that it is not much above or below that of the rectum, administration of the solution or mixture under low pressure, which means that the surface of the column of the liquid should not be more than 20 cm (8 in.) above the anus; and manual pressure over the rectum with a cellucotton compress, or other suitable material, after the catheter is removed. If possible the patient should refrain from using the bedpan for several hours after the treatment; otherwise the whole, or a portion, of the feeding may be expelled. He should be kept comfortable and quiet following the treatment, the bed protection left undisturbed to avoid moving him and to prevent soiling the bed in case the enema is expelled or there is seepage from the anus. In some cases, when the patient finds it difficult to retain the fluid, it is helpful to clamp the catheter but leave it inserted in the rectum for 15 or 20 minutes after the completion of the treatment.

7. MEDICATED RETENTION ENEMAS

Definition. A medicated enema is the rectal injection of a fluid drug. The drugs prescribed vary with the purposes for which the treatment is given.

Therapeutic Uses. When given for their systemic effect, or effect after absorption, the medicated enemas used are: (1) sedatives, such as paraldehyde; (2) analgesics and anesthetics, as, for example, tribromoethanol (Avertin) and ether; and (3) stimulants, such as coffee (now seldom used). Medicated enemas that are prescribed for local effects are: (1) oils to soften fecal matter and aid in its expulsion; (2) salts to draw fluid from the tissues in edema, or to stimulate peristalsis; (3) anthelmintics to kill or paralyze pinworms; (4) emollients to relieve irritation of the rectum; and (5) astringents to check bleeding.

Equipment and Suggested Procedure. All enemas to be retained are given in the same manner, and therefore the equipment needed for the administration of a medicated enema is the same as that for a nutritive enema. The same factors aid in retention and absorption. The physician prescribes the amount and kind of solution. When irritating drugs are given, such as anthelmintics, they are sometimes siphoned off after a stated period or removed by a cleansing enema. Sedatives and analgesics also are removed in some cases as soon as the desired sedation or analgesia is reached. Such drugs as tribromoethanol, the purpose of which is to produce a partial anesthesia, usually preceding the administration of an inhalation anesthetic, are given by an anesthetist. (Formulas for enemas are given in Appendix I. Most hospitals have nursing manuals that specify the particular mixtures and quantities used in their institutions.)

8. RECTAL SUPPOSITORIES

Definition. Rectal suppositories are concentrated food, soap, glycerin, plain or medicated cocoa butter, prepared in the shape of a cone. They retain this shape at ordinary room temperatures, but when introduced into the rectum are dissolved by body heat. Drugs contained in them are then set free.

Therapeutic Uses. (1) Soap and glycerin suppositories are used to stimulate defecation. They are particularly valuable when the feces are in the lower bowel or rectum, but are not expelled because the anal sphincter will not relax. The presence of the suppository acts as an irritant that stimulates the rectum to expel its contents. Glycerin suppositories for adult use are naturally larger than those for infants and young children. Soap suppositories may be purchased, but may easily be made by taking a splinter of white soap and holding it in hot water until smooth and rounded to the required length and shape. It should be cone-shaped and from 2.5 to 7.5 cm (1 to 3 in.) long. Soap is very irritating to the mucous membrane and should not be used very often or without a doctor's prescription.

2. Astringent suppositories of tannic acid, belladonna, and glycerin are prescribed in dysentery and diarrhea to contract the tissues, check bleeding, relieve pain, and dry up the secretions. Bismuth suppositories are also used; it forms a coating on the rectal mucosa and protects it from irritation.

3. Ice suppositories are sometimes used to check local bleeding or to relieve local inflammation. An ice suppository may be made in the same way as the soap suppository. It must be smooth and of a suitable shape and size.

4. Anodyne or local sedative suppositories are prescribed for hemorrhoids, dysentery, diarrhea, rectal abscesses, or postoperative conditions in which it is necessary to keep the rectum at rest. Drugs commonly used are cocaine, opium, and belladonna added to cocoa butter. Cocaine relieves pain and, by contracting the blood vessels, checks bleeding if it occurs. Opium and belladonna relieve pain, check peristalsis, and dry up secretions.

5. Suppositories containing opium or barbital (Veronal) are used for a general sedative effect if for any reason it is inadvisable to give medication by mouth.

6. Specific suppositories. In treating malaria, large doses of specifics may cause gastric disturbances. To prevent this, quinine has been given in the form of a suppository.

Suggested Procedure. Lubricate a suppository with petroleum jelly before inserting it. Carry it to the bedside in a piece of paper (Celluwipe). Wear a glove and insert the suppository as far as the finger will reach. Then apply pressure over the anus for a short time, until all desire to expel the suppository has passed. A patient should not insert a suppository because it is too difficult for him to do it properly.

Suppositories should always be kept in a cool place to prevent melting. It is necessary to keep glycerin suppositories under refrigeration.

9. IRRIGATION OF A COLOSTOMY

Nature of a Colostomy.   Colostomy is performed for the purpose of making an artificial anus in the anterior abdominal wall, the location of the opening being determined by the nature of the pathology in the colon. This surgical procedure is carried out when there is an acute obstruction of the large intestine (colon, sigmoid, or rectum) that prevents the passage of fecal contents. Other reasons for a colostomy are: to divert the fecal contents under certain circumstances associated with benign lesions of the colon, such as diverticulosis and ulcerative colitis; to promote repair of a traumatic wound of the colon; and as the first step in resecting a part of the colon.[31]

A colostomy may be a permanent or temporary opening. When it is necessary to resect the rectum and anus because of a malignant growth, the colostomy is permanent. Should the procedure be elective prior to a second operation on the more distal colon, as in diverticulitis, the opening may be temporary. The interval between operation and closure of a colostomy varies; some of the factors to be considered are: the patient's general condition, causative pathology, presence of infection that necessitates use of appropriate chemotherapeutic agents to control the infection, and healing of the operative wound in the distal portion of the colon.[32]

Preparation of the Patient for a Colostomy.   Many persons having symptoms that suggest a growth in the intestine postpone a medical examination because they fear an operation and the possibility of a colostomy. The most difficult task of medical personnel may be getting the patient to accept this temporary or permanent condition. The emotional shock of having to change a function so fundamental as defecation should not be underestimated. The person who accepts this cheerfully is usually a good actor.

It is the surgeon's responsibility to explain the procedure to the patient and help him accept the operation that may be essential for life; the nurse also plays an important role in this process. The patient will need encouraging, sympathetic assistance to face and accept the many adjustments that a colostomy will necessitate. The nurse supplements the physician's explanation and answers the patient's many questions. She may help him to see how he can adapt to this condition by showing him the devices that are used for irrigating, etc.

If it is possible in the preoperative period for the patient to talk with someone who has a colostomy and has learned to regulate daily elimination, such a conversation will be very reassuring to the patient.[33] If this is not possible to arrange, he might read, or have read to him, some of the articles written by patients who are leading a normal life in spite of the inconveniences of a colostomy.

In an emergency when such mental preparation is not possible, the physician and nurse must give the patient such assistance in the postoperative period.

Because colostomy is often performed on patients having cancer, who are generally anemic, malnourished, and in poor physical condition, the preoperative treatment is especially important. During this period, dehydration and electrolyte imbalance (see pp. 392 ff.) are corrected by feeding and, if indicated, by the intravenous administration of various solutions as prescribed by the physician. Protein hydrolysates, glucose, salts, and vitamins may be given parenterally. Frequently blood transfusions are given to combat anemia. In obstruction with vomiting, parenteral therapy is lifesaving.

Intubation of the small bowel by means of a gastrointestinal suction tube makes possible the deflation of the distended intestinal tract in obstruction.

When the obstruction is partial and the patient free from nausea, a drug such as one of the sulfonamides may be given to retard the growth of bacteria in the colon and to help prevent infection postoperatively. Drugs used for this purpose are those that are not absorbed from the gastrointestinal tract.[34]

Postoperative Care. If the rectum is not resected, the postoperative care of these patients does not differ from any other type of abdominal surgery except in the care of the colostomy itself. At operation a single loop of bowel is brought out on the abdomen.* The dressings protecting the operative site are not changed until after the colostomy has been opened by the surgeon. If the obstruction was not complete, the loop of gut is usually not opened until the abdominal incision has healed; this prevents infection of the wound from contamination by fecal drainage. However, if the obstruction was complete and the patient's condition poor, the surgeon will probably open the loop of bowel and insert a catheter to drain off fecal matter.[35] This type of drainage helps to prevent contamination of the abdominal wound, and with a complete obstruction it is essential to empty the intestine. (In such cases intubation has probably been instituted to drain the upper part of the alimentary tract.)

When the patient returns to the nursing unit from the operating room, the catheter is connected with a drainage bottle. The tubing leading from the catheter to the bottle is fastened to the mattress with a safety pin to prevent undue pull on the catheter; kinking of the tubing is thus avoided. The nurse observes the drainage; if the catheter seems to be clogged, distention may result. To ensure patency, the catheter may be irrigated with normal saline as ordered by the doctor.

Accurate record of fluid intake, urinary output, and fecal discharge is important in the postoperative period since these data are essential to the surgeon when he evaluates the fluid needs of the patient. Fluids are given intravenously as indicated. Oral feedings are withheld until the colostomy is opened with cautery by the surgeon. At the time of operation the laparotomy wound is protected by a covering of moistureproof material which is sealed around the edges to keep the wound clean (see Fig. 200).

As soon as the artificial anus is opened, the dressings should be changed fre-

---

* When a colostomy is performed prior to a second operation, the surgeon constructs a double-barrel loop on the abdominal wall. The nurse must know that the upper, or proximal, loop is the one irrigated daily. The lower, or distal, loop is irrigated only when ordered by the physician as a preliminary measure to the next surgical step.

quently to prevent disagreeable odors, excoriation of the skin, and discomfort to the patient. Because this is not a sterile procedure, the skin can be cleaned gently with soap and warm water and pieces of gauze (gauze that has been washed for re-use is economical) or absorbent cotton. A light coat of talcum may be desirable.

Ointments such as aluminum paste, Desitin ointment, or zinc oxide have been commonly used in the past to protect the skin from contact with feces. Virginia C. Dericks and Kathryn A. Robeson[36] report that in their study of patients with

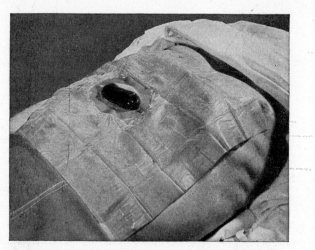

Figure 200. Colostomy stoma immediately after surgery and prior to the application of the final dressing. Waterproof cellulose film is cemented to the skin an inch or so from the stoma; soft, loose absorbent gauze and then a cellulose pad are placed over the stoma; the dressings are enclosed in the cellulose film, the edges of which are folded on themselves to make a waterproof package. Skin irritation and soiling of clothing and bedding are reduced to a minimum with this dressing. (Courtesy of Scotch Brand Cellophane Tape, Minnesota Mining & Manufacturing Co., St. Paul, Minn.)

colostomies simple cleanliness gave best results, especially since the removal of a tenacious ointment is itself irritating.* If a waterproof dressing is applied around the stoma until bowel movements are regulated and if evacuations occur during irrigation thereafter, the surrounding skin should never get excoriated. If it does, however, ointments should be tried out until one is found that relieves the condition. ("Kerodex"† is a recently developed coating to protect the skin from a wide variety of chemical irritants; it may prove helpful to colostomy patients during certain periods.) During a bout of diarrhea, or with high colostomies or ileostomies, Dericks and Robeson recommend cementing a waterproof envelope or bag to the

---

* If an ointment has been applied to the abdominal wall, it must be removed when an x-ray has been ordered. This is done by wiping the area gently with cotton dipped in mineral oil until *all* of the ointment, such as aluminum paste, has been removed. A protective dry dressing is then applied.
† Ayerst Laboratories Inc., New York, N. Y.

skin around the stoma *before* the skin is irritated. The digestive enzymes in the bowel contents are irritating to the skin, and it should be protected from them.

Soft absorbent dressings are held in place with Montgomery straps and an abdominal binder as well, if the latter is indicated. The dressing should be abundant and loosely applied to soak up any discharge through the stoma. This is likely to run out from under a tight or compact dressing. When the nurse is changing the dressing, she must not in any way show that the procedure is unpleasant; a calm, matter-of-fact manner will be very reassuring to the patient who is doubtless sensitive about the colostomy and embarrassed by the fecal liquid drainage that he is unable to control.

The absorbent material in the colostomy dressing should be enclosed in a waterproof jacket that is fixed to the skin around the stoma to prevent soiling of the clothing and linen. Sister Dolores Mary in a communication to "The Trading Post"* recommends the use of 5½-in. × 10-in. cellulose film refrigerator bags. She advocates closing the top and cutting a hole on the side to fit over the stoma. Barbara Haviland describes a similar dressing.[37]

As soon as the colostomy has been opened, the nurse explains to the patient the special skin care and discusses the type of dressing in the hospital and the type of protection he will apply at home, and how he will be able to control elimination by daily irrigations. She also discusses diet with him. During such conversations the nurse will have many opportunities to answer questions the patient will ask; the following list illustrates some of the usual queries.

How will a colostomy change my way of living, and working, and other everyday activities, such as a tub bath?

Can regularity of elimination really be established and what about odor?

What equipment will I need for self-care and where can it be bought?

What kinds of food should I eat and will my diet have to be different from that served my family?

How can I explain to the younger members of my family what a colostomy is?

By study and by observing experienced workers the nurse should prepare herself to help patients with the solution of these and other problems.

When the incision has healed and the patient's general condition has improved, the surgeon opens the colostomy and tells the nurse which loop is to be irrigated, indicating whether there are any restrictions on the amount of irrigating solutions and whether there are any unusual deviations in the intestinal passage.

Colostomy Irrigation.   When the colostomy is irrigated, the procedure is carried out by the nurse. (The surgeon may irrigate during a dressing to establish the patency of the opening.) The nurse begins at once to explain the steps of the procedure to the patient and excourages him to participate. As soon as the patient is ambulatory, the nurse helps him carry out the procedure. This hastens the patient's rehabilitation. A patient who chooses to remain anonymous wrote an excellent article entitled "No One Knows I Have a Colostomy,"† describing her

* *Am. J. Nursing,* **52:**877, (July) 1952.
† *Am. J. Nursing,* **51:**703, (Dec.) 1951.

inadequate preparation for self-care, her later search for understanding, and her very effective rehabilitation. She urges nurses to see that all patients are prepared before they leave the hospital to select the necessary equipment, irrigate the colostomy, and regulate bowel activity.

The nurse discusses the equipment with the patient and explains the various items included in the irrigating setup. The following items are needed:[38]

1. Irrigating set consisting of: 2-qt can or bag, tubing, glass connection, catheter (size #16 or #18 French), clamp, and colostomy irrigator
2. Solution thermometer
3. Solution (tap water or normal saline), 37.8° to 40.6° C (100° to 105° F), up to 2000 cc
4. Lubricant for catheter (e.g., petroleum jelly)
5. Soft toilet tissue or cotton to clean around opening before and after the irrigation
6. Paper bag or piece of newspaper for soiled dressings
7. Irrigating pole on which to hang the irrigating can
8. Clean dressings to apply after the irrigation

Suggested Procedure.* If possible, have the patient sit on the toilet for the irrigation since he will do so at home during the daily irrigation.

1. Arrange articles conveniently within reach of the patient.
2. Assemble irrigating equipment: attach tubing to can; close clamp, and attach glass connector and catheter.
3. Fill the can with solution.† Prepare a pitcher of slightly warmer solution in case more is needed.
4. Suspend the can from an irrigating pole so that it is between 45 to 60 cm (18 and 24 in.) above the colostomy opening. A patient describing a method she had found successful says that the bottom of the can should be 10 cm (4 in.) below the shoulder. At this height 1500 cc (1½ qt) of liquid will flow into the colon in 20 minutes.
5. Assemble the colostomy irrigator by placing the drainage sheath over the lower portion of the irrigator cup; later this is put over the colostomy opening and held in position by a belt with snap fasteners.
6. Remove the dressing and clean the skin with toilet tissue that can be discarded into the toilet or with soap and warm water should a more thorough cleansing be indicated.
7. Insert the catheter through the opening in the back of the irrigator cup; lubricate the catheter tip; allow a small amount of solution to run through the tubing to remove air.
8. Insert the catheter gently into the colostomy opening from 7½ to 15 cm (3 to 6 in.) with full flow of water through the catheter. The cup is held firmly against the abdomen by the belt; outlet tubing hangs between the legs into the toilet.
9. Allow 500 to 750 cc (½ to ¾ qt) enter the colon; if cramps result, pinch the tube and lower the irrigating can so that the force of the flow is not so great. Then tighten the clamp so that solution will return through the outlet sheath into the toilet. If this amount of solution does not induce an effective evacuation, it may be desirable to

* Based on *Booklet of Instructions for Persons with a Colostomy,* rev. Cornell University, New York Hospital, New York, 1952, pp. 8-11.
† In the home the patient may use plain tap water or water to which is added 1 tsp of salt to every quart of solution used.

use as much as 2000 cc (2 qt) or even 3000 cc (3 qt), providing the patient is tolerating the irrigation well. After the patient has become adjusted to larger amounts of solution, the catheter is inserted from 15 to 20 cm (6 to 8 in.).

One patient reports that if the tube is inserted for 37.5 cm (15 in.), there is little tendency for the fluid to return, or leak from the colostomy. She reports best results with thorough filling of the colon and with the use of sufficient liquid to get a clear return.* The author has been told by other patients that as little as a pint of water will bring about satisfactory evacuation.

The amount of solution to be used will vary with each patient; however, sufficient solution must be used to prevent drainage between irrigations. If the can needs to be refilled, do this while waiting for the return flow of the solution instilled. The bowel may be sluggish after surgery and require a greater quantity of fluid to induce an evacuation than is later needed. The nurse and patient should experiment to determine his particular needs.

10. After the irrigation has been completed, detach the sheath and place the collection bag over the lower opening of the irrigator cup. At this point the patient should be encouraged to massage the abdomen, lean forward and from side to side, and even stand up once or twice. Activity hastens bowel discharge. Let the collection bag remain in place until the patient thinks all drainage has ceased. (The nurse may suggest that he read a magazine or newspaper while he is waiting.)

11. When reasonably sure drainage has ceased, clean the skin around the colostomy opening and dry it thoroughly. Apply a clean dressing.

12. The equipment is cleaned immediately after use. It is first rinsed in cold water, then washed with soap and warm water. Special attention must be given the irrigator cup and the outlet sheath so that they are thoroughly cleaned. Rubber items are scrubbed on the outside and then inverted so that the interior may also be scrubbed.† The equipment is rinsed again in cold water and dried with a cloth or hung to dry. After the equipment is dry, it is stored in a convenient place until it is to be used again the next day. Immediate cleaning of equipment is the best preventive against odor. Cornstarch or talcum powder may be dusted on the rubber parts to prevent sticking.

Charting.   Note and record the time the treatment was given, the amount and kind of solution used, whether the nurse administered the treatment or whether the patient carried out the procedure and how capably he managed self-care. Progress in rehabilitation of the patient with a colostomy should be as carefully noted as that for an amputee or a paraplegic.

Self-care and Rehabilitation.   In the home, a hook or nail at the correct level should be inserted in the wall near the toilet so that the can or bag of solution may be suspended from it. The patient may need to keep in the bathroom a small table on which to assemble the equipment for the procedure or an orange crate may be used since the partition serves as a tray. After the irrigation has been completed and the equipment cleaned, the patient can store the items in the orange crate and turn the open side toward the wall.

Although it may take some time, the diet can be regulated so that frequent bowel movements are avoided. Following the opening of the colostomy, the patient is

---

* "Letters Pro and Con," *Am. J. Nursing,* **52:**666, (June) 1952.

† A disposable plastic sheath is now available. After the irrigation, it is removed from the irrigator cup and dropped into the toilet bowl.

given a liquid diet which is increased to a soft diet; it is then progressively increased toward a regular diet. Dericks and Robeson in the study cited report best results when solid foods are given early after operation. They do not consider a low-residue diet necessary in many cases;* others recommend such a diet.

By adhering to the diet the patient has found best for himself, he will be able to control frequent loose stools and should be able to have a regular well-formed stool once a day. If diarrhea occurs, the patient should wear a colostomy bag, and pay special attention to the diet in an attempt to determine the food or foods that had a laxative effect. Fluid intake can be temporarily reduced at this time. If diarrhea persists, he should consult his physician. Laxatives are *not* to be taken unless the physician specifically orders them. Constipation as well as diarrhea can be controlled usually by diet. Patients will vary in their need for amounts of roughage. Until the bowel movements are again well regulated, the patient should wear a bag over the opening to prevent embarrassment from unexpected bowel movements. Ointment on the skin to prevent excoriation may be needed until regularity of elimination has been re-established and the patient can successfully get along with only a small gauze dressing over the opening. The gauze dressing is held in place by an elastic belt or girdle.

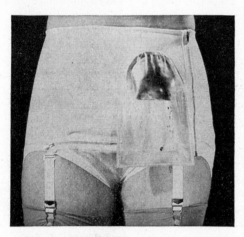

Figure 201. Special colostomy pants to wear with a colostomy bag when use of the latter is indicated. (Courtesy of Ferguson Manufacturing Co., Grand Rapids, Mich.)

Some people may feel more secure if they wear a colostomy dome which is a round saucer, sometimes made of plastic, that fits over the colostomy opening and is held in place with a belt. Most patients find this difficult to conceal under clothing and learn to control bowel movements so that this is unnecessary. One patient recommends a dressing of first a paper handkerchief, next a piece of waxed paper, and then a thin gauze dressing. Figure 201 shows a girdle and pants designed to be worn by a patient with a colostomy.

Because of individual variations, each patient with a colostomy must learn what is best for him to eat and what type of dressing he feels most secure with. Conferences with his physician to discuss problems of care and activity will be needed from time to time. When a "routine" has been established, the patient is much more content since his general work and home activities can be carried on as they were before his operation.†

* Dericks and Robeson recommend the elimination of those foods that cause the patient to have diarrhea, gas formation, or constipation.

† Most colostomy dressings have been worked out by patients. One man, an industrial engineer who has well-regulated bowel movements through the colostomy opening and who finds a small dressing adequate protection, is annoyed by the odor of fecal gases. J. W.

Before leaving the hospital, the patient should clearly understand the regulation of diet, change of dressing, irrigation and care of equipment, and care of the skin. The adjustments that the patient faces necessarily are many, and any help that can be given him will make the adjustment period less trying.

REFERENCES

1. Alvarez, Walter C.: *An Introduction to Gastro-Enterology*, 4th ed. Paul B. Hoeber, New York, 1948, p. 608.
2. Bastedo, Walter A.: *Pharmacology, Therapeutics and Prescription Writing for Students and Practitioners*, 5th ed. W. B. Saunders Co., Philadelphia, 1947, p. 211.
3. Todd, Thomas W.: *Behavior Patterns of the Alimentary Tract*. Williams & Wilkins Co., Baltimore, 1930, pp. 72-75.
4. Hertz, Arthur F.: "The Passage of Food Along the Human Alimentary Canal," *Guy's Hosp. Rep.*, **61:**389, 1907.
5. Hirschman, Louis J.: "Enemas; Some of Their Uses and Abuses," *J.A.M.A.*, **89:**1039, (Sept). 1927.
6. Morse, Frederick H.: "The Therapeutics of Colonic Irrigation and Physical Methods," *Arch. Phys. Therap., X-ray, Radium,* **12:**355, (June) 1931.
7. Evans, Charles A. L.: *Starling's Principles of Human Physiology*, 9th ed. J. & A. Churchill, Ltd., London, 1945, p. 860.
8. Fulton, John F. (ed.): *Howell's Textbook of Physiology*, 16th ed. W. B. Saunders Co., Philadelphia, 1949, p. 995.
9. Cutting, Reginald A.: "Absorption of Dextrose and Water by the Small Intestine and the Colon," *Arch. Surg.*, **29:**643, (Oct.) 1934.
10. Ebeling, W. W.: "Absorption of Dextrose from the Colon," *Arch. Surg.*, **29:**1039, (Dec.) 1934.
11. Corkhill, A. B.: "The Value of Rectal Administration of Glucose," *M. J. Australia*, **23:**807, (June) 1936.
12. Smith, Austin: *Technic of Medication*. J. B. Lippincott Co., Philadelphia, 1948, p. 131.
13. Walkling, Adolph: "Rupture of the Sigmoid by Hydrostatic Pressure," *Ann. Surg.*, **102:** 471, (Sept.) 1935.
14. Grant, Russell B., and Douglas, Murray S.: "Perforation of the Sigmoid following Enema," *Surgery*, **24:**867, (Nov.) 1948.
15. Houston, William R.: *The Art of Treatment*. The Macmillan Company, New York, 1936, pp. 106-7.
16. Stevens, Arthur A.: *The Practice of Medicine*, 3rd ed. W. B. Saunders Co., Philadelphia, 1931, p. 1097.
17. Bastedo, Walter A.: "Colonic Irrigations; Their Administration, Therapeutic Application and Dangers," *J.A.M.A.*, **98:**734, (Feb.) 1932.
18. Bastedo, Walter A.: *Pharmacology, Therapeutics and Prescription Writing for Students and Practitioners*, 5th ed. W. B. Saunders Co., Philadelphia, 1947, p. 213.
19. Snyder, R. G., and Fineman S.: "A Clinical and Roentgenologic Study of High Colonic Irrigations as Used in the Therapy of Subacute and Chronic Arthritis," *Am. J. Roentgenol.,* **17:**27, (Jan.) 1927.

Hirshfield and H. B. Sutton have described "A New Colostomy Protector," designed by this patient which is a plastic chamber equipped with a deodorizing filter that eliminates the odor from gases. It also fits so tightly to the skin that it prevents leakage from liquid stool. (*Am. J. Surg.*, **84:**126, [July] 1952.)

Lela Jaffe, a patient with an ileostomy where liquid stools are more likely to be a problem, advocates the girdle with an opening to admit the pouch worn over the colostomy and sealed to the skin. This patient also reports complete rehabilitation. ("The Patient and His Ileostomy," *Am. J. Nursing*, **54:**68, [Jan.] 1954.)

20. Shaine, Mark S.: "High Enemata and Irrigations," *M. J. & Rec.,* **123:**735, (June) 1926.
21. Hare, Hobart A.: *A Textbook of Practical Therapeutics,* 21st ed. Lea & Febiger, Philadelphia, 1930, p. 610.
22. Kellogg, John H.: *Rational Hydrotherapy; A Manual of the Physiological and Therapeutic Effects of Hydriatic Procedures and the Technique of Their Application in the Treatment of Disease.* Modern Medicine Publishing Co., Battle Creek, Mich., 1928, p. 897.
23. DuBois, Eugene F.: *Fever and Regulation of Body Temperature.* Charles C Thomas, Publisher, Springfield, Ill., 1948, p. 31.
24. Blumgarten, A. S.: *Textbook of Materia Medica, Pharmacology, and Therapeutics,* 7th ed. The Macmillan Company, New York, 1937, p. 105.
25. Bacon, Harry E.: *Anus, Rectum, Sigmoid, Colon; Diagnosis and Treatment.* J. B. Lippincott Co., Philadelphia, 1949, Vol. 1, p. 283.
26. Case, James T.: "Fundamentals in Roentgenology of the Colon," *Am. J. Surg.,* **8:**844, (Apr.) 1930.
27. Bastedo, Walter A.: "Colon Irrigations; Their Administration, Therapeutic Application and Dangers," *J.A.M.A.,* **98:**734, (Feb.) 1932.
28. Cantor, Meyer O.: *Intestinal Intubation.* Charles C Thomas, Publisher, Springfield, Ill., 1949, p. 199.
29. "The Harris Drip" (editorial), *Am. J. Nursing,* **28:**1212, (Dec.) 1928.
30. Titus, Paul: *The Management of Obstetric Difficulties,* 3rd ed. C. V. Mosby Co., St. Louis, 1945, p. 920.
31. Cutler, Elliott E., and Zollinger, Robert M.: *Atlas of Surgical Operations,* 2nd ed. The Macmillan Company, New York, 1949, p. 120.
32. Cutler, Elliott E., and Zollinger, Robert M.: *op. cit.,* p. 124.
33. Secor, Sophie M.: "New Hope for Colostomy Patients," *Nursing Outlook,* **2:**642, (Dec.) 1954.
34. West, John P.; Keller, Manelva W.; and Harmon, Elizabeth: *Nursing Care of the Surgical Patient,* 5th ed. The Macmillan Company, New York, 1950, p. 250.
35. West, John P.; Keller, Manelva W.; and Harmon, Elizabeth: *op. cit.,* p. 257.
36. Dericks, Virginia C., and Robeson, Kathryn A.: "Problems of Colostomy Patients," *Pub. Health Nursing,* **41:**16, (Jan.) 1949.
37. Haviland, Barbara: "Effective Colostomy Dressing," *Am. J. Nursing,* **49:**154, 1949.
38. *Booklet of Instructions for Persons with a Colostomy,* rev. Cornell University, New York Hospital, New York, 1952, p. 8.

Additional Suggested Reading

Cameron, Charles C.: "Professional Attitudes and Terminal Care," *Pub. Health Rep.,* **67:**955, (Oct.) 1952.
Christopher, Frederick (ed.): *A Textbook of Surgery,* 5th ed. W. B. Saunders Co., Philadelphia, 1949.
DuBois, Eoline: "Hints on the Management of a Colostomy," *Am. J. Nursing,* **55:**72, (Jan.) 1955.
Ewing, M. R.: "Colostomy; The Patient's Point of View," *Postgrad. Med.,* **26:**584, (Nov.) 1950.
Frohman, I. Phillips: "Constipation," *Am. J. Nursing,* **55:**650, (Jan.) 1955.
Gross, J. M.: "Preparation for Sigmoidoscopy in a Cancer Detection Center," *J. Internat. Coll. Surgeons,* **23:**34, (Jan.) 1955.
Sutherland, Arthur, et al.: "The Psychological Impact of Cancer and Cancer Surgery (Adaptation to the Dry Colostomy)," *Cancer,* **5:**5, (Oct.) 1952; also *Pub. Health Rep.,* **67:**1139, (Nov.) 1952.
Tinklepaugh, Irene: "A New Colostomy Set," *Am. J. Nursing,* **51:**675, (Nov.) 1951.
Wiggers, Carl J.: *Physiology in Health and Disease,* 5th ed. Lea & Febiger, Philadelphia, 1949.
Wright, A. D.: "Complications of Rectal Injections," *Proc. Roy. Soc. Med.,* **43:**263, (Apr.) 1950.

CHAPTER 31. DRAINAGE, IRRIGATION, AND MEDICATION OF THE URINARY BLADDER

1. BASIC PRINCIPLES UNDERLYING TREATMENTS OF THE BLADDER

The bladder is a highly elastic musculomembranous sac in the pelvic cavity behind the symphysis pubis. When distended, it reaches above the symphysis pubis and may be felt, and its outline seen if the abdominal wall is not obese. It functions as a reservoir for the urine that is constantly secreted by the kidneys and carried from them to the bladder in very small amounts by peristaltic waves that pass over the ureters every few seconds. With a cystometer the tone of the bladder wall can be estimated. T. C. Ruch, writing in John F. Fulton's text,[1] says that the normal bladder holds its contents under very low pressure, usually less than 10 cc of water. Increasing volumes of urine change the pressure very little and healthy persons, especially in youth, can train the bladder to increase its *capacity*. Oswald S. Lowsley and Thomas J. Kirwin[2] say the bladder is capable of great distension without rupture. While the bladder may be distended to hold 2000 cc (2 qt) or more, the accumulation of 240 to 300 cc (8 to 10 oz) elicits the desire to micturate or empty the bladder. This desire is a vague sensation in the penis or perineum and is thought to be initiated by rhythmic contraction of the bladder walls which is in turn initiated by stretching or distension of the bladder. After infancy the act of voiding is under the control of the will in healthy persons.[3, 4] The mechanism of micturition is discussed in Chapter 14. This and the subject of retention should be reviewed as a basis for understanding tidal drainage, particularly.

As was pointed out in Chapter 14, emotion may give rise to an almost constant desire to void, and this must be understood to interpret correctly the physician's directions for catheterization. Inflammation of the bladder results in this same symptom of "urgency," and it is important to determine its true origin. Treatment should be designed to eliminate the cause; either relief of mental stress or inflammation. This last may be the result of infection or a very acid urine.[5]

Retention, or failure to empty the bladder normally, must often be relieved by catheterization, for undue *distention* of the bladder wall with consequent reduction of the blood supply is believed to predispose to infection. It is generally thought that normal voiding empties the bladder completely. Charles H. Best and Norman B. Taylor say: "It is well known that the bladder can be emptied [in micturition] though it contains only a few cubic centimeters of urine."[*] This suggests that the complete emptying of the bladder by catheterization would be safe. *The amount of urine to remove* by catheter has, however, been a perennial subject of discussion. When it is thought that the bladder is distended, nurses are sometimes directed to remove "half the contents" as if the abdominal and bladder walls were transparent, enabling the nurse to make such a judgment. In some hospitals it is routine to withdraw the catheter after collecting, or removing, 500 cc (1 pt). Some physicians approve complete emptying but prescribe the instillation of 30 to 60 cc of a sterile solution to prevent a sudden change in vesicular pressure. It is believed that this sudden change may result in engorgement of the blood vessels made almost toneless by the thinning of the wall during retention. Lowsley and Kirwin[6] say that in "long-standing" retention the bladder should be slowly decompressed, but Charles D. Creevy,[7] reporting his experience and a published record of 300 cases of urinary retention in which the bladder had been completely emptied, says that no unfavorable reaction was observed in any case; other urologists refer to the fractional emptying of the bladder as a moot question. Therefore, since it is an unsolved problem in therapy, the nurse should determine the physician's wishes in relation to this aspect of the procedure. *The amount of solution to introduce into the bladder* at a single injection during irrigations should vary with patients and their conditions and with the physician's plan of treatment. Since the objectives of the treatment are to clean, medicate, and sometimes to distend the bladder wall, the amount is usually sufficient to get rid of the folds in the lining of the bladder and varies from 150 to 400 cc (5 to 13 oz). Larger quantities, of course, are used in the total process of the irrigation.

In describing bladder irrigations, all the urologists whose methods have been examined state that the fluid should be introduced slowly, under *gentle pressure.* Water introduced into a closed cavity exerts equal pressure in every direction, so that this force, if great enough, could carry the bladder contents up into the ureters. The total force of a liquid on a surface is equal to the area of the surface times the depth of the liquid times the density of the liquid. Applying this principle, it can readily be seen that reducing the depth of the liquid, which in this instance is the same thing as the height of the column of the irrigating fluid, reduces the force. The top of the column of the irrigating fluid should not be more than 15 to 20 cm (6 to 8 in.) above the meatus.

The cause of infections associated with catheterization has been given a great

---

* Best, Charles H., and Taylor, Norman B.: *The Physiological Basis of Medical Practice,* 5th ed. Williams & Wilkins Co., Baltimore, 1950, p. 485.

deal of attention in medical literature. _Catheter cystitis_ is a term often used in the past, and this expression implies that the infection was caused by the catheter. Victor C. Marshall, discussing the irritating effect of an indwelling catheter in genitourinary infections, says: "Even in the gentle and so-called aseptic catheterization, trauma results and urethral organisms move higher up. There is no such thing as a perfectly atraumatic catheterization."* There seems to be an increasingly large group of clinicians, however, who believe that the cystitis occurring among catheterized patients is caused by the overdistention of the bladder walls before catheterization rather than by the introduction of bacteria by the catheter. This opinion is expressed by Creevy, Lowsley and Kirwin, and others. Richard W. TeLinde and C. Bernard Brack,[8] writing in Carl H. Davis' text, urge that following gynecological operations, especially, great emphasis be placed on frequent emptying of the bladder both for the patient's comfort and the prevention of infection. If the patient is not kept comfortable by voiding, they advise catheterization 12 hours postoperatively and every 8 hours thereafter until the patient voids 100 cc or more at one time. Even then, if she has the sensation of pressure, catheterization is continued, for they believe there is less hazard in the procedure than in the distended bladder.

Hugh Cabot and Mary D. Giles say: "The introduction of bacteria into the normal bladder has repeatedly been shown incapable of producing inflammation . . . inflammation will occur only in the presence of abnormality of the bladder wall consequent upon overdistention, sudden relaxation on emptying, with the congestion, edema, and lowered vitality of the tissues."†

Hugh C. Ilgenfritz[9] and other writers mention the administration of 1 cc of 1:4000 solution of neostigmine (Prostigmin) given hypodermically before and after operations to stimulate voiding and elimination of gas from the intestines. If used, it is often unnecessary to catheterize the patient.

It seems to be generally accepted that the bladder is not a sterile cavity, although to prove this is difficult, since to collect a specimen of urine for bacteriological examination the catheter must be introduced through an external orifice for which there is no known method of sterilization. Urine collected by a catheter may therefore contain bacteria normally present in the bladder or those introduced by means of the catheter. Hugh H. Young et al.[10] say that there are organisms in the outer portion of the urethra in normal individuals; Edward L. Keyes and Russell S. Ferguson[11] say that the genitourinary tract is "emphatically" not sterile. E. Perearnau[12] and William H. Park and Anna W. Williams[13] say that coli organisms appear to be taken to the bladder by the blood stream as well as by way of the urethra. Young et al. reported that, in 600 cases of bladder infections, 351 were infected by the colon group. Other microorganisms found in cystitis are the proteus, typhoid, and tubercle bacilli, the gonococcus, and strains of the staphylococcus and streptococcus. None of these microorganisms are spore-bearing, which indicates that sterilization of the equipment for catheterization by boiling, which is effective in the

---

* Gold, Harry (ed.): _Cornell Conferences on Therapy,_ Vol. IV. The Macmillan Company, New York, 1951, p. 298.

† Cabot, Hugh, and Giles, Mary D.: _Surgical Nursing,_ 4th ed. W. B. Saunders Co., Philadelphia, 1940, p. 415.

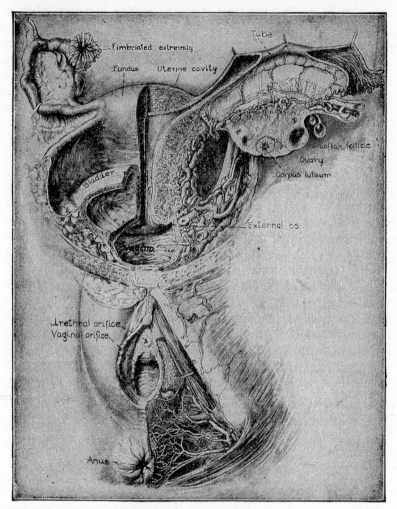

Figure 202. Female generative tract showing internal and external organs. Note normal position of urethral orifice between the clitoris and the vaginal orifice. (Reproduced from Frohse Life-size Anatomical Charts. Courtesy of A. J. Nystrom & Co., New York City.)

destruction of vegetative forms, may be an adequate method of sterilization. Whether pathogenic spore-formers are a menace to the bladder, however, is difficult to say with any certainty. Edwin O. Jordan and William Burrows[14] state that the spore-producing *Clostridium welchii* has been found in infections of the genitourinary tract. Since such infections, though rare, are nearly always fatal, sterilization of the equipment by steam under pressure is desirable.

Although the bacterial agent is the direct cause of infection, injury to the mucous membrane is the predisposing factor. Urologists repeatedly state that the normal bladder and urethra with intact mucous surface can protect themselves from infection, but that trauma produces a vulnerable spot upon which otherwise helpless invaders can gain a foothold. The importance of maintaining the integrity of the tissues suggests that smooth, pliable, and unbreakable catheters not too large in size, should be used; that they should be well lubricated and skillfully handled. Although metal, glass, and rubber catheters all are used, medical opinion favors a pliable catheter. Of 26 urologists in 14 states, 19 advocated the use of rubber catheters by physicians and nurses for all types of cases; the remainder advocated metal catheters for female patients. Twenty-four physicians thought glass catheters contraindicated in general practice. Traumata thought to be caused by catheters were reported in greater numbers from glass and metal than from rubber instruments. Ten urologists had known of more than one case in which a portion of a glass catheter was left in the bladder; only one case of a broken-off rubber catheter was reported. By comparative studies of the reaction of more than 50 women in a series of catheterizations with metal, glass, and rubber instruments, it was shown that there was little if any difference in the sensations aroused by the insertion of the three different types. The insertion of the catheters caused no appreciable discomfort except where there was some urethritis. After considering the safety of the patient, his comfort should be the next most important factor in determining the type of catheter to use.*

Too much emphasis cannot be placed on the skillful handling of the catheter. It can be manipulated more sensitively if grasped in the fingers rather than by a forcep. If a stiff catheter is used, it may be held with a clean hand far enough from the tip to make its introduction bacteriologically safe, but a rubber catheter has to be held much nearer the tip and the worker should therefore wear a sterile glove.

Since the meatus cannot be sterilized and should not be irritated, an effective cleansing is probably all that should be attempted. The removal of the bacteria with a neutral detergent may be more effective than the use of antiseptics that can inhibit or destroy few bacteria in so short a period of contact. Cotton sponges are recommended because they are less likely to irritate. In order to reduce the bacteria on the area as much as possible, sterile sponges are used and are manipulated with a sterile instrument which keeps the worker's hand clean for holding the catheter.

Catheter lubricants may be one of the hydrocarbons, such as mineral oil or petroleum jelly, one of the vegetable oils, or a lubricating jelly with a water base. Although the oily substances are more effective as lubricants, the water-soluble jellies are preferred by many physicians. They are absorbed by the tissues and leave the urethra closed, whereas oils, particularly inorganic oils, tend to remain on the surface of the mucous membrane and provide a pathway over which microorganisms gain access to the bladder. Another reason for using water-soluble lubricants is that they do not destroy rubber catheters as the oils, especially the hydrocarbons, do.

The *distance to insert the catheter* depends upon the length of the urethra; George A. Piersol[15] gives the average length in the female as about 3.5 cm (1½ in); and 17½ cm (7 in.) in the male, there being much more variation in the male than in

---

* Studies referred to above were made in the Department of Nursing Education, Teachers College, Columbia University, 1934 and 1935. (Unpublished.)

the female. The urine begins to flow as soon as the eye of the catheter reaches the bladder. If the catheter is inserted too far toward the end of the catheterization the opening may be occluded by the superior bladder wall that descends to the base of the bladder as the organ is emptied; withdrawing the catheter slightly frees the opening and allows the operator to completely empty the cavity. The catheter should not be inserted too far, because it is possible to injure the lining of the bladder, and even to puncture the wall with a stiff catheter if enough force is exerted.

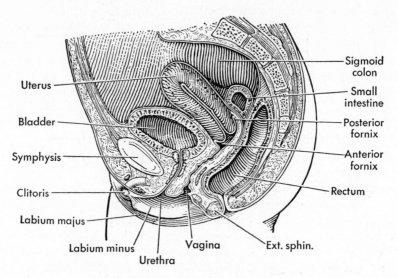

Figure 203. Median section of the female pelvis. Note the direction a catheter should take to follow the normal curve of the urethra. (Kimber, D. C.; Gray, C. E.; Stackpole, C. E.; and Leavell, L. C.: *Textbook of Anatomy and Physiology,* 13th ed. The Macmillan Company, New York, 1955.)

Introduction of the catheter is often made difficult by abnormalities in the meatus and urethra. The orifice varies in shape and position in the female, but is usually a sagittal slit in the center of the papilla just above the opening of the vagina and about 2½ cm (1 in.) below the clitoris. In some cases it is in the anterior vaginal wall and cannot be seen. The meatus is often difficult to find in children, or if the area is inflamed and swollen, or if the vagina is packed postoperatively. Packing in the vagina tends to displace the surrounding parts.

Since a living organism involuntarily protects itself from harmful objects, there is a natural withdrawal of the body and a contraction of the urethral orifice when an attempt is made to insert a catheter. Strong emotions and chilling, interfering with relaxation of the urethra, make the introduction of the catheter difficult. In preparation, the nurse should see that the patient is warm and, if possible, free from fear and excitement. Embarrassment over exposure and fear of being hurt are frequent causes of stress. Assurance of privacy, adequate draping, and the use of gloves or finger cots for the necessary handling of the genitalia may reduce the patient's embarrassment. A careful and truthful explanation of the procedure will relieve the patient's fear of pain if he or she has confidence in the nurse. The treatment should be expeditious and so arranged that the patient is not left alone. The area should be well lighted so that there is no doubt as to whether the catheter is in the meatus. After the tip of the catheter is inserted, a few moments should be allowed for relaxation of the sphincter before introducing the catheter farther.

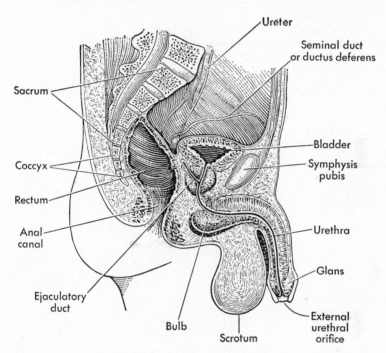

Figure 204.   Median section of the male pelvis. Note the curve in the urethra that should be modified during the introduction of a catheter. (Kimber, D. C.; Gray, C. E.; Stackpole, C. E.; and Leavell, L. C.: *Textbook of Anatomy and Physiology,* 13th ed. The Macmillan Company, New York, 1955.)

If the patient concentrates on deep breathing, looks about the room, or does anything that takes his mind off the introduction of the catheter, relaxation is fostered. The catheter should be inserted by the operator in an upward and backward direction in the female; this is the course of the urethra with the patient lying in the dorsal recumbent position.

Introduction of a catheter in the male is more difficult than in the female, because the urethra is longer and contains several curves. Where it passes through the prostate gland and at various other points, there may be constriction caused by contraction of the surrounding tissue. In order to straighten the passageway as much as possible, the penis is held at an angle of 60 deg. Ralph M. LeComte[16] says

How the Drainage System Operates

Fluid flows from flask to reservoir at rate prescribed by physician.

When the reservoir is filled, fluid flows through tubing 10 to bladder and rises simultaneously in glass manometer 11 and rubber tubing 2C. This continues until fluid fills the curve of tubing. At this point the liquid begins to flow down into the drainage bottle thereby creating suction, the loop acting as a siphon to empty the reservoir of solution and to drain the bladder of its contents.

When the reservoir is emptied, air enters the system through the manometer tube, thus breaking the siphonage system and starting a new cycle.

Note: The top of the reservoir must be 12 in. below the level of the symphysis pubis. The size of the reservoir influences the length of the cycle, and the distance of the loop above the bladder determines the maximum pressure to which the bladder is subjected.

This distance between the bottom of the irrigating bottle and the lower surface of the stopper in the reservoir bottle should be 40 in.

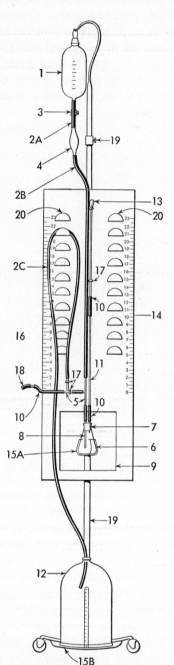

Parts of Apparatus

1. Irrigating bottle of sterile solution as ordered by physician
2A. Pressure tubing (5/32-in. bore), 12 in. long
2B. Same type of tubing, 18 in. long
2C. Same type of tubing, 72 in. long
3. Compression clamp to regulate flow
4. Drip bulb (no air vent)
5. Glass T tube, ¼-in. diameter
6. Glass reservoir, 4-oz capacity
7. Two-hole rubber stopper
8. Glass tube with fused end
9. Window in board
10. Rubber tubing, 5/32-in. bore
11. Glass tube, 28 in. long, ¼-in. diameter
12. Drainage bottle, 4 qt
13. Gauze filter over top of manometer tube
14. Calibration to facilitate regulation of bladder drainage (marking on each side for convenience only)
15A. Rack to hold reservoir
15B. Platform with attached calibrated metal strip on which drainage bottle rests
16. Level of symphysis pubis must be marked or recorded on board
17. Clamps to hold apparatus in position
18. Tubing to catheter, 5/32-in. bore
19. Adjustable standard
20. Metal carriers for rubber tubing

Note: Catheter must have a lumen at least twice that of the fused tube 8.

Figure 205. Diagram showing apparatus for tidal drainage of the urinary bladder. (Adaptation of Munro's apparatus by Helen Gillies, New York City.)

it should be drawn forward and upward from the body to stretch it slightly and in so doing straighten the anterior urethra.

Because the introduction of an instrument into the bladder is accompanied by danger of injury and infection, the nurse should use all her skill and ingenuity to get the patient to void normally in cases of retention. Such measures have been discussed in Chapter 14. If catheterization is unavoidable, the procedure must be performed in as aseptic a manner as possible and with the utmost gentleness in order to reduce the danger of trauma.

To prevent the necessity for repeated catheterization in cases where the neuromuscular mechanism is out of order, as in injuries to the lower part of the spinal cord, a retention catheter is left in the urethra. This may be opened periodically for drainage, or it may be attached to an apparatus which empties the bladder when the pressure within it approaches that which stimulates normal micturition. Periodic emptying with or without accompanying irrigation is more nearly physiological than allowing the bladder to drain constantly. Tidal drainage, as this is called, is described in this chapter.

2. CATHETERIZATION OF THE URINARY BLADDER

Definition.   The word *catheter* comes from a Greek word meaning a thing put down. Catheterization of the bladder is the introduction of a tube into the bladder, the tube being passed through the external opening or meatus. The general purpose of the treatment is to drain the bladder.

Therapeutic Uses.   Catheterization is performed for the following reasons: (1) to get as clean a specimen of urine as possible for diagnostic purposes; (2) to determine whether the failure to void at all or to void a normal amount is due to inability to expel urine from the bladder (retention), or to failure of the kidneys to secrete urine (suppression); (3) to empty the bladder or remove a portion of the urine when a condition of retention is thought to exist; and (4) to prevent the patient's voiding voluntarily or involuntarily if there are surgical wounds, bedsores, or other conditions that make it important to keep the genitalia and surrounding area clean and dry.

Equipment.   Several catheters usually are brought to the bedside in case one is accidentally contaminated, or the instrument has to be removed and reinserted. A pliable catheter, made of plastic or rubber, is the safest type, and should always be used for male patients, for children, for patients who are irrational and cannot be relied upon to keep still during the procedure; for obstetrical cases before delivery; for patients who have a urethral stricture or for those subject to urethral spasm; for patients who have had pelvic operations; and when the vagina is packed. Woven silk catheters are fairly pliable, but are not very satisfactory because they are destroyed by sterilization with heat. Commercially sterilized, disposable, plastic catheters are now available and highly recommended. The caliber of the catheter is determined by the size and condition of the urethra. Plastic and rubber catheters range from #10 to #22 French.

If a pliable catheter is used, sterile gloves should be added to the equipment; otherwise the nurse must scrub her hands immediately before handling the catheter. Unless the scrubbing facilities are in the room or the nurse has an assistant, this necessitates leaving the patient, which is to be avoided if possible. If a stiff catheter is used, rubber finger cots may be worn on the thumb and first finger of the left hand when they are used to separate the labia. A sterile lubricant is essential. Lubricating jelly may be sterilized by boiling the tube each time it is used, or by autoclaving individual portions in small jars with screw tops. A small amount of

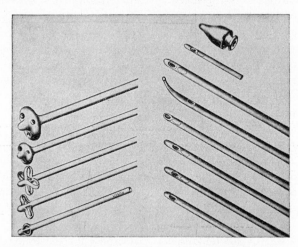

Figure 206. Various urological catheters. (*Left, top to bottom*) Pesser catheter, 30-mm head, 3 eyes, natural rubber latex with reinforced tip; Pesser catheter, smaller size, 3 eyes, natural rubber latex with reinforced tip; four-wing Malecot catheter, natural rubber latex with reinforced tip; two two-wing Malecot catheters, natural rubber latex with reinforced tips. (*Right, top to bottom*) Urethral tip, natural rubber; female catheter, solid tip, 2 eyes; Robinson catheter, hollow tip, 2 eyes; Tiermann catheter, coudé solid tip, olivary, 1 eye; whistle-tip catheter, 1 eye; Robinson catheter, red rubber, hollow tip, 2 eyes; Robinson catheter, amber, hollow tip, 2 eyes; Nélaton catheter, red rubber, solid tip, 1 eye. (Courtesy of Clay-Adams Co., New York City.)

warm detergent or antiseptic prescribed by the physician, such as pHisoHex or benzylkonium (Zephiran), with large cotton balls and forceps to apply it, will be needed for cleaning the meatus and surrounding area.

Several low, covered containers should be provided for the collection of urine. In an initial catheterization, provision should be made for the collection of 2000 cc (2 qt) of urine, as in retention patients may have this amount in the bladder. Since the nurse cannot leave the patient to get another vessel, she is in a very awkward situation if the containers she has provided are inadequate. A paper bag or other type of receptacle should be provided for dry waste. A small rubber square with cotton cover or a waterproof paper pad is used to protect the bed. No sterile draping is necessary, although with a male patient it may be convenient to have a sterile fenestrated sheet or several sterile towels with which to surround the penis after the glans and meatus have been cleaned.

All this equipment, with the exception of the bed protector which may be kept in the patient's unit, should be brought to the bedside on a covered tray or cart, together with the catheter, lubricant, gloves, and cleansing material. Moistureproof wrappers, covered trays, or small drums are used to keep the equipment sterile.

Before preparing the equipment, the catheter should be scrutinized for defects. Only perfect instruments should be used; rubber catheters that have lost their resiliency and cracked or roughened instruments should be discarded.

Preparation of the Patient. Gain the patient's cooperation by explaining the necessity for the treatment. As in all such cases, what is said to the patient depends upon his intelligence, former experience, and condition. It is most desirable that he accept the treatment; an unreceptive attitude inevitably hinders relaxation and thereby increases discomfort and possible danger.

Have the patient lying on his back near the side of the bed most convenient for the nurse. In catheterization of a female patient, the knees should be flexed, the feet flat on the bed, and the legs well separated while the meatus is cleaned and the bladder emptied. If the patient is weak or irrational, the legs should be supported in this position with rubber-covered pillows. In order to keep the irrational patient in the desired posture, restraining devices or several assistants may be necessary. Place the waterproof protector over the bedding between the legs and slightly under the buttocks; arrange the clothing in neat folds above the hips; replace the upper bedclothes with two treatment blankets folded in half lengthwise. Both these blankets remain over the chest and arms, but are separated over the lower abdomen so that the genitalia are exposed and each leg is wrapped or covered with one of the folded blankets. In hot weather very thin blankets or cotton sheets should be used for this draping. See that the room is warm; and, if the patient shows signs of being cold, place hot-water bottles at the feet. It is important for the patient to be warm, not only for his comfort and welfare but also as a means of promoting relaxation of the urethral musculature.

In the preparation of a male patient, the chest may be covered with a folded treatment blanket, and the upper bedclothes turned down to the pubes and covered with a waterproof square. The patient should be protected from unnecessary exposure, and a clean area provided around the penis by using sterile towels or a fenestrated sheet. A pillow under the knees promotes relaxation.

A good light must be directed on the area. A standing lamp with a flexible neck is satisfactory. In case the lighting in the room is not adequate, a flashlight, if available, may be substituted. *It is essential that the nurse see the meatus before attempting to insert the catheter.*

If a catheterized specimen is required, a sterile covered vessel should be added to the equipment. A 300-cc (10-oz) glass bottle with an open mouth covered by a metal screw cap or a fluted paper cap is commonly used. More than 180 cc (6 oz) of urine is rarely required for examination. The physician ordinarily wants this collected after the urine has begun to flow freely. If for any reason the whole amount, or a sample from the whole amount obtained, is required, the covered pans used to receive the urine must be kept sterile or a very large sterile bottle used for the collection of the urine. It is undesirable to transfer the specimen from one container to another as it might be contaminated in the process.

All equipment should be within easy reach of the worker and on a table beside the bed rather than on the bed itself. Materials placed on the bed may be accidentally contaminated, solutions upset, or the patient's movements limited.

Suggested Procedure for Catheterization of a Female Patient. If a rubber catheter is used, put on a pair of sterile rubber gloves; if these are not available, scrub the hands under running water as in preparation for any aseptic procedure. Should a stiff catheter be used, wash the hands before bringing the equipment to the bedside. When gloves are not worn, it is desirable to protect the thumb and forefinger of the left hand with rubber finger cots. Holding the sponges with forceps in the right hand, moisten them in the detergent or antiseptic solution and clean the genitalia; remove any secretion from the labia majora, separate and lift upward the labia minora with the thumb and forefinger of the left hand, exposing the meatus; clean the area around the meatus with particular care. It is desirable, but not necessary, to remove the detergent with sterile water; the area should then be dried. Throughout this cleansing process, use a gentle but firm downward motion and take a fresh sponge for each stroke. The last sponge may be left in the vaginal orifice to keep any vaginal secretions from spreading upward over the meatus. (When this is done, care should be taken that the sponge is placed in the orifice and not packed in the vagina, as this would cause pressure on the urethra and interfere with the passage of the catheter.) Without removing the fingers of the left hand from the labia, place the receptacle for the urine in position on the bed, dip the tip of the catheter into the lubricant, and insert the catheter into the urethral meatus without allowing anything to touch that portion that is to come in contact with the urethra. If a pliable catheter is used, it must be grasped near enough the tip to control its direction; if the catheter is rigid, it may be held as much as 4 in. from its eye without any loss of control by the operator. After relaxation has followed the initial contraction of the urethra, introduce the catheter about 4 cm (1½ in.), or until the urine begins to flow. Since the bladder may in some cases be empty, the rule "until the urine begins to flow" must not be followed too literally. The catheter should not be introduced much more than the supposed length of the urethra without consulting a physician. When introducing the catheter, bear in mind the upward and backward direction of the urethra. If a catheterized specimen is desired, keep the outer end of the catheter sterile until after the specimen is collected. This is received in a small sterile glass bottle after the urine begins to flow freely. If the physician wants to examine the whole amount, or a sample taken from the whole amount, collect the urine in a large sterile bottle or vessel that can be sent to the laboratory.

As soon as the urine ceases to flow freely, or drips from the end of the catheter, withdraw the instrument slightly to see whether any more urine will flow with the eye of the instrument nearer the urethral outlet. Withdraw the catheter slowly, and when the bladder appears to be empty, remove the catheter gently. If only a prescribed amount of urine is to be removed, the nurse should have some way of determining when this has been withdrawn. The procedure can be stopped at any time by removing the catheter from the bladder. After the removal of the catheter, clean the meatus of any excess lubricant. Rearrange the clothing and bedding, remove the equipment, and leave the surroundings in order.

Send a specimen, if requested, to the laboratory, labeling it with the patient's name, address (nursing unit and service in the hospital), and date and hour collected. Indicate the kind of specimen, and the type of examination desired. In some cases the diagnosis is noted, and almost always the name of the attending physician is included.

Recording the Treatment. Chart the treatment, the time, pain or discomfort occasioned; also the amount, appearance, and any unusual odor of the urine withdrawn.

Suggested Procedure for Catheterization of a Male Patient. The operator should wear rubber gloves or prepare the hands as for any aseptic procedure. With the left hand retract the foreskin, exposing the meatus, situated in the center of the glans. Using the forceps in the right hand to keep this hand uncontaminated, clean the area surrounding the meatus. After lubricating the catheter insert it into the meatus, gently stretching the penis with the left hand and lifting it to an angle of about 60 deg in order to straighten the urethral canal as much as possible. The catheter is inserted approximately 17½ cm (7 in.) or until the urine begins to flow. The same precaution should be taken with the male patient as with the female patient—not to insert the catheter an unreasonable distance. The bladder may be empty, and it is possible to injure its lining by forcing a catheter along its walls. Since the length and size of the penis vary in different individuals, the size of the catheter and the length of the insertion will therefore have to be determined in each case. The passage of an instrument through the male urethra is often a difficult procedure. Before attempting it, the operator should get a clear picture in his mind of the structure and position of the urethra and surrounding tissues; this is essential for an intelligent direction of the course of the catheter and for manipulation of the parts in such a manner as to eliminate as far as possible the urethral folds and curvatures.

The physician usually passes the catheter in the male patient or supervises its passage. Exposure and handling of the genitalia in medical treatment and nursing care are generally less embarrassing to men and women if members of their own sex are in attendance upon them; for this reason the catheterization of a male patient is usually performed by a man physician in order to reduce the embarrassment, which is not only unpleasant for the patient but may interfere with relaxation. In some hospitals men nurses or special technicians are taught to give this treatment. Any professional woman nurse should be prepared to carry out the procedure when need arises and a physician or man nurse is not available.

3. IRRIGATION OF THE URINARY BLADDER

Definition. The term *irrigation* scarcely needs interpretation. Irrigation of the bladder is similar to irrigation of any other body cavity. It consists of several injections of 150 to 400 cc (5 to 13 oz) each, with provision made for emptying the bladder through the catheter after each injection. This is commonly referred to as a "hand irrigation" in contrast to the more mechanical tidal irrigation described on page 887.

Thrapeutic Uses. Irrigations are given for the following reasons: (1) to clean the bladder; (2) as a means of applying heat to the mucous lining (this is rarely desired, for the inflamed bladder and urethra are highly sensitive, and temperatures above that of the body are likely to cause pain); and (3) to medicate the lining of the bladder for which usually an antiseptic, an astringent, or an anticoagulant is used. Cystitis is now more often treated with systemic drugs than with local applications. Penicillin and the sulfa drugs are particularly effective although methena-mine (Urotropin), mandelic acid, acriflavine, and other drugs are often used.[17]

Selection of Method. ① An irrigation of the bladder may be given with a reservoir, such as a plastic or glass container, or an irrigating can, filled with solution and attached to a two-way, or Y-shaped, catheter. The fluid flows into the bladder through one arm of the catheter and out through the other. ② The fluid may also be introduced through a funnel attached to the catheter, inverting the funnel to empty the bladder, and repeating these alternate steps until the prescribed amount of solution has been used or until the return is clear. ③ A third method is to inject the solution through the catheter with a large syringe, detaching the syringe and emptying the bladder by lowering the catheter, and repeating this process until the treatment is completed.

If a large amount of solution is prescribed, or if it is ordered for its thermal effect, the reservoir method is probably best, since it maintains the solution at a fairly uniform temperature. Because the equipment is simple and available in most cases, and is easily transported by nurses caring for patients in their homes, the funnel method is often used. The disadvantages of this method are that the solution cools quickly, and unless the worker is very skilled, the instruments are contaminated, air is introduced with the liquid, and the bedding is soiled. The syringe method is easy, the equipment is not difficult to procure, and it can be transported in a small space. The temperature of the solution probably remains more constant when the syringe is used than when the funnel is employed, and there is less risk of injecting air and soiling the bedding.

Equipment. To the articles collected for catheterization should be added a sterile calibrated container for the prescribed amount of solution and either a glass-and-rubber syringe or a funnel for injecting it. If an irrigating can is used, the solution may be carried to the bedside in it; for a female catheterization a two-way catheter, which has a short piece of rubber tubing and a clamp on the outflow arm, is needed. Clamps should likewise be provided for the inflow tube. In case a rubber catheter is used, a glass Y tube is inserted into the open end of the catheter to provide a passageway for the inflow and outflow.

A fairly large shallow pan, which can be placed on the bed near the meatus, must be provided for the return flow. A covered pail, large enough to hold the entire amount of fluid used in the treatment should be conveniently placed for emptying this pan each time it fills.

The *irrigating fluids* commonly used are physiological sodium chloride solution; boric acid 1:50; mercury compounds in low concentrations, such as bichloride of mercury 1:10,000, mercuric oxycyanide 1:5000, and merbromin (Mercurochrome) 1:100; silver preparations in low concentrations as, for example, silver nitrate 1:8000 and protein silver (Protargol) 1:10,000; acriflavine 1:4000 to 1:8000; and potassium permanganate in a strength of 1:5000 to 1:30,000. Sodium citrate 1:8000 is sometimes used to prevent the formation of clots.[18] The nurse is not responsible for selecting the kind of solution or the strength. She should know that high concentrations of irritating drugs are not ordinarily prescribed for the bladder, and if she should see an order written for such a treatment she is justified in questioning the physician as to whether there may not have been some error in the writing of the order or misinterpretation in reading it. If, as sometimes happens, the physician orders a bladder irrigation without specifying the kind of solution and the nurse is unable to communicate with him, she could safely use physiological saline.

Unless otherwise ordered, the solution should be administered at body temperature, that is, it should be around 37.2° C (99° F) as it enters the bladder. Lowsley and Kirwin say temperatures ranging from 37.8° to 43.3° C (100° to 110° F) may be used according to the tolerance of the patient. In cystitis and urethritis the mucous membrane is highly sensitive to temperatures varying appreciably from that of the body. It is, therefore, important to regulate accurately the temperature of the solution. At room temperatures—around 25° C (77° F), 1000 cc (1 qt) of solution should be prepared at approximately 42° C (107.6° F) to allow for the cooling that takes place while the patient is catheterized and the solution injected.

Suggested Procedure.   Catheterize the patient in the usual manner, keeping the outlet of the catheter uncontaminated. The irrigation may be done in any of the following ways, according to the type of equipment used:

No. 1. Using an irrigator: Hang or support the reservoir so that the surface of the liquid is not more than 15 to 20 cm (6 to 8 in.) above the level of the meatus. Attach the tubing to one arm of the two-way catheter or, if a rubber catheter is used, attach the tubing to the catheter by a glass Y-shaped tube. Expel the air from the tubing before attaching the catheter. Place the basin to receive the return under the outflow tube; clamp the outlet tube. Open the inflow tube and inject the solution in such an amount as to get the degree of distention prescribed by the physician. The amount introduced at one time varies from 30 to 500 cc (1 to 16 oz), according to the condition of the bladder and the purpose of the treatment. The physician may direct that the treatment be given so that the bladder is distended with increasingly large amounts. Between these injections of fluid, the bladder is drained by opening the outflow tube. The order for the treatment may stipulate that a definite amount of solution is to be used, or the physician may request that the irrigating process be kept up until the return from the bladder is clear. At the termination of the irrigation, clamp the tubing, remove the catheter gently, and complete the treatment according to the directions for catheterization on page 882.

No. 2. Using a funnel: Attach the funnel to the catheter with the uncontaminated right hand. Place the basin for collection of the return on the bed conveniently near the meatus. Hold the funnel with one hand and with the other pour the desired amount of solution from the calibrated container down the side of the funnel. The amount of solution to be introduced at one time varies, as just stated. The physician may want the same amount introduced at each injection, or he may request that the amount be increased with each injection. When introducing the solution, do not allow the funnel to empty. If the tubing is allowed to empty, air will be sucked into the bladder. To empty the bladder between injections of the irrigating solution, pinch the tubing, lower and invert the funnel over the basin for the return. The alternate processes of filling and emptying the bladder are kept up as directed above, and the treatment terminated in the same manner as under method No. 1.

No. 3. Using a syringe: Clamp or pinch the catheter used to empty the bladder so that it will not drain dry, fill the Asepto syringe from the calibrated container of solu-- tion; attach the syringe tip to the catheter, being careful not to contaminate either, and inject the solution slowly into the bladder. If more than one syringeful is to be injected before emptying the bladder, pinch the tubing, detach and refill the syringe, and proceed as above. In order to empty the bladder, pinch the tubing, detach the syringe, lower the tubing over the basin for the return and remove the pressure on the tubing. Repeat these alternate processes of filling and emptying the bladder and terminate the procedure as directed under method No. 1.

Recording the Treatment. Chart the treatment and the time at which it was administered; any pain or discomfort experienced; the kind, concentration, and amount of solution used; the appearance of the return—whether it contained mucus, pus, blood-tinged particles, or other substances indicative of the condition of the bladder. Record the amount of urine withdrawn before the irrigation and describe its appearance.

4. INSTILLATION OF THE URINARY BLADDER

Definition. An *instillation* of the bladder is the introduction of a small amount of sterile water or some medication into the bladder through a catheter. The general purpose of the treatment is to distend the bladder walls or to medicate the mucous membrane. Therefore, the patient is encouraged to retain the solution for several hours or until the next normal voiding or appointed catheterization.

Therapeutic Uses. Some reasons for bladder instillations are: (1) to keep diseased bladder walls apart; and (2) to apply medications, such as antiseptics, astringents, anticoagulants, or neutralizing solutions, to the lining of the bladder. Some hospitals have standing orders for the instillation of a specified solution following every catheterization.

Equipment. Everything listed as necessary for catheterization is needed for bladder instillation and, in addition, a small funnel and glass and rubber connections to attach the funnel to the catheter. A glass-and-rubber syringe may be used in place of the funnel. A calibrated container, such as a measuring glass or cup, should be provided for the drug to be instilled. It is desirable to have the drug near body temperature, but chemicals whose composition is altered by heat should not be warmed. The drugs for irrigation (p. 884), as well as mild silver protein (Argyrol, 5 per cent), are used. Urinary antiseptics given systemically in many cases may be used locally. The antibiotics and sulfa drugs, for example, are sometimes instilled.

Suggested Procedure. Catheterize the patient in the usual manner, completely emptying the bladder but not draining the catheter. Attach the funnel to the catheter and, holding the funnel about 12½ cm (5 in.) above the level of the meatus, pour into the side of the funnel the liquid to be instilled. Pinch the rubber attachment, or the rubber catheter if one is used, when the funnel empties; remove the catheter gently. Before giving the treatment the nurse should learn whether the physician wants the drug retained for several hours or whether he wishe the drug to be retained for a short period only. When irritating antiseptics are used, some physicians direct that the drug be immediately siphoned from the bladder.

Recording the Treatment. Chart the treatment, the time at which it was given, any attendant pain or discomfort, and the nature, strength, and amount of the drug. Record the catheterization preceding the instillation in the usual manner.

5. TIDAL IRRIGATION (TIDAL DRAINAGE)

Definition.   Tidal irrigation, also called tidal drainage, is a mechanically controlled method of gradually filling the bladder with an irrigating solution, in addition to the urine, and then periodically emptying it. The apparatus enables the operator to control the pressure exerted on the bladder wall and the intervals at which the vesicle is emptied.

Therapeutic Uses.   Tidal irrigation has the following therapeutic uses: (1) to empty the bladder periodically when injuries of the spinal cord or surgery of the bladder interfere with normal functions; (2) to combine with periodic emptying the gradual distention of the bladder within physiological limits to prevent retention and increase the tone in an atonic bladder and to distend and prevent continuous emptying of a hypertonic bladder; (3) to combine with the preceding the action of antiseptic, astringent, anticoagulant, or neutralizing solutions used in periodic filling of the bladder or that used in additional flushings; and (4) to prevent bed wetting and maceration of the skin of an incontinent patient.[19, 20, 21]

As is usual in therapy there is difference of opinion on the value of tidal drainage. It is most often recommended as an intermediate step in rehabilitation of the patient with "a cord bladder." This term is used for a bladder which does not respond normally to pressure within because the spinal cord has been injured and nerve pathways, supplying the bladder, destroyed. If there is incontinence following such an injury and the bladder is continually emptying itself, or if retention (usually with overflow) exists, some physicians believe that an automatic function can be more rapidly established if tidal drainage, with its gradual filling and periodic emptying of the bladder, is instituted. H. Carey Bumpus et al.,[22] describing the successful treatment of a series of patients with cord injuries, say that tidal drainage was used in a few cases. They believe that the person's inability to control bladder function, however, is due chiefly to thickening of the musculature at the mouth of the bladder. They suggest that this may be the result of the unusual effort required to empty the organ following paralysis. They report success with surgical removal of some of the tissue at the internal sphincter, or mouth. After operation, with this impediment to emptying removed, they find most patients could train the abdominal muscles and external sphincter to take over the control of the bladder contents. Tidal drainage was used by Bumpus and associates postoperatively in conjunction with bladder irrigation "by hand." They say: "It was found that irrigations at least 3 times a day and once at night with piston syringe kept the bladder cleaner than did tidal drainage alone."*

P. W. Nathan,[23] reporting a series of suprapubic cystostomies with indwelling catheters, and discussing the experience of others, concluded that chemotherapy was

---

* Bumpus, H. Carey, et al.: "Urologic Complications in Injuries of the Spinal Cord," *J.A.M.A.*, **33**:366, (Feb.) 1947.

more effective than irrigations, including the tidal variety, in controlling infection. Wilson Stegman,[24] discussing experience with 200 consecutive bladder operations, urges the "total avoidance" of bladder irrigations postoperatively. He makes the following points: (1) tissues should not be disturbed postoperatively since the collection of fibrin should be encouraged; (2) suction may remove a clot and start bleeding; (3) the solution used in irrigation might conceivably enter the vascular system; (4) irrigations are likely to be painful; and (5) they may introduce infectious material. His surgical patients are treated with simple drainage from indwelling catheters. A. Lloyd Stockwell, discussing Stegman's report, urges a sterile closed system of gravity drainage, using large tubing. Obstructions in catheters can often be removed by squeezing them or by applying suction with a hand syringe. Both these physicians urge that the drainage tubes be less than 1 meter (39.4 in.) in length and that the drainage bottle be hung well above the floor. A long tube exerts so much suction that it draws blood clots into the lumen and obstructs the tube.

Donald Munro, who has done so much to develop tidal drainage, values it highly in rehabilitation of patients with cord injuries affecting bladder function. He thinks the incidence of urinary sepsis almost five times as great without tidal drainage as with it. Basing his judgment on his own experience and a survey of medical opinion, George C. Prather[25] says that tidal drainage is an excellent way of draining and irrigating the bladder but that it is not essential for the optimum rehabilitation of the paralyzed bladder.

Selection of Equipment and Method.   All the methods the writer has seen, or seen described, combine periodic emptying of the bladder by siphonage with the gradual filling of the bladder by secreted urine mixed with a sterile solution which flows by gravity from a reservoir and tubing. The rate of the solution's flow is controlled with clamps and a drip bulb. Arthur E. MacNeill complains that there is confusion in the use of the terms "tidal drainage" and "tidal irrigation." In criticism of the procedure as an irrigating method MacNeill says: "Regardless of their efficiency, the nearest such apparatus can come to irrigating the bladder is mixing of irrigating fluid with considerable quantities of urine."* He thinks all such apparatus should make it possible to irrigate the bladder with clean solution as frequently as is desired. He mentions "a complex apparatus" that is to his knowledge the only one that provides this feature. William F. McKenna in 1948 and O. A. Nelson and A. W. Kretz in 1950 describe similar methods, although the latter offer some improvements.

Nelson and Kretz outline the following "requirements" of a satisfactory instrument:

1. The action of the apparatus must be positive so that siphonage invariably takes place as soon as the level of the fluid reaches a certain height.

2. The bladder should be completely empty before each siphonage action ceases.

3. The apparatus must be so constructed that the intravesical pressure can be varied at will.

* MacNeill, Arthur E.: "Urologic Complications" (correspondence), *J.A.M.A.*, **133**:1237, (Apr.), 1947.

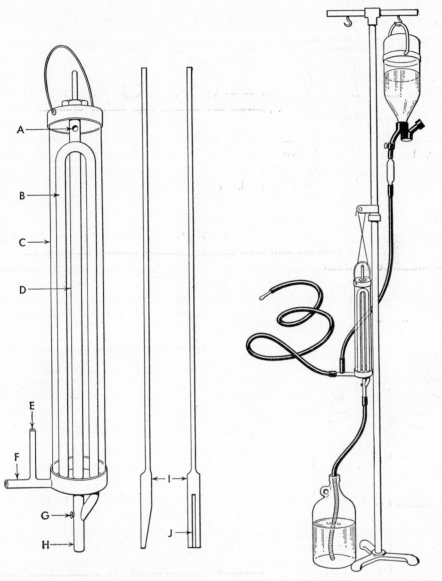

Figure 207. (*Left*). Apparatus with essential measurements for a tidal irrigator. (*A*) Hole in pipe; (*B*) inverted U-shaped tube; (*C*) exterior container, a glass tube; (*D*) central pipe; (*E*) connection for irrigating solution; (*F*) connection for catheter; (*G*) set screw, to position sluice gate; (*H*) connection for waste container; (*I*) sluice gate and stem; (*J*) groove in sluice gate. (Courtesy of Dr. O. A. Nelson.)

Figure 208 (*right*). Tidal irrigator with apparatus for essential measurements in position. (Nelson, O. A., and Kretz, A. W.: "Improved Tidal Irrigator," *Northwest Med.*, **49**:374, [June] 1950.)

4. Fluid remaining in the apparatus, after the siphonage has ceased, should not be washed into the bladder.

5. As far as possible, the apparatus should be simple to operate, easy to clean and sterilize.

6. The only adjustment necessary should be the placing of the high-tide point of the apparatus at the proper height in relation to the bladder and also to regulate the rate of drip of irrigating fluid.*

These authors go on to say their instrument meets all these requirements. They describe it as consisting of:

An inverted U-shaped metal tube, placed inside a glass cylinder [Figs. 207 and 208 in this text]. Each end of the cylinder is covered by a metal cap. In the top cap are three holes. Two small ones serve as air vents and a large one admits a screw-threaded truss rod which is attached to the bottom cap. A nut on top of the rod, when tightened, draws each metal cap against the respective ends of the glass cylinder, thus holding the apparatus together.

Between the bottom end of the glass cylinder and the metal cap is a rubber gasket. Through the bottom cap is placed the tube from the bladder and also the outlet arm of the inverted U-tube or siphon. The lower end of the last-mentioned tube has three features essential to the proper function of the apparatus. First, a constriction in the tube; second, an air vent; and, third, the lower end of the tube is enlarged so as to fit a sizable rubber tube which conveys the fluid to the waste container.†

Such improved equipment is not always available. Nurses must learn how to operate many kinds of tidal drainage apparatus. Figure 205 shows a setup in common use. The principles underlying all tidal drainage devices are similar.

As McKenna points out, tidal drainage should depend upon "natural phenomena" and not on "forcing mechanical instruments." The mechanism is essentially a siphon. The fluid flows into the bladder by gravity; therefore, the reservoir must be hung above the level of the bladder. Atmospheric pressure supports the column of liquid in a siphon that empties when the pressure within the bladder exceeds the atmospheric pressure, supporting the column of fluid. The pressure exerted on its contents (urine and/or the solution from the reservoir) by the bladder wall depends upon its elasticity, the strength of its muscle contraction, and the push on the pelvic organs during abdominal contraction. The height of the siphon determines the force required to push the column of liquid through it.

It is essential that doctor and nurse understand how to operate tidal drainage apparatus; it is almost equally important in some cases that the patient and his family understand it. His rehabilitation depends largely on re-establishing bladder control of which this is the first step.

The physician must always initiate tidal drainage and prescribe (1) the nature of the solution, (2) the rate of flow for the solution (drops per minute), and (3) the height of the reservoir and the siphon in relation to the symphysis pubis and the opening of the drainage or outlet arm of the tubing.

* Nelson, O. A., and Kretz, A. W.: "Improved Tidal Irrigator," *Northwest Med.*, **49**:374, (June) 1950.

† Nelson, O. A., and Kretz, A. W.: *op. cit.*

Solutions used to irrigate, medicate, and regulate pressure within the vesicle are similar to those listed for irrigation of the bladder "by hand." Since contact with the solution is protracted, irritating chemicals must be diluted. H. I. Suby and Fuller Albright[26] advise the use of a citrate solution containing magnesium when, during constant urinary drainage, there is a tendency to form phosphatic calculi, or stones.

The *rate of flow* usually varies from 40 to 60 drops per minute. At the latter rate, McKenna says the average bladder will fill in about an hour taking the patient's secretion into account; at 200 drops per minute, the bladder will empty every 10 minutes. Emptying is dependent not only on the solution's rate of flow but also on the *height of the siphon*—or the distance between the outlet to the bladder and the height of the column of liquid. The equipment is usually adjusted with the outlet to the bladder (a tubing connected to the catheter) 2 to 3 cm (about 1 in.) below the level of the anus, and the arch of the siphon about 10 cm (4 in.) above the level of the base of the bladder. With this adjustment, McKenna says: "The pressure within the bladder will not exceed that amount [10 cm]. This degree of bladder pressure is well within the limit of natural tissue elasticity of an intact bladder. . . ."*

The lower end of the drainage tube must not be too long because sufficient negative pressure may be created therein, during the drainage aspect of the cycle, to pull the bladder wall into the eye of the catheter. The drainage bottle should be suspended off the floor and *the end of the drainage tube kept above the level of fluid in the bottle*. Siphonage will not occur if the end of the drainage tube is in the fluid. McKenna recommends that all tubing be of approximately the same caliber. Authorities differ on the *size and kind of catheter*. Indwelling catheters are often used. If a balloon type is prescribed, it must be tested with 5 cc of sterile water or air before inserting it. After insertion it is inflated with 3 cc of air or sterile water to hold it in place. A balloon in poor condition can rupture and leave fragments in the bladder. Even a soft catheter makes pressure on the bladder wall, and for this and other reasons tidal drainage is discontinued periodically. To keep the balloon from pushing against the neck of the bladder, the tubing is so pinned or clipped to the bedding that it is never taut. The catheter is fixed to the leg with a narrow strip of adhesive for this same reason, or in the case of an ordinary catheter to keep it from slipping out of the urethra.

Even with the greatest care organisms will be carried into the bladder and the tissues irritated by tidal drainage. *Strict asepsis* must be observed throughout. The entire apparatus is exchanged for a fresh sterile setup every 4 to 6 days or oftener.[27]

Preparation of the Patient.   Since this is a step in the patient's rehabilitation, it is particularly important that he understand and accept it. When his cooperation is gained he can assume considerable responsibility for the management of the apparatus, and the procedures may interest rather than horrify him. The nurse must realize, however, that it is difficult for him and his family to accept so un-

---

* McKenna, William F.: "A Simple Efficient Automatic Tidal Drainage Apparatus," *Urol. & Cutan. Rev.,* **52:**18, (Jan.) 1948.

natural a means of performing a body function and she must be sympathetic if they move slowly in this direction. As in all such therapy, the nurse amplifies and reinforces the doctor's original explanation and instruction. Eleanora A. Seidel recommends giving the patient a demonstration with a dummy setup, using a balloon for a bladder, before starting the procedure. To understand tidal drainage one must know bladder psysiology, at least to some extent. Bladder capacity was discussed in the beginning of this chapter, and micturition, incontinence, and retention in Chapter 14. [All bladder therapy is aimed at the ultimate goal of making it possible for the patient to control the emptying of the bladder, to void painlessly, and to hold comfortably in the bladder sufficient urine to enable him to carry out normal daily activities without undue interruptions.] Assessment of the individual patient's capacity for storing urine, or the response of the neuromuscular elements of the bladder on filling, is made with a manometer. Since tidal drainage involves cystometry this diagnostic procedure should perhaps be discussed before continuing the description of tidal drainage. These measurements are made by the physician before prescribing the conditions of tidal drainage.

Cystometry. Measurement of pressure exerted by the bladder wall on its contents is called cystometry. The process is based on the same physical principles as those in measuring the pressure of the vessel walls on the contained blood or the pressure of the meninges on the spinal fluid. Liquids in a membranous sac behave the same way all over the body, the pressure exerted upon them depending upon the contractile elements in the walls of the sac and the pressure exerted on the outside of the sac by the surrounding structures. If a vertical tubular outlet is provided for the fluid, on which pressure is being exerted equally in all directions, the fluid will rise in the outlet to a level equivalent to the pressure exerted on the contained fluid. The level will fluctuate in the outlet with fluctuations in pressure on the fluid within the sac or cavity. Pressure on the bladder contents varies with muscular contractions of the bladder and the contractions of the diaphragm and abdominal muscles in breathing, coughing, sneezing, laughing, sighing, groaning, and, of course, defecating and voiding. The purpose of cystometry is primarily to measure the strength and frequency of bladder contractions; other pressure fluctuations are largely disregarded. The patient is asked to breathe naturally and uninterruptedly, therefore, throughout the test. Excursions of the fluid in the manometer (cystometer) caused by respiration can then be clearly seen[28, 29] and differentiated from those due to bladder contraction.

Equipment needed for cystometric measurements is that used for a bladder irrigation with the addition of a cystometer. This is nothing more than a water manometer, or a calibrated glass tube. The manometer must be supported on a fixed standard so that the heights to which the fluid rises in it above the level of the bladder can be exactly measured. Most tidal drainage sets incorporate what is, in effect, a cystometer as can be seen if Figures 205 and 208 are studied. Fluid used in these measurements may be normal saline or any of those listed for bladder irrigation (see p. 884).

The *procedure* of cystometry is as follows: Empty the bladder with a rubber catheter attached by a glass T tube to the cystometer and to a drainage tube, or outlet. Attach the cystometer to a reservoir of fluid so that measured amounts may be allowed to flow into the bladder. Provide clamps for the inlet and outlet tubes. Empty or catheterize the bladder as described on page 882; clamp the out-flow tubes and see that the attached cystometer is registering zero. Start the flow of solution; usually at the rate of 120 drops per minute to approximate a normal rate of bladder filling by urine. After each 50 cc of fluid is introduced, stop the flow and record the corresponding intravesicular pressure. Record the fluctuation of pressures, indicating the occurrence of emptying contractions. An abrupt excursion of the fluid with a slow return to a point near which it started represents a con-traction of the detrusor muscles. The level from which the rise started and the peak should be noted. Record the first discomfort and any increase, or pain, there-after; record at what point there is a desire to void and any leakage around the catheter. Intravesicular pressure varies in the normal bladder from 0 when it is empty to about 12 to 20 cm (water) when the bladder holds 500 cc. At this pressure it empties. Great modifications in these figures occur in disease.

Suggested Procedure for Tidal Irrigation. Having gained the patient's cooperation, collect the equipment for the cystometric tests and tidal drainage. Prepare the bed and drape the patient as described for catheterization; then proceed with the catheterization or leave this for the physician who, with the nurse, will make the cystometric measure-ments. The catheter inserted for emptying the bladder should serve also for cystometry and tidal drainage so it is desirable for the physician to perform all the functions that require gloved or scrubbed hands and for the nurse to be free to handle unsterile objects. Unless otherwise specified by the doctor select Foley catheters (#16 to #18 for women; #18 to #22 for men.) After draining the bladder into a covered vessel or into the drainage bottle, adjust the tubing so that a measured amount of fluid can flow from a calibrated reservoir into the bladder and fix the catheter to the patient's thigh with a narrow strip of adhesive. Distend the Foley catheter with 5 cc of air or sterile water injected with a sterile syringe. The inlet and drainage tubes should be closed at the start of the procedure. Adjust the height of the cystometer so that the outlet (zero point) is level with the symphysis pubis. After eliminating the air in the system of tubes, attach the inlet tube to the catheter and allow the fluid from the reservoir to flow at the specified rate and in the specified amounts. The nurse may record the findings as the cystometric tests proceed or the physician may prefer to do so. He, having now assessed the condition of the bladder, may immediately prescribe the rate of flow for the tidal irrigation and the height of the siphon. He will adjust the mechanism to the patient's condition and will test the effectiveness of the adjustment before leaving it to others.

To prevent kinking of the excess tubing, keep it coiled and fixed to the bedding with tapes or safety pins. See that it is not collapsed by the patient's leg. Leaking around the catheter (a wet bed) may be caused by an obstructed drainage tube or by blood clots or sloughing tissue in the catheter. If the tubes are unobstructed, the doctor will decrease the height of the siphon, since contractions of the bladder may be sufficient to empty it but the pressure insufficient to carry the fluid over the siphon loop.

If fluid escapes from the air vent, check the patency of the drainage tube; be sure that the end of the drainage tube is above the level of the liquid in the drainage bottle.

Check all connections to prevent the introduction of air into the system. Bubbles can occlude the tubes in various places.

To control urethral irritation Seidel recommends daily removal of encrustations of dried exudate on the catheter. She suggests that after thorough cleaning of the surrounding area the catheter be withdrawn until the resistance offered by the inflated balloon is felt. Using strict asepsis the exposed part should be wiped free of secretions with a lubricant.

As long as tidal irrigation is functioning, check the tubing and general operation of the apparatus. Replenish the solution when necessary, usually every 8 hours.

To discontinue the irrigation while the patient is sitting up, walking about, or for any other reason, clamp the inlet and outlet tubes and detach the catheter from the glass T connection, draining both ends into a waste basin without contaminating them. Place them on a sterile surface—a towel or a sterile vessel. Wrap the ends of the catheter and glass connection with sterile gauze or paper, fixing the protectors with rubber bands. Fasten the catheter to the patient's thigh with a small adhesive strip taking care to vary the skin area to which it is applied. Put the equipment aside until it is again connected.

If possible, keep tidal drainage out of sight, especially while the patient has visitors. The drainage bottle can be hung on the bed under the covers, and a screen may be placed around the standard with the irrigating fluid and the siphon.

The physician will discontinue the treatment from time to time to test the patient's ability to retain urine and void spontaneously. He will probably want the patient catheterized after voiding in order to know whether he is emptying the bladder. It is wise to use the kind of catheter for this procedure that will be needed if it is necessary to re-establish tidal irrigation.

Recording the Treatment. Many hospitals have special forms for tidal irrigation records. Intake and output forms may be modified to include the following information: (1) the total intake of fluids, by mouth and by vein, or any other parenteral route; and (2) total output by the urinary route. Estimate this by subtracting (3) the amount of solution used from (4) the total drainage. Also record (5) the amount in the reservoir and (6) amount in the drainage bottle.

Record the initiation of the procedure and the physician who did it, the solution used, the rate of flow, and the height of the siphon in relation to the symphysis pubis. Record significant remarks of the patient showing acceptance or aversion to the treatment and any physiological or mechanical difficulties encountered.

REFERENCES

1. Fulton, John F. (ed.): *Textbook of Physiology,* 16th ed. W. B. Saunders Co., Philadelphia, 1949, p. 1210.
2. Lowsley, Oswald S., and Kirwin, Thomas J.: *Clinical Urology,* 2nd ed. Williams & Wilkins Co., Baltimore, 1944, p. 948.
3. Starling, Ernest H.: *Principles of Human Physiology,* 9th ed. J. & A. Churchill, London, 1945, p. 987.
4. Best, Charles H., and Taylor, Norman B.: *The Physiological Basis of Medical Practice,* 5th ed. Williams & Wilkins Co., Baltimore, 1950, p. 485.
5. Gershenfeld, Louis: *Urine and Urinalysis,* 3rd ed., Pierson Romaine, Publishers, Inc., New York, 1948, p. 37.
6. Lowsley, Oswald S., and Kirwin, Thomas J.: *op. cit.,* pp. 883, 1159.
7. Creevy, Charles D.: "Sudden Decompression of the Chronically Distended Urinary Bladder; a Clinical and Pathologic Study," *Arch. Surg.,* **25:**356, (Aug.) 1932.

8. Davis, Carl H. (ed.): *Gynecology and Obstetrics.* H. F. Prior Co., Hagerstown, Md., 1951, Vol. 3, p. 70.

9. Ilgenfritz, Hugh C.: *Preoperative and Postoperative Care of Surgical Patients.* C. V. Mosby Co., St. Louis, 1948, p. 331.

10. Young, Hugh H., et al.: "Infections in the Genito-Urinary Tract, and Complications," *J.A.M.A.,* **98:**715, (Feb.) 1932.

11. Keyes, Edward L., and Ferguson, Russell S.: *Urology,* 6th ed. D. Appleton-Century Co., Inc., New York, 1936, p. 125.

12. Perearnau, E.: "Infection of the Urinary Apparatus with the Colon Bacillus," *Brit. J. Urol.,* **2:**138, (June) 1930.

13. Park, William H., and Williams, Anna W.: *Pathogenic Microorganisms,* 11th ed. Lea & Febiger, Philadelphia, 1939, p. 488.

14. Jordan, Edwin O., and Burrows, William: *Textbook of Bacteriology,* 15th ed. W. B. Saunders Co., Philadelphia, 1949, p. 583.

15. Piersol, George A.: *Human Anatomy,* 9th ed. J. B. Lippincott Co., Philadelphia, 1930, pp. 1923, 1924.

16. LeComte, Ralph M.: *Manual of Urology,* 4th ed. Williams & Wilkins Co., Baltimore, 1948, p. 20.

17. Lowsley, Oswald S., and Kirwin, Thomas J.: *op. cit.,* p. 1008.

18. Lowsley, Oswald S., and Kirwin, Thomas J.: *op. cit.,* pp. 1007, 1161.

19. McKenna, William F.: "A Simple Efficient Automatic Tidal Drainage Apparatus," *Urol. & Cutan. Rev.,* **52:**18, (Jan.) 1948.

20. Munro, Donald: "Rehabilitation of Patients Totally Paralyzed Below the Waist, with Special Reference to Making Them Ambulatory and Capable of Earning Their Living; Tidal Drainage, Cystometry and Bladder Training," *New England J. Med.,* **236:**223, (Feb.) 1947.

21. Seidel, Eleanora S.: "Tidal Drainage—Its Present Status," *Am. J. Nursing,* **50:**702, (Nov.) 1950.

22. Bumpus, H. Carey, et al.: "Urologic Complications in Injuries of the Spinal Cord," *J.A.M.A.,* **133:**366, (Feb.) 1947.

23. Nathan, P. W.: "Treatment of the Bladder after Suprapubic Cystostomy," *Lancet,* **2:**47, (July) 1947.

24. Stegman, Wilson: "Total Avoidance of Postoperative Bladder Irrigation; Results and Conclusions from 200 Consecutive Cases," *J. Urol.,* **63:**882, (May) 1950.

25. Prather, George C.: *Urologic Aspects of Spinal Cord Injuries.* Charles C Thomas, Publisher, Springfield, Ill., 1949, p. 66.

26. Suby, H. I., and Albright, Fuller: "Dissolution of Phosphatic Urinary Calculi by the Retrograde Introduction of a Citrate Solution Containing Magnesium," *New England J. Med.,* **228:**81, (Jan.) 1943.

27. Munro, Donald: *op. cit.*

28. DeGutierrez-Mahoney, Carlos G., and Carini, Esta: *Neurological and Neurosurgical Nursing.* C. V. Mosby Co., St. Louis, 1949, p. 372.

29. Munro, Donald: "Activity of Urinary Bladder as Measured by New and Inexpensive Cystometer," *New England J. Med.,* **214:**617, (Mar.) 1936.

Additional Suggested Reading

Harrison, Francis G., and Warres, Herbert L.: "Present Day Therapy of Anuria," *Am. Pract. & Digest Treat.,* **1:**584, (June) 1950.

Lenkowski, Michael F.: "Catheterization of the Male Patient," *Am. J. Nursing,* **51:**401, (June) 1951.

Schwartz, M. S., and Stamton, A. H.: "A Social Psychological Study of Incontinence," *Psychiatry,* **13:**399, (Nov.) 1950.

Youngblood, V. H., and Fort, Chester A.: "A Practical Method of Handling a Paralyzed Urinary Bladder," *North Carolina M. J.,* **11:**557, (Oct.) 1950.

CHAPTER 32. IRRIGATION AND MEDICATION OF THE VULVA, PERINEUM, AND VAGINAL CANAL

1. BASIC PRINCIPLES UNDERLYING THE SELECTION OF METHOD

Certain *anatomical and physiological factors* have a definite bearing on the selection of method in cleaning and medicating the vulva and vaginal canal. For example, structural characteristics influence the length and direction of the insertion of irrigating tips or of suppositories; temperature tolerance determines, to a large extent, the heat of irrigating solutions, and resistance to bacteria determines the preparation of equipment.

Skin covers the labia majora and gradually merges into a modified mucous membrane on the labia minora. The mucous lining of the vagina is arranged in folds, which makes a thorough cleansing of the canal difficult. A delicate sheet of mucous membrane, the hymen, may entirely or partially occlude the vaginal orifice in the virgin. If such an occlusion exists, the condition is referred to as an *imperforate hymen,* and an operation is indicated to allow egress of the vaginal flow. It is, of course, impossible to give a vaginal irrigation if an imperforate hymen exists. In giving this treatment for the first time, the nurse should examine the orifice carefully in order to be sure that the condition is a normal one. The physician rarely prescribes an irrigation without having made this examination himself.

An especially important anatomical feature of the female reproductive tract is the fact that the mucous membrane of the external genitalia is continuous with the lining of the uterus and through the Fallopian tubes with the peritoneum, or the serous lining of the abdominal cavity. This makes it possible for an infection of the vagina to spread by direct extension to the peritoneum. Since peritonitis is a highly serious condition, physicians try to prevent any possibility of its occurring and rarely irrigate the uterus. There is general agreement that *vaginal irrigations should be given under low pressure* to avoid the possibility of forcing infectious material into the uterus.

896

The uterus opens into the Fallopian tubes; the tubes, into the peritoneal cavity. For this reason an infection of the uterus can by direct extension spread throughout the abdomen.

Except during menstruation and the later stages of pregnancy, the internal and external openings of the cervix (the neck of the uterus) are normally closed. This, to some extent, protects the body of the uterus from bacteria always present in the vagina. Most authorities advise against vaginal irrigations during both menstruation and pregnancy, because there is more likelihood at these times of forcing material into the uterus. The downward and outward flow of the menstrual discharge and lochia tends to wash pathogenic bacteria from the vaginal tract. Any reversal of the flow is contraindicated.

The vaginal secretion contains lactic acid that, according to Dugald Baird,[1] Jacob P. Greenhill,[2] J. Bernard Bernstine and Abraham E. Rakoff,[3] and other authorities, discourages the growth and decreases the virulence of organisms resident in the vagina and cervix. Benjamin P. Watson, writing in Arthur H. Curtis' book,[4] says that following delivery the uterine cavity is invaded with pathogenic organisms. Varying degrees of immunity to this invasion exist.

There seems to be general agreement that under ordinary circumstances *the intact vaginal mucosa discourages the growth of pathogenic organisms;* however, the generative tract is peculiarly susceptible to infection during the late stages of pregnancy, at delivery, and during the post-partum period. This lowered resistance may be explained by the stretching and injury of tissues, or by the change that occurs in the chemical nature of the secretions, or to both circumstances. Undoubtedly, the introduction of foreign strains of microorganisms is especially dangerous to the obstetrical or surgical patient. The low incidence of infections in home deliveries as compared to those in the hospital, when both groups receive comparable medical and nursing care, suggests the hazard of exposing a woman to a large group of attendants and to a new bacterial environment to which she has not developed immunity.

Apparently the reproductive tract is much more susceptible to infection from one type of organism than another. It is well to know that all human feces contain strains of colon bacilli and that most persons harbor welchii bacilli in the colon. Fecal organisms have easy access to the vagina, and if infections do not occur it must mean that there is natural protection. Andrew A. Marchetti[5] in 1934, in a careful study of medical literature over a long period, found only 56 cases of welchii bacillus infections reported. Coralie Rendle-Short[6] brings this review up to 1942 and remarks on the rarity of welchii infections. In comparison it is estimated that the streptococcus caused the majority of puerperal infections and that puerperal infections cause approximately one fourth of the total number of maternal deaths. A large number of healthy persons are found to have streptococci in the throat. Such groups as the Committee on Public Health Relations of the New York Academy of Medicine,[7] studying maternal mortality in New York City, therefore, strongly recommend that attendants giving perineal care mask the nose and mouth.

In spite of the fact that infections by spore-forming organisms are rare, sterilization by steam under pressure is the method of choice for the preparation of sterile supplies for the postoperative or obstetrical patient.

Many physicians believe that at any age and under any circumstances resistance to infection in the vagina is lowered by irrigations that wash away secretions offering a natural protection. Such treatments should be used only under the direction of a physician.

The length of the vagina varies markedly in the child, the adolescent, and in the fully developed woman. Abnormalities of the vagina occur occasionally. The average length of the anterior wall is 6¼ to 7½ cm (2½ to 3 in.) and that of the posterior wall 7½ to 8¾ cm (3 to 3½ in.) in the woman. The intravaginal portion

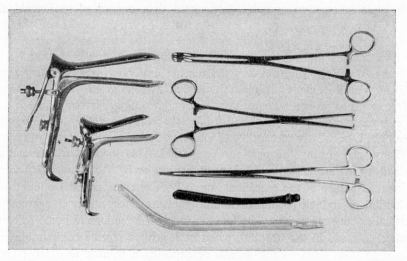

Figure 209. Equipment used during a vaginal examination or treatment. (*Left*) Vaginal speculums, two sizes; (*right, top to bottom*) sponge forceps, tenaculum, clamp, and two douche tips (one hard rubber, one glass). (Courtesy of Clay-Adams Co., New York City.)

of the cervix projects into the vagina at such an angle that a sort of pocket is formed between the cervix and the posterior wall of the vagina. In suppurative vaginitis, or following the rupture of a pelvic abscess, pus may collect in this pocket. Irrigations to clean the vagina under such circumstances should be so administered that the solution comes in contact with this area.

The direction in which the tip or nozzle is inserted largely determines whether the solution reaches all parts of the vagina, as it should. By studying Figure 203, it can be seen that in the standing position the direction of the vagina is upward and backward. With the recumbent patient, the vaginal tip should be directed upward and backward at an angle of about 35 deg. Since a reasonable amount of vaginal dilation causes no discomfort or irritation, the tip may be gently rotated without danger to the tissues.

The *position* of the patient also should favor the entrance of the irrigating solution into the upper part of the vagina. Elevating the hips and lowering the head helps to distend the vaginal walls with the irrigating fluid.

There is normally a small amount of mucous *discharge from the vagina* between the menstrual periods. A profuse or purulent discharge is an indication of pathology. Like most body discharges, the vaginal secretions contain protein substances that on decomposition have a strong odor. Frequent cleansing of the vulva with soap and water is esthetically essential to prevent an accumulation of these secretions in the mucous folds. After using the bedpan, a patient should be given the necessary articles for bathing this area; or, if she is too ill to make the effort, the nurse should do it. Under normal conditions vaginal irrigations are not necessary and may be harmful for reasons that have just been given (p. 897).

Deodorizing powders, such as sodium borate, may be used after cleaning the vulva, but solutions having characteristic odors as, for example, a carbolic compound, should never be used. The odor of the drug is itself disagreeable and comes to be associated with the odor it is intended to correct. In carcinoma of the uterus, oxidizing agents are sometimes used as deodorants but are not very effective. Motor-driven devices placed under the bed act in the same manner as an air-conditioning mechanism and are helpful. *Antiseptics,* such as silver nitrate 1:200, bichloride of mercury 1:1000, boric acid 1:50, or potassium permanganate 1:2000, are used in treating vaginal infections, but must be ordered by the doctor. Bernstine and Rakoff say that many women, using strong antiseptics and disinfectants in douches, do not realize that dangerous irritation, sensitivity, and burns may result. *Astringents* such as tannic acid, acetic acid, and alum are used to check secretions. Many irrigations are ordered purely for the heat effect, in which case water or physiological saline is most often used. If the physician prescribes an irrigation and fails to stipulate the kind of solution and he cannot be reached, it is always safe for the nurse to use water or sodium chloride 1:100.

During the puerperium, there is a growing tendency to consider cleanliness the sole object of so-called *perineal care.*[8] Everett D. Plass[9] in 1935 recommended this simplified care. Many hospitals and visiting nurse organizations are giving up chemical antiseptics in this procedure and substituting sterile or tap water and sterile soap solution applied with sterile or clean sponges, handled aseptically. Thelma A. Casper and Marie Cawley[10] describe the self-care given by ambulatory patients in two obstetrical hospitals. The nurse cleans the vulva during the first 12 hours following delivery; after this, the patient does it. In both hospitals patients use shower baths daily or as desired. In one institution, the vulva is cleaned with a cloth, kept for this purpose in the patient's bedside stand, after voiding, and/or defecation; in the other, the patient uses sterilized gauze which, with sterile vulva pads, are given her in paper bags. In both cases the nurse teaches the mother how to carry out the procedure so that material from the anus is not brought forward over the vulva.

Generally speaking, mucous membrane is less sensitive to high and low *temperatures* than is the skin. The vaginal mucosa tolerates irrigating solutions too hot to be borne by the skin. Since any solution injected into the vagina immediately runs out over the vulva, temperatures must not be used that cause discomfort to the skin. The fact that temperatures above 46.1° C (115° F) are destructive to tissue cells must be borne in mind. The temperature of the fluid must never go above this point. Bernstine and Rakoff advocate temperatures ranging between 39° and 40.6° C (102.2° and 105° F). In preparing the solution allowance must be made for the cooling effect as the solution flows through the tubing. If tissues are tender or injured, as they are likely to be following childbirth or an operation, a solution at body temperature causes least discomfort. Application of an oil to the skin helps to reduce irritation from high temperatures.

Exposure of the genitalia is embarrassing to the average person, and so the nurse should make every effort to reduce it to a minimum, to ensure privacy during the treatment, and to work expeditiously.

2. IRRIGATION OF THE VULVA AND PERINEUM (PERINEAL CARE)

Definition. An aseptic irrigation, or sponging, of the vulva and perineum given after voiding or defecation in a specified period following delivery, or an operation on the birth canal, perineum, urinary meatus, or anus is termed *perineal care*.

Therapeutic Uses. Special attention is given to the external genitalia, perineum, and anus when any condition makes these areas susceptible to infection. The object of the treatment may be merely to clean the skin and mucous membrane under aspetic conditions or to discourage the growth of bacteria by application of antiseptics and to encourage healing with protective substances.

Equipment. Ordinarily the physician prescribes the solution, any one of a number of antiseptics or cleansing fluids; in addition, an oily drug, such as balsam of Peru, may be prescribed to form a waterproof covering over stitches in the perineum. The amount of solution needed to clean the parts thoroughly varies, but it is more convenient to adopt a standard practice and use 500 cc (1 pt) of cleansing solution, to avoid confusion in estimating the quantity of urine voided. A convenient container for the cleansing solution is a covered calibrated pitcher or cup with a lip. If two liquids, for example, a detergent and water, are used, a second small container is necessary. The detergent should be neutral and non-irritating. Unless otherwise ordered, the irrigating fluid should be prepared at a temperature of about 42° C (107.6° F).

Cotton and gauze sponges are both used. Gauze cleans more effectively because it is rougher, but cotton is less likely to catch in sutures and irritate the tissues. While the number of sponges needed varies according to whether the patient has voided or defecated, again it is more satisfactory to provide a specified and adequate number, so that it is never necessary to return to a workroom for an additional supply. In order to prevent contamination of the sponges, they must be handled with sterile forceps or scrubbed hands. The former practice is preferable, because skin disinfection is doubtful at best and is very time consuming. In home nursing, where instruments are not readily available, the latter practice is usually taught. A paper bag should be provided to facilitate disposal of soiled dressings.

A dressing is usually applied over the genitalia for protection and to absorb discharge. This dressing should be soft and aseptic. It should be held in place by pinning it to a belt. If possible, the belt should be elastic so that it gives with the movements of the body. If an elastic one is not available, it is essential that the belt be adjustable in size. On the theory that a perineal pad makes the discharge "back up" in the vagina, some obstetricians forbid its use. In such cases the patient lies on a large absorbent pad of cellucotton that must be changed frequently as it is soon soiled.

Since a number of articles must be brought to the bedside at once, a small tray is a convenience. A bedpan or douchepan is necessary. To prevent soiling of the bed linen, an impervious paper square or rubber treatment sheet covered with a piece of absorbent paper or muslin should be placed under the bedpan. The upper bedding must be folded down to expose the area to be treated and covering provided for the upper part of the body and, ideally, for draping the thighs. In most cases the upper sheet is used to drape the legs.

Suggested Procedure.   Gain the cooperation of the patient by an explanation of the purpose and nature of the treatment. Before preparing the equipment, mask the nose and mouth and wash the hands carefully. Screen the patient or make provision for privacy, fold the upper bedding midway of the body, and cover the upper half of the body with a treatment blanket. Place a clean bedpan in position, remove the soiled dressing, and put it in a paper bag; allow time for the use of the bedpan before returning to the bedside. If the hands are contaminated, wash them before returning to the patient. Expose the pubic-anal region as much as is necessary to allow the worker to see the condition of the parts. Pour a portion of the cleansing solution over the genitalia from above downward. Handling the sponges with sterile forceps, moisten them with the detergent solution and clean the vulva and perineum; use each sponge once only and stroke from above downward, making as little pressure as possible on the tissue. Work from the median line outward. Rinse the soap off by pouring the remainder of the cleansing solution over the area. Pat the vulva and perineum dry with sterile sponges. Remove the bedpan and at the same time turn the patient on her side. Dry the anal region and buttocks with the remaining sponges. In applying the dressing, avoid touching the surface that comes in contact with the vulva and perineum; pin the compress to the belt or binder. Dispose of the soiled dressings, note the contents of the bedpan and estimate the urine by subtracting the known quantity of the cleansing solution from the total amount of liquid in the bedpan. All equipment is washed and sterilized before it is stored or used again.

In giving perineal care to a group of patients, it saves time and effort to have the clean supplies on a movable cart. These supplies must be touched only after the hands have been washed, and no contaminated materials should be returned to the cart.

If in home nursing it is impossible to provide sterile forceps and aseptic dressings, reasonable protection is afforded the patient by using clean cotton dressings and solutions and by scrubbing the hands immediately before handling the sponges. In teaching the patient or a member of the family to give this treatment, simplify the procedure as much as possible and then stress the essentials.

Recording the Treatment.   Note the character and amount of discharge, the appearance of the wound and of sutures if visible; record giving the treatment and the nature and quantity of the elimination.

3. VAGINAL IRRIGATION

Definition. A vaginal irrigation is sometimes called a *vaginal douche,* but the former term is correct, because a douche implies that a stream of water is directed against a part with force. A vaginal irrigation should be the introduction of a liquid at low pressure. It is similar to the irrigation of any open cavity, such as the external auditory canal, from which the liquid immediately returns.

Therapeutic Uses. Vaginal irrigations may be prescribed to: (1) discourage growth of bacteria by the application of an antiseptic, (2) remove a foul or irritating discharge, (3) apply heat or cold in the treatment of inflammation or possibly to control hemorrhage, and (4) clean the vagina in preparation for surgery. Vaginal douches are now less often used than in the past. The physician is able to control a large number of vaginal infections with chemotherapy and antibiotics given systemically. Bernstine and Rakoff say specifically that while the antibiotics and sulfanilamides have proved very useful in gonococcal and other infections, effective agents for the treatment of trichomoniasis and moniliasis are unknown. Heat in the form of diathermy has to some extent replaced the use of hot irrigations.

Equipment. Articles required are: a douchepan or bedpan to receive the return flow; a reservoir for the solution (an irrigating can, rubber bag, or plastic or glass bottle), with a convenient length of tubing and a clamp attached; a douche tip, a small container for this tip; soft paper squares or a treatment towel for drying the patient; and a waterproof protector for the bed. The protector must be covered with muslin or crepe paper.

Vaginal "douche tips" are made of glass, plastic, or hard rubber. Glass has the advantage of being easy to clean; hard rubber, the merit of being difficult to break. Metal tips are unsuitable, because they conduct heat too readily and would be painful to the patient if used for a hot irrigation. Tips come in various sizes suitable for children and adults. Before using a tip, it must be examined to see that it is intact and has a smooth surface.

The prescribed solution in the required amount, usually 2000 cc (2 qt), is brought to the bedside in the reservoir. The temperature must be regulated with a thermometer, according to the physician's prescription, allowing about 2° C or 5° F for cooling before the solution reaches the vagina. If neither the temperature nor the kind of solution is specified, it is safe to use water, sodium chloride 1 per cent, or sodium bicarbonate 2 per cent at 40.6° C (105° F).

The articles just listed must be *clean* or "medically aseptic" in preparation for most vaginal irrigations. Following an abortion, a delivery, or a surgical operation, the treatment must be given with *sterile* equipment and must be handled with surgical asepsis. In administering a clean douche, it is convenient to bring the reservoir, tubing, tip, and treatment towel to the bedside in a clean douchepan or bedpan;

if giving a sterile douche, it is more convenient to use a tray for these articles and to provide rubber gloves for manipulating the tip, and cleaning and separating the labia. As in all such treatments, it is important to cover the equipment in transporting it to and from the bedside.

Suggested Procedure. Gain the cooperation of the patient by a thorough and appropriate explanation. If the treatment is given for the first time, and especially if the patient is a child or a young girl, this explanation must be made with the greatest tact. (The treatment should never be administered to a responsible patient unless she understands it and is willing to have it.) Ensure privacy with signs on the door, screen the bed, and drape the patient to avoid unnecessary exposure.

Place the patient on the bedpan or douchepan. Support the back with a pillow and cover the seat of the douchepan with a pad. It is desirable to support the flexed legs. If the irrigation is given as slowly as it should be, the patient tires in this position unless care is taken to make her comfortable.

Replace the upper bedding with two treatment blankets. Arrange these so that they separate and drape each leg, leaving the pubic region exposed. Hang the reservoir so that the base is about 30 cm (12 in.) above the vaginal meatus; this keeps the solution at low pressure, slows the rate of flow, and makes the treatment last long enough to produce a temperature effect. Allow a small amount of the solution to flow over the vulva to remove any gross discharge. If the temperature of the solution is uncomfortable and there is no therapeutic indication for giving it at this temperature, make the necessary change before continuing. Examine the nozzle carefully for cracks and nicks and, if intact, attach it to the tubing. Insert the nozzle very gently into the vagina; the patient may prefer to do this herself, and if the effort is not injurious to her, she should be helped to do so. (In cases where there is an infection such as gonorrhea, do not allow the patient to handle the tip or tubing as it is desirable to prevent contamination of a bed patient's hands. Without access to running water, it is difficult for her to get her hands clean, and there is always danger of infecting the eyes. In addition to other steps taken to maintain medical asepsis, the nurse should wear glasses to protect the eyes from accidental splashing. Gloves are not necessary for the protection of the nurse, the gonococcus being easily killed with soap and hot water, but a gown should be worn. The nurse should mask in postoperative or obstetrical cases.) Directing the nozzle upward (toward the head) and backward (toward the sacrum) tends to keep the stream of water from forcing its way into the mouth of the cervix. Openings at the side and not at the end of the nozzle also help to prevent this. With the proper amount of force, the liquid should fill and distend the vagina.

After the administration of the prescribed amount of fluid, allow the patient to remain on the bedpan for a few minutes to drain the vagina. Dry the postoperative or obstetrical patient with sterile sponges, handled aseptically; other patients may be dried with toilet paper or with the folded treatment towel used to pad the seat of the douchepan.

Before emptying the douchepan, note the character of the return. Discard soiled sponges or paper squares, send used linen to the laundry, wash and return the treatment sheet to the patient's unit, and boil all other articles of equipment before returning them to storage space. In homes, or in private-hospital rooms equipped with running water, the articles required for a vaginal irrigation may be washed and kept separate for the use of the patient. This avoids the necessity for concurrent sterilization. If sterile irrigations are ordered, it saves time and effort to sterilize the equipment after use and store it in a covered container ready for the next treatment. It is often most convenient to wrap the articles in paper and sterilize them with steam under pressure in a central supply department.

Recording the Treatment.   Note the time the treatment was given, the kind, amount, and temperature of the solution, the character of the return flow, and the reaction of the patient. Vaginal irrigations are sometimes continued when no longer necessary if the nurse fails, for example, to state that the fluid returns clear.

4. VAGINAL SUPPOSITORIES

Definition.   Vaginal suppositories are cones of cocoa butter or paraffin impregnated with a drug; they are made to approximate the length and diameter of the vaginal cavity.

Therapeutic Uses.   Local applications of an astringent, an antiseptic, or other types of drugs can be made by the introduction of a suppository. Actually, this form of therapy is rarely practiced, because drugs are more easily applied in other ways.

Suggested Procedure: Cool and harden the suppository in a refrigerator. In hospitals, suppositories are kept stored in refrigerators. Explain the nature and the purpose of the procedure to the patient. Place the patient in the dorsal recumbent or left lateral (Sims') position. Drape the patient to expose only the vaginal orifice. Lubricate the suppository with a vegetable jelly. Gently insert the full length of the suppository into the vagina. The nurse may wear a rubber glove or finger cots on the thumb and forefinger of the hand that manipulates the suppository.

Recording the Treatment.   Note the time at which the suppository was inserted, its nature, and any significant reaction, such as pain or discomfort, experienced by the patient.

REFERENCES

1. Baird, Dugald (ed.): *Combined Textbook of Obstetrics and Gynaecology, for Students and Practitioners,* 5th ed. E. & S. Livingstone, Edinburgh, 1950, p. 764.
2. Greenhill, Jacob P.: *Principles and Practice of Obstetrics* (originally by Joseph B. DeLee), 10th ed. W. B. Saunders Co., Philadelphia, 1951, p. 803.
3. Bernstine, J. Bernard, and Rakoff, Abraham E.: *Vaginal Infections, Infestations and Discharges.* Blakiston Co., New York, 1953, pp. 59, 60.
4. Curtis, Arthur H. (ed.): *Obstetrics and Gynecology.* W. B. Saunders Co., Philadelphia, 1933, Vol. 2, p. 194 ff.
5. Marchetti, Andrew A.: "Intrapartum Gas Bacillus Infection," *Am. J. Obst. & Gynec.,* **26:** 612, (Apr.) 1934.
6. Rendle-Short, Coralie: "Clostridium Welchii Infection of the Uterus, Complicating Delivery," *J. Obst. & Gynaec. Brit. Emp.,* **49:**581, (Dec.) 1942.
7. New York Academy of Medicine, Committee on Public Health Relations: *Maternal Mortality in New York City, 1930-32.* Oxford University Press, New York, 1933, pp. 75-76.
8. Davis, M. Edward, and Sheckler, Catherine E.: *DeLee's Obstetrics for Nurses,* 15th ed. W. B. Saunders Co., Philadelphia, 1951, p. 398.
9. Plass, Everett D.: "Simplified Obstetric Care," *Minnesota Med.,* **18:**768, (Dec.) 1935.
10. Casper, Thelma A., and Cawley, Marie: "Early Ambulation and Postpartum Care," *Am. J. Nursing,* **52:**1210, (Oct.) 1952.

Additional Suggested Reading

Bowes, Kenneth (ed.): *Modern Trends in Obstetrics and Gynecology.* Paul B. Hoeber, New York, 1950.

Brady, Leo, et al.: *Essentials of Gynecology,* 2nd ed. The Macmillan Company, New York, 1949.

Curtis, Arthur H., and Huffman, John W.: *A Textbook of Gynecology,* 6th ed. W. B. Saunders Co., Philadelphia, 1950.

Eastman, Nicholson J.: *Williams' Obstetrics,* 10th ed. Appleton-Century-Crofts, Inc., New York, 1950.

Heardman, Helen: *Physiotherapy in Obstetrics and Gynaecology.* E. & S. Livingstone, Edinburgh, 1951.

Meigs, Joe Vincent, and Sturgis, Somers H. (eds.): *Progress in Gynecology,* Vol. 2. Grune & Stratton, New York, 1946.

Miller, Norman F., and Hyde, Betty: *Gynecology and Gynecologic Nursing,* 2nd ed. W. B. Saunders Co., Philadelphia, 1949.

Novak, Emil: *The Woman Asks the Doctor,* 2nd ed. Williams & Wilkins Co., Baltimore, 1944.

Novak, Emil, and Novak, Edmund R.: *Textbook of Gynecology,* 4th ed. Williams & Wilkins Co., Baltimore, 1952.

Smout, Charles F. V.: *Gynecological and Obstetrical Anatomy,* 2nd ed. E. Arnold & Co., London, 1948.

Young, James: *A Textbook of Gynecology for Students and Practitioners,* 8th ed. A. & C. Black, London, 1951.

CHAPTER 33. IRRIGATION AND MEDICATION OF THE EYE, EAR, NOSE, AND THROAT

1. IRRIGATION OF THE CONJUNCTIVAL SAC

Definition. An eye irrigation is the washing out of the conjunctival sac by a stream of liquid.

Therapeutic Uses. Irrigations are given in various forms of inflammation of the conjunctiva (conjunctivitis) for cleansing, antiseptic purposes, and temperature effects.

Selection of Method. The conjunctiva is a continuous, thin, transparent layer of mucous membrane lining the eyelids and covering the anterior surface of the eyeball. It is exposed to infection and irritation from wind, smoke, and dust and other foreign bodies. It has a rich supply of blood vessels, and lymphatics. It is also supplied with mucous and lacrimal glands. The conjunctiva is liable to congestion and swelling, and an increase in secretions when irritated or infected, the lids becoming tender, edematous, adherent, and difficult to separate. An abundant nerve supply makes the conjunctiva sensitive to minute irritation, and the resulting conjunctivitis is very painful. Secretions of the conjunctival sac drain through the lacrimal, or tear, duct into the nasal cavity.

The conjunctiva is never free from live organisms although its normal condition is not conducive to their growth. The lacrimal secretion contains lysozyme which dissolves many air bacteria. Normal tears contain comparatively few live organisms.[1] Phillips Thygesen, writing in Conrad Berens' text,[2] comments on the relative immunity of the mucous membrane of the eye in comparison with that in other parts of the body. It is, however, susceptible to infection by the gonococcus, staphylococcus, streptococcus, the viruses of inclusion-conjunctivitis of the newborn, trachoma, and the bacilli of Koch-Weeks and Morax-Axenfeld. The meningicoccus and pneumococcus; the colon, diphtheria, and tubercle bacilli; the treponema of syphilis; and some other organisms are rarer causes of conjunctivitis. Foreign proteins, animal parasites, and growths produce hyperemia of the eye covering. Nutritional deficiencies and endocrine imbalance are contributing factors.

Willis S. Knighton, also writing in Berens' text,[3] says that the layman's name for any conjunctivitis, "pink eye," is dangerous because it suggests a mild condition that can be cured with home care.

Infective agents are usually brought to the conjunctiva from the environment, that is, they are exogenous. Endogenous infection brought by the blood or lymph occurs less often. Thygesen calls attention, however, to our limited knowledge of many conjunctival disorders.

Health regulations, enforcing protective treatment for the eyes of the newborn, and the effectiveness of the antibiotics and chemotherapy have greatly reduced the incidence of conjunctivitis where modern medicine is practiced. Both types of agents may be given systemically or administered locally in the form of drops or ointments. Antitoxin may also be used systemically or locally. Penicillin is particularly effective in the control of eye infections. It has largely replaced silver preparations in the prevention of gonorrhea neonatorum. The sulfa drugs are very effective in trachoma and other types of conjunctivitis.

When irrigations are used for any type of conjunctival infection, every precaution should be taken to control the spread of the disease. *Antiseptic solutions for irrigations and instillations should be chosen for their effect upon the causative organisms.* In a series of studies on antiseptic solutions commonly employed in the treatment of eye infections, Frederick Ridley[4] found a wide variation in their effectiveness on staphylococci and hemolytic streptococci. Boric acid (2 per cent) had no effect on the organisms; mercuric oxycyanide (1 per cent) and Argyrol (25 per cent) had slight effect; however, acriflavine (1 per cent) inhibited the growth of the bacteria, and silver nitrate (1 per cent) was germicidal. Sir Stewart Duke-Elder says that silver nitrate is not "strongly bactericidal" but that the organisms are caught in the coagulum that it forms and are removed with it. He says that most eye lotions cannot be used in sufficient strength to act as "efficient antiseptics." If the organism, however, is susceptible to the action of penicillin, it is very effective when dropped into the eye. He recommends 1500 to 2000 units of penicillin per milliliter.[5]

If irrigations are given for mechanical cleansing or for temperature effects, it seems reasonable to use a sodium chloride solution, which is nonirritating. In a series of tests made on normal subjects the writer found that there was less sensation of burning or smarting with a 1.0 per cent sodium chloride solution than with plain water or a 2.0 per cent boric solution. George V. Hosford and Avery M. Hicks[6] believe that the sensation when substances are instilled in the eyes is intimately associated with the hydrogen ion concentration. The pH of tears is 7.35, approximately the hydrogen ion concentration of blood and lymph. This suggests that for comfort the solutions used for eye irrigations should be approximately neutral in reaction.

(Ordinarily, the irrigating solution is specified by the physician. If he fails to do so, and the nurse cannot reach him, it would be safe in most cases to use a physiological saline solution.)

The *temperature* of the solution varies according to the effect desired, and should be prescribed by the physician. Irrigations are most comfortable if given at or near body temperature. In treatment of inflammatory conditions, they may be prescribed as hot as the patients can tolerate them. The writer has found that solutions at a temperature of 43.3° C (110° F) are uncomfortably hot for normal subjects. Cold irrigations are rarely ordered; cold compresses, however, are common. Any increase in the rate or force of the solution intensifies the temperature sensation.

All the authorities consulted seem to agree that the *pressure* or force of the liquid should be reduced to that which is necessary to maintain a steady flow.

The *amount* of solution also varies with the effect desired, and may range from 30 to 1000 cc (1 oz to 1 qt). When larger quantities of solution are ordered, it is desirable to use a reservoir rather than a syringe.

Equipment.   For an eye irrigation the articles required are: the prescribed solution, an irrigator, a basin for the return, eye cotton pledgets, a paper bag, a waterproof protector, and towel to cover it. The fluid may be delivered from a flask or an irrigating can, saturated absorbent cotton, an eye dropper, a soft rubber bulb, or an undine. Everything that comes in contact with the eye should be sterile. A good light is essential.

Solutions commonly used are boric acid (2 per cent) or sodium chloride in physiological concentration (0.9 per cent); bichloride of mercury (1:10,000) or mercuric oxycyanide (1:5000) is sometimes ordered but is used with caution. Other disinfectant solutions, such as formalin (1:2000), potassium permanganate (1:5000), merbromin (1 to 2 per cent), and acriflavine (1:2000) are occasionally employed in purulent conjunctivitis. Solutions of silver nitrate (1:100 to 1:1000) are used in many eye infections, but, like zinc sulfate, mild silver protein, sodium ethyl mercurithiosalicylate (Merthiolate), benzethonium (Phemorol), benzalkonium (Zephiran), and other potent drugs they are mostly administered by drops or instillations. The solution should be prepared so that it is at the prescribed temperature when it reaches the eye.[6, 7]

Suggested Procedure.   Have the patient sit comfortably or, if in bed, lie on his back with his head turned slightly to the side to be irrigated. When the patient is a small child, it may be necessary to wrap him firmly in a sheet in order to keep his hands away from his eyes and to prevent interference with the treatment with possible injury to the eyes from sudden, violent movements. Arrange the light in such a way that it is sufficient for the operator but does not shine in the patient's eye. Protect the patient's shoulder with a towel. Incline his head to the side being irrigated, tilted slightly backward and support it if the patient is sitting up and the nurse standing behind him. Show the patient how to hold the basin to the side of his face to receive the return flow.

Before irrigation, carefully clean the eyelids to remove any secretions or particles of dust adhering to the lashes, which would otherwise be carried into the sac. Separate the lids very gently with the thumb and fingers of the left hand so that the fluid will reach all parts of the membrane. In separating the lids, pressure is exerted on the cheek and brow, never on the eyeball. Use just sufficient force in irrigating to dislodge the secretions.[8] Direct the fluid from the inner angle of the eye so that it will flush the sac and discharge the secretions from the outer angle. The fluid should not flow down the lacrinal duct to the nose; this might spread the infection. Never touch the eye with the irrigator. Dry the lids as soon as the sac has been thoroughly flushed and all secretions removed.

In acute infections, irrigations must be given with care to prevent spread of infection to the nurse and other patients or to the nonaffected eye. Duke-Elder recommends a waterproof transparent protective dressing for the uninfected eye (called a Buller's shield). It is made with a watch crystal and adhesive, or with Scotch tape and cellophane. If by accident a drop of pus should spurt into one of the nurse's eyes, immediate steps should be taken. Only a short time is sufficient to cause serious damage, and neglect may result in loss of sight. The conjunctiva lining the upper and lower lids should be exposed and the sac thoroughly irrigated with one of the germicidal solutions previously mentioned. A few drops of mild silver protein, a 2 per cent solution of silver nitrate, or a penicillin suspension should be instilled into the eye; the other eye should be protected until all danger of infection has passed. The nurse may protect her eyes from such accidents by wearing glasses or goggles.

Recording the Treatment. Chart the type of solution used, its concentration and temperature, and the hour at which the treatment was given. Report any unusual reaction or any change in the condition of the eyes.

2. EYE INSTILLATIONS

Definition. An instillation means the introduction of a liquid into a cavity by drops.

Therapeutic Uses. Various drugs are instilled into the eyes for purposes of examining the eye, for the treatment of disease, and for local anesthesia.

Suggested Procedure. An eye dropper is generally used for the instillation of drops. In drawing up the solution from the bottle, do not draw up more than required, since excess solution must not be returned to the bottle for fear of contamination and mistaken drug identity.

To instill the drops, tilt the head of the patient slightly backward; wipe away any secretions and place the soiled cotton in a paper bag; then gently separate the lids, draw down the lower lid with the left hand, ask the patient to look up, and allow the

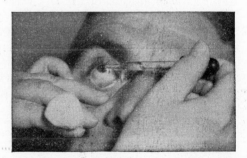

Figure 210. Instillation of eye drops. (Courtesy of Clay-Adams Co., New York City.)

drop to fall on the center of the everted lower lid.[9] (See Fig. 210). The drop should never be allowed to fall on the sensitive cornea; that would be startling and disagreeable. The dropper should never touch the lashes, lids, or eyeball, lest this result in injury. When the lids are closed, the drops are distributed over the surface. Hold a cotton pledget over the inner angle of the eye so that the drug will not be lost down the lacrimal duct. Wipe from the lids and cheek any overflow of the drug or secretion.

The same dropper should not be used for two patients or for different solutions. All drugs to be instilled in the eyes should be inspected for changes in the color or for the formation of a sediment.

3. EVERSION OF THE EYELIDS

Skill in eversion of the eyelids is necessary in examinations, irrigations of the conjunctival sac, the removal of foreign bodies, and in the application of remedies to the conjunctiva and eyeball. Eversion of the lower lid is quite a simple matter; eversion of the upper eyelid is more difficult and requires considerable practice. In all cases precautions should be taken to avoid injury to the lids or eyeball, but

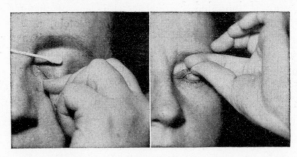

Figure 211.   Eversion of upper lip in search for foreign body; (*left*) placing an object over which cartilage in lid can be turned, and (*right*) showing everted upper lid. (See Fig. 264, Chapter 43, that shows removal of a foreign body with a sterile moistened applicator.) (Courtesy of Clay-Adams Co., New York City.)

particularly in diseases of the eyes when the lids are likely to be tender, swollen, very sensitive, and easily injured.

The following instructions are from a manual prepared in the Manhattan Eye, Ear, and Throat Hospital of New York City.

Suggested Procedure.   *Eversion of the lower lid* is a very simple matter. "Place a finger or thumb upon the lower lid, just below the lashes, direct the patient to look upward and at the same time press downward with the finger; the edge of the lid will roll outward exposing the conjunctival sac.

"*Eversion of the upper lid* is more difficult and requires some practice. To evert the lid direct the patient to look downward without inclining the head forward, grasp the lashes of the upper lid between the thumb and forefinger of one hand, and with the other hand place a small pencil or applicator horizontally along the upper part of the lid and at the same time press downward. [See Fig. 211, *left*] If there is no pencil or applicator at hand the finger may be substituted. The patient should be instructed to look downward without moving the head and continue to do so as long as it is necessary to keep the lid everted. If the patient should look upward even after the lid has been turned successfully, the lid will return to its normal position."* (The continuity of the conjunctiva over both lids and the front of the eyeball explains why movements of the latter affect the lids.)

4. EYE MEDICATIONS

Application of Ointments.   Antiseptic, irritant, or caustic ointments are frequently applied to the eyes in inflammatory diseases of the eyelids, conjunctiva, or cornea.

In *applying* the ointment, the eyelids should first be cleaned of all secretions or discharges and scales or crusts removed. A solution of borax (about half a teaspoonful in a cupful of hot water) will soften the crusts and aid in cleansing. The ointment may then be applied to the margin of the lids with a glass rod or spatula or cotton applicator. If intended for the conjunctiva or cornea, the ointment may be applied to the everted lower lid; in this way it is introduced into the conjunctival sac. Gentle massage of the lids will help to spread the ointment over the surface of the eyeball.[10] Ointments may be obtained in tubes and, for individual use, applied directly.

Application of Solutions.   Antiseptic, astringent, caustic, and disinfectant solutions are painted or brushed on the everted lids in inflammatory diseases of the conjunctiva or applied directly to infected corneal ulcers. This is usually done by the physician.

5. EAR IRRIGATIONS

Definition.   An ear irrigation is the washing out of the external auditory canal with a stream of liquid.

Therapeutic Uses.   Ear irrigations are used for their cleansing, antiseptic, or temperature effects in disease of the external auditory canal or the middle ear, and for the removal from the canal of cerumen and some types of foreign bodies.

Selection of Method.   The difference in the structure of the auditory canal in the infant and the adult must be borne in mind when irrigating the ear.

In an *infant* the auditory canal is mostly cartilaginous and is nearly straight, but because the drum membrane at the end of the canal (separating it from the middle ear) is in an oblique position, the floor of the canal is in contact with it. When irrigating, it is necessary to draw these two surfaces apart so that the fluid can reach and clean all parts of the canal; in order to do this, the auricle of an infant is drawn gently downward and backward.

In an *adult* the canal is about 2 to 2.5 cm (¾ to 1 in.) in length; only its outer third remains cartilaginous, the inner two thirds of its walls being composed of bone. It takes a spiral course inward, forward, and upward. Lifting the ear (or

* Webster, David H., et al.: *Nursing in Diseases of the Eye, Ear, Nose and Throat,* 8th ed. W. B. Saunders Co., Philadelphia, 1948, p. 22.

pinna) upward and backward straightens the canal, according to David H. Webster and William W. Morrison.[11]

Other anatomical factors to keep in mind are the position and function of the tympanic membrane, the nerve supply, and the surrounding structures. The latter suggests the serious complications that may result from injury or spread of infection into the mastoid cavity or the Eustachian tube.

Irrigations were most often used in the past to remove an accumulation of discharge from the external auditory canal when there had been a rupture or a puncture of the drum, and drainage from the infected middle ear into the canal. This procedure is now rarely followed. Lawrence R. Boies[12] (1951) does not, for example, mention the use of irrigation following a myringotomy. He advocates teaching the patient to promote drainage by dry wiping with sterile applicators. Like many other authorities he comments on the reduction in otitis media since the development of sulfonamides and antibiotics. Miriam H. Rutherford,[13] admitting the value of drug therapy for the control of the respiratory (usually streptococcal) infections, says that they may have lulled the physician into a false sense of security. Establishment of drainage is urged when the infection threatens the ear structures, with resulting deafness.

After the drum ruptures or is incised, the infection is usually a mixed one. Since the growth of an organism may be stimulated and its virulence increased by the presence of another strain, it is important to use only sterile equipment when irrigating an ear with a punctured or incised drum. The initial infection spreads from the mouth and nose by way of the Eustachian tube when the drum is intact. Figure 212 shows the avenues by which infection can travel from one mucous-lined cavity to the other in the head and, in fact, throughout the respiratory and intestinal tracts.

There seems to be general agreement among otologists that, if used, ear irrigations should be given with minimal *force,* unless the drum is intact. The danger of driving infectious material into the mastoid cells by forceful irrigation has led some physicians to discontinue the use of this treatment altogether. Others advocate the irrigation and suction of the external auditory canal with an eye dropper, because they believe that it is not possible to use enough force with this device to make the solution enter the middle ear from the external auditory canal.

When a reservoir is used, the level of the solution should not be more than 15 cm (6 in.) above the level of the ear. Irrigations to remove plugs of cerumen (wax) are given with a fair amount of force, but in this case the drum is intact and there is no question of driving material from the auditory canal into the middle ear. A metal syringe is commonly employed in this type of irrigation, and force is exerted by manual pressure on the solution.

Irrigations are usually prescribed at 3- to 4-hour periods during the day; sometimes less frequently.

Solutions used for ear irrigations are, on the whole, similar to those prescribed for irrigations of the eye. The point is made repeatedly that the kind of solution is immaterial; the benefit to be derived from an irrigation is that, by washing the

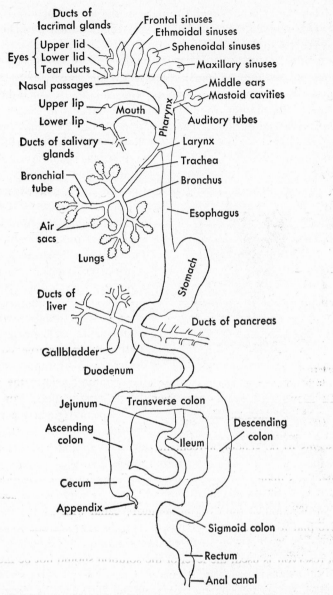

Figure 212. Diagram showing the continuity of the gastropulmonary mucous membrane. Note the possibilities of extending infection by improper methods of irrigating the ear, nose, and throat. (Kimber, D. C.; Gray, C. E.; Stackpole, C. E.; and Leavell, L. C.: *Textbook of Anatomy and Physiology,* 13th ed. The Macmillan Company, New York, 1955.)

discharge from the external canal, drainage of the ear is encouraged. If irrigations are used for the removal of cerumen, a 1 per cent solution of sodium bicarbonate softens and breaks up the wax plug.

For the comfort of the patient the *temperature of the irrigating solution* should be near that of the body. Temperatures below or above set the endolymph in motion, and this can cause dizziness and nausea.[14] According to George B. McAuliffe,[15] this motion of fluid within the inner ear causes the nystagmus that is sometimes seen during an ear irrigation. In order to allow for cooling as it flows from the irrigating can or the syringe, the solution should be prepared at about 40.6° C (105° F). Cold solutions are rarely used except for diagnostic ("caloric") tests.

The *amount of solution* varies with the purpose of the treatment. In some cases the irrigation is stopped as soon as the return flow is clear, indicating that the canal has been thoroughly cleaned. Varying amounts of solution are therefore needed. If the effect of heat is desired, as much as 1000 cc (1 qt) should be used. An irrigating can is a satisfactory device to use for the administration of the solution because, if a syringe is used, the patient is annoyed by the unavoidable repeated starting and stopping of the flow. A plastic container of a commercially prepared sterile solution is recommended.

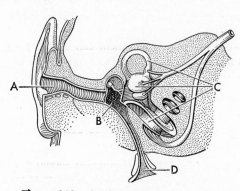

Figure 213. Section through the ear, showing the condition in cases of acute otitis media. (*A*) The external ear; (*C*) the internal ear; (*D*) the Eustachian tube; and (*B*) the middle ear, shown filled with pus which causes the eardrum to bulge outward. (Burdon, Kenneth L.: *Textbook of Microbiology*, 4th ed. The Macmillan Company, New York, 1958.)

After the irrigation is completed, the patient should lie on the affected side, to allow the ear to drain on a cellucotton pad. A gauze wick, sometimes impregnated with a drug, may be inserted in the canal by the physician, but the meatus should not be plugged with cotton as this tends to dam discharges in the middle ear.

Equipment. The following articles are required: a treatment tray with the prescribed solution, an irrigator, a towel to cover the patient's shoulder, several sterile applicators, a paper bag, a curved basin for the return, a larger waste container into which the contents of the emesis basin may be emptied, and petroleum jelly if the skin is excoriated by the discharge. A good light is essential. The irrigator may be a glass or plastic bottle, a soft rubber bulb syringe, a glass syringe, or an irrigating can with tubing and glass tip; the syringe or reservoir and tubing and the glass tip should be sterile. After the treatment they should be cleaned and decontaminated.

Solutions used are similar to those listed for eye irrigations although the ear can probably tolerate a more irritating drug (see p. 908).

The *temperature* of the solution should be such as to give a sensation of comfort; it may vary in the reservoir from 40.6° to 43.3° C (105° to 110° F). A solution that feels either cool or uncomfortably hot to the patient should never be used; it may cause mild discomfort or a severe earache that lasts for hours. If the patient has a high temperature, remember that the solution of a given temperature is likely to feel cooler than when the body temperature is normal.

Suggested Procedure.   Carefully explain the treatment to the patient before starting, relieve his apprehension if possible, and elicit his cooperation. If his condition permits, seat him comfortably in a chair or support him in an upright position. The dorsal recumbent position also may be used, with the ear brought to the edge of the pillow. When necessary, two persons should give the treatment.

Protect bedding and clothing with waterproof material. The patient can usually hold the curved basin just below the auricle and against the neck, but the nurse should see that it does not overflow and that the patient's fingers are not contaminated, for the discharge often contains virulent organisms.

When straightening the canal, take firm but gentle hold of the cartilaginous part of the auricle; do not grasp or pull on the tip of the ear—this is useless and uncomfortable. Place the tip of the syringe at the opening of the canal, or barely within, so as not to block the passage of the return flow.

In irrigating, use a *gentle* flow of the solution. The stream of solution should also be steady and continuous. When irrigating with the small rubber bulb, it is wise to use two, so that one fills while the other is in use. Air must be removed from the bulb so that bubbles will not be forced into the ear; they produce loud sounds and cause great discomfort. If the irrigation is painful or occasions dizziness, faintness, or nausea, it should be stopped and the doctor consulted.

As soon as the canal is thoroughly cleaned, the external area should be carefully dried with clean cotton; petroleum jelly should be applied if the skin is excoriated. It is important in using an applicator to protect it with cotton in order to avoid injury to the delicate tissues; such an applicator keeps the cotton from slipping off in the ear where its removal might be difficult.

Recording the Treatment.   The amount and character of the discharge and any nausea, dizziness, or any other discomfort should be recorded.

Removal of Cerumen (Ear Wax) and Epithelial Plugs.   Ear wax and epithelial scales may collect in the auditory canal, obstruct the passage, and harden against the drum membrane. This condition is fostered by pushing a cloth into the meatus when washing and drying the ear; the wax, instead of being thrown off in the normal way, is forced inward. Impacted ears are more common in the aged because the external meatus usually flattens in later life. The symptoms of an impaction are deafness, dizziness, a sense of fullness, sometimes pain, and a reflex cough from irritation of a nerve that supplies the lungs.

The treatment of this condition is to soften the mass and remove it by syringing. Before syringing, it is desirable and sometimes necessary to instill a few drops of warm hydrogen peroxide, sweet oil, or a mixture containing sodium bicarbonate (1.6 gm), glycerin (4 cc), and water (30 cc). Webster et al. suggest using the described mixture a day before the removal of wax. Hydrogen peroxide and oil may soften the wax in 10 minutes, or it may be necessary to repeat the instillation at intervals. Lying on the unaffected ear encourages absorption of the "cerumen drops."

Wax is sometimes removed with instruments; however, this method should be used only by a surgeon and then as a last resort.

A 1 per cent soap or sodium bicarbonate solution is most often used for the irrigation. The large metal Pomeroy or Neumann ear syringe is most satisfactory, but a rubber or rubber-and-glass instrument may be substituted. Considerable practice is necessary before these metal syringes can be manipulated with safety or skill; they are heavy, difficult to handle without injury to the ear and to operate so as to get a steady stream with little force. It is a wise precaution to cover the syringe tip with a piece of rubber tubing since there would be less danger of injury if it accidentally hits the ear. In some hospitals where it is impossible for all nurses to have sufficient practice in the use of these metal syringes, nurses are not allowed to give irrigations with them. After use they are easily cleaned and sterilized, as they can be taken apart.

Equipment used in the irrigation of an ear with an intact drum membrane should be clean (sterilized after it is used) but need not be sterile.

A good light is essential. The doctor must direct the stream of solution between the wax and the canal at different points so as to separate it and force it outward. The canal should be inspected from time to time so that syringing will not be continued after the wax is removed.

After the irrigation, the canal is dried. The physician may inject air into the middle ear through the Eustachian tubes if the drum is retracted. He usually fills the canal very loosely with absorbent cotton and tells the patient to remove it in 12 to 24 hours.

Removal of Foreign Bodies.   Webster et al. say that foreign bodies can "in nearly every case" be removed by syringing and that "no one but an experienced otologist should ever attempt their removal in any other way."* Insects may often be smothered by filling the canal with oil, and in any case this may facilitate the removal of the object by irrigation.† Beans, or any object that will absorb water, are best removed by alcohol irrigation.

6. NASAL IRRIGATIONS

Definition.   A nasal irrigation is the washing out of the nasal cavity by a stream of liquid.

Therapeutic Uses.   In some medical texts nasal irrigations are advocated to apply heat, to clean the nose, and to combat the disagreeable odor connected with chronic rhinitis in which there is a purulent discharge or the formation of crusts. Because there is danger of forcing infectious material into the sinuses communicating with the nose, the treatment is used only when the condition fails to respond to less hazardous methods.

---

* Webster, David H., et al.: *op. cit.,* p. 103.
† The writer has been told that a live insect will often follow a beam and crawl out of the meatus if a flashlight is held to the ear.

Selection of Method.   Because of the dangers involved, nasal irrigation must be given with great care, preferably by a physician. If administered by a nurse at the request of the physician, he should specify the kind of solution, its amount, temperature, and force, and the position of the patient.

The *solution* may be any one of the mild antiseptics used on the mucous membrane; physiological saline solution is commonly advocated. Morrison mentions a 1:4000 solution of potassium permanganate to reduce odor in atrophic rhinitis. Webster et al. recommend a temperature of 43.3° C (110° F), but this may be uncomfortably hot to some patients. Solutions tolerated by the mucosa of the mouth and pharynx are painfully hot if applied to the nose.

The greater the *pressure* or *force* of the solution, the greater the possibility of driving material from the nose into the sinuses. The reservoir should be so adjusted that the stream from the nozzle is a gentle steady flow when the tip of the nozzle is held at the level of the patient's head. Fluid flows from the tip into one nostril, around the posterior border of the septum and out of the other. If less force is used and if the tip does not fill the nostril, the fluid can be limited to one side.

The *amount* of solution varies according to the condition under treatment but usually ranges from 500 to 1000 cc (1 pt to 1 qt), because less than this does not loosen crusts or give the desired temperature effect.

Any *position* assumed by the patient must favor the return flow of the solution from the open nostril; therefore, the head must be held forward. The patient must be told to breathe through his mouth and not to speak or swallow. Changes in pressure within the nasal or aural cavity may draw material into the Eustachian tube and sinuses. Since the patient may feel impelled to speak, cough, or swallow, it is desirable to teach him how to hold the tip in the nose and how to remove it. The nurse can shut off the flow as necessary, or the patient may learn to control the flow himself.

Equipment.   Articles used vary with the method. The irrigation may be given with a Douglas syringe or with an irrigating bottle, rubber tubing, nasal irrigating tip, and a basin for the return. Paper handkerchiefs, a waterproof bib, a cotton cover to protect the clothing, and a receptacle for waste should be provided. The equipment need not be sterile but must be clean (sterilized after it is used and handled with clean hands).

Preparation of the Patient.   Before starting the treatment it must be carefully explained to the patient, and he must understand what he should do during the irrigation. Any lack of cooperation on his part increases its danger.

Suggested Procedure.   Have the patient sitting in a chair or in bed and bending over a sink or basin with his head well flexed on his chest. Maintain a copious, gentle, and uniform stream of solution up one nostril, back into the nasopharynx, and around the septum, allowing it to run out the opposite nostril. Direct the patient to keep his head forward, to breathe through his mouth, and not to speak or swallow. Conversation by the nurse or doctor with the patient or with others is unwise, as the patient is tempted to say something while the irrigation is flowing.

Insert the irrigating tip or nozzle in the nostril just tightly enough to prevent the return of fluid from that nostril, unless the aim is to irrigate only this side. Support the irrigator so that the surface of the liquid in the reservoir is not more than 20 cm (8 in.) above the level of the nose. If the patient coughs or chokes, check the flow, as coughing usually indicates that the solution, owing to some obstruction, is not returning properly. In case one nostril is more obstructed than the other, some authorities say that the stream should be directed first up the unaffected side; this washes out the discharge from the obstructed side without so much danger of forcing material into the unaffected side or into the Eustachian tubes. Other authorities advise injecting the fluid only into the narrow, obstructed side; in this method the unobstructed nostril allows free passage for the exudate. The nurse should ask the physician which method he prefers.

Patients should be warned not to blow excess fluid from the nose for several minutes after the procedure, as this may force discharges into adjoining cavities. They are also advised to stay in a warm temperature for an hour or more, since the blood vessels of the nose are dilated and more subject to chilling.

Recording the Treatment.   Chart the treatment, the nature, temperature and amount of solution used, the character of the return, and any symptoms of middle-ear disturbance, such as dizziness or a feeling of fullness in the ears.

7. NASAL INSTILLATIONS

Definition.   The introduction of a liquid into the nose, drop by drop, constitutes a nasal instillation.

Therapeutic Uses.   Nasal instillations are used as a means of coating the nasal mucosa with: (1) an antiseptic drug, (2) a soothing substance, (3) an astringent, and (4) a local anesthetic.

Selection of Method and Suggested Procedure.   The drug is administered from an eye dropper. The patient's head should be tilted backward; otherwise the liquid will run out of the anterior nares as soon as it is injected. If the patient is in bed, it is desirable to have him in the supine position with the head over the side of the bed or with the pillows removed and the head tilted backward, sometimes called the Proetz position.[16] The dropper should not be inserted in the nose more than 1 to 1½ cm (about ½ to ⅔ in.). Some of the solution will run into the mouth, and since drugs used often have a disagreeable taste, a waste basin should be provided for expectoration. Paper handkerchiefs and a paper bag for waste should be available.

If drops are put into the nose of an infant, a young child, or an irrational person who is struggling against the treatment, protect the tip with a short length of rubber tubing. Particles of mineral oil or any drug not absorbed by the tissues, passing from the nose through the larynx and trachea into the lung, may cause an abscess or pneumonitis. Health departments have warned the public against the use of such drugs. Nasal instillations should be avoided unless prescribed by the physician.

8. SPRAYING THE NOSE AND THROAT

Therapeutic Uses.   Sprays are used in acute or chronic inflammation as a means of covering the mucosa with a film of antiseptic, astringent, soothing, or anesthetic drug. Estrogenic sprays are used in some diseases of the nose.[17]

Selection of Method. Drugs may be applied to the mucous lining of the nose or throat by means of a hand atomizer; the solution is forced out through the perforated tip by air pressure, produced by squeezing the attached rubber bulb. The instrument should give a generous stream of droplets; a very forceful spray is injurious. There should be separate tips for watery and oily sprays, because a larger opening is necessary for heavy liquids.

Prescribed solutions vary according to the condition and results desired; if warmed to a temperature of 37.8° C (100° F) they are likely to be more comfortable. When the treatment is painful, it should be reported to the physician who may order a weaker or a different solution.

Suggested Procedure. A spray is frequently administered by the patient, but the nurse should be sure that he carries out the treatment effectively. The end of the nose should be raised and the tip of the atomizer placed just within the nostril. Less force should be used in spraying the nose than in applying a drug to the throat. To carry the drug to the larynx, the tip should be turned downward.

9. THROAT IRRIGATIONS

Definition. A throat irrigation is the washing out of the oral pharynx by a stream of liquid.

Therapeutic Uses. The purposes of the irrigation are: (1) to soften the mucus and to remove accumulated secretions; (2) to stimulate the circulation and absorption of inflammatory products; (3) to relieve congestion, swelling, and pain; and (4) to stimulate and bring to a head the inflammatory process of suppuration, so that the abscess may be incised and the pus removed. A throat irrigation is ordered in place of a gargle if gargling is painful or if a more continuous and prolonged effect is desired. Webster et al. say that a gargle "is of doubtful value beyond the tonsillar region."* However, it is not easy to persuade patients to allow solutions to pass beyond this point during an irrigation.

Selection of Method. The *solution* used for a throat irrigation may be any one of those ordered as gargles and they are numerous indeed. In some cases drugs that act as a mild local anesthetic may be in the irrigating solution. The benefits are probably the result of heat and mechanical cleansing; therefore, it is doubtful whether one solution is much more desirable than another. Since the treatment is unpleasant if a solution has a disagreeable taste, plain hot water or physiological saline solution would seem to be the choice for cleansing purposes and temperature effect. The nurse would be safe in using either of these if the physician failed to specify the solution and she was unable to communicate with him.

Solutions of a *temperature* not tolerated by other parts of the body feel comfortable in the mouth. A throat irrigation is often ordered as hot as the patient can stand it; however, temperatures above 49° C (120.2° F) might cause tissue damage.

If the irrigation is ordered for a temperature effect, the duration of the treat-

* Webster, David H., et al.: *op. cit.,* p. 175.

ment is of some importance, and it is necessary to use from 1000 to 1500 cc (1 to 1½ qt). The *amount* of the solution may or may not be specified by the physician. In any event the treatment should not tire the patient unduly, and if an ill person shows signs of exhaustion before the entire amount has been administered, the treatment should be stopped.

To get the desired results from a throat irrigation, a continuous stream of the solution must reach the affected parts without making the patient gag. If this occurs, he will probably swallow or aspirate some of the irrigating fluid. The *position* of the head must allow the solution to flow freely in and out of the mouth; the head must tilt forward so that the solution can flow over the lower lip or tilt to one side in such a way that the solution can flow from the corner of the mouth. If the patient directs the stream of liquid himself he feels less nervous about the treatment. The purpose of the irrigation and the method of giving it should be carefully explained to the patient. He is told to hold his breath while the solution is flowing, to prevent aspiration of the fluid, but he should realize that the irrigation can be stopped at any time so that he can rest or breathe. This treatment is comforting, and after he is once taught to take a throat irrigation, the average person will cooperate fully.

If the patient is able to sit up, the return flow is most satisfactorily received in a large basin, placed on a table under his chin. The irrigation can be even more comfortably given with the patient lying down, his head turned so that the cheek is on the edge of the pillow. In order to clean the entire throat, the patient shifts his position in the middle of the procedure and lies on the other side. If the irrigation is given in this position, the return flow is received in a curved or rectangular basin placed under the cheek and mouth. The bedding must be protected with a waterproof cover.

Equipment.   Articles required are an irrigating pole, irrigating can, tubing with clamp, an irrigating tip, the solution, a large pail for the return, a waste basin in which to collect the solution as it runs from the mouth, protection for the chest and shoulder of the patient, paper handkerchiefs, and a receptacle for used handkerchiefs. Equipment must be clean but need not be sterile.

Suggested Procedure.   Explain the procedure thoroughly to the patient. Place him in a sitting or recumbent posture, according to his condition and preference. Protect the clothing or bedding with suitable materials, such as rubber sheeting, oiled silk, or cellulose film; cover the part that goes around the patient's neck with a towel or piece of soft crepe paper. Give the patient a paper handkerchief. Place in position the basin for the collection of waste. Support the irrigating can so that the level of the solution is approximately 30 cm (12 in.) above the level of the mouth. If the treatment is new to the patient, allow the solution to flow for a very short time, remove the tip, and discuss any difficulties he may have had. As he acquires more confidence, he can direct the flow of solution, hold his breath for longer periods, and make the solution reach farther into the pharynx. At frequent intervals empty the waste basin into the pail to prevent spilling. If it is necessary for the nurse to look at the pharyngeal mucosa, the usual care must be taken in depressing the tongue, so as to prevent gagging and injury.

Recording the Treatment. Chart the treatment, the time it was given, the kind, amount, and temperature of the solution, and the patient's reaction to it.

10. GARGLES

Gargles are sometimes used in the same conditions of the throat as those in which sprays or irrigations are used. Solutions employed may be cleansing, soothing, or antiseptic, and either hot or cold. The patient must be cautioned against swallowing the solution, although antiseptics used are rarely toxic if swallowed in small quantities. Gargling is likely to be fatiguing and is often painful. Its value is questioned by many doctors, who feel that the rigid control of the throat and breathing are so difficult for the already sensitive, painful, and swollen throat that the effort may be quite inadequate to bring the solution into contact with all parts of the inflamed mucous lining. For this reason, many physicians prefer sprays that may be applied directly to the diseased part, or irrigations if a temperature effect is desired.

REFERENCES

1. Duke-Elder, Sir Stewart: *Parsons' Diseases of the Eye,* 12th ed. The Macmillan Company, New York, 1953, p. 127.
2. Berens, Conrad (ed.): *The Eye and Its Diseases.* W. B. Saunders Co., Philadelphia, 1949, p. 363.
3. Berens, Conrad, (ed.): *op. cit.,* p. 997.
4. Ridley, Frederick: "The Use of Antiseptics in Opththalmology," *Proc. Roy. Soc. Med.* **25:**480, (Feb.) 1932.
5. Duke-Elder, Sir Stewart: *op. cit.,* p. 133.
6. Hosford, George V., and Hicks, Avery M.: "Hydrogen Ion Concentration of Tears," *A.M.A. Arch. Ophth.,* **13:**14, (Jan.) 1935.
7. Duke-Elder, Sir Stewart: *op. cit.,* pp. 137, 143.
8. Berens, Conrad (ed.): *op. cit.,* p. 372.
9. Webster, David H., et al. *Nursing in Diseases of the Eye, Ear, Nose and Throat.* W. B. Saunders Co., Philadelphia, 1948, p. 25.
10. Webster, David H., et al.: *op. cit.,* p. 25.
11. Morrison, William W.: *Diseases of the Ear, Nose and Throat.* Appleton-Century-Crofts, Inc., New York, 1948, p. 42.
12. Boies, Lawrence R., and associates: *Fundamentals of Otolaryngology.* W. B. Saunders Co., Philadelphia, 1951, p. 66.
13. Rutherford, Miriam H.: "Proper Use of Antibiotics in Treatment of Acute Otitis Media," *California Med.,* **75:**98, (Aug.) 1951.
14. Parkinson, Roy H.: *Eye, Ear, Nose and Throat Manual for Nurses,* 6th ed. C. V. Mosby Co., St. Louis, 1949, p. 133.
15. McAuliffe, George B.: *The Essentials of Otology.* Oxford University Press, New York, 1927, p. 90.
16. Morrison, William W.: *op. cit.,* p. 280.
17. Morrison, William W.: *op. cit.,* p. 262.

Additional Suggested Reading

Barnhill, John F., and Mellinger, William J.: *Surgical Anatomy of the Head and Neck,* 2nd ed., Williams & Wilkins Co., Baltimore, 1940.

Berens, Conrad, and Posner, Adolph: *The Eye and Its Importance in Relation to General Disease.* Commission for the Blind, State Department of Social Welfare, New York, 1949.

Denison, Abby-Helen, and Eklund, Lyyli: *A Textbook of Eye, Ear, Nose, and Throat Nursing,* 2nd ed. The Macmillan Company, New York, 1937.

Fabricant, Noah H.: *Modern Medication of the Ear, Nose and Throat.* Grune and Stratton, New York, 1951.

Garland, Phyllis: *Ophthalmic Nursing,* J. B. Lippincott Co., Philadelphia, 1952.

Kirby, Daniel B.: *Surgery of Cataracts.* J. B. Lippincott Co., Philadelphia, 1950.

Lederer, Francis L.: *Diseases of the Ear, Nose and Throat.* F. A. Davis Co., Philadelphia, 1952.

Meek, Raymond E.: *Eye Hazards and Eye Injuries.* Commission for the Blind, State Department of Social Welfare, New York, 1949.

Seltzer, Albert P.: *Diseases of the Eye, Ear, Nose and Throat; a Textbook for Nurses.* McGraw-Hill Book Co., New York, 1950.

Town, Arno: *Ophthalmology.* Lea & Febiger, Philadelphia, 1951.

Vail, Derrick, and Lindsay, John R. (eds.): *The 1951 Year Book of the Eye, Ear, Nose and Throat.* Year Book Publishers, Chicago, 1952.

CHAPTER 34. FACTORS INFLUENCING TREATMENT AND NURSING CARE

Adaptation of Treatment and Nursing Care to the Needs of the Patient. Those who see the skill and confidence of successful physicians and nurses often marvel at their ability to adapt treatment and nursing care to the particular needs of their patients, no matter how ill they are, what disease they have, or what age they may be. Obviously, even those medical workers with the widest experience have not always seen similar physical conditions, and each personality is unique. Their success must therefore lie in a knowledge of guiding principles and in their ability to study the patients and provide the treatment that each demands. The development of this ability should be the major aim of every nursing curriculum. Nursing faculties are constantly trying to find satisfactory answers to the questions: How much and what kind of experience is necessary to enable the graduate to adapt nursing care to particular patients and situations? What method of attack should the student nurse use to get the best results? These questions must occur also to anyone writing a text of this kind.

In presenting "Common Problems in Nursing Practice," as the last section of this text is entitled, a selection must be made of what seems most important, since it is certainly not within the scope of a general nursing text to cover the whole field of even medical and surgical nursing. The purpose of this chapter is to present briefly the bases for selection of conditions discussed and some factors influencing treatment and nursing care everywhere.

Classification of Subject Matter and Its Influences upon Medical and Nursing Thought. Clinical courses in nursing and medicine in the past have been based on anatomical classifications of disease. For example, units of study were and still are entitled "Treatment and Nursing Care of Diseases of the Respiratory System," or of the genitourinary system or the nervous system. A great effort was formerly made to enable medical and nursing students to see as many diseases as possible and to take part in the care of patients with the diseases if opportunity was afforded. It is no wonder that students of both professions, brought up under such an educational plan, have committed the crime of referring to "the pneumonia in Room 15," or "the cardiac in Bed 2." With the emphasis placed on the disease rather than on the individual with certain symptoms and difficulties, it is not surprising that these students were likely to assume that all persons with the same disease should be similarly treated.

Recently, there has been a marked effort to emphasize factors other than the diagnosis that may be pinned (sometimes incorrectly) upon the patient. For example, a course entitled "Nursing of Children" places the emphasis on age as the common factor among patients rather than disease diagnosis. "Nursing Care of the Chronically Ill" would emphasize the duration of the illness and the consequent restriction of living as the common factor rather than the particular organs involved. William R. Houston in his medical text, *The Art of Treatment,* has made a radical departure from the usual arrangement of subject matter. He places patients in the following groups, the common factor being the "principal method of therapy employed," as he terms it:

1. Patients who are to be treated chiefly by nursing care
2. Conditions for which there are known or "specific" remedies
3. Conditions in which the chief therapeutic method is psychotherapy, or guidance
4. Diseases which impose a limitation upon life as the condition of treatment
5. Disorders in which physiological considerations guide treatment
6. Conditions in which treatment is tentative and experimental*

In the discussion of the treatment of each disease, the special elements of therapy are presented, but the common elements are emphasized throughout. The author builds up for the reader a set of guiding principles for the treatment of each group rather than a set of rules for the treatment of each disease. By constant reference to experimental work and the experience of others, this text, like many others in the medical field, impresses the student with the importance of studying the disease; on the other hand, equal emphasis is placed on the importance of considering the patient's problems and upon the individual differences likely to occur in reaction to the same disease.

In psychiatry, especially, the emphasis is changing. It is no longer on the treatment of a diagnosed disease but on a study of the patient and an effort to help him recognize and deal effectively with his particular problems. Many curriculum studies are in progress. Most of them are concentrating on the development of the psychosocial aspects of medicine and nursing because it is believed that they were neglected in the first half of the century during which period there was such a phenomenal development in the physical aspects of medical science. Greater economy and satisfaction in learning are also sought in curriculum revision.

There is pretty general agreement that it is more important for a medical student to be skilled in general methods of diagnosis and to be able to study the patient and work out a rational plan of therapy than to have a more varied, but less thorough, experience in seeing all sorts of diseases. The National League of Nursing Education[1] in large measure accepted this principle in its recommendations for the basic nursing curriculum in 1937. The problem-solving attitude is stressed

* Houston, William R.: *The Art of Treatment.* The Macmillan Company, New York, 1936, p. 80.

throughout, and emphasis is placed upon a wise selection of clinical experience for the student rather than upon a great variety of cases.

A committee of this organization published a list of diseases and conditions with which it recommended that the student nurse should become familiar during her basic professional course. Each disease or condition was judged important for several or all of the following reasons: because (1) it is prevalent in this country; (2) it is a serious disease that may result in death or crippling of the patient's abilities; (3) nursing care is an important factor in recovery; (4) nursing involves either fundamental nursing measures or specific procedures difficult to learn outside the hospital. Using these standards as a basis for selection, the committee was faced with such a long list that it was found necessary to make groups of diseases in which nursing care was thought to be similar, with the recommendation that the student have experience in taking care of a patient with at least one of these conditions.

So in nursing, as in medicine, many members of the profession are coming to think that emphasis should be placed on developing the reasoning capacity of the student rather than on learning the symptoms, treatment, and rules for medical or nursing care in a long list of conditions. It is assumed, for example, that if the student demonstrates the ability to take care of a patient with one acute eruptive febrile disease, and recognizes the problems involved, he or she should be able to develop an effective plan of care for a patient with a similar condition or a patient having like symptoms. If this is true, it would seem that *a nursing text should attempt to group diseases according to the type of nursing care required.*

Certainly, the anatomical classification does not do this. There is more similarity in the nursing care needed by two chronically ill middle-aged men, regardless of the organs involved, than there is in the nursing care of asthma and pneumonia, although both are diseases of the lungs. The nursing care of two sick infants has more in common, regardless of the diagnosis, than the care of an infant with bacillary dysentery and the care of a young adult with the same disease. To further illustrate the point that other factors have more influence upon the kind of nursing care needed than do the anatomical structures involved, attention may be called to the mood of the patient as a conditioning factor. A patient with a manic-depressive psychosis requires one type of nursing care when he is depressed and suicidal, and another when he is euphoric and hyperactive.

Other examples might be given to show that the duration of the illness, age, helplessness, and mental state of the patient may have far more to do with the kind of nursing care required than the system or the organs affected by the disease. In teaching nursing students and in trying as a practicing nurse to develop some basic principles of nursing care, it would seem desirable to organize the nursing care of diseases and conditions under such headings as the following:

Unit 1. The ambulatory patient; the mildly ill with a self-limiting disease; the chronically ill.

Unit 2. The infant; the child; the adolescent; the young adult; the middle-aged; the aged.

Unit 3. The hypoactive depressed (suicidal) patient; the hyperactive euphoric patient.

Unit 4. The helpless rational patient; the irrational; the unconscious; the patient in shock; the dying.

Unit 5. Patients handicapped by limited vision, speech, hearing, equilibrium, or motor ability.

Unit 6. The patient with an acute communicable disease; an acute local infection; extensive burns; extensive skin disease.

Unit 7. Preoperative nursing care; postoperative nursing care; special needs of patients in regional surgery, such as eye, chest, abdominal, and brain surgery.

If a nursing curriculum were constructed along such lines, the emphasis would fall on solving the outstanding nursing problems presented by patients everywhere rather than on treatment of diagnosed conditions, which is the major problem of the physician. Moreover, if such units as those listed above were studied as the core of the clinical program, a great deal of duplication would be avoided and more time would be available on each service for consideration of the specific needs of patients found there.

In the present revision of this text a complete regrouping of diseases and conditions according to this concept is not attempted. An effort has, however, been made to emphasize the general principles underlying the nursing care of groups of patients thought especially representative. No claim is made to cover a complete list of the conditions that might be placed in each group. It is the hope of the writer that this section will give the nurse specific help in the care of a few types of patients and in conjunction with the remainder of the text, and particularly Chapter 4, will serve as a guide to studying, planning, and executing the nursing care of any patient.

REFERENCE

1. National League of Nursing Education, Committee on Curriculum: *A Curriculum Guide for Schools of Nursing.* The League, New York, 1937, p. 567.

CHAPTER 35. NURSING IN THE CARE OF
THE DYING AND THE DEAD

1. **ATTITUDE OF THE NURSE**
2. **SIGNS OF APPROACHING DEATH**
3. **NURSING CARE OF THE DYING AND COOPERATION WITH THE FAMILY, THE MINISTER, AND THE PHYSICIAN**
4. **NURSING CARE OF THE BODY AFTER DEATH**
5. **PUBLIC HEALTH REGULATIONS ON THE DISPOSITION OF THE BODY AFTER DEATH**

1. ATTITUDE OF THE NURSE

It is natural that in a culture where the young are so often protected from the sight and talk of death many adults are uneasy in the presence of a dying person. Montaigne, writing in the sixteenth century, said that we should not make death a stranger but should think of it daily and without fear, directing our thoughts toward the prolongation of our services rather than life itself.

The end of our cariere is death, it is the necessarie object of our aim; if it affright us, how is it possible we should step one foot farther without an ague? The remedie of the vulgar sort is not to thinke on it. . . . Let us learne to stand, and combat her with a resolute minde. . . . Let us remove her strangeness from her, let us converse frequent, and acquaint ourselves with her, let us have nothing so much in minde as death. . . . He who hath learned to die hath learned to serve. There is no evill in life for him who hath well conceived, how the privation of life is no evill. To know how to die doth free us all from subjection and constraint. . . . I would have a man to be doing and to prolong his lives offices as much as lieth in him, and let death seize upon me, whilst I am setting my cabiges, careless of her dart, but more of my unperfect garden.

For the aged and for the hopelessly ill death is, indeed, as he says, "no evill"; for the religious who believe in life hereafter, there is no fear or dread. Doctors, nurses, and ministers of wide experience tell of many who are happy and exalted in death. Death can be made beautiful by the courage with which the person, and those around him, face it. Montaigne, quoting Epaminondas, implies that dying well is the ultimate test of a man. He says: "Epaminondas being demanded which of the three he estemed most, either Chabrias, or Iphicrates, or himselfe; '*It is neces-sary,*' said he, 'that we be seene to die, before your question may be well resolved. Verily we should steale much from him, if he should be weighed without the honour and greatness of his end.' "*

Literature is full of instances of those who, in their manner of dying, showed an unsuspected strength of character that changed men's former judgments of them. There is, perhaps, a universal desire in man to die well, unshaken in whatever faith supports him. Most men are comforted by the presence of their minister and those for whom they have greatest affection. Russell L. Dicks shares with the less experienced the insight he has acquired through his association with the dying. Nurses will profit by a study of his and Richard C. Cabot's texts.[1, 2] Plato's[3] descrip-tion of Socrates' noble death has helped to rid some persons of their fear of it. All medical workers who think that it is part of their function to help their patients die as they would wish, will find themselves fortified by any reading, or experience, that increases their belief in the ultimate goodness of the scheme of the universe. Since medicine is the one service that knows no bounds set by nation, creed, or race, the workers' understanding and sympathy should be equal to the demands this makes upon them.

No rules can be laid down for the nurse's behavior with the dying person and his family because no two situations are alike. Even though this is her first contact with death, however, she need not fear self-consciousness and embarrass-ment if she turns her entire attention to the task of helping them. A great deal depends upon the nurse's sensitiveness to people, her taste and judgment; in other words, the kind of person she is. Nursing skills can be learned that will lessen the physical discomfort of the patient and, consequently, the distress of the family, but everyone concerned will sense the nurse's willingness, or unwillingness, to go beside them through this experience with death, which is not a skill to be learned but an attitude. If the nurse measures up in this test, all are sustained by her professional knowledge, by what strength of character she possesses, and by her sympathy, ex-pressed in thoughtful actions rather than in words.

2. SIGNS OF APPROACHING DEATH

There are many kinds of death, and many variations in the way in which its approach is manifested. George Draper, a student of the personality, says: "And finally at the end, because his passage on earth is determined according to the patterns of his individual constitution, each man dies in a notably personal way."† Death may come suddenly, a few moments after the individual seemed in good health; in other cases a person may be on the borderline between life and death for weeks. In sudden death there is no time for the failing circulation to bring about

* Montaigne, Michel E. de: *Essayes.* Modern Library, Random House, New York, 1928, pp. 47-56.
† Draper, George, et al.: *Human Constitution in Clinical Medicine.* Paul B. Hoeber, Inc., New York, 1944, p. 74.

those changes in the appearance and behavior that occur when death comes at the end of an illness. Alfred W. Worcester[4] has given a striking description of the process of death when it comes slowly and the care that should be given the dying. He does not believe that it is possible to say in any case just when the process of dying begins. He comments on the "multifarious" ways in which "death triumphs," and cautions the young doctor against expecting every patient to follow the text-book description. Certain signs do serve, however, as indications that life is approaching its end. First, there is a general slowing of the circulation shown by the fact that the feet, especially, and later the hands, ears, and nose are cold to the touch. Usually there is excessive sweating; the skin is pale or mottled from congestion of blood in the veins. Because the muscles are losing their tone, the body assumes a supine position; the jaw sags while the dying man breathes through his mouth, with the flaccid lips and cheeks sucked in and blown outward with each respiration; the reflexes gradually disappear; the pupils fail to react to light; the ability to swallow is lost. The unswallowed mucus in the throat and drying of the upper part of the tract, due to the open mouth, cause noisy breathing and, at the last, what is spoken of as *the death rattle*. The respirations may be rapid and shallow, or abnormally slow. The eyes are often sunken and half closed. Sometimes they appear to have a film over them. Speech is difficult—it is usually mumbled and confused in character. Hearing is thought to be dulled in most cases, but since the dying may lose their ability to speak or move while their hearing is intact, *it is not known when they cease to hear*. The patient may give evidence of anxiety or distress, such as restless, tossing movements, pulling at the bedclothes, crying, moaning, and talking incoherently. Shakespeare's description[5] of Falstaff's death put in the mouth of Mistress Quickly is a classic and accurate picture of the dying.

Some of the distressing signs of death are indicative of either mental or physical suffering that can often be relieved by proper care. When the physician is convinced that there is no longer hope for the patient's recovery, the prescribed treatment is directed toward the relief of discomfort rather than the prolongation of life. The nurse should be alert to changes in the patient's condition in order that she may report them to the right persons and record them on the patient's chart; also, because the nursing care will be altered by the knowledge that death is near.

3. NURSING CARE OF THE DYING AND COOPERATION WITH THE FAMILY, THE MINISTER, AND THE PHYSICIAN

Most patients seem to have a realization that they are going to die even before signs of death are apparent to their medical attendants, although in many instances they are surprisingly unaware of their condition up to the last. This foreboding of death, when it is present, produces as profound changes in the mental outlook of the individual as in the physical functions of the body. Tolstoy's story,[6] "The Death of Ivan Ilych," gives a good picture of the dying man's state of mind. While the nurse's particular usefulness lies in relieving any physical distress there may be in the process of dying, she is inevitably placed in positions where she can contribute toward the patient's peace of mind. The family, the friends, the minister, and the physician depend upon the nurse to tell them when the patient wants to see them, and it is her responsibility to report any changes that indicate that death is near.

The physician decides when the family should be told that the person's condition is critical but in his absence the nurse may have to take this responsibility. In hospitals, nurses should make every effort to provide privacy for the patient and his distressed family. When private rooms are not available, screens give some semblance of seclusion. Dying ward patients are often moved into nearby rooms, not only out of consideration for them, but because the sight and sounds of death affect the other patients. The hospital activities cannot be stopped because a person is dying, but the air of bustle and the preoccupation of nurses and doctors in their other duties are likely to make the family feel that the staff is indifferent to their suffering. Everyone should try to show genuine concern for them and to protect them from sights or sounds that might seem unsympathetic. The sensitive nurse will attempt to keep those who disturb the patient away from him and those who comfort him nearby, although tact and good judgment are needed to avoid seeming officious. She should make herself inconspicuous and sense the patient's desire to be left alone with his family, a minister, or his physician.

In many cases the dying ask the nurse questions about their condition, but they rarely do so unless they are prepared to hear the answer. The nurse should always avoid being untruthful; she can generally satisfy the patient by asking him what his doctor has told him. When all hope for his recovery is lost, difficult though it may be, most physicians feel that it is their duty to tell the person the medical opinion if he wants to know it. It is also usual for the physician to discuss the imminence of death with the patient's family and to notify them of his death when it actually occurs.

The dying often want to make or change a will. State laws require wills to be signed in the presence of two or three witnesses.[7] The nurse may be asked to serve as a witness and to get one or more persons to serve in this capacity with her. It is unwise for medical personnel to act in the role of witnesses or to help a patient to write a will. There may be subsequent litigation, and they will be taken from their more important work to appear in court.[8]

There are certain observances in most religions that bring comfort to persons of each faith. Ministers of all denominations are prepared to give the services of their church to the dying, and will administer them at the patient's request. In some religions there are no sacraments; in others they are of vital significance. This is, therefore, not the only, or chief, reason why every sick patient wants to see his minister. If a helpful relationship exists between them the patient's faith is strengthened; he has a friend and confidant who will face the fact that he is dying and will discuss with him his hopes and fears, his plans for his family, and the consequences of his death. It is easier for the minister to help the patient if he has been seeing him throughout his illness. If there are resident chaplains in the hospitals their visits are made routinely; if not, the family, the doctor, or the nurse should help to find a clergyman who will give the patient spiritual comfort. (Working with the clergy has been discussed at some length in Chapter 4.) The patient should know that the minister is coming to see him. If the nurse has any reason to believe that the patient does not realize the seriousness of his condition, and may fear that a visit from a clergyman means that he is thought to be dying, she may assure him, in an indirect way, that all patients are visited by clergymen regularly on all hospital services. As much privacy as possible should be provided by screens or curtains in an open ward, or by signs placed on doors of private rooms. The nurse should meet the clergyman and tell him as much as she can that she thinks will be helpful about the patient's physical condition, his problems, and his need, unless she believes the clergyman has this knowledge. The minister, priest, or rabbi may prefer to go to the patient unaccompanied, but the nurse should offer to take him to the bedside and, if the patient does not know him, to introduce him. It is very desirable for this visit to be so timed that the patient is awake and rational. Among Christians the Catholics—Roman, western non-Roman, and Eastern Orthodox—attach the greatest importance to the sacraments. The Episcopalian, Lutheran, and Moravian are spoken of as "bridge faiths" between Catholicism and Protestantism and have some sacraments and rituals in common. If the patient belongs to any of these groups it is desirable to have ready the few simple things the clergyman will need for the administration of the sacraments. He will usually want a table covered with a white cloth and on it a glass, a small bowl of water, a spoon, and a linen napkin or a small towel. A glass, a tube, and fresh drinking water should be on the bedside table. The Catholic priest brings the oil if he expects to give Extreme Unction. If not, he may ask the nurse for oil in a small bowl; he will also need about six cotton balls, which the nurse supplies. The minister or priest provides whatever else he needs. However, in denominational hospitals sacred objects such as holy oil and crucifixes are kept in a special place ready for use. If a nurse of the same faith is available she may be of especial help to the patient, his family, and the clergyman.

The sacraments have been described in Chapter 4, but it might be repeated here that the Roman Catholics especially believe that the sacraments are essential to a "state of grace" and admission to heaven. The sacraments administered to the dying are Baptism (if the person has not been baptized), Penance (Confession), Holy Eucharist (Communion), called Viaticum when received by a dying person, and Extreme Unction. If the dying person is a Roman Catholic and has not been baptized (as in the case of an infant), the nurse should make every effort to get a priest to baptize the person; if this is not possible a Roman Catholic member of the staff should be asked to administer the sacrament, or in the last resort the non-Catholic should do so.[9, 10, 11]

It is not possible to describe the ministrations of the spiritual adviser to the various Protestant, Catholic, Jewish, Hindu, Mohammedan, and other faiths, but nurses should know something about all the great religions. Their understanding would be broadened by reading such works as Joseph Gaer's *How the Great Religions Began* or even Florence M. Fitch's *One God: The Ways We Worship Him,* written for children. Books on the relationship of religion and health are included in the references for this chapter. The nurse serves the dying patient best by seeing that the proper representative of his church is present and then by providing the clergyman as nearly as she can with the conditions he indicates as essential to or helpful in his ministry. Dicks warns those who attend the dying person against trying to make him conform to their theological beliefs. Visits of clergymen should be charted, the name of the person administering the sacraments, and the time at which it was received.

The nurse should realize that the patient's state of mind will influence his physical reaction to death and also the kind and amount of care she should give him. This is a time, above all others, when the wishes of the patient himself, and those of his family, should be considered of paramount importance, and no treatment should be forced upon a dying man. Nursing measures suggested here should be used only if they seem to give comfort.

Attention has been called to the changes that occur as the circulatory mechanism begins to fail. It is customary to try to warm the cooling extremities by the application of blankets and hot-water bottles. This should be done with great care. Worcester attributes much of the restlessness and pulling of the bedclothes, seen in the dying, to the fact that they themselves feel hot although the skin may feel cold to the touch. If the patient can respond he should be asked whether he would like additional warmth. The bedding should be light in weight. A gown if wet with perspiration should be changed. Rubbing the skin gently with alcohol has a refreshing effect.

The dying patient is often seen lying on his back, which is probably the *least* comfortable position for him. In this posture the tongue falls against the pharynx, mucus collects in the mouth, and the effect of both is to close off the respiratory passage and cause strangulation. If the patient is turned on his side, the tongue falls forward and the mouth drains more satisfactorily. Since there is little muscular control left, the body must be well supported by pillows. The patient often prefers to have his head elevated, feeling that he can breathe more easily in this position. Several writers of long experience in medical practice say that the dying wish to be turned toward the light and that the room should never be darkened because of the patient's dimming vision and his natural desire to see until the end of his life. The room should be airy as well as light, for the patient breathes more easily if the air is in movement.

The mouth should have special care. The excessive dryness caused by mouth breathing can be relieved by coating the mucous membrane with a thin layer of oil applied with a cotton applicator or with an atomizer. Water, or some refreshing liquid, should be given in small amounts at short intervals to keep the mouth moist. By putting the finger over one end of a drinking tube after it is in a glass of water, suction is created and water is held in the tube. Small amounts can be given the patient from this tube. It is well known that the dying suffer from dehydration. In some cases they can drink enough to control it; in others, infusions are given until death is believed near. Since transfusions and infusions delay death, it is difficult for the doctor to decide when it is kind and when it is unkind to prolong the irreversible process. When mucus collects in the mouth, it may be removed with cotton sponges held with forceps. It is most efficiently removed with a suction apparatus, if one is available.

Because the patient's hearing becomes less acute, the nurse should stand near him and speak distinctly. *Nothing should be said in the room that he should not hear, for no one knows how much the seemingly unconscious person can hear. Whispering especially should be avoided; the patient may see the lips move and be distressed that he cannot hear what is said.*

As the muscles lose their tone, leakage may occur from the bladder and rectum. To avoid this embarrassment to the patient, the bedpan and urinal should be put in position periodically. Even though the patient has too little strength to ask for them, he may be able to use them. The bed should be protected by soft pads of cellucotton that have a waterproof paper base. These can be changed frequently without much inconvenience to the patient. In some cases the bladder becomes distended from a failure to void, and the physician will order catherization to relieve the sensation of pressure.

Every effort should be made to prevent disagreeable odors in the room. If anything is used to mask unavoidable odors, it should have an aromatic smell, like that of ammonia or camphor, rather than either an acrid or sweet smell. For the sake of the patient and his family whatever makes for beauty in the environment should be kept until the end. It is possible that music might help many who are dying. Certainly we should try to keep the person surrounded with what he would like to see at the last.

Most physicians prescribe narcotics for the dying in sufficiently large doses to relieve all pain and discomfort. In some cases the individual asks that nothing be given him that will cloud his consciousness at the end. They may feel as Robert Browning expressed it in *Prospice:*

> I would hate that death bandaged my eyes and forebore,
> And bade me creep past.

A request of this kind should be respected, and the patient made as comfortable as possible without the aid of drugs. When drugs are used, they are occasionally given in a vein, if the processes of absorption have slowed up to such an extent that a subcutaneous injection would have little effect.

The nurse stays with the patient as long as he shows signs of life except for short periods when he may want to be left with a friend, a member of the family, the physician, or the minister. Cessation of breathing is generally considered the ultimate sign of death, and the exact time when this occurs should be reported and recorded on the patient's chart. The heart may beat after respiration has ceased, but the physician, who is the one to pronounce death, bases his decision on the latter sign. Edmund V. Cowdry, writing on the aging process, says:

A human being is pronounced dead when the circulation fails, consciousness is lost, and there is no longer a possibility of resuscitation. But he is then not wholly dead because some of his cells continue to live for varying periods. . . . Death is always piecemeal for humans. . . . Death is disorganization of living matter which makes permanently impossible any and all vital phenomena. . . .*

In cases of asphyxia or drowning, every effort is made to re-establish the respiration as long as the heart functions; however, this is not desirable when the patient is hopelessly ill, and it is only a question of prolonging life for a few hours or days.

When the patient ceases breathing, the nurse reports this fact immediately if the physician is not present. After the physician certifies the death of the patient, and the family is ready to leave the body in her hands, the nurse prepares the body for the undertaker, who is notified as soon as possible.

4. NURSING CARE OF THE BODY AFTER DEATH

In hospitals where a physician is present or can be gotten immediately to pronounce death, the nurse takes no steps toward caring for the body until this has been done. In home nursing, hours may elapse before the physician's visit, and certain precautions must be observed to prevent distortions of the face or body. The patient is not legally dead until the physician has certified his death, and nothing should be done that would interfere with life, as there is always a possibility of life remaining in the body. The undertaker, for example, cannot accept the body or prepare it for burial before this official pronouncement has been made.

Custom varies in relation to the nursing care of the body after death, but certain principles should be kept in mind. Bodies are usually embalmed, or chemically preserved, and made to look as natural as possible. Congestion and clotting within the blood vessels before or after death interfere with the embalming process. Distortion, discoloration, or scarring of the body is distressing to the family and friends, and should therefore be prevented. The body itself should be clean and wrapped in clean covering when sent to the undertaking establishment, and should be plainly marked to avoid mistakes in identity.

In order to keep the normal position of the features and form, the eyes are closed immediately, as in sleep, and the body is straightened with the arms laid at the sides; the mouth is closed and any dentures that have been removed for the patient's comfort are replaced; the head is elevated on one pillow, and a folded towel is used to prop the chin in position for a short time until the process of death stiffens the features. (Bandages have been used to hold the jaw firm, but at the present time many undertakers prefer to have this omitted because the bandage, if too tight, may discolor the skin.) All of this may be done before the physician's certification of death, if it is impossible for him to see the patient for several hours or more after the nurse believes that death has occurred.

Before proceeding with any necessary bathing of the body, all rings (including wedding rings), earrings, bracelets, beads, or other articles worn should be removed and placed in a separate package with other articles of value, such

* Cowdry, Edmund V. (ed.): *Problem of Aging: Biological and Medical Aspects,* 2nd ed. Williams & Wilkins Co., Baltimore, 1942, pp. 364-65.

as money, jewelry, receipts, eyeglasses, letters, keys, and any emblem of sacred or religious meaning. If the death has occurred in the hospital, an itemized list of such valuables should be made, and later, together with the package, taken to the administrative office. Nothing is too small to be listed. What may seem of trivial value to the nurse may be, on account of its association, of untold value to a family. When earrings or rings cannot be removed, a note to this effect should be made on the list of valuables. When it is requested by members of the family that a wedding ring, or like article, remain on the body, it should be securely tied on with a bandage. In institutions it is wise to have requests of this kind in writing, and such written requests should be left in the main office.

Soiled dressings should be replaced with fresh dressings. Adhesive marks should be removed with benzine. In hospitals a pad of cellucotton, lined on one side with waterproof paper, and a diaper of old muslin are applied to prevent the escape of urine and feces from the relaxed meatus and anus. In some hospitals a mortuary gown is put on the body; in others it is omitted. A tag containing the patient's name, the clinical division, and the date is attached to one wrist. When the toilet is complete, the body is wrapped in a shroud that is usually made of a very large square of muslin. This square is arranged diagonally. A tag is attached to the outside bearing the same information as that attached to the wrist. A stretcher is prepared, and the body is placed on it and covered in such a way that it cannot easily be distinguished from a living person. It must be securely fastened to the stretcher. In the hospital the removal of the body from the clinical division to the morgue should be conducted inconspicuously and with respect and dignity. As far as possible all the details of the death, aftercare, and removal of the body should be spared other patients.

All clothing and other personal property of the patient should be listed, wrapped neatly in a bundle, properly tagged, and taken to the office or given to the family according to the regulations of the institution.

In homes the body is left dressed in some soft gown until the undertaker comes. A large sheet should be provided for wrapping the body if it is to be removed from the dwelling to be prepared for burial.

5. PUBLIC HEALTH REGULATIONS ON THE DISPOSITION OF THE BODY AFTER DEATH

The death certificate, which is sent to the local health department, is made out by the physician, the undertaker, and the pathologist if an autopsy is performed. Figure 215 shows a death certificate properly made out. The form was developed by the federal government and is used by most states. To facilitate compilation of international statistics, the World Health Assembly in 1948 recommended the specific medical information requested on the certificate of death. These recommendations have been accepted by all states in this country.[12, 13] In hospital practice, some of these data are gotten for the physician by other personnel; in homes,

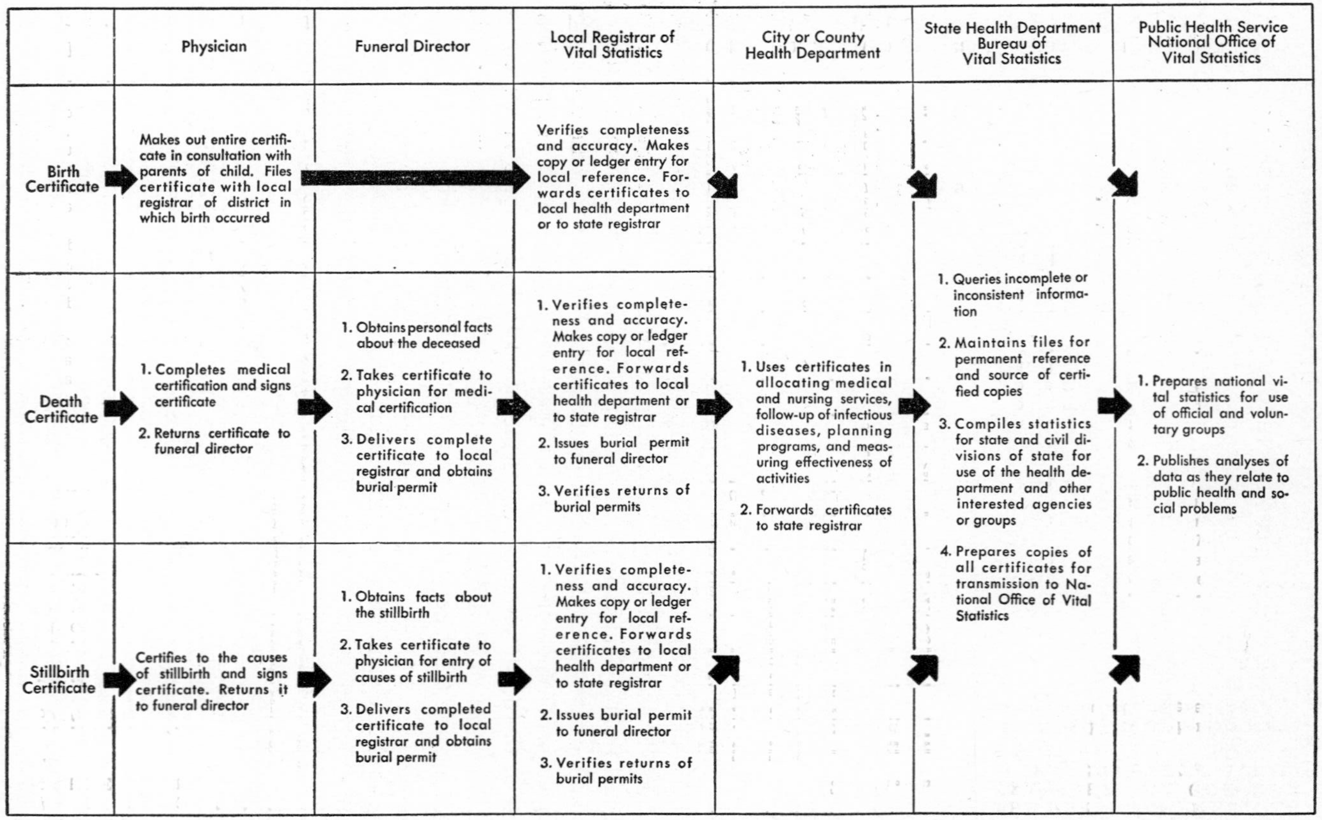

	Physician	Funeral Director	Local Registrar of Vital Statistics	City or County Health Department	State Health Department Bureau of Vital Statistics	Public Health Service National Office of Vital Statistics
Birth Certificate	Makes out entire certificate in consultation with parents of child. Files certificate with local registrar of district in which birth occurred		Verifies completeness and accuracy. Makes copy or ledger entry for local reference. Forwards certificates to local health department or to state registrar			
Death Certificate	1. Completes medical certification and signs certificate 2. Returns certificate to funeral director	1. Obtains personal facts about the deceased 2. Takes certificate to physician for medical certification 3. Delivers complete certificate to local registrar and obtains burial permit	1. Verifies completeness and accuracy. Makes copy or ledger entry for local reference. Forwards certificates to local health department or to state registrar 2. Issues burial permit to funeral director 3. Verifies returns of burial permits	1. Uses certificates in allocating medical and nursing services, follow-up of infectious diseases, planning programs, and measuring effectiveness of activities 2. Forwards certificates to state registrar	1. Queries incomplete or inconsistent information 2. Maintains files for permanent reference and source of certified copies 3. Compiles statistics for state and civil divisions of state for use of the health department and other interested agencies or groups 4. Prepares copies of all certificates for transmission to National Office of Vital Statistics	1. Prepares national vital statistics for use of official and voluntary groups 2. Publishes analyses of data as they relate to public health and social problems
Stillbirth Certificate	Certifies to the causes of stillbirth and signs certificate. Returns it to funeral director	1. Obtains facts about the stillbirth 2. Takes certificate to physician for entry of causes of stillbirth 3. Delivers completed certificate to local registrar and obtains burial permit	1. Verifies completeness and accuracy. Makes copy or ledger entry for local reference. Forwards certificates to local health department or to state registrar 2. Issues burial permit to funeral director 3. Verifies returns of burial permits			

Figure 214. The registration system in the United States; flow chart of birth, death, and stillbirth certificates. (*Physician's Handbook on Death and Birth Registration,* 10th ed. National Office of Vital Statistics, US Public Health Service, US Government Printing Office, Washington, D. C., 1949.)

THE STANDARD CERTIFICATE OF DEATH

This is a permanent document. Type or use permanent black ink. Do not use ball-type pen.

THE FUNERAL DIRECTOR IS TO COMPLETE ITEMS 1-3, 5-17, 24, 25.

To be filled in by Vital Statistics Office.

Differentiate between urban and rural areas (i.e., within or outside city or town limits).

Use such terms as White, Negro, Indian, etc.

Complete both 10(a) and 10(b) for all persons 14 years and over, even though disabled, retired, unemployed or institutionalized.

In 10(a) give occupation followed during most of working life. Use specific terms, such as welder, farm laborer, carpenter, etc.

In 10(b) give business or industry in which occupation named in 10(a) was followed. Use specific terms, such as coal mine, cotton mill, automobile factory, farm, etc. Do not use company or organization names.

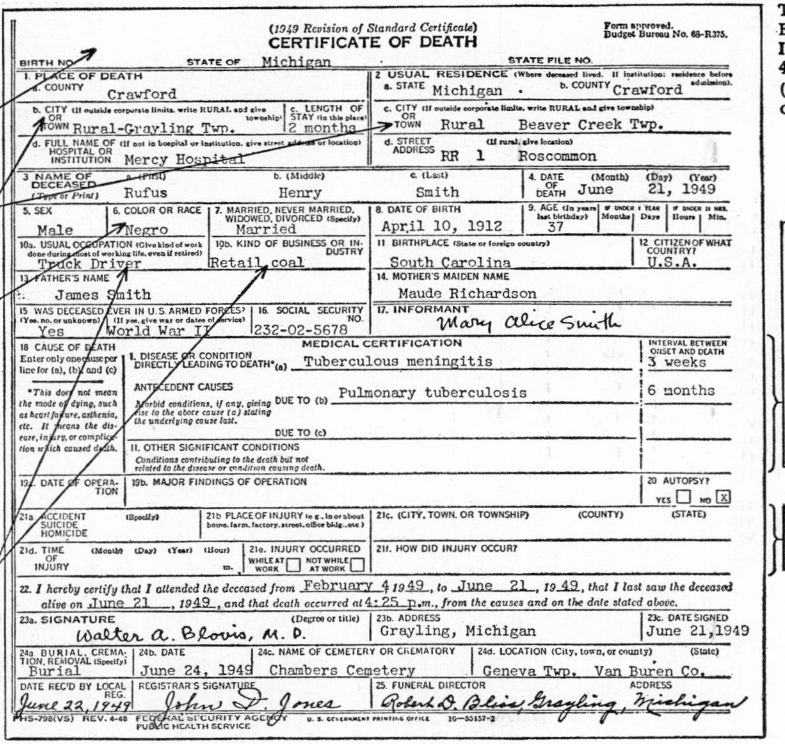

(1949 Revision of Standard Certificate)
CERTIFICATE OF DEATH
Form approved. Budget Bureau No. 68-R375.

BIRTH NO. — STATE OF Michigan — STATE FILE NO.

1. PLACE OF DEATH a. COUNTY Crawford
b. CITY OR TOWN (If outside corporate limits, write RURAL and give township) Rural-Grayling Twp. | c. LENGTH OF STAY (in this place) 2 months
d. FULL NAME OF HOSPITAL OR INSTITUTION (If not in hospital or institution, give street address or location) Mercy Hospital

2. USUAL RESIDENCE (Where deceased lived. If institution: residence before admission) a. STATE Michigan b. COUNTY Crawford
c. CITY OR TOWN (If outside corporate limits, write RURAL and give township) Rural Beaver Creek Twp.
d. STREET ADDRESS (If rural, give location) RR 1 Roscommon

3. NAME OF DECEASED (Type or Print) a. (First) Rufus b. (Middle) Henry c. (Last) Smith
4. DATE OF DEATH (Month) June (Day) 21, (Year) 1949

5. SEX Male | 6. COLOR OR RACE Negro | 7. MARRIED, NEVER MARRIED, WIDOWED, DIVORCED (Specify) Married | 8. DATE OF BIRTH April 10, 1912 | 9. AGE (In years last birthday) 37 | If under 1 year: Months, Days | If under 24 hrs.: Hours, Min.

10a. USUAL OCCUPATION (Give kind of work done during most of working life, even if retired) Truck Driver | 10b. KIND OF BUSINESS OR INDUSTRY Retail coal | 11. BIRTHPLACE (State or foreign country) South Carolina | 12. CITIZEN OF WHAT COUNTRY? U.S.A.

13. FATHER'S NAME James Smith | 14. MOTHER'S MAIDEN NAME Maude Richardson

15. WAS DECEASED EVER IN U.S. ARMED FORCES? (Yes, no, or unknown) Yes (If yes, give war or dates of service) World War II | 16. SOCIAL SECURITY NO. 232-02-5678 | 17. INFORMANT Mary Alice Smith

MEDICAL CERTIFICATION

18. CAUSE OF DEATH Enter only one cause per line for (a), (b), and (c)
I. DISEASE OR CONDITION DIRECTLY LEADING TO DEATH* (a) Tuberculous meningitis — INTERVAL BETWEEN ONSET AND DEATH 3 weeks
ANTECEDENT CAUSES Morbid conditions, if any, giving rise to the above cause (a) stating the underlying cause last. DUE TO (b) Pulmonary tuberculosis — 6 months
DUE TO (c)
*This does not mean the mode of dying, such as heart failure, asthenia, etc. It means the disease, injury, or complication which caused death.
II. OTHER SIGNIFICANT CONDITIONS Conditions contributing to the death but not related to the disease or condition causing death.

19a. DATE OF OPERATION | 19b. MAJOR FINDINGS OF OPERATION | 20. AUTOPSY? YES ☐ NO ☒

21a. ACCIDENT SUICIDE HOMICIDE (Specify) | 21b. PLACE OF INJURY (e.g., in or about home, farm, factory, street, office bldg., etc.) | 21c. (CITY, TOWN, OR TOWNSHIP) (COUNTY) (STATE)
21d. TIME OF INJURY (Month) (Day) (Year) (Hour) m. | 21e. INJURY OCCURRED WHILE AT WORK ☐ NOT WHILE AT WORK ☐ | 21f. HOW DID INJURY OCCUR?

22. I hereby certify that I attended the deceased from February 4 1949, to June 21, 1949, that I last saw the deceased alive on June 21, 1949, and that death occurred at 4:25 p.m., from the causes and on the date stated above.

23a. SIGNATURE (Degree or title) Walter A. Blovis, M. D. | 23b. ADDRESS Grayling, Michigan | 23c. DATE SIGNED June 21, 1949

24a. BURIAL, CREMATION, REMOVAL (Specify) Burial | 24b. DATE June 24, 1949 | 24c. NAME OF CEMETERY OR CREMATORY Chambers Cemetery | 24d. LOCATION (City, town, or county) (State) Geneva Twp. Van Buren Co.

DATE REC'D BY LOCAL REG. June 22, 1949 | REGISTRAR'S SIGNATURE John D. Jones | 25. FUNERAL DIRECTOR Robert D. Bliss | ADDRESS Grayling, Michigan

HS-798(VS) REV. 4-48 FEDERAL SECURITY AGENCY PUBLIC HEALTH SERVICE U.S. GOVERNMENT PRINTING OFFICE 16—55157-2

THE PHYSICIAN, MEDICAL EXAMINER, OR CORONER IS TO COMPLETE ITEMS 4, 18-23.

(See pp. 4-14 for further discussion of what should be entered here.)

In part **I**, give the sequence of events that led to death, specifying last the underlying cause which initiated the train of events. Do not report symptoms or mode of dying.

In part II, report other important diseases or conditions, if any, that contributed to the death but were not related to the causes given in part I above.

Complete items 21(a) - 21(f) if death was due to violence or external causes.

Figure 215. The standard certificate of death. Form follows the recommendations of the World Health Organization that were made in 1948. Two similar certificates are used to report births; one for live births, the other for stillbirths.

he usually assumes responsibility for all items in the report except those the under-taker and pathologist are responsible for.

State laws regulate the disposition of both unidentified and identified bodies. In getting permission for autopsies when an unidentified person dies in a hospital, the local health department is notified, and this agency assumes responsibility for trying to determine the identity of the body and for making arrangement for burial. Some states rule that bodies may be available for study and research by a recog-nized medical group, if they are not identified within a stated period, usually 48 hours, after death. When a person has a family or is in the custody of friends, most state laws require that the permission of the nearest of kin or the custodial friend be obtained before an autopsy is performed. If there is a question of poisoning, however, or any other circumstance in connection with the death that necessitates a coroner's inquest, the state is permitted to conduct an autopsy, without the consent of the relatives of the deceased.[14]

The local health departments set up special regulations governing the treatment of bodies of persons who die of certain communicable diseases. The Sanitary Code of New York City[15] stipulates that undertakers must not expose or hold the bodies of persons who die of cholera, bubonic plague, diphtheria, poliomyelitis, scarlet fever, or smallpox. Such bodies must be placed in the coffin, which is sealed im-mediately.

SUMMARY

The care of the dying patient is an experience that exacts a good deal from the physician and the nurse. It is a part of their work and a responsibility that they should not want to escape. At no other time are their services more appreciated, nor is there greater opportunity for the exercise of good judgment, consideration, and true kindness. The nurse should be alert in observing signs that indicate the approach of death; she should feel responsible for notifying those who are con-cerned about the patient's condition and should cooperate to the fullest extent with the physician, the family, and the patient's religious advisers. It is her particular function to relieve the physical discomforts that accompany the process of dying and to use effectively the measures prescribed by the physician for the relief of pain. It is her responsibility to care for the body after death in such a manner as not to interfere with the processes the undertaker uses in preparing the body for burial. The protection of the patient, his family, and his friends from needless suffering is difficult when death occurs in the hospital. Every effort should be made to surround them with a sense of privacy and to give them the assurance that the hospital staff is sincerely interested in them and anxious to do everything within its power to help them.

Certain public health and institutional regulations govern the way in which deaths are reported, and permits obtained for autopsies and burial rights. The nurse who is informed on such matters is able to cooperate more intelligently with others who are concerned in the care of the dying and the dead.

REFERENCES

1. Cabot, Richard C., and Dicks, Russell L.: *The Art of Ministering to the Sick.* The Macmillan Company, New York, 1936, pp. 298-315.
2. Dicks, Russell L.: *Who Is My Patient?* The Macmillan Company, New York, 1941, pp. 299, 303, 305, 308, 314.
3. Livingstone, R. W.: *Portrait of Socrates; Being the Apology, Crito and Phaedo of Plato in an English Translation with Introduction and Notes.* Oxford University Press, London, 1938.
4. Worcester, Alfred W.: *The Care of the Aged, the Dying and the Dead.* Charles C Thomas, Publisher, Springfield, Ill., 1935, pp. 34, 37-51.
5. *The Works of William Shakespeare.* Oxford University Press, New York, 1938, p. 493.
6. Tolstoy, Lev. N.: *Short Novels.* Dial Press, New York, 1949, p. 409.
7. Lesnik, Milton J., and Anderson, Bernice E.: *Legal Aspects of Nursing.* J. B. Lippincott Co., Philadelphia, 1947, p. 268.
8. Hayt, Emanuel, and Hayt, Lillian R.: *Legal Guide for American Hospitals.* Hospital Textbook Co., New York, 1940, pp. 40, 41, 46, 362, 364, 635, 658, 660.
9. Day, Sister Mary Agnita Claire: *Principles and Techniques of Nursing Procedures.* C. V. Mosby Co., St. Louis, 1943, pp. 151-67.
10. Montag, Mildred L., and Filson, Margaret: *Nursing Arts,* 2nd ed. W. B. Saunders Co., Philadelphia, 1953, pp. 404-26.
11. Nagle, Richard A., et al.: "The Patients' Spiritual Needs," *Am. J. Nursing,* **50:**64, (Feb.) 1950.
12. US National Office of Vital Statistics: *Physicians' Handbook on Death and Birth Registration* (prepared under the supervision of Halbert L. Dunn), 10th ed. US Government Printing Office, Washington, D.C., 1949.
13. Maxcy, Kenneth F. (ed.): *Rosenau's Preventive Medicine and Hygiene,* 7th ed. Appleton-Century-Crofts, Inc., New York, 1951, p. 1348.
14. Hayt, Emanuel, and Hayt, Lillian R.: *Law of Hospital, Physician and Patient.* Hospital Textbook Co., New York, 1947, p. 450.
15. New York City: *Rules and Regulations of New York City Agencies . . . 1938-1946.* Law Department of the City of New York, New York, 1946, p. 181.

Additional Suggested Reading

Draper, George, et al.: *Human Constitution in Clinical Medicine.* Paul B. Hoeber, New York, 1944.
Fitch, Florence M.: *One God: The Ways We Worship Him.* Lothrop, Lee and Shepard Co., New York, 1944.
————: *Their Search for God: Ways of Worship in the Orient.* Lothrop, Lee and Shepard Co., New York, 1947.
Gaer, Joseph: *How the Great Religions Began,* rev. ed. Dodd, Mead & Co., New York, 1951.
Hiltner, Seward: *Religion and Health.* The Macmillan Company, New York, 1943.
Lansing, A. I. (ed.): *Cowdry's Problem of Aging: Biological and Medical Aspects,* 3rd ed. Williams & Wilkins Co., Baltimore, 1952.
Lawton, George (ed.): *New Goals for Old Age.* Columbia University Press, New York, 1943.
Wise, Carroll A.: *Religion in Illness and Health.* Harper & Brothers, New York, 1942.

CHAPTER 36. NURSING CARE OF PATIENTS WITH LOCALIZED INFECTIONS

1. TYPES OF WOUNDS

Definition. A wound is defined as "a disruption in continuity of an external or internal surface of the body."

Classification. Wounds are classified according to the part wounded, their cause, and their size and shape. They are also classified as clean or infected and poisoned wounds, but this perpetuates the misconception that a wound can be completely protected from bacteria. It is safe to say that all wounds are infected to some extent. Infection that threatens the general health and delays wound healing is rightly considered a special problem; in this sense the classification of clean and infected wounds is helpful. Breaks in tissue continuity made by animals and insects are sometimes put in the special category of poisoned wounds. Surgery produces a wound which must be treated in the same way as an accidental wound except that it is less exposed to infection. This suggests the classification, surgical and accidental wounds.

For purposes of treatment the wounded in any catastrophe might be divided into two groups—those who are seriously wounded, showing signs of shock, and those who are not. They might be further divided into those with wounds of the head, the chest, abdomen, or extremity; into those with obvious fractures or those with injuries of soft tissues. Injuries from burns might be still another classification; they may be caused by heat, electricity, x-rays, radioactive substances, and caustic chemicals. Since burns are included in the definition "a disruption in continuity . . ."

wounds are sometimes classified as mechanical, electrical, irradiated, or chemical injuries. Burns are discussed in the chapter on emergencies.

Terms Used in Describing Accidental Wounds.   Accidental wounds may be stab, incised, punctured, contused, lacerated, or poisoned wounds. They are all considered infected.

A *stab wound* is caused by a sharp, cutting, pointed instrument, such as a dagger or knife.

An *incised wound* is caused by a sharp, cutting, pointed instrument, such as a razor, which severs the tissues, causing them to gape open.

A *punctured wound* is made by a sharp, narrow, pointed instrument, such as a needle, splinter of wood, or a nail. A rusty nail is more dangerous because, being rough, it injures the tissues more and also holds more dirt and bacteria. A *gunshot wound* is also a punctured wound.

A *contused wound* is made by a blunt instrument. The skin is ruptured, crushed, or split, and the surrounding tissues are bruised.

A *lacerated wound* is one in which the tissues are torn apart—the edges are roughened and jagged, and there is more or less contusion around it. Examples are the bite of an animal, torn knuckles caused by striking the mouth and teeth, a hook drawn through the tissues, and wounds caused by machinery.

Poisoned wounds may be caused by the bites of poisonous snakes or spiders, a rabid dog, and insect bites and stings.

2. REACTION OF THE BODY TO TRAUMA. THE NATURE OF INFLAMMATION

The reaction of the body to trauma is the same wherever it occurs although it varies so much in degree that the condition of the mildly and seriously injured may pose very different problems. Henry K. Beecher, urging that what has been learned about the military wounded be applied to civil life, says:

The consequences to the human body are the same whether an artery is severed by a shell fragment or a broken windshield. . . . There is a universality in these cause and effect relationships, a universality, too, in the principles of treatment that makes them apply to thousands of victims of atomic violence as well as to a child whose tonsillectomy wound [continues to] bleed.

. . . . It will be tragic if medical historians can look back on the World War II period and write of it as a time when so much was learned and so little remembered.*

Bleeding.   The immediate and visible response to injuries is bleeding. If capillaries only are injured, in very superficial wounds blood will edge away from the surface; if larger vessels, or veins are severed, blood will stream from the wound; while it will spurt from an artery. Bleeding results in formation of a clot, unless there is an uncontrolled and, therefore, fatal hemorrhage. Bleeding and control methods are discussed later in this chapter.

* Beecher, Henry K: *Early Care of the Seriously Wounded Man.* Charles C Thomas, Publisher, Springfield, Ill., p. 1.; also *J.A.M.A.,* **145:**196, (Jan.) 1951.

Local Inflammatory Reaction to Injury.   Local response to trauma has been partially understood since man could analyze the *subjective symptoms* and the *visible changes*—redness, heat, swelling, pain, and disturbance of function. Hippocrates named the process, characterized by the first four signs, inflammation. With the development of the microscope it became possible to describe the minute

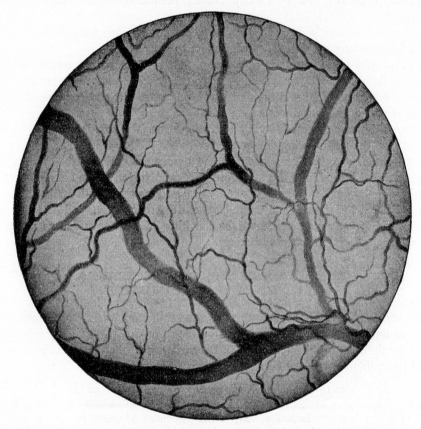

Figure 216.   Portion of a normal diaphragm to show relatively few visible blood channels. (McCollum, W. G.: *Textbook of Pathology.* W. B. Saunders Co., Philadelphia, 1936.)

structural changes: the immediate vasoconstriction followed by vasodilation with slowing of the current; increase in permeability of capillaries; resulting accumulation of intercellular fluids; increase in the number of blood cells, particularly certain types of white cells; emigration of white cells from the capillaries and engulfing of foreign particles, including bacterial, by white cells (phagocytes, *phagein* = to eat, and *kytos* = a cell); laying down of fibrils, and the development of normal cells (proliferation) to fill in, or bridge, the break in the continuity of tissue.

If the process of inflammation is observed microscopically it will be seen that, although the vessels remain dilated, more resistance seems to be made to the flow of blood and the stream slows down. (The nature of this resistance is not understood, but is thought to be some change in the endothelial lining of the blood vessels.) With the slowing of the stream, white cells are carried by their own weight to the sides of the vessels; in the venules they are seen rolling along close to the walls, then adhering to them, and finally passing through by active ameboid movements into the tissue spaces. Here they are called "wandering cells" and are chiefly of the *polymorphonuclear* type.

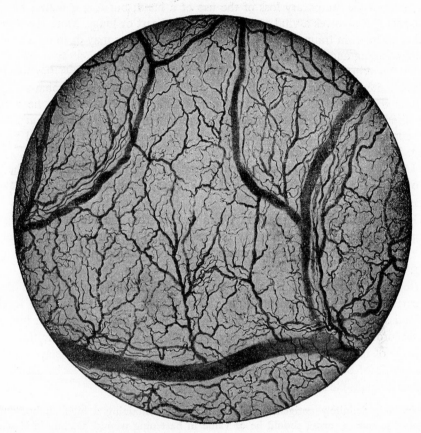

Figure 217.   Portion of inflamed diaphragm to show the abundant dilated blood channels. (McCollum, W. G.: *Textbook of Pathology.* W. B. Saunders Co., Philadelphia, 1936.)

Red cells in varying numbers also are found outside the vessels. How they get out is unknown. It is thought that they have no power of motion, but they are compressible and may passively follow the leukocytes, a process called diapedesis. The red cells are soon destroyed if they escape from the blood vessels. The breakdown of red blood cells is indicated by the discoloration of the part. Outside the blood stream these cells swell or shrink, clutter up the zone, and are picked up and carried away by the white blood cells.

At the same time, and probably before the passage of cells, fluid oozes out into the tissues; the lymphatics and lymph spaces, before invisible, are seen to be engorged with fluid (edema) distending the tissues, crowding the cells, and causing pressure on the sensitive nerve endings. Thus the third physical symptom—*swelling,* and the fourth symptom—*pain* are explained. The swelling of the injured part, pain, and, more important, nature's effort to avoid increasing irritation and pain by movement, together cause the fifth symptom—*loss of function.* This loss of function, although a matter of inconvenience, may not be very serious if it merely involves a finger or even the temporary loss of the use of a hand; but it is a matter of great seriousness if it involves a vital organ, such as the heart or lungs. More recently the chemical changes in trauma have been studied. The findings may open up a new era of understanding and treatment.

Valey Menkin discussing the biochemistry of inflammation says the local reaction is limited by disturbance in the fluid exchange between the lymphatics, blood vessels, and tissue cells. The increased permeability of the capillaries he regards as an important change. In studying the *chemistry of response to trauma* he and other contemporary scientists have isolated and described five chemical factors having, in brief, the following action:

1. Leuckotaxine: it increases the local permeability of the capillaries and the passage of white blood cells (diapedesis of leukocytes) from the capillaries into the intercellular space.

2. Leukocytosis-promoting factor: When carried from the site of trauma to the bone marrow, it induces the marrow to produce and discharge a greater number of blood cells of special types (immature leukocytes, granulocytes, and megakaryocytes).

3. Necrosin: a toxic substance which breaks down or splits protein. It acts locally and, carried in the blood stream, it may affect distant areas. It raises the level of the blood sugar, presumably by stimulating the liver to convert glycogen into glucose. According to Lucian Szmyd injured cells also produce glucose. He thinks the knowledge of those two chemical actions of value in explaining the delayed healing characteristic of diabetes. Szmyd thinks that necrosin may prove to be useful as a therapeutic agent. He says:

Necrosin is definitely antigenic, yielding a serum containing a high antibody titer; theoretically, such a serum should be of value in hastening wound healing, in lessening the toxic or injurious manifestations of numerous inflammatory on infectious processes. It is conceivable that the gradual development of resistance to infections occurring with age may in part be due to a subliminal immunization to necrosin liberated as a result of previous wounds or infections.*

4. Pyrexin: a substance, thought to be a glycopeptide, that induces fever. It is believed to act on the heat-regulating center in the hypothalmus. Its action can be reduced or neutralized by antipyretic drugs.

5. Leukopenic factor: a substance that reduces the number of leukocytes in the

* Szmyd, Lucian: "Modern Concepts of the Dynamics of Inflammation," *Mil. Surg.,* **108:**45, (Jan.) 1951.

peripheral blood. Menkin says they are apparently "trapped in lungs, liver, and spleen."*

Nurses will soon see these chemicals used in the treatment of wounds and participate in their administration. With better understanding of the way in which chemicals produced at the site of injury affect the whole body a more effective effort can and will undoubtedly be made to eradicate inflammatory processes, or "foci of infection."

Szmyd thinks that:

The research of Menkin and his associates has given rise to the following immediate clinical implications:
1. Ability to alter the level of circulating leukocytes
2. Utilization of the antigenic properties of necrosin
3. Revision of our views on so-called focus of infection
Bernier states that the inflammatory process is an irreversible one which cannot be stopped, but may be influenced. Additional research on the problem of inflammation will provide the therapist with sufficient means to exert a greater influence on this irreversible process.†

Inflammation has long been regarded as a protective process. The more that is known about it the more certain this seems. It represents the struggle of nature to overcome an injurious agent. Brought to a successful termination it results in healing, but healing may never occur and the systemic effects of unresolved inflammation may be fatal.

Differentiation of Trauma, Inflammation, and Infection. Trauma is defined as "a wound or injury" and in psychiatry as "an emotional shock leaving a deep psychological impression"; inflammation as "the reaction of the tissues to injury"; and infection as "the implantation of an infective agent" or "the communication of disease from one subject to another." Trauma is therefore an all-inclusive term applied to any injury, whereas inflammation is a specific response to injury although extreme fear or psychic trauma with no visible injury to the tissues initiates a physical response that may be more fatal than inflammation. Trauma from mechanical objects causes inflammation. The traumatic effect of sunlight and other forms of heat is inflammatory. (The effect of electrical, x-ray, and radioactive burns is not a typical inflammation and might be considered separately and represents a specialized body response.) Infection following trauma occurs only when a living organism finds its way into a traumatized tissue. Microorganisms may enter through the skin or mucous membrane, or they may be brought to the area by the circulating fluids from other parts of the body. If there is a high degree of resistance in the tissues there may be no visible signs of infection—that is, the body defenses may immediately destroy the invading organisms; if, on the other hand, the resistance is low or the invaders strong and numerous, symptoms of inflammation will soon appear. Those factors that go to make up susceptibility to infection are the *predisposing* causes. Some of these are traumatized tissue; a decreased blood supply;

---

* Menkin, Valey: "Biochemistry of Inflammation," *Lancet*, 1:660, (May) 1947.
† Szmyd, Lucian: *op. cit.*

blood that is lacking in protective elements, such as a specific agglutinizing substance or a normal number of white blood cells; and metabolic diseases that result in an undernourished condition of the tissues. Friction and pressure from the outside or presence of an insoluble foreign body inside the tissues destroys and irritates cell bodies, thereby lowering their resistance to infection. Nature may in some cases wall off a foreign body with fibrous tissue in such a way as to protect the surrounding structures; more often the object is forced to the surface of the body or to the wall of a cavity, breaks through it, and is ejected from the body. If this process occurs, it is often accompanied by infection even before it ruptures the skin or mucous membrane, and always at this point. The predisposing cause of the infection is irritation of the tissues, and the direct cause is the bacteria that may have been present on the foreign body or that later enter the wound from the skin or mucous surface.

Termination of Inflammation and the Healing Process.   If the injury has been slight, the inflammatory reaction will be mild. Fluid that oozes out from injured vessels will quickly cause the sides of the wound to grow together; leukocytes will carry away dead cells; and digestive enzymes will liquefy the dead tissue that will then be absorbed. When the area is cleared of debris in this manner, inflammation is said to end by *resolution,* and the tissues are said to be resolving.

Injury to the tissues may be so severe, or the wounded area so extensive, that the damaged tissues can neither be revitalized nor carried away fast enough by the process of resolution. The same tissue will then die and form a slough that will separate by degrees from the living tissues, leaving an ulcer that must be filled in by the formation of new tissue.

If the irritated or injured area is invaded by bacteria there are living cells opposed to each other, and struggling for existence. If the tissue cells are weak, or if the bacteria are very virulent, or attack in great numbers, they destroy large numbers of living cells. Serum and fibrin permeate the devitilized tissue; ferments from dead leukocytes and cells gradually liquefy it, forming a zone of thick, yellowish fluid (pus). Finally, the whole mass is liquefied into a circumscribed collection of pus, or an abscess. When this occurs the inflammatory process is said to progress to *suppuration.*

Suppuration terminates in various ways according to the extent of the process, the virulence of the organisms, and other factors. Some of the exudate and toxins are absorbed into the lymph stream by resolution; or the abscess, if superficial, may rupture on the body surface and drain; in a boil, it may rupture the skin; in the lung, some of it will be coughed up. If the abscess is deep it may form a sinus or tract to the surface; or it may have to be incised and the fluid withdrawn by drainage or aspiration. The pressure may help to form an outlet of discharge for the pus, or may force it into the tissues, pushing it along the lines of least resistance. An extension of the inflammatory process into a large surrounding area is known as cellulitis.

All inflammatory exudates caused by bacteria are not purulent, however. Microorganisms that cause pus formation are called pyogenic microorganisms. Because of their significance, from a diagnostic and prognostic standpoint, physicians have given names to exudates that indicate their chief characteristics. The adjectives commonly used are serous, mucoid, fibrous, and purulent; all of them except the last, which has been defined, are self-explanatory.

The *reparative process* depends upon the nature, extent, and location of the injury and the types of cells injured. It also depends upon the age and vitality of the host. Healing may take place either by primary or by secondary union.

The wound made in a surgical operation, if infection does not already exist, is a clean, incised wound. It is made by a sterile, sharp, cutting instrument, and the tissues are cleanly divided without tearing or laceration. When the edges of such a wound are brought together, it should heal by direct primary union, or "first intention." This means that the cut edges grow together or heal, with the slightest inflammatory reaction and with the minimum of new tissue.

When, for any reason, the edges of a wound cannot be brought together, and a gap remains between them that must be filled in, repair is said to take place by indirect union. The new tissue is called granulation tissue.

Granulation tissue consists of abundant blood vessels and young connective-tissue cells spread apart by fluid and fibrin. When healthy it is soft, gray or grayish red, gelatinous, and translucent, with an irregular, velvety surface, bleeding readily, but quite insensitive to pain because it contains no nerves. Although the surface of a healthy granulating wound offers great resistance to bacterial invasion, this resistance may be broken down by very slight injuries, such as probing, or the removal of a dressing, particularly a dry dressing that sticks to the surface. Skin edges also tend to turn inward and may act as a wick, carrying infection into the wound. Many surgeons now use so-called closed dressings on even badly infected wounds because they want to avoid injury to the granulating tissue. The dressing on a compound fracture or a burn may be left undisturbed for days, or maybe weeks. The pus that forms under it acts as a water cushion and protects the delicate young cells.

Sometimes healing is delayed or indolent. When this occurs the tissue is pale, dry, shrunken, flabby, and unhealthy looking. Sometimes it grows too fast, and is soft and bleeds easily. It is then said to be redundant. Granulation should form from the bottom and sides of the wound, until even with the surface, but sometimes it grows above the surface and must be removed; or sometimes there is a tendency to close in at the top leaving an open channel, or sinus, underneath. A wick or drain in the wound prevents healing from the top because it keeps the wound open.

When the gap in a surface wound is nearly filled, a thin, grayish-blue film of epithelium may be seen spreading from the edges to cover the surface. The epithelial cells behind divide, multiply, and push the others forward until the surface is finally covered. At first the tissue looks bluish or purplish under the pearly epithelium because of the abundant blood vessels; later many of the new blood vessels are pressed shut and disappear, and the part becomes hard and very white because of the lack of specialized pigment cells. At this stage it is called a cicatrix or scar. Specialized structures, such as secreting glands, hair, and pigment cells, are not formed. When a wound is extensive, or the formation of new epithelium is slow, a graft of living tissue is usually applied.

Repair by indirect union may be a mere patchwork; it may be quite unsightly and fail to restore the function of the part because several kinds of tissue are injured, and tissues vary greatly in their power to regenerate themselves. Connective and epithelial tissue form the bulk of new material for repair. The connective tissue produced by the body in the healing process is of fibrous tissue that is strong but not elastic and poorly supplied with blood vessels. Because the tissue is inelastic it causes a contraction of the part. Extensive scar tissue causes deformity, or a partial loss of function unless this is prevented.

To summarize, wounds may heal cleanly and neatly by first intention when there is a minimum of infection present; seriously infected areas heal with one or more of the following results or complications: (1) An ulcer—a raw surface caused by necrosis of skin or mucous membrane resulting from such conditions as poor circulation, poor nutrition, and from interference with the nerve supply; (2) an abscess with sinus formation—a channel extending from an abscess to the skin, mucous membrane, or wound; (3) scar formation, with deformity and loss of function; and (4) keloid—an actual tumor formed in the surface of a scar due to overactivity of the connective tissues. All treatment of wounds is designed to promote complete healing without appreciable derangement of function or disfigurement.

Systemic Reaction. The effect of trauma on the total organism can scarcely be discussed without dividing it into the immediate and later reactions, and without considering separately the effect of slight trauma and the profound effect of a severe injury. The immediate response is determined by the blood and other fluids lost, the extent and location of tissue damage, the emotional component, the exposure to cold, and the person's general condition, all of which contribute to the degree of shock. The systemic effect during the later stages of injury depends of course upon all these factors, the kind of treatment he receives, and his response to it, but his fate often hangs on the severity and nature of the infection that is so likely to invade traumatized tissue. A discussion of the systemic reaction to injury may involve the reaction to hemorrhage and shock and the response to large areas of devitalized tissue (gangrene) and infected tissue. Special sections are therefore devoted to these topics.

3. IMMEDIATE CARE OR FIRST AID TO THE WOUNDED

Beecher says that treatment of wounded men falls into three main channels: (1) treatment of reduced blood volume, (2) treatment of the local wound, and (3) treatment of pain and mental stress. Since the seriously wounded will require surgical treatment and are unable to walk, transportation is also an important aspect of first aid.

Since deterioration in the patient's condition is in direct relation to the blood loss, according to some authorities, the first step is the control of hemorrhage. The only other aspect of first aid that takes precedence over it is the establishment of an airway; deprived of oxygen the subject will, of course, suffocate in a very short time. Turning the patient into the prone position may allow the relaxed tongue to fall forward or it may drain obstructive fluid from the mouth; or turning the head to one side may be sufficient. Movement should be limited until the nature of the injury is known. If there are fractures, some splinting is desirable before any gross body movement and always before transportation. If the patient is in shock, transportion with the head lowered is desirable unless there are signs of pulmonary edema or cranial hemorrhage. If fluid collects in the mouth or if there is nasal bleeding, the patient should be transported face downward.

Hemorrhage should be controlled by pressure dressings directly over the wound, by manual pressure over the bleeding points, by the position of the bleeding area, and by tourniquets. (See p. 952.) "Sucking" chest wounds must be closed with the best dressing material available. In the military services plasma is provided for immediate administration by field personnel. Morphine is available to all soldiers in case of severe pain following injury, and they are taught how to give it to themselves and others. Beecher and others say that morphine should be used with great care and in the smallest effective doses. If given intramuscularly, it may be very slowly absorbed and if repeated can produce delayed poisoning with the characteristic depression of respiration. Barbiturates are recommended as treatment of the anxiety and hysteria sometimes seen in the wounded. When pain is severe, morphine is indicated, and Beecher thinks it should be given intravenously for rapid and sure absorption. He recommends a dosage of morphine sulfate 10 mg ($\frac{1}{6}$ gr) and never more than 15 mg ($\frac{1}{4}$ gr). He thinks "stimulants," the vasoconstrictors, of little use and contraindicated in large dosage. Pain can often be relieved if clothing is loosened or cut over swollen areas. When Thomas splints are adjusted over shoes, the latter should be unlaced and split.

It is stressed repeatedly that surgery is an essential part of treatment for the seriously wounded. Nothing should be done, therefore, while giving first aid or treatment for shock to make surgery dangerous or difficult. When the wounded person arrives at the clinic or hospital, he will be treated for shock and prepared as rapidly as possible for surgery, where vessels will be ligated, debris removed, bones set, wounds closed, and aseptic dressings applied. The wounded, who are dehydrated by sweating, possibly vomiting, and loss of blood, suffer acutely from thirst. They may rinse the mouth, but should be given nothing by mouth because the stomach should be empty in preparation for surgery. The danger of insufflation of fluid and food particles is so great that vomiting should be induced and, unless there is a possibility of gastric perforation, the stomach should be washed out before an anesthetic is administered. Glucose and saline solutions given intravenously relieve thirst; however, they do not restore blood volume and raise the blood pressure as do plasma and whole blood. Beecher stresses the importance of the latter in the resuscitation of the wounded in military and civil life alike.

He writes:

The patient who is in poor condition from blood loss with low blood volume and probably low hematocrit will often be seriously endangered if his blood . . . volume is increased by plasma without hemoglobin being added.*

* Beecher, Henry K: op. cit., p. 115.

He says that while blood must not be wasted, it may be necessary to give as much as 6000 cc before a man in *severe* shock is ready for surgery. It is suggested that the wounded man is ready for surgery when he has "*a rising blood pressure* (80 mm Hg or above), *falling pulse rate,* a *warm skin,* and *good color* of the mucous membranes." Delaying surgery beyond this point Beecher thinks inadvisable since the inevitable infection progresses, and resuscitative measures must be continued up to the time of operation. Jonathan E. Rhoads, writing in Frederick Christopher's text, says that the question of the use of tetanus antitoxin should be raised in connection with every traumatic wound. In the case of a penetrating or dirty wound received under circumstances at all likely to cause the introduction of the tetanus organism, the use of antitoxin must be insisted on. This is especially necessary in the case of gunshot wound or a puncture wound in the sole of the foot. Rhoads thinks the family and physician should share the responsibility for taking the risk if the decision not to give antitoxin is reached. He recommends 1500 units as a prophylactic dose for an adult. This should be repeated in 10 days if the likelihood of tetanus is great. Tetanus antitoxin is available in both horse and bovine serum. Before giving the dose of antitoxin, a few drops should be injected intradermally. If the patient is sensitive to the serum, there will be a reddened area around the wheal. Persons sensitive to horse serum may tolerate the bovine preparation.

Beecher found in his study of the military wounded, that, to his great surprise, only 23.7 per cent of a total of 215 seriously wounded men had "bad pain." Only 27.0 per cent wanted relief therapy; 32.1 per cent said they had no pain. Beecher concluded that morphine is often unnecessary and should never be given except for severe pain since its effect as a respiratory depressant and its tendency to nauseate make the anesthetic more hazardous. Morphine dulls the appetite, is constipating, and delays recovery from surgery in various ways. The suffering of the wounded is not confined to pain, and relief should be aimed at its source. What is said to give reassurance is of great importance for anxiety over the outcome of the wound is often extreme. For this reason the chaplains who went among the wounded on the battlefield and who saw them as they came to the hospitals in the combat zone gave great comfort. Civil hospitals should be equally ready to meet this need. It is generally accepted that there is a psychogenic factor in shock; that fear and excitement preoperatively predispose to shock postoperatively. Since hemorrhage and shock are specific problems in the immediate care of the wounded, they are treated in some detail in the following sections.

4. HEMORRHAGE AND GENERAL METHODS OF TREATMENT

Classification According to Time.   A *primary* hemorrhage is one that occurs at the time of injury. An *intermediate* or *recurrent* hemorrhage occurs in from 12 to 48 hours after the injury. A *secondary* hemorrhage is one that is delayed for a few days, occurring from two days up to the time of complete healing.

Classification According to Source.   *Arterial* hemorrhage is most dangerous because it is very difficult to control. It may be recognized by the bright red color of the blood; the escape of blood in spurts; and by the fact that in an extremity the pulse below may be obliterated, and pressure above the wound (between it and the heart) controls the hemorrhage.

In a *venous* hemorrhage, the blood is darker in color. It flows steadily, and bleeding is more easily controlled because the blood pressure is very low in the veins.

A *capillary* hemorrhage is one in which there is general oozing of blood from the surface. It neither spurts nor flows steadily, but wells up in the wound, and the surface seems to weep.

In some instances, hemorrhage occurs from all three sources at once.

Classification According to Cause and Location. Trauma is usually responsible for hemorrhage but an ulcer or any lesion that destroys the integrity of blood vessels may cause hemorrhage. *External* hemorrhage takes place when blood escapes from the skin or soft parts. *Internal* or *concealed* hemorrhage is one in which blood escapes into a body cavity as in the rupture of a Fallopian tube, into the stomach from an ulcer or growth, into the peritoneal cavity from ulceration and perforation of the intestine, or into the chest (hemathorax).

A *subcutaneous* hemorrhage occurs when the blood flows into the soft tissues beneath the unbroken skin as in a hematoma, a contusion or bruise where bleeding occurs from many small blood vessels; ecchymoses, or black and blue marks, hemorrhages too small to form a tumor. Some persons bleed abnormally, or for none of the usual causes. *Purpura hemorrhagica* consists of small hemorrhages under the skin. Pinpoint bleeding points are called petechiae. The spots are at first bright red but get darker as the hemoglobin disintegrates. Daniel M. Enerson and J. Garrott Allen say this condition is attributed to "hypersplenism" because the removal of the spleen often controls the symptom. They think, however, that the basic cause of the disease is unknown. Purpura occurs in some infectious diseases and may be associated with empyema, septicemia, leukemia, and in purpura hemorrhagica, in which there may also be epistaxis, hematuria, and bleeding of other surfaces.

Hemophilia is a hereditary disease that occurs in men, but is transmitted along the female line. Apparently normal women transmit it to their sons. Enerson and Allen say:

> Despite innumerable attempts to delineate the coagulation abnormality, there is still no general agreement on this point. It has been proposed that the principal defect may be an increased stability of the blood platelets . . . .*

In other words, the clotting time is delayed when blood platelets that are exposed to air and rough surfaces (conditions accompanying a wound or hemorrhage) do not disintegrate normally to set free a substance, known as tissue extract, considered essential for normal clotting time.

Men suffering from hemophilia are called *bleeders*. Their blood fails to clot so that bleeding from a slight wound may be impossible to control. There are other

---

* Enerson, Daniel M., and Allen, J. Garrott: "Treatment of the Bleeding Patient," *M. Clin. North America,* **35**:267, (June) 1951.

less well-established types of abnormal bleeding whose etiology is equally obscure. A deficiency of any of the factors in the physiological chain action of clotting can delay or prevent it. Deficiencies are found in prothrombin, fibrinogen, bile, and vitamin K. Overdoses of heparin, an anticoagulant, may cause bleeding.

Classification According to Severity and Danger. Hemorrhage may be *slight, severe,* or *profuse,* according to the extent of the injury, the size and number of vessels cut, and the amount of blood and rapidity with which it is lost. A severe hemorrhage from a large artery or vein is always accompanied by shock. Beecher found that the degree of shock was in direct proportion to the blood lost. He believed this is the only factor that demonstrably affected shock. A sudden loss is much more dangerous than a gradual loss, because the body has insufficient time for the necessary adjustment; however, gradual loss, as from hemorrhoids, may cause a very severe anemia.

Nature's Method of Reacting to Loss of Blood. When a small vessel is cut, its walls contract, making its lumen smaller, and at the same time it shrinks within its outer elastic sheath, which then partially or completely closes over the opening. The blood, meeting this resistance and coming in contact with air, soon begins to coagulate, forming clots around the opening and extending into the lumen so that bleeding is checked before a serious loss occurs. If this natural response did not take place, the merest untreated scratch would be fatal.

Clotting occurs very quickly in small vessels, especially the veins, because their walls collapse more readily than those of the arteries and thus prevent a serious loss of blood. When large vessels are injured, clots cannot form at first because of the force of the blood current. As blood continues to escape, however, the volume is so depleted that the blood pressure is lowered. As the force of the current is reduced, the blood is usually able to clot and plug the opening before death occurs.

Later the blood-forming organs manufacture and deliver to the blood an increased number of cells to make up for those lost, but nature's reaction alone is not in many cases sufficient to check a hemorrhage nor to repair rapidly the damage caused by a serious loss of blood. To prevent loss of life, the following methods must be promptly applied.

Local Treatment of Hemorrhage. Hemorrhage may be controlled by pressure, position, extreme heat or cold, astringents or styptics, ligation, torsion, sutures, and cautery.

Pressure may be made with the fingers (digital pressure), a tourniquet, compresses or packing, and a tight bandage. The bleeding must be controlled by whatever means are at hand. Pressure with the fingers along the course of the bleeding vessel will control a hemorrhage temporarily, even from a large vessel. Lay persons as well as medical workers are being taught to know exactly where and how pressure may be made on large vessels, such as the facial, cartoid, subclavian, axillary, brachial, and femoral arteries. They may learn this by feeling their own bodies to discover where each artery approaches the surface and where it lies against a bone —that is, where its pulse may be most easily felt and compressed.

So-called pressure points for the control of hemorrhage, or for counting pulsations of the artery, include: (1) temporal artery, for wounds in region of the temple; (2) facial artery, for wounds of the face below the temple; (3) carotid artery, for wounds in upper part of the neck; (4) subclavian artery, for wounds of the shoulder and upper part of the arm; (5) brachial artery, for wounds in the arm below this point; and (6) femoral artery, for wounds in the leg.

Bleeding from the forearm can be checked only by pressure on the vessels in front of the elbow or on the brachial artery, because the radial and ulnar arteries are too deeply embedded in the tissues to be easily compressible. Their branches also anastomose freely. The same is true of bleeding from the lower leg.

In bleeding from an artery, pressure must be made above the wound—that is, between it and the heart. In bleeding from a vein, digital pressure must be made below the bleeding point—that is, between it and the periphery. Also, all tight constricting bands (tight clothing, elastic garters, etc.) between the bleeding point and the heart must be removed to allow the blood to return by the deep veins.

The *tourniquet* is one of the most successful means of controlling bleeding from a large artery in an extremity, but because it is dangerous it is a last resort. It is applied above the bleeding point, but as low as possible on the extremity. The especially constructed tourniquets are made either of rubber or of heavily braided material. Improvised tourniquets may be used—rubber tubing, a folded handkerchief, a necktie, or a leather strap serves the purpose. In all cases the tourniquet must be of sufficient width not to cut the skin, and pressure must never be made on nerve trunks. A hard, firm compress is placed over the line of the artery (where digital pressure is made). A tourniquet must be tight enough to control the hemorrhage, if necessary tight enough to obliterate the pulse. It is never left on longer than necessary. Loosening the tourniquet at hourly intervals may save the extremity. Prolonged pressure causes severe pain and results in severe injury. Since the region below the tourniquet is deprived of all circulation, gangrene may set in. A tourniquet is used only when a pressure dressing and other methods of control have failed; therefore, it usually must remain on the extremity until the bleeding vessels can be ligated on the operating table, even though gangrene results.

Systemic Treatment of Hemorrhage. The patient should be kept as quiet as possible and in the recumbent position with the head lowered and the trunk and extremities elevated to increase the blood supply to the brain. Direct transfusions should be started as soon as possible. (When a populace is threatened, everyone should have his blood typed so that in a catastrophe blood tranfusions can be started with the least possible delay.) In capillary hemorrhage, continuous transfusions are sometimes given to make up for the constant loss of blood.

Transfusion is indicated as treatment for bleeding from known causes but it is also used to control the hemorrhage of hemophiliacs and others with bleeding of obscure origin. Enerson and Allen say that in hemorrhagic jaundice where a prothrombin deficiency delays clotting that transfusion should be used until enough vitamin K can be absorbed to control the bleeding. (Decrease in bile decreases prothrombin formation, and this lowers the rate of absorption of vitamin K, essential to clot formation.) When bleeding is caused by overdoses of heparin (anticoagulant) protamine sulfate is recommended by Enerson and Allen. They say that protamine inactivates heparin in ratios of 1:1. In other words the excess heparin is estimated, and an equal amount of protamine sulfate given. Until the mechanism of clotting is thoroughly understood, knowledge of how to treat bleeding will be partially experimental. It has recently been observed that the blood from victims of accidental death reliquefies a few hours after withdrawal from the veins (such blood can be used in a transfusion without an anticoagulant). The possibility that nature has more than one mechanism for maintaining hemostatis (stagnation of the blood) is suggested. Enerson and Allen say:

. . . . It is established that many hemorrhagic states are associated with a decreased capillary tolerance to pressure and that this capillary tolerance is restored to normal when the normal hemostatic mechanism is re-established. In other words, the walls of the capillaries may be directly or indirectly influenced by parts of the mechanisms of coagulation. . . .

In general, it would appear that the integrity of the walls of the small vessels depends in some way on the clotting mechanism of the blood, including the platelets, and that abnormal and spontaneous bleeding result when these general hemostatic phenomena are disordered. . . .

. . . . Since the ultimate fate of neither the platelets nor fibrin is known, the physiology of abnormal bleeding remains obscure even when a clotting abnormality is demonstrated and when an effective means for its correction is available.*

The administration of calcium salts has been used to decrease clotting time when there is slow bleeding. Harry Sobotka and Nathan Adelman[1] report that "T.A.L.," a water-soluble adrenochrome derivative, is a potent hemostatic agent. They say the administration of 10 mg shortened the bleeding time an average of 38 per cent in 32 subjects.

Bleeding from Special Areas and Methods of Control. Epistaxis, or bleeding from the nose, is a capillary hemorrhage from a deeply congested mucous membrane.

The great vascularity of the nose accounts for the frequency of nasal bleeding and for occasional difficulty in controlling it.

The *causes of epistaxis* are *local*—traumatism, ulceration, foreign bodies, new growths, and picking and scratching with the fingers; or *constitutional*—hemophilia, the onset of certain infectious diseases, venous congestion in cardiac or pulmonary or cerebral diseases. Nasal bleeding is seen in puberty in some children, especially those with a rheumatic tendency. There may be a hereditary tendency to epistaxis.

Epistaxis may occur during sleep, the blood swallowed being vomited later and thus confused with hematemesis; or the blood may be coughed up and so confused with hemoptysis.

In the *treatment* of epistaxis the patient's head should be kept erect or elevated, or the head of the bed elevated, in order to aid the venous return. He should not bend over a basin. The clothing, especially the collar, should be loosened. Raising the arms above the head will lessen the blood supply to the nose.

* Enerson, Daniel M., and Allen, J. Garrott; *op. cit.*

The blood tends to clot and thus spontaneuosly check the bleeding. The patient should be warned not to blow his nose or in any way loosen the clot until control of bleeding is established. Pressing the outer aspect of the nares against the septum for 5 minutes usually arrests bleeding. Ice or ice compresses may be applied to the forehead, the bridge of the nose, and the back of the neck. Ice may be pressed against the nose.

Compression may be made on the facial artery by pressure on the superior maxilla near the nose on the bleeding side. The anterior nares may be packed with sterile gauze or cotton, but this should be lubricated with petroleum jelly so that it will not disturb the clot when it is removed. It is obvious that the blood must not be allowed to run down into the throat. This is one reason why patients with face injuries are transported in the prone position which allows fluids to drain from the mouth.

When first-aid measures fail to control nasal bleeding and a physician is called in, he may carry out the following "routine" that is based on an article by Ross A. Goodsell:[2]

1. Reassurance with or without sedation and "removal . . . from the patient's room of anxious friends and relatives."

2. Removal of clots by blowing the nose, "hawking," or suction, if available, so that the bleeding vessel can be seen and exposed to the vasoconstrictor epinephrine (Adrenalin) and local anesthetic (0.5 per cent cocaine or 0.25 per cent phenylephrine [Neosynephrine]) that is sprayed on, or applied to, the spot. Goodsell says that suction is almost essential as preparation for seeing the bleeding spot.

3. If bleeding persists, the application of a lubricated pack, or gauze in petrolatum. He mentions salt pork, once used for this purpose, as having the same effect.

4. After control of the hemorrhage, when the mucous membrane is dry, the area subject to bleeding may be cauterized. In incontrollable nasal bleeding occlusion of the arterial blood supply is necessary.

Hemorrhages of the stomach and *of the lung* are considered together because they are often confused. The term *hematemesis* refers to the vomiting of blood; *hemoptysis* means the spitting of blood from the larynx, trachea, or lungs.

The *causes of gastric hemorrhage* may be *local* or *constitutional*. Local causes include: (1) cancer, ulcer, diseases of blood vessels (miliary aneurysms and varicose veins), acute congestion, and operations on the stomach; (2) passive congestion, caused by obstruction of the portal system as in cirrhosis of the liver, thrombus in the portal vein, and enlarged spleen, or pressure on the portal veins from without by tumors; and (3) traumatism from wounds and corrosive poisons. Hemophilia and severe anemia are constitutional causes of gastric hemorrhage.

The *causes of lung hemorrhage* are: (1) diseases of the lungs—pulmonary tuberculosis, pneumonia, cancer, abscess, gangrene, and ulceration of the bronchi, trachea, or larynx; (2) certain diseases of the heart, particularly mitral lesions that dam blood in the left atrium, then into the pulmonary vessels and cause marked pulmonary congestion; and (3) erosion of an aneurysm of a large blood vessel.

It is often difficult to differentiate the symptoms of gastric hemorrhage from those of pulmonary hemorrhage. The vomiting of blood is not always a sign of bleeding from the stomach, because blood from the nose, throat, or lungs may be swallowed and later vomited.

When red blood cells stay in the stomach for a short time, they are disintegrated by the action of gastric juice, setting free the hemoglobin. Hemoglobin is in turn disintegrated forming hematin, a brown pigment. The same result occurs in the intestines. This accounts for the clotted, dark-brown or coffee-ground vomitus and also for the tarry stool when the hemorrhage has occurred some time before. Blood from the stomach will have an acid reaction.

Table 14. Differentiation between Hematemesis and Hemoptysis (Osler)

HEMATEMESIS	HEMOPTYSIS
1. Previous history points to gastric, hepatic, or splenic disease.	1. Cough or signs of some pulmonary or cardiac disease precedes, in many cases, the hemorrhage.
2. The blood is brought up by vomiting, prior to which the patient may experience a feeling of giddiness or faintness.	2. The blood is coughed up, and is usually preceded by a sensation of tickling in the throat. If vomiting occurs, it follows the coughing.
3. The blood is usually clotted, mixed with particles of food, and has an acid reaction. It may be dark, grumous, and fluid.	3. The blood is frothy, bright red in color, alkaline in reaction. If clotted, rarely in such large coagula, and mucopus may be mixed with it.
4. Subsequent to the attack the patient passes tarry stools, and signs of disease of the abdominal viscera may be detected.	4. The cough persists, physical signs of local disease in the chest may usually be detected, and the sputa may be bloodstained for many days.

In the treatment for gastric hemorrhage, the patient should lie quietly. Morphine is often prescribed, but a barbiturate that does not predispose to nausea and other undesirable effects is preferable. Nothing should be given by mouth unless it is prescribed by the physician. Cold compresses, an ice bag, or an ice coil may be applied to the epigastrium. Coagulant drugs may be prescribed hypodermically. No stimulants are given because of the danger of increasing the hemorrhage. Blood transfusions are indicated if there is appreciable blood loss.

In pulmonary or lung hemorrhage, the patient is usually frightened. The attendant should reassure and encourage him. According to Osler, death seldom occurs in hemoptysis from tuberculosis.

The patient should be turned on the affected side, if this can be determined, as the blood is then less likely to enter the unaffected lung. If he wants to sit up, however, and can breathe more easily and is less anxious or alarmed when in that position, it is better to allow him to do so. To lessen the nervous excitement one of the barbiturates is usually prescribed. Some physicians allow the patient to suck pieces of ice, but when immediate surgery is possible oral intake is contraindicated.

An ice bag is sometimes applied over the sternum or over the part where the bleeding is thought to be.

If food is permitted, it should be very light.

An extensive or prolonged hemorrhage of any sort is always treated with whole blood if available.

Menorrhagia is a profuse or prolonged menstrual flow; *metrorrhagia* is loss of blood in the intervals between menstruation; a *post-partum hemorrhage* is one occurring after childbirth or a miscarriage. Lesions, tumors, foreign bodies, displacements, and systemic disorders and visceral diseases, such as diseases of the heart, may cause vaginal bleeding.

Any irregular bleeding from the uterus or unusually profuse menstrual flow, particularly after the age of thirty-five, should be reported to a surgeon *without delay*. It may result from cancer in which the only hope of control is an early diagnosis and surgical interference. If such a condition is brought to the attention of the nurse, she should urge an immediate medical examination. People are usually alarmed at the sight of blood or a hemorrhage from the nose, lungs, stomach, or any other organ, but women are likely to be confused as to the cause of bleeding from the uterus and so ignore the early symptoms of disease. Nurses share with doctors the responsibility for teaching the lifesaving effect of early treatment.

The immediate treatment of vaginal bleeding depends upon the cause. In all cases of marked bleeding the patient should be put to bed and kept quiet. The buttocks should be elevated and an ice bag applied to the lower abdomen. Ergot or oxytocic substance (Pitocin) may be prescribed to contract the uterus. Hot vaginal or intrauterine douches at 47.8° to 48.9° C (118° to 120° F) are sometimes, but rarely, given with or without astringents. Vaginal tampons or uterine tampons are frequently inserted to check bleeding by pressure. In giving douches or in packing the vagina or uterus, everything must be sterile. Packing the uterus is never attempted by a nurse, except as a last resort after all other measures have failed and only when it is impossible to secure the services of a doctor.

Surgical treatment consists in removal or correction of the causes, such as tumors, foreign bodies, or displacements, by operative procedure and/or radium therapy. Systemic treatment is the same as in all severe hemorrhage.

Cerebral hemorrhage is discussed in the section devoted to head injuries (see pp. 1143 ff.).

Primary bleeding generally occurs at the time of trauma or operation. It may be a steady oozing from capillaries which involve a large operative area, or it may occur from the small blood vessels which were tied off in surgery.

Intermediate or *recurrent* bleeding occurs normally within a few hours after trauma or operation, when the circulation and blood pressure have returned to normal. At the time of operation, owing to the depressing effect of the anesthetic upon the circulation, bleeding from the capillaries may be very slight and easily controlled by the normal clotting of blood; bleeding from small blood vessels may be so slight as to be overlooked by the surgeon and not be tied off; or a ligature around a large vessel may be tied too near the cut edge, or not tied securely. As the depressing effect of the anesthetic wears off, the heartbeat becomes stronger and the blood pressure is increased, so that blood clots are easily displaced and bleeding begins from the capillaries and small blood vessels. The increased blood pressure may cause a ligature to slip, so that bleeding may occur from a large vessel. Restless movements of the patient increase the rate and force of the heartbeat, and raise the blood pressure, thus increasing the danger of hemorrhage.

Secondary bleeding may occur any time after the first 24 hours up to the time of complete healing of the wound. A secondary hemorrhage is likely to be severe, as it usually occurs from a large vessel, the smaller vessels being occluded after the first 24 to 48 hours. In surgery it may occur from the slipping of an insecurely tied ligature, and should be watched for, particularly in infected wounds, where there is sloughing of the tissues, sloughing or slipping of ligatures, or erosion of the walls of blood vessels.

Local or external hemorrhage occurs at the site of a visible wound. Direct pressure or tying the offending blood vessel with a ligature is usually sufficient to control this. Internal bleeding occurs within the body, as, for example, when a wound is closed or tightly packed, with no means of drainage, the blood will flow into the tissues or into a body cavity, causing systemic symptoms and eventual shock, with little or no local evidence. It is comparatively easy to observe and report on a patient's visible blood loss, but it requires keener observation on the part of the nurse to detect the signs which may be indicative of early internal bleeding.

In general both the local wound area and the patient's systemic condition should be taken into account when observing for hemorrhage. The nurse should be familiar with the character and amount of drainage expected with various types of surgery, so that she can differentiate between normal postoperative bleeding and hemorrhage. In some cases external evidence of bleeding is minimal or absent. Other manifestations of hemorrhage must then be relied upon. These are restlessness, apprehension, rapid pulse, weakness, and thirst. If prolonged or severe, hemorrhage produces shock, with a fall in blood pressure, weak rapid pulse, cold clammy perspiration, and apathy. If bleeding is severe, death follows rapidly. It has been said that death will occur if one half the volume of blood is lost; but a hemorrhage of a smaller amount, accompanied by other complications, may also be fatal.

Summary.   Since hemorrhage is the cause of shock and loss of life in accidental trauma and surgery, it is essential for the nurse to understand its physiology and be able to recognize early the signs and symptoms.

It is estimated that a healthy man weighing 75 kg (165 lb) may lose blood amounting to 3 per cent of the body weight and still recover. Blood loss can usually be treated successfully, and the patient's life saved, provided the hemorrhage is noticed in time.

Since blood transfusions are so commonly used, it is the practice of most hospitals to type the blood of the surgical patient before the operation is performed, so that a transfusion may be given in as short a time as possible, should the need arise. Since the advent of the blood bank, it is possible for friends and relatives of prospective surgical patients to donate blood for future use.

Control of hemorrhage is the immediate concern of all present. The patient should be kept quiet, and a sedative administered. Local treatment may include inspection of the wound and ligation of a blood vessel, applying a pressure dressing, elevating the bleeding extremity, packing the wound, or the use of styptics or vasoconstrictors. The head of the bed is usually lowered to prevent shock; and blood loss is estimated and replenished by blood transfusions. When a blood transfusion is not immediately possible, intravenous solutions of plasma, saline, or glucose may be used as substitutes, but they are less effective and in some cases contraindicated. If the site of the hemorrhage is deep-seated or if bleeding is difficult to control, it may be necessary to reopen a surgical wound and ligate the blood vessels in the operating room. In slow bleeding, preparations which encourage the clotting of blood, such as calcium and vitamin K and newer drugs such as "T.A.L.," are given. Cold applications are also used to control capillary bleeding. Intense heat contracts blood vessels, but its effect is less reliable and is briefer than that of cold. Bleeding areas are in a few cases cauterized. Prevention and control of shock are discussed fully in Chapter 40.

5. NATURE AND TREATMENT OF SHOCK

Shock is a complex of symptoms that results from injury and other causes. It must be included in any complete discussion of wounds because the patient's life depends upon a reversal of the physiological changes in the shock syndrome. However, because the circulatory collapse typical of traumatic shock is believed to be so similar to the circulatory collapse that occurs in many diseases, and because the treatment and nursing care of the patient in shock is highly specialized, Chapter 40 is devoted to this subject. It should be studied in conjunction with the treatment and nursing care of wounds (Chapter 37).

6. LATER CARE OF THE WOUNDED

First aid of the wounded has been discussed. It is assumed that, if indicated, all clothing has been removed, the extent of the injury assessed, and asphyxia, hemorrhage, or shock resulting from the wound controlled or treatment instituted. Now the medical team turns its attention to repair of the wounded area, preventing infection, and building up the individual's general health, if the wound is a threat to it. The local treatment of a deep or extensive injury may require major surgery. In such cases the patient must be prepared as for any emergency operation; slight injuries often require additional treatment besides the first-aid treatment that has been described. Some wounds may appear to be insignificant and yet demand special caution. The particular dangers of even slight head injuries are discussed on page 1112. Injuries that destroy nerves may cause paralysis, and signs of nerve injury must be watched for; stabs and punctures are particularly dangerous because microorganisms are driven into the deeper tissues. Anaerobic bacilli of gas gangrene and tetanus multiply rapidly in tissues without access to air as "anaerobic" indicates. The patient must be specially treated to reduce this hazard. A pinprick can be lethal if it carries into the tissues a sufficient number of deadly organisms. Wounds made by gunshot, needles, or fishhooks are often x-rayed to locate a bullet or a piece of the mutilating object if there is any reason to believe that it has been left in the body. (Sometimes when a fishhook is embedded in the tissues it can only be removed by further trauma.) Contused and lacerated wounds may require excision of hopelessly injured tissue that, potentially necrotic, will act as a foreign body in the wound. Living tissue tends to protect itself from alien material by walling it off in a fibrous capsule or by forming pus around it. When the abscess drains, the foreign body is extruded from the wound. Nature's care is obviously a long-drawn-out process during which the patient may die. Thorough cleansing and surgical debridement are an essential part of the treatment of many wounds. Poison wounds require care. Treatment of the bites of snakes, insects, and rabid animals is discussed in Chapter 43.

7. WOUNDS

Treatment by a surgeon should be sought at once, especially for dangerous or disfiguring wounds. When this is impossible for hours or days, steps must be taken to clean the wound after bleeding has been controlled. The operator should scrub his hands in the usual way for a sterile procedure if no sterile instruments are available for handling articles that come in contact with the hand. The wound should be covered with sterile gauze, and the area around it should be shaved if necessary and cleaned with a detergent. The wound itself should then be gently irrigated with a sterile saline solution or a very mild antiseptic. Some surgeons recommend peroxide of hydrogen 1:3 because with its bubbling effect and its penetrating quality it brings dirt to the surface. Disinfecting solutions strong enough to destroy bacteria are likely also to destroy the tissue cells; however, dressings impregnated with the sulfonamides and antibiotics are well tolerated and have markedly increased the speed with which wounds heal. The local application and systemic administration of these drugs has made it possible to leave the initial dressing applied after debridement (with perhaps a cast over it) undisturbed for days or weeks.

General Therapeutic Measures and Nursing Care.   With the development of the sulfa drugs and antibiotics the practice of giving them routinely to prevent or control threatened infection has grown up. Some surgeons give penicillin in all major surgery as a protective measure and for the same reason would employ it in treating accidental wounds. Some authorities believe that this trend is regrettable for the following reasons: (1) the surgical team may be lulled into a false sense of security and therefore relax its efforts to make the surgical procedure really aseptic; (2) bacteria that are now sensitive to antibiotics may develop strains resistant to drugs too commonly encountered; and (3) therapeutic agents should be prescribed on a specific rather than a general basis. Of the known antibiotics and chemicals used to combat infection no one substance is equally effective against all bacteria. On the contrary they are the drugs that are highly selective in their action. Another way of putting it is that strains of organisms infecting wounds vary greatly in their resistance to therapeutic agents. Medical literature abounds in reports on the relative merits of the known sulfa compounds and antibiotics. Almost any opinion cited is, however, out of date before it can be published. New agents are developed so rapidly that it is impossible to keep abreast of knowledge in this field. Statements that any one preparation is *the* most therapeutic agent should be considered tentative.

In order to apply what is known about specific action of the sulfonamides and antibiotics the doctor should know the organism, or organisms, he is attempting to control. Ideally, cultures are made and drugs ordered on the basis of the laboratory findings. This is essential in the selection of antisera. In some cases the facilities for making cultures are not available, and often the physician or surgeon believes that he can judge the probable nature of the threat of infection from the location of the wound. It is common practice, therefore, to give one of the antibiotics to the wounded in protective doses. When an elevation of body temperature and other symptoms indicate that a wound is seriously infected, most surgeons think it is gross neglect to fail to discover, if possible, the chief invading organisms.

All physicians are confronted daily with the problem of the selection of an antibiotic for a specific patient. To use these agents with the greatest efficiency and with the lowest cost to the patient, it is essential that a proper etiologic diagnosis be made and the best drug selected and used. This is not always an easy problem, but it is well to know the relative merits of each antibiotic.*

Chester S. Keefer goes on to discuss the uses of penicillin, streptomycin, chlortetracycline (Aureomycin), chloromycetin, and oxytetracycline (Terramycin). Had he been writing now he might have added several others to his list of commonly used preparations.

In Chapter 41, "Nursing Care of Patients with Systemic Infections," there appears a table on the current use of major antibiotics and sulfonamides in systemic infections (see pp. 1074-75).

Penicillin Administration. Using penicillin as an example of the antibiotics it might be well to discuss its administration in some detail. It was the first antibiotic to be used and it is still the agent of choice in many infections. The fear that its widespread use would lead to resistant strains of common bacteria is not so far substantiated according to Sir Alexander Fleming. He says:

Some bacteria are highly resistant to penicillin; some are extremely sensitive, and a few are midway. It was found early that in the laboratory a few sensitive organisms could be made resistant by continued exposure to sub-lethal doses, and it was feared that the misuse of penicillin would lead to a widespread dissemination of resistant forms. Fortunately this has not materialized, except perhaps with the staphylococcus. . . .

It is impossible to say, however, that resistant strains cannot be induced by inadequate treatment; . . . there are other antibiotics which can deal with the situation, so this problem is of less practical importance.†

Penicillin has proved so far to be remarkably nontoxic. Some persons develop dermatitis, and other allergic reactions have been reported but these are rare.

* Keefer, Chester S.: "Evaluation of Antibiotic Therapy," *Postgrad. Med.,* **9:**101, (Jan.) 1951.
†Fleming, Sir Alexander: "Modern Penicillin Therapy," *Practitioner,* **165:**639, (Dec.) 1950.

The antibiotics are applied locally to wounds, but in combating infection with marked systemic symptoms they may be given intravenously, intramuscularly, or by mouth in sufficient amounts and in such a way that a therapeutic level of the agent is maintained in the blood stream. Fleming says:

In considering the dosage scheme it is well to know the penicillin content of the blood after different sized doses. . . . A dose of 1500 units lasts three to four hours or less; a dose of 1,000,000 units lasts for about twelve hours (in the blood stream). Thus an increase in the dose of almost 70 times only increases the period of detectable penicillinaemia some four times. These figures show that the most economical way to use penicillin is the method of small doses frequently repeated, of which the continuous drip is the extreme example.*

He goes on to say that unless the patient is hospitalized more than two daily injections are impractical and that many patients can be successfully treated with 100,000 units twice daily, or in dealing with "septic organisms" 500,000 units.

Several methods have been adopted since 1945 to make it possible to reduce the number of injections of penicillin without reducing its effectiveness. The first was giving it in oil and beeswax to slow the rate of absorption. This had technical difficulties. If the preparation was cold it was too thick to be drawn into or forced out of a syringe through the needle; if it was overheated in the liquefying process it was inactivated. Fortunately procaine penicillin developed since then does not have this disadvantage.

Procaine added to penicillin was found to cause a fine precipitate but this was soon discovered to be as effective and longer lasting than the unprecipitated preparation. Later the two drugs were deliberately combined, and now it is used by preference in water or oil suspensions. It forms a "penicillin depot" in the tissues on which they draw during the 24-hour period. The usual dose is 300,000 to 400,000 units as a suspension in 1 cc of oil or water. Aluminum monostearate still further delays absorption, and so this is often added. Many times sodium penicillin (100,-000 units) and procaine penicillin (300,000 units) in 1 cc are combined in a commercial solution so that it acts both long and quickly.

Some drugs given by mouth prolong the action of penicillin. Of those reported up to 1950 Fleming thinks "carinamide" the most effective. It is not toxic but causes "pentosuria." The following table gives Fleming's figures for blood and exudate levels of penicillin when it is given intramuscularly in three different forms:

DOSE: 30,000 UNITS INTRAMUSCULARLY	TIME DURING WHICH PENICILLIN DETECTABLE IN	
	Blood	*Exudate*
Aqueous penicillin	3 hours	8 to 9 hours
Oil-wax penicillin	12 hours	18 hours
Procaine penicillin	24 hours	31 hours

* Fleming, Sir Alexander: *op. cit.*

Oral penicillin was not too effective in its first preparation. The gastric juice destroyed so much of it that 10 times the intramuscular dose was advocated. The newer preparations are coated with a substance that protects them from the secretions of the stomach. The effectiveness of these new forms for oral administration promise to revolutionize penicillin therapy. Most of the antibiotics can now be given by mouth, if the patient is not nauseated and vomiting, and if the more rapid effect of parenteral administration is not indicated. Giving these agents by mouth spares the patient the discomfort of injections, and the nursing service the inordinate expenditure of time that has been devoted to antibiotic therapy in the past. When parenteral administration cannot be avoided the commercially prepared disposable units are recommended as timesaving and as providing optimum protection from infection.

Promoting Drainage and Closure in Infected Wounds.   The sulfonamides and antibiotics have worked miracles in the control of infections associated with wounds. Conditions that would have taken months to control heal in a few days or weeks with the "wonder drugs." Sometimes, however, even they fail, and a life is lost or the wound continues to drain. In such cases hot wet dressings, irrigations, or suction of the wound may be prescribed; the surgeon may incise walled-off pockets of pus, or he may remove the abnormal tissue around the wound and attempt a fresh closure or a plastic repair.

Specific Aspects of Treatment and Nursing Care.   Processes of repair are greatly influenced by diet, as has been repeatedly emphasized in this text. A high-caloric, high-protein, high-vitamin diet with increased mineral content is stressed. If, for any reason, the patient's oral intake is inadequate it must be supplemented by nutritious parenteral fluids. There is no greater service the nurse can render the patient than accurately observing and reporting what he eats. It is often necessary to feed a severely wounded person. This need is obvious if his hands are injured, or if his position makes eating difficult; it is not so obvious when he fails to eat because the effort of getting the food to his mouth is so great that he decides "it isn't worth it." The nurse is the person who should take the initiative; few patients will ask to be fed.

A high fluid intake is important. If they are diluted, chemicals produced in the healing process are less irritating to all tissues, and particularly to the kidneys that excrete them. While serious infections are usually prevented with modern treatment, few patients run a completely afebrile course. A high fluid intake replaces the fluid lost in sweating associated with fever and the dehydrating effect of drainage from the wound, when this is appreciable. The care of a person who is running a high temperature is described in more detail in Chapter 41. Exercise should be specifically prescribed for the seriously wounded. The dangers of immobility were discussed in Chapter 15 and elsewhere in this text. The wounded have special need of therapeutic exercises to combat contractures, or deformity. Such measures are prescribed by the surgeon. They are initiated by the physical therapist, if one is available. Usually the exercises must be continued by the nurse and, of course, the patient. In some cases the nurse must assume the function of the physical therapist.

Rest and sleep, induced by a good hygienic regime rather than drugs, are, of course, important. Without variety, occupation, and some satisfaction of emotional

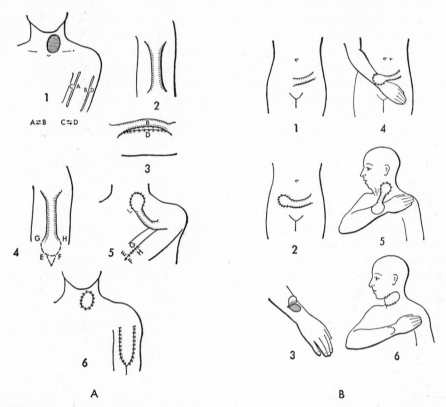

Figure 218. (*A*) Method of making a tubed pedicle skin flap on the arm attached to a defect on the neck and replacing the pedicle. (*1*) Parallel incisions on the arm. The tube is formed by approximating the skin edge *A* to *B* about the subcutaneous tissue with the skin covering the tube. Closure is made by drawing the skin edges *C* and *D* together. (*2*) The skin tube from above. (*3*) The skin tube from the side showing closure. (*4*) Showing outline of flap, *GH*, to be raised and skin, *EF*, to be excised. (*5*) The flap is transplanted into the defect on the neck, and closure of the denuded area is completed after undermining. (*6*) Division of the flap and replacement of the pedicle on the arm.

(*B*) A delayed tubed pedicle flap from the abdomen to the neck—caterpillared by an intermediate stage to the forearm. (*1*) Formation of tubed pedicle. (*2*) Delaying the flap by raising it and suturing it back in place. (*3*) Raising of a flap on the forearm. By such a flap a bed of twice the size of the tissue included in the incision is made available for nourishment. (*4*) The tubed flap attached to the forearm flap. (*5*) The pedicle flap of the iliac region attached to a defect on the neck. (*6*) The remainder of the neck contracture is excised, and the defect covered by the unrolled pedicle flap. The forearm flap has been returned to its normal position.

(Christopher, Frederick (ed.): *A Textbook of Surgery*, 5th ed. W. B. Saunders Company, Philadelphia, 1949, p. 1407.)

needs from congenial companionship, relaxation is difficult to achieve. Each patient's program should provide an opportunity for diverting, and productive or creative, activities and for association with friends, family, and other patients, according to his tastes and needs.

Rehabilitation of the wounded may involve very little or a complicated program requiring the cooperation of almost every type of medical worker. Patients with wounds that leave functional handicaps or ones whose mutilating effects are visible demand particular care. The plastic surgeon, the maker of prostheses, the vocational expert, and often the psychiatrist and psychologist must be added to the regular members of the medical team. The rehabilitation program should be started, ideally, on the patient's admission to the hospital; otherwise he may have much to unlearn and many an unnecessary physical handicap to overcome.

REFERENCES

1. Sobotka, Harry, and Adelman, Nathan: "Shortening of Bleeding Time by a Water-Soluble Adrenochrome-Derivative," *Proc. Soc. Exper. Biol. & Med.,* **75:**789, (Dec.) 1950.
2. Goodsell, Ross A.: "Nosebleed," *Ann. West. Med. & Surg.,* **4:**814, (Dec.) 1950.

Additional Suggested Reading

Beaumont, G. E.: "The Medical Treatment of Threatened Gangrene," *Practitioner,* **164:**502, (May) 1950.

Christopher, Frederick (ed.): *Textbook of Surgery,* 5th ed. W. B. Saunders Co., Philadelphia, 1949.

Felter, Robert K., et al.: *Surgical Nursing,* 6th ed. F. A. Davis Co., Philadelphia, 1952.

First Aid Textbook (prepared by the American Red Cross), 3rd ed. Blakiston Co., New York, 1945.

Fleming, A.: "Current Therapeutics. XXXVI—Modern Penicillin Therapy," *Practitioner,* **165:**639-45, (Dec.) 1950.

Gold, Harry (ed.): *Cornell Conferences on Therapy,* Vol. V. The Macmillan Company, New York, 1952, pp. 27-44.

Goodman, Louis S., and Gilman, Alfred: *The Pharmacological Basis of Therapeutics,* 2nd ed. The Macmillan Company, New York, 1955.

Graham, Evart A. (ed.): *Year Book of General Surgery.* Year Book Publishers, Chicago, 1952.

Johnson, A. E.: "Antibiotics," *Am. J. Nursing,* **50:**688-90, (Nov.) 1950.

Keefer, C. S.: "Evaluation of Antibiotic Therapy," *Postgrad. Med.,* **9:**101-5, (Feb.) 1951.

Kolmer, John A.: *Penicillin Therapy,* 2nd ed. Appleton-Century-Crofts, Inc., New York, 1947.

Waksman, S. A. (ed.): *Streptomycin.* Williams & Wilkins Co., Baltimore, 1949.

Weinstein, L.: "The Newer Antibiotics," *Ohio M. J.,* **46:**246–53, (June) 1950.

West, John P.; Keller, Manelva W.; and Harmon, Elizabeth: *Nursing Care of the Surgical Patient,* 6th ed. The Macmillan Company, New York, 1957.

CHAPTER 37. CARE OF WOUNDS, INCLUDING SURGICAL DRESSINGS

1. FUNCTIONS OF THE NURSE IN CARE OF WOUNDS
2. PRINCIPLES OF ASEPSIS APPLIED TO SURGICAL DRESS-
   INGS
3. TYPES OF DRESSINGS USED IN CARE OF WOUNDS
4. EQUIPMENT FOR SURGICAL DRESSINGS
5. SUGGESTED PROCEDURE FOR DRESSING WOUNDS IN
   HOSPITALS
6. PRINCIPLES UNDERLYING THE SELECTION AND APPLI-
   CATION OF BANDAGES AND BINDERS

1. FUNCTIONS OF THE NURSE IN CARE OF WOUNDS

Preventing Infection and Promoting Healing. The surgeon prescribes the dressing for a wound and usually applies it. In some cases he delegates the dressing to
a nurse, to the family, or the patient himself. Protection of the wound is essential,
and is the joint responsibility of the surgeon and the nurse. If healing is to take place
as rapidly and as completely as possible, the nurse must prevent strain that might
rupture or tear open the wound. She should see that dressings are never displaced,
and that they are kept clean and dry. With modern surgery, rupture of wounds is
rare, and more and more surgeons have discarded the use of binders over wounds.

The patient's diet, his surroundings, general health, and mental attitude influence
the healing of wounds as discussed earlier.

Interference with the circulation, whether from high blood pressure, arteriosclerosis, or pressure from tight bandages or adhesive straps interferes with healing.

Position and *pressure* are frequently used to regulate and to promote circulation. In treating ulcers of the leg, for instance, the part is usually elevated and
a tight bandage applied to prevent congestion in a dependent part and to aid the
return of venous blood. Too much pressure or prolonged pressure, however, must
be avoided. For maintenance of conditions that promote healing and for reporting
conditions that retard it, nurses are largely responsible.

Preparing and Assisting with Dressings. In many situations the nurse is responsible for preparing dressing materials and the carriage that contains them;

966

preparing for the round of dressings in the clinical division; and planning the dressing sequence and procedure that will provide for asepsis, for the comfort of patients, and for such assistance as ensures that wounds may be dressed by the surgeon with the greatest ease and efficiency.

To plan and to assist with dressings, a nurse should know the nature and results of the operation concerned: the kind of wound (whether clean or with drainage), the type of dressing and any special equipment required, when the first dressing after operation is likely to be done, and the time scheduled for dressings. The dressing on a clean wound may not be changed until the fifth or seventh day or even later, when the skin stitches or clips are removed. Wounds with drainage are usually dressed by the surgeon the first day after operation and daily thereafter. Sometimes when soiled, the outer dressings are changed by the nurse as frequently as necessary—saturated with drainage, such dressings are a source of great discomfort. In present-day practice there is a tendency to leave wounds undisturbed. Compound fractures are treated with the closed method. Plaster casts are put over dressings which are not changed unless they are too foul to be tolerated. With the administration of antibiotics and the sulfa compounds, patients with infected wounds are not so likely to develop septicemia as they were several decades ago. Special protection for the bed should be provided, and other equipment that may be required. Every need of the surgeon and of the patient should be foreseen as far as possible.

Observing the Patient for Local and Systemic Symptoms.   The local symptoms of infection (tenderness, heat, swelling), the systemic symptoms (an elevated temperature, increased pulse), and signs of the rupture of the wound must be reported as soon as they are noted. A nurse should always watch closely for bleeding (staining of dressings, bandage, or bed). A line may be drawn around a bloodstain to see whether it remains the same size or increases.

2. PRINCIPLES OF ASEPSIS APPLIED TO SURGICAL DRESSINGS

Sterilization and Aseptic Handling of Equipment and Supplies.   Everything that comes in direct contact with a wound should be sterilized by steam under pressure, if this is available. The fairly prevalent organisms that cause the dreaded wound infections of gas gangrene and tetanus are spore-forming, and to kill these spores it is necessary to employ temperatures above that of boiling water. It is possible to secure high temperature with boiling oil and heated air, but moist heat is more effective than dry heat; therefore, autoclaving is the preferred method of sterilization as was noted in Chapter 7. Sterilizing in boiling water for a long period, if this is possible, is probably the best substitute for steam under pressure.

Equipment that would be destroyed by high temperatures should be soaked for adequate periods in the most effective chemical disinfectants available. Recent developments suggest the possibility of using ultraviolet rays to sterilize equipment that is injured by moisture and chemical disinfectants.

Handling Equipment and Supplies Used in Surgical Dressings. In order to maintain the sterility of objects that come in contact with the wound, it is necessary to handle them with sterile forceps or sterile gloves. Hands cannot be made sterile by scrubbing, and since the process, besides being questionable bacteriologically, is time consuming, either sterile gloves or sterile handling forceps are used when available. Manipulation with instruments is by far the most efficient way of handling sterile surgical materials. It must be remembered, however, that instruments used for one dressing cannot be used for another with safety, until they have been resterilized. The efficiency of chemicals as a means of sterilizing instruments in a short time has not been satisfactorily demonstrated.

There is always danger of contamination of articles exposed to the air, especially air exhaled by human beings. For this reason, dressings put up in large jars that are opened and closed frequently during the day, but sterilized only once in 24 hours, are not so likely to be sterile as those wrapped in individual packages; in fact, the former practice should be discontinued. To prevent infection of wounds from the exhaled air of surgeons and nurses, some authorities recommend that these workers wear masks.

Sterile draping around the wound is not essential, if unsterile bedding does not come in contact with the wound or in close proximity to it. Clean draping that protects the bedding and clothing is desirable. The bed may be protected from cleansing and irrigating solutions by the proper use of basins and pads made of cellucotton and impervious paper. Squares of rubber, covered with soft paper, are also used. Dressing rubber should not be taken from one patient to another without being adequately disinfected each time that it is used. If a patient has a wound, the dressing of which requires protection of the bedding, it is an economy of time and effort to leave a rubber protector in his unit until there is no longer any use for it —then it may be thoroughly sterilized before being placed in the unit of another patient.

Unsterile articles, such as binders and pins, used to hold dressings in place, bandages, scissors, and basins for the collection of waste should be handled with clean hands. To prevent infection of the wound, it is necessary to keep unsterile objects from coming in contact with it. To prevent the spread of disease generally, it is important that clean and contaminated equipment be kept separate and that all medical attendants wash their hands after every service to the patient that requires handling the body discharges, clothing, or bedding.

3. TYPES OF DRESSINGS USED IN CARE OF WOUNDS

Dry Dressings. So-called *clean wounds* are dressed by the application of eight or more layers of gauze, folded into a suitable size and shape. This dressing is held in place by strips of adhesive, a bandage, or a binder. In some cases the wound and the surrounding area are cleaned with solvents, such as alcohol, ether, sterile soap, or neutral detergent solutions. Drugs such as benzylkonium, nitromersol, iodine, or acriflavine may be applied for their antiseptic value. Sulfa preparations and antibiotics may be applied as preventives against possible infection. Many surgeons believe, however, that if a wound shows signs of healing satisfactorily, the less that is done to it the better, and they make no other effort than to keep the gauze protection dry and clean. There is a possibility that liquids used to clean the wound may at the same time infect it by carrying contamination from the skin into the deeper areas of the incision or puncture.

Pressure Dressings. When there is danger of bleeding or when there may be seepage from a wound, the surgeon is likely to use a pressure dressing. This is a thick sterile pad made of gauze or gauze and cellulose applied with a firm bandage or binder. The latter is often attached to the dressing so that it can be applied speedily.

Wet Dressings. If wounds are infected, the dressings used are sometimes designed to soften the discharge and hence promote drainage. There may be a further effort to hasten the suppurative process that localizes the infection into an area that can be incised and drained. Wet dressings tend to have both these effects. If the wet compresses are also hot, they are thought to stimulate the suppurative process. When dressed, such wounds are thoroughly cleaned with sponges saturated in saline solution or in a mild antiseptic; they may be irrigated with a syringe, and the surgeon may want to probe the wound with an instrument or to insert a wick or packing. Wet dressings or compresses are made of many layers of gauze or a pad of cellucotton covered with gauze. An impervious material, such as rubber tissue, rubberized silk,

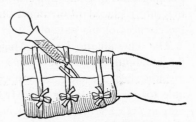

Figure 219. Diagram showing one method of irrigating infected wounds, using the Carrel-Dakin technique. (After Mason, R. L.: *Preoperative and Postoperative Treatment.* W. B. Saunders Co., Philadelphia, 1937.)

cellulose film, or moistureproof paper, should be used to hold the dressing in place. Obviously, the protector must itself be sterile. The skin around the wound area is sometimes protected with strips of gauze impregnated with petroleum jelly or some other oily substance that prevents maceration of the skin by the wet dressing.

Carrel-Dakin Dressings. During World War I, a technique for treating deep infected wounds was developed by Alexis Carrel and H. D. Dakin; this technique is still used occasionally. The object of this type of dressing is to provide either frequent or constant flushing of the wound. A tube, closed at the end and having fine holes along the sides, is inserted in the wound; the irrigating solution is then introduced through this tube, which is held in the wound by gauze packed lightly around it. Soft thick compresses are laid over the wound to absorb the drainage; these must be changed frequently in order to avoid soiling the clothing and bedding. Usually, the area around the wound is protected with strips of gauze, saturated with petroleum jelly.

Various types of solutions are used for irrigating the wound, but the one used by Carrel was a preparation of sodium hypochlorite developed by the chemist Dakin.

When it is fresh, the chlorine that it liberates is believed to be destructive to bacteria and only slightly irritating to the tissues of the wound. Some question remains as to whether the good results that are seen in the use of this technique are the result of the mechanical cleansing of the wound or of the antiseptic value of the solution. Any fluid used for irrigation may be introduced periodically with a syringe inserted into the end of the tube, which lies outside the dressing (see Fig. 219), or continuously by attaching the end of the tube to a reservoir, such as a cylinder or Kelly flask.

Dakin's solution deteriorates when exposed to light; therefore, it must be kept in dark bottles and, because it is very unstable, must not be used after 2 or 3 days at the most. When this type of dressing is used, the tubes and packing are usually replaced daily, since the purulent material from the wound tends to saturate the packing and clog the holes of the drainage tubes. As the compresses get soggy, they are replaced from time to time throughout the day, as often as necessary for the comfort of the patient.

The Therapeutic Use of Maggots in Wounds.   Maggots (grown from eggs of the bluebottle fly), have been applied to sloughing, suppurative wounds in osteomyelitis, because they are supposed to digest dead necrotic material and they are able to differentiate the dead from the living tissues, more minutely than can the human eye. The flies are kept in cages in the laboratory and fed entirely on sterile food. Their eggs are placed in a sterile culture medium and allowed to hatch in an incubator kept at 38° C (100.4° F). Maggots thus produced are kept for 24 to 48 hours, during which time cultures are taken from the medium in which they are living. If cultures prove to be positive for any organism, particularly the tetanus and gas bacilli, the maggots are discarded.

The maggots are inserted into the wound every four days, the first insertion following eight days after the infected area has been cleaned as far as possible by the surgeon. A shield made of wire is used to protect the wound; a cradle is placed over the area and an electric light bulb suspended from the roof of the cradle. Since maggots turn from the light, this is used to keep them from working out of the incision, or to regulate their position in relation to the wound. A severe constitutional reaction follows, generally about 24 hours after the application. For this and other reasons, many surgeons do not use this method of treatment.

The nurse's responsibilities consist in constant supervision of the patient, in the aspiration or withdrawal of the large amounts of secretion in the wound that follows the use of maggots, in the provision for drainage of the wound, and in the adjustment of the bedding, screen, cradle, and light. This treatment is now extremely rare. Sulfa drugs, antibiotics, and improvements in surgery reduce the need for such treatment, which is at best difficult for the patient and not always successful.

Miscellaneous Dressings.   Some wounds, as, for example, tuberculosis lesions, are treated by exposure to light and air. Dressings are omitted, except prehaps for a single layer of gauze, and the wound is exposed to the rays of the sun or to artificial light. Great care must be taken to keep contaminated objects from coming in contact with the wound, and the bedding under the part must be protected from drainage. Areas that show irritation, due to pressure or excoriation from body discharges, are sometimes treated in this manner. (For a detailed discussion of pressure sores, or bedsores, see Chapter 15.)

Dressings for burns are very different from those applied to incised wounds. Dressings commonly used for burns are discussed in Chapter 43.

Ointments and oils of various kinds, and resinous substances, such as balsam of Peru, are used on excoriated surfaces to prevent the access of moisture, which may carry microorganisms to the wound.

4. EQUIPMENT FOR SURGICAL DRESSINGS

Hospital Practice. Materials used in hospitals for surgical dressings are usually kept on a wagon or carriage, so that they can be brought to the bedside with the least possible effort. The use of a carriage involves at least two workers; one who remains uncontaminated and handles clean objects stored on the carriage, and the other who removes the old dressing and applies a new one. While the manipulation of the dressing itself is done with forceps, the handling of the bandage or binder and the patient's clothing and bedding necessarily contaminates the hands of one worker; therefore this person cannot safely touch clean materials on the cart. Since the use of dressing carts requires the services of two persons for dressing wounds, and because a number of doctors and nurses may want the equipment at the same time, some institutions have individual dressing trays, either for all dressings or for those that a doctor or nurse can apply without assistance. The use of a cart saves effort in conveying materials by hand, and if proper care is taken to prevent contamination of its contents, this is in many cases more efficient than the use of trays. On the other hand, if each surgeon and each nurse dresses the wounds of patients assigned to his or her care, the tray method is more desirable.

Contaminated articles are not returned to the cart containing clean and sterile supplies. Discarded dressings, used sponges, and soiled instruments may be collected on a cart used solely to convey contaminated equipment and waste to workrooms, where it is cleaned and sterilized, or the soiled equipment may be carried directly from the bedside to the workroom after each dressing.

Dressing carriages or trays contain: sterile towels; gauze-and-cotton sponges; dressings of various sizes; gauze packing of different widths; drains made of tubing, rubber tissue, and other materials; rubber tubes and syringes for irrigating wounds; flasks and bottles of solutions; cups and bowls of different sizes; instruments, such as forceps, scissors, scalpels, and probes, ointments, strips of gauze impregnated with petroleum jelly; and other items such as wooden spatulas, applicators, bandages, binders, adhesive, pins, and paper bags for the reception of waste. Obviously, it is easier to provide a wide choice in such supplies for the surgeon if a cart is used than if an attempt is made to assemble what is needed for each dressing on an individual tray. If the nurse is sufficiently familiar with the needs of the patient and the preferences of the surgeon, however, she should be able to assemble what is required without difficulty.

Supplies are kept sterile in covered metal or glass containers, or put up in packages. It is convenient to sterilize dressings and instruments in drums of suitable sizes and shapes, but Carl W. Walter questions their use, suggesting that in opening and closing drums the contents are likely to be contaminated. If drums are used, a special shelf for their conveyance may be attached to the dressing carriage, if there is not room for them otherwise. It is desirable to have the lids of drums operated with a pedal that leaves the hands free for other operations.

In *home nursing* the equipment used by the nurse, or provided for the surgeon dressing a wound, is necessarily much simpler. Since autoclaves are not available, dressings must be purchased already sterilized or brought from hospitals or clinics in small packages. Visiting nurses and doctors carry in their bags sterile dressings that have been autoclaved. Sponges for cleaning may be made nearly sterile in a pressure cooker or by boiling in a pan in the kitchen of the home; they may be used directly from the container in which they are sterilized. The pan in which instruments are boiled can be allowed to serve as a sterile tray after the water has been poured out. In emergencies, when a dry sterile dressing is not available, a substitute can be made by ironing pieces of soft and absorbent fabric of suitable sizes, not allowing anything that has not also been subjected to some sterilizing process to touch the dressing between the time it is ironed and applied to the wound. Since the presence of moisture aids in the destruction of bacteria, it is desirable to wet the cloth before ironing. A moist cloth laid over a hot iron and allowed to dry is perhaps the cleanest dry dressing that can be produced in the home. A visiting nurse can apply a surgical dressing with the simple equipment that the patient can provide in addition to what she carries in her bag. The instruments used for the dressing are boiled in an enamel tray, and a sterile dressing can be removed from its paper wrapper. The essentials of asepsis are observed, although the procedure is very simple and the protection not so complete as that afforded in hospitals when all sterile articles used in the dressing are autoclaved.

5. SUGGESTED PROCEDURE FOR DRESSING WOUNDS IN HOSPITALS

Hospital Routines in Relation to Surgical Dressings. It is customary in hospitals to dress all wounds that require attention during certain hours in the morning, usually between 9 and 11 A.M. If dressings are performed by individual surgeons and the nurses assigned to their patients (which seems to be altogether the most desirable practice), the nurse prepares the patient, assembles equipment, assists the surgeon, readjusts binders and bandages, makes the patient comfortable, and takes care of the equipment afterward. In large hospitals, however, the surgical team, composed of a surgeon and two nurses, changes all or most of the dressings in a clinical division or ward. The surgeon cleans the wound and applies the dressings, keeping his hands free from contamination by using forceps or wearing sterile rubber gloves. Usually one of the more experienced nurses assists the physician by handing him supplies from the cart. This nurse keeps sterile objects aseptic by handling them with sterile forceps; her hands remain clean because she touches only uncontaminated equipment and supplies. The second nurse prepares the first patient for the dressing, washes her hands, and then prepares a second patient. The first patient, having had his wound dressed in the meantime, is ready to have a bandage or binder applied, the clothing readjusted, and his unit put in order. The finishing of the dressing is done by the second nurse after she has again washed her hands. In other words, the nurse who handles contaminated equipment, clothing, and dressings, must safeguard the patients and herself by washing her hands each time after preparing a wound for a dressing or completing the process. In some institutions used instruments and soiled dressings are cleaned and properly disposed of in workrooms by nurses, aides, or attendants.

Preparing a Patient for a Dressing.   Before dressings are begun, the patient's unit or room should be in order, with screens in readiness for use, the patient in bed, the bed in order with no unnecessary articles in the way, and the preparation of the dressing carriage completed. The individual concerned should know what is to be done. Since anticipation may cause more suffering than the dressing itself, the explanation should often be postponed until immediately before the dressing, but it is important to gain the patient's cooperation and to relieve unwarranted anxiety.

His position depends upon the area to be dressed, but is most frequently the dorsal recumbent. The patient should be made as comfortable as possible and free from all strain; for instance, he should not be obliged to raise his head or an extremity for the application of a dressing or bandage without support. At the same time, the position should be a convenient one for the person applying the dressing. The hands should be out of the way and in no danger of contaminating or interfering with the dressing. Usually, it is wise to suggest to the patient that he turn his head away to prevent the sight of the wound from increasing the fear and discomfort or intensifying the possible pain present. Sometimes, when the pain is very great, the patient is helped by holding tightly to the sides of the bed or to the hand of the nurse. In case a wound is to be irrigated, the patient should be drawn to the side of the bed. When extra pillows, a back rest, or Gatch frame interferes with the dressing, the pillows should be removed or the back rest lowered.

The arrangement of the clothing will depend upon the area to be dressed, but in all cases the following principles should be observed: with the exception of the top sheet, the upper clothing should be turned back neatly and smoothly so as to allow a free area around the wound for the dressing, with no bulky folds to interfere with it; the upper sheet should then be turned back forming one thin flat fold at the margin of the area. Avoid any unnecessary exposure and chilling of the patient. If the dressing is on an abdominal wound, the spread and blanket should be turned back neatly and smoothly to the thighs. If the weather is cool, or if there is any danger of chilling, a chest protector, or folded bath blanket should first be placed across the chest. The sheet is folded down to expose the area to be dressed; the patient's gown is tucked back out of the way. If drainage from the wound is free, or if the wound is to be irrigated, dressing rubbers are used to protect the bed and bedding, and suitable basins are provided to collect the discharge.

The bandage or binder confining the dressing is then removed; cast or splints and other appliances also are removed when necessary. The adhesive strapping is loosened on one side or both. In case a daily dressing is necessary, sometimes tape strapping (adhesive to which tape is fastened and tied over the dressing) is used. When removing adhesive, pull it on each side toward the wound to prevent pain and strain on the sutures or wound. Saturating the adhesive with a hydrocarbon, such as benzine, or with ether, makes its removal painless. Removing adhesive quickly is much less painful than removing it slowly. Removal of adhesive is most painful if hairs were not shaved from the skin before its application. The old dressing is never removed until the doctor is ready to apply a fresh one.

Completing the Dressing and Making the Patient Comfortable. Dressings are held in place by the application of Scotch tape, adhesive strapping, binders, or bandages.

In order to apply Scotch tape or adhesive strapping over the dressing, first remove any adherent particles of adhesive with benzine or alcohol—these particles are unsightly and irritating. If the skin is abraded, hot water may be used.

Adhesive strapping is applied to hold dressings in place, to draw the edges of the wound together and relieve strain on sutures, and to give support to the muscles of the abdomen, especially if thick and pendulous.

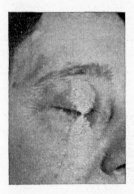

Figure 220. A "butterfly" dressing made with a small piece of bandage and collodion. This keeps the eye shut and protects it when the corneal reflex is absent. (Courtesy of Neurological Institute of the Columbia-Presbyterian Medical Center, New York City, and Clay-Adams Co., New York City.)

For a dressing on the abdomen, the straps should be wide enough and should be applied tightly and firmly enough to give support and prevent the pull of the muscles on the wound and sutures. Narrow strips cut the skin, give no support, dry up, and peel off quickly. The straps must be long enough to extend well around to either side. It may be necessary to pad prominent hipbones where the skin is thin. The first strip should usually be across and over the lower border of the dressing, partly on the skin and overlapping the dressing, so that the lower border is completely sealed, so that neither the fingers nor any foreign matter can get under it, and also in order that the discharge cannot escape to spread infection. The other strips are applied in the same way from below toward the waist. To apply the strap, first fasten securely on the opposite side, then draw it toward you over the dressing with one hand and with the other gently but firmly press the abdominal wall toward the wound (away from you), and quickly and securely fasten the adhesive in place. This draws the edges together, relieves strain, and gives support, so that the patient is more comfortable, does not feel as though he were falling apart, and is not afraid to move. Do not apply adhesive over an abraded skin. When a daily dressing is necessary, to prevent irritation of the skin and pain and discomfort to the patient caused by the daily removal of adhesive, tape strapping is sometimes fastened on either side and tied over the dressing. This is useless when support of the part is necessary. If used, the tapes should be removed as soon as they are soiled, the edges are curled, or adhesion is lost.

Binders and bandages are frequently used to secure dressings in place and for support. They are discussed and different types illustrated in the next section of this chapter.

A liquid adhesive is available that is convenient for certain dressings. It is said to be less irritating than adhesive tape. A cellulose film product, Scotch tape, is often used to hold face dressings in place because it is transparent and therefore inconspicuous. As soon as the dressing has been fixed in position, the dressing rubber and towels are removed, the bedding straightened, pillows adjusted, and bedside table replaced, if moved. Light anesthetics are given for some very painful dressings. In such cases the patient may require special aftercare. Soiled linen is placed in the hamper, and the dressing rubber is removed to be cleaned and dried; if used by other patients, it must be disinfected as well. Soiled instruments are collected in a basin; used dressings are placed in a paper bag and immediately disposed of in a waste container in the workroom.

Sterilization of Equipment between Dressings.   Frequently, when a number of dressings are to be done, there is not a sufficient supply of sterile instruments, basins, and other articles to complete the dressings without resterilizing them between dressings. In this case, equipment must be cleaned and sterilized by boiling, unless the clinical division is equipped with a very efficient autoclave. Methods of preparing different types of surgical equipment for aseptic procedures have been discussed fully in Chapter 8.

Before attempting to assist the surgeon, the nurse should make herself thoroughly familiar with the contents of the dressing carriage and the position of different articles on it, in order that she may anticipate and promptly supply the needs of the doctor, or another nurse, she assists and to avoid any movement that would contaminate articles coming directly or indirectly in contact with the wound.

The articles should always be in the same place and arranged according to the frequency with which they are used and in the order in which they are ordinarily required. A jar containing sterile forceps in an antiseptic solution, to be used for passing sterile dressings and the like to the doctor or nurse doing the dressing, is always kept on the top shelf of the dressing carriage.

Suggested Procedure for Surgical Dressings When Using a Dressing Cart.   Wheel the carriage to the lower side of the bed, where the person dressing the wound will stand. Arrange sterile and unsterile articles in the most convenient position, on the individual tray, pan, or other container provided for each dressing. Open packages of sterile towels, dressings, basins, and so on (if kept in packages), and pour solutions ready for use as soon as the wants of the operator are known. (Never put stoppers where their inner surfaces will come in contact with an unsterile object.)

During the dressing, assist the operator by passing (with sterile forceps from the jar of antiseptic solution), as required, sterile instruments, syringes, tubings, dressings, and by pouring cleansing and antiseptic solutions as needed. If an irrigation is necessary, arrange the irrigating can with tubing attached and pour in the solution. (The lower end of the tubing is usually handled by the person doing the dressing.) Or hand the operator a syringe and a container of irrigating fluid.

Both the operator and the assistant handling the supplies on the cart should attempt to keep their hands clean by manipulating contaminated objects with forceps. If it is necessary for either the operator or the assistant to touch the patient or the soiled dressings or his clothing, the contents of the cart must not be touched by that person until the hands have been washed.

During the dressing, any conversation should be of such a nature as to reassure the patient, to make him feel that he is the center of attention and care at this time, and that everything possible is being done to make the dressing effective and free from unnecessary discomfort.

6. PRINCIPLES UNDERLYING THE SELECTION AND APPLICATION OF BANDAGES AND BINDERS

Purposes for Which Bandages Are Used.   Bandages are used in first-aid treatment, and in orthopedic and general surgery. They are applied for the following purposes: (1) to hold surgical dressings, medicinal applications, or splints in place; (2) to apply pressure on various parts in order to control bleeding, to support weak-walled blood vessels, to relieve congestion, to promote the absorption of fluid or exudates, and to prevent or reduce edema or swelling; and (3) to immobilize a part, to afford support and protection to injured limbs and joints, and to correct deformity.

Materials of Which Bandages Are Made.   Various materials are used, the most common being crepe paper, gauze, muslin, elastic webbing, rubber, woven cotton, Canton flannel, flannel, and crinoline impregnated with plaster of Paris or other substances. The material selected must be suitable for the purpose for which the bandage is applied.

Crepe paper is cheap, light, smooth, and readily adjusted. It is suitable for bed patients and for home use.

Gauze is thin, light, soft, porous, and cool. It can be readily adjusted with an even pressure and is suitable for holding dressings and splints in place. It is always used to retain wet dressings in place, and is usually preferred to muslin in applying bandages to children. Gauze is more pliable and stays on better, but it should be remembered that the soft tissues of children can tolerate little pressure.

Unbleached muslin is heavier and firmer and may be used to apply pressure, to give support, to limit motion, and to hold splints in place. Sometimes sheet wadding is first wrapped around the limb when muslin bandages are applied for pressure and support.

Canton flannel is used under splints and plaster-of-Paris bandages to protect the skin. It is also used for abdominal, and many-tailed, bandages or binders.

Flannel is soft and elastic, and may be applied smoothly and with even pressure using simple spiral turns; it is warm and absorbent. Flannel is applied to painful joints and extremities in rheumatism and gout, for comfort. It is sometimes used to apply even pressure in varicose veins and to reduce swelling.

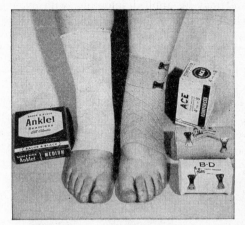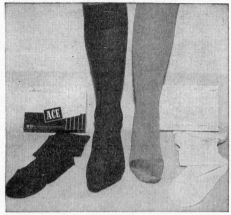

Figure 221. (*Left*) Cotton elastic bandage applied to an ankle and elastic anklet, both used for support of a sprained ankle. (*Right*) Elastic stocking, knee length and full length; worn when circulation in the extremity is poor or for varicosities. (Courtesy of Clay-Adams Co., New York City.)

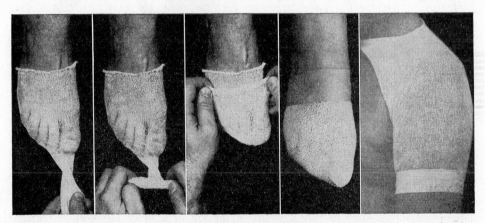

Figure 222. Application of Surgitube to foot. Surgitube may be used as a clean dressing when applying ointments or it may be used over a sterile dressing instead of a roller bandage to hold it in place. (*Right*) Completed dressing of the same material, applied to the shoulder. (Courtesy of Surgitube Products Corp., New York City.)

The *rubber (Esmarch) bandage* is used to give support and apply pressure over varicose veins and to control hemorrhage. It may be applied smoothly, with even pressure by making simple spiral turns. It is expensive and is hot and uncomfortable because it does not allow for evaporation from the skin.

The *woven rubber bandage* is made of an elastic network covered with silk or cotton. It is used for the same purposes as the Esmarch bandage, and is preferable, as it allows for evaporation.

The *elastic cotton bandage* is made so that it will stand considerable stretching. It may be used for the same purposes as the rubber elastic bandages. It has the advantages of being lighter, less expensive, and easily laundered. It makes even pressure, permits evaporation, and has no odor. It is especially good for home use.

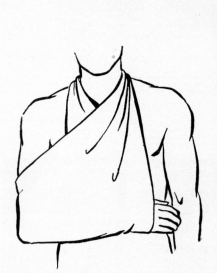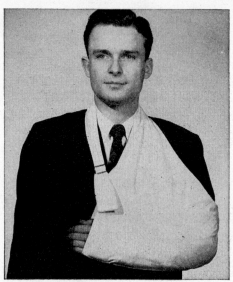

Figure 223. (*Left*) Sling made with triangular bandage; it is usually applied over the clothing. (*Right*) Teare arm sling (courtesy of the M. M. Teare Co., Buffalo, N. Y.).

Crinoline impregnated with starch, plaster of Paris, or plastics is used to immobilize a broken limb or joint. It is also used as a means of support in diseases of bones or joints, such as osteomyelitis of the leg or a tuberculous ankle. Space is left to allow for dressings.

Types of Bandages and Their Uses. (1) The *triangular bandage* is used as a sling to support the hand and arm, and may be used to hold dressings in place on the shoulder, hand, foot, hip, breast, or buttocks.

2. The *cravat bandage* is a triangular bandage in which the apex is first folded to the base and the material then rolled or loosely folded to the base, thus making a bandage of the desired width. It is used as a sling to support the hand and in first-aid treatment to hold dressings in place on such parts as the axilla, groin, or back of the neck.

A *sling* is a swinging bandage most commonly used to support the hand, forearm, and elbow. It may be made of a roller bandage, a cravat, or a triangular bandage.

The *triangular bandage* is the sling generally used. It may be made of any firm, pliable material, but is usually made by folding a piece of muslin a yard square into a triangle.

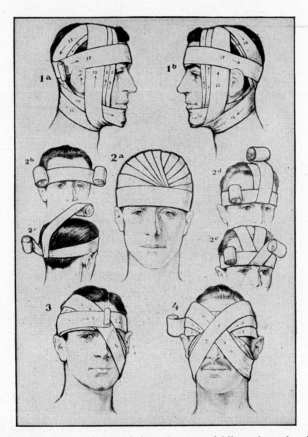

Figure 224. Head, forehead, lateral eye, and bilateral eye bandages.

Before applying the sling, the injured arm is extended horizontally across the body, in the semiprone position—that is, with the thumb up. The triangle is placed under the injured arm so that the hand rests on the base and the apex extends beyond the elbow. The corner of the base of the triangle that rests against the body is carried up over the shoulder of the injured side while the other portion is carried up over the opposite shoulder. The two ends are then tied around the neck. The apex at the elbow is then folded neatly and pinned securely to the body of the bandage. Some surgeons prefer to pin it to the posterior portion while others pin it to the anterior portion.

The cravat sling is used when it is necessary to support the wrist and hand only.

3. The *handkerchief bandage* is made of thin, pliable material cut in squares of different sizes, folded in the shape of a triangle or cravat, and readily adjusted to different parts of the body. The ends can be securely tied or pinned. The handkerchief bandage has been used for centuries. It is especially useful to secure temporary

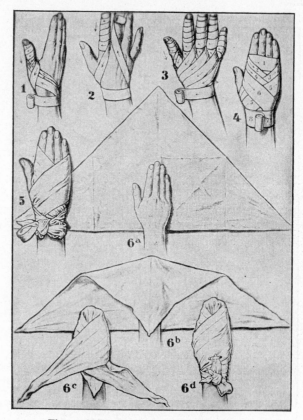

Figure 225. Hand and finger bandages.

dressings on the head, hand, foot, knee, or elbow in first-aid and emergency work and for applications that require frequent attention.

4. *Tailed bandages* consist of a body and one or many tails. The most commonly used are the *single-T,* or the *double-T* bandage, the *four-tailed, six-tailed,* and *many-tailed* bandages. They are used to retain dressings and other applications, such as poultices, on various parts of the body. They are particularly useful if the patient is confined to bed, if a dressing requires frequent attention and changing, or if it is applied to a part that must be disturbed as little as possible, as in the treatment of a wound in a fractured limb. The body of the bandage is used to cover the dressing, and the tails are used for fastening.

The *single-T bandage* or *binder* consists of a single upright strip that extends at right angles from the middle of a horizontal strip, thus forming the shape of a letter *T*. It is sometimes made of Canton flannel, but is usually made of double unbleached muslin stitched around the edges. It is used to hold dressings in position over the rectum and external genitals, and occasionally for pressure.

A single-T binder is used for female patients. The belt or horizontal strip that fastens around the waist should be wide enough for comfort. The upright strip that passes between the thighs over the external genitals must be wide enough

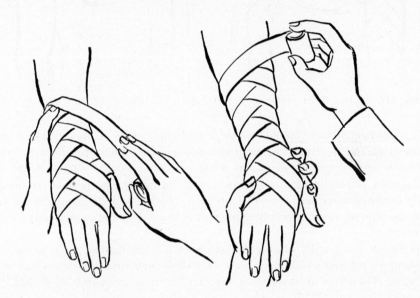

Figure 226. (*Left*) Spiral-reverse bandage of the forearm, showing effective position of the hands in reversing the bandage; (*right*) figure-of-eight bandage of the forearm, showing the oblique direction the bandage should take.

to cover the dressing and hold it securely in place in such a way that the dressing or wound will not become infected from external sources. This strip should be fastened securely to the belt with safety pins.

These binders must be changed immediately when soiled or dampened from perspiration or discharge from the wound.

Double-T binders are made of the same material and in the same way as the single binder, but they have two upright strips instead of one. They are used for the same purposes as the single-T binder and are nearly always used for male patients.

The *four-tailed bandage* is used to retain dressings or applications on the head, chin, or knee.

The *six-tailed bandage* (sometimes called the Galen or poor-man's bandage) is an excellent bandage for covering a dressing to the entire scalp.

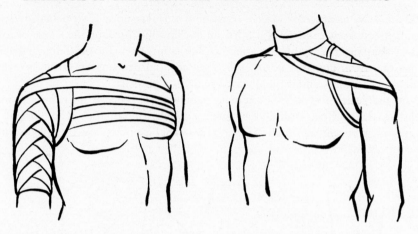

Figure 227. (*Left*) Spica of the shoulder; (*right*) bandage of the neck and shoulder.

The *scultetus,* or *many-tailed, binder* is frequently used on the abdomen to re-tain dressings and to give added support following abdominal operations. It is used particularly after extensive operations if the muscle walls are thick or flabby or if the abdomen is pendulous, and the patient is inclined to be restless. It prevents tension on the sutures and wound. If properly applied, it adds greatly to the com-fort of the patient. If not properly applied, it is loose, hot, and untidy, and a source of discomfort.

The binder is made by placing five strips of Canton flannel, three inches wide and about a yard and a half long, together so that each strip overlaps a half of the one below. The strips are then sewn together for about a quarter of a yard. This

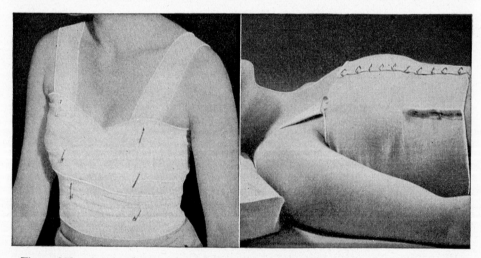

Figure 228. Ace bandage used as breast binders. (Courtesy of Johnson & Johnson, New Brunswick, N. J.)

forms the body of the bandage, the balance being the tails. In applying the bandage, the center is placed under the patient so that its lower border will come well down over the hips but not interfere with the use of a bedpan. The strips are then brought one by one from either side obliquely over the abdomen, so that they cross each other directly in the midline. Considerable traction is used in order to give firm support, the patient's comfort determining the degree of traction used. There must be no wrinkles over the hips, and strips must not end on these prominences, as the ends are likely to cause discomfort from pressure if the patient lies on his side. When a binder is applied in a surgical case, the pressure is usually made from below upward; that is, the lowest tails are applied first. Following childbirth, the tails are sometimes applied from above downward, to make pressure on the uterus. (See Fig. 229.)

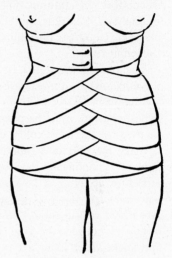

A many-tailed bandage may be used also on other parts of the body, such as the chest or extremities, if it is necessary to inspect or change dressings frequently without moving the part.

5. The _roller bandage_ is the one most commonly used. It is made by cutting or tearing any of the above-mentioned materials into long narrow strips and rolling them into a compact cylinder. The width and length of the bandage will depend upon the part of the body to which it is to be applied.

Figure 229. Scultetus, or many-tailed, bandage used as an abdominal binder. Note the oblique direction given the tails as they cross in the midline of the abdomen.

Variations in Width and Length of the Roller Bandage. The width and length will usually vary as follows:

	WIDTH (INCHES)	LENGTH (YARDS)
Finger	¾ to 1	1 to 5
Hand	1 to 2	3
Arm	2 to 2½	7 to 9
Head	2 to 2½	6
Eye	2	3
Foot	1½ to 3	3
Leg	2½ to 3	9
Body	3 to 6	9 to 10

To make a roller bandage by hand, fold one end of a bandage upon itself again and again until a small stiff roll is formed, firm enough to grasp between the thumb and finger without bending. If this roll, or core, is not tight, it will be impossible to make a well-rolled bandage. This roll is then grasped between the thumb and index finger of the left hand, and the free end is held tightly and firmly between the thumb and index finger of the right hand. The cylinder is revolved by the left hand, the right hand holding the free end firmly and acting as a guide to keep the bandage even. Some may find it easier to reverse this order, holding the roll in the right hand and the free end between the thumb and index finger of the left hand.

Principles to Observe in the Application of Bandages. Bandaging requires much practice to acquire the necessary skill and dexterity. In applying the bandage, comfort and durability should receive first attention. A bandage should never cause discomfort. In addition, the aim should be to acquire ease in applying, economy in time and materials, and a neat, finished appearance. Only clean bandages should be used. Comfort, durability, and neatness can be attained only by observing the following rules:

The patient must first be placed in a comfortable position and convenient for the nurse, who, in most cases, must stand *directly in front of the patient* in applying the bandage. Parts that are elevated while being bandaged, such as a foot, leg, pelvis, or head, must be properly supported. Sandbags, pillows, or special rests may be used for the heel, ankle, elbow, or pelvis.

Place the part in a functional position and apply the bandage. For instance, in applying a bandage to the elbow, the arm should be flexed at the elbow, not extended.

Before applying a bandage see that the part is clean and dry. Dust it lightly with powder. Two skin surfaces must never be allowed to come in contact. Absorbent cotton should be used, for example, under the breasts, between the toes or fingers, between the arms and body, and behind the ear. Joints, bony prominences, and angles, such as in the axilla, groin, bend of the elbow or of the knee, where the bandage is likely to press or cut, should always be padded. Hollows should also be padded.

In applying a bandage, the roll is always held uppermost. The outer surface of the initial extremity is placed on the part to be bandaged and is held in place by the fingers of the left hand and the body of the bandage is held by the right hand. Never unwind more bandage than is absolutely necessary (unwind gradually as required), and bandage from right to left if right-handed. Always anchor a bandage securely by making two circular turns around the part. The second turn fixes, or anchors, the first.

In bandaging an arm or a leg, begin at the extremity and work toward the trunk. This is in order to avoid congestion, swelling, and possible death of the part below. Fingers and toes are usually left exposed so that they may be observed from time to time as a guide to the condition of the circulation. If they become pale, cold, blue, tingling, or numb, the bandage is applied too tightly and must be removed.

Each turn of a bandage should be applied with even pressure or tension. The comfort of the patient and durability of the bandage depend to a large extent on the tension used. Good judgment is required in each case in order to know just how much pressure to make, and considerable practice in bandaging is necessary before good judgment can be achieved. The patient's comfort is one of the best guides. Always question the patient as to the comfort of the bandage, both during the procedure and after its completion.

Pressure should not be used over inflamed, painful tissues, and especial care should be taken in applying bandages to infants and young children. Care should be taken also in bandaging wet dressings in place, for this bandage when dry will shrink and become unbearably tight. The bandage should be tight enough to ensure permanency but not tight enough to interfere with the circulation.

In bandaging, avoid useless turns. This makes the part uncomfortably hot, wastes the bandage, and makes the pressure uneven—each turn over the same region nearly doubles the pressure. Use a second bandage if necessary to complete a bandage, but do not make extra turns just to use all the bandage. Each turn should overlap

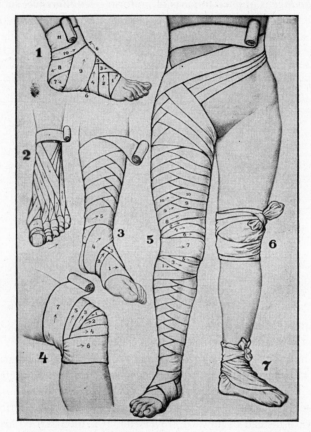

Figure 230.   Feet, toes, ankle, leg, and knee bandages.

exactly the same area of the preceding turn; the area covered is usually one half or two thirds. Reverses and crosses should always be even or in a straight line. Portions of skin (gaps between the turns) should never be left uncovered.

If the preceding rules are observed, the desired pattern and a finished appearance will follow.

Fundamental Bandages.   These are the circular, spiral, spiral-reverse, figure of eight, spica, and recurrent. These, together with combinations or modifications of these turns, are the basis for the greater number of bandages used. The form chosen will depend upon the part of the body to be bandaged and the purpose of the bandage.

The *circular bandage* consists of several circular turns of a roller bandage around a part, each turn exactly covering the preceding one. It is used to retain dressings on such parts as the neck, wrist, or forehead, and one or two circular turns are always made to anchor the initial end of a bandage; each turn holds the preceding one firmly in place.

The *spiral bandage* is applied to parts of uniform circumference, such as the upper arm, fingers, or trunk. It consists of simple oblique turns around the part, each turn ascending (or sometimes descending) higher than the preceding one and overlapping it one half or two thirds.

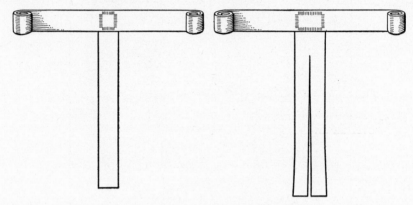

Figure 231. Single-T and double-T bandage or binders, used to hold dressings over pubic and anal regions.

The *spiral-reverse bandage* consists of the spiral bandage in which reverses are made; by means of these the bandage may be made to fit parts that are tapering or of uneven circumference, such as the forearm or leg. When it is necessary to make a reverse in order to have the bandage fit, place the thumb of the left hand on the bandage where the reverse is to be made; with the right hand holding the roll, unwind the latter about 6 in. The hand is then pronated so that the bandage is directed downward instead of upward (reversed). It is then carried around the limb with firm traction. The turns are continued, making sure that the reverses are uniform and in line and that each turn covers the same area as the preceding one; otherwise the bandage will be uncomfortable and will not fit or stay on, and the pressure will not be even. Reverses should not be made over bony prominences or joints, as they increase the pressure.

The bandage is used to retain dressings or splints in place and to apply pressure and afford support. It is used chiefly on the arms and legs.

The *figure-of-eight bandage* consists of oblique turns that alternately ascend and descend after encircling the part. Each turn crosses the preceding one in front, making a figure of eight, and overlaps it one half or two thirds. This bandage is used to retain dressings in place, to apply pressure and afford support, and is particularly useful in immobilizing joints, such as the elbow, ankle, knee, wrist, thumb, hip, neck, and axilla, or the head and neck. In affording support to a limb, it is often combined with the spiral-reverse.

The *spica bandage* derives its name from the fact that the turns are supposed to resemble the arrangement of the husks of an ear of corn. It is applied to the thumb, shoulder, groin, and foot. Each turn follows the preceding turn, covering two thirds of it and either going higher or lower, according to whether the bandage is an ascending or descending spica. The turns cross each other, forming an angle or spica.

The *recurrent bandage* is used chiefly to retain dressings on the ends of the fingers, the head, or the stump of an amputated extremity. It consists of a series of turns, the first turn usually being in the middle and the following turns passing back and forth over the part, first on one side, then on the other, each time returning (or recurring) to the starting point, until the whole area is covered. Each turn covers one half to two thirds the preceding one. The ends are bound down firmly with several circular turns.

Method of Securing a Bandage. A bandage may be secured by pinning, sewing, tying, or by adhesive strapping. It should never be pinned or tied in the following places: (1) over an injured part or inflamed surface; (2) over a bony prominence, or on the inner surface of a limb; (3) over a part that the patient may lie on; (4) over a part where there is likely to be friction or where it may cause discomfort in any way. Body bandages should be pinned in front, and head bandages over the temple.

Small safety pins are preferable to large ones. Pins should be inserted in the long axis of the bandage so that friction or straining will not remove but rather make it more secure. To tie a bandage: tear the terminal end the required distance, which depends upon the circumference of the part, twist or tie the ends to prevent further tearing, and pass them around the part in opposite directions and tie at the starting point.

Method of Removing a Roller Bandage. The bandage may be cut with bandage scissors if necessary to avoid pain or fatigue, to save time in an emergency, or when the bandage is soiled. In all cases where the bandage is to be used again, unfasten the terminal end and unwind, gathering the loose turns as unwound and passing them from hand to hand; otherwise, the bandage will become entangled about the limb. This method also saves time and prevents the bandage from getting soiled.

The Use of Woven Tubing as a Substitute for Roller Bandages. "Surgitube," shown in Figure 222, is available in widths to fit almost any body area. It is easily and quickly applied, and as surgeons, nurses, and the public learn about it, such tubing replaces the roller bandage as a means of holding a dressing in place.

"Band-Aids" for Small Dressings. Commercially sterilized dressings, backed by adhesive and ready for application, are available in many shapes and sizes. Flesh-colored adhesive is used to make these dressings inconspicuous. Because the public is so familiar with this convenient and efficient product, it is not illustrated in this text. Their use for minor wounds is highly recommended, however.

Suggested Reading

Christopher, Frederick (ed.): *Textbook of Surgery,* 5th ed. W. B. Saunders Co., Philadelphia, 1949.

Felter, Robert K., et. al.: *Surgical Nursing,* 6th ed. F. A. Davis Co., Philadelphia, 1952.

Graham, Evart A. (ed.): *Year Book of General Surgery.* Year Book Publishers, Chicago, 1952.

Levenson, S. M., et al.: "The Healing of Soft Tissue Wounds; the Effects of Nutrition, Anemia, and Age," *Surgery,* **28:**905-35, (Nov.) 1950.

Meleney, Frank L.: *Clinical Aspects and Treatment of Surgical Infections.* W. B. Saunders Co., Philadelphia, 1949.

Menkin, V.: *Newer Concepts of Inflammation.* Charles C Thomas, Publisher, Springfield, Ill., 1950.

Pratt, D.: *Antibiotics.* J. B. Lippincott Co., Philadelphia, 1950.

Walter, Carl W.: *The Aseptic Treatment of Wounds.* The Macmillan Company, New York, 1948.

West, John P.; Keller, Manelva W.; and Harmon, Elizabeth: *Nursing Care of the Surgical Patient,* 6th ed. The Macmillan Company, New York, 1957.

CHAPTER 38. PREOPERATIVE NURSING CARE

1. PROGRESS IN SURGERY

Inactive nurses often say that they would be "afraid" to nurse surgical patients because their care has changed so greatly in the last decade. This fear is justified to a large extent, and to get an overview of these changes it might be helpful to mention the developments that have made modern surgery one of the marvels of the century. Sir Cecil Wakeley,[1] discussing "The Changing Face of Surgery," thinks that scientific surgery is based on the knowledge of the human body acquired by dissection. This opportunity has been available to the surgeon for a relatively short time historically. Asepsis came several centuries later with anesthesia, another cornerstone of effective surgery. With these developments all of us are familiar. Few of us, however, can, or even try to, keep up with the enormous change in physiological concepts on which are based our present practices in maintaining electrolyte, acid-base balance or in maintaining normal nutrition through parenteral therapy and improved oral feeding. The expanded use of x-rays, radium, and radioactive elements in diagnosis and therapy necessitates the use of new preoperative and postoperative techniques with which the nurse must be familiar. The multiplicity of the sulfonamides has given way to the elaboration of antibiotic treatment of infections, and it is almost impossible for anyone outside the specialty to know the latest arrival in the antibiotic family; methods of administering them are moving toward simplification—fortunately. Those unfamiliar with hospital care during the last ten years are amazed to see that a high value is set on activity, particularly walking, and exercise in the recumbent position, for the same patients who would formerly have been kept in bed and moved with care. Rehabilitation and the phrase "early ambulation" come easily; both have had wide publicity, but the older nurse finds it difficult to believe that the patient who has had his stomach removed is expected to flex and extend his legs the night of the operation, turn himself freely and be prepared to get on his feet, and perhaps walk, the same or the next day even though he may have an intubation tube in his nose and a cannula in a vein ready for the next blood transfusion. New ways of treating wounds are developing as more is learned about the chemistry of inflammation and healing. Emphasis on the use of whole blood and plasma and of antibiotics and pressure dressings has hastened the process of repair in wounds and burns and in many places revolutionized the dressing carts of yesterday. Study of resuscitation of the shocked and wounded in military medicine has demonstrated the uselessness of some established procedures and the importance of others, particularly the value of whole blood and early surgery. The technique and tools of the surgeon have been improved generally so that the percentage of patients who survive surgery is far higher than it has been in the past. At the same time, the surgeon is attempting increasingly difficult feats with spectacular advances in cardiac and nerve surgery.

Nurses must work hard to keep up with surgical progress; on the other hand, they can undertake the care of the patient with a hope of his recovery not possible a few decades ago.

2. SOCIAL AND PSYCHOLOGICAL ASPECTS OF PREOPERATIVE CARE

Reception.   Every patient should be received with kindness and courtesy. The importance of first impressions was discussed in Chapter 6. Persons admitted for surgery, especially for major operations, are in need of particular consideration since they are nearly always fearful. People rarely express their anxiety in words, but it is safe to assume that they feel apprehensive.

Anxiety Associated with Surgery.   In some clinical divisions it is customary for a representative from the religious and social services to visit every patient scheduled for major surgery. It is assumed that an operation will raise problems that have to do with cost, the care of dependents, return to previous occupation, provision for convalescence, and aftercare or possible disability and death. Very often the immediate family or intimate friends share the anxiety, and if the medical team can give them help, reassurance, or confidence, they will make the patient feel more hopeful. The nurse helps to establish this confidence by the effectiveness of her service and by a sympathy that is manifested in thoughtful acts rather than in words.* Morton A. Seidenfeld,[2] however, in discussing the psychological aspects of illness, stresses "therapeutic answers" to patients' questions; he thinks that what the nurse says, as well as what she does, is important. He believes that such simple

* Kahlil Gibran says in *The Prophet,* "Work is love made visible." He might have said the same of sympathy. (Alfred A. Knopf, Inc., New York, 1923.)

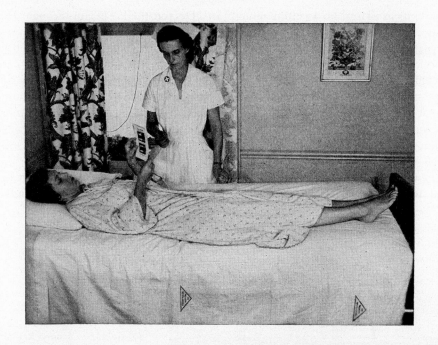

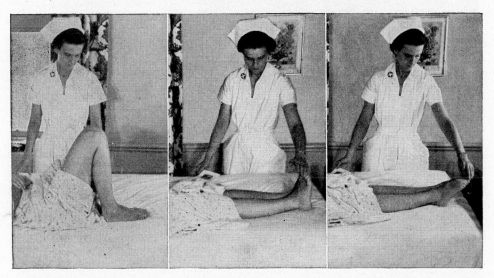

Figure 232. (*Top*) A patient looking at illustrations of the exercises she will be asked to do postoperatively. (*Bottom*) The nurse supervises: the first exercise—flexion of the knees; the second exercise—flexion of the ankles and toes; and the third exercise—extension of the ankles and toes. (Courtesy of Columbia-Presbyterian Medical Center, New York City, and Clay-Adams Co., New York City.)

questions as "How am I getting along?" or "Do you think I'll pull through, Doc?" may represent "a wealth of emotional disturbance" and that fear will not be dissipated by a guarded or superficial reply. He thinks people want specific information, even statistics sometimes on their "chances." Nurses, who are with the patient so much more than the surgeon, are in a particularly favorable position to recognize signs of fear and their sources. Ordinarily, the nurse doesn't answer questions about diagnosis or prognosis, but she can bring these questions to the attention of the surgeon in written or oral reports, and there are many queries she can answer fully and helpfully. Listening and showing interest in what the patient says is itself therapeutic.

Few surgeons have, or take, the time for detailed explanations of preoperative and postoperative procedure. Within surgical departments committees composed

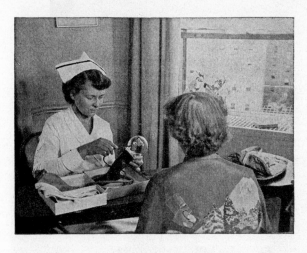

Figure 233. A nurse explaining a colostomy irrigation to a patient who knows she is to have a colostomy and who has asked questions indicating her interest. (Courtesy of Columbia-Presbyterian Medical Center, New York City, and Clay-Adams Co., New York City.)

of surgeons, anesthetists, nurses, social workers, physical therapists, nutritionists, and chaplains should develop a preoperative teaching program that would eliminate unnecessary fear of surgery and prepare the patient to participate more effectively in the postoperative program. In some hospitals leaflets offering explanations and directions are used as teaching aids. Patients with recent surgical experience can often contribute helpful suggestions. For example, the writer heard a man who had seemed calm the day after operation tell the participants in a nursing clinic much later that he had on that day thought he was dying because he had found himself in a room rather than in his accustomed place on the clinical division when he awaked to consciousness after the operation. He said that had someone thought to tell him before the operation that he would be put there to be near the night nurse, he would have been spared this mental anguish.

It should be explained to patients and their families that blood transfusions, intubations, or other procedures that may be fearsome to them, are used routinely in operations such as theirs; that such treatments do not indicate that the patient has "gone bad." If procedures such as using the bedpan or doing postoperative exercises are explained and practiced preoperatively, there is far less resistance postoperatively; if a patient is shown side rails and told that they will probably be put on his bed the first night, he may not be frightened by looking through bars in one of his first conscious moments. Likewise, if the patient is to be put in a recovery room, its nature and advantages should be explained because he may be badly frightened by the sight of other patients; indeed, if he is awake in the recovery room, there may be no way to keep him from being frightened by what he sees.

Anesthetists often comment on the difficulty of anesthetizing the frightened patient. They think that many patients dread the anesthetic more than the operation. In one or more visits to the patients they try to establish rapport with him while, at the same time, they assess his condition as a basis for deciding what anesthesia to give, and what risks are entailed. In such visits the anesthetists can enhance the help given by the surgeon and the nurse; or he can simply duplicate it. Preoperative care that reduces anxiety to a minimum necessitates joint planning and a nice coordination of the work of many persons.

Continuity of Nursing Care in Surgery. Continuity of care by the same personnel will go a long way toward eliminating the anxiety, strangeness, and loneliness of hospital experience. When the patient uses the expression "my doctor" or "my nurse" and shows trust in them, it is a sure sign that his load is lightened. As one surgeon puts it, confidence is the "sheet anchor" for the patient, and once this is established he "ceases to worry."[3] He cannot, however, establish this relationship of trust with "a battalion of workers," as Seidenfeld says. It is very desirable, therefore, to have the same nurses assigned to the patient for the preoperative and postoperative periods, and highly desirable to have one of them go with the patient to the operating room. (Postoperative care is simplified for the nurse if she can watch the operation, but there is seldom enough personnel to make this possible except in private nursing practice.) In medical practice this principle of continuity of medical care is so thoroughly established that it needs no comment here.

Attention paid the family and explanation of rules and routines that may seem unpleasant or unreasonable react favorably on the patient who may be as unhappy on their account as on his own. From the beginning, an effort should be made to prevent misunderstanding about the visiting hours or the number of visitors likely to benefit the patient. The family also should feel that their convenience is taken into account. Time may be as precious to them as to hospital personnel. When a long treatment is to be done or a lengthy examination made, it is thoughtful to tell visitors who are waiting; this enables them to go out for a meal or make some other use of their time, and it relieves impatience. The smaller the nursing circle, the easier it is for them to form friendly and helpful relationships with the family. Relatives are always happier when they are assured that at least a few of the patients' attendants know him and are interested in him as a person.

Occupation and Companionship in the Preoperative Period. The preoperative period is often made unnecessarily difficult by unreasonable routine practices that may have a depressing effect. For example, while the patient may feel entirely well and natural, his clothes are taken away and he is put to bed, feeling perhaps like a punished child, at best like the little boy in Stevenson's verse who sadly "had to go to bed by day." In many cases it would be far better to encourage the patient to be up and about and to keep himself occupied. His clothing can be such that it is easily removed or adjusted for necessary tests, examinations, and treatments, but at least he will not be lying in bed all day looking at a blank ceiling and "stewing in his own juice." Very often, preoperative treatment is designed more for the convenience of the staff than for the patient's benefit. Reading, playing games, or making something interesting might convert this period of waiting into a less boring or fearful experience. For some persons companionable occupation is definitely desirable; others will prefer solitude. Patients who are going to have a dreaded operation such as a colostomy or an amputation may be comforted by talking to a convalescent patient who has made a good adjustment to a similar problem. This sort of help from one patient to another is not always easy to plan and must be arranged with care and delicacy. Nurses, who are chiefly young, healthy men and women, need considerable imagination in working with the individual who is about to have mutilating surgery. Virginia Dericks and others have wisely remarked that the person must be permitted a period of grief. It is a mistake to try to jog them out of it with a superficial cheerfulness.

A brief discussion, such as this, of the psychological or emotional preoperative problems is obliged to be superficial and almost misleading. Nurses are face to face with the fear of death, disfigurement, disability, separation from family and friends, the dread of unconsciousness, of pain, of temporary loss of freedom, and all the unknown and, to many, frightening experiences of hospitalization. A mature and dominating executive may suddenly realize that temporarily at least he will be helpless and his very life will depend on the judgment of nurses and doctors who may look to him both young and inexperienced. Even the best medical team, with the greatest good will cannot dispel all preoperative anxiety; they can, however, minimize it and in so doing set the stage for an easier anesthesia, a better operation, and a more rapid recovery.

3. SURGICAL "PERMISSIONS"

A physician can be sued for malpractice if the patient can prove that he has been operated on against his knowledge or desire. If the patient is a minor, his parents or guardian will make the charges. No reputable doctor or hospital board wants such things to happen; therefore, it is routine in most institutions to have the patient or his guardian sign an operative permit. (See Fig. 234.) Emanuel Hayt points out that this does not necessarily protect the surgeon from charges of malpractice, but he thinks that in case the operation leads to litigation, there is less room for controversy. The following excerpts are taken from a recent article by this authority on medical jurisprudence.

From a legal standpoint, *consent* is defined as a unity of opinion in which there is an accord of the minds of two or more persons. . . .

The main purpose of consent is to protect the physician against claims of unauthorized operations and to protect the patient against unsanctioned surgery. Written acquiescence is safest, because there is less room for controversy about the contemplated treatment or for denial that permission was granted. Authorization may be the best legal defense.

It is difficult for consent to be disproved when it is in writing with a witness to the signature. . . .

Consent does not imply that the surgeon may perform unnecessary surgery. No matter how broad or general the authorization may be, the burden is upon the physician to be reasonably certain the operation was pathologically indicated.

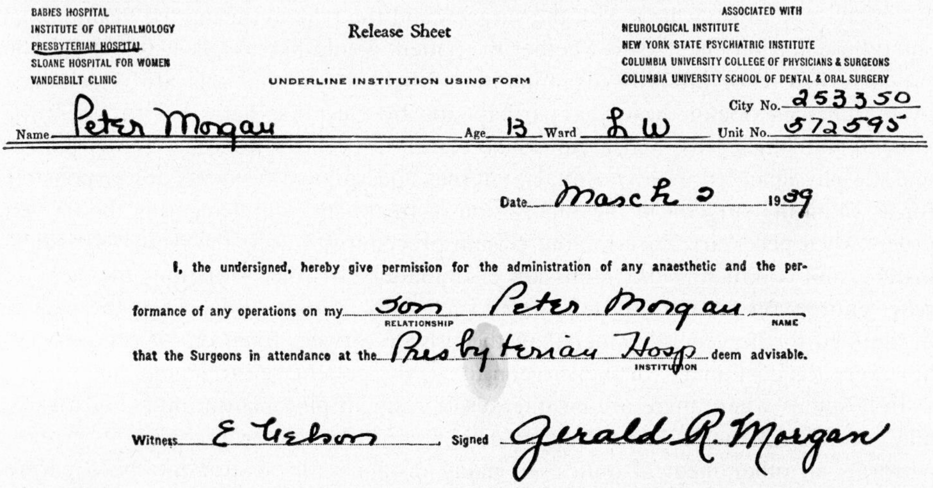

BABIES HOSPITAL
INSTITUTE OF OPHTHALMOLOGY
PRESBYTERIAN HOSPITAL
SLOANE HOSPITAL FOR WOMEN
VANDERBILT CLINIC

Release Sheet

UNDERLINE INSTITUTION USING FORM

ASSOCIATED WITH
NEUROLOGICAL INSTITUTE
NEW YORK STATE PSYCHIATRIC INSTITUTE
COLUMBIA UNIVERSITY COLLEGE OF PHYSICIANS & SURGEONS
COLUMBIA UNIVERSITY SCHOOL OF DENTAL & ORAL SURGERY

Name _Peter Morgan_   Age _13_ Ward _L W_   City No. _253350_
Unit No. _572595_

Date _March 2_ 19_39_

I, the undersigned, hereby give permission for the administration of any anaesthetic and the performance of any operations on my _Son   Peter Morgan_
RELATIONSHIP   NAME
that the Surgeons in attendance at the _Presbyterian Hosp_ deem advisable.
INSTITUTION

Witness _E Gibson_   . Signed _Gerald R. Morgan_

Figure 234. "Release slip" or form that the patient, or his guardian, is asked to sign before an anesthetic is given, or an operation is performed. (Courtesy of Columbia-Presbyterian Medical Center, New York City.)

There are situations, of course, in which it is either impractical or unnecessary to obtain consent. An emergency to save life or prevent irreparable injury serves in lieu of authorization, either express or implied.

Generally speaking, unless an immediate operation is urgently and reasonably necessary a surgeon has no right to perform such [an] operation without the patient's consent, express or implied. . . .*

4. PREOPERATIVE EXAMINATION

The Medical Examination and Its Purpose.   The surgeon sees the patient as soon as possible after his admission to the hospital, in order to encourage and reassure him, but also to assess his condition. No matter how thorough the diagnostic

* Hayt, Emanuel: "A Signed Permit for Surgery Is Safest," *Hospitals,* Journal of the American Hospital Association, **24**:56. (June) 1950.

examination, this does not take the place of the immediate preoperative evaluation. George Crile, Jr., and Franklin L. Shively, Jr.,[4] cite a number of instances in which patients' lives have been saved by this practice or lost by its omission. Some of the conditions that affect the risk of surgery are pulmonary and cardiac disease; metabolic and endocrine disorders such as diabetes, Addison's disease, or hyperthyroidism; mouth infections; blood disorders such as anemia and hemophilia; dehydration; and malnutrition with especial reference perhaps to vitamin C and protein deficiency. In some cases the findings of a thorough examination immediately before the scheduled operation may indicate that the operation should be postponed until the surgical risk can be reduced by treatment; they may also indicate that surgery would be fatal, in which case the operation is postponed indefinitely. The nurse who is with the surgeon and the patient during the examination should use her judgment as to whether the patient would like to talk with his surgeon privately before or after the examinations. Medical examinations are often made by the unaided doctor; however, participation by the nurse helps her to assess the patient's nursing needs, and it can make certain aspects of it easier for the patient and the physician. In many hospitals, internes and surgical residents are responsible for assisting the surgeon in the supervision of treatment: supplementing the written orders when necessary, carrying out certain procedures, taking the patient's medical history, and conducting the admission examination. In some situations the surgeon relies entirely on the interne staff for all such work. This is usual when the patient is admitted to the general rather than the private service. Even on "ward" service, however, it is customary for the surgeon to see the patient before he operates.

In hospitals where there are no internes or resident physicians, a nurse or a clerk may record the general data for the medical record; the doctor in charge of the case performs all other medical duties. In many instances the doctor has been caring for the patient before admission and has the history of the case on file except for the immediate preoperative data.

As soon as the patient is admitted, the interne on the service is notified. The necessary assistance is given in getting the patient ready for the physical examination. (See Chapter 18.) The interne takes a complete history and makes a thorough examination of the patient. The history and laboratory reports are completed as soon as possible, so that they may be ready for the surgeon to review. In surgical emergencies all of this must be done with the greatest dispatch. If the patient is hemorrhaging internally or if there is severe intercranial pressure, it may be necessary to omit most of the preoperative routine. The usual *blood tests* include: complete cell counts, hemoglobin estimate, tests for syphilis, coagulation time, and blood grouping.*[5] If there is a likelihood that blood transfusion will be needed, the patient's blood should be crossmatched with available blood. (See Chapter 26.) Crile and Shively say that if there is any evidence of nephritis, and particularly with elderly patients, the level of blood urea should be checked. If there is any evidence of malnutrition, an estimate should be made of the serum protein. Blood sugar estimates are made routinely by many surgeons and always when diabetes is sus-

---

* Robert L. Mason and Harold A. Zintel say that a positive test for syphilis is probably not a threat to the operative team if no primary or secondary lesions exist.

pected or known to exist. Lucian Szmyd,[6] reviewing "Modern Concepts of the Dynamics of Inflammation," says that healing is influenced by the pH of the tissues and suggests that the lowering of the pH below optimum levels, typical of uncontrolled diabetes, may be the explanation of retarded healing in such cases. R. J. Minnitt, writing particularly for fellow anesthetists, has the following recommendation:

Operations on diabetics do not now entail the risk of former years. Pre-operative administration of glucose and insulin after the patient has been standardized has made possible even the giving of ether as the anesthetic agent. When an urgent operation is necessary and diabetes has only been discovered before-hand, and when ketonuria is excessive, an intravenous infusion of 10% glucose in saline at the rate of one pint per hour, accompanied by 50 units of insulin, would be the kind of treatment to administer during anesthesia.*

A more complete study of the blood is prescribed for some patients who show signs of cardiac, kidney, or liver damage, marked dehydration, or malnutrition.

Urinalysis is so routinely done preoperatively that the nurse should always save an admission specimen. Chest x-rays are made routinely for all admissions in some hospitals; they have a particular value in detecting conditions that would contraindicate inhalation anesthesia. Operations for the removal of suspected tumors, for fractures, and for many other conditions are always preceded by x-rays except in direst emergencies.

Few surgeons operate until a thorough study has been made of the patient although this may not immediately precede surgery.

Blood Pressure and Other Vital Signs. As part of the medical examination the physician will measure the temperature, the pulse and respiratory rates, and the blood pressure; or he may ask that these measurements be made by the nurse. Since she will be making some of these estimates at frequent intervals postoperatively, it is desirable for her to know their preoperative characteristics as a basis for comparison. J. M. Finney, Jr.,[7] in Frederick Christopher's text, says that the surgeon is not "playing fair with the patient or himself" if he doesn't make every effort to reduce operative hazards to a minimum *before the operation.* This may entail a much more extensive list of diagnostic tests and longer preoperative treatment than is suggested in this chapter.

5. ANESTHESIA

Much of the progress in modern surgery has been possible because of the advances in anesthesia. Not only have new agents been found, but the number of physicians with special training in anesthesia is increasing. Their cooperation with surgeons and the discovery of new drugs have made many operations possible that were impossible before and have improved pre- and postoperative care. Except in

* In another part of this article Minnitt suggests that *any* patient who has had glucose preoperatively be given 5 units of insulin to prevent postanestheic nausea and other toxic signs. He says, "This treatment has not gained the notoriety it deserves." Minnitt, R. J.: "Some Aspects of Modern Anesthesia," *M. Press,* 225:159, (Feb.) 1951.

cases of emergency, administration of an anesthetic lies outside the nurse's province; however, it seems desirable for her to have a practical knowledge of anesthetic agents and their relative merits. In most states there are laws prohibiting the administration of an anesthetic by anyone other than a trained person, except in extreme emergencies. There have been and still are many nurse anesthetists who have special preparation, but it is becoming more common for physician anesthetists to take charge of this work. The physician anesthetist can be of great assistance to the surgeon by assuming part of the responsibility for the patient's condition during the operation and also by ordering the immediate postoperative care. Henry K. Beecher,[8] Minnitt,[9] and John B. Dillon[10] stress the importance of the anesthetist's preoperative evaluation as a basis for selecting the anesthetic and minimizing its risks. This theme is emphasized in everything one sees in current books and articles. While the anesthetist studies the patient's record and uses the opinions and findings of other medical personnel, he makes certain tests and measurements himself and assesses the person's emotional make-up and attitude toward the operation and the anesthetic. When he is prepared to assume the major share of responsibility for the patient's general condition during the operation, the surgeon is able to give his complete attention to the intricacies of the operation itself.

Patients who can recall taking an anesthetic twenty-five years ago, on taking one today, are amazed at the ease with which they "go under." They often have no recollection of the anesthetic. Premedication makes them drowsy, and in this state they are taken in their bed to the operating suite, where an anesthetist induces anesthesia with an intravenous injection which they scarcely feel. In their next conscious moment, very often, they realize that the operation is over and that many hours have elapsed. In some cases the anesthetist brings the drugs used for induction of anesthesia to the patient's room, and in this case the patient cannot even remember going to the operating room. Minnitt believes that subjectively this represents the greatest advance in anesthesia.

Giving different drugs by different routes has greatly reduced the risks of anesthesia. One drug may be a respiratory depressant, another may be toxic to the kidneys. Obviously, when they are combined, less is needed of each one and the danger of each reduced. Patients often notice that the effects of anesthesia are briefer and milder.

Inhalation Anesthesia. Ethyl ether used by William Morton in 1846 was the first successful anesthetic. John A. Paulson and John S. Lundy[11] in 1950 and Beecher[12] in 1952 say that it is still the safest agent for most patients in the hands of most anesthetists. Ether may be inhaled from a cone or mask on which the liquid is dripped or from a vaporizing machine. Often its vapor, mixed with air or oxygen, is insufflated from a tube passed into the pharynx or trachea although these mixtures may also be breathed in through masks over the nose.*

* Intratracheal anesthesia is desirable when the surgeon must work around the patient's head and neck, making it almost impossible for an anesthetist to hold a mask in place. Nurses often notice that following brain surgery tracheotomies are necessary. One reason is that the pharynx and trachea have been irritated by the tube as well as by the anesthetic, and the resulting swelling and accumulation of mucus block the airway.

Vinyl ether, ethylene, and *cyclopropane* are substitutes for ethyl ether. Vinyl ether is highly recommended by Ralph J. Knight in Christopher's text for short surgical procedures where a quick pleasant induction and a rapid recovery are needed. He thinks except for its inflammability it has taken away all need for *chloroform.* Knight says that vinyl ether has the same advantages but is not so likely to injure the kidneys. *Nitrous oxide* gas produces an anesthesia quickly and easily and has been called "laughing gas." Like *ethyl chloride* and *ethylene* it is used for short surgical procedures where complete relaxation is unnecessary. Cyclopropane has had ardent advocates and is still used but it has serious disadvantages. The period of induction is shorter and pleasanter than that of ether, and there is no suffocation or falling sensation. It is not a circulatory depressant and the respirations are not labored, making it especially desirable for upper abdominal and chest surgery. Recovery from cyclopropane anesthesia is rapid and usually uncomplicated. It has a major disadvantage in that, since so much oxygen is given, the patient's color remains good regardless of his condition. Other common symptoms, such as changes-in-the-eye reactions, are obscured, and for these reasons only a highly experienced person should administer cyclopropane. Cyclobutane, cyclopentane, and cyclohexane are comparable anesthetics whose value can be assessed only after a longer period of use.[13]

Rectal or Colonic Anesthesia. Tribromoethanol (Avertin) is the most popular and probably the most successful of the rectal anesthetics. It is often administered in conjunction with some form of inhalation. Ether was used when rectal anesthesia was introduced, but it is irritating and the determination of dosage difficult. Rectal anesthesia is most often used to produce unconsciousness in an apprehensive child or in an excitable adult, as, for example, the hyperthyroid. Since most patients are accustomed to rectal injections, the anesthesia can be induced in this way without their realization. There is a difference of opinion as to whether deceiving the child or "stealing the goiter," as it is called, is desirable. Minnitt and Knight say that dosage should be based on weight and colonic requirement. In rare cases the nurse injects rectal anesthesia, but only those with special preparation should anesthetize the patient by any method. She may often, however, prepare the patient by preliminary enemas or colon irrigation. These should be given a few hours before the anesthetic; otherwise the colon, stimulated to contract by these treatments, will not retain the anesthetic mixture.

Spinal Anesthesia. *Procaine, dibucaine (Nupercaine), pipercocaine (Metycaine), tetracaine (Pontocaine),* and 10 per cent solution of procaine *(Spinocain)* are anesthetics injected into the spinal canal. The equipment and process used are similar to that described under lumbar puncture followed by a medication (p. 810). The duration of spinal anesthesia is difficult to control. Vasopressin (Pitressin), epinephrine, and other vasoconstrictors may be given with the anesthetic to prolong the effect, or spinal anesthesia may be supplemented by intravenous anesthetics or analgesics.[14, 15]

Intravenous Anesthesia. *Hexobarbital (Evipal), thiopental (Pentothal), amobarbital (Amytal* and *Thioethamyl), thiamylal (Surital),* and *pentobarbital (Nem-*

butal) are some of the drugs given intravenously to produce a shorter or longer period of unconsciousness. While Paulson and Lundy classify them as "analgesic and sedative drugs," Knight says that thiopental has proved so useful that it is given either alone or in combination with other anesthetics and methods in 30 to 35 per cent of all cases.

Muscle Relaxants. A recent development in anesthesia is the simultaneous administration of drugs such as *curare, mephensin (Myanesin), decamethonium iodide,* or *gallamine (Flaxedil)* to relax muscles. When relaxation required by the surgeon can be accomplished with such drugs, the amount of anesthetic required is reduced. The drugs are very toxic, and their administration must be carefully controlled.[16]

Hazards of Explosion. Catastrophes in recent years in some of the most reputable medical centers have made everyone more aware of the danger of explosion from anesthetics. Knight says: "Explosion may occur when a mixture of ether, ethylene, or cyclopropane with nitrous oxide or oxygen is exposed to a flame or spark within the respiratory tract, breathing tubes or bags, or tanks, or within about 2 feet of any point of escape therefrom."*

Control methods include: (1) avoiding static spark by having a relative humidity above 55 per cent; (2) keeping electric and hot instruments away from the explosive mixtures; (3) combining explosive gases with helium and nitrogen in such ratio as to make them nonexplosive; (4) using "closed systems" or apparatus from which the gas cannot escape; and (5) grounding with metal, or metal and water, all persons and objects in the room. Operating room personnel are required to wear special shoes or to pull nonconductive covers over regular shoes. They are also required to wear cotton, rather than rayon or nylon, clothing because the latter conduct static electricity. Nurses who go with patients to and from the operating room must also regard this regulation.

Beecher, in his text on resuscitation and anesthesia of wounded men, says that ether should be stored in the refrigerator, or when this is not possible kept in a wet cloth bag.

Nerve Block and Regional Anesthesia. Almost every body area can be made insensitive by injecting the sensory nerve supplying the area with an anesthetic or by injecting the drug locally. Small areas can be desensitized by application of certain substances. Moist mucous membrane will absorb a sufficient quantity of an anesthetic to make a procedure bearable that would be otherwise very painful. Crile and Shively say that nerve block or regional anesthesia is often the most satisfactory kind from the standpoint of the surgeon and patient. They think it particularly suitable for the older cooperative patient; unsuitable for the child and the nervous adult. Edward M. Livingston and Constantine Oden summarize its advantages as follows in Christopher's surgical text:

. . . . 1. The conscious cooperation of the patient is retained, alertness being but slightly dulled through judicious use of premedication given to alleviate apprehension.

* Christopher, Frederick (ed.): *Textbook of Surgery.* 5th ed. W. B. Saunders Co., Philadelphia. 1949. p. 1507.

It is highly advantageous that the patient be able to move a limb, to breathe deeply, or to cough at the direction of the surgeon. 2. The surgeon, if he so desires, can work without the aid of a special anesthetist, a consideration of moment in certain emergencies, either military or civil. 3. The airways remain patent, and sensitive respiratory mucous membranes sustain no pathologic injury. 4. Medullary centers are protected. 5. Damage to liver, kidney, and other vital organs is minimal. 6. The injurious inflow of noxious sensory stimuli from the periphery or operative site is cut off. This is not the case under inhalation or intravenous anesthesia, where the patient is rendered incapable of response while such a bombardment continues. 7. The patient often is able to walk from the surgical amphitheater and to help himself, to take nourishment promptly, to co-operate in the frequent postural changes important in the prevention of thrombosis and embolism; all in all, operations are shorn of much of the character of dreaded ordeals.*

The benefit of blocking off painful stimuli is believed so desirable that some surgeons use a local anesthetic even when the patient is completely unconscious from the effect of ether. Nerve block and regional anesthesia are used in conjunction with minimal doses of anesthetics by other routes.

Nerve block is used diagnostically to determine the cause of pain; it may also be used to see (prognostically) what would happen if the injected nerve were severed surgically. Nerve block is used to control intractable pain. Samuel Monash[17] says that local anesthesia can be maintained for weeks by the subcutaneous injection of procaine in water or ethyl alcohol 50 per cent or procaine penicillin. Adding the antibiotic to a local antiseptic reduces the risk of infection; adding a vasoconstrictor, such as epinephrine, tends to prevent dispersion of the drug or to localize its effects. Some local anesthetics are, however, themselves vasoconstrictors.[18]

Cocaine was first used in 1884, but because it is so toxic and habit forming, *procaine* (*Novocaine*) soon displaced it. Local anesthetics have developed so rapidly in recent years that it is impractical to try to list all of them here. *Tetracaine* (*Pontocaine*), *butamben* (*Butesin*), *novocol, dibucaine* (*Nupercaine*), *phenacaine* (*Holocaine*), and *diperodon* are a few substitutes for cocaine and procaine (*Novocaine*).

Ethyl alcohol is used for nerve block. *Ethyl chloride* sprayed on the skin reduces its temperature with a resulting anesthesia of short duration. It is seldom used except in preparation for manipulation of a painful area. Solid carbon dioxide acts in the same way. Phenol is an ingredient in some lotions to control itching, but it is a protoplasmic poison and must be used with caution. It is not prescribed in preparations for surgery.[19]

Local anesthetics may be applied with a dropper, an atomizer, on cotton applicators, or injected with a needle and syringe. These drugs are toxic, and idiosyncrasies to them are not uncommon. The writer has seen a patient die from this almost before the surgical team realized what was happening. A fragment of the therapeutic dose should be given first to test the individual's response to the drug. From 5 to 10

* Christopher, Frederick (ed.): *Textbook of Surgery,* 4th ed. W. B. Saunders, Philadelphia, 1945. p. 1446.

minutes should elapse between the injection of the local anesthetic and surgery to allow time for the drug to act.[20]

Because the nurse often assists the surgeon in the use of a local anesthetic, and may prepare it, she should realize its dangers and have some knowledge of dosage. Most of the drugs mentioned are used in concentrations of from 0.5 to 2.0 per cent, but she must use every means of checking the desired strength and dosage in each case.

Refrigeration Anesthesia. It has long been known that lowering the temperatures of tissues makes them insensitive. It is "an anesthesia of protoplasm instead of a mere anesthesia."* In recent years some surgeons have advocated ice anesthesia. When, for any reason, general anesthesia is contraindicated and local anesthetic or nerve block impracticable, they refrigerate the tissue and operate with no other means of controlling pain except an analgesic, such as morphine. This method has been advocated for amputation when there is threatened gangrene, especially when the subject is an elderly person who will tolerate anesthetics poorly.

Ludwig H. Segerberg[21] in 1943 reported a lowered mortality with this refrigeration anesthesia in arteriosierotic and diabetic gangrene. Bertram Cook[22] in 1950 wrote that he uses it in severe accidents with a view to "stalling" until he can get the patient ready for radical surgical treatment. Ice anesthesia procedure is seen so rarely that one must conclude that it is either not generally accepted as the best method or that it is thought impractical. Cynthia Van Blarcom, discussing the nursing care, says," . . . the postoperative course of these patients is astounding . . . postoperative nursing care is simplified one-hundred fold."† Segerberg reports that such operations do not produce shock because the loss of blood is minimal and the limb has been gradually separated, metabolically, from the body. Little pain is suffered after the operation; the patient may eat a meal immediately on return to the clinical unit. Wounds are said to heal normally in spite of tissue refrigeration.

The *technique* of ice anesthesia as described is briefly this: After the usual systemic preparation of the patient, including an analgesic, and the local skin cleaning and shaving, elevate the head of the bed and protect the mattress with a full-length waterproof sheet. Van Blarcom suggests a cotton blanket over this sheet and under the patient. Put a layer of chipped ice 2 in. deep in the bottom of a galvanized tank or rubber trough, large enough to hold the arm or leg, first having removed the sharp edges from the chipped ice by passing it through water. Gently lift the limb onto the ice. Surround the limb up to the groin or armpit with ice. Use a sponge-rubber cuff at the proximal end of the limb. (The amount of ice required for anesthetizing the leg is about 150 lb.) Elevate the head of the bed so that the water from the ice, as it melts, will drain away from the body. (Use of a zippered boot or an electrical refrigeration unit reduces the expendi-

* Allen, F. M.: "Reduced Temperature in Surgery; Surgery of Limbs," *Am. J. Surg.,* **52**:225, (May) 1941.

† Van Blarcom, Cynthia: "Nursing Care in Ice Anesthesia," *Am. J. Nursing,* **43**:799, (Sept.) 1943.

ture of time and energy and results in more complete anesthesia of the upper third of the thigh, when this is important.[23]) If the leg is under treatment, protect the genitalia and the unaffected leg with bath towels and hot-water bottles. About 2 hours before the operation, the surgeon applies a tourniquet, protecting the skin under it with a folded towel. Ice bags may be applied over the area exposed in this process. Transport the patient to the operating room in his bed about 4½ hours after the application of the ice.

On the return from the operating room icecaps are placed around the stump for 24 to 48 hours so that return to normal tissue temperatures is gradual. Frequently, a rubber tourniquet and a Kelly clamp are kept at the bedside for several days postoperatively, because of the danger of hemorrhage.

The pain caused by refrigeration is said to be surprisingly little, lasting only about 20 minutes after the beginning of the treatment.

6. PHYSICAL PREPARATION OF THE PREOPERATIVE PATIENT

Preoperative Orders. The surgeon's and anesthetist's orders usually relate to feeding, or its omission; evacuation of the contents of the stomach, bowel, and/or bladder; the administration of parenteral fluids; and the use of hypnotics or analgesics. Laboratory tests and the preparation of the operative site are usually included. In many hospitals there is a routine procedure for preparation of patients undergoing certain operations, and if no deviation from this program is indicated in the surgeon's orders, the staff is expected to follow it. Some practices in preoperative care are so universal that every nurse is supposed to know them, and no surgeon includes them in his written orders. Grave emergencies may reduce the immediate preoperative care to almost nothing. In the following discussion it is assumed that time is available for optimum preparation. According to the patient, the anesthetic, and the operation, this may be a period of hours, days, or weeks.

Oral Intake. Except for emergency surgery the emphasis has shifted from restricting the preoperative diet to building the patient up with a diet low in fat but high in carbohydrate, protein, vitamin, and in calories. Morris J. Nicholson,[24] discussing the patient who goes into shock in the operating room, says that a consistent effort should be made to bring the protein content of the blood to normal before surgery. He speaks of the anemic patient with low blood protein as being in a state of "chronic shock." D. P. Cutherbertson,[25] who has made a study of diet in relation to trauma, believes that there is a characteristic "catabolic" response to injury that accounts largely for the unavoidable nitrogen loss following surgery. Sidney C. Werner[26] and his associates, studying postoperative nitrogen loss, believe that if surgery is not complicated by infection, the utilization of foods is the same following surgery as at any other time. They indicate that if surgical patients are not depleted before surgery, and if their protein intake is kept constant, there is no significant increase in nitrogen output as a result of the operative process. Nutritional needs of the patient are based on such studies as those described in

Chapter 13. At no time is a careful estimate of more importance than preceding surgery.

To keep the intake of nutrients constant up to and immediately after surgery, parenteral therapy is necessary because the stomach should be empty when the patient is taken to the operating room. This is particularly true when inhalant anesthetics are used because they stimulate coughing, choking, and vomiting with the accompanying danger of aspirating the stomach contents.

Some surgeons allow patients who are having general anesthesia to take foods and fluid by mouth up to six hours before operation. Anesthetists are, by and large, inclined to be more cautious. Beecher makes the following comment and recommendation.

. . . . The commonest preventable fatal accident to occur in any operating room is probably the aspiration of vomitus under anesthesia. It ought not to happen. It would not happen if stomachs were properly emptied. In most cases this can be accomplished only by carefully withholding all food or fluids for 12 to 18 hours preoperatively. In emergency cases it can be accomplished only by taking active steps to empty the stomach by inducing vomiting. Aspiration through the largest tube which can be inserted into the stomach should not be neglected, but the size of chunks of food individuals ordinarily swallow can often not be aspirated through the largest tubes employed for the purpose.*

If all food and fluid is withheld for 18 hours prior to operation, the patient will be dehydrated unless water and nutrients are given parenterally. Surgeons differ considerably in their methods of supplying food and fluid preoperatively. It is the nurse's responsibility to see that the doctor's wishes are carried out. She should, however, understand the physiology of water and electrolyte balance and be prepared to discuss the patient's needs with the doctor if she thinks they are not being met.

Parenteral Therapy. Electrolyte and water balance with maintenance of adequate nutrition by parenteral injection has been discussed in Chapters 13 and 26. Nurses might be reminded, however, that anything inhibiting the normal body urges or the patient's ability to satisfy them upsets this balance. With food and drink prohibited and with a period of anxiety, inactivity, and, usually, unconsciousness forced on the patient, he will inevitably suffer from imbalance unless the medical staff prevents it. Articles or texts by Ralph E. Homann,[27] Ariel M. Irving and Arnold J. Kreman,[28] Henry T. Randall et al.,[29] John H. Bland,[30] Beecher,[31] and many others discuss in detail parenteral methods of supplying nutritional needs. Water and electrolytes are nearly always given; protein hydrolysates and glucose are often added. The value of whole blood, and in fact the demand for it preoperatively when the oxygen-carrying elements of the blood are low, is stressed throughout the literature. Nicholson urges that insulin accompany any glucose given preoperatively. He believes this controls postoperative nausea. A total of 2000 to 4000

* Personal communication. Henry K. Beecher, Department of Anesthesia, Massachusetts General Hospital, Boston, March, 1953.

cc or more (2 to 4 qt) of parenteral fluids in the 24 hours preceding operation is said to be needed by many (adult) patients.

Bland, discussing parenteral fluids for surgical patients, emphasizes that in preoperative care nutritional deficits must be met and shock prevented with fluids and electrolytes. He says:

Fluid and electrolytes by mouth is the most physiologic of all methods and should be used as much preoperatively as is practicable and as soon postoperatively as possible. There remains enough unknown about fluid and electrolyte balance by parenteral means to make it necessary to provide insofar as is possible calories, water and electrolyte in the most physiologic manner we know, and a return to full and normal diet should be stressed. . . . The caloric and protein requirements particularly should be calculated. . . . If oral feedings are not sufficient to make up necessary caloric and protein requirements, parenteral protein hydrolysate may be used to make up the difference. If the caloric and protein requirements must be met entirely by the parenteral route, this may be accomplished by using protein hydrolysate, whole blood, glucose solutions and human serum albumin; alcohol has recently been added. . . . The vitamins, particularly ascorbic acid, thiamine hydrochloride, nicotinic acid, riboflavin and vitamin K, should be provided. . . . Parenteral therapy is always second best and is to be used either when the oral route is contraindicated or as an emergency measure.*

He thinks most preoperative patients are grossly "undertreated" although in some cases they may be given more water than they need. He thinks potassium depletion particularly common and believes it accounts for a great deal of the postoperative lassitude.

No aspect of preoperative care is more important than supplying water, nutrients, and oxygen-carrying blood elements as needed. This helps to prevent shock, nausea, thirst, and many other dangers and discomforts of surgery. There may be considerable loss of blood during the operation and in many cases water loss through sweating and vomiting.

Elimination. A *cathartic* is sometimes ordered on the day preceding the operation, but this practice has been discontinued by many surgeons for the following reasons: free catharsis depletes the patient's strength, robs the tissues of water, relaxes and lowers the tone of the intestinal muscles, thus predisposing the patient to postoperative distention. D. M. Dunlop comparing past and current opinion on preoperative purging says: "I remember as a house surgeon . . . how surprised we were that emergency cases, which had not had the benefit of our eliminative ministrations, progressed so relatively well after operation."† Crile and Shively believe that castor oil may be given 48 hours before the operation when the patient has taken large quantities of Amphojel or barium; these substances if left in the intestine might solidify and form impactions postoperatively.

A *cleansing enema* is usually given to empty the lower bowel and prevent the

* Bland, John H: *The Clinical Use of Fluid and Electrolyte.* W. B. Saunders Co., Philadelphia, 1952, pp. 145-49.

† Dunlop, D. M.: "Modern Trends in Therapeutic Dietetics," *Brit. J. Nutrition,* 4:225, (Feb.) 1950.

conditions mentioned in the preceding paragraph. If the result is not satisfactory, it may be necessary to repeat the enema; sometimes, particularly for operations on the vagina, colon, or perineum, enemas are given until the return is clear, showing a thorough cleansing. The enema is usually given 6 hours before an operation to allow peristalsis to subside; in an emergency operation, the enema is often omitted.

Vomiting is induced, a *gastric lavage* is given, or *gastric drainage* established according to the recency of the last meal and the nature of surgery.

Beecher has urged the importance of inducing vomiting with the gastric tube in preparation for emergency operations in order to reduce the danger of aspirating vomited food during and after surgery. Gastric lavage may be indicated unless there is a possibility of perforating the stomach. Gastric drainage is used in preparation for operations on the stomach.

Elimination from the bladder usually takes care of itself, but if there is any possibility of urinary retention the patient is *catheterized*. Some surgeons suggest that the patient be sent to the operating room with a clamped-off indwelling catheter, or an ordinary catheter held in position with adhesive. The bladder can then be emptied immediately before the operation and the catheter removed after the operation is completed. As preparation for bladder operations, cleansing and antiseptic irrigations are often prescribed.

The general anesthetic relaxes all the muscles of the body. The patient's control of the sphincter muscles, which normally guard the passage of feces from the rectum and urine from the bladder, is therefore lost so that the contents of the rectum and the bladder may be expelled on the operating table. This contaminates the draping, which must be changed, and causes serious delay when the life of the patient may depend upon the speed with which the operation is performed. Full organs are obviously more easily punctured than empty ones, and for this reason it is essential to see that the stomach, intestines, and bladder are not distended when the patient goes to the operating room.

Mouth Hygiene. A clean mouth will obviously reduce the risks of postoperative infections, particularly those of the lungs and salivary glands. A prophylactic treatment by the dentist or oral hygienist is desirable if time is available; if not, the nurse can supplement the patient's efforts as indicated by his particular needs. The principles and technique of mouth cleansing are discussed in Chapter 12.

Bathing and Care of the Hair. For esthetic reasons it is desirable that the patient have a bath either the night before or the morning of the operation. Encrusted dirt should be removed, and skin irritations or lesions of any sort cleared up before the operation. This is particularly important if afterward the patient must be inactive. The nails should be cleaned and nail polish removed so that the anesthetist and surgeon can detect color changes in the nail bed. Fastidious persons usually have a shampoo before admission for an operation. To those not so careful the nurse may suggest one. Since washing the hair may be uncomfortable for some time postoperatively, this seems a reasonable procedure. Baths and shampoos are of course contraindicated when the patient is in shock or when he is being prepared for an emergency operation.

Preparation of the Area of Operation.   The location and extent of the local *skin area* to be prepared depend upon the operation to be performed. *Most surgeons want an extensive area shaved:* for example, when an abdominal operation is to be done, whether the incision is made in the upper or lower portion, the entire abdomen is prepared. Precise specifications are helpful to the inexperienced nurse

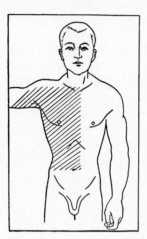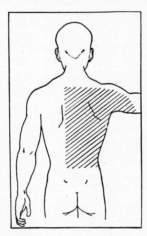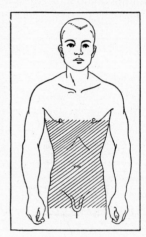

Figure 235. (*Left and center*) Site to be prepared for thoracic surgery. (West, John P.; Keller, Manelva W.; and Harmon, Elizabeth: *Nursing Care of the Surgical Patient*, 6th ed. The Macmillan Company, New York, 1957.)

Figure 236. (*Right*) Site to be prepared for abdominal surgery. (West, John P.; Keller, Manelva W.; and Harmon, Elizabeth: *Nursing Care of the Surgical Patient*, 6th ed. The Macmillan Company, New York, 1957.)

or one uninitiated in the preferences of the surgeon. In head surgery an effort is made not to disfigure the patient. Eyebrows, for example, are rarely shaved. Crile and Shively say that pubic hair should be shaved only when necessary because the discomfort of the short stubble hair growing back outweighs the advantage of its removal. They say: "Hair that is carefully washed with soap and water and prepared with an antiseptic solution need not be considered a major source of contamination."* However, this opinion is not shared by all surgeons, for many insist on the rule of a clean shave. Figures 235, 236, 237, and 238 suggest areas that are often specified. The technique of shaving is described in Chapter 12. There are a number of points reiterated by surgeons because they find them neglected. The skin should be shaved thoroughly, but it must not be abraded. Sometimes when the abdominal hair is heavy, it is necessary to inspect the area an hour or so before operation, if the preparation has been made the night before, to be sure that the area is still free from hair. Experience has shown that iodine should not be applied

* Crile, George, Jr., and Shively, Franklin L., Jr.: *Hospital Care of the Surgical Patient*, 2nd ed. Charles C Thomas, Publisher, Springfield, Ill., 1946, p. 125.

to skin recently moistened; therefore, a dry shave is indicated in preparation for emergency operations. Until fairly recently the operative site was disinfected and a dressing applied the night before the operation. Surgeons now believe that as the skin perspires under the dressing deep-lying organisms may come to the surface and multiply. They think also that the skin may be softened by the dressing and that the patient may sleep better without it. When hexachlorophene is used to disinfect the operative site, the skin is thoroughly washed every day for 2 or 3 days with this solution because it has a cumulative action.

Thorough cleaning of the umbilicus with cotton swabs saturated with a fat

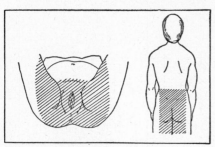

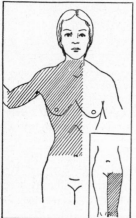

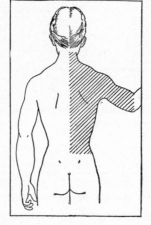

Figure 237. Site to be prepared for perineal surgery. (West, John P.; Keller, Manelva W.; and Harmon, Elizabeth: *Nursing Care of the Surgical Patient,* 6th ed. The Macmillan Company, New York, 1957.)

Figure 238. Site to be prepared for mastectomy. Inset shows area on thigh to be prepared when skin graft is contemplated. (West, John P.; Keller, Manelva W.; and Harmon, Elizabeth: *Nursing Care of the Surgical Patient,* 6th ed. The Macmillan Company, New York, 1957.)

solvent, such as gasoline or ether, and inspection of the unshaved pubis for lice are two more points emphasized by surgeons. It is often difficult to clean thoroughly the skin of patients who have not bathed for a long time, but irritating substances and stiff brushes must not be used. The abraded skin is likely to be irritated by antiseptics employed in the operating room. Skin disinfection was discussed at length in Chapter 7, and the opinions of numerous experts cited. While there is still difference of opinion, many surgeons favor the combined use of neutral detergents and hexachlorophene for preliminary or final cleansing. Benzalkonium (Zephiran) and iodine are the skin disinfectants most often used in the operating room for immediate skin disinfection.*

---

* Attention has been called to the desirability of substituting other skin antiseptics for iodine because its use for this purpose may render invalid the findings in studies of radioactive iodine or iodine isotopes.

George K. Coonse, writing in Robert L. Mason and Harold A. Zintel's text, states that in orthopedic operations a more stringent preparation should be made over a 48-hour period. As a final step in the procedure, he advocates that 3½ per cent iodine be used to paint the part, which is then covered with sterile gauze and sterile towels.

In the past, nurses on the clinical division were asked to include skin disinfectants as part of the preparation for abdominal surgery. Quite generally at the present time, if any disinfectant is used, it is applied by the surgeon in the operating room.

In surgery of the eye, nose, throat, and genitourinary and alimentary tracts, where mucous membrane predominates, the problem of preparing the site of operation is one of trying to make the operative field clean rather than sterile. The surgeon writes specific directions for the preparation of these areas, or a routine is set up on these special services for particular operations. Intestinal antiseptics may be given by mouth for several days before operations on these tracts.[32]

Promoting Sleep and Rest. Preoperative medication is a much discussed subject. It is generally agreed that a good night's rest before the day of operation is important. Sometimes pain may interfere with sleep, but in most cases the control of anxiety is all that is necessary. Minnitt and Nicholson recommend one of the barbiturates the night before the operation. Morphine, if used at all, is reserved for preanesthetic medication. Beecher and others call attention to the harmful effects of morphine, and urge the substitution of other drugs unless control of pain is the first and foremost consideration. Nurses should use every art at their disposal in promoting sleep and rest preoperatively. Chapter 15 discusses these arts; a repetition here seems unnecessary (see pp. 500-505).

7. CARE OF THE PATIENT IMMEDIATELY BEFORE TRANSFER TO THE OPERATING ROOM

Immediate Personal Care of the Operative Patient. On the morning of the operation, the temperature, pulse, and respiration are taken and recorded as usual. If the temperature is elevated, it is reported through the head nurse to the doctor. When she takes the temperature, the nurse should look for any sign of a cold, sore throat, or obstruction in breathing. The doctor will postpone the operation, even at the last hour, if there are symptoms of an upper respiratory infection.

More than the usual degree of nervousness and emotion, which must be estimated in terms of the particular patient's average reaction, should be reported. There are a number of things that must be done to prepare the patient for his removal to the operating room. One of the duties of the operating room nursing staff should be to report immediately any changes in the hour set for operation. Perhaps no other single factor makes a patient so nervous and fearful as waiting in the anterooms or corridors of the operating suite for an undue length of time.

The nurse in charge of the preoperative patient knows that her patient is scheduled for surgery at a particular time; she should plan her work accordingly. Early morning hours are considered desirable for operations, but it is not possible to give everyone this advantage. Patients should not be made ready too far in advance of a midmorning or afternoon operation. Judgment and experience are required for accurate timing of nursing procedures, and consideration of the patient should have precedence over hospital routine.

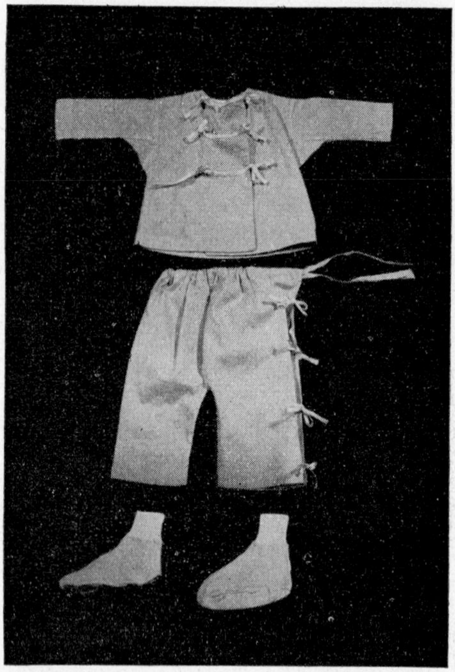

Figure 239. Garments designed for the operative patient. The jacket, which comes midway of the thighs may be worn to open front or back; the pants may be opened on either leg, and the opened leg drawn across the body to expose the pelvis. Knitted cuffs hold the socks on the feet. (Courtesy of Clay-Adams Co., New York City.)

Ordinarily the patient has his preoperative bath the day before the operation, but additional bathing, which does not interfere with the prepared area or unduly tire the patient, often makes him feel more relaxed.

Long hair should be carefully combed and arranged in two snug braids, securely fastened at the ends. All pins, combs, and clips must be removed because of the danger of their sticking into the patient when she is unconscious. As a rule, both men and women have some kind of cap to cover their hair completely while they are in the operating room. A stockinette cap is soft, adjustable, and easily kept in place, or, if not available, a towel may be used.

While the hair is being combed, even though an inspection for head lice has previously been made, further examination is indicated in some cases. This can be done tactfully and without the knowledge of the patient. Ether is known to make pediculi visibly active, which means that, if any part of the body is infested, the pediculi are likely to make their presence known by crawling over the skin, possibly the operative area. It is not safe to depend on the social position of a person as a criterion for the necessity of this inspection. Even well-groomed persons may accidentally become infested.

Practices vary with regard to clothing worn to the operating room; but a short nightgown and laparotomy stockings are often used. (See Fig. 15.) To avoid exposure of the pubic area, a T binder or other covering may be applied. Clothing should be loose and easy to remove and change, but improvement in hospital garments for patients is overdue. The pajamas in Figure 239 are designed for protection of the patient and the convenience of the surgical team.

Protection of Valuable Belongings.   Although it is the policy in most divisions in a hospital to request the patient to keep as few valuable articles as possible in his unit, nevertheless there are several things to safeguard while he is in the operating room. His money, even small change, watch, and rings, for example, must be protected. Since most patients who wear a wedding ring wish to keep it on, the common practice is to secure it by slipping a tape through the ring, knotting it, and then bringing the ends up around the wrist and again tying them securely.

All other valuable articles should be placed in an envelope on which is written the patient's name, room number or unit, and the date. In some cases the envelope is left with the head nurse, who places it in a locked drawer or cabinet in her office. In other instances it is placed in the hospital safe until the patient can again assume responsibility for his possessions.

Valuable articles are lost in hospitals from time to time; their loss and replacement cause great embarrassment and expense to the personnel and hospital authorities. Every precaution should be taken to prevent such occurrences.

Before a patient is anesthetized, false teeth, detachable bridges, plates, and chewing gum must be removed. This should be done when the mouth is cleaned shortly before the patient is transferred. Some anesthetists now prefer that plates be left in the mouth because, when the cheeks are filled, the mask used in administering the anesthetic fits more snugly, and the anesthetic is given more easily. An occasional patient will have artificial teeth that look removable but actually are not. This should be recorded on the chart and called to the attention of the anesthetist, since a valuable denture may be broken if the anesthetist tries to remove it when the patient is too drowsy to explain or protest. The presence of loose teeth also should be noted on the chart.

Good care should be taken of false teeth, and glass eyes too, which also must be removed before an operation. Artificial teeth and eyes are costly. The latter should be wrapped and labeled in the event that the patient is to be transferred to another unit postoperatively. If the patient is to return to his original unit, these articles should be left in suitable containers. Dentures are often placed in a covered paper cup. If the glass eye also is taken care of in this way, gauze or cotton must be used in the receptacle to prevent chipping or breaking. All articles in the room or unit that might be damaged or lost or that might injure the patient while he is unconscious are removed. A satisfactory explanation should be given the patient, so that he will understand why his wrist watch, for example, is taken away from him temporarily. Since little things of this kind seem to make a great difference, every effort should be made to consider the patient's wishes.

Removal of Urine from the Bladder. The bladder should be emptied 5 to 15 minutes before the patient leaves the ward, to prevent both the possibility of the individual's voiding on the operating table and an accidental puncture of a distended bladder in an abdominal operation.

Sometimes the patient is unable to void shortly before his transfer to the operating room, largely on account of nervous reaction. In this case it may be necessary for the nurse to catheterize a woman or call an interne to catheterize a man. To prevent delay in getting the patient to the operating room, it is well to determine the necessity for catheterization in advance of the appointed time for transfer. Instead of performing the catheterization in the clinical division, some surgeons prefer to carry out the procedure in the operating room, so that they may be perfectly sure of the state of the bladder. The use of an indwelling catheter to make it easy to empty the bladder just before operation was discussed on page 1006.

Preliminary Medication.   The most commonly given preanesthetic analgesic is morphine. Beecher thinks that morphine should be reserved for the person in severe pain. He says:

Morphine is not to be used to treat the restlessness arising from fear, apprehension, a confused mental state, anoxia, anemia, low blood volume, low blood pressure, hemorrhage or shock.

. . . . The outstanding effect of overdose with morphine is respiratory depression with anoxia. This is followed by circulatory damage. Less severe poisoning than the above, even therapeutic doses, often complicates treatment of the patient. Morphine by causing anorexia, nausea and vomiting limits the intake of food and fluids by mouth and increases fluid loss in vomitus and sweat. (Its needless use in shock is to be condemned.) Severe constipation is produced.*

Beecher goes on to say that if the circulation is sluggish absorption of morphine given intramuscularly or subcutaneously may be delayed and its action may be most marked during surgical operations when depression of the respiration is decidedly dangerous. He advocates the intravenous administration of morphine when pain demands it and suggests that not more than 15 mg (¼ gr) be given. He thinks its maximum analgesic effect is produced by 10 mg (⅙ gr). Another objection to morphine is the well-known idiosyncrasy that the very young and elderly have to this drug. Nurses will find surgeons substituting for morphine preoperatively such drugs as pentobarbital (Nembutal), amobarbital (Amytal), secobarbital (Seconal), or meperidine (Demerol). There is general agreement that some drug that makes the patient less aware of what is happening should be used. In this detached state, the anesthetic can be given much more easily; also, his memory of events preceding the operation will not be so vivid. Atropine, which depresses the secretory function, lessens the amount of saliva and mucus in the mouth and throat and creates a freer airway. With the analgesic it is usually given about 30 minutes before the operation.

Nurses should remember that the preoperative medication may make the patient lightheaded or dizzy and therefore uncertain of himself when he is on a narrow stretcher. A most disagreeable sensation is experienced by the patient who is feeling this way, when he is wheeled down a corridor, when his stretcher is pushed into an elevator, or when it accidentally bumps into something. There is no remedy for the sensation, but it helps to have stretchers that can be easily steered, handled by attendants strong enough to manage them, and moved at an even pace. Sudden stops should be avoided. The elevator should be precisely at floor level, and neither started nor stopped with a jerk. Whenever the stretcher must be

* Beecher, Henry K.: *Early Care of the Seriously Wounded Man: The Management of Traumatic Shock.* Charles C Thomas. Publisher, Springfield, Ill., 1949, p. 23, 24.

pushed up or down an incline, the patient should be warned, if he is awake, and in any event he should be steadied. It is a regulation in most hospitals that the patient be strapped to the stretcher in going to or returning from the operating room.

If morphine is given it may cause nausea; therefore, the nurse who accompanies the patient to the operating room should provide squares of soft paper and a basin. Celluwipes also are useful, if the patient perspires excessively, as is often the case when morphine is administered. A paper bag for waste should be at hand.

Modern hospital construction and equipment allow the patient to be transferred to the operating room in his bed—a very comfortable, expedient method. In such cases the bed can be warmed and protected while the operation is proceeding, and at its completion the patient need be moved only once.

The nurse should not discuss the operation with the patient while transferring him, nor talk to him if he obviously wishes to be undisturbed; she should, however, explain what will happen during the transfer step by step. Unexpected motion is disagreeable enough when one is fully conscious, and may be highly disturbing to the confused mind of the drugged patient. In most hospitals, orderlies transport patients to the operating room, but it is desirable to have a nurse or an anesthetist whom the patient knows in constant attendance.

Hospital facilities should include, when possible, waiting or anesthesia rooms that can be quiet and comfortable. Even if such provision has not been made, a thoughtful nurse can do a great deal to bring about these conditions wherever the patient must wait in the operating suite.

Whenever possible, the nurse should watch the operation performed on her patient in order that she may be better prepared to care for him. Complications may be encountered; emergencies may occur. The operative findings will be known to her, which may mean that she can take more intelligent care of the patient since the diagnosis is often changed after the surgeon's exploration.

In many cases, unavoidable periods of waiting occur in an operating unit. A long time may pass before the operation is begun; a more extensive operation may be performed than was expected. It is a period of almost unbearable waiting for the relatives who come to the hospital. Every minute seems like an hour; they cannot gauge time or find any but tragic explanations for the delay. One of the kindest things a nurse can do is to learn how things are progressing so that she may encourage those who are waiting. If they realize that the 20 minutes already passed include a 10-minute delay before the operation was started, they are relieved of some suspense. It does not matter so much whether the floor supervisor, head nurse, special nurse, or student does this so long as it is accomplished in a kind and effective manner. Hospital regulations and duties may determine who will do it. Tact, good judgment, and real sympathy are needed. Some hospitals have gone so far as to allow a member of the family or a close friend to go to the operating suite with the patient. They also provide a sitting room where the family can wait during the operation, and members of the operating room staff see that reports are relayed from time to time on the progress of the operation and the patient's condition.

THE PRESBYTERIAN HOSPITAL IN THE CITY OF NEW YORK
THE SLOANE HOSPITAL FOR WOMEN

OPERATIVE SLIP

Date 3/2/39
Name Peter Morgan Age 13
Address 601 West 175 St. Unit No. 572595
Medicine on Ward
Floor 2 Ward West
Into Oper. 11 35 P.M Out of Oper. 12 15/pm.
Condition good P. 104 R. 22
Drains None
Medicine on Table # 712 0/3 ml @ 10 50 pm.
Rx Medium head & knee gatch when conscious
Magendie 0/2cc (H) q4h SOS ad iii
Rectal taps 200cc q4h
Poultice & Rectal tube p.r.n.
Clysis 1000cc. Saline
Clear fluids tomorrow
L. Brown
House Surgeon
S443

Figure 240. Postoperative orders written by the surgeon and sent with the patient to the clinical division from the operating room. (Courtesy of Columbia-Presbyterian Medical Center, New York City.)

8. PREOPERATIVE AND OPERATIVE RECORDS

Recording the Preparation of the Patient. All significant procedures entering into the preparation of the patient for operation are recorded on his chart: for example, the nurse notes a cleansing enema, *if given;* the time and amount of last voiding; the way in which the area of operation was treated; the administration of prescribed medication; and the time at which the patient was taken to the operating room. She also notes the presence of dentures in the mouth and records any symptoms or reactions of the patient that might influence the administration of the anesthesia or the operative procedure. The patient's record is sent to the operating room with him.

Recording the Operation. All reputable hospitals require anesthetists to make a full written report of the administration of the anesthetic and all surgeons to make an equally detailed report of the operative procedure. Throughout the operation, data are recorded by appointed members of the departmental staff, and immediately after the operation the anesthetist and the surgeon incorporate them into a formal written report. A sample form of an operative report is shown in Figure 240. The surgeon's postoperative orders and the patient's chart are sent to the clinical division with him; the operative report is added to the patient's record within a few hours. The medical and nursing staff assigned to the care of the patient should be familiar with the contents of these reports if they expect to give him the most intelligent medical and nursing service.

REFERENCES

1. Wakely, Sir Cecil: "The Changing Face of Surgery," *Lancet,* **249:**6641, (Dec.) 1950.
2. Seidenfeld, Morton A.: *Psychological Aspects of Nursing Care.* Charles C Thomas, Publisher, Springfield, Ill., 1946, p. 123.
3. Wakely, Sir Cecil: *op. cit.*
4. Crile, George, Jr., and Shively, Franklin L., Jr.: *Hospital Care of the Surgical Patient,* 2nd ed. Charles C Thomas, Publisher, Springfield, Ill., 1946, p. 123.
5. Mason, Robert L., and Zintel, Harold A. (eds.): *Preoperative and Postoperative Treatment.* W. B. Saunders Co., Philadelphia, 1946, p. 7.
6. Szmyd, Lucian: "Modern Concepts of the Dynamics of Inflammation," *Mil. Surgeon,* **108:**45, (Jan.) 1951.
7. Christopher, Frederick, (ed.): *A Textbook of Surgery,* 4th ed. W. B. Saunders Co., Philadelphia, 1945, p. 1456.
8. Beecher, Henry K.: *Resuscitation and Anesthesia for Wounded Men: The Management of Traumatic Shock.* Charles C Thomas, Publisher, Springfield, Ill., 1949, p. 138.
9. Minnitt, R. J.: "Some Aspects of Modern Anesthesia," *M. Press,* **225:**159, (Feb.) 1951.
10. Dillon, John B.: "The Importance of Preoperative Evaluation of the Patient for Premedication and Choice of Anesthesia," *Arizona Med.,* **7:**28, (Oct.) 1950.
11. Paulson, John A., and Lundy, John S.: "Anesthesia," *Ann. Rev. Med.,* **1:**303, 1950.
12. Beecher, Henry K.: *Early Care of the Seriously Wounded Man.* Charles C Thomas, Publisher, Springfield, Ill., 1952, p. 26.
13. Paulson, John A., and Lundy, John S.: *op. cit.*
14. Paulson, John A., and Lundy, John S.: *op. cit.*
15. Christopher, Frederick (ed.): *op. cit,* p. 1444.
16. Paulson John A., and Lundy, John S.: *op. cit.*
17. Monash, Samuel: "Prolonged Use of Anesthesia by Injection with Procaine Base," *J. Invest. Dermat.,* **14:**79, (Feb.) 1950.
18. American Medical Association, Council on Pharmacy and Chemistry: *New and Nonofficial Remedies.* J. B. Lippincott Co., Philadelphia, 1950, p. 50.
19. American Medical Association, Council on Pharmacy and Chemistry: *op. cit.,* p. 49.

20. Christopher, Frederick (ed.): *op. cit.,* p. 1448.

21. Segerberg, Ludwig H.: "Ice Anesthesia," *Am. J. Nursing,* **43:**797, (Sept.) 1943.

22. Cook, Bertram: "Experience with Refrigeration Anesthesia in General Practice," *M. J. Australia,* **1:**467, (Apr.) 1950.

23. Dzubay, Rose Marie Weidorn: "Here's an Idea," *Am. J. Nursing,* **50:**555, (Sept.) 1950.

24. Nicholson, Morris J.: "Preoperative Preparation and Premedication," *S. Clin. North America,* **30:**635, (June) 1950.

25. Cutherbertson, D. P.: "Diet and Trauma," *Brit. J. Nutrition,* **4:**232, (Apr.) 1950.

26. Werner, Sidney C., et. al.: "Postoperative Nitrogen Loss," *Ann. Surg.,* **130:**688, (Oct.) 1949.

27. Homann, Ralph E.: "Fluid and Electrolyte Therapy in Surgical Patients," *Am. J. Surg.* **81:**10, (Jan.) 1951.

28. Ariel, Irving M., and Kreman, Arnold J.: "Compartmental Distribution of Sodium Chloride in Surgical Patients Pre- and Postoperatively,"*Ann. Surg.,* **132:**1009, (Dec.) 1950.

29. Randall, Henry T., et al.: "Sodium Deficiency in Surgical Patients and Failure of Urine Chloride as a Guide to Parenteral Therapy," *Surgery,* **28:**182, (Aug.) 1950.

30. Bland, John H.: *The Clinical Use of Fluid and Electrolyte.* W. B. Saunders Co., Philadelphia, 1952, p. 147.

31. Beecher, Henry K.: *Resuscitation and Anesthesia for Wounded Men: The Management of Traumatic Shock.* Charles C Thomas, Publisher, Springfield, Ill., 1949, p. 56.

32. Crile, George, Jr., and Shively, Franklin L., Jr.: *op. cit.,* p. 134.

Additional Suggested Reading

Cabot, Richard C., and Dicks, Russell L.: *The Art of Ministering to the Sick.* The Macmillan Company, New York, 1936.

Varco, Richard L.: "Preoperative Dietary Management for Surgical Patients," *Surgery,* **19:**303, (Mar.) 1946.

CHAPTER 39. POSTOPERATIVE NURSING CARE

1. GENERAL CONSIDERATIONS

Postoperative nursing care requires skilled nursing which provides supportive care through the various phases of a patient's recovery from an operation. It is designed to care for the unconscious patient, the disoriented patient, care in physical emergencies, and prevention of postoperative discomfort and complications. It begins when the patient is transferred from the operating room to the recovery unit, and ends in two stages: first, the recovery from anesthesia and from the trauma produced by surgery; and, second, the rehabilitation of the patient to as wide a range of normal activities as possible.

2. TRANSPORTATION FROM THE OPERATING ROOM

When surgery is completed, the patient is returned to his own room or to a special recovery room designed and equipped to care for patients during the immediate postoperative period. The patient's own bed or a stretcher may be used as a conveyance. Using the patient's bed minimizes the amount of lifting and unnecessary moving of an unconscious patient; it enables the operating team to place the patient in a desirable position immediately after surgery; it also increases the element of safety during transportation. Transfer of the patient to his bed or to a stretcher should be accomplished with as little jarring and strain on the patient as possible to avoid overtaxing the circulatory system and prevent undue strain on the operative area. The body should be kept straight, with the extremities, head, and trunk well supported. At the same time there should be no undue strain on those who lift him. This is easily and quickly accomplished by several persons who support the patients' weight against their chests, or by means of a lifting sheet that extends the full length of his body. Once the patient is comfortably placed in bed, the top covering is tucked in as usual, and the cap and stockings worn in the operating room removed. With a woman patient it may be preferable to leave the cap in place longer so that the hair is protected from vomitus.

The patient's position should be one to permit relaxation of the body and prevent strain. The bed is usually flat, or occasionally the head slightly lower than the feet to promote an adequate blood supply to the vital centers of the brain as well as to permit drainage of mucus and vomitus from the mouth. The lateral position is preferred because it further facilitates this drainage.[1, 2] In this position one knee is flexed, a pillow may be placed between the knees, and the arms are flexed in front of the body (see Fig. 241B). It is desirable for the anesthetist to accompany the patient to the recovery unit in order to observe his condition during the transfer and before relinquishing his care to the nurse. When this is not possible, a nurse should accompany the patient from the operating room. If an infusion is running, a special standard designed so that the base may be tucked under the mattress is useful for supporting the bottle during transportation.

3. THE RECOVERY UNIT AND BED

The unit for receiving the patient should be prepared in anticipation of the patient's postoperative needs. The environment should be quiet, moderately warm, and adaptable to very frequent observation. Constant care is essential for all patients postoperatively whether they are returned to their own room or to a special recovey unit where it is possible for several patients to be observed by one nurse.

It is the nurse's responsibility to see that all equipment needed to administer postoperative care is assembled and ready for use before the patient arrives. This should include a sphygmomanometer, equipment for administering infusion and transfusion, shock blocks, side boards, suction apparatus, mouth wedge, emesis basin, tissue wipes, and provision for note taking. Emergency equipment, such as oxygen, airway, tracheotomy set, dressing tray, and stimulant tray should also be accessible for immediate use.[3, 4]

The bed for the reception of the postoperative patient differs very little from the ordinary bed. The foundation is the same except for an additional strip of rubber or plastic sheeting covered by a cotton drawsheet that is placed across the

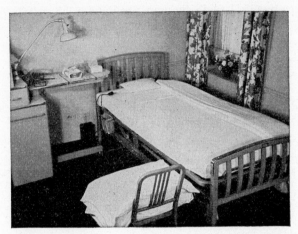

Figure 241A. Clinical unit prepared for the postoperative patient. Note the protection of the bedding, the fanned bedclothes, and the pillows to be used to keep the patient in a desirable position. A blood pressure apparatus, a record for vital signs, emesis basins, water and drinking tubes, and paper handkerchiefs are on the bedside stand. Nearby are several plastic airways. (Courtesy of Columbia-Presbyterian Medical Center, New York City, and Clay-Adams Co., New York City.)

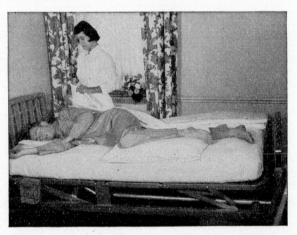

Figure 241B. Postoperative position that favors drainage from the mouth as well as abdominal relaxation. A pillow can be placed against the abdomen to support the patient's left arm and to expand the chest. A pillow at the patient's back tends to keep him from rolling over but is contraindicated in operations on the spine. (Courtesy of Columbia-Presbyterian Medical Center, New York City, and Clay-Adams Co., New York City.)

upper part of the mattress to protect it from any vomitus, mucus, or blood which may drain from the mouth. Usually the upper bedding is not tucked in, but is folded to the edge of the mattress on one side so that the patient may be easily transferred. In cold weather, hot-water bottles may be added to the bed to ensure warmth; but if the room is adequately heated this is unnecessary.

Provided the room is adequately heated and free from drafts, the postoperative patient needs no more covering than the average patient. Placing him between warm blankets or in a room above average temperature only causes profuse perspiration and general discomfort. In addition to an increased fluid loss, this results in a greater burden on the circulatory system or the vital centers, and in many instances does more harm than good.[5, 6]

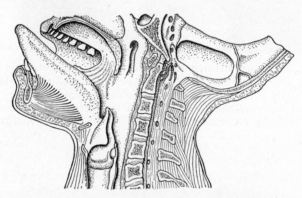

Figure 242.   Median section of portion of head and neck showing that upward traction on the tip of the tongue draws the epiglottis away from the glottis opening and permits free ingress of air. (Redrawn from Hare, H. A.: *Practical Therapeutics.* Lea & Febiger, Philadelphia, 1927.)

4. POSITION AND MAINTENANCE OF AIRWAY

The position of the patient will, of course, vary with the kind of operation performed and with his condition. As stated earlier, the patient is usually kept flat, or in some cases of hypotension the foot of the bed may be elevated 25 to 45 cm (10 to 18 in). Unless contraindicated, the patient should be placed on his side as shown in Figure 241 B, until the swallowing and gag reflexes return. For additional support a pillow may be placed along the back, against the abdomen, or between the knees, making fuller relaxation possible. Leaving the patient on his back while he is unconscious is hazardous because with diminished swallowing and gag reflexes he may aspirate mucus or vomitus into the bronchi, or the breathing may be obstructed if the relaxed tongue falls back into the throat ("swallowing the tongue"). With the patient in the lateral position, the tongue drops to the side of the mouth, air passes above it, and the respirations are improved. If, for some reason, it is advisable for the unconscious patient to remain on his back, the danger of aspiration can be lessened by turning the head to one side when he vomits, suctioning the secretions or vomitus from the throat as required, and observing for respiratory obstruction so that the proper measures may be employed promptly.

Because there is a constant danger of the patient's aspirating secretions, blood, or vomitus into the lungs when he cannot voluntarily expectorate, it is desirable to suction this material from the throat at frequent intervals as it accumulates. This may be accomplished by means of a whistle-tip catheter connected to an electric or wall suction or other suitable type of negative pressure. The catheter should be inserted into the pharynx through the mouth, but occasionally if the patient's mouth cannot be opened it may be inserted through the nostril. If the nostril is used, care should be taken to pinch off the catheter during insertion and removal so that the nasal mucosa will not be damaged. The catheter should be left in place only long enough to suction the secretions, and then removed.

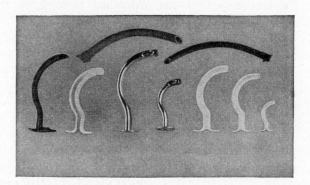

Figure 243. Plastic, hard- and soft-rubber, and metal airways in a variety of sizes. (Courtesy of Clay-Adams Co., New York City.)

Often, as an added precaution, the patient will have an artificial airway inserted before or after going to the recovery unit. The purpose is to hold the tongue forward by means of a hollow tube and thus ensure unobstructed breathing. (Types of airways are illustrated in Fig. 243.) Suctioning can be carried out by inserting the catheter directly through the airway. When the patient begins to gag or push the airway out with his tongue, it can usually be removed, as this indicates a return of the swallowing and gag reflexes.

If the patient is in the proper position and the breathing unobstructed, the rate of respirations will be fairly constant, probably ranging from 12 to 24 per minute. The rhythm and depth of the respirations should be uniform. Any obstruction in breathing will be evidenced by a change in the character of the respirations and possibly by the appearance of cyanosis. Frequently, the falling back of the tongue into the pharynx is the cause of obstruction. This can be relieved by correctly pressing on the angle of the lower jaw, and pushing it forward, at the same time keeping the teeth separated. If an unobstructed air passage cannot be maintained in this way, it may be necessary to insert an artificial airway. On certain occasions, grasping the tongue and pulling it forward will allow for a free passage of air (a gauze square covers the nurse's fingers and enables her to hold the tongue firmly).

Use of a mouth wedge whenever it is necessary to take hold of the patient's tongue or force the teeth apart will safeguard the nurse's fingers against injury. Most wedges are made of wood, soft enough to lessen the possibility of the patient's breaking a tooth if his jaws should tighten. A satisfactory mouth wedge may be made by wrapping several tongue blades together, and padding them with gauze and adhesive tape.[7, 8]

The patient's position should be changed frequently to ensure good expansion of the lungs and prevent postoperative pulmonary complications. Turning the patient every hour is usually recommended.

As the patient begins to regain consciousness and the possibility of aspiration is decreased, he may be placed on his back. When he is fully conscious he is usually more comfortable if the head of the bed is elevated about 15 to 25 cm (6 to 10 in.). With the elevation of the head and shoulders, respirations are easier, and there is less tension on the abdominal muscles. In the past, Fowler's position was widely used. This includes not only elevation of the head, but also flexion of the knees by means of a pillow or knee Gatch. Although this posture does provide comfort, various authorities[9, 10] now advise against its use because it predisposes to venous stasis and thrombosis by accentuating a dependent position of the pelvis and by compressing the femoral and popliteal veins in the legs. Some surgeons have discontinued the routine elevation of the head of the bed, preferring the horizontal position in the immediate postoperative period. If the patient's condition improves satisfactorily, he may soon assume any position desired, providing it is changed frequently.

5. RESTLESSNESS AND CONFUSION

Most patients reacting from a general anesthetic undergo a period of restlessness and mental confusion before consciousness is fully regained. With some anesthetics, such as cyclopropane,[11] the degree of restlessness may be more pronounced than with others. Preoperative fear and resistance to the induction of anesthesia may also bring about increased restlessness.

Another factor which has a bearing on postoperative restlessness and confusion is sound. Many persons who have undergone an operation will attest that the faculty of hearing returns before the ability to make a verbal response. Every effort should be made to eliminate noise, confusion, and unguarded conversation, which may be misinterpreted or exaggerated by the patient who is semiconscious. While a familiar voice can offer much reassurance to one who is confused and bewildered, visitors, as a rule, are excluded from the recovery unit. Within recent years, however, many pediatricians are advocating that the mother be present before a child is taken to the operating room, and also when he reacts from the anesthetic.[12, 13] Thus, the child hears his mother's voice in the interval preceding surgery, and again as he regains consciousness. This principle may also be employed with adults, by having a nurse who is familiar to the patient care for him before and after surgery.

In general, while the patient is recovering from anesthesia, minor movements should not be discouraged. Restraining the patient only increases restlessness, and should not be employed unless it is necessary for his protection. If he is receiving an infusion, there is the possibility that he may injure himself by uncontrolled movements of the extremity; and during this time some form of minor restraint is indicated until he is sufficiently conscious to benefit by explanations and reassurance. The patient's arm or leg may need to be tied to the side of the bed in order to prevent dislodging the needle, or a padded arm board may be used to prevent flexion of his elbow or wrist. Care should be taken to pad the extremity before tying it, and to release the restraint at frequent intervals, so as to provide for a change in position. To safeguard the patient from falling out of bed, the use of side boards should be employed. These are usually left in place through the first postoperative night in case the patient is still under the effects of the anesthetic or is confused by narcotics.

Usually, with attentive care and repeated explanations, the above methods will afford the patient adequate protection. If restlessness is very severe, it may be necessary to employ a more limiting type of restraint, for it seems more sensible to provide this than to expect a nurse of ordinary strength to prevent a large and vigorous patient from falling out of bed or otherwise injuring himself.

6. RELIEF OF PAIN

As the effects of the anesthetic wear off, the patient will become increasingly aware of pain, discomfort, and outside stimuli. During this period there may be an inclination to talk and express some of the fears, confusion, or pain that the patient naturally experiences. Reassurance and explanations given repeatedly will do much toward alleviating his concern and reducing his response to pain.

In order to relieve operative pain and ensure rest it is often necessary to administer a narcotic as soon as the patient reacts from the anesthetic, or shortly thereafter. Robert Elman says that the practice of keeping the patient asleep or in a dozing (i.e., depressed) condition for the first 48 hours after operation is now thought undesirable. The objective should be to eliminate pain and discomfort, preferably by physical or psychologic means, aided by mild sedatives and analgesics. It follows then that narcotics, when used, should not be administered routinely, but only as required for pain which cannot otherwise be prevented or relieved. This will enable the body to function as normally as possible without the influence of depressing drugs. Most surgeons will make provision for administering a narcotic such as morphine or meperidine hydrochloride, every four hours as required for pain for the first day or two following surgery. The frequency with which it is given is usually left to the discretion of the nurse. Untoward effects of narcotics should be carefully observed, especially respiratory depression, continued nausea and vomiting, and an abnormal dependence on drugs. The nurse must be judicious in their use, knowing when to administer them, and when to employ other measures than drugs to relieve pain.

In the administration of analgesics and narcotics it is reasonable to give them prior to the activities which tend to make the pain more severe, such as turning the patient or getting him out of bed. The writer has had experience in a number of cases where no analgesic or narcotic was required or desired after major surgery. In these instances the patient was given careful instruction as to what his role would be in the postoperative recovery period, and emphasis was placed on turning and having the patient exercise the extremities and breathe deeply every one or two hours during the first 24-hour period, both day and night. Aside from inducing early mobilization, this regime prevents the severe pain which results from the motion of muscles which have been abnormally splinted in an unchanged position for hours at a time. Thus the patient is prepared for getting out of bed with a minimum of weakness and discomfort.

Pain should always be regarded as an individual matter, however, and depends largely on the patient's tolerance, the type and extent of surgery performed, and the complications encountered. Good nursing care can do much to minimize pain. Frequent changes of position, the use of pillows, correct anchorage of drainage tubing, and similar nursing measures all contribute greatly to the patient's general comfort.

7. OBSERVATIONS AND CHARTING

An extremely important part of the postoperative nursing care is observation of the patient. Since this care is a continuation of that received at the time of operation, the nurse should know what operative procedure was performed as well as how the patient withstood the procedure. It may not be possible for the nurse to be present at the operation, but she should familiarize herself with the records kept by the anesthetist and surgeon. This information will enable her to give postoperative care more specifically adapted to the needs of the patient.

As soon as the patient is brought to the recovery unit, the nurse should check the patient's condition with the anesthetist or nurse who transferred him. This should include the patient's color, and body warmth, as well as his blood pressure, pulse, and respirations.

In the beginning, the patient's face is usually flushed and the skin moist and warm, because most anesthetics dilate the superficial capillaries. The appearance of cyanosis indicates lack of oxygen which may be caused by inadequate respiratory movement or obstruction of the air passages. The blood pressure, pulse, and respirations are taken immediately, and at short intervals thereafter (usually every 15 to 20 minutes) until the patient has fully reacted, and then every hour or less often as his condition improves and if the blood pressure stays fairly constant. (For normal figures, see p. 302.) Any marked variation from the average blood pressure is reported to the surgeon, for it may indicate a complication, such as shock or hemorrhage. In order to determine whether or not the blood pressure is abnormally low or high, the nurse should know what the patient's blood pressure was prior to surgery. This may be determined from the notes on the chart. Usually a drop in blood pressure can be expected postoperatively due to the loss in blood volume and to the effect of the anesthetic and depressant medications. If the blood pressure was within normal range or above before surgery, a drop of 20–30 mm of mercury might indicate oncoming shock. In patients with hypotension, however, the range of safety is considerably less. A systolic blood pressure of 90 mm should be considered dangerous, and "any patient with a blood pressure lower than 80 mm of mercury is in grave danger, and urgently needs resuscitation before irreversible lesions occur in the nerve centers."* Evaluation of the blood pressure changes should always remain on an individual basis, depending on the patient's general condition and pre-existing pressure.

The pulse and respiratory rates are also indicators of the patient's condition that may be determined easily and quickly. They are generally taken at the same interval with the blood pressure, but in some cases more frequently. After surgery the pulse is usually more rapid and sometimes weaker with a regular volume and rhythm. Excessive increase in pulse rate or weakness in volume may indicate shock or hemorrhage.

The respirations are often noisy until the patient is conscious. Any change should be noted, such as excessively shallow, rapid, or difficult breathing. If the difficulty is due to an obstructed air passage, immediate measures, such as those discussed previously, should be instituted. If the character, rate, or rhythm of the respirations continues to be inadequate, the surgeon should be notified. It may be that the lungs are poorly ventilated and oxygen is needed.

Unless the surgeon fears a disturbance in the body's heat mechanism, the temperature is ordinarily not measured in the immediate postoperative period. In most cases, it is taken every four hours for the first 24 hours, and then less frequently if it is not elevated to an unusual degree. A slight elevation in body temperature usually exists for about the first three days after an operation. According to Robert L. Mason and Harold A. Zintel, the exact cause of this postoperative rise in temperature has not been determined, but it is believed to be the result of absorption of blood and lymph at the incision and the subsequent repair of the tissues affected by surgery. The routine administration of antibiotics, such as penicillin and oxytetracycline, in surgical patients plays a tremendous role in reducing the incidence of postoperative infections, and hence fever due to this cause is much less frequent than formerly. If an elevation of temperature persists beyond the third postoperative day, it is probably caused by one of the postoperative complications that will be discussed subsequently (pp. 1037-41). If the temperature is below normal, additional warmth may be necessary to help raise it, or it may exist concomitantly with the complication of shock or hemorrhage.

Since hemorrhage is a constant danger during the first 24 hours, the dressings should be observed at frequent intervals during this period. The nurse should be familiar with the character and amount of drainage expected with various types of surgery, so that she can differentiate between normal drainage and hemorrhage. Blood will, of course, flow by gravity to the lowest point, so that the upper dressing

* Trueta. J.: *The Principles and Practice of War Surgery.* C. V. Mosby Co.. St. Louis. 1943. p. 134

may not be stained although the bed beneath the patient may be. Should a dressing become stained with blood, the size of the stain should be observed frequently to determine whether or not it increases. This can be observed easily by measuring the stained area or outlining it with a pencil and noting any increase in size. If this does occur, the doctor should be immediately notified. A small amount of bleeding may occur from the superficial capillaries and therefore be of no significance; on the other hand, a severe hemorrhage may occur at the operative site. The dressings are only reinforced by the nurse if there is an appreciable amount of drainage, because the surgeon usually prefers to have the original dressing kept in place until his arrival.

The length of time required for the patient to regain consciousness and the way he reacts from the anesthetic are also important observations. During the unconscious phase, the patient does not respond to questioning or painful stimuli. As he passes into the semiconscious phase, he often responds to painful stimuli by restlessness and moaning or loud talking. With the return of the gag and swallowing reflexes, vomiting and expectoration of mucus often occur. In order to determine when the patient has fully reacted, it is necessary to be sure that he is oriented to his surroundings. He should be able to answer questions related to his identity, time, and familiar happenings. It should be remembered, however, that, in determining reaction from anesthesia, it is necessary to compare the expected mental and physical response postoperatively with the response displayed in the preoperative period. It is desirable to allow the patient to return to consciousness naturally rather than jog him or talk loudly in an effort to hasten his return to consciousness. Speaking distinctly, close to the ear, and at the same time pressing on his arm or hand usually suffice to elicit a satisfactory response if he is reacting.

The nurse's postoperative notes should include a concise record of the observations discussed, in order to give a progressive picture of the patient's postoperative recovery. Since the nurse remains with the patient constantly until he reacts from the anesthetic, she is in an excellent position to make notations. In summary, concurrent notes should be kept on the vital signs, color, body warmth, condition of the dressing, presence of nausea and vomiting, reaction from the anesthetic, and evidences of pain or discomfort. A written record of the treatments administered should also be made. Fluids administered, medications, irrigations, and similar treatments should all be included in the postoperative record. In general the record for the postoperative patient is not unlike that for any other patient except that notes are made more frequently in accordance with the patient's condition.

8. FLUID AND ELECTROLYTE BALANCE

Within recent years much emphasis has been placed on the importance of fluid and electrolyte balance in the management of surgical patients.

The average patient who undergoes surgery is a notable candidate for dehydration and electrolyte imbalance, as well as nutritional deficiency. Often he has been unable to ingest or digest foods because of the disease process requiring the surgery;

and, preoperatively, oral intake may be further restricted in preparation for the operation. In addition, there may be considerable loss of fluids and electrolytes by bleeding, vomitus, perspiration, and drainage. These should be replaced in accordance with the body's physiological response to surgery. In a study of the preoperative and postoperative tolerance of sodium chloride, Irving Ariel and Arnold J. Kremen demonstrated a varying response in the distribution of chloride administered to the same individual before and after surgery. They say: "In the postoperative state a larger portion is delivered to the interstitial space, and a disproportion between plasma and interstitial volume develops. Therefore, the interstitial electrolyte is apparently not as readily delivered to the kidney for excretion," and hence more is retained. They believe that there can be "serious complications from relatively slight excesses of saline solution," and "the sequelae which result . . . may contribute to the demise of the patient."*

Recent authorities[14, 15, 16] have also demonstrated that immediately following extensive surgery large amounts of potassium are lost from the traumatized muscles and excreted in the urine; this loss parallels the degree and extent of the trauma. Other electrolytes, such as sodium and bicarbonate, may be also retained or excreted in abnormal amounts. If provision is not made to counteract such trends, serious complications may ensue.

For the above reasons, the surgeon will be vitally interested in the patient's intake and output. Through a study of these relationships, and by tests on the blood and urine, he is able to prescribe the parenteral feedings needed. In general, the patient is supported by intravenous feedings until he is able to take a full-liquid diet by mouth. As he gradually increases his oral intake, he is given less by vein. The nurse gives an invaluable service when she keeps an accurate record of the patient's oral and parenteral intake, as well as his urinary output and the fluid loss through vomitus, feces, and drainage from any body area.

Because of the increased need for fluid postoperatively, and because it cannot always be administered simultaneously with the body's natural urge to drink, the patient frequently experiences thirst. This sensation is caused by the body's physiologic response to the need for fluids. If there is an inadequate amount present, water is drawn from the tissues to compensate, leaving the mouth dry and coated. The nurse should realize, however, that thirst can be quenched with the administration of fluids by the parenteral route as well as the oral. It is, of course, more desirable to give as much of the fluid as possible orally, for it is the natural, and likewise the most pleasant and comfortable, way of receiving it. Frequent attention to mouth care will also help to alleviate a dry mouth, as will be discussed later (pp. 1029-30).

It is apparent from the foregoing discussions that a large proportion of the nursing care of surgical patients will, of necessity, focus around the care of a patient receiving infusions, transfusions, and blood tests, as well as the need for measuring and recording intake and output. Simple explanations of the tests per-

* Ariel, Irving, and Kremen, Arnold J.: "Compartmental Distribution of Sodium Chloride in Surgical Patients," *Ann. Surg.*, **132**:1009, (Dec.) 1950.

formed and instructions regarding the necessity for measuring fluids and excreta will contribute much toward a wholesome and relaxed attitude on the part of the patient. In addition, provision should be made for rest and change of position while infusions are running. The use of a padded arm board should be employed whenever the needle is injected at a site where the joint should not be moved, such as the elbow or wrist. Even when these sites are used, there is no reason why the arm should be completely immobilized. With caution, the patient may be instructed to tighten and relax the muscles in his arm and to flex the uninvolved joints at periodic intervals. He should also be encouraged to change his position from side to side. When his condition permits, the nurse can assist him to walk by protecting his involved arm as he gets out of bed, and by supporting the solution bottle as she walks with him.

9. EXERCISE AND EARLY AMBULATION

Within recent years there has been increasing emphasis on mobilizing the patient immediately after surgery. This is in an effort to aerate the lungs and speed the circulation, which in turn helps prevent pulmonary and circulatory complications heretofore so prevalent in the postoperative period. Through exercise and ambulation, the body is quickly restored to its average physical performance, which was interrupted by the surgical procedure.

Because it is only natural for the average person to feel reluctant about performing exercises, and, in addition, getting up and walking following an operation, the nurse should begin her education of the patient well in the preoperative period. She should not wait, as did one nurse who said to her patient postoperatively: "I will help you get up now," and the patient replied: "Certainly not. Don't you know I've had an operation?"

As soon as the patient has fully recovered from the anesthetic, he is encouraged to move his arms and legs, breathe deeply, and change his position frequently. To accomplish this the nurse should assist him with a program of exercises which emphasize flexion and extension of the extremities; expansion of the chest with deep breathing, coughing, and raising sputum; and turning from side to side. These should be carried out as often as every one or two hours for the first 24 hours (when the vital capacity is lowest) and later several times a day. With this regime the patient is usually able to walk for the first time with a minimum of discomfort. He should be helped out of bed and encouraged to walk with assistance on the operative or first postoperative day or later, depending on the type of surgery performed. He is often weak, but can derive much support and encouragement from the nurse, enabling him to walk at least a few steps. Occasionally the patient will feel faint, in which case it is advisable to help him back to bed and attempt ambulation again later in the day.[17, 18, 19]

For the first day or two after an operation many surgeons advise against sitting in a chair, except for very short periods, such as required for making the bed.[20] This is to prevent compression of the popliteal and femoral veins and a dependent position of the extremities, which predisposes to venous stasis and thrombosis.

In general, it is more desirable for a patient to be either walking or in bed. After a few days, he is usually able to get about freely by himself, and should be encouraged to do so.

In the past an abdominal binder was usually applied when the patient was walking, but this is no longer considered essential. With adequate suturing, the wound is sufficiently strong to withstand the ordinary activities of postoperative ambulation. Moreover, various authors mention the use of abdominal binders and tight dressings as a cause for venous stasis by increasing the intra-abdominal pressure. To prevent venous stasis many surgeons will prohibit wearing an abdominal binder postoperatively except when the patient is very obese or the wound defective; and some advocate the use of elastic bandages on the lower extremities to aid venous return.[21]

The program for postoperative exercise and early ambulation should be carried out under the nurse's supervision either individually or in a group. The important aspect is to describe the program in sufficient detail, and to give each patient individual consideration. In addition Elman suggests the use of a printed form with which surgical patients may become familiar soon after admission. He also points out how a resourceful nurse can enhance such a program by promoting diversional therapy for her patients, since the psychologic effect of diversion is an important incentive for increasing physical activity.

With many types of surgery the patient will have one or more tubes attached to the body for urinary or other type of drainage, or for the infusion of parenteral fluid. In walking these patients, the nurse must use caution to prevent dislodging the tube or allowing the drainage to soil the patient's clothing. When there is a catheter or open drainage tube in place it may be attached to a small bottle or other appropriate receptacle for walking. When an infusion is running the nurse can support the bottle in her hand as she walks along with the patient.

It should be remembered that, although a postoperative patient is "up and about" and "can bathe himself," his wound and general physical condition will not always permit a full range of activities. If he has a sterile dressing on the body, he cannot take a shower or a tub bath (unless some means is provided for keeping the dressing dry) (Fig. 57, p. 332); hence he is often dependent on the bed bath or sponge bath at the hand basin. With many types of surgery it is difficult or painful for the patient to reach certain body areas, such as the back, feet, and genitalia. Also, the patient may require help in reaching or lifting articles from his table. For example, his water pitcher may be entirely too heavy for him to do any "forcing" of fluids without some practical assistance. Plastic tubing that reaches into the supply of drinking water may be indicated in some cases. A wise nurse will take dependency factors into consideration while caring for ambulatory patients, and provide whatever help and guidance are required.

10. CLEANLINESS AND MOUTH CARE

Following surgery the patient usually perspires excessively, and in addition may experience vomiting and an uncontrolled flow of secretions from the nose and mouth. Discomforts due to uncleanliness and a disagreeable taste in the mouth may often be relieved by thoughtful attention to hygienic measures.

During the unconscious and semiconscious phases of recovery, the nurse should keep the patient as clean as possible, changing the gown and linen as necessary, and wiping the secretions and perspiration from the face. After the patient has regained consciousness, the mouth should be cleaned thoroughly in order to eliminate the unpleasant taste of vomitus and anesthetic. Since for a number of hours following consciousness the patient may be nauseated and may vomit which increases with motion, it is better to wait to give a complete bath until this phase has subsided. Later, the patient is more likely to benefit from the relaxing as well as cleansing effects of a bath.

Postoperatively, mouth care is an important hygienic need of the patient. When fluids cannot be taken orally, or if the patient is on a nonchewing diet, the salivary flow is decreased, the mouth becomes dry, and the tongue coated. In many instances there is also a foul odor to the breath. Bernard J. Ficarra[22] explains the high incidence of mouth odor in surgical patients on the basis of possible pathology such as pyorrhea, dental caries, bronchiectasis, or rhinitis, and on the postoperative dehydration that aggravates a pre-existing odor. In other cases halitosis may indicate the onset of a complication such as parotitis, gastric dilation, intestinal obstruction, or lung abscess. In order to keep the mouth comfortable after surgery, and also as a preventive against parotitis, special care should be given. Several times a day the tongue and teeth should be cleaned with a toothbrush, and the mouth rinsed at frequent intervals with a mouthwash or plain water. Many surgical patients who are fed nothing by mouth say that in order to obtain relief from dryness it is advisable to rinse the mouth every hour. It is also helpful to chew gum following surgery. This stimulates the salivary glands to activity, and keeps the mouth moist, which lessens mouth odor. This may not be feasible, however, for patients with a nasopharyngeal tube. If the tongue should become coated, a mixture of hydrogen peroxide and water, 1 part to 4, may be used to loosen the coating. Carbonated water or a sugar-free carbonated drink used as a mouthwash has a similar action and is more palatable. (For a general discussion of mouth care, see pp. 339 ff).

For the first few days following an operation, the patient usually requires considerable help with his hygienic needs. Gradually, as he regains strength and increases his scope of activities, he should be encouraged to help himself as much as possible. The transition should not be sudden, however, but progressive in accordance with the patient's physical condition and his mental acceptance of the need for acquiring independence.

11. VOIDING AND RETENTION OF URINE

Postoperatively, the bladder tends to hold the urine which has accumulated in it for longer periods of time than under ordinary conditions. If the urine is allowed to accumulate without provision for its release at normal intervals, it will result in urinary retention. Besides causing the patient considerable discomfort and restlessness, retention of urine also predisposes to the development of cystitis. Several reasons are given why urinary retention tends to occur postoperatively. Most authorities[23, 24] agree that diminished sensitivity after general anesthesia permits the bladder to fill more completely than under ordinary circumstances, and also that psychic phenomena play a definite role. Besides this, Vernon S. Dick suggests that overdistention of the bladder may occur more quickly than is realized following surgery because of the rapid administration of fluids. This in turn causes a decrease in muscle tone of the bladder with later difficulty in urination.

Adding to these circumstances is the fact that the voluntary abdominal and perineal muscles play a much greater part in the act of micturition than many people realize, and if the operative site is so located that pain is produced by effort to contract these muscles, further interference of vesical emptying is produced.*

It is well known that nervous apprehensive patients are more likely to be unable to void than those who are relaxed and made comfortable. Frequently a patient will suffer from retention as long as he remains on bed rest, and be relieved immediately when allowed to get up and assume the normal position for voiding. In a study of postoperative urinary retention Charles W. McLaughlin, Jr., and John R. Brown studied 1964 young men undergoing surgery. In one group the patient was not permitted to stand to void but received doses of neostigmine (Prostigmin). The incidence of urinary retention under these conditions was 3 per cent. When injections of saline were substituted for neostigmine the incidence remained essentially the same. In the second group the patient was permitted up to void and received the same doses of neostigmine as the first group. Under those conditions the incidence was only 0.76 per cent, and did not significantly change when saline was substituted for the neostigmine. With early ambulation, then, and with conditions simulating a normal atmosphere for the function of elimination, urinary retention is not as common a problem as it was when patients were kept in bed for longer periods of time. However, it is still an important function of the nurse to safeguard the patient against this untoward development, for it is through intelligent and sympathetic nursing that the incidence of urinary retention and its complications can be reduced.

To be observant of urinary retention, the nurse should be familiar with the amount and frequency of normal voiding in health (see p. 449) and also with the normal deviation following surgery. The amount of urine voided following an operation is not great. Hugh C. Ilgenfritz has said that "the average patient will void 200 to 400 cc. of urine within six to eight hours after operation; if not, he should be examined for evidence of urinary retention. . . ."† If the patient receives no parenteral fluids the day following the operation, his fluid intake is generally inadequate; in addition, fluids may be lost by routes other than the kidneys (e.g., diaphoresis and vomiting). However, when the daily intake averages 3000 cc, the

* Dick, Vernon S: "Management of Postoperative Urinary Retention," *Lahey Clin. Bull,* **7:**57-62, (Oct.) 1950.

† Ilgenfritz, Hugh C.: *Preoperative and Postoperative Care of Surgical Patients.* C. V. Mosby Co., St. Louis, 1948, p. 329.

patient should void 1000 cc or more of urine daily. An infusion that is administered rapidly will have a diuretic effect, and the patient often voids 300 to 400 cc in several hours. Since vesical sensation and reflexes are decreased in the postoperative period, the bladder may become distended without the usual sensations of urgency; as a result the patient may be restless and uncomfortable, and aware only of a persistent, lower abdominal pain.

In some cases retention may be accompanied by overflow, in which instance the patient voids frequently and in small amounts, usually 50 to 100 cc. If there is doubt as to whether or not a patient has urinary retention, several measures may be employed by the nurse as a guide: (1) recording each time the amount that the patient voids is essential in a comparative study between intake and output, (2) pressing gently upon the suprapubic area to note a discomfort or an intensified desire to void, and (3) palpating the abdomen for distention just above the symphysis pubis. Generally the bladder is not demonstrable above the symphysis pubis by either palpation or percussion until it contains at least 500 cc of urine. Other measures which may be employed by the surgeon include percussion and rectal or vaginal examination.

Most surgeons will make provision, in case a patient is unable to void, for catheterizing him within 8 to 10 hours after the operation. Some allow a shorter period of time, and others, a longer interval; but the aim is always to catheterize the patient before the bladder becomes distended, provided other measures are unsuccessful. Various authorities[25, 26] agree that when the bladder is allowed to become overdistended, and is then decompressed, there is congestion and edema of the mucous membrane, and the tendency to develop cystitis increases. The residual urine then serves as a culture medium for the growth of bacteria upon introduction of a catheter. Also, stretching of the vesical wall may induce atony and interfere with later resumption of normal tone and voiding. Since a healthy bladder mucosa is highly resistant to infection, cystitis rarely follows catheterization, if careful technique is used, before considerable distention occurs. If, however, overdistention does occur, the possibility for cystitis increases tremendously even with one catheterization, although the patient is able to void spontaneously later on.

Should the patient continue to have difficulty with urination, the surgeon may prescribe a drug to stimulate the parasympathetic nervous system. Two drugs which are used for this purpose are carbachol (Doryl) and bethanechol (Urecholine).

12. BOWEL ELIMINATION AND GAS PAINS

The surgical patient's ability to expel flatus and have a bowel movement spontaneously indicates that normal function has returned to the gastrointestinal tract. The first time either occurs following surgery is an important observation which the nurse should report. Although flatus may be expelled earlier, a spontaneous bowel movement does not usually occur until about the fourth or fifth postoperative day.[27] This delay is due to the temporary paralysis of the gastrointestinal tract following surgery and anesthesia, and to the lack of bulk in the intestines. To aid defecation some surgeons prescribe an enema or cathartic on the second or third postoperative day. Others prefer to wait for a natural movement, provided the delay is not prolonged. Elman says that it is unwise to hasten defecation by artificial means, such as enemas, cathartics, or peristaltic stimulants. This is because postoperative cessation of peristalsis serves as a physiologic protective mechanism to keep the gastrointestinal tract at rest, just as immobilization of an injured arm is a voluntary protective mechanism to keep the arm at rest. He considers that a delay in defecation of four or five days following surgery produces no harmful effects, and that methods of routine postoperative purging may not only produce harm, but are "just as illogical as whipping a tired horse," besides causing needless pain and distress to the patient. If proper attention is paid to postoperative exercise, ambulation, nutrition, and to the patient's physical and psychogenic needs, such as privacy, normal position, and timing with the urge to defecate, there is generally no problem.

In cases where the feces tends to remain in the rectum longer than usual, as can be determined on rectal examination, or the patient feels the urge to defecate without being able to expel adequate amounts, some assistance is usually required. This occurs more frequently with elderly patients and children. The simplest methods of aiding evacuation may be tried first, such as mild cathartics, the introduction of a thin glycerin suppository, or a small oil retention enema followed by a small cleansing enema. If the feces should become impacted, more drastic measures may need to be employed, such as digital removal or instrumental removal through an anoscope. The occurrence of very small bowel movements or of diarrhea should be noted and reported to the surgeon, for it may indicate the presence of fecal impaction.

Abdominal distention and gas pains occur very commonly after an operation, and in some cases cause more discomfort than the operation itself. Although cutting and burning the intestine produce no painful sensation, stretching it, as occurs with gas distention, is extremely painful.

Usually gas pains develop after the first 24 hours, and last only a few days, or until the patient is able to regain more normal activity. It is estimated that about 70 per cent of all gas reaching the gastrointestinal tract comes from swallowed air.[28] Under normal conditions its expulsion is aided by peristalsis and daily exercise. Postoperatively, however, peristalsis is decreased and the patient's activity is limited. The accumulation of gas, therefore, may stretch the intestine to an enormous size, and all attempts to expel it may be unsuccessful. Segments of the bowel often undergo spastic contractions, causing the pain to be intermittent and cramplike in character.

Distention with gas may be due to a variety of causes. According to a study by Edward J. Ottenheimer[29] on 400 surgical patients, the average incidence of gas pains in 300 abdominal operations was 70 per cent. Two factors were especially noted. Rest of the gastrointestinal tract, with the patient taking nothing by mouth following surgery, tended to decrease the incidence; and the degree of trauma during surgery was in direct proportion to its occurrence postoperatively. Although the more obvious and frequent cause is extensive exposure and handling of the gastrointestinal tract, Ottenheimer's study showed that the incidence of gas pains in 50 herniorrhaphies was 50 per cent and in 50 extra-abdominal operations 23 per cent. Thus, it may occur as a reflex phenomenon following other types of surgery besides gastrointestinal. Other factors which increase distention are certain drugs and anesthetic agents, postoperative inactivity, and inflammatory processes, such as peritonitis. Diet can be an important source of gas production. According to a study by Jacob Fine and Walter S. Levenson[30] on the effect of foods on postoperative distention, drinks that are high in glucose content, such as orange juice, cause considerable distention. The more slowly they are absorbed, the more gas is produced, owing to the greater time interval for bacterial fermentation. Also, milk is a prolific generator of gas. Other carbohydrate and protein foods, especially semisolids such as toast, cereal, and eggs produce very little gas.[31] There is some belief that extremely cold liquids lessen peristalsis and thereby increase distention.

Gas pains can usually be minimized, and in many cases prevented, or relieved by conscientious nursing. Eliminating gas-forming foods from the diet and instructing the patient to swallow less air, especially while drinking, are helpful measures. Frequent changes in position and ambulation will do much toward preventing the accumulation of gas, and will also help in its expulsion. With the doctor's permission, inserting a tube in the rectum is often sufficient to start the expulsion of gas. Application of heat to the abdomen may give relief, and can be used alone or in conjunction with a rectal tube. Occasionally the surgeon will prescribe drugs which stimulate the contraction of the intestinal muscles, such as vasopressin (Pitressin), surgical vasopressin (surgical Pituitrin), and more recently bethanechol (Urecholine), usually in combination with a rectal tube. In some cases it may be necessary for the surgeon to introduce a tube nasally to decompress the stomach or intestines. If the cessation of peristalsis continues for many days or for weeks, this is known as paralytic ileus, and is discussed on page 1040.

13. NAUSEA AND VOMITING

Almost invariably nausea and vomiting follow surgery with general anesthesia; and occasionally they follow local and regional anesthesia as well. Nausea usually procedes vomiting, but it may also occur alone. This sensation, which occurs at the back of the throat or pit of the stomach, is caused by an increased tension upon the walls of the stomach or duodenum, or by distention of the lower end of the esophagus. Vomiting occurs as a reflex movement in which the abdominal muscles forcibly contract against the stomach and eject its contents. The condition producing nausea and vomiting can be local trauma, action of drugs, or a strong emotion. Postural changes of the viscera, as occurs with motion, may also produce it. Sometimes, when the stomach is empty, and the muscular contractions are violent without being able to produce vomiting, retching occurs.[32]

Postoperative nausea with or without vomiting usually occurs when the gag reflex returns, and may continue from one to several hours after the patient regains consciousness. This may be due to various reasons, including the effects of the anesthetic or drugs, especially ether and morphine, or to the local trauma produced with abdominal surgery. Sometimes temporary paralysis of the stomach and intestines, accompanied by the swallowing of air with resultant distention, is the responsible mechanism. Certain nervous persons vomit more readily and may continue to do so for a longer period of time than others. It is estimated that women vomit about twice as frequently as men.[33] In general, vomiting does not usually persist beyond the first day. If it does, more serious complications may be the cause, such as peritonitis or intestinal obstruction.

Nausea and vomiting cause considerable discomfort, and may, with certain types of surgery, be hazardous because it strains the suture line or causes undue fluid and electrolyte loss. In cases where vomiting is hazardous to the success of the operation, or to the condition of the patient, the surgeon usually introduces a tube into the stomach preoperatively or immediately following surgery. This is to provide drainage and to keep the area at rest.

Various measures may be used to prevent or relieve postoperative nausea and vomiting. The nurse should realize that nausea tends to increase with motion. Thus it sometimes presents a conflict with early mobilization. In changing the patient's position it should be done slowly and with extreme gentleness. Oftentimes the administration of a sedative such as phenobarbital will decrease nausea by inducing rest. On the other hand narcotics such as morphine may increase it. Carl J. Rudolph and others[34] have reported excellent results in the management of postoperative nausea and vomiting with the use of dimenhydrinate (Dramamine), which is also used for motion sickness. (See p. 1166 for a discussion of its action.) They believe that a toxic labyrinthitis develops from high concentrations of the anesthetic agent in the blood stream during anesthesia. The prophylactic dose is 100 mg (1.7 gr) administered orally ½ hour before surgery; and the therapeutic dose is 100 mg (1.7 gr) in 20 cc saline administered by rectum. R. J. Minnitt suggests the use of insulin (5 units), given as a prophylactic dose before surgery or therapeutically in the postoperative period. Drinking fluids, although they may temporarily increase vomiting, will at the same time remove the anesthetic from the stomach and eventually stop it. Some additional considerations are discussed by Elman.

In a few patients solid foods will be tolerated better than liquids. Anything very much desired by the patient is not apt to produce nausea. A patient who is allowed up and about early is not as likely to suffer nausea and vomiting as much as one who must remain in the horizontal position.*

Instructing the patient to breathe deeply is another means which often proves helpful.

For the patient who is vomiting, the head should be turned to one side and an emesis basin conveniently placed. By supporting the patient's head firmly, the nurse

* Elman, Robert: *Surgical Care: A Practical Physiologic Guide.* Appleton-Century-Crofts, Inc., New York, 1951, pp. 308-9.

can prevent excessive movement and relieve some of the strain involved. It is undesirable to keep an emesis basin within sight of the patient, because the power of suggestion may in itself induce vomiting. The basin should, however, be easily reached. The face should be kept clean and dry, and the room well ventilated and free from odor. If nausea and vomiting continue, it may be necessary to put the gastrointestinal tract at rest by insertion of an intragastric tube, if one is not already present, or by the resumption of parenteral feedings. Excessive vomiting causes dehydration and loss of electrolytes, which in turn causes further nausea and vomiting as well as hindering the body's reparative process. Since the fluid will need to be replaced by the parenteral route, it is important for the nurse to observe and record the type, amount, and frequency of vomitus, as well as the amount of fluid taken by mouth.

Reassurance and measures of cleanliness are definitely indicated with patients who are nauseated or vomiting, since the psychogenic element is important. Thoughtful nursing can contribute greatly to a more rapid alleviation of the symptom. Although it is not always possible to differentiate the psychogenic causes from the physical, it should nevertheless be realized that emotional response to factors such as a disagreeable odor, foul-tasting mouth, fear, or resentment can certainly aggravate or perpetuate an "upset stomach" no matter what the original cause. It is therefore wise for the nurse to use a combination of physical and psychological measures in caring for patients with this disturbing symptom.[35, 36]

14. DIET

The postoperative diet is prescribed by the doctor in accordance with the type of operation and the condition of the patient. Usually water may be given as soon as nausea and vomiting cease, and, in some instances, even before that clear liquids such as tea and bouillon are frequently given as soon as the patient is able to tolerate them. Milk and cocoa are generally avoided for the first day or so because they are retained in the stomach for a relatively long period of time and because they produce gas. Other foods known to cause gas distention should also be avoided. (These are mentioned on p. 1034.) The fluids administered should be cool, not ice cold or tepid. It is believed that very cold fluids cause distention by lessening peristalsis, and that ice chips increase the patient's thirst. Tepid water may act as an emetic, increasing nausea and vomiting.

If there has been no abdominal incision or surgical involvement of the gastrointestinal tract, a regular diet is usually prescribed as soon as the effect of the anesthetic disappears. If there was surgery on the gastrointestinal tract, diet is advanced more slowly. Soft solid foods, such as cereals, eggs, and custard, are usually given for a day or two preceding the regular diet. It is often easier for the patient to retain solid food which he enjoys, than a liquid diet to which he is unaccustomed.[37]

Flexibility in the diet to conform with the patient's preferences helps to increase the patient's comfort and promote his recovery. This alone may not suffice in many instances, however. Since patients often cannot eat or do not relish all the foods served on a hospital diet, the foods consumed by the average postoperative patient tend to be deficient in protein and vitamins, so necessary for tissue healing. It should be realized that blood loss and wound drainage result in loss of protein, and excessive perspiration in loss of vitamin C; both of these are necessary for healing and body repair. Consequently, the role of blood transfusions, diet, and dietary supplements are of major significance. Often it is necessary to administer protein and vitamin supplements parenterally when satisfactory levels cannot otherwise be maintained. The nurse, then, should consider the dietary intake of her patient as conscientiously as she considers the administration of an important medication. Effort should be made to serve foods and supplements that are palatable, and the value of protein and vitamins in wound healing explained to the patient.[38, 39]

15. POSTOPERATIVE COMPLICATIONS

Following operations, various conditions may develop which delay the patient's recovery from the surgical procedure and may prolong his convalescence. It is a responsibility of the nurse attending the surgical patient to know the signs and symptoms of the more common postoperative discomforts and complications and to report them promptly. Accurate observation and detailed recording, as well as verbal reporting, help to ensure early treatment of complications. Prompt treatment often keep them from becoming major hazards.

There are two main groups of complications: (1) general conditions and (2) other sequelae relating to breathing and maintenance of the circulation, nutrition, and elimination.

General Postoperative Complications. One of the most serious complications is *shock* which may develop during or following an operation. This condition is discussed in detail in Chapter 40.

Another complication is *hemorrhage* which may occur at the time of operation or later on, after the patient has returned to the clinical unit. Hemorrhage is discussed in Chapter 36.

As mentioned earlier in this chapter (p. 1023), relief of *pain* in the immediate postoperative period is very important. As the patient regains consciousness, he is increasingly aware of pain and discomfort; both may be further aggrevated by outside stimuli.

If the postoperative patient is a diabetic, for example. careful skin care is indicated to prevent the development of *bedsores*. Frequent changes of position are necessary to avoid a local anemia from continued pressure on bony prominences. Surgery, however, rarely necessitates sufficient immobility to promote the formation of bedsores. For a detailed discussion of the prevention of decubiti, see Chapter 15.

Wound *infection* is indicated by an increased pulse rate and an elevated temperature. The nurse observes the vital signs closely and takes and records them as ordered by the physician, usually every four hours day and night for the first 24 to 48 hours postoperatively. The treatment and nursing care of patients with wounds and localized infections are discussed in Chapter 36.

Postoperative Respiratory Complications.   Two common pulmonary complications which may occur postoperatively are *atelectasis* and *pneumonia*. A primary cause is incomplete aeration of the lungs with the formation of a mucous plug that closes one of the bronchi entirely; this, in turn, causes atelectasis or a collapse of the pulmonary tissue beyond the plug. The nurse should watch the depth of the patient's respirations as well as the rate, and she helps him turn from side to side at intervals of not more than an hour unless he is getting needed sleep. Frequent change of position helps the patient breathe more deeply and occasionally may induce coughing that dislodges the mucous plug. Patients will avoid coughing because it shakes the body and causes discomfort so that the nurse should persuade them of its value. The physician may order a blow bottle to stimulate deeper respirations. In this treatment the patient exhales into a piece of tubing, equipped with a wooden mouthpiece; he must exhale with enough force to create bubbles in the blow bottle.* The patient is encouraged to use the blow bottle every hour or as ordered by the physician; this procedure may be continued until the patient is ambulatory. In some cases, the doctor may prescribe carbon dioxide inhalations.

If the mucous plug is not dislodged and inadequate aeration of the lungs persists, the patient may develop bronchopneumonia. Treatment usually consists of forcing fluids and a highly nutritional diet, continuing bed rest, and using appropriate chemotherapy; in addition, the physician may prescribe an expectorant. Abdominal distention must be watched for and prevented if possible since it increases respiratory embarrassment.

Older patients who have sustained a fractured femur or pelvis which necessitates a long stay in bed may develop *hypostatic pneumonia*. Early physical signs include a slight elevation of temperature, increased pulse and respiratory rates, and occasionally a slight cough. It is important for the nurse to help or encourage the patient to change his position at least hourly. It is also important that the posture allow for full chest expansion (see Chapter 15). In most cases the person breathes more easily if the head and shoulders are elevated.

Bronchitis is a complication that may develop and is effectively treated by steam inhalations (see Fig. 159). For a discussion of this treatment see Chapter 25.

Pulmonary embolism may occur during convalescence, most frequently during the second week after the operation. A pulmonary embolism is a foreign body in the blood stream that is carried to the heart and is forced into one of the pulmonary arteries or one of its branches by the circulation. Signs that this has happened occur suddenly, and the patient has sharp, stabbing pains in the chest and is breathless and anxious. Treatment includes placing the patient in an upright position with proper support, administering an opiate such as morphine to quiet the patient and reduce his panicky apprehension, and the administration of oxygen to ease his breathing and prevent anoxia.

---

* Water pressure against which the patient blows is established by the insertion of a piece of bent glass tubing (in a two-hole rubber stopper) to a depth of 37½ cm (15 in.) in a large bottle filled with water.

It is apparent, after a study of the subject, that most postoperative respiratory complications result from inadequate pulmonary ventilation. As a preventive, postoperative exercises in bed and early ambulation are useful. The physician evaluates the patient's general condition and postoperative progress, and allows the patient to be up as soon as possible following the surgical procedure.

Postoperative Circulatory Complications. *Thrombophlebitis* (or *femoral phlebitis with thrombosis*) is a postoperative complication that occurs more frequently after operations on the lower abdomen or in severe septic diseases such as peritonitis. A primary cause is venous stasis which tends to occur more in the elderly, in persons with varicose veins, and among those who are prone to muscular inactivity, as, for example, patients who sit for a long time in Fowler's position or in a chair with the knees flexed.

The first symptom may be a pain or cramp in the calf which the patient reports to the nurse during morning care. When this happens, the nurse has the patient remain in bed until the doctor has examined him.

In thrombophlebitis, it is important to keep the leg at rest, since even slight movement or exertion may be sufficient to dislodge the thrombus. Straining of any kind, as during defecation, should be avoided. On no account is the leg to be massaged. Elevation of the leg, on soft pillows, slightly flexed at the knee, aids the return flow of blood. Support of the bedclothes by a cradle prevents pressure on the affected area. If heat is prescribed, the cradle is equipped with light bulbs.

In addition to the above measures, the physician may institute anticoagulant therapy. Anticoagulant drugs include heparin, which is given intravenously and has prompt action, and bisdihydroxycoumarin (Dicoumarol), which may be given orally and has a delayed (24 hours) but prolonged action. The drugs may be used alone or in combination. Because these drugs depress prothrombin activity which is necessary for blood coagulation, determinations of prothrombin levels, as well as clotting time, are made frequently. The dosage, prescribed by the physician, is determined by these findings. During anticoagulant therapy, the nurse must be alert to observe and report at once any tendency to hemorrhage (e.g., nosebleed). Although the therapy does not decrease the size of the original thrombus, it does prevent continued development of the thrombus and/or other thrombi while inflammatory changes subside and the clot is given an opportunity to resolve.

If the above regimen does not prove adequate, the surgeon may ligate the femoral vein to prevent the breaking off of the thrombus or thrombi which might result in a pulmonary embolism.

The patient is restricted to bed rest until his temperature has returned to normal and has remained there for several days. Increase in the patient's activity and ambulation are determined by the physician. To aid venous flow, the physician may have the patient wear cotton elastic stockings.

Postoperative Gastrointestinal Complications. *Nausea and vomiting* are perhaps the most frequent postoperative gastrointestinal symptoms; they are discussed earlier in this chapter (pp. 1034-36).

Thirst, a sign of dehydration, is another troublesome symptom after anesthesia. Dryness of the mouth and pharynx is frequently aggravated by a preoperative injection of atropine, which dries secretions. Intravenous fluids and mouth care allay thirst to a large extent. They are discussed on pages 1026 ff. and pages 1029 f.

Dryness of the mouth should be prevented since, in debilitated patients, it can cause *parotitis*. For a day or two after operation the diet is largely liquid; this means the jaws are not used for mastication, and there is little or no stimulation of parotid secretion. If the mouth is not kept meticulously clean, the inactive glands may be exposed to a massive invasion of microorganisms from the mouth through the parotid duct. The resulting parotitis may be unilateral or bilateral.

Abdominal distention and gas pains occur following an operation, especially on the abdomen, and can cause the patient a good deal of discomfort. For a more complete discussion of these postoperative symptoms, see pages 1032-34.

Abdominal distention also occurs in other conditions, such as peritonitis, where it may be a much more serious symptom, requiring drastic treatment.

Acute dilatation of the stomach and *paralytic ileus* result when the muscular walls of the stomach and small intestine are temporarily paralyzed. There is rapid enlargement of the organs through the accumulation of gas and fluid which the stomach and small intestine are unable to pass along because of atony of the walls. The stomach may also be dilated when trauma or some other factor causes a paralysis of the small intestine. Almost immediate relief is obtained by intubation which drains the affected part of the alimentary canal. For a discussion of intubation and the importance of recording the fluid intake and output, see pages 823 ff.

Disturbances of Metabolism.   Whenever physiological processes are as profoundly upset as they are likely to be by general anesthesia and surgery, problems in metabolism result. Although they range greatly in their severity, such problems include *dehydration* and *acidosis*. The reader is referred to the discussion of fluid and electrolyte balance which appears on pages 329 ff.

Hiccup (Singultus). Carl Muschenheim[40] in Russell L. Cecil and Robert F. Loeb's text describes hiccup as diaphragmatic spasm, which is only "medically important" when it is persistent. The cause is usually obscure, but protracted hiccup is associated with serious illness. According to Muschenheim, the reflex center controlling the spasm is believed to be in the upper part of the cervical cord. Both central and/or peripheral stimuli are believed to produce hiccup. The list of possible causes includes the following: gastric, intestinal, pleural, mediastinal, pericardial, or diaphragmatic irritation; or the reflex center in the cord may be stimulated by uremia, encephalitis, or other neurological conditions. Persistent hiccup as a result of surgery is not apparently understood. It is said to occur as often with operations on the abdomin and pelvis as with chest surgery. When respiratory stimulation with carbon dioxide fails, Muschenheim recommends gastric aspiration or gavage.*

Persistent hiccup rarely responds to the measures used effectively to stop a mild attack. Muschenheim advocates first trying firm traction on the tongue or pressure on the phrenic nerve in the neck. If neither of these measures is effective, he sug-

* C. E. Friedgood and C. B. Ripstein report that chlorpromazine (Thorazine) was effective in the treatment of severe hiccups in forty-six patients out of fifty. It is effective given orally or parenterally, but acts more rapidly if injected intravenously. ("Chlorpromazine [Thorazine] in the Treatment of Intractable Hiccups," *J.A.M.A.,* **157:**309, [Jan.] 1955.)

gests the use of carbon dioxide. The simplest way to give carbon dioxide is to have the patient rebreathe the air he expires into a paper bag held over his face. If the condition is not under control after this procedure, gastric lavage may remove a possible source of irritation. If hiccup still persists, the administration of 3 to 10 per cent carbon dioxide in oxygen with a mask is indicated. Overdosage induces convulsions and unconsciousness; therefore the mask should be applied for periods of not more than 5 to 10 minutes. Dizziness indicates that the treatment should be stopped. This procedure is dangerous except in the hands of a physician, an anesthetist, or a specially prepared nurse.

When all other methods fail and hiccup threatens to exhaust the patient, the surgeon may recommend an operation in which the phrenic nerve is injected in order to block the efferent impulses to the diaphragm.

Postoperative Urinary Complications. *Urinary retention* may occur after any operation, but is most frequent following operations on the lower abdomen and adjacent structures. See pages 1030 ff. for a discussion of urinary retention.

Anuria, or *suppression of urine,* is a condition in which the kidneys have ceased to excrete urine. It occurs more often after operations on the kidney, but may follow other surgical procedures. It is important to distinguish between anuria and retention of urine; generally this is possible only after a catheter has been passed into the bladder. Immediate efforts to stimulate the kidneys to function are important; fluids are forced by mouth if possible and if necessary are given intravenously. Diuretic drugs may also be prescribed by the physician. Unless anuria is corrected promptly, it results in uremia, a serious condition in which urinary constituents (waste products) are retained in the blood because the kidneys fail to excrete them.

Incontinence of urine may occur at any age but is most common postoperatively in the elderly. In some instances, an indwelling catheter may be inserted. The incontinent patient requires meticulous care to prevent the development of bedsores (see Chapter 15).

16. SPECIAL CARE OF THE TRACHEOTOMIZED PATIENT

Nature of a Tracheotomy. Tracheotomy is an operation in which a vertical incision is made in the trachea to permit the insertion of a double tracheotomy tube through which the patient breathes.

Indications. Tracheotomy may be performed as an emergency procedure when sudden, complete obstruction of the airway results from aspiration of a foreign body; edema of the larynx; infections and/or edema about the throat following operation, or occasionally for primary infections such as diphtheria; or complete postoperative vocal cord paralysis due to injury to both recurrent laryngeal nerves. Tracheotomy is also performed as a preliminary step to laryngectomy for malignant disease.[41]

Preparation of the Patient. In an emergency it may be necessary to perform this operation without any preparation. If time permits, the skin from the top of the larynx to the sternum should be carefully cleaned with appropriate antiseptic solutions, and sterile towels draped around the wound site. In both elective and emergency cases, local infiltration anesthesia is used.[42] For children and nervous, hysterical patients, a general anesthesia may be preferred; however, when there is marked dyspnea, a general anesthesia is contraindicated.

If the patient is able to comprehend, he should be told he will lose his voice temporarily following the operation and that he will breathe by means of the tube to be placed in the trachea. He should be assured that he will be able to breathe easily through the tube and therefore will be more comfortable. Knowing that someone will be with him constantly until he can assume responsibility for suctioning the tube reassures the patient and helps him relax. A calm and quiet manner on the part of the nurse also helps to lessen the patient's apprehension.

Postoperative Care.   When local anesthesia is used, the patient is placed in semi-Fowler's position; such a semisitting position makes breathing less difficult, reduces throat irritation from the tube, and helps to prevent intense, prolonged coughing. No opiate or atropine is given; morphine would depress respirations and the cough reflex, and atropine would dry secretions. However, one of the barbiturate sedatives may be given if necessary.[43]

It is desirable that a patient with a tracheotomy be in a single room. Because he will need constant nursing care until he is able to assume responsibility for suctioning the tube, everything required for his care should be assembled in the room; by so doing, the nurse, without leaving the patient, will be able to meet all nursing needs and any emergency that may arise. Special equipment includes:

1. Simple suction set: medium-sized tray covered with a face towel containing the following equipment which is clean but not sterile: (a) solution bowl with tap water (if mucus is tenacious, normal saline may be substituted); (b) 2 glass jars: one containing the obturator for tube in trachea, and the second containing 4 x 4 sterile gauze squares without cotton filling for dressings (cut to center on one side); (c) whistle-tip catheter to fit inside tracheotomy tube (cut extra holes near tip); (d) catheter tray with tap water in which catheter is placed when not in use; (e) pointed irrigating tip to attach catheter to wall suction tubing; (f) Kelly clamp (to clamp off suction when not in use); (g) small jar with unsterile mineral oil; (h) pipe cleaners (autoclaved but not kept sterile) and small brush for cleaning inner tube; (i) drainage bottle (to which 60 cc of water has been added).

2. Treatment towel containing sterile equipment which is used by the doctor when he changes the tube daily: a second tracheotomy tube (outer tube, inner tube, obturator—same size as tube in patient's throat), three-pronged tracheal dilator, 4 x 4 gauze squares without cotton filling cut down side to center, Kelly clamp.

3. Package of sterile gloves (for doctor when changing tube and dressing).

4. Complete sterile tracheotomy set (usually packaged and autoclaved by a central supply service or, occasionally, by the operating room).

5. Small tank of oxygen equipped with a catheter (when given, oxygen is administered by catheter directly into tracheotomy tube).

6. Steam inhalator to moisten air in unit; uncut 4 x 4 gauze squares without cotton filling to cover opening of tube.

7. For use of patient: (a) paper wipes; (b) paper bag pinned to bed within easy reach; (c) mirror; (d) pencil and paper or "magic" slate; (e) tap bell or signal cord to call floor nurse, when private nurse is no longer necessary.

Care of the tracheotomy tube is an important factor in the postoperative period. Tubes may be made of sterling silver or silver plate as well as rubber and plastic. The type selected will be determined by the length of time the tube is to remain in the trachea, the cost, and the preference of the patient and the doctor. Double tubes are used so that when the inner tube is to be inspected for mucus and cleaned, it may be removed by releasing the key, cleaned with cold running water* and pipe

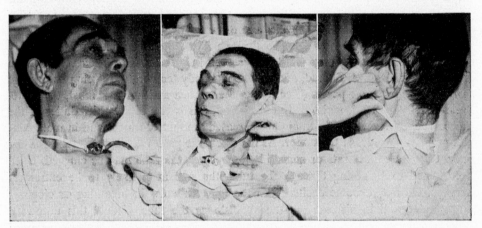

Figure 244. (*Left*) Nurse reinserts moistened inner cannula when suctioning has been completed. (*Center*) Nurse replaces gauze square beneath top of outer tube. Note that the square has been cut partially to permit easy replacement. Such protection of the skin of the patient's throat is important. (*Right*) Final step is the placement of a bib over the tube. The bib tape is tied on the opposite side from the knot in the tapes which hold the outer cannula in place. A bow knot is used for the bib tape; a square knot for the tube tape. (Courtesy of Bellevue Hospital, New York City, and Clay-Adams Co., New York City.)

cleaners or a small brush, and reinserted. The outer tube is held in place with tapes, tied with a square knot, that encircle the neck; it is important that the tapes be securely, but not too snugly, fastened. The outer tube is removed only by the doctor when he is changing the tube daily; it is never removed by the nurse. A layer of soft sterile gauze is placed between the plate of the outer tube and the skin; it is inserted by pulling gently the cut gauze square from below upward. The uncut area of the gauze below the tube will protect the skin of the neck from irritating mucous discharges; when soiled, the gauze square is changed by the nurse. In addition, whenever discharges are profuse, a towel may be placed across the chest, below the tube.

Careful handling of tracheotomy tubes is important; when they are made of a

---

* If the mucus is particularly tenacious, the inner tube is placed in a bowl to which hydrogen peroxide has been added to the tap water.

soft metal, they can be easily dented. A dented inner tube does not slip readily into the outer cannula. A part of one tube is not interchangeable with a similar part of another set of tubes; therefore, each set of three parts must be kept intact. Each tube consists of: (1) an outer cannula to which the retaining tapes are fastened; (2) an obturator, an olive-tipped curved rod, that is used to guide the outer cannula into the tracheal opening; and (3) an inner cannula that is inserted into the outer cannula after the obturator has been withdrawn. The two tape ties are usually about 16 in. long and 1 in. wide. To avoid knots that might press on the front of the patient's neck, the following method is recommended: (1) make a horizontal slit about 1 in. from the end of each tape; (2) slip the ends of the tapes through the vertical openings in the plate of the outer tube; and (3) thread the uncut ends of the tapes through the horizontal slits and draw smoothly and snugly into place.

As the patient must now breathe through this tube and is entirely dependent upon it, the greatest vigilance must be observed in his care. The *inspired air,* which is normally moistened, filtered, and warmed to body temperature during its passage through the nose, now passes directly into the trachea and lungs. It must, therefore, be artificially warmed, moistened, and filtered; this is one of the chief duties of the nurse. The *expired air* will contain an increased amount of mucus and in malignancies perhaps particles of the tumor. As the discharge passes through the tube and the patient cannot expectorate or control it in any way, the tube may be clogged. Until accustomed to breathing through the tube, the patient is likely to be extremely nervous. He may become excited with the least difficulty in breathing or clogging of the tube, and in his excitement may dislodge the tube. Should this untoward event occur, the nurse keeps the tracheal incision patent with a three-pronged dilator until the doctor arrives to insert a second tracheotomy tube that is kept in the unit, ready for use. Immediate action is essential to prevent asphyxiation.

In order artificially to moisten, filter, and warm the inhaled air to body temperature, the following methods are used: (1) Gauze squares, dampened with warm sterile water or normal saline, are kept over the mouth of the tube; they are held in place by another piece of tape (36 in. long) and suspended bib-fashion over the opening of the tube; they are changed when dry or when soiled. There must never be any loose threads in the gauze, as they might accidentally get into the tube and trachea and strangle the patient. It is important that the room be meticulously clean to reduce dust in the air. The temperature of the room is kept at about 26.7° C (80° F) if possible. (2) A steam inhalator, with or without a croup tent, that warms and moistens the air gives great comfort to the patient. Chilling drafts are to be avoided for there is always danger of pneumonia. Too saturated an atmosphere is also to be avoided.

The patient is never left alone if there is danger of a clogged inner tube. The inner tube is removed and cleaned as often as indicated; this may be every few minutes, every hour, or every two or three hours, depending upon the condition of the patient. Any manipulation about the wound during suctioning or when inserting the inner tube or applying a clean gauze dressing must be done gently to prevent irritation since violent coughing attacks could dislodge the tube and such attacks always make it difficult for the patient to breathe.*

Any secretion from the mouth of the tube is wiped away quickly to prevent its aspiration into the cannula. Immediately after operation, the mucus may be slightly blood-tinged. This should disappear gradually. Bloody mucus that persists may indicate hemorrhage. The nurse suctions the outer tube frequently, every 15 minutes the first day, or more often. Suction should be gentle to avoid injury to mucous membranes. The size of the whistle-tip catheter is determined by the size of the tracheotomy tube. The catheter should also have numerous openings near the tip to make adequate suctioning possible. Deeper aspiration is performed only by the physician.

Suggested Procedure for Suctioning Tube. (1) Remove catheter from catheter tray. (2) Loosen Kelly clamp to turn on wall suction. (3) Place catheter tip in solution basin to draw water through catheter. (4) Pinch catheter to shut off suction temporarily; place tip in mineral oil and touch to clean gauze square to remove excess oil; release suction. (5) Pinch catheter and insert about 5 in. through outer tube into trachea; release pressure on catheter and suction gently, moving catheter slightly in and out. Remove catheter from trachea as necessary to keep patient's respiratory rate at a regular rhythm. Reinsert catheter and continue suctioning until outer tube is clean. (6) Tip of catheter is placed in solution basin and solution sucked through catheter until it is clean. Catheter is clamped and placed in catheter tray; it is fastened to the towel on the tray with the Kelly clamp.

Note: When the subject is a child, tip the head back by placing a quilted pad under the shoulders (a child may be uncooperative or may not be able to hold his head back as instructed).

Charting. Record the amount and character of the mucus, frequency of suctioning, any bleeding through and around the tube, and condition of the skin of the neck. Also record any observed changes in the patient's breathing, color, pulse rate, and temperature; noting the patient's mental outlook is important too.

Daily Care and Rehabilitation. As the patient's condition improves, the nurse helps him learn how to suction the tube. She explains the parts of the tube and how they work, and helps him carry out the procedure several times, or oftener if necessary, before the patient is asked to do it unaided but with the nurse watching him. Only when the patient has carried out the procedure satisfactorily on a number of occasions can the physician and the nurse be certain he clearly understands it.

A mirror enables the patient to see the tube in his throat, to wipe away secretions, and to suction the tube, first with the nurse's assistance and later on by himself. When the patient assumes responsibility for the suctioning, he may ask that the moistened gauze square over the tube be omitted; he may feel more confident about the suctioning if he does not have to remove the square to see the opening and to manipulate the catheter.

Keep about 60 cc of water in the drainage bottle; the water prevents the

---

* Depending upon the patient's general condition, the physician may instruct the patient to cough *gently* every 5 to 10 minutes to help him dispel mucous secretions and so keep the inner tube patent.

tenacious mucus from adhering to the inside, which makes it difficult to clean the collection bottle. The suction apparatus should be thoroughly cleaned at least once a day (more often as indicated) by washing with soapy water, rinsing well, and then boiling the articles of which it is composed. Another suction setup should be in the patient's room so that he is never left without this equipment.

Every time the inner tube is removed for aspiration it is inspected for adherent discharges and, when soiled, cleaned before reinsertion. The tube is cleaned with cold running water and pipe cleaners or a small brush; occasionally it may be necessary to moisten and draw a gauze square through the tube with a Kelly clamp. Cotton or a cotton-tipped applicator is *not* used since there is great danger of the cotton tip being retained in the narrow tube, thereby asphyxiating the patient. Final inspection of the inner tube's lumen is essential before it is reinserted by the nurse.

After the daily changing of tubes by the doctor, they are cleaned and sterilized. If the silver is tarnished, it is polished before sterilizing the individual parts. Sterling silver or silver plate tubes are boiled in water for 10 minutes or autoclaved; plastic tubes may be boiled, autoclaved, or immersed in cold germicidal agents.* The inner and outer tubes and the obdurator are then packaged in a sterile towel, labeled, and returned to the unit.

The patient's diet, his comfort, rest, sleep, and all other factors that keep up his strength demand the most scrupulous attention. Oral feedings can usually be started immediately after the operation when the anesthesia has been local; infrequently nasal feedings may be necessary. After the patient has become accustomed to the tracheotomy tube, the liquid diet is supplemented with soft solids that are easily swallowed. The mouth is cleaned before and after each feeding.

The mental attitude of the patient plays an important part in his adjustment to this unnatural, and at first possibly alarming, situation. Actually, the tube in the trachea cannot interfere with swallowing, because the cartilaginous rings do not completely encircle the esophagus; therefore, there is no pressure of the trachea upon the esophagus that might interfere with deglutition. If the patient is apprehensive about swallowing liquids and soft foods, the nurse can suggest he lean forward slightly. Because the patient can carry out this action easily, he will feel more relaxed.

Another source of distress to the patient is difficulty in speaking or inability to speak. Even though the patient is provided with pencil and paper or a "magic" slate for communication with the nurse, he may still not feel relaxed and may try to speak. The nurse should anticipate his needs, and especially in the immediate post-operative period when the physician may prescribe complete silence to rest the edematous tissue and promote healing. However, after the patient is ambulatory and able to care for the tracheotomy tube, he should be encouraged to speak. Placing a finger over the mouth of the tube while talking will enable him to speak (this

---

* Several examples of such agents include benzalkonium chloride (aqueous Zephiran chloride) and 70 per cent alcohol; the parts of the tube are rinsed with sterile normal saline after immersion for the prescribed period.

method is generally demonstrated by another tracheostomy patient). Although the speech of patients with a permanent tracheostomy tube (or laryngostomy tube) is altered, they can be understood without much difficulty. It is important for others to make an effort to understand what the patient is saying so that he does not have to repeat. Such a situation is embarrassing since many patients are sensitive about the tube in the throat and the way their voice sounds.

When the tracheotomy tube is removed before the patient leaves the hospital, it is done gradually to permit the patient to become accustomed to breathing normally. The method of gradual withdrawal of the tube is called *decannulation.* It may be accomplished by partially obstructing the airway with a cork. If the patient tolerates a small cork without untoward respiratory signs, larger corks may be used progressively until the entire opening has been closed off.[44] When the patient tolerates complete obstruction of the tracheotomy tube, it is removed by the surgeon, and the opening permitted to heal. As a rule the corks are fastened to the tracheotomy tube with a thread.

Before the patient is discharged with a tracheostomy tube in place, the physician and nurse must be certain that the patient understands all details for caring for the tube and that he has had ample experience in self-care. If the patient is a child, the mother or some other responsible adult must be carefully instructed in all details of care. So far as appearance is concerned, the nurse suggests to a woman patient that a scarf or similar tie can be worn to cover the tube in the throat. Generally a man's shirt collar will cover the tube.

Danger of aspirating water through the opening in the throat is also discussed with the patient, and he is told that because of this danger he must *not* go swimming and that he must be cautious in taking a shower. Since a laryngostomy opening is about ½ to ¾ in. in diameter and is located below the cough reflex area, a patient could drown should he fall asleep in the tub; for this reason, a daily shower is strongly recommended instead of a tub bath.

Explanations to members of the patient's family are needed so that each individual will do his utmost to assist the patient in returning to and maintaining a normal way of living. Persons who have made a good adjustment to laryngostomies can be very helpful to others who have the same problem. In some large cities such persons have formed clubs (affiliated with a national organization), since they find comfort and encouragement in the society of those who thoroughly understand their difficulties.

REFERENCES

1. Mason, Robert L., and Zintel, Harold A. (eds.): *Preoperative and Postoperative Treatment,* 2nd ed. W. B. Saunders Co., Philadelphia, 1946, p. 97.
2. Macintosh, R. R., and Bannister, Freda B.: *Essentials of General Anesthesia,* 5th ed. Blackwell Scientific Publications, Oxford, Eng., 1952, pp. 288-89.
3. Conboy, Catherine F.: "A Recovery Room," *Am. J. Nursing,* **47:**686-87, (Oct.) 1947.
4. Carnahan, Julie M.: "Recovery Room for Postoperative Patients," *Am. J. Nursing,* **49:**581-82, (Sept.) 1949.

5. Tourish, William J., and Wagner, Frederick B.: *Preoperative and Postoperative Care.* F. A. Davis Co., Philadelphia, 1947, p. 43.

6. Elman, Robert: *Surgical Care: A Practical Physiological Guide.* Appleton-Century-Crofts, Inc., New York, 1951, p. 287.

7. Ilgenfritz, Hugh C.: *Preoperative and Postoperative Care of Surgical Patients,* 2nd ed. C. V. Mosby Co., St. Louis, 1948, pp. 112-14.

8. Minnitt, R. J.: "Some Aspects of Modern Anesthesia," *M. Press,* **225**:159, (Feb.) 1951.

9. Spalding, J. E., and Lord, M. S.: "Fowler's Position," *Lancet,* **1**:643-45, (May 4) 1946.

10. Ilgenfritz, Hugh C.: *op. cit.,* pp. 114-16.

11. Flagg, P. J.: *The Art of Anesthesia.* J. B. Lippincott Co., Philadelphia, 1939, p. 426.

12. Winkley, Ruth: "When a Child Must Go to the Hospital," *Child,* **17**:34-36, (Nov.) 1952.

13. Jessner, Lucie, and Kaplan, Samuel: "Observations on the Emotional Reactions of Children to Tonsillectomy and Adenoidectomy." A Preliminary Report in *Problems of Infancy and Childhood* (Transactions of the Third Conference, May 7-8, 1949), Josiah Macy, Jr. Foundation, New York, pp. 97-156.

14. Winfield, James M.; Fox, Charles L., Jr.; and Mersheimer, Walter L.: "Etiologic Factors in Postoperative Salt Retention and Its Prevention," *Ann. Surg.,* **134**:626-40, (Oct.) 1951.

15. Moore, F. D.: "Adaptation of Supportive Treatment to Needs of the Surgical Patient," *J.A.M.A.,* **141**:646-53, (Nov. 5) 1949.

16. Danowski, T. S.: "Newer Concepts of the Role of Potassium in Disease," *Am. J. Med.,* **7**:525-31, (Oct.) 1949.

17. Goodall, J. W. D.: "Early Ambulation: A Survey of Hospital Practice," *Lancet,* **1**:43-46, (Jan. 6) 1951.

18. Burch, J. C., and Fisher, H. C.: "Early Ambulation in Abdominal Surgery," *Ann. Surg.,* **124**:791-98, (Oct.) 1946.

19. Leithauser, Daniel J.: "Early Ambulation," *Am. J. Nursing,* **50**:203-6, (Apr.) 1950.

20. Elman, Robert: *op. cit.,* p. 154.

21. Ilgenfritz, Hugh C.: *op. cit.,* pp. 385-86.

22. Ficarra, Bernard J.: "Postoperative Fetor Oris," *Rev. Gastroenterol.,* **17**:1151-52, (Dec.) 1950.

23. Ilgenfritz, Hugh C.: *op. cit.,* p. 328.

24. McLaughlin, Charles W., Jr., and Brown, John R.: "Postoperative Urinary Retention," *U.S. Naval M. Bull.,* **42**:1025-32, (May) 1944.

25. Crile, George, Jr., and Shively, Franklin L., Jr.: *Hospital Care of the Surgical Patient,* 2nd ed. Charles C Thomas, Publisher, Springfield, Ill., 1946, pp. 99-100.

26. Ilgenfritz, Hugh C.: *op. cit.,* pp. 330-31.

27. Mason, Robert L., and Zintel, Harold A. (eds.): *op. cit.,* p. 113.

28. Cantor, Meyer O.: *Intestinal Intubation.* Charles C Thomas, Publisher, Springfield, Ill., 1949, p. 78.

29. Ottenheimer, Edward J.: "Postoperative Gas Pains," *New England J. Med.,* **213**:608-14, (Sept. 26) 1935.

30. Fine, Jacob, and Levenson, Walter S.: "Effect of Foods on Postoperative Distention." *Am. J. Surg.,* **21**:184-203, (Aug.) 1933.

31. Fine, Jacob, and Starr, Arnold: "Intestinal Distention," *Rev. Gastroenterol.,* **6**:419-22, (Sept.-Oct.) 1939.

32. Best, Charles H., and Taylor, Norman B.: *The Physiological Basis of Medical Practice,* 5th ed. Williams & Wilkins Co., Baltimore, 1950, pp. 603-4, 821-22.

33. Harris, T. A. B.: *The Mode of Action of Anesthetics.* E. and S. Livingstone, Ltd., Edinburgh, 1951, pp. 632-33.

34. Rudolph, Carl J.; Park, D. Davis; and Hamilton, Charles: "Treatment of Postanesthesia Nausea and Vomiting," *J.A.M.A.,* **144**:1283, (Dec. 9) 1951.

35. Felter, Robert; West, Frances; and Zetzsche, Lydia M.: *Surgical Nursing,* 6th ed. F. A. Davis Co., Philadelphia, 1952, pp. 124-25.
36. West, John P.; Keller, Manelva W.; and Harmon, Elizabeth H.: *Nursing Care of the Surgical Patient,* 5th ed. The Macmillan Company, 1950, pp. 119-20.
37. Cooper, Lenna F.; Barber, Edith M.; Mitchell, Helen S.; and Rynbergen, Henderika J.: *Nutrition in Health and Disease,* 12th ed. J. B. Lippincott Co., Philadelphia, 1953, Chapter 32.
38. Levenson, Stanley M., et al.: "The Healing of Soft Tissue Wounds: The Effects of Nutrition, Anemia and Age," *Surgery,* **28:**905, (Nov.) 1950.
39. Wolfer, John A., et al.: "An Experimental Study in Wound Healing in Vitamin C Depleted Human Subjects," *Surg., Gynec. & Obst.,* **84:**1-15, (Jan.) 1947.
40. Cecil, Russell L., and Loeb, Robert F. (eds.): *A Textbook of Medicine,* 9th ed. W. B. Saunders Co., Philadelphia, 1955, p. 1074.
41. Cutler, Elliott E., and Zollinger, Robert M.: *Atlas of Surgical Operations,* 2nd ed. The Macmillan Company, New York, 1949, p. 20.
42. Cutler, Elliott E., and Zollinger, Robert M.: *op. cit.,* p. 20.
43. West, John P.; Keller, Manelva W.; and Harmon, Elizabeth: *op. cit.,* pp. 165, 168.
44. West, John P.; Keller, Manelva W.; and Harmon, Elizabeth: *op. cit.,* p. 169.

Additional Suggested Reading

Bird, Brian: "Psychological Aspects of Preoperative and Postoperative Care," *Am. J. Nursing,* **55:**685, (June) 1955.
Brookes, H. S., and Castile, Pearl: *A Textbook of Surgical Nursing,* 2nd ed. C. V. Mosby Co., St. Louis, 1940.
Cabot, Richard C., and Dicks, Russell L.: *The Art of Ministering to the Sick.* The Macmillan Company, New York, 1936.
Eliason, E. L.; Ferguson, L. K.; and Sholtis, L. A.: *Surgical Nursing,* 9th ed. J. B. Lippincott Co., Philadelphia, 1950.
Stanton, Joseph R.: "Venous Thrombosis and Pulmonary Embolism," *Am. J. Nursing,* **55:**709, (June)1955.
Tracy, M. A., and others: *Nursing—an Art and a Science,* 3rd ed. C. V. Mosby Co., St. Louis, 1949.

CHAPTER 40. TREATMENT AND NURSING CARE OF THE PATIENT IN SHOCK

1. DEFINITION

There has been a tendency in the past to designate a related group of symptoms following injury as "shock" and to describe a similar bodily state as "collapse" when it is not associated with accidents or surgery. Currently, the term "shock" is applied to the syndrome characterized by acute prostration and circulatory collapse from almost any cause. Five surgeons in different sections of Frederick Christopher's textbook[1] of surgery discuss traumatic shock, and there are many other references to the condition; there is as much emphasis on "shock" in Russell L. Cecil and Robert F. Loeb's *Textbook of Medicine*[2] with more space devoted to the treatment of shock from specific causes. In the index of the medical text "collapse, circulatory" is followed by references to pages that deal with "shock" or "circulatory collapse and shock."

Eugene A. Stead, Jr., under the latter title says: "The terms 'circulatory collapse' and 'shock' are used to describe the clinical appearance of patients with circulatory insufficiency in which the usual signs of congestive heart failure are absent."* He describes the "shock syndrome" as produced by six types of pathology although he says repeatedly that several or all of these changes in body function may be involved and that there are still unknown factors in shock. Alfred Blalock discussing traumatic shock says:

The word shock is applied to practically all types of acute peripheral circulatory failure, regardless of cause or of multiplicity of causes. The grouping together under one term of a variety of conditions, some of which have little relationship to one another,

---

* Cecil, Russell L., and Loeb, Robert F. (eds.): *Textbook of Medicine,* 9th ed. W. B. Saunders Co., Philadelphia, 1955, p. 1261.

has made definition unsatisfactory and classification difficult. Attempts to substitute more exact terminology have resulted in failure.*

While the medical dictionaries consulted associate "shock" with injury oι trauma, in contradistinction to "collapse" or circulatory impairment from other causes, usage does not support these differentiations. "Electric shock" and "insulin shock" are common medical and lay terms, and none of us would hesitate to say that a friend was so "shocked" by bad news that she fainted. In none of these cases is the cause physical trauma in the ordinary sense. In the first case it is an electric charge, in the second a chemical, and in the third a psychic stimulus. It might be helpful in summary to point out that "shock" is the more general term used to describe a depressed bodily state of varying severity and duration; symptoms may vary from sensations of weakness, dizziness, and nausea, typical of fainting, to the disturbance of consciousness and the profound prostration of all vital functions seen in a person who has been hemorrhaging, in one who has been thrown from a moving vehicle, or in the diabetic whose early signs of insulin shock have been unrecognized and untreated. In each case a "shock syndrome" is observed as the vital organs are deprived of circulating fluids of physiological quantity, or quality.

For nurses as well as doctors it is essential to think in terms of the causes of shock and circulatory collapse. A rational system of treatment depends upon a knowledge of the cause and the resulting physical changes.

2. CAUSES

There is one undisputed cause of shock—blood loss. It is generally agreed that shock may result from loss of whole blood, as in hemorrhage, or loss of plasma that seeps from burns, or multiple contusions. John H. Bland says, however, that a shift in blood fluids can have the same effect as bleeding:

Traumatic shock with its immobilization of electrolyte and extracellular water is indistinguishable from medical shock due to actual loss of water and electrolyte. This chemical pathologic change should be taken into account preoperatively. In the presence of lack of circulatory integrity or impairment by shock or exposure to physical cold, the intracellular fluids of the muscles gain sodium and lose potassium. . . . In tissue anoxia from any cause, the same shift of extracellular sodium for potassium intracellulary occurs. . . . We are in the habit of thinking in terms of external losses of fluid and electrolyte and are apt not to think in terms of immobilization of water and electrolyte or internal shifts from one compartment to another. . . .†

Most authorities agree that psychic trauma alone can cause a fleeting type of shock, but rarely a profound and serious circulatory failure. As a contributory cause of secondary or profound shock all authorities agree that psychic trauma (fear,

* Christopher, Frederick (ed.): *Textbook of Surgery,* 5th ed. W. B. Saunders Co., Philadelphia, 1949, p. 1313.
† Bland, John H.: *The Clinical Use of Fluid and Electrolyte.* W. B. Saunders Co., Philadelphia, 1952, pp. 143-44.

grief, acute anxiety) is important. A great deal of work has been done to demonstrate that an increase in the permeability of the capillaries is present in shock. A number of workers believe that absolute proof of this theory is lacking. Other theories on the etiology of shock are also questioned so that Henry K. Beecher's suggestion to treat the patient on the basis of established causative factors seems wise. In a study of traumatic shock in the military services, he found that the severity of shock was in direct proportion to the amount of blood lost, and the treatment of the wounded soldier in shock was based squarely on this factor. Since what

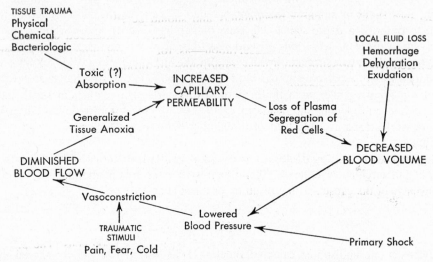

Figure 245. Process of shock. (White, Paul D.: *Heart Disease,* 4th ed. The Macmillan Company, New York, 1951.)

we call shock occurs without hemorrhage, other causes must be studied. Any factor which causes dilatation of the peripheral blood vessels, such as spinal anesthesia, operations on the sympathetic nervous system, or severe emotional trauma, may also cause a drop in blood pressure by increasing the size of the vascular bed. It is repeatedly stated, for example, that patients who are frightened preoperatively are more likely to experience shock than those who are not. Shock is said to develop more often in the old or in the very young, in the weak or poorly nourished, in those with some organic disease, in those exhausted by physical and mental strain, and in patients with heart disease or in the emotionally unstable—than in young healthy adults. It commonly follows extensive injuries, such as burns and multiple wounds where there is minimum bleeding; operations in which there has been prolonged exposure or excessive handling of the abdominal viscera; and exposure to cold. In the following pages the symptoms, treatment, and nursing care are discussed in general terms. Tabulated material on pages 1054 ff. is an effort to show some prevailing concepts on the etiology of shock and to suggest the way in which the cause explains the severity and particular character of the shock syndrome and how both of these suggest specific treatment. The material in this chapter is based largely on books edited or written by: Russell L. Cecil and Robert F. Loeb, Frederick Christopher, Robert Elman, John H. Bland, and Henry K. Beecher. It seems impractical to try to further identify the many sources of information that have been consulted. World Wars I and II have made shock one of the most extensively discussed subjects in medical literature.

3. SYMPTOMS, GENERAL TREATMENT, AND NURSING CARE

Because shock may occur precipitately and should be treated with utmost dispatch, the nurse should know its signs, and when there is likelihood of shock the patient should be under constant observation—as, for example, after major surgery. A lowered blood pressure and a weak rapid pulse are probably the most important signs. The systolic and diastolic blood pressures are indicative of the degree of shock from which the patient is suffering. A systolic pressure below 90 mm of mercury should be considered dangerous. The vital centers are considerably damaged if the systolic presure remains below 50 mm for long. Such a condition is usually terminated by death. When the systolic pressure is as low as 80 mm, it is often impossible to determine the diastolic pressure, but the lower the diastolic reading, the more profound the state of shock. Other signs of shock are apathy, pallor, and cold, moist skin. Generally, the patient is quiet and listless, but he may be anxious and apprehensive. This is particularly true if he knows his life is threatened by hemorrhage. The temperature is frequently subnormal, and the respirations may be rapid and shallow, or deep. Cyanosis may follow marked loss of blood cells. The patient does not usually lose consciousness, but may if the shock is severe or prolonged.

If sufficient precautions are taken, shock can usually be prevented in surgery. As can be seen by the study of tabulated material on pages 1054 ff., it is an inevitable accompaniment of some accidents and the terminal stage of certain diseases.

Treatment of the condition, once it develops, depends on the underlying cause. Since reduction of blood volume, by one means or another, is by far the most common cause of shock, it is essential that the volume of blood be restored as quickly as possible. A quick and easy method for supplying more blood to the vital centers is elevation of the foot of the bed, which assists venous return by gravity. The nurse may take this step if medical help is not immediately available. She must, however, remember that patients with head injuries should remain horizontal. Restoration of blood volume can be accomplished by blood transfusions, or if that is not immediately possible, by intravenous solutions of plasma, albumin, or substitutes such as dextran.* In catastrophes it is necessary for many persons to know how to give this treatment. Since the circulation is very unstable in shock, the patient should not be turned or moved and his head should not be raised during the time his blood pressure is very low, or fluctuating within a low range. The application of heat by means of hot-water bottles, extra blankets, etc., is advised now by very few

---

* Macrodex is a trade name for dextran in this country. It is made by Pharmacia Laboratories, New York City.

(*Text continued on p. 1059.*)

CAUSE	SIGNS AND SYMPTOMS	TREATMENT AND NURSING CARE
1. *Small blood volume with failure of venous return* due to: (a) Hemorrhage, internal or external, following accidents, surgery, and disease that rupture blood vessels—"hematogenic shock."	1. Patient appears ill and progresses from anxiety and fearfulness to unconsciousness unless condition is arrested.	1. Place in a recumbent position with the head lowered so that blood is concentrated in the vital organs of the heart and brain. Give barbiturates for anxiety. Medical and often religious reassurance needed.
	2. Pain may or may not be present in shock from trauma.	2. Give morphine intravenously in small doses for pain but withhold in brain injuries.
	3. Skin is pale and damp or bathed in sweat and feels cool or cold to the touch.	3. Put blanket under the patient and cover him, but do not apply extra warmth that will cause sweating and dilate the peripheral vessels. (Vasoconstriction is nature's method of maintaining hemostasis.)
	4. If conscious, he complains of thirst; nausea and vomiting are common.	4. Allow the patient to rinse his mouth but give nothing by mouth if there is a possibility that surgery is indicated. Thirst is relieved somewhat by intravenous injections. Vomiting should be encouraged in preparation for surgery. Head turned to the side, and suction used if available.
	5. Radial pulse varies greatly and even in severe traumatic shock it may be slow, but it tends to increase in rate and decrease in size with loss of blood and depth of shock, until it gets thready and running, or uncountable.	5. Keep a record of the pulse taken at intervals of 5 minutes if possible. A falling or steadying of the pulse rate is a sign that the patient is improving.
	6. Respirations may be rapid, and sighing and cyanosis are present when sufficient hemoglobin is lost.	6. Artificial respiration, oxygen administration, or use of a respirator may be indicated.
	7. Systolic and diastolic blood pressure vary with the vigor of the individual, but both fall in proportion to the loss of blood and depth of shock. Beecher gives the	7. Keep a blood pressure cuff on the arm and record the pressure at 5-minute intervals unless the patient's condition is obviously improving. (It is assumed that steps have been taken to control hemor-

CAUSE	SIGNS AND SYMPTOMS	TREATMENT AND NURSING CARE

following rough averages for vigorous wounded soldiers:

Degree of Shock	Systolic Pressure	Diastolic Pressure	Pulse Pressure
Slight	109	66	44
Moderate	95	58	36
Severe	49	25	24

Cardiographic studies show that cardiac output falls.

8. Laboratory blood analysis shows lowering of the plasma proteins and hematocrit (per cent of cells) in relation to the depth of shock although the two may progress independently.

rhage [discussed on p. 952]. Blood is given until the systolic blood pressure is rising and has reached at least 80 mm of mercury. (Robert T. Vaughn says that rapid transfusions delay clotting in hemorrhage. Most authorities urge immediate replacement in spite of this risk.)

8. Give whole blood since patient has lost whole blood. Plasma and albumin are its best substitutes. The need for blood is based to some extent on plasma protein concentration and hematocrit when these laboratory findings are available.

(b) Plasma lost from circulating fluids as in burns.

A patient in shock caused by seepage of plasma from the burned area (the secondary shock of burns) presents the picture just described, but the blood findings differ from shock caused by loss of whole blood.

Here the hematocrit is raised; or the cell count and hemoglobin are high in relation to the blood plasma, although there is loss of cells. The total volume of circulating fluid is reduced to as dangerous a point as in massive hemorrhage.

Since plasma loss is in direct relation to the area burned, and it progresses at an established rate, secondary shock in burns can usually be prevented by the parenteral administration of plasma and whole blood in appropriate quantities (see p. 1177), and water and electrolyte solutions by mouth if the patient is not vomiting. If he is, they must also be given parenterally. Secondary shock will occur in severe burns unless the patient is so treated within 2 hours of the accident. (Oliver Cope.)

(c) Dehydration or loss of water and electrolytes as in continued vomiting, diarrhea, acidosis, and a crisis in Addison's disease.

Here the volume of circulating fluid is low due to loss of water and electrolytes; blood analysis shows a high hematocrit. The nature of electrolyte loss depends upon whether fluid is lost from the stomach or intestines.

In acute adrenal cortical insufficiency (likely to occur when the person with a

Shock caused by dehydration without the conflicting factor of endocrine deficiency is treated chiefly by plasma intravenously and water and electrolytes by mouth or vein until blood findings approach normal values. Control of this type of shock is relatively simple.

Addisonian crisis demands "massive substitution therapy." (George W. Thorn.)

CAUSE	SIGNS AND SYMPTOMS	TREATMENT AND NURSING CARE
	chronic deficiency is exposed to a traumatic experience) the circulatory collapse is the result of water and electrolyte loss, low blood sugar, and vasodilation due to deficiency of the constrictor enzyme of the adrenal cortex. Typical changes are seen in the differential blood count. Thorn says in effect that in the presence of shock, gastrointestinal symptoms, and hypoglycemia, an insufficiency of the adrenal cortex should be suspected; particularly when these symptoms develop in the presence of severe stress or an overwhelming infection.	Epinephrine is given intravenously if systolic blood pressure is below 90 mm of mercury; desoxycorticosterone intramuscularly; and plasma or albumin, sodium chloride (.85 per cent) with dextrose (5 per cent) intravenously. Plasma is recommended to avoid the danger of homologous serum jaundice. Adrenal cortex extract is given intravenously and then intramuscularly. Continued effort to prevent hypoglycemia is urged, and also prevention of infection with antibiotics.
2. *Failure of the heart* or decreased cardiac output as in myocardial infarction (cardiac thrombosis) or in pericardial effusion of such magnitude as to keep the heart from filling with blood.	Massive myocardial infarction produces shock because it decreases the heart's output. Venous pressure may be normal, if there has been no previous congestive failure. Often the pulse rate is slow. In congestive heart failure, patients show signs of shock in the last days or hours before death. Pallor, sweating, narrow pulse pressure, and confusion increase as the output of the failing heart decreases. Venous pressure is elevated as it is in shock produced by stab wounds of the heart or conditions that cause serous or purulent effusions of the pericardium.	When shock is produced by heart failure, rapid digitalization and diuretics are often of value. Pericardial aspiration may be indicated if there is evidence of marked effusion. Surgery is often indicated when shock follows stab wounds of the chest.
3. *Blocking of the main arterial pathways with a blood clot or pressure.* As seen in pulmonary, myocardial, and mesenteric infarction; malignancies of the lung and spontane-	A patient with a massive pulmonary embolus or multiple smaller emboli that blocks the pulmonary arteries or with a growth in the lung affecting the capillary circulation will go into shock. The acuteness of the onset de-	When shock results from emboli, anticoagulants are given to prevent the formation of more clots. Venous ligation is resorted to in some cases.

CAUSE	SIGNS AND SYMPTOMS	TREATMENT AND NURSING CARE

ous pneumothorax with emphysema into the mediastinum.

pends upon the size, number, and location of the blocking clot or necrotic tissue.

---

4. *Changes in the tone of small blood vessels* as seen in "primary shock" following psychic trauma which may or may not be associated with physical trauma, as, for example, burns. The common faint is a form of primary or "neurogenic shock." Vasodilation occurs with the loss of tone resulting from psychic stimuli. A blow in the stomach by reflex stimulation can produce the same effect. Healthy athletes are often "knocked out" in games by this. Vasodilation may result from the action of histamine on blood vessel walls, from the action of foreign proteins as in anaphylactic shock; it can result from the action of alcohol or other toxic substances. This may be termed "vasogenic shock."

In neurogenic shock:
(a) The person suddenly appears ill, anxious, fearful, and weak; this state may progress to unconsciousness. In some cases he has a "blackout" at the onset.
(b) The skin is pale and damp to the touch.
(c) If conscious the person is likely to say he is nauseated and may vomit.
(d) The radial pulse tends to increase in rate.   :
(e) Respiratory rate may or may not be affected, and cyanosis is seen only in rare cases.
(f) A drop in blood pressure would usually be found if it were measured.
In vasogenic shock the symptoms listed above may be much more severe with marked cyanosis and in some cases rapid progression to a fatal end. Death may result from unchecked anaphylaxis, but it is possible that interference with cell metabolism or hemoconcentration from capillary damage produces the circulatory failure.

Primary neurogenic shock is rarely fatal, and the patient usually recovers without treatment. Full consciousness and relief of symptoms are hastened by the horizontal position or lowering the upper part of the body. Fainting sometimes follows standing in one position overlong. The cause has not been determined, but movement from time to time prevents the accident. Drugs are unnecessary.
If primary shock is occasioned by physical trauma that threatens to materially decrease blood volume, immediate steps must be taken to prevent the more serious secondary shock that will inevitably follow.
Vasogenic shock caused by vasodilating drugs or foreign proteins is effectively treated with vasoconstricting substances such as epinephrine if given soon enough to prevent the fatal outcome of severe anaphylaxis; similarly, the toxic effect of vasodilating drugs may be neutralized.

---

5. *Failure of cell metabolism.* Circulatory insufficiency is noted for days in patients dying from uncontrolled infections, from burns, renal or liver disease.

Dying patients may exhibit the shock syndrome without an appreciable loss of blood volume and with no demonstrable increase in capillary permeability to protein. The signs of shock are attributed to loss in tone of the arterioles and veins and to

The shock syndrome in the dying patient is considered "irreversible" unless the underlying cause of disturbed cell metabolism (an infection, for example) can be controlled. Shock caused by failure of cell metabolism is said not to respond to the administration of blood or plasma.

CAUSE	SIGNS AND SYMPTOMS	TREATMENT AND NURSING CARE

disturbance in the metabolic activities of all body cells. Shock produced in dogs by hemorrhage shows irreversible changes in the liver so that the liver is no longer able to inactivate vasodepressor materials as it normally does. Severe and prolonged shock produces irreversible changes in brain tissue. If, in such cases, the patient's life is saved, he may live the remainder of his life in a vegetative state.

6. *Hypoglycemia* (low blood sugar), "insulin shock."

So-called "insulin shock" is not automatically produced by any specific blood sugar level. Loeb says that if the blood sugar is over 70 mg per 100 cc the diagnosis of insulin shock is in doubt. Symptoms vary markedly in different persons but usually follow the same pattern in each individual. The common symptoms according to Loeb are:
(a) Trembly feeling inside
(b) Empty feeling in the epigastrium
(c) Profuse sweating
(d) Pallor
(e) Rapid pulse
(f) Weakness and fleeting loss of memory
These symptoms may develop in 15 to 30 minutes or the "shock" may have an abrupt onset with:
(a) Disorientation
(b) Confusion
(c) Delusions
(d) Aphasia
(e) Ataxia
(f) Loss of consciousness or general convulsions. With protamine zinc insulin, the

All diabetics should carry identification including the insulin dosage and the type used. It is essential that insulin shock and diabetic coma be differentiated for purposes of treatment. Insulin shock occurs most often when the patient delays eating more than 30 minutes after taking insulin. With protamine zinc insulin which is slowly absorbed, Loeb says the reaction may appear as much as 48 hours after the last dose, particularly if it is a large one. If the diabetic patient is unconscious (and unable to swallow) and if the cause may be hypoglycemia or acidosis, Loeb advocates giving 1000 cc of 5 per cent glucose and 0.5 to 1 cc of epinephrine (after taking a blood sample) as an emergency measure.

All diabetics should be taught to keep a lump of sugar in a pocket and take it, or a small glass of orange juice, at the first sign of approaching "shock."

4. TABULATION OF SPECIFIC TREATMENT BASED ON SPECIFIC CAUSE (cont.)

CAUSE	SIGNS AND SYMPTOMS	TREATMENT AND NURSING CARE
	onset and progression are likely to be insidious with headache, nausea, and vomiting.	

physicians because peripheral vasoconstriction is one means of raising the blood pressure and sweating dehydrates. The aim should be to keep the patient sufficiently warm to protect him from heat loss alone. In the very early stages of shock morphine is advocated by most authorities for the relief of pain, but it markedly depresses the vital centers and predisposes to nausea, vomiting, and later to constipation and other undesirable reactions. Nervousness should be treated by reassurance and by barbiturates. Circulatory stimulants, as a rule, are ineffective in shock, and most authorities believe now that they are contraindicated. Digitalis, however, may be used when shock is due to inadequacy of the heart. Special cases like this are discussed in the tabulated material that precedes. There is no better test of the nurse's ability to act effectively under pressure than the first aid she gives the patient during incipient shock and the care she gives him later under the direction of the doctor's prescribed treatment.

REFERENCES

1. Christopher, Frederick (ed.): *Textbook of Surgery,* 5th ed. W. B. Saunders Co., Philadelphia, 1949.
2. Cecil, Russell L., and Loeb, Robert F. (eds.): *Textbook of Medicine,* 8th ed. W. B. Saunders Co., Philadelphia, 1951.

Additional Suggested Reading

Beecher, Henry K.: *Resuscitation and Anesthesia for Wounded Men: The Management of Traumatic Shock.* Charles C Thomas, Publisher, Springfield, Ill., 1949.

Bland, John H.: *The Clinical Use of Fluid and Electrolyte.* W. B. Saunders Co., Philadelphia, 1952.

Crile, George, Jr., and Shively, Franklin L., Jr.: *Hospital Care of the Surgical Patient,* 2nd ed. Charles C Thomas, Publisher, Springfield, Ill., 1946.

Eliason, E. L.; Ferguson, L. K.; and Sholtis, L. A.: *Surgical Nursing,* 9th ed. J. B. Lippincott Co., Philadelphia, 1950.

Elman, Robert: *Surgical Care: A Practical Physiological Guide.* Appleton-Century-Crofts, Inc., New York, 1951.

Felter, Robert; West, Frances, and Zetzsche, Lydia M.: *Surgical Nursing,* 6th ed. F. A. Davis Co., Philadelphia, 1952.

Ilgenfritz, Hugh C.: *Preoperative and Postoperative Care of Surgical Patients,* 2nd ed. C. V. Mosby Co., St. Louis, 1948.

Mason, Robert L., and Zintel, Harold A. (eds.): *Preoperative and Postoperative Treatment,* 2nd ed. W. B. Saunders Co., Philadelphia, 1946.

Tourish, William J., and Wagner, Frederick B.: *Preoperative and Postoperative Care.* F. A. Davis Co., Philadelphia, 1947.

West, John P.; Keller, Manelva W.; and Harmon, Elizabeth H.: *Nursing Care of the Surgical Patient,* 6th ed. Macmillan Co., New York, 1957.

CHAPTER 41. NURSING CARE OF PATIENTS WITH SYSTEMIC INFECTIONS

1. PREVENTION
2. TREATMENT AND NURSING CARE
3. SUMMARY TABLE OF DATA

1. PREVENTION

Current Concepts. In the history of medicine there are no more exciting chapters than those that tell of the conquest of infectious disease. This is often said to be modern medicine's greatest accomplishment. Epidemiologic methods of studying and eradicating these diseases have been developed which, if universally practiced, would control, if not eradicate, diseases caused by living organisms. So dramatic are the results of these methods that they have come to be the basis for controlling other conditions, as, for example, nutritional deficiencies, vascular disease, cancer, mental disorders, and accidents. The program for the elimination of communicable disease is the cornerstone of modern medicine. As the approach developed in this field has been adapted to others, however, it has also been modified so that, at the present time, there is equal emphasis on conditions within and without the human organism. At the beginning of this century the emphasis was on sanitation. Hugh R. Leavell and E. Gurney Clark, discussing the present inclusive concept of epidemiology, define it as: "*A science concerned with the study of factors that influence the occurrence and distribution of disease, defect, disability, or death in aggregations of individuals.*" They go on to say: "It should be pointed out in this connection that it is impossible to draw a sharp line between the aggregations of individuals and the individuals that make up the aggregation, for whatever affects one is obliged to be reflected in the other."* While the "epidemiologic unit" is "an aggregation of individuals" rather than one individual, which is the "clinical unit," the emphasis in epidemiology is no longer on the environmental factors affecting the patient but rather on the interaction between the host and the disease agent.

Present-day epidemiologic studies include the incidence of the defect, disability, or disease and the distribution according to climate, geography, sex, age, race, and socioeconomic status. Some studies have included detailed physical measurements

* By permission from *Textbook of Preventive Medicine* by Hugh R. Leavell and E. Gurney Clark. Copyright 1953, McGraw-Hill Book Co., Inc., New York, p. 31.

that might serve as a basis for typing the individuals or temperaments susceptible to poliomyelitis, influenza, hypertension, or schizophrenia, for example.

Modern epidemiology not only tells us what diseases are found where and in what quantity, but it goes further in suggesting diagnostic procedures and treatment. Just as these studies led to the recognition of the mosquito as the carrier of malaria or typhus fever, the epidemiologic studies of lung cancer are suggesting its relationship to smoking and the respiratory irritants in urban life; research in schizophrenia offers some clues to the social conditions that may produce it, and studies of accidents point to internal states that make the individual "accident prone."

Prevention of disease follows a similar pattern regardless of the cause although modern man has been most successful in preventing the infectious diseases because his knowledge of their causes is most specific. Prevention depends upon identification of the agent of the disease, and the conditions within the environment and the host that make it possible for the agent successfully to invade and attack the host. After this identification a program can be launched (1) that removes or destroys the agent or (2) that renders the host immune to its attack. Most programs are a combination of these measures. One disease after another has been brought under control. In this country we no longer fear diphtheria, smallpox, or typhoid fever, chiefly because we have immunized the host against the agent of the disease through the use of vaccines; dysenteric disease, hookworm, and malaria, as examples, are, on the other hand, less feared because the conditions in the environment that enabled the agent to invade the host have been modified by improved sanitation.

In Chapters 2 and 7 it was pointed out that in 1900 pneumonia, tuberculosis, diarrhea and enteritis, and diphtheria were included in the ten leading causes of death, whereas in 1948 only the respiratory infections—pneumonia (including influenza)—and tuberculosis remain in the list and in order of rank these are preceded by heart disease and cancer.[1] Even with so great an accomplishment to the credit of the medical worker, however, there are many thousands of preventable deaths caused by infectious diseases or their sequelae. We need not only an extension of knowledge but also a more thorough application of measures whose values have been demonstrated. Nor can science ever rest on its laurels. There is evidence that flies and other insect vectors are acquiring an immunity to DDT, and it is generally believed that according to the laws of adaptation microorganisms will learn to survive in the presence of the therapeutic agents that now seem so deadly to them.[2] All this means that the struggle against disease is an unending one and that it is probably a mistake to think of any disease as conquered once and for all. T. H. Ingalls, discussing in hopeful terms the control of mongolism, says that there is never a single cause of any disease, that disease is "a complex process that depends upon an injurious agent, a susceptible patient, and a particular environment."* The control of any disease, therefore, would depend upon epidemiologic and clinical research, the implementation of these findings, and public education. Nurses are taking an increasingly active part in all aspects of this program. For example, they

---

* Ingalls, T. H.: "Mongolism," *Scient. Am.*, **186**:60, (Feb.) 1952.

played a major role as workers in the research on the BCG* vaccine in the control of tuberculosis; the public health nurse's success in finding persons infected with tuberculosis or syphilis is admittedly second to none, and her daily contact with individuals everywhere has done more to teach the average citizen the means of controlling infection than any other form of education. A part of the successful care of the infectious patient is the protection of others. In this country the nurse is the person who, more than any one else, enforces a rigid aseptic technique.

The nurse must continually extend her knowledge as the causes of disease are discovered and as methods of prevention and treatment are developed. This is such a rapidly developing field that health agencies are urged to designate and, if necessary, prepare one or more doctors and nurses to act as specialists and to direct the periodic revision of control practice within the agency.

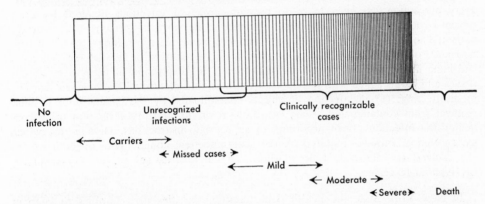

Figure 246. Spectrum of disease. (Anderson, Gaylord W., and Arnstein, Margaret G.: *Communicable Disease Control,* 3rd ed. The Macmillan Company, New York, 1953.)

Aspects of Prevention.   Among the measures used in the control of infectious disease the following should be stressed. They demand the establishment of laws and public health regulations to enforce many of them.

1. The provision of a sanitary environment including clean food, milk and water, and safe disposal of sewage and waste
2. Reporting infectious disease, the isolation of the patient, the quarantine of "contacts," the administration of protective vaccines and sera, and the use of effective concurrent and terminal disinfection
3. Health education in homes, industry, schools, and health agencies
4. Epidemiologic research and a system of records and statistics
5. A program of detection or case finding, with emphasis on recognition of early symptoms
6. Health promotion through adequate nutrition, protection from excessive fatigue and emotional strain

* *Bacillus Calmette-Guérin.*

The provision of a sanitary environment has been discussed in Chapters 5 and 7, and they might be reviewed in conjunction with the study of this chapter. Reporting infectious disease is the responsibility of the doctor who makes the diagnosis, but the nurse (in fact, any citizen) is negligent if she does not report to him or a public health official a patient who, she has reason to believe, is suffering from an untreated communicable condition.

Isolation is the separation of infected from noninfected persons and may be strict or modified. Leavell and Clark describe strict isolation as follows:

Isolation is defined as separation of infected persons from noninfected persons for the period of communicability, under conditions which will prevent the transmission of the infectious agent. *Strict isolation* requires (a) a separate bed in a room protected from vectors; (b) exclusion from the sick room of all persons except those caring for the patient; (c) avoidance of contact with others by persons caring for the patient until every precaution has been taken to prevent spread of infectious material from the patient's room; (d) a washable outer garment to be worn by persons caring for the patient, hands to be washed with soap and hot water after handling patient or contaminated objects in room, and outer garment to be removed on leaving the sick room and hung in the patient's room until disinfected; (e) deposition in paper bags of soft tissues and cloths soiled with discharges from nose and mouth, with subsequent burning or disinfecting; (f) disinfection of objects contaminated by the patient prior to their removal from contaminated areas; (g) disposal of the patient's feces and urine containing the infectious agent according to appropriate instructions. Diseases for which strict isolation is usually required are (a) acute infectious conjunctivitis of the newborn, (b) cholera, (c) diarrhea of the newborn, (d) diphtheria, (e) plague, (f) smallpox, (g) typhoid fever.*

In New York State the health department authorities urge families to keep at home those with the most highly communicable diseases (examples are measles, chickenpox, and smallpox), if they are uncomplicated by conditions that demand hospitalization.[3]

Modified isolation varies with the disease and the conditions under which the patient is treated. There is a trend away from strict isolation to a modified form. If the general measures used to protect all patients in a health agency from unrecognized infection are as effective as they should be, very little need be added when a patient is admitted with the less readily transmitted infections; some infectious diseases are so hard to communicate that isolation is not required. Leprosy, for example, is communicable only after months or years of close contact. It is only in certain states that lepers are isolated. Where they are, public opinion forces on the victim a deprivation of his liberty, which is dictated by fear rather than scientific knowledge. In this country we have established leprosaria in southern states in spite of the data showing that patients have a poorer chance of remission and survival in a warm climate than they would in a cold one.[4, 5] Generally speaking, the public health regulations on isolation need revision in terms of the newer knowledge of communicable disease. For example, it has been learned that persons with the same

* Leavell, Hugh R., and Clark, E. Gurney: *op. cit.,* p. 87.

diagnosis may be infected with different strains of the same organism and should therefore be placed in separate rooms rather than grouped (this is especially true in the streptococcal infections), and also the use of the newer drugs and antibiotics has shortened the period of communicability.

Quarantine is a term derived from the practice of keeping offshore for forty days a ship suspected of carrying infection. Now it is used to mean limiting the freedom of a person who has been exposed to a communicable disease until the incubation period has expired. Some state laws require quarantine for more diseases than others. California confined its list in 1952 to smallpox, cholera, plague, and diphtheria.[6] The New York State Department of Health's authorities say quarantine for chickenpox is urgently indicated and they advocate quarantine for measles with "completely preventive doses of gamma globulin or convalescent serum" to "exposed susceptibles."*

Learning the supposed incubation periods of communicable diseases is difficult. Frank Fenner, discussing "The Significance of the Incubation Period," says that the incubation depends upon the capacity of the parasite to:

(a) . . . produce a lesion by local multiplication, (b) to multiply in phagocytes and thus overcome the barriers of lymph nodes and spleen-liver-bone marrow + (c) on the rate of multiplication of the parasites and what we may call its critical concentration—this is, the degree of multiplication which must occur in any organ before lesions are produced.†

The length of the incubation period depends upon the nature of the parasite, the strength of the invading agent, and the response of the host. Fenner points out that where the reaction is a local one, as in an infected wound, the incubation is relatively shorter than when the reaction is a general one as, for example, secondary syphilis, for in this case many more body defenses have been broken down. A large invasion decreases the incubation period; inoculation by a few organisms increases the incubation period. (The incubation periods shown in Table 17 are, of course, approximations.) Fenner makes the point, however, that "underneath the endless diversity of symptomatology of the infectious diseases there is unity in the mechanism of infection, which, with certain exceptions, is essentially the same for the smallest viruses and the largest bacteria."‡

Immunization to communicable disease is so generally practiced in most countries that the average adult has some knowledge of the procedure even though he may not understand the biological process involved. Each of the infectious diseases is a *specific disease*; that is, each has a specific cause and the organism causing it has its own characteristics, its definite mode of attack, its mode of living, and means of transmission. Protection of the individual from each disease, whether by natural immunity or acquired by artificial means, is also specific. A newborn baby

* New York State Department of Health, Bureau of Epidemiology: *Guide for the Handling of Communicable Diseases in General Hospitals.* The Department, Albany, 1950, p. 7.
  † Fenner, Frank: "The Significance of the Incubation Period," *M. J. Australia,* **2:**813, (Dec.) 1950.
  ‡ Fenner, Frank: *op. cit.*

(*Text continued on p. 1069.*)

Table 15. Immunization Measures*

METHOD	CHARACTERISTICS	USES
I. Active immunization	Preferable to passive immunization, since it gives the individual a lasting protection that guards against potential future exposures	Active immunization, if applied to a large enough fraction of a population and extended to new generations, gives a more lasting protection than any other method except in certain types of environmental control, such as water sanitation and insect eradication
A. Antigens	Any substance that stimulates the body to produce its own antibodies is called an antigen†	
1. Living antigens	Organisms, during the process of infecting the body, stimulate it to produce antibodies. However, preparation, storage, and degree of virulence are not easily determined; therefore, using an antigen that has no capacity for multiplication involves less risk even though living antigens are said to be "attentuated"	Smallpox vaccine is the only living antigen commonly used in human beings. Yellow fever vaccine, the original Pasteur antirabic vaccine, and the recently developed influenza vaccine are also in this group
2. Nonliving antigens	Derived from microorganisms	
a. Bacterial extracts	Some bacteria during growth secrete antigenic substances that may be separated by filtration; they are then purified or modified before use	Example: Diphtheria bacilli, during growth in a suitable medium, produce a toxin, the same as that which develops in the course of the disease. The final product is antigenic though relatively nontoxic. Since it is a modified toxin, it is referred to as a "toxoid"

* Anderson, Gaylord W., and Arnstein, Margaret G.: *Communicable Disease Control*, 3rd ed. The Macmillan Company, New York, 1953, pp. 58-70.

† A vaccine is a type of antigen and consists of either living or dead organisms. Although some persons use the term "vaccine," as synonymous with the term "antigen," vaccine does not correctly include bacterial extracts or their derivatives—this excludes the toxins and toxoids.

Table 15. Immunization Measures (cont.)

METHOD	CHARACTERISTICS	USES
b. Dead organisms	In some cases, it is not possible to separate any active component from the living organisms; yet a suspension of killed organisms is found to be antigenic. In these instances, the antigen consists of dead organisms	Examples: Typhoid fever vaccine, whooping cough vaccine
II. Passive immunization*	An emergency measure designed to carry an individual through a limited period of increased hazard	Any substance that contains antibodies may be given to confer passive immunity, the degree of resistance depending upon the ultimate concentration in the blood stream
A. Specific therapeutic serum	Usually derived from a horse actively immunized for a specific disease	Advantage: Specific serum has a high antibody content. Disadvantage: Since it contains a protein foreign to the human body, it may cause a serum reaction
B. Hyperimmune serum	Derived from humans rather than from other animals	At present, only hyperimmune serum of practical importance is that for whooping cough (this has the advantage of not containing a foreign protein)
C. Convalescent serum	Blood serum from a person who has recently recovered from the disease in question (therefore, such serum contains antibodies)	Application is limited because of the difficulty of obtaining an adequate supply

* Methods used for passive immunization may also be used to modify a disease (e.g., a combination of passive immunization and normal infection—example, tetanus).

1067

Table 15. Immunization Measures (cont.)

METHOD	CHARACTERISTICS	USES
D. Adult serum	Blood serum of adults selected at random from the general population (method little used in this country)	Its use depends on the assumption (usually correct) that the donors have developed a resistance; a weaker form of convalescent serum, its main advantage is that it can be obtained in larger quantity
E. Parental whole blood	Injections of whole blood from one of the parents of the child to be protected depends on the same assumption as that for adult serum	Use of parental whole blood has been found to be practical only with respect to measles and even here is of limited application
F. Placental extract ("immune globulin human")	Obtained from normal human placenta	Material effective, but its use has been curtailed by occasional reactions not encountered with convalescent serum
G. Gamma globulin (human immune serum globulin)	A by-product of human serum production. Antibodies in any human serum contained in that part of the blood serum protein are referred to as the gamma globulin fraction. It represents the most highly refined and purified source of human antibodies	Gamma globulin is available as a dried powder, readily dissolved in salt solution to prepare it for injection*

* Prevention of measles which is a severe disease in babies and preschool children is important. When gamma globulin is given within four days after initial exposure to infection, *measles* will not develop; however, the child will possess passive immunity only, which fades within a few weeks. Gamma globulin is also administered to pregnant women who develop *German measles* or who have been exposed to the disease during the first three months of pregnancy; otherwise the embryo will develop some severe physical or mental defect (e.g., congenital cataracts, mental deficiency, etc.). (Smillie, Wilson G.: *Preventive Medicine and Public Health,* 2nd ed. The Macmillan Company, New York, 1952, pp. 221–23.)

Since gamma globulin also contains antibodies of other diseases, studies have been made as to its effectiveness in *poliomyelitis.* (Mustard, Harry S.: *An Introduction to Public Health,* 3rd ed. The Macmillan Company, New York, 1953, p. 112.) Use of gamma globulin in this instance is being replaced by the vaccine developed by Dr. Jonas Salk and associates.

Gamma globulin has been administered to nurses and children in institutions and to personnel in military units in which there are cases of *hepatitis.* Gamma globulin provides sufficient passive resistance to guard against severe infection, but not enough to preclude a mild infection which leaves the individual with an active and more durable resistance. (Anderson, Gaylord W., and Arnstein, Margaret G.: *op. cit.,* p. 231.)

is born with immunity, or antibodies derived from its mother's body fluids that protect it from some diseases. Examples of these are believed to be diphtheria, scarlet fever, rubella (German measles), mumps, and poliomyelitis. It is highly susceptible to the ordinary pyogenic infections, the upper respiratory infections, tuberculosis, syphilis, erysipelas, smallpox, chickenpox, and whooping cough. On the basis of this fact placental extracts have been used as prophylactic agents and as treatment in these diseases.

In giving vaccines and sera one must decide whether active or passive immunity is desired. Vaccines or actual attacks of the disease excite the body to form agents that protect it against the bacteria, while antisera introduce the bacteria-destroying agents into the body and immunity is not dependent upon the reaction of the body to the organism.

The nurse works with the doctor in giving tests, noting reactions to the various tests, helping to break down ignorance and prejudice toward the tests, and developing an interest and a desire for prophylactic measures. Immunization practice is changing, and nurses must be able to interpret the changes. Grandmothers, for example, will often oppose inoculation of young infants and may persuade mothers to disregard medical advice unless they can be helped to understand the reasons for these changes. E. Albert Moody, discussing the subject, urges immunization against pertussis (whooping cough) between the ages of four and six weeks, which to many older persons seems a radical procedure. While he admits that the very young infant does not respond to the process of active immunization as well as the older infant, he thinks it should have "at least partial protection against pertussis at an age when its mortality is the highest."*

Table 15 summarizes information about immunization measures. For persons who are traveling from one country to another and who wish to know what protection they should seek, a booklet has been prepared by the US Public Health Service entitled *Immunization Information for International Travelers.* This booklet is available for a nominal sum from the Department of Health, Education, and Welfare in Washington, D.C. It shows the required and recommended procedures as agreed upon in that committee of the World Health Organization concerned with communicable disease control.

If the reader wishes more detailed information on immunization than is provided in Table 15 he should consult one of the texts listed at the end of this chapter.

The nurse is often responsible for giving immunizing agents and, in some cases, examining the patient to see what local reaction has occurred. Explicit directions for their administration accompany most biological preparations. It is important that they be fresh, and that they be stored in a refrigerator, but that freezing is avoided since this may destroy their potency. They must, likewise, not be heated before they are administered, but they should be given at room temperature because they are more viscid and less irritating than when they are injected cold.

Education of the public in the control of disease has progressed to such a point

* Moody, E. Albert: "Present-Day Concepts of Immunization of Infants," *Northwest Med.,* **50**:30, (Jan.) 1951.

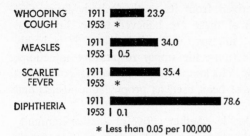

WHOOPING COUGH   1911   ▉▉▉▉ 23.9
                  1953   *

MEASLES   1911   ▉▉▉▉▉ 34.0
                  1953 | 0.5

SCARLET FEVER   1911   ▉▉▉▉▉ 35.4
                  1953   *

DIPHTHERIA   1911   ▉▉▉▉▉▉▉▉▉ 78.6
                  1953 | 0.1

* Less than 0.05 per 100,000

Figure 247A. Standardized death rates per 100,000 from four communicable diseases among children between the ages of 1 and 14 years, showing the dramatic effect of control measures. (Courtesy of Metropolitan Life Insurance Co., Industrial Department, New York City.)

in this country that even school children are aware of the dangers of using drinking vessels in common, or of failing to protect a wound. Teachers, biologists, doctors, nurses, and nearly all categories of medical workers have contributed toward the public awareness, but probably none of them is called upon more consistently than the nurse for specific information and particularly for personal instruction and demonstration of control measures. Federal, state, and local public health agencies have a wealth of teaching materials as do the private health agencies devoted to the control of particular communicable diseases such as tuberculosis and poliomyelitis. A number of life insurance companies spend large sums on educational materials. The nurse is most effective when she has command of a large body of information that enables her to answer accurately the questions that patients and their

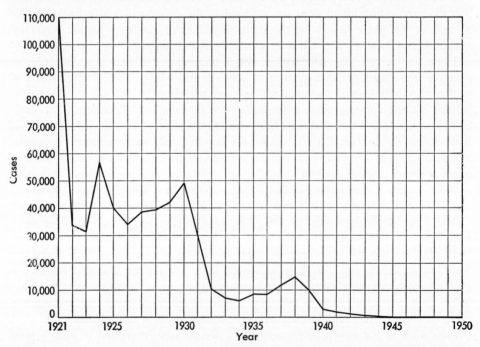

Figure 247B. Cases of smallpox reported in the United States, 1921-1950. (Dublin, Louis I.: *The Facts of Life from Birth to Death*. The Macmillan Company, New York, 1951.)

families ask; since, however, she cannot hope to have all the data they need at the tip of her tongue, nor has she time to impart it, she should be able to use and suggest to others the printed and audio-visual sources of information that are available.

There is a division, or department, of research in every health agency concerned with communicable disease control, although the programs range from very limited to very extensive ones. All nurses employed in these agencies contribute to these programs through the records they keep; some nurses are employed full time on research projects. There is a great need for nurses trained to take an active part in this kind of research.

Case finding or detection is an integral part of all communicable disease programs. Interviewing is a skill that is particularly important for nurses who are trying to find persons who have been exposed to tuberculosis and syphilis; actually, it is a tool that every nurse should possess.[7, 8]

Finally, communicable disease, as is the case with all disease, must be controlled by improving the individual health status. It is the theory of the "organic gardener" that the production of healthy plants, rather than insect control, is the key to good crops. While it is debatable whether healthy plants and animals can always resist invasions of parasitic organisms, the resistance of the host is a major factor in all infections. The known susceptibility of certain pathogenic microorganisms to the slightest change in the pH of laboratory culture media suggests the basis on which overindulgence in sweets, for example, may predispose a person to infection. The known relationship between disease and dietary deficiencies has been discussed in Chapter 13 and elsewhere. The provision of an adequate diet is the cornerstone on which every health program rests. Another body state that affects susceptibility to all disease, including those produced by microorganisms, is fatigue, whether it is caused by lack of sleep, overexertion, or nervous tension. The effects of these conditions have been discussed in Chapter 15 and elsewhere in this text and will not be elaborated upon here. Every student of physiology is probably ready to accept the existence of a relationship between physical and emotional fatigue and almost every classification of disease.

2. TREATMENT AND NURSING CARE

General Principles. Therapy in communicable diseases has many common elements because the diseases have a common causation—a living organism. Therapy is aimed at killing or destroying the potency of such organisms. When the causative organism has been isolated and/or when a therapeutic agent has been discovered, the plan of therapy is relatively simple; when the organism is unknown and when there is no effective therapeutic agent, treatment can be only symptomatic. Organisms producing disease in man vary so greatly in their character and in the tissues they effect that the symptoms, or the pathological changes, have a wide range. They can, however, be categorized into local tissue changes and the systemic manifestations produced by the toxic products of the causative organism. These toxins are carried throughout the body in the circulating fluids. "Symptoms" of infection are interrelated and are most realistically seen as syndromes. Of these groups of related symptoms fever is the most common. Unchecked infections of certain organisms may produce septicemia and finally pyemia with multiple local abscesses.

When an effective therapeutic agent is known and available, therapy is usually simple and recovery rapid. Nursing care in such cases is relatively less important than when recovery depends upon supporting nature in her defensive mechanisms. The number of infections that fail to respond to drugs and antibiotic agents is rapidly diminishing, and this is one reason why the character of nursing care is undergoing rapid change. In William Houston's text *The Art of Treatment,*[9] published in 1936, he listed the common cold, acute tonsillitis, influenza, acute tuberculosis, leprosy, smallpox, typhus, yellow, malta, typhoid, and dengue fevers, chickenpox, measles, mumps, whooping cough, and plague among those diseases "treated chiefly by nursing care." If he were writing this text today he would discuss most of these diseases in the chapter entitled "Specific Measures," in which category he at that time placed diphtheria, tetanus, cerebrospinal meningitis, and rabies, among others. The development of chemicals and antibiotics that have a specific effect upon pathogenic organisms has not only shortened the duration of illness but has cut down the period of communicability of the disease so that most of our isolation and quarantine regulations are open to question. Few state or local health departments have yet applied all the new developments in clinical microbiology, and there is considerable confusion, with wide variation in public health regulations. While this lag in the application of knowledge may be inevitable, it can be reduced by constructive criticism and suggestion. Informed nurses in administration are helping to change the regimen of tubercular patients in sanatoria and homes. The newer drugs and antibiotics are so lethal to the tubercle bacilli that in a short time many patients with pulmonary tuberculosis have so-called "negative sputum" and can take part in communal living with no danger to the nontubercular.

Regardless of the nature of the infection, the following principles apply to treatment and nursing care:

1. Identifying the invading organism, if possible.
2. Administering a therapeutic agent that kills, destroys, or decreases the pathogenicity of the organism, if the organism is identified and a specific agent is available. (The therapeutic agent may be applied locally or given by mouth and/or parenterally.)
3. Identifying and relieving symptoms, particularly those of fever.
4. Giving supportive care essential in any illness when the patient is unable to provide for his needs.
5. Preventing the transmission of the patient's infection to other persons, animals, or insects.

The responsibility for carrying out the foregoing is shared by the members of the medical team, the patient, and his family as discussed in Chapter 4. Diagnostic methods were discussed in Chapter 19, and to some extent in Chapter 18. Details of tests for a particular disease can be found in texts listed at the end of this chapter.

Because it plays such a prominent role in the program of communicable disease control, and because it is a new and confusing subject, the use of chemotherapeutic agents and antibiotics is summarized in the following pages.*

Use of Antibiotics and Sulfonamides in Treatment of Infections. Louis S. Goodman and Alfred Gilman *define* antibiotics as "chemical substances produced by various species of microorganisms (bacteria, fungi, actinomyces) which suppress the growth of other microorganisms and may eventually destroy them." Although the total number of antibiotics now extends into the hundreds, less than a score have been developed to the stage where they are of value in the therapy of infectious diseases.

Some of the major antibiotics and sulfonamides are summarized in Table 16,† and their *current uses,* alone or in combination, are indicated. Each of the four main categories in this table will be discussed briefly.

1. *Penicillin,* discovered by Fleming in 1928, is now available in four major natural penicillins (in England designated by Roman numerals, and in the United States by the capital letters F, G, X, and K). Because penicillin G is the master standard for unit dosage and because all major classes of penicillin preparations contain mainly, or only, penicillin G, the penicillin category in Table 16 has been so headed. Penicillin G is very effective in the treatment of streptococcal and staphylococcal infections, lobar pneumonia, meningitis, anthrax, gas gangrene, gonorrhea, syphilis, and Vincent's angina. It is useful in the treatment of diphtheria, particularly for the carrier state and to prevent suppurative complications.

2. *The streptomycins* include streptomycin, the parent material, and dihydrostreptomycin. Streptomycin was discovered in 1944 by Schatz, Bugie, and Waksman. Dihydrostreptomycin is obtained by catalytic hydrogenation of the parent material. The streptomycins are very effective in the treatment of tuberculosis and have proved effective in leprosy, urinary tract infections, and meningitis.

3. *The tetracyclines* are effective in rickettsial and some viral diseases as well as in various bacterial diseases. The first antibiotic in this group was discovered in 1948 and was named Aureomycin, but it is now referred to as *chlortetracycline.* In 1950 Terramycin was developed; in current terminology it is now called *oxytetracycline.* Two years later, in 1952, *tetracycline* was prepared; it is a semisynthetic tetracycline (achromycin, tetracyn, polycycline). The tetracyclines are very effective in the treatment of staphylococcal and urinary tract infections, meningitis, chancroid, and amebiasis; they are effective in the treatment of a number of diseases such as streptococcal infections, lobar pneumonia, diphtheria, anthrax, bacillary dysentery, gonorrhea, and syphilis.

4. *The sulfonamides* include a number of derivatives of para-amino-benzene-sulfonamide (sulfanilamide). More than 5400 congeneric substances were synthesized and studied in the 10-year period following the discovery of sulfanilamide, which was first prepared in 1908. However, less than a score of the sulfanilamides have attained any therapeutic importance, and of these *sulfadiazine* is the sulfanila-

---

* The summary is based on Chapters 56-60 in *The Pharmacological Basis of Therapeutics,* 2nd ed., by Louis S. Goodman and Alfred Gilman. The Macmillan Company, New York, 1955.

† Disease entities selected from the original table include those that respond effectively or very effectively to one or more of the major antibiotic groups.

(*Text continued on p. 1076.*)

Table 16. Current Use of Major Antibiotics and Sulfonamides in Systemic Infections

(Based on Table 57 from *The Pharmacological Basis of Therapeutics*, 2nd ed., by Louis S. Goodman and Alfred Gilman. The Macmillan Company, New York, 1955, pp. 1322–23.)

MAJOR DISEASE	Penicillin G		The Streptomycins		The Tetracyclines		The Sulfonamides	
	Very eff.	Eff.	Very eff.	Eff.	Very eff.	Eff.	Very eff.	Eff.
Streptococcal infections (β-hemolytic)	x					x		x
Staphylococcal (pyogenic) infections	x[1]				x[1]	(x)[2]		
Lobar pneumonia: meningitis	x[3]					x		x[3]
Gonorrhea	x					x		x
Epidemic meningitis	x[3]					x	x[3]	
Diphtheria		x[4,5]				x[4,5]		
Anthrax	x					x		
Tetanus	—[4,6]							
Gas gangrene	x[4]							
Urinary tract infections (*A. aerogenes*)				x	x[1]			
Typhoid fever[7]								
Paratyphoid fever[7]								
Bacillary dysentery						x	(x)[2]	

1074

Table 16. Current Use of Major Antibiotics and Sulfonamides in Systemic Infections (cont.)

MAJOR DISEASE	AGENT							
	Penicillin G		The Streptomycins		The Tetracyclines		The Sulfonamides	
	Very eff.	Eff.	Very eff.	Eff.	Very eff.	Eff.	Very eff.	Eff.
Meningitis				x[8]	x[9]			
Pertussis								
Chancroid					x		x	
Syphilis	x					x		
Vincent's angina	x							
Tuberculosis			x[10]					
Leprosy				x[10]				
Amebiasis					x[11]			

[1] Strain susceptibility and "acquired" resistance markedly affect the therapeutic results obtained with the indicated agent.
[2] The alternative ratings given in parentheses ( ) are based on differences in clinical opinion or differences in susceptibility of various strains of the microorganism in question.
[3] In coccal meningitides, combined penicillin and sulfadiazine therapy is usually indicated.
[4] Also antitoxin therapy.
[5] Does not cure; useful in carrier state and to prevent suppurative complications.
[6] Penicillin is primarily of value in controlling secondary infections, but also promotes eradication of Clostridium.
[7] Chloramphenicol is agent of choice in therapy of typhoid fever and paratyphoid fever.
[8] Streptomycin and sulfadiazine give better results than does either alone.
[9] Tetracycline and sulfadiazine together represent treatment of choice and give better results than does either alone.
[10] Streptomycin is used in combinations with other agents. . . . .
[11] Intestinal amebiasis only.

mide most widely employed at present. Sulfonamides have a wide range of anti-microbial activity against both gram-positive and gram-negative organisms. They are very effective in epidemic meningitis, bacillary dysentery, and chancroid, and are effective in streptococcal infections, lobar pneumonia, and gonorrhea.

Miscellaneous antibiotics include the following: (1) *Chloramphenicol,* first isolated in 1947, is used mainly for the treatment of typhoid fever. Its restricted use is due to the fact that serious blood dyscrasias may result following its administration. (2) *Erythromycin,* discovered in 1952, resembles penicillin in its field of use-fulness. (3) *Carbomycin,* an orally effective antibiotic, has been used to advantage against enterococcal infections (especially of the urinary tract); however, its general use still must be confirmed. (4) *Polymyxin B,* discovered in 1947, may be given orally, intramuscularly, intrathecally, or topically. It is used in a variety of infections caused by gram-negative bacteria. (5) *Neomycin,* discovered in 1949, is used mainly for topical application and intestinal antisepsis prior to surgery of the large bowel. (6) Use of *bacitracin,* isolated in 1943, is limited largely to topical application (ophthalmic ointment for styes, acute and chronic conjunctivitis, keratitis, etc.) and local infiltration. It must be used with caution because, when given systemically, it exerts a nephrotoxic action. Bacitracin is also used in oral dosage in intestinal amebiasis and pinworm infestations. (7) *Tyrothricin,* the first antibiotic to follow the isolation of penicillin, was discovered in 1939. It is, therefore, of historical interest. However, because its systemic toxicity is great, its use is limited to topical application for the control of localized or surface infections.

Other Drugs Used in Systemic Infections. The dramatic effect of the antibiotics and sulfanomides should not be emphasized to the exclusion of old and new drugs in other categories. The use of vitamins and their derivatives in the treatment of infections is a very important development. Nydrazid (*isonicotinic acid hydrazide*), used so effectively in tuberculosis, is a striking example of a drug in this category. The general effectiveness of vitamins in preventing infections and hastening recovery from avitaminoses characterized by infections was stressed in Chapter 13. Here we might call attention to some recent reports of the "ameliorative" action of flavonoid-ascorbic acid mixtures on upper respiratory infections, chiefly of viral origin.[10]

Antimalarial drugs have appeared in rapid succession (quinacrine [Atabrine], chloroquine [Resochin], and chloroquanide [Paludrine] to replace quinine, and there is reason to hope that there will continue to be improvements in comparable specifics which will increase their toxicity to the invading organism and decrease the danger to the host. Few nurses can keep abreast of the research in therapeutics, but they can grasp every opportunity to participate in it and to learn about it, particularly as it relates to the care of their patients. While doctors prescribe, nurses must usually administer the therapeutic agent, or teach the patient to take it, and this cannot be done intelligently without knowledge of the nature and effect of the agent.

Symptomatic and Supportive Care—"Fever Nursing." *The treatment and nursing care of local manifestations of infection*—inflammatory and suppurative processes—were dealt with in Chapter 36. One or both of these are present in many acute systemic infectious diseases. Examples are the inflamed and sometimes necrotic pharyngeal tissues of tonsillitis and diphtheria, the skin lesions of erysipelas, chickenpox, smallpox, and impetigo, and the lesions of tuberculosis and syphilis that are present on either the exterior or interior of the body, sometimes both. In a few of the acute generalized infections the local manifestation is the only troublesome symptom, as, for example, the pustules of impetigo or chickenpox; in others it is a rash of very limited duration that demands no local treatment except, perhaps, a soothing bath, lotion, or ointment. Such rashes are seen in scarlet fever and measles. It has been stated by a number of investigators that infections are typified by capillary hemorrhage either produced by their dilation or by a "fragility" of the wall that is the result of infection.[11, 12] The citrus flavonoids are claimed by these authors to reduce this "fragility" which is the cause of the petechial type of skin eruption. Local treatment of petechial rashes is rarely used except to allay itching. Very smooth bedding and clothing reduce irritation. Cellulose film sheeting is helpful for this purpose; it is placed under the irritated area and covered with cotton sheets to protect a mattress when there is seepage from eruption.

Lesions of erysipelas and impetigo are treated as infected wounds. It is common practice to remove the crusts from impetigo pustules because they protect the organisms from the action of the prescribed antiseptic ointment or lotion.

Inflammation of the mucous membranes of the eyes, ears, nose, and throat is common in many acute systemic infections. When the eyes are inflamed, as in measles and some upper respiratory conditions, they should be kept at rest and protected from bright lights with an eyeshade or eyeglasses. The physician may prescribe sprays, irrigation, or other types of applications for the throat, etc. (see Chapter 33).

Symptomatic and supportive care in most infections is directed toward *combating the harmful effects of fever.* While it is now realized that fever is one of the body's means of making itself uninhabitable to the invading microorganisms, it is generally believed that if this reaction is prolonged or very severe, the body tissues as well as the invading organisms may suffer. Artificially produced fever (fever therapy) was used in the 1930's and 1940's in the treatment of gonorrhea and other infections, but is seldom used now. In 1948 Eugene F. DuBois in his classic monograph on fever says that it is: ". . . not without danger . . . and will probably be used less and less as the antibiotics . . . come into more general employment."* This prophecy is borne out in fact, and we seldom hear of this treatment; however, we also seldom see drugs, baths, and packs used for the specific purpose of reducing temperature, as would have happened early in the century. DuBois says:

A temperature of 41° C (105.8° F) may be harmful and temperatures over 42° C (107.6° F) dangerous if prolonged a few hours. It is doubtful if a temperature of 40° C (104° F) even over a period of days can be considered harmful in itself, though of course it is usually an indication of severe infection accompanied by many other

* DuBois, Eugene F.: *Fever and the Regulation of Body Temperature.* Charles C Thomas, Publisher. Springfield, Ill., 1948, p. 41.

deleterious factors. Fever is only a symptom and we are not sure that it is an enemy. Perhaps it is a friend.*

The fever chart was until recent years a diagnostic aid because each infectious disease had a somewhat characteristic pattern of temperature fluctuation. Current drugs and antibotics arrest the disease so quickly, however, that the daily or weekly record of body temperature is no longer of much help to the physician in identifying the infection. Improved laboratory methods more than compensate for the loss of the fever chart as a clue to diagnosis.

Most of us have experienced fever or have watched someone else with it. Knowledge of its effect on body functions suggest the nursing needs. The following is a picture of a typical febrile patient.

The respiratory rate is increased, as is the pulse rate; there is a vague or marked feeling that something is wrong; there may be headache and nausea, so the victim instinctively seeks rest and seclusion; he feels groggy and seems to sleep a great deal, but he has wild dreams and when the fever is highest he has a sense of unreality; he is not sure whether it is night or day, and his dreams merge into waking fantasies so that we say he is "delirious." His skin feels hot and dry when the fever is at its height and he kicks off the bed covers, but with fevers that fluctuate and just before the onset of a sudden fever, there is a sensation of chilliness or a shaking chill that is not relieved by external warmth. Profuse sweating occurs preceding a drop in the body temperature; the clothing and even the sheets may be soaking wet. The appetite is usually poor and food is sometimes repugnant, but thirst is a prominent feature.

Since fever weakens the patient and dulls his judgment, he may become severely dehydrated, and if neglected he loses weight rapidly. His lips are parched or cracked, and crusts form on them and in his nose. His nasal air passages are occluded, and the patient breathes through his mouth; his tongue is coated, often swollen, and if the fever persists, and its effects are not successfully combated, his gums swell and bleed easily and the margins may be discolored and discharge pus. A febrile patient is usually irritable; he loses interest even in those he loves. In a delirium he asks questions that no one can answer satisfactorily, and this adds to his confusion. If the fever is not too intense or prolonged, the brain damage is only temporary. Unless the patient is competently nursed, the urine is scanty because there is excessive water loss through sweating. Constipation or diarrhea may be present according to what the patient eats and the effect of the infection on the alimentary canal.

Many of these symptoms can be identified as signs of a neglected febrile patient; they can be forestalled and the picture greatly modified by effective care, especially adequate feeding. DuBois, discussing "the management of fever patients," says, "In the first place a good nurse is required."†

If the foregoing is an accurate description of the febrile state, the following symptomatic nursing care is suggested:

* DuBois, Eugene F.: *op. cit.,* p. 57.
† DuBois, Eugene F.: *op. cit.,* p. 55.

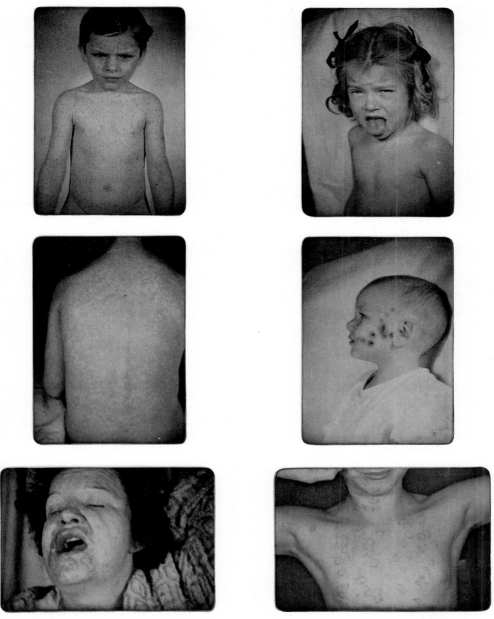

Plate IV. Skin lesions of common communicable diseases. (*Left, top to bottom*) Chicken-pox: face, trunk, and upper extremities, first day of eruption (courtesy of Franklin H. Top, M.D.); measles, close-up of back (courtesy of Franklin H. Top, M.D.); syphilis: primary and secondary (mixed), chancre of mouth and face (courtesy of Frank C. Combes, M.D., et al.). (*Right, top to bottom*) Scarlet fever: upper half of body, third day of rash (courtesy of Franklin H. Top, M.D.); impetigo, lesions of the face (courtesy of Franklin H. Top, M.D.); generalized tinea (ringworm) of body (culture, *Microsporum lanosum*) (courtesy of Nathan Pensky, M.D., and Natalie D. Goldberg, M.D.). (Courtesy of Clay-Adams Co., New York City.)

Bed rest is indicated when there is sufficient rise in temperature to affect appreciably the respiratory and pulse rates. It is usually prescribed when the adult's oral temperature exceeds 38° C (100.4° F), although a persistent temperature of even less than this suggests the need for more than the average amount of rest and sleep.

Quiet surroundings are indicated by the tendency to headache, nausea, and irritability and by the need for extra sleep. If there is photophobia, dark glasses, an eyeshade, or a silk scarf tied over the eyes is welcome. This is to be preferred to darkening the room, although the latter may be desirable in some cases. A dark, gloomy room is depressing and particularly so to the confused or the delirious. It is also more difficult for the nurse to give effective care if she cannot see the patient's response to treatment or see clearly the equipment with which she is working.

Sleep should be encouraged by removing the sources of discomfort, if possible. Sedatives may induce sleep but they increase the patient's mental confusion and depression and, as in all cases, tend to develop a dependence upon drugs. A skillfully given sponge bath, a back rub, a cool, smooth bed, relief of thirst, and cleaning the mouth and removal of any crusts that obstruct the nose will induce a more natural, restful sleep than medications.

Reassurance should be given the anxious and delirious patient. The presence of anyone he trusts is reassuring, but if the nurse can anticipate his needs and discover the sources of his worries and in what way he is disoriented, she can reduce his anxiety appreciably. He may, for example, mistake a robe thrown over a chair for a person sitting in it and feel frustrated if the nurse, not seeing what he sees, tells him there is no one with him except herself. A little effort might enable the nurse to distinguish between optical illusions and hallucinations and to understand the fears that often accompany fever. Restraint of the febrile patient may be necessary in understaffed hospitals, but it is never desirable. The disoriented person struggles against restraint and thus increases the tax on his heart. Reducing the patient's physical discomfort usually reduces restlessness. For example, the nurse should be sure that the bedclothes are not too warm or restricting, or that he is not thirsty or feeling the urge to urinate or defecate. The room of a febrile patient should be cool but free from drafts.

Reducing extremes of body temperature is a responsibility shared by the physician and nurse. While he ordinarily prescribes the measures to be used, the physician expects them to be adapted to the patient's needs by the nurse. Antipyretic drugs, so commonly employed in the first part of the century, are rarely given unless they have some other therapeutic effect for which they are prescribed. Aspirin (acetylsalicylic acid), for example, reduces the temperature slightly and it is often used, but for its mildly sedative rather than its antipyretic action. Sponge baths are still used routinely in many services for protracted fevers of 39° C (102.2° F) and over. While temperatures of less than 40.6° C (105° F) are not likely to cause permanent injury to nerve tissue, they are likely to produce intense discomfort and delirium. Sponge baths and other forms of cooling therapy are given, therefore, every three or four hours during high temperatures or until there is a temperature reduction. These procedures are described in Chapter 21. They are discontinued, of course, if the patient responds unfavorably. If the patient has a low-grade fever and is ambulatory, ordinary clothing is appropriate. It is often wise to dress a sick child so that he does not have to stay under the bedclothes for warmth. The restriction may do him more harm than good.

The profuse sweating that accompanies fever demands frequent cleansing baths and changes of clothing. Alcohol applied to the skin has a cooling effect, and the odor is refreshing to most persons. During a chill extra covers and external heat are welcomed by the patient, but they may have no effect on the paroxysm. Absorbent cotton clothing is likely to feel less clammy than silk, but personal preferences should be considered.

Combating water loss and electrolyte imbalance and other forms of malnutrition is the nurse's major task in fever nursing. The febrile patient usually eats reluctantly and, if nauseated, cannot even tolerate fluids while, as was pointed out in Chapter 13, fever speeds up metabolism. DuBois refers to the "so-called toxic destruction of protein" demonstrated in typhoid fever patients by the elimination of two or three times the normal amount of nitrogen in the urine. He found that when nurses were available who could see that the patient ate and drank a diet that provided at least 2000 cc (2 qt) of fluid, ample protein, and 2000 to 4000 calories (according to individual needs) a "level of resting metabolism" could be maintained during the protracted temperature elevation in typhoid fever.*

During brief periods of fever there is little probability of dangerously increasing the toxemia with a lowered intake. Infants and young children are, however, very susceptible to this form of toxemia, and even with adults it is unwise to allow the urinary output to fall below 1000 cc (1 qt). Since a diet complete in all food elements except fat can be given parenterally there are few cases in which a fever patient in the hospitals of this country need be exposed to the danger of an inadequate diet. Where he must depend upon mouth feeding, the nurse's skill may be taxed to the utmost, and if vomiting is persistent, extraoral feeding is essential. Vomiting may be induced by coughing. This is a particular problem in pertussis (whooping cough). It is helpful in this disease to feed the patient after a paroxysm, to avoid overloading the stomach, and to reduce tension during feeding periods as much as possible.

No effort should be spared in providing the nutritional requirements during the febrile period. It is well known that starvation in itself can produce fever and that a poor appetite is one of the signs of a vitamin deficiency. The cracked lips, the swollen gums, and furry tongue (sordes), so common in protracted febrile states in years past, were unquestionably signs of a vitamin lack since it was customary to "starve a fever." Malnutrition starts a vicious cycle, which, once established, is hard to interrupt.

Elimination by the skin, bowels, and bladder should be observed by the nurse, and her observations reported. The excessive sweating, as has been noted, often

---

* DuBois, Eugene F.: *op. cit.*, pp. 48–55.

reduces the elimination by the kidneys to a dangerous point. The nurse keeps a record of intake and output so that the physician can prescribe parenteral fluids if there is an inadequate intake by mouth. The nurse herself should, however, realize that for an adult an output of less than 1000 cc is a danger signal, as is concentrated urine, which is evidenced by its dark color. Bowel elimination is regulated by diet, if possible. Cathartics increase the tendency to nausea and they hurry food through the intestines before optimum absorption has occurred. Suppositories, enemas, and irrigation of the colon may be prescribed for constipation when diet is ineffective and carthartics contraindicated. With the present-day recognition of the "dangers of bed rest" most doctors are likely to permit patients "bathroom privileges" even though they have a fever. The use of the bedpan is, however, necessary in most cases because a private bathroom is essential while the patient can transmit his disease to others.

Skin care, or bodily cleanliness, is a special problem because excessive sweating may keep a fastidious person feeling "unclean." Frequent baths are often desirable for their refreshing as well as their antipyretic effect. Starch baths are soothing in eruptive diseases, such as measles and scarlet fever, but unless there is a private bathroom available to the patient it is difficult to provide a comforting starch bath without subjecting others to the disease.* When immersion baths are contraindicated by the existence of skin lesions that the physician thinks will be adversely affected by water, the nurse should bathe those portions of the body where lesions are not present, particularly the face and hands, the axillae, pubic area, and feet. If such body aspects are bathed the patient feels very much as he might if the whole body had been bathed.

Care of the eyes, nose, mouth, and ears is a simple or difficult problem according to the age of the patient, the duration of the fever, and the effect of the specific infection on the mucous membrane. If the microorganism causing the fever does not also produce lesions of the mucous membrane, the care of the eyes, nose, and mouth may not differ from that given in health although the cleansing processes may be required at more frequent intervals. Because sordes accompanied fever more or less regularly in the past, mouth lesions were looked upon as inevitable, and it was customary to replace the toothbrush with cotton applicators that were believed to clean more gently. With adequate feeding and with persistent and effective use of the toothbrush, sordes can be prevented. The writer doubts whether the teeth are ever thoroughly cleaned unless a brush is used. A refreshing mouthwash is helpful, and the lips should be lubricated with cold cream or its equivalent. Sprays, gargles, and irrigations may be prescribed by the doctor when there is an infection of the mouth or pharynx.

Crusts should be removed from the nose with a cotton-tipped applicator that has been slightly moistened with an emollient, such as vegetable oil. The eyes may need cleaning frequently if there is a discharge. If this is tenacious and has a tendency to dry and hold the lids closed, a small amount of petroleum jelly on the lid margins will help.

* Aveeno is a patented preparation of starch available in a convenient form for this purpose.

The ears require no special care unless the infection invades them. The nurse should be alert to the early symptoms of an ear involvement since this complication occurs frequently in many of the acute systemic infections unless they respond to treatment in their early stages.

Providing companionship, diversion, and occupation is a major problem in fever and communicable disease nursing. During the acute phase when there is prostration, physical discomfort, and anxiety the patient needs someone with him almost

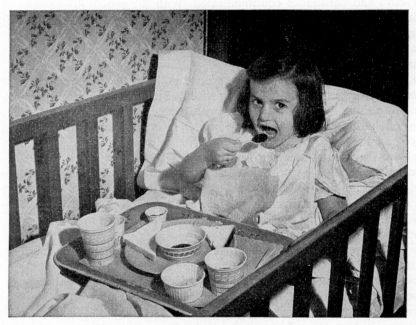

Figure 248. Child convalescing from a communicable disease in the home. Paper dishes are used since they may be discarded and burned. (Courtesy of Field Research Division, Paper Cup and Container Institute, Inc., New York City.)

constantly in order to supply him with water, nourishment, and other bodily wants, as well as to provide reassurance. As he recovers and is able to do more and more for himself, the seclusion forced on him by the communicability of his disease may be depressing and, to the small child, frustrating. The companionship of other patients with the same disease is usually helpful but not always available. In any event, the nurse should consider the provision of diversion and occupation a part of the responsibility she shares with the family and other members of the medical team. *The rehabilitation* of the person with tuberculosis, leprosy, or poliomyelitis should begin during the early stages; however, the special problems involved cannot be discussed adequately in this text.

Preventing the Transmission of the Patient's Infection to Other Persons, Animals, or Insects. Medical and surgical asepsis was discussed in Chapters 7 and 8 and has been stressed throughout this text. The tabulated data that follow will, it is hoped, give the reader the specific information needed in providing controls for the more common communicable diseases. It should be clear from these data that the recommended measures depend upon the avenues through which the infection enters and leaves the body. A group of procedures is advocated for the control of diseases in which the invading organism enters the body through the mouth and leaves it in the urine and feces; another group of precautions is necessary when the invading organism is transmitted by an insect vector, and so on. The reader will find a general discussion of this subject in earlier chapters of this text and for more details should refer to books and articles listed at the end of the chapter.

In summary it might be said that nursing the patient with an acute infectious disease rarely presents new problems. It demands an understanding of the effect of fever and it requires the nurse to practice and teach others to practice a more rigid aseptic technique than is necessary elsewhere. The distressing symptoms of infection are seen on all services and they are relieved by measures the nurse uses quite commonly. Effective care in communicable disease depends upon prompt diagnosis and treatment and upon anticipating the patient's nursing needs. Complications such as nephritis, otitis media, pneumonia, and hemorrhage are rarely seen in the reputable hospitals of this country. Avoidance of complications is not, however, the ultimate goal. As with all categories of disease, the medical team should not feel satisfied until the patient has been rehabilitated and has assumed an effective place in the life of the community.

REFERENCES

1. Dublin, Louis I. *The Facts of Life from Birth to Death.* The Macmillan Company, 1951, p. 105.
2. Leavell, Hugh R., and Clark, E. Gurney: *Textbook of Preventive Medicine.* McGraw-Hill Book Co., New York, 1953, p. 445.
3. New York State Department of Health, Bureau of Epidemiology: *Guide for the Handling of Communicable Diseases in General Hospitals.* The Department, Albany, 1950.
4. Maxcy, Kenneth F. (ed.): *Rosenau's Preventive Medicine and Hygiene,* 7th ed. Appleton-Century-Crofts, Inc., New York, 1951, p. 321.
5. Kluth, Fred C.: "The Epidemiology of Hansen's Disease," *Nursing Outlook,* 2:77, (Feb.) 1954.
6. Leavell, Hugh. R., and Clark, E. Gurney: *op. cit.,* p. 88.
7. Federal Security Agency, Public Health Service, Division of Venereal Disease of the Bureau of State Services: *Nursing in Venereal Disease Control.* Public Health Service Publication No. 198, US Government Printing Office, Washington, D.C., 1952.
8. Hall, Reina F.: "Interviewing as a Nursing Procedure," *Am. J. Nursing,* 52:707, (June) 1952.
9. Houston, William R.: *The Art of Treatment.* The Macmillan Company, 1936, p. 85.
10. Biskind, Morton, and Martin, William C.: "The Use of Citrus Flavonoids in Infections. II," *Am. J. Digest. Dis.,* 22:41, (Feb.) 1955.
11. Sokoloff, B.: "The Capillary Syndrome in Viral Infections, Treatment with Citrus Flavonoids," *Am. J. Digest Dis.,* 22:7, (Jan.) 1955.
12. Klenner, F. R.: "The Use of Vitamin C as an Antibiotic," *J. Appl. Nutrition,* 6:274, (Mar.) 1953.

("Additional Suggested Reading" appears on p. 1108.)

3. SUMMARY TABLE OF DATA

Table 17. Presenting in Simplified Form the Important Aspects of Control in Communicable Diseases*

DISEASE	NUMBER OF STATES REPORTING IN 1934 (AND 1949†)	CAUSATIVE ORGANISM	PORTAL OF ENTRY AND MODE OF TRANSMISSION	INCU-BATION PERIOD	PERIOD OF COM-MUNICA-BILITY	IM-MUNITY AFTER RE-COVERY	IMMUNIZATION	RESISTANCE OF ORGANISM	CONTROL BY ASEPTIC MEASURES	HOUS-ING
			DISEASES SPREAD MAINLY THROUGH DISCHARGES FROM THE MOUTH AND NOSE							
A. Caused by Bacilli										
1. Diph-theria	48 (49)	Coryne-bacterium diph-theriae (Klebs-Loeffler bacillus)	Eyes, nose, mouth (may also infect wounds). Di-rect contact by kissing. Drop-let infection. Indirectly by articles soiled with dis-charges from mouth, nose, or wound. In milk or other food. By car-riers	2–7 days	Variable, un-til virulent bacilli have disappeared from the se-cretions and lesions. Usu-ally 2 weeks or less, sel-dom over 4 weeks	Usually immune	Every child should be im-munized by 2 injections at one-month intervals, with alum-precipi-tated toxoid, beginning after 3 months of age. One fur-ther injection should be given before school entrance and at any time thereafter that diphtheria ap-pears in the community	Resists dry-ing if pro-tected by al-buminous material. Re-sists freez-ing. De-stroyed at 60° C (140° F) in 30 minutes. Killed by boiling at 100° C (212° F) in 10 minutes	Isolate for period of communica-bility. Individual bedside equip-ment. Attendants wear moisture-proof masks and gowns to protect clothing. (Authorities dif-fer on the advisa-bility of using masks.) Boil dishes and uten-sils 10 minutes. Boil linen 10 minutes. Auto-clave or destroy books	Room: recom-mended; ward: not recom-mended

* General references referred to for compilation of Table 17 are listed in "Additional Suggested Reading," page 1108.
† Figures within parentheses in this column are 1949 figures, taken from *Statistical Abstracts of the United States*, 1951. p. 85.   District of Colum-bia counted as a state.

		Causative organism	Mode of transmission	Incubation period	Period of communicability	Immunity	Immunization	Resistance of organism	Precautions	Isolation
2. Tuberculosis (pulmonary)	33 (49)	*Mycobacterium tuberculosis*	Nose, mouth, gastrointestinal tract. Direct contact with sputum, discharge from tubercular lesion anywhere in body, urine, or feces. Droplet infection. Inhalation of contaminated dust. In milk and water. On fingers and soiled personal objects	Probably not less than 1 month and may be much longer	Until disappearance of organism from sputum and other secretions	Disease is arrested; infection remains active or dormant throughout life	BCG vaccination is recommended by some for groups of tuberculin nonreactors who are relatively more exposed to tuberculosis. Duration of protection still unknown	Resists drying in sputum three months. Destroyed at 60° C (140° F) in 30 minutes. Destroyed by boiling at 100° C (212° F) in 10 minutes	As in diphtheria for acute respiratory infections. As in amebic dysentery for intestinal infections. As in boils, abscesses, etc., for wound infections. (Precautions may be less rigid in tuberculosis sanatoria where patients have an active infection and members of the staff arrested infections)	Room: recommended; cubicle: permissible; open ward: not recommended
3. Vincent's angina (trench mouth) (ulcerative stomatitis)	Not reportable	*Bacillus fusiformis* and *Borrelia vincentii* are considered to be causes	Mouth. Direct contact with nose and throat discharges. Droplet infection. Indirectly by contact with soiled dishes, linen, and personal articles. Carriers	Unknown	Until smears from nose and throat are negative	Not immune. Recurrence is very likely		Destroyed by boiling at 100° C (212° F) in 10 minutes	Precautions as in common cold. Isolation of the patient is not necessary, but proper care of the discharges and soiled utensils are essential	Open ward: permissible
4. Whooping cough (pertussis)	48 (49)	*Hemophilus pertussis*	Nose, mouth. Direct contact with nose and throat discharges. Drop-form-	7-21 days; almost uniform-	From appearance of catarrhal symptoms until 3 weeks	Immune	Give vaccine starting at 3 to 4 months of age; 3 doses, usually given	Destroyed by boiling at 100° C (212° F) in 10 minutes	Isolate for period of communicability. Precautions as in diphtheria. (Because	Room: recommended; open ward:

Table 17. Presenting in Simplified Form the Important Aspects of Control in Communicable Diseases (cont.)

DISEASE	NUMBER OF STATES REPORTING IN 1934 (AND 1949)	CAUSATIVE ORGANISM	PORTAL OF ENTRY AND MODE OF TRANSMISSION	INCU-BATION PERIOD	PERIOD OF COMMUNICA-BILITY	IMMUNITY AFTER RE-COVERY	IMMUNIZATION	RESISTANCE OF ORGANISM	CONTROL BY ASEPTIC MEASURES	HOUS-ING
DISEASES SPREAD MAINLY THROUGH DISCHARGES FROM THE MOUTH AND NOSE (CONT.)										
A. Caused by Bacilli			let infection. Indirectly by articles soiled with discharges from the mouth or nose. Human carriers may be more impor-tant than was formerly sus-pected	ly within 10 days	after the first whoop		with 1-month interval; boost-er dose advis-able 6 to 12 months follow-ing completion of initial in-jections. Vac-cine is made from *Hemo-philus pertussis,* Phase I organ-isms. Recent tendency is to combine whooping cough vaccine with diphtheria toxoid or with diphtheria and tetanus toxoids		this is often a mild and long-drawn-out dis-ease, the patient is allowed to mix with immune persons but kept away from the general public)	not recom-mended

1086

B. Caused by Cocci

		Causative organism	Source and mode of transmission	Incubation period	Period of communicability	Immunity	Prophylaxis	Destruction of organism	Isolation period	Room or ward
1. Epidemic meningitis (cerebrospinal fever)	45 (49)	*Neisseria intracellularis*	Nose, mouth. Direct contact with nasal secretions, spinal fluid, or urine of infected person. Droplet infection. Indirectly by contact with contaminated articles. Flies. Carriers	1–10 days, usually 7 days	Until organisms disappear from nasal secretions and urine	Not immune, but second attacks are rare	None	Readily destroyed by drying. Destroyed by boiling at 100° C (212° F) in 10 minutes	Isolate for 14 days or until end of febrile period or until cultures are negative	Room: recommended; open ward: not recommended; cubicle: permissible
2. Pneumonia (pneumococcal)	22 (48)	Pneumococcus	Nose, mouth (may also infect wounds). Direct contact with nose and throat discharges. Indirectly by contact with contaminated articles. Carriers	Believed to be short, usually 1–3 days. Not well determined	Unknown, presumably until discharges of mouth and nose no longer carry infectious agent in an abundant amount or in a virulent form	Not immune	In experimental stage	Destroyed by boiling at 100° C (212° F) in 10 minutes	Isolate for period of communicability. Precautions are similar to those outlined for the care of the patient with diphtheria	Room: recommended; open ward: not recommended
3. Scarlet fever and streptococcal	48 (49) 29	Several known strains of hemolytic strepto-	Nose, mouth (may also infect wounds). Direct contact with nose,	2–7 days; usually 2–5 days	From beginning of symptoms until all lesions have	Usually immune, but only to specific	Of questionable value	Destroyed at 60° C (140° F) in 30 minutes. Destroyed	Isolate for period of communicability. Precautions are the same as those	Room: recommended; open ward:

DISEASE	NUMBER OF STATES REPORTING IN 1934 (AND 1949)	CAUSATIVE ORGANISM	PORTAL OF ENTRY AND MODE OF TRANSMISSION	INCUBATION PERIOD	PERIOD OF COMMUNICABILITY	IMMUNITY AFTER RECOVERY	IMMUNIZATION	RESISTANCE OF ORGANISM	CONTROL BY ASEPTIC MEASURES	HOUSING
B. Caused by Cocci										
	DISEASES SPREAD MAINLY THROUGH DISCHARGES FROM THE MOUTH AND NOSE (CONT.)									
sore throat		coccus (the causative organism is closely related to that of erysipelas)	throat, and ear discharges. Indirectly by contact with contaminated articles. Milk and ice cream. Undiagnosed, mild cases; carriers, man and cow		healed and all abnormal discharges have stopped, and until throat cultures are negative (average 2 weeks)	type of organism causing disease		by boiling at 100° C (212° F) in 10 minutes	outlined for the care of the patient with diphtheria	not recommended
C. Caused by Filtrable Viruses										
1. Common cold	Not reportable	Two filtrable viruses. (May be aggravated by secondary invaders—pneumococci, strepto-	Eyes, nose, mouth. Direct contact with discharges from nose and throat. Droplet infection. Indirectly by articles freshly soiled with discharges from	From 1–6 days according to type of virus	May be infectious during incubation period before evidence of symptoms; continues as long as discharges from nose, mouth,	Not immune	None	Survives anaerobically 13 days. Destroyed by boiling at 100° C (212° F) in 10 minutes	Desirable to isolate for period of communicability. Individual toilet articles. Burn discharges from nose, mouth, eyes, and ears. Boil dishes. Air mattress and blankets in sun-	Room: recommended; cubicle: permissible; open ward: not recommended

	cocci, or staphylococci)	nose, mouth, or eyes		eyes, or ears contain the virus			light 6 hours. Wash unit with soap and water		Room: recommended; open ward: not recommended
2. Enceph-alitis	37	5 forms established, all attributed to viruses	Probably as in colds for type A, other types by insect bites. Type A probably transmitted by droplet infections from humans; animals are believed to be hosts to other types, and transmitted by insect bites	From 1–21 days according to type, usually 5–15 days; unknown for type A	Unknown for type A. Other types probably not communicable from man to man	Usually immune but only to virus causing illness	In experimental stage	Screening from insects is important, for all types but type A	Destroyed by boiling at 100° C (212° F) in 10 minutes	Room: recommended; open ward: not recommended
3. German measles (rubella)	28	Unknown, presumably a virus	Nose, mouth; mode of transmission as in common cold	10–21 days, usually about 18 days	From onset of catarrhal symptoms for at least 4 days, but not more than 7; the exact period is undetermined	Usually immune	None	Isolate for 5 days from beginning of rash. Precautions are the same as those outlined for the care of patients with diphtheria	Destroyed by boiling at 100° C (212° F) for 10 minutes	Room: recommended; open ward: not recommended
4. Influ-enza	33 (46)	2 viruses, each with many strains	Nose, mouth; same as in colds	Short, usually 24–72 hours	Undetermined, possibly in the prodromal as	Immune about 6 months against strain	In experimental stage	Isolate for period of communicability. Precautions are the same as those	Destroyed by boiling at 100° C (212° F) for 10 minutes	Room: recommended; open ward:

Table 17.   Presenting in Simplified Form the Important Aspects of Control in Communicable Diseases (cont.)

DISEASE	NUMBER OF STATES REPORTING IN 1934 (AND 1949)	CAUSATIVE ORGANISM	PORTAL OF ENTRY AND MODE OF TRANSMISSION	INCUBATION PERIOD	PERIOD OF COMMUNICABILITY	IMMUNITY AFTER RECOVERY	IMMUNIZATION	RESISTANCE OF ORGANISM	CONTROL BY ASEPTIC MEASURES	HOUSING
C. Caused by Filtrable Viruses										
DISEASES SPREAD MAINLY THROUGH DISCHARGES FROM THE MOUTH AND NOSE (CONT.)										
					well as in the febrile stage	causing disease			outlined for the care of patients with diphtheria	not recommended
5. Viral pneumonia (primary atypical pneumonia)		Probably a virus	Nose, mouth; same as in colds	7–21 days, usually 11 days	Undetermined	Questionable	None	Destroyed by boiling at 100° C (212° F) in 10 minutes	As in diphtheria	Room: recommended: open ward: not recommended
6. Measles (rubeola)	48 (49)	Filtrable virus	Nose, mouth; as in colds	About 10 days from date of exposure to onset of fever; 13–15 days	From onset of catarrhal symptoms until cessation of discharges from eyes, nose, pharynx, and ears	Immune	Children between 6 months and 5 years should be given gamma globulin injections. This completely protects younger children and allows modified	Dies quickly when exposed to air. Destroyed by boiling at 100° C (212° F) for 10 minutes	Isolate for period of communicability, as in diphtheria	Room: recommended; open ward: not recommended

1090

	No.	Cause	Mode of infection	Incubation period	Immunity	Prevention	Destruction of organism	Isolation	Ward
				to appearance of rash; uncommonly longer or shorter. If passive immunization has been attempted too late, incubation period may be 21 days		measles in older ones. 2 cc of gamma globulin suffices. Adults can be also protected from severe attacks with gamma globulin. Convalescent human serum also effective, but there is risk of serum hepatitis			Room: recommended; open ward: not recommended
7. Mumps (parotitis)	39 (46)	Filtrable virus	Nose, mouth. Usually by direct contact or droplet infection; rarely indirectly	12–26 days, most commonly 18 days	Immune; second attacks rare	In the experimental stage	Destroyed by boiling at 100° C (212° F) for 10 minutes	As in diphtheria. Isolate for period of communicability	Room: recommended; open ward: not recommended
8. Polio-myelitis,	48 (49)	3 viruses so far	Nose, mouth. As in colds.	Usually 7–14	Usually im-	Vaccines against all 3	Destroyed by boiling	As in diphtheria and dysentery.	Room: recom-

Table 17. Presenting in Simplified Form the Important Aspects of Control in Communicable Diseases (cont.)

C. Caused by Filtrable Viruses

DISEASES SPREAD MAINLY THROUGH DISCHARGES FROM THE MOUTH AND NOSE (CONT.)

DISEASE	NUMBER OF STATES REPORTING IN 1934 (AND 1949)	CAUSATIVE ORGANISM	PORTAL OF ENTRY AND MODE OF TRANSMISSION	INCUBATION PERIOD	PERIOD OF COMMUNICABILITY	IMMUNITY AFTER RECOVERY	IMMUNIZATION	RESISTANCE OF ORGANISM	CONTROL BY ASEPTIC MEASURES	HOUSING
acute anterior (infantile paralysis)		demonstrated	Feces, food, milk, flies. Dust (?)	days; may be 3–35 days	cubation period through acute illness, possibly longer	mune; second attacks rare and may be caused by a virus of a different strain	types of polio have been developed and used safely and successfully in preliminary tests. Gamma globulin seems to confer temporary immunity	at 100° C (212° F) for 10 minutes. Strong oxidizing agents such as potassium permanganate and hydrogen peroxide, as well as ultraviolet radiation, also destroy virus	Discharges from nose and throat of patient are infectious early in the disease, and tissues used should be placed in a bag and burned. Feces are infectious for a long period, and patient's bedpan should not be used by others until sterilized. Isolate for period of communicability	mended; open ward: not recommended
9. Smallpox (variola)	37 (49)	Filtrable virus	Nose, mouth, wounds; direct contact with secretions from nose or mouth or skin lesions. Indirectly by	7–21 days, usually 12 days	From first symptoms until all scabs disappear; most communicable in the early stages	Immune	Vaccination with cowpox virus confers immunity. WHO and US consider immunity from vaccination	Preserved by drying. Destroyed by boiling at 100° C (212° F) for 10 minutes	As in diphtheria. Burn discharges from lesions. Isolate for period of communicability	Room: recommended; open ward: not recommended

		contaminated articles. Dust. Flies		of the disease	valid for 3 years. Vaccination in early infancy, revaccination of children on entering school, and of entire population when disease appears in severe form are necessary public health measures			

DISEASES SPREAD MAINLY THROUGH DISCHARGES FROM THE SKIN AND MUCOUS MEMBRANES

No.	Disease	Etiologic agent	Mode of transmission	Incubation	Communicability	Immunity	Immunization	Destruction of agent	Prevention	Isolation
23	1. Chancroid	Hemophilus ducreyi	Genitourinary tract; direct contact with genital ulcer during sexual intercourse. Indirectly on towels, instruments, or dressings soiled with discharge from ulcer	From 1–12 days, usually 3–5 days	As long as the etiologic agent persists in the original lesion or regional lymph nodes	Not immune	None	Dies at room temperature. Destroyed by boiling at 100° C (212° F) for 10 minutes	Personal cleanliness. Abstinence from sexual intercourse during course of the disease. Individual toilet articles. Boil contaminated linen 20 minutes. Burn dressings soiled with discharge from lesion	Room: not recommended; open ward: permissible; cubicle: recommended
48 (48)	2. Chickenpox (varicella)	Filtrable virus	Nose, mouth. Direct contact with watery vesicles on the mucous membranes and	14–21 days	Several hours before eruption appears until 6 days after ap-	Immune	None	Destroyed by boiling at 100° C (212° F) for 10 minutes	Isolate for duration of disease. Precautions are the same as for patient with diphtheria	Room: recommended; open ward: not

Table 17. Presenting in Simplified Form the Important Aspects of Control in Communicable Diseases (cont.)

DISEASES SPREAD MAINLY THROUGH DISCHARGES FROM THE SKIN AND MUCOUS MEMBRANES (CONT.)

DISEASE	NUMBER OF STATES REPORTING IN 1934 (AND 1949)	CAUSATIVE ORGANISM	PORTAL OF ENTRY AND MODE OF TRANSMISSION	INCUBATION PERIOD	PERIOD OF COMMUNICABILITY	IMMUNITY AFTER RECOVERY	IMMUNIZATION	RESISTANCE OF ORGANISM	CONTROL BY ASEPTIC MEASURES	HOUSING
			skin or with discharges from the nose and throat. Indirectly by contact with articles contaminated with these discharges		pearance of first crop of vesicles					recommended
3. Ringworm (epidermophytosis) (one form of ringworm: athlete's foot)	Not reportable	Microsporon, trichophyton, epidermophyton, and other species of fungi	Skin, especially moist skin between the toes. Direct contact with skin lesions. Indirectly by contact with gymnasium floors, swimming pools, shower floors, contaminated stockings or shoes	Unknown	As long as lesions remain	Not immune	None	Destroyed by boiling at 100° C (212° F) for 10 minutes	Keep affected area covered to protect others. Personal cleanliness to prevent autoinoculation. Individual toilet articles. Boil linen which has been in contact with lesions for 1 hour. In public places: Provide antiseptic foot baths in showers.	Room: not recommended; open ward: permissible; cubicle: recommended

Disease	No.	Causative organism	Source and mode of transmission	Incubation period	Period of communicability	Immunity		Resistance of organism	Control measures		Admission
4. Gonorrhea (including gonorrheal conjunctivitis)	44 (49)	Neisseria gonorrhoeae	Genitourinary tract, eyes. Direct contact during sexual intercourse. Indirectly on hands, bed linen, clothing, towels, bathtubs, and toilet seats possibly; and to babies' eyes during passage through birth canal	1–14 days, usually 3–5 days	As long as organism is present in discharge. May be years	Not immune	None	Slight resistance to light and heat. May live in a thick layer of pus on linen for several weeks if protected from light and heat. Destroyed by boiling at 100° C (212° F) in 10 minutes	Isolate during acute stage and protect others from contact with gonorrheal discharges at all times. Individual bedside equipment. Burn discharges from genitourinary tract and eyes. Boil linen 10 minutes. Boil dishes and utensils 10 minutes. Burn books or papers if contaminated with discharges. Air mattress and blankets in sunlight 6 hours. Wash unit with soap and water. Silver nitrate 1 per cent in eyes of the newborn	Clean floors thoroughly. Admit sunlight and air to public bathrooms if possible	Room: not recommended; cubicle: recommended; open ward: permissible
5. Impetigo con-	7	Probably staphylo-	Skin. Direct contact with	2–5 days	As long as lesions re-	Not immune	None	Destroyed by boiling	Isolation during acute stage. Per-		Room: not

Table 17. Presenting in Simplified Form the Important Aspects of Control in Communicable Diseases (cont.)

DISEASES SPREAD MAINLY THROUGH DISCHARGES FROM THE SKIN AND MUCOUS MEMBRANES (CONT.)

DISEASE	NUMBER OF STATES REPORTING IN 1934 (AND 1949)	CAUSATIVE ORGANISM	PORTAL OF ENTRY AND MODE OF TRANSMISSION	INCUBATION PERIOD	PERIOD OF COMMUNICABILITY	IMMUNITY AFTER RECOVERY	IMMUNIZATION	RESISTANCE OF ORGANISM	CONTROL BY ASEPTIC MEASURES	HOUSING
tagiosa		cocci and streptococci	lesions. Auto-inoculation by scratching. Indirectly on hands, instruments, and linen		main un-healed			at 100° C (212° F) in 10 minutes	sonal cleanliness to prevent auto-inoculation. Individual toilet articles. Burn discharges from lesions. Boil used instruments 10 minutes. Boil linen in contact with lesions 10 minutes. Air mattress and blankets 6 hours in sunlight. Wash unit with soap and water	recommended; cubicle: recommended; open ward: permissible
6. Scabies (itch)	37	*Sarcoptes* or *Acarus scabei* (itch mite)	Skin. Direct: man to man and animal to man. Auto-inoculation by scratching. Indirectly by contact with contaminated	Length of time for the itch mite to burrow into the skin	Until itch mite and ova are destroyed	Not immune	None	Destroyed by boiling at 100° C (212° F) in 10 minutes	Individual toilet articles. Boil linen and clothing 10 minutes. Dry-clean bedding and clothing that cannot be boiled, using care to avoid	Room: not recommended; cubicle: recommended; open ward:

			clothing, bed linen, and towels	and lay ova					contamination of other clothing	permissible
7. Syphilis	44 (49)	*Treponema pallidum*	Genitourinary tract, mucous membrane of mouth, abrasion in skin. Direct contact with primary sore during sexual intercourse or kissing (first stage). Direct contact at site of contact. Indirectly on drinking cups, linen, and instruments	10–90 days, average 3 weeks; after exposure chancre appears at site of contact. 4–6 weeks to 1 year after appearance of chancre secondary stage occurs with mucous patches and papules. After	Throughout primary and secondary stages and during mucocutaneous relapses. Disease may be transmitted from mother to fetus during secondary and tertiary stages	An infection appears to confer immunity against further infection. However, if the infected person is treated in the early stage and cured, reinfection may occur	None	May live in moist secretion on linen 12 hours. Destroyed by drying. Destroyed by boiling at 100° C (212° F) in 10 minutes	Isolate during primary and secondary stages until lesions heal. Individual bedside equipment. Burn discharges from lesions. Attendants wear rubber gloves when handling dressings. Boil linen 10 minutes. Boil dishes and utensils 10 minutes. Air mattress and blankets in sunlight for 6 hours. Wash unit furnishings, and contaminated surfaces with soap and water and expose to air and sunlight	Room: not recommended; cubicle: recommended; open ward: permissible

Table 17. Presenting in Simplified Form the Important Aspects of Control in Communicable Diseases (cont.)

DISEASE	NUMBER OF STATES REPORTING IN 1934 (AND 1949)	CAUSATIVE ORGANISM	PORTAL OF ENTRY AND MODE OF TRANSMISSION	INCUBATION PERIOD	PERIOD OF COMMUNICABILITY	IMMUNITY AFTER RECOVERY	IMMUNIZATION	RESISTANCE OF ORGANISM	CONTROL BY ASEPTIC MEASURES	HOUSING
Diseases Spread Mainly through Discharges from the Skin and Mucous Membranes (cont.)										
				4 years or more tertiary stage occurs with systemic manifestations						
Diseases Spread Mainly through Discharges from the Gastrointestinal Tract										
1. Amebic dysentery	36 (49)	*Endamoeba histolytica*	Mouth. Direct contact with infected feces, urine, or pus from liver abscess. By carriers; often food handlers. Indirectly in water, on uncooked vegetables grown	Variable; usually 3–4 weeks; from 2 days in severe infections to	During course of infection and until repeated microscopic examination of feces shows absence of *Endamoeba histolytica*	Not immune; second attacks and relapses are quite common	None	First stage (trophozoite) frail; not infective. Second stage (cysts) highly resistant; may live in water 4 weeks. Killed in less than a	*In public places:* Examine food handlers for presence of disease organisms in feces. Screen patient from flies. Supply individual toilet equipment. Disinfect bowel discharges and	Room: not recommended; cubicle: recommended; open ward: permissible

1098

Disease	Mode of transmission	Incubation period	Period of communicability	Immunity	Prophylaxis / vaccines	Viability of organism	Disinfection and precautions	Isolation
(continued)	in soil contaminated with infected feces. Flies	several months in subacute and chronic cases	(either trophozoites or cysts)			minute in water above 80° C (176° F)	urine with 5 per cent chlorinated lime. Boil dishes and utensils, also linen, 10 minutes. Burn discharges from liver abscess. Air mattress and blankets in sunlight 6 hours. Wash unit furnishings and contaminated surfaces with soap and water; expose to air and sunlight. Decontaminate drinking water with triglycine hydroiodide	
2. Bacillary dysentery (shigellosis) — *Shigella dysenteriae* and *paradysenteriae*	Mouth. Direct contact with infected feces, or urine, Indirectly in water, milk, food. On uncooked vegetables grown in soil contaminated with infected feces. By carriers; flies	1–7 days; usually less than 4 days	During the acute phase of the disease and until the microorganism is absent from the feces. Feces usually become negative in a few weeks without specific therapy	Not immune. Recurrences are not uncommon	Vaccines have not been used because they are toxic and do not seem to offer much protection	May live in feces 1–2 days. May live for months when moist or frozen. Destroyed at 60° C (140° F) in 20 minutes. Destroyed by boiling at 100° C (212° F) in 10 minutes	Observe same precautions as for patients with amebic dysentery	Room: not recommended; cubicle: recommended; open ward: permissible

Table 17. Presenting in Simplified Form the Important Aspects of Control in Communicable Diseases (cont.).

DISEASES SPREAD MAINLY THROUGH DISCHARGES FROM THE GASTROINTESTINAL TRACT (CONT.)

DISEASE	NUMBER OF STATES REPORTING IN 1934 (AND 1949)	CAUSATIVE ORGANISM	PORTAL OF ENTRY AND MODE OF TRANSMISSION	INCUBATION PERIOD	PERIOD OF COMMUNICABILITY	IMMUNITY AFTER RECOVERY	IMMUNIZATION	RESISTANCE OF ORGANISM	CONTROL BY ASEPTIC MEASURES	HOUSING
3. Paratyphoid fever	48 (49)	Bacilli paratyphosus A and B	Mouth. As in bacillary dysentery; also in sputum of infected person; sea food	Usually 1–10 days; sometimes longer	From onset until 2 negative stool specimens have been obtained not less than 24 hours apart	Usually immune	A mixed vaccine containing typhoid, paratyphoid A, and paratyphoid B used for combined immunization against all 3 diseases. Given in 3 doses at weekly intervals; lasts 2–3 years	May live in feces several months. May live in water 3 days. Destroyed at 60° C (140° F) in 20 minutes	Observe same precautions as those listed in the care of patients with amebic dysentery	Room: not recommended; cubicle: recommended; open ward: permissible
4. Typhoid fever	48 (49)	Eberthella typhosa	Mouth. As in bacillary dysentery	Usually 7–14 days, but may be 3–40 days	As in paratyphoid fever; also as long as typhoid bacilli appear in the feces or urine, and for a varying period of time after cessation of all symptoms	Usually immune	See paratyphoid column above	As in paratyphoid	Observe same precautions as for patients with amebic dysentery	Room: not recommended; cubicle: recommended; open ward: permissible

| 1. Anthrax | 16 | *Bacillus anthracis* (spore former) | *Wounds:* Direct contact with lesion; also abrasions in the skin contaminated by handling hides, hair, or fleeces of cattle, sheep, horses, and swine. *Respiratory tract:* Inhalation of spores that float in air as wool is sorted. *Gastrointestinal tract:* Ingestion of infected meat or food contaminated by unclean hands. Rarely transmitted from man to man. 95 per cent through wounds and 5 per cent through respiratory tract. (Gastrointestinal tract: cases rare) | Within 7 days; usually less than 4; may be within 24 hours in pulmonary cases | During febrile stage of the disease and until lesions have ceased discharging | Not immune; second attacks have occurred within less than 1 year | No vaccine for humans; livestock can be vaccinated with a spore vaccine (Carbozoo), as illness is in almost all cases transmitted by livestock | Very resistant to drying and sunlight. Destroyed by steam at 120°C (248° F) in 20 minutes. Destroyed by dry heat above 160° C (320° F) in 1 hour | Isolation of patient until all lesions are healed. Supply individual bedside equipment. Burn discharges from lesions. Protect nurses' and doctors' hands with gloves when handling contaminated dressings or instruments. Sterilization of instruments, utensils, and linen whenever possible by steam under pressure. If not available, use fractional sterilization by boiling or by streaming steam. Sterilize blankets. Burn waste food or disinfect with 5 per cent chlorinated lime. Burn books. Autoclave mattress if possible; otherwise place in air and sunlight for 3 days. | Room: recommended; cubicle: recommended |

Table 17. Presenting in Simplified Form the Important Aspects of Control in Communicable Diseases (cont.)

DISEASES TRANSMITTED TO WOUNDS BY ORGANISMS FROM VARIOUS SOURCES (CONT.)

DISEASE	NUMBER OF STATES REPORTING IN 1934 (AND 1949)	CAUSATIVE ORGANISM	PORTAL OF ENTRY AND MODE OF TRANSMISSION	INCUBATION PERIOD	PERIOD OF COMMUNICABILITY	IMMUNITY AFTER RECOVERY	IMMUNIZATION	RESISTANCE OF ORGANISM	CONTROL BY ASEPTIC MEASURES	HOUSING
									Wash unit with soap and water. Expose to air and sunlight	
2. Boils, abscesses, and suppuration	Not reportable	*Staphylococcus aureus, Staphylococcus albus*	Wounds. Direct contact with discharges from infected lesions. Indirectly by contact with contaminated hands, dressings, instruments, or sutures. Flies	Questionable	As long as discharge continues	Not immune	Vaccines have been used with partial success	Killed by moist heat at 60° C (140° F) in 30 minutes. Destroyed by boiling at 100° C (212° F) in 10 minutes	Keep area covered. Burn discharges. Boil used instruments 10 minutes	Open ward: permissible in most cases
3. Erysipelas	16	Hemolytic streptococcus (distinct species; questionable)	Abrasions of wounds in skin or mucous membrane. Direct contact with lesion. Indirectly by contact with	2–10 days; usually 2–3 days	As long as lesions remain and as long as there are purulent discharges; at least, and probably, for	Not immune. Recurrences are frequent	None	Lives for months in dried blood or pus at room temperature. Destroyed by boiling	Isolate for period of communicability. Supply individual bedside equipment. Burn discharges from affected area, and nose	Room: recommended; cubicle: permissible; open ward:

Disease	Reporting	Source / mode of transmission	Incubation period	Period of communicability	Immunity	Resistance of organism	Control measures	Isolation
		articles contaminated with discharges from lesion or with nose and throat discharges		several days thereafter		at 100° C (212° F) in 10 minutes	and throat (if respiratory tract is involved). Attendants wear moistureproof masks. Boil linen 10 minutes. Boil dishes and utensils 10 minutes. Autoclave or burn books. Air mattress and blankets in sunlight 6 hours. Wash unit and furnishings with soap and water and expose to air and sunlight	not recommen
4. Gas gangrene	Not reportable	*Clostridium welchii* (alone or with other species of clostridia; spore formers)	Wounds. In feces of man and domestic animals. Introduction of contaminated soil into wounds. Contact with discharges from wound. Improperly sterilized sutures, instruments, and dressings. Flies. Soil is normal habitat	3–6 hours usually; may be several days, if gas bacilli are "terminal invaders"	As long as open lesions remain	Questionable; if any, slight and temporary following recovery	Gas gangrene antitoxin is used prophylactically and therapeutically	Resistant if protected from air. Destroyed by steam at 120°C (248° F) in 20 minutes. Destroyed by dry heat above 160° C (320° F) in 1 hour	Observe same precautions as for patients with anthrax	Room: not recommended; cubicle: recommended

Table 17. Presenting in Simplified Form the Important Aspects of Control in Communicable Diseases (cont.)

DISEASE	NUMBER OF STATES REPORTING IN 1934 (AND 1949)	CAUSATIVE ORGANISM	PORTAL OF ENTRY AND MODE OF TRANSMISSION	INCUBATION PERIOD	PERIOD OF COMMUNICABILITY	IMMUNITY AFTER RECOVERY	IMMUNIZATION	RESISTANCE OF ORGANISM	CONTROL BY ASEPTIC MEASURES	HOUSING
			DISEASES TRANSMITTED TO WOUNDS BY ORGANISMS FROM VARIOUS SOURCES (CONT.)							
5. Puerperal sepsis	13	Usually *Streptococcus hemolyticus.* May be caused by *Streptococcus viridans,* or *Staphylococcus* or *S. aureus albus*	Denuded area within the uterus or birth canal. From the nose or throat discharges of the patient or her attendants to the birth canal by droplet infection, on hands, instruments, or dressings. Rarely transmitted from inflamed vagina or Fallopian tubes	1–3 days, rarely longer	As long as lochia contains organism	Not immune	None	Lives for months in dried blood or pus at room temperature. Destroyed by boiling at 100° C (212° F) in 10 minutes	Observe the same precautions as for patient with erysipelas. The vaginal secretions to be treated as discharges from lesions of erysipelas	Room: recommended; cubicle: permissible; open ward: not recommended
6. Tetanus (lockjaw)	25	*Clostridium tetani*	Wounds. As in gas gangrene; also imperfectly sterilized gelatin, vaccines, and	4 days to 3 weeks, possibly longer	As long as organisms are present in wound discharges	Not immune	Active immunization with tetanus toxoid recommended in infancy, preferably	Killed readily when exposed to air. Lives in dry soil for years. De-	As in gas gangrene if wound is discharging; otherwise isolation is not necessary	No special precautions necessary as

other substances injected under the skin. Animals such as horses may remain permanent carriers		combined with pertussis and diphtheria vaccination. After initial injections a booster dose should be given within a year and renewal doses at time of each injury from which there is danger of tetanus. Reinjections recommended at 5-year intervals. Passive immunization for about 10-days' duration can be relied upon from use of tetanus antitoxin for people who have not been actively immunized	stroyed by steam at 120° C (248° F) in 20 minutes. Destroyed by dry heat above 160° C (320° F) in 1 hour	and only ordinary cleanliness is maintained	it is not considered to be spread from patient to patient

Table 17.   Presenting in Simplified Form the Important Aspects of Control in Communicable Diseases (cont.)

DISEASES SPREAD MAINLY BY INFECTED ANIMALS

DISEASE	NUMBER OF STATES REPORTING IN 1934 (AND 1949)	CAUSATIVE ORGANISM	PORTAL OF ENTRY AND MODE OF TRANSMISSION	INCUBATION PERIOD	PERIOD OF COMMUNICABILITY	IMMUNITY AFTER RECOVERY	IMMUNIZATION	RESISTANCE OF ORGANISM	CONTROL BY ASEPTIC MEASURES	HOUSING
1. Malta fever (brucellosis; undulant fever)	46 (49)	*Brucella melitensis* (goats); *Brucella abortus* (cattle; *Brucella suis* (hogs)	Mouth, abrasions in skin or mucous membranes; respiratory tract (questionable); direct contact with urine or feces of infected animal (goats, sheep, cattle, swine) or man; tissues, blood, unpasteurized milk, or dairy products of infected animals. Inhalation of contaminated dust (questionable)	6–30 days or more; average 14 days	Probably not communicable from man to man; if so, from onset of symptoms until urine is negative for the organism: a period of from 20 days to 1 year	Doubtful	None	Very resistant to drying. Destroyed at 60° C (140° F) in 30 minutes	Observe same precautions as for patient with bacillary dysentery. Protect small cuts in skin	Same as for tetanus
2. Rabies	24	Filtrable virus	Bite of rabid animal, and scratches in the skin. Rabid de-	10 days to 7 months, de-	In the dog for 3–7 days before onset of clinical	Always resulting in death	Vaccination of bitten people is usually effective; im-	Lives 4–8 days when dried and in absence of	Observe same precautions as for patient with erysipelas	Same as for tetanus

animals mostly dogs, but may also be cats, vampire bat, wolves, foxes, cattle, horses, skunks, rabbits, sheep, coyotes, swine, goats. Contact with nose and throat discharges of infected person (questionable)	pend-ing on amount of virus trans-mitted and place of bite in re-lation to rich-ness of nerve supply and length of nerve path to brain	symptoms until death; rarely, if ever, com-municated from man to man	munity lasts probably from 6-12 months. Prompt anti-rabic vaccina-tion of per-sons bitten by or intimately exposed to saliva of rabid animal is recommended. Treatment may be dis-continued if laboratory ex-amination proves animal not to have had rabies. Chance of in-fection is to be weighed against very small chance of developing paralysis due to treatment. An occasional death results due to post-vaccinal en-cephalitis	heat or light. Destroyed at 60° C (140° F) in 30 minutes. Destroyed by boiling at 100° C (212° F) in 10 minutes

Additional Suggested Reading

American Public Health Association: *The Control of Communicable Diseases in Man,* rev. ed. US Government Printing Office, Washington, D. C., 1950.

Banks, H. Stanley (ed.): *Modern Practice in Infectious Fevers.* Paul B. Hoeber, New York, 1951.

Christopher, Frederick (ed.): *Textbook of Surgery,* 5th ed. W. B. Saunders Co., Philadelphia, 1949.

Greenberg, Morris, and Matz, Anna V.: *Modern Concepts of Communicable Disease.* G. P. Putnam's Sons, New York, 1953.

National Foundation for Infantile Paralysis: *Isolation Techniques and Nursing Care in Poliomyelitis.* The Foundation, New York, 1952.

New York State Department of Health: *Guide for the Handling of Communicable Diseases in General Hospitals.* The Department, Albany, 1950.

Pillsbury, Mary E., and Sachs, Elizabeth J.: *Nursing Care of Communicable Diseases,* 7th ed. J. B. Lippincott Co., Philadelphia, 1952.

Pullen, Roscoe L.: *Communicable Diseases.* Lea & Febiger, Philadelphia, 1950.

Statistical Abstract of the United States, 1951. US Government Printing Office, Washington, D.C., 1951.

US Public Health Service: *Reported Incidence of Communicable Diseases in the United States 1950.* US Government Printing Office, Washington, D.C., 1951.

US Public Health Service, Foreign Quarantine and International Health Division: *Immunization Information for International Travel.* US Government Printing Office, Washington, D.C., 1951.

CHAPTER 42. NURSING CARE OF PATIENTS WITH SKELETAL INJURIES

1. SPRAINS
2. DISLOCATIONS
3. FRACTURES
4. SUPPORTS USED IN SKELETAL INJURIES

1. SPRAINS

Cause and Results.   A sprain is an injury to a joint caused by a sudden, violent movement—a wrench, twist, or strain that bruises the synovial membrane, ruptures or stretches the ligaments, tendons, and muscles that support the joint; with bleeding into the tissues, often into the synovial sac. An inflammatory reaction follows with an exudation in the ligaments, tendons, muscles, subcutaneous tissue, and sometimes in the synovial sac.

Symptoms.   There is first severe pain, sometimes so severe as to cause fainting, or nausea and vomiting. The joint swells quickly, is extremely tender to the touch, and is soon discolored if the surface blood vessels have been injured. Discoloration from rupture of the deeper vessels may not appear for a day or two. When the inflammatory reaction begins, there is heat and increased swelling, tenderness, and pain on motion.

Treatment.   A fracture may be very easily mistaken (and sometimes is) for a sprain. X-ray examination is necessary for a correct diagnosis. It is unwise to attempt to "walk off" a sprain of the ankle.

The treatment depends upon the severity of the case and varies with the surgeon. Efforts are first made to relieve pain, to arrest hemorrhage and serous effusion, to aid its absorption, and so to reduce swelling. Sometimes cold applications in the form of ice compresses are used with the part elevated and at rest. This relieves pain, contracts blood vessels, and lessens hemorrhage and effusion. The part is then bandaged or strapped firmly enough to give support and relieve strain without preventing movement, and the patient encouraged to move the part freely. A certain amount of exercise increases the circulation, reduces swelling, and prevents stiffness. For severe sprains, splints or molded plaster casts are sometimes employed. For a sprained wrist, the arm may be supported by a sling. Elasticized bandages, in various widths, and supports for arms, hands, legs, and feet are available and very satisfactory (see Fig. 221, *left*). To increase the circulation about and in the joint, local applications of heat (baking, electric light, high-frequency current, hot water), massage, and passive movements are used after the swelling has subsided.

Adhesive strapping is sometimes applied for support and uniform pressure. Adhesive plaster is made of rubber, petroleum, and either lead acetate or zinc oxide spread on linen. It is applied directly to the skin. The warmth of the body is usually sufficient to make it adhere; if not, the adhesive may first be flamed over an alcohol lamp.

Before applying plaster, the skin must be clean and dry and, if necessary, shaved to prevent irritation and pain on removal of the adhesive. Painting the skin with tincture of benzoin is said to have an adhesive and antiseptic action. The physician applies the adhesive, while the nurse supports the injured part in proper position throughout the procedure. The strips are applied so that the pressure and support are given where most needed; the success of the application depends upon this. In applying plaster, care must be taken to make it fit the surfaces smoothly, without wrinkles; snipping the margin at intervals will help to accomplish this. Adhesive should never be applied tightly enough over soft parts to cut into the tissue. When adhesive is soiled, curling, or peeling at the edges, it should be removed using benzine, carbon tetrachloride (Carbona), or ether for adherent portions. The part should then be washed with soap and warm water and dried gently and thoroughly. If necessary the physician restraps the injured area.

A sprain, if not too severe, will heal without treatment. Therapy as just described is aimed at the relief of pain and discomfort. Hyaluronidase (discussed on p. 735) injected into the soft tissues stimulates absorption of fluid and relieves pain by reducing swelling.

Ethyl Chloride Spray. This has been used to relieve pain in a number of musculo-skeletal conditions. Among these are sprains of the ankle and wrist, as well as the "frozen" shoulder syndrome. The treatment can be easily applied by the physician in his office. After several sprayings with ethyl chloride, the patient limping with a sprained ankle should be able to walk without discomfort. The pain in the "frozen" shoulder syndrome is generally so alleviated that the person can move his arm freely.[1, 2]

2. DISLOCATIONS

Cause and Results.   A dislocation is the separation of the articular surfaces of two or more bones entering into the formation of a joint. It may be caused by an injury which stretches or tears ligaments, or by disease of the articulating structures, or it may be congenital. Injury to blood vessels, nerves, and soft tissues usually results. The dislocation may be compound—that is, an external wound leads to the injured joint. A severe hemorrhage producing a hematoma sometimes occurs, and a fracture of one or more bones may take place at the same time.

Symptoms.   First there is sickening pain, greatly increased by motion of the part. Deformity with a lengthening or shortening of a limb occurs, depending upon the line of displacement; there is limited motion in the part. Swelling of the surrounding tissues may occur. Some degree of shock is nearly always present.

Treatment. *First-aid* treatment consists primarily in preventing shock or treating it if present. The limb should be put at rest in the position most comfortable for the patient. For a dislocation of the shoulder, elbow, or wrist, apply a splint or bandage and support the arm in a sling (see Fig. 223). For a dislocation of the hip, knee, or ankle, put the patient to bed and apply a splint as in a fracture of the femur. To combat pain and swelling, ice compresses may be applied.

The *importance of early treatment* by an expert cannot be overemphasized. Reduction of a dislocation requires both knowledge and skill, and should never be attempted by an inexperienced person if the services of a surgeon are available, even after a lapse of many hours. Permanent injury may result from improper manipulation. A general anesthetic is frequently necessary to relax the muscles and relieve pain before reduction is even possible. Because the injury is followed by a marked inflammatory reaction with considerable exudation, early reduction is very desirable. If the dislocation is not reduced, this exudate later forms fibrous material that fills up the socket or adhesions that bind the bone in its abnormal position. The attached muscles contract which also limits the function of the joint.

Surgical treatment is usually indicated. X-ray examination is necessary to determine the extent of the injury. The dislocation is reduced by manipulation and extension (usually under an anesthetic), or by open operation, and the joint is immobilized for several weeks with bandages and splints. After the restraint has been removed, gentle passive motion is used to restore function and later massage, baths, and electrotherapy.

Compound dislocations exposing the larger joints are extremely serious and demand an extensive operation. Injury to surrounding tissues, blood vessels, and nerves is usually severe and results in shock. The danger from infection is great; amputation may be necessary in extreme cases.

3. FRACTURES

Definitions. A fracture is an injury that produces a solution of the continuity of a bone—that is, a break or violent separation of a bone into two or more parts. Most fractures result from external violence, either direct or indirect. When direct, the fracture occurs at the point of impact. When indirect, the impact transmitted through one or more bones causes a fracture at a distance from the site of the impact. Because their bones have become brittle due to loss of some of the mineral content, a fracture in elderly people may result from relatively slight injuries.[3]

The varieties of fracture include the following:

A *simple fracture*—the bone is broken, but the skin and surrounding tissues are unbroken.

A *compound fracture*—a wound in the skin and surrounding tissues which exposes or leads to the ends of fragments of the broken bone.

A *comminuted fracture*—the bone is crushed, splintered, or broken into a number of small fragments, the lines of the break communicating with one another.

An *impacted fracture*—one fragment of bone is forcibly driven into another and remains more or less fixed in that position.

A *greenstick fracture*—the shaft is bent and cracked, but not completely broken through. This type is common in children, because their bones are not fully calcified, but are still elastic like a green twig.

The terms *single, double,* and *multiple* refer to the number of breaks; and *recent, old, united,* and *nonunited* to the time of the injury and the degree of repair.

Fractures are also classified into (1) fractures of the *epiphyses* (extremities) in which the articulations are frequently involved and (2) fractures of the *diaphyses* (shafts). The breaks may be longitudinal, transverse, or spiral. In fractures of the shaft, motion is felt at a point where there should be none, the broken ends of the bone tend to overlap (because of the weight of the limb and the pull of muscles), and shortening of the limb results.

A *Colles' fracture*—fracture of the lower end of the radius and of the styloid process of the ulna. (It is named after an Irish surgeon who first described the condition.)

A *Pott's fracture*—fracture of the lower end of the fibula and of the internal malleolus of the tibia. (It is named after the surgeon who first described it.)

Symptoms.   A fracture may be recognized by the (1) subjective and (2) objective symptoms.

1.The *subjective symptoms* are pain and loss of function. Following an accident, if the injured person complains of severe pain on attempting to use the part, one should suspect a fracture and treat accordingly. Usually there is loss of function, but this is not always the case. If a man falls and is unable to get up or to walk or if he is unable to use an arm or hand, one or more bones involved are probably fractured. He may be able to walk and still have a fracture of the fibula, however, because this bone gives little support and the tibia will act as a splint for it. Again the ability or inability to use the fingers is not a safe test, as has been supposed, of a suspected fracture of the bones of the forearm. They may still be used, though with great pain, even if these bones are broken.

Following an injury to the pelvic region, inability to stand or sit, a feeling of "coming apart," or bleeding from the rectum or bladder indicates a fracture. Severe pain on breathing or coughing, or bloody expectoration following a chest injury, suggests that one or more ribs are broken. Symptoms may be absent or very slight in fractures of the skull. Headache and mental confusion may be the only symptoms the patient complains of, or there may be unconsciousness and paralysis with a slow pulse and slow respirations. Because head injuries producing comparatively mild symptoms can produce delayed and perhaps fatal pathology, it is wise to keep the victim quiet and recumbent until an x-ray is taken.

2. The early *objective symptoms* are localized tenderness and abnormal mobility —that is, movement where there should be none, as, for instance, between the shoulder and elbow. Displacement of the broken ends usually produces deformity, and injured blood vessels hemorrhage into deep tissues; soft parts may be swollen and discolored. The pull of the muscles attached to the fragments causes displace-

ment. Overlapping of the broken ends may cause one limb to be shorter than another, and it is often in an unnatural position. Crepitus is "the grating of fractured bones." This may be felt and sometimes heard, but should not be searched for, because the slightest movement of the ragged bone fragments adds further injury to the surrounding tissues.

In a fracture of the base of the skull, the tympanic membrane may rupture with bleeding (or serosanguinous drainage) from the ear. Blood may pass from the ear into the Eustachian tube, escape through the nose, or run into the mouth where it may be swallowed. This may not be discovered until later when it is vomited. Blood may escape also into the orbit, turning the white of the eye red. Cerebrospinal fluid may be mixed with the blood if the dura and arachnoid membranes are ruptured. Cranial nerves emerging from the base of the brain may be injured. Trauma of the facial nerve results in facial paralysis, and injury of the auditory nerve in deafness.

X-ray examination is ordinarily the only means of making an accurate diagnosis. In fractures of the spine or skull, the diagnosis is also dependent upon observation of symptoms, for they indicate the location and extent of injury. An exploratory operation is sometimes necessary. The fluoroscope also is used as an aid to diagnosis and in setting a fracture.

Systemic symptoms are present in all severe injuries. Fractures of the skull, spine, pelvis, and femur are especially likely to be accompanied by prolonged shock. Gastric disturbances, general malaise, and a slight rise in temperature frequently occur.

Complications. The injury and bruising of surrounding tissues that cannot be gauged in a superficial examination are said by experts to be "of greater importance to future function than the more obvious deformity of the bone"* in many cases. Nerves may be torn, bruised, or stretched; internal organs, such as the lungs, pleura, or bladder, may be perforated, or the brain, spinal cord, or large blood vessels injured.

Infection may develop, and should be guarded against in all compound fractures, particularly those of the skull, nose, or jaw. The nose and mouth are never free from pathogenic organisms. In fractures of the base of the skull, the nose and ears must be kept clean. Sterile cotton is usually placed in the ears. Infection may cause meningitis or septicemia, either of which was likely to prove fatal before the various antibiotics, now used to control infections, were available.

Ischemic (anemic) paralysis sometimes occurs. This is a form of paralysis and deformity caused by pressure that temporarily shuts off the supply of arterial blood from the part. Permanent loss of function may result. Pressure may be produced by circular plaster casts, bandaging, or splints applied so tightly to a fresh fracture that they do not allow for the increased blood supply, exudation, and swelling that always occur in an injured part. If the ischemia is unrelieved for six or more hours,

* Knocke, Frederick J., and Knocke, Lazelle S.: *Orthopaedic Nursing.* F. A. Davis Co., Philadelphia, 1952. p. 212.

such marked degenerative changes are produced in the muscles and nerves that paralysis, contraction of muscles, and, in some instances, gangrene follow.

The symptoms of ischemia due to pressure are pain, coldness, numbness, edema, and cyanosis of the extremity. In order that the symptoms may be readily recognized, the fingers and toes are usually left exposed. Sometimes, to make the patient more comfortable, a sock is placed over the toes. When this is done, the nurse should remove it frequently to check the appearance and to feel the foot. If any symptoms appear, they should be reported immediately so that the bandage, splint, or cast may be loosened or removed.

Sometimes fat globules from the marrow of the broken bone enter the blood stream. They may be first arrested in the pulmonary, cranial, or other visceral capillaries where they form a plug, *or a fat embolism*. This shuts off the circulation, a condition that is likely to prove fatal.

Restlessness, insomnia, and *delirium tremens* may be present in alcoholics following an accident. Habitual drinkers have a great deal of discomfort if suddenly deprived of alcohol for any reason; therefore, the physician should know if he has an alcoholic patient. If the accident occurs during or after a state of intoxication, injury is likely to be more severe since alcohol is a powerful depressant.

Later complications are limitation of motion and paralysis from injury to a nerve trunk or from pressure of the callus. Poor circulation may cause atrophy of muscles with resulting weakness and lack of use. Delayed union, nonunion, or vicious union (union with deformity and loss of function) may take place. If the ends of bones are not approximated, fibrous tissue, which will not function normally, grows between the fractured ends.

Treatment.   Two factors are of utmost importance in the treatment of fractures: *reduction* (placing the broken ends of the bone in apposition, or proper alignment) and *immobilization* of the broken bone. The part played by nature in the repair and treatment of a fracture should not be overlooked, however. In all cases repair depends on the extent of injury to the bone, periosteum, nutrient blood vessels, nerves, and surrounding tissues, as well as the presence or absence of infection, the general condition of the patient, and the treatment given. If the broken ends are accurately replaced and kept completely at rest, repair and healthy union will take place rapidly (in from 3 to 6 weeks) provided the part is free from infection, is well supplied with blood, and the injury to the periosteum is not too great.*

If, however, the bones have not been set properly—the fault of the surgeon, or if set and then disturbed by any movement—the fault of the nurse, nature will do her best to bridge the gap; but the repair will be slower, the building will be sprawling, so to speak, and will take up an area belonging to the muscles and thus will greatly interfere with their function.

Infection or poor circulation may cause death of bone tissue, and this results in a greatly delayed union or in nonunion. Dead bone fragments, or sequestra, may

---

* Periosteum is essential because its inner vascular layer contains the active bone-forming cells or osteoblasts that must rebuild the new bone.

lead to the formation of sinuses, which do not close but continue to discharge until all the dead bone has been removed.

Delayed union or nonunion may be caused also by other factors, such as a faulty position, constant slight movement, removal of too much bone, plugging of the medullary cavity with callus, or to a systemic condition of the patient that interferes with healing.

Treatment may be considered under four main headings: first aid; closed reduction, or setting, and immobilization; open reduction; and after-treatment.

1. *First-aid treatment* is extremely important; it may affect the duration of the handicap, the restoration of function, the loss of an injured part of the body, and even the life of the patient.

The most important things to remember are to prevent further injury, shock, and pain; to control bleeding if present; and to prevent infection. If a doctor can be summoned quickly, and the injured person has fallen but is in a place of safety, it is best for an inexperienced person (or even a nurse) merely to make him comfortable where he lies (with pillows, blankets, and similar means) and to disturb the part as little as possible. The treatment of shock is discussed in Chapter 40.

Before moving the patient, the injured part should be put at rest or immobilized in order to relieve pain and prevent further displacement of ragged edges of bone and tearing of soft tissues, blood vessels, or nerves. The affected member should be placed in a position that tends to cause relaxation of muscles, the contraction of which is causing pain and displacement. A patient will often instinctively do this for himself—for instance, in a fractured clavicle he inclines his head to the injured side, raises his shoulder, and supports his elbow; in a fracture of the upper extremity he will support his elbow, forearm, wrist, or hand. An extremity must never be allowed to dangle, and, even after bandages or splints are applied, a patient should never be allowed to attempt to use an injured part.

The injured should be handled as little as possible and then with care and gentleness. In lifting a limb it should always be supported under the broken ends and under the joints above and below the break. Movement at either joint will further displace the fragments. It is best to apply an even support to the whole limb before lifting. Careless handling may change a simple fracture into a compound one, with danger of infection, loss of a limb or even of life. One should watch for discoloration and note whether the pulse in an extremity is present and normal. One should watch also for symptoms of internal injury to the brain, spinal cord, lungs, bladder, or rectum. Clothing should be removed with the utmost care—it should always be removed from the uninjured side first, and cut away if necessary. If the patient is to be sent to the hospital it is better to wait until he gets there to undress him.

Swelling of the part should be prevented by applying ice, by proper support, and elevation when possible. Swelling not only adds to the pain but also greatly hampers a proper reduction of the fracture. It was formerly thought that pain was to be avoided as it not only caused distress but was believed to be one of the factors in the development of shock. Morphine was commonly given routinely to the seriously injured, but research during World War II has shown this to be unwise (see p. 950). If a wound is present, bleeding should be checked. To prevent infection, the wound and surrounding skin should be cleaned, covered with a sterile pad, and bandaged (see p. 960).

All patients suffering from shock or painful contusions, from fractures of the skull, pelvis, or lower extremity should be carried on a stretcher, with as little jolting as possible, to their homes or, preferably, to a hospital. If the patient is unconscious it is wise to transport him in the prone position to favor drainage from the mouth. If a cervical injury is suspected, the neck should be extended; patients with fractures of the thoracic or lumbar vertebrae should be in a supine position with the back extended.

First-aid methods of immobilization involve the application of bandages, adhesive strapping, and splints, according to the location of the fracture and the available facilities.

Bandaging is used chiefly in the following cases: A four-tailed bandage or a Barton bandage may be used for a fractured jaw; a Velpeau bandage for a fractured clavicle. If it is not possible to secure any sort of splint, a fractured arm may be bandaged to the side (the axilla and side being first well padded); and a fractured leg to the other leg, in this way utilizing the patient's own body as a splint. A bandage or tight binder is sometimes applied for fractured ribs, but must not be left on too long as it restricts the expansion of the thoracic cage which in turn will restrict the action of the lungs. A triangular bandage in the form of a sling is used to support the forearm in fractures of the clavicle, arm, or hand. A tight binder may be applied around the hips and the knees bandaged together to give support and immobilize the hips in a fractured pelvis. (For discussion of bandages and binders, see Chapter 37.)

Adhesive strapping is usually applied in fractures of the ribs to limit the motion of the chest during respiration. This relieves pain and may promote healing by limiting the expansion of the affected side of the chest and approximating the edges of the broken bones. Accidents that injure the chest so severely that the viscera are affected threaten life itself, but simple fractures of the ribs are fairly common and will usually heal satisfactorily even without treatment.[4] When applying adhesive the chest wall should be shaved first. Occasionally tincture of benzoin is applied to the skin prior to the application of the tape by the physician.

Splints are used in fractures of long bones and should be firm enough to give support. Many objects will serve this purpose. An umbrella, cane, or folded pillow may be used in an emergency; but splints of a lightweight metal rod are best. They should be long enough to fix the joints above and below the fracture and should provide a means of applying traction. For instance, in a fractured femur the outer splint should extend from the axilla to below the foot, and in a fracture of the lower leg the splints should extend from above the knee to below the foot. If metal splints are not available, two or more wooden splints may be needed to support an arm or leg.

Splints must always be padded, especially over the tender areas or bony prominences, and also in hollows, such as the axilla, flexed elbow, knee, or groin. A pad in the palm of the hand supports the hand, prevents discomfort, and maintains its normal arch. Splints are held in place by some sort of bandage. If they are not well padded or if tied on too tightly, the pressure causes swelling, pain, blisters, ulcers, sloughing of tissues, and may result in a permanent impairment of function.

All ambulances, doctors' offices and cars, and hospital emergency rooms should be fitted with a set of hinged-ring arm splints (Murray-Jones) and Thomas type leg splints. In communities where such services are available, the treatment of fractures should be materially improved by proper handling immediately after the injury.

In the first-aid treatment of fractures of an extremity, it is important to immobilize the part before moving the person. Shock can be prevented or treated during the process. Temporary traction should be applied and maintained until the splint has been adjusted; in the hospital should traction be the method of treatment selected, an orthopedic bed will be used and traction maintained with the use of weights. Traction is stressed because it prevents movement of the broken ends of the bones that may damage the soft tissues and cause further bone destruction. Widespread knowledge, among not only medical workers but also the public as well, of the proper technique to be used in applying emergency splints is essential. Figure 256 shows the Keller-Blake hinged splint applied with triangular bandages to the leg. The bandages are used to make a hammock for the extremity and the ends brought up and tied over the leg to hold it in position. The ring is held firmly against the buttock by straps so that traction can be made against the fixed point of the splint.

2. *Closed reduction, or setting, and immobilization* are surgical measures that should be started in all fractures as soon as possible in order to prevent overlapping of the broken ends and further injury to the periosteum and other tissues. Frequently pain, swelling, or muscular rigidity makes it difficult to determine the exact position and nature of the fracture, so that reduction must be done under a general anesthetic and under guidance of an x-ray. Later x-ray examinations may be made to verify the position and to observe the process of repair.

Reduction of the fracture may sometimes be accomplished by gentle manipulation; and fixation secured with bandages, strapping, wood or metal splints, or casts. Continuous traction is another method of immobilization (see pp. 1130 ff.). Splints or bivalved casts are generally used when it is difficult to keep the part at rest and absolute fixation is necessary, as in a fracture of both bones of the forearm or leg. Molded casts that cover the extremity are often applied when the injury is extensive. Leg casts are usually equipped with a foot piece that enables the patient to walk while wearing the cast. A shoulder spica is frequently used for a fractured arm, a hip spica for a fractured femur, and a body cast or jacket for a fractured spine or pelvis.

Many fractures cannot be reduced or the bones maintained in their proper position by simple manipulation. In such cases, reduction and fixation must be accomplished with traction, or traction combined with suspension. Traction is the extension of the member in the direction or position believed by the surgeon to promote healing and optimum function later. It is used when the broken ends of bones are overlapping. The object is to prevent this overlapping and resulting deformity. It is accomplished by the use of weights (metal, or bags of sand or shot) and pulleys, by utilizing the weight of the patient, and by the use of splints.

3. *Open reduction of fractures* is resorted to if a satisfactory reduction cannot be made and maintained by the preceding methods. In open reduction there is, of course, danger of infection. Incisions must be made, and some internal means of fixation, such as plates, sutures, wires, screws, nails, bolts, or an inlay of bone graft, may be used. These procedures are carried out in the operating room.

The metal internal means of fixation are usually made of Vitallium or Ticonium* because they are noncorrosive and nonirritating (do not act like a foreign body). Sometimes the metal item is removed after bony union has resulted; occasionally it is left in place.

If bone is used to splint the fracture, the graft may be taken from one of the segments of the broken bone itself or from another part of the body, such as the tibia. The patient's bone is ordinarily used for such a graft since it has a better chance of remaining vital and affecting a permanent incorporation in a bony union.

4. *After-treatment and the responsibility of the nurse* cannot be overemphasized. The nurse should have an understanding of the physiology involved in tissue repair and of the doctor's plan of therapy. She should use her expert knowledge and skill to help the patient recover from the immediate effects of injury and help him with the more drawn-out process of rehabilitation.

Much depends upon the patient's general health, mental and physical. In many cases the long-enforced absence from work and home requires financial or social adjustment. The cooperation of the social service department is often needed. Anxiety and depression, with accompanying physical derangement, should be combated. In Chapter 16 rehabilitation in orthopedic nursing was discussed briefly. In this service the nurse must work closely with the physical, occupational, and recreational therapists as well as with the social worker and the physician.

The hygienic care is, of course, important. A diet rich in vitamins, protein, and calcium is usually prescribed. Motion is often restricted by casts and traction devices, and it is the nurse's responsibility to see that the position is changed frequently and discomfort relieved by massage and supports; every precaution must be taken to avoid skin irritation due to pressure from splints, casts, or other appliances, or from lying too long in one position. Pressure sores and pneumonia are to be guarded against, particularly in elderly persons.

The patient must be observed frequently for signs of discomfort, irritation from

---

* Trade names for super-heat-resistant alloys:

1. Vitallium is made of cobalt, molybdenum, and chromium. Since it has no electric potential in tissues, it is inert. This alloy cannot be machined and must be cast and ground to shape. Because casting defects occur somewhat frequently and interfere with its strength, it is not completely satisfactory.

2. Ticonium is composed of nickel, cobalt, chromium, and molybdenum. It is also corrosive resistant and is well tolerated when implanted in tissue.

appliances, and interference with the circulation in the extremities. A great deal depends upon the maintenance of the prescribed range of position, and the nurse must observe and correct or report to the physician too great deviations from this. Support must be provided for the entire body to relieve strain and to further the process of repair.

It is often necessary to use cradles over an extremity and to supply heat to the part.

Active motion of the adjacent joints (by the patient), which does not endanger the proper position of the fragments, is of the greatest importance in stimulating repair and in preventing atrophy of the muscles and stiffness of joints. It is usually begun after the first 24 hours following closed reduction; when the fracture has been reduced by open reduction the surgeon will indicate when active motion of adjacent joints is to be started.

Massage is one of the best means of stimulating repair and of preventing atrophy of muscles and stiffness of joints and tendons. The surgeon prescribes it; if a physical therapist is available he or she may initiate it; the nurse may both initiate and follow through on the physician's prescription. Massage is often given daily, as soon as union is established and there is no danger of displacement. If repair is delayed, *dry heat* in the form of baking or an electric pad is sometimes used to stimulate the circulation. *Radiant light* and heat as well as diathermy are other physical agents that stimulate the vital activity of cells and hasten recovery (see Chapters 23 and 24).

4. SUPPORTS USED IN SKELETAL INJURIES

Plaster Casts.   These bandages are made by rolling and rubbing plaster of Paris into meshes of crinoline;* they are usually machine-made and ready for use. Plaster of Paris is gypsum, or hydrated calcium sulfate. When water is added, it returns to a crystalline form and when applied and allowed to dry it forms a cast. It may be a circular cast—that is, completely encircles the limb, or a molded cast which fits the limb but does not completely cover it. The molded cast is bandaged in place with a gauze or Ace bandage. It supports and immobilizes the part and allows for frequent inspection. It does not interfere with the circulation and the

---

* In making plaster-of-Paris bandages, the crinoline is first cut into strips of the desired width and length and rolled into roller bandages. A large flat surface will be necessary upon which to make the bandages. The table and floor should be protected. The required amount of plaster is placed on the table. The plaster should be fresh, free from lumps, and of a good quality that will dry quickly. The crinoline bandage is placed on the table opposite the operator, with the body uppermost and the initial end drawn toward the operator. The plaster is spread over the crinoline freely and is rubbed smoothly and evenly into all its meshes. A spatula may be used for this purpose, but the best method is to rub the plaster in with the heel of the hand. A rubber glove may be worn if desired. The strip is loosely rolled as each portion is finished. It is advisable to wrap each bandage separately and securely in waxed paper as soon as it has been prepared. Then the bandages are stored in an airtight box or container; this will prevent the bandages being handled individually until they are to be used. The wrapper helps to prevent deterioration of the plaster from exposure to the moisture of the air and prevents the sifting out of the plaster which is undesirable.

nutrition of the part as the circular cast, if not properly applied, is in danger of doing; also, it is more convenient if dressing the part is required. In the circular cast a hole is made over the wound by means of which dressings may be changed.

The bandages are *applied* by the surgeon. The nurse's responsibility is to prepare the patient and articles required and to assist with the application. First, the part to be bandaged is shaved, washed, dried thoroughly, and powdered. The bed or table and floor should be protected. A rest should be provided to elevate and sup-

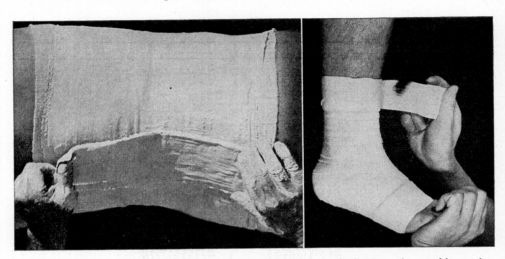

Figure 249. (*Left*) A body plaster-of-Paris cast being applied. Note the stockinette between the body and the cast to protect the skin. The stockinette will be turned over the edges of the cast to protect the patient from the rough edges. (Courtesy of Johnson & Johnson, New Brunswick, N. J.)

(*Right*) Sheet wadding being used to cover an extremity and to protect the skin prior to the application of a cast. (Courtesy of Bauer & Black, Chicago, Ill.)

Stockinette and sheeting wadding are sometimes used in combination when applying a cast.

port the part, which must be kept in the proper position—that is, the position in which it is to remain after the application is completed. (Frequently casts are applied in the operating room and special tables used that support the body but leave the affected parts accessible to the surgeon.)

The articles required are rubber gloves and a gown for the doctor, plaster bandages, the number and size depending upon the part to be bandaged and the desired strength of the cast,* stockinette and sheet wadding bandages, which are first applied to protect the skin, sheets of felt to pad bony prominences, and a deep basin or pail full of tepid water. Plaster bandages are applied while wet. They are removed from a vessel of water in which they are immersed as soon as bubbles

---

* Occasionally light wooden splints, wire netting, or other strengthening materials are incorporated into a cast as reinforcements over joints and other areas likely to be subject to more than average strain. The size as well as the placement of the cast are determining factors.

cease to rise. They should not be squeezed as that removes the plaster. Salt, 4 cc to 1000 cc, is sometimes added to the water to hasten the drying of the plaster. Two or three sandbags may be required to steady the limb. Some surgeons require a basin of dry plaster, which they rub over the bandages after they are applied. This is moistened with water and spread over the whole surface, giving it a smooth, even, and finished appearance. In applying the plaster bandages a portion of the stockinette and sheet wadding is left uncovered, so that it can be turned back to form a cuff over the rough edges of the plaster in order to protect the skin. (In some

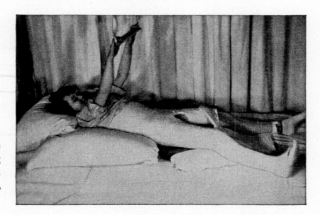

Figure 250. Patient with a plaster cast on the bedpan. Note the adequate support by using pillows. (Courtesy of Frederick J. Knocke and Lazelle S. Knocke, and Clay-Adams Co., New York.)

cases the plaster is put directly over the skin, but this is done when there is no danger of swelling under the cast.[5]) The quality of plaster varies; many surgeons have special preferences, but a plaster that makes as light a cast as possible should be used.

The patient's position must be maintained after the cast is applied until it is dry. Sandbags are placed at either side to prevent movement. The cast is left uncovered. The bedclothes should be arranged to keep the rest of the body warm and comfortable. A cradle is sometimes placed over the cast, and an electric light suspended from it to supply heat to hasten the drying of the plaster. An electric drier that blows warm air over the cast is sometimes used. Properly placed pillows are an aid when a cast is fresh; it is important to protect such casts from pressure and strains which might indent or bend the soft plaster. A bed board under the mattress will help to prevent the cracking of large casts during this stage.

It must be remembered that the water in which the plaster bandages were moistened should never be discarded into the sink or toilet, because the plaster residue hardens and blocks the pipes. Such water is discarded into a hopper which has a trap in the waste pipe. The trap collects the plaster and protects the plumbing.

Other types of casts are made by impregnating muslin or fiber-glass bandage with a plastic substance (cellulose acetate) that is soluble in acetone and other solvents. These bandages are easily molded to the part which may or may not be padded.

Advantages of this bandage are that it is easily applied, waterproof, very light, and is transparent to x-ray; its disadvantages are that it dries slowly, is slightly more expensive, and gives less support than a plaster cast.

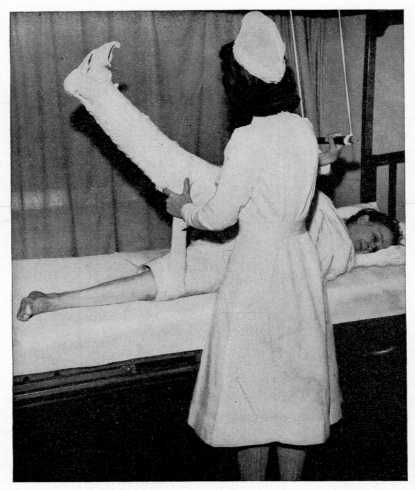

Figure 251.   Turning a patient in a body cast. Patient assists by use of hand trapeze. (West, John P.; Keller, Manelva W.; and Harmon, Elizabeth: *Nursing Care of the Surgical Patient,* 6th ed. The Macmillan Company, New York, 1957.)

Extensive casts, particularly those confining the body, are very uncomfortable. Skin around and under the edges of the cast requires constant observation and care to prevent irritation, chafing, and pressure sores. Plaster casts are never applied as tightly as other bandages, because they shrink as they dry. The parts below the cast should be observed for symptoms of poor circulation, such as pain, pallor, a bluish color, tingling, numbness, or coldness. Any sign of pressure must be reported early, because gangrenous areas (ulcers), which may develop if the circulation is impaired, are painless after the first stage of tissue destruction. Frederick J. Knocke and Lazelle S. Knocke advocate splitting a circular cast immediately when it is put over a recent injury; later on, should circulatory impairment occur, the cast can then be spread easily and without delay.

Studies made of the reaction of adults to body casts have shown the following to be among the common complaints: a feeling of being restricted; a sense of helplessness, of dependence on others; a fear of falling out of bed on turning; oppression at the thought of the time required by the treatment; fear that the injured part is not healing properly; a physical sensation of pressure in some areas; itching underneath the cast; excoriation of the skin around the groin; and a sense of uncleanliness, and fatigue that is caused by the restricted position.

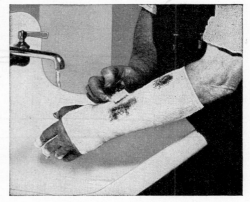

Figure 252. A cast made of Aire-Cast is light in weight and not damaged by water; therefore, it has some advantages over plaster of Paris for convalescent casts. (Courtesy of Tower Co., Seattle, Wash.)

With skillful care most of these difficulties can be overcome. A thorough explanation of the necessity for keeping the broken ends of bones in apposition may reconcile the patient to being in a cast and may give him a sense of security. To make him feel less helpless, a trapeze can be suspended from the Balkan frame over the bed; this will enable him to lift himself.

The type of skeletal injury will determine the selection and use of special equipment such as Crutchfield tongs, traction with a chin strap, and a Stryker frame. In spinal injuries, skeletal traction may be applied, or traction may be carried out either with *Crutchfield tongs* or with a chin strap. When Crutchfield tongs are introduced into the skull, the wounds are protected by small dressings; these wounds must be examined at least daily for signs of infection. A patient with tongs is turned "log" fashion, with at least two, preferably three, assistants when the patient is an adult. (See Figs. 255 A-D for procedure in turning a patient with a cervical cord injury.) It is essential that when the patient is turned body (spinal column) alignment is maintained. When a *chin strap* is used, turning is not permitted. Since the skin under the chin tends to break down because of the traction, careful observation and constant care are indicated. With the increasing use and availability of the *Stryker frame* (see Figs. 254 A-E), care of patients with spinal injuries is greatly facilitated. Nursing care can be more easily given, and the patient can be turned by one nurse. In addition the patient can carry out various activities, such as reading and playing checkers, without assistance; therefore he should be able to maintain a good mental attitude and should feel more optimistic and cheerful.

Overhead mirrors that enable the person in bed to see himself and to see anyone who is coming into the room help to make a restrictive position less onerous. Overbed tables with reading desks also make him more independent; pockets for writing materials, toilet articles, and other objects hung on the bed within his reach add greatly to the patient's comfort. Wisely selected occupational therapy does more than any other one thing to make time pass quickly. Patients with crippling orthopedic conditions often learn a useful trade from the occupational therapist. During the convalescent period, special forms of occupation and recreation may be prescribed for their value in muscle training. For its effect on the mental outlook of the patient, some form of occupational therapy is desirable for all patients whose physical condition permits it.

Pressure is relieved by frequent change of position. A small pillow under one shoulder or one hip may alter the distribution of weight sufficiently to accomplish this. When a sensation of pressure persists, it should be reported to the surgeon who may find it necessary to remove and reapply the cast.

Discomfort from itching is partially prevented by thoroughly cleaning and shaving the skin before application of the cast. Scratchers should always be provided. They are made in the following manner: Strips of gauze or cotton bandage are placed in a longitudinal direction over the skin to which the cast is to be applied. These strips should extend for some distance above and below the cast so that when it is completed the ends of the bandage can be tied together over the cast. When itching occurs under the cast, these ends are untied and the bandage moved about to create friction. These strips may be replaced at any time by tying a clean piece of bandage to one end of the used piece and drawing it under the cast into position. Gauze saturated with alcohol and drawn under the cast in this fashion further alleviates itching. There is some doubt as to whether scratchers should be used for children, because it suggests to them putting all sorts of things under the cast.

Irritation of the skin around the edge of a cast at the groin or the axilla is prevented to some extent by keeping the cast clean. Plaster may be protected in various ways. It can be made waterproof with paint or varnish, after which it may be washed with soap and water; or the exposed edges may be covered with oiled silk or some sort of cellulose film, which is successfully held in place with Scotch tape, another cellulose product. Elevating the head of the bed slightly when the patient uses the bedpan helps to prevent soiling. The patient in a cast must be properly supported with pillows when on the bedpan (see Fig. 250).

In removing a plaster cast, it is first moistened in a straight line where the opening is to be made. Solutions of sugar and water, peroxide of hydrogen, vinegar, or bichloride of mercury may be used for this purpose; however, none of these substances is much more effective than water. The cast is then cut with a plaster knife, saw, or scissors. When the cast is applied, special devices which facilitate removal can be inserted that leave a line of perforations at the place where the surgeon expects to cut the cast. A strip of material, such as hard rubber or felt, is sometimes placed under the cast so that when the cast is removed the skin is protected from the cutting instrument.

In treating fractures it is essential that a position be maintained that keeps the broken ends of bones fixed and in proper alignment. Special beds are manufactured for this purpose. Fracture beds are improvised in hospitals and in homes, but the essential features are the same no matter where they are found.

The Fracture Bed. The first essential of a bed for a patient with a fracture of the trunk or leg is that it is flat. Sagging is prevented by the use of a firm mattress that rests on a bed board or wooden frame which is placed on the bedsprings under the mattress. Commercial fracture beds have canvas straps stretched across the metal framework to support the patient. A firm mattress and wire springs are placed directly under such canvas straps. Each canvas strap can be tightened with a special device at the side, or loosened and removed. A middle section of the mattress can be lowered without affecting the upper and lower sections. These features make it possible to remove the straps under the buttocks, lower the mattress, and introduce the bedpan without necessitating a change in the patient's position and without removing the support from the rest of the body.

Plaster casts may be used to keep the ends of broken bones in apposition or pins of different kinds driven into the bone, but traction is frequently employed for this purpose. When the surgeon adopts the latter method, it is necessary to have some sort of framework from which weights attached to the leg can be suspended. This framework is usually referred to as a *Balkan frame*. It may be made of wood or metal. Such a frame enables the surgeon to apply traction at any part of the body and in any plane. It also provides a means of suspending appliances, such as a trapeze or a wooden handle on ropes, over the patient, which helps him to lift and turn himself. Patients with certain types of fractures should be provided with such a bed, even when it is not required for traction, because of the comfort it is to them and the assistance to the nurse in giving care.

The Bradford Frame. This is used in the treatment of fractures and diseases of the spine, hip, and other joints. It may be used to relieve pressure on bedsores or wounds of the back, and to protect dressings on the back and thighs from soiling by the involuntary passage of urine and stool. The *Whitman frame* is a curved Bradford frame used when hyperextension of the spine is indicated. The Deckert bed may also be used for hyperextension and is much more satisfactory.

The frames are made of gas piping, and vary in length and width according to the size of the patient. They should always be about a foot longer than he is and wide enough to avoid contact with the shoulders. Two pieces of canvas are stretched across the frame and stitched or laced securely to it. (Sometimes one piece of canvas with an opening to allow for toilet care is used.) A space is left between the upper and lower strips, wide enough to leave the buttocks free and allow the use of a bedpan. The frame and canvas are covered with a sheet. The patient is placed on the protected canvas with the buttocks directly over the space. If restraint is necessary, strips of canvas (or other stout material) can be fastened to either side of the frame and laced, pinned, or buckled over the body, but, needless to say, restraint is avoided if possible. When used, friction and pressure must be guarded against. The frame may be fastened to the sides of the bed. When used for an infant to prevent soiling of dressings from urine and stool, the frame is suspended from the sides of the crib and the bedpan is left on the bed under the buttocks.

The lower canvas and mattress should be protected by a waterproof material. If used to prevent pressure, the frame is suspended and the canvas adjusted so as to leave the wound or tender spot free from contact with the canvas or bed. The patient is covered with the usual bedclothes.

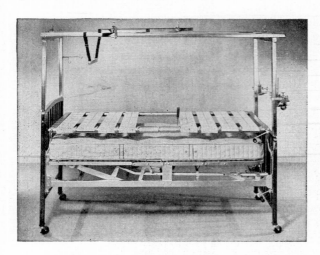

Figure 253. Bed with a Bradford frame which is removable and adjustable; it is used as a substitute for a Stryker frame when the latter is not available. Note also the Balkan frame from which a hand trapeze is suspended. (Courtesy of Simmons Co., New York City.)

The Bradford frame may also be used to facilitate the care of obese adults.

Within the past few years, Bradford frames have been replaced by Stryker frames and Foster orthopedic beds, however.

The Stryker Frame. *Nature and Uses.* The Stryker frame is a modification of the Bradford frame. Both are named after doctors who designed them to facilitate the care of patients with neuromuscular disorders. The more recent device is shown in Figures 254 A-E. It is obvious that the Stryker frame has many advantages over its predecessor. The chief ones are: (1) with it one nurse can turn a heavy patient, and (2) the Stryker frame is lighter and, when mounted on its own carrier, more mobile than the Bradford frame which is used on a bed. Three or four persons are needed to turn an adult on a Bradford frame. Both frames are designed to facilitate nursing care and at the same time to keep the body in good alignment. Both make it possible to place a bedpan under the patient without lifting him. With both frames, but particularly with the Stryker frame, the patient can feed himself, read or occupy his time with manual skills when he is prone. A patient can be transported on a Stryker frame, and many are taken home on it. Without this device effective home care would be almost impossible for certain injured persons. Patients with spinal fractures, with tuberculosis and other diseases that attack the vertebrae, and with cord lesions benefit from the use of this mechanism. The skin of the paraplegic patient, so susceptible to pressure sores, can usually be kept in good condition because it is an easy matter to turn him frequently.

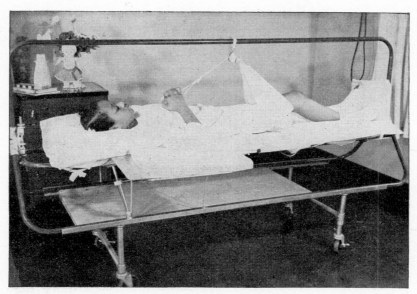

Figure 254A. The Stryker frame. The patient is in the supine position with the arms supported on rests and the feet maintained in a position to prevent foot drop. (The sling around the thigh is used to enable the patient to exercise an injured leg; it is not part of the Stryker frame.)

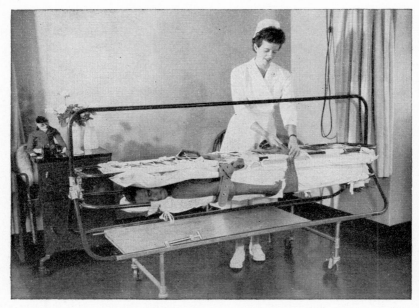

Figure 254B. The nurse is preparing to change the patient from the prone to the supine position. She is sandwiching the patient between the upper and lower frames.

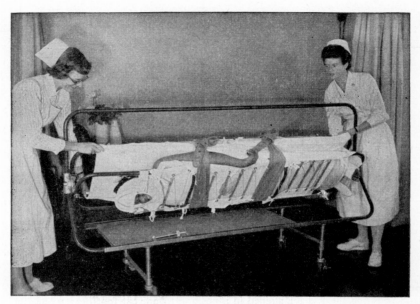

Figure 254C. While one nurse can turn the patient, it gives the patient more confidence to have a second nurse at the head of the frame the first few times the patient is turned.

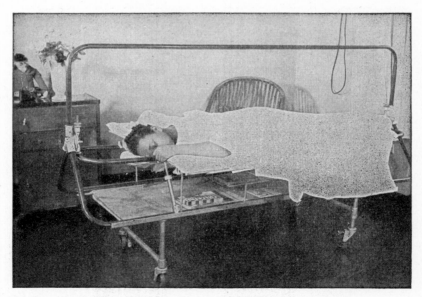

Figure 254D. The patient is in the prone position for sleeping, with the arm rests adjusted. The head is supported on a covered rubber ring, suspended between the bars of the frame.

Study of Figures 254 A-E shows that there are two frames between which the patient is sandwiched as he is turned. The frame on which he lies prone is called the anterior frame, that on which he lies supine the posterior frame. Both are fitted with sectioned canvas covers laced on tightly. Both frames have middle sections that can be removed for the use of the bedpan. (The middle section for the anterior frame can be merely fenestrated for the male patient.) The upper section of the canvas on the anterior frame extends from the shoulder girdle to the symphysis

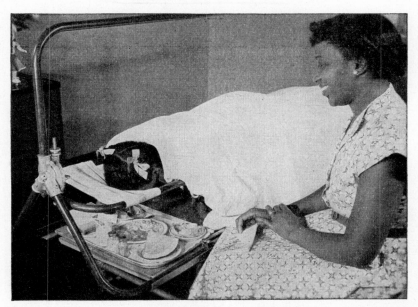

Figure 254E. In the prone position with the arm rests removed, the patient is able to feed herself, to read, or to play such games as checkers. Note the use of a towel pinned over the frame as a head support. Many persons prefer this to the rubber ring.

(Figs. 254 A-E, courtesy of Columbia-Presbyterian Medical Center, New York City, and Clay-Adams Co., New York City.)

pubis, allowing the face and head freedom, and the lower section of the canvas extends 4 in. below the symphysis pubis to the internal malleolus, leaving the feet free. The forehead is supported by a padded canvas strip, a folded towel pinned tightly to the frame, or a head piece made by the manufacturer.

The patient should have a thorough explanation of the frame before he is placed on it. When he is turned he should be secured between the frames with the canvas strips provided for this purpose and should be told to grasp the rod underneath the frame. He should know when the quick turn will be made and in which direction. Until he feels very secure it is wise to have two persons in whom he has confidence adjust the frames and operate the swivel.

The Foster orthopedic bed is a modification of the Stryker frame and is preferred by some operators under certain conditions.

Sandbags.   Different sizes and shapes of sandbags are used for support in maintaining certain positions or for restraint. They are placed also around a part of the body to limit motion, and to relieve pain caused by muscle twitching. They are sometimes covered with stout ticking, but when they are, waterproof covers must be provided to facilitate washing and disinfecting. Cotton or Canton flannel

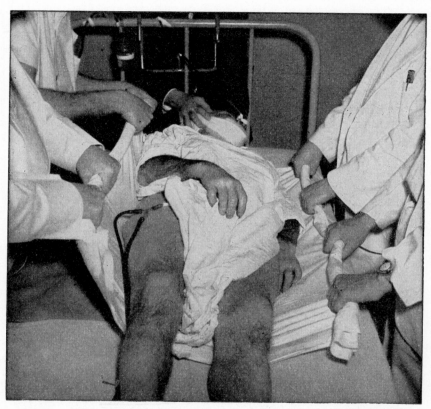

Figure 255A. Turning a patient with a cervical cord injury to his left side with the aid of a draw sheet (in four steps; Figs. 255 A-D). *Step 1:* The draw sheet is pulled tight beneath the patient. (Munro, Donald: *The Treatment of Injuries to the Nervous System.* W. B. Saunders Co., Philadelphia, 1952.)

cases are used as an outer covering and changed when soiled. A part of the body may be restrained by covering it with a towel and placing sandbags over the ends of the towel, at the same time fitting them snugly against both sides of the restrained part. This prevents both lateral and upward movement.

Traction, Suspension, and the Use of Splints.   The broken ends of bones may be brought into alignment and held in position by exerting a pull, or traction, on the two parts. In a leg fracture, a weight is attached to the extremity below the break and countertraction exerted against the leg above the fracture by the use of a splint that is fixed to the body. Weights used in traction may be attached to a rope that is fastened in some way to either the bone below the fracture or to the skin. Skeletal or bone traction may be exerted against a Vitallium pin driven into the bone, a device similar to Crutchfield tongs, or by drilling a hole in the bone through which

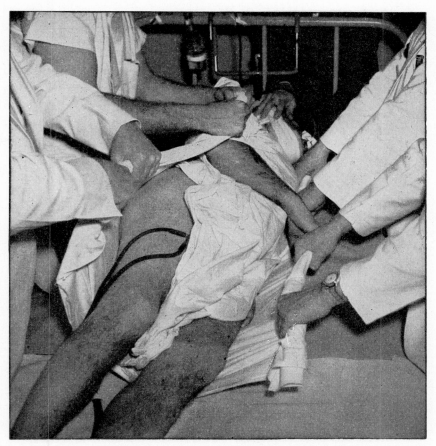

Figure 255B. *Step 2:* The patient is rolled toward his left. (Munro, Donald: *The Treatment of Injuries to the Nervous System.* W. B. Saunders Co., Philadelphia, 1952.)

wire is introduced. Application of traction on the skin, which is probably less generally used now, is referred to as *Buck's extension*. With it, a heavy adhesive or moleskin is applied to the skin of the arm or leg, which has been cleaned and shaved; tincture of benzoin may be applied to the skin before the adhesive. The ends of the moleskin are brought down beyond the foot, or arm, and fixed to a board to which weights can be attached. As in all types of traction, the extremity is supported by a splint and countertraction exerted by means of this device. Weights are always supported on ropes that pass over pulleys attached to the framework of the bed in such a way that force is exerted on the body in the proper plane and the part kept at the prescribed angle in relation to the rest of the body.

Traction exerted on the skin is usually less desirable than skeletal traction, be-

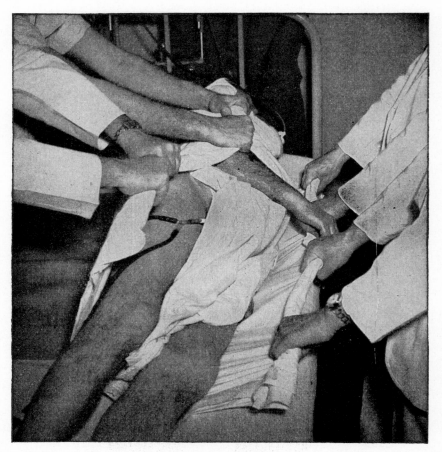

Figure 255C. *Step 3:* The patient is turned on his left side at the edge of the bed. (Munro, Donald: *The Treatment of Injuries to the Nervous System.* W. B. Saunders Co., Philadelphia, 1952.)

cause the adhesive or moleskin is often displaced and many individuals develop a dermatitis under the adhesive. The introduction of Smith-Peterson or Steinmann pins, tongs, or wire into the bone may cause a local infection, but it has been found that such infection, if it does occur, rarely has serious consequences. The pins which are made of a noncorrosive and nonirritating alloy such as Vitallium are driven into the bone under aseptic conditions; the wounds are then covered with sterile dressings.

Splints of various kinds are used when treating a fracture with traction. Some of the most common types are the Thomas and Murray-Jones splints, their modifications, aeroplane splints, and the Bahler frame. These splints are light in weight,

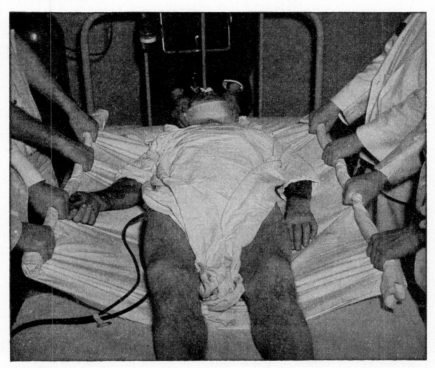

Figure 255D. *Step 4:* The patient is moved to the center of the bed. (Note the attendant turning the patient's head, throughout procedure.) (Munro, Donald: *The Treatment of Injuries to the Nervous System.* W. B. Saunders Co., Philadelphia, 1952.)

having a slender metal framework and a ring that is padded and covered with leather. Because this ring is held against the groin or the axilla, it should be protected from soiling by a waterproof fabric covered with soft absorbent cotton material. The leg or arm is supported on a hammock made by weaving a Canton flannel bandage or cravat bandages over the metal framework (see Fig. 256). Weights used in maintaining traction must drop from a point beyond the framework of the bed, and attendants must take care not to knock against them as this jerks the patient's leg and causes pain.

Occasionally splints are used without traction; for example, if a bone in a finger has been broken. Small plastic splints in varying sizes are available; after the fracture has been reduced and the dressing applied, such splints are slipped over the finger and held in place with bandage or a special cover which ties around the wrist.

There are several advantages of the open traction method of treatment over the use of plaster casts. Having the arm or leg exposed ensures better circulation, and therefore promotes healing and lessens the danger of decubiti. Some surgeons believe that the patient has less pain and is generally more comfortable. Traction allows motion in the joints without interfering with alignment of the broken ends of bone and so prevents stiffness of the joints and loss of function. The patient may be propped up in the vertical or semirecumbent position and by means of the hand grasps or trapeze may turn and lift himself so that the linen

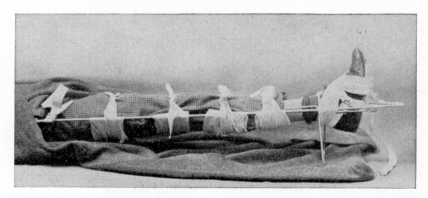

Figure 256.   Emergency splint applied to the leg, with cravat bandages supporting the leg, and traction exerted by a strap attached to the foot piece. (Gildersleeve, G. H.: "First Aid Treatment of Fractures," *Am. J. Nursing,* **38:**627, [June] 1938.)

may be easily changed and the back massaged and properly cared for; the danger of pneumonia is also lessened; and dressings or other treatments are more easily done. The fact that the patient can help himself by systemic exercise of the joints has a particularly beneficial effect.

In nursing a patient in traction, it is essential to understand what the surgeon is trying to do, the positions he intends the patient to assume, the amount of activity he wants him to have, the line of traction, and the force to be exerted in terms of weight to be applied to the bone or skin, according to whether skeletal or skin traction is used.

For skeletal traction, the patient is ordinarily taken to the operating room, since pins, tongs, or wire must be introduced into the bone under aseptic conditions. When the patient returns to the clinical division, the proper appliances should be in readiness. In most hospitals an orthopedic cart is used. In its many compartments may be found rope, weights, pulleys, padding, adhesive, bandage, and all the other common items of orthopedic equipment.

Buck's extension or skin traction is not used so frequently as in the past, but a nurse may have to collect the necessary articles. Briefly, they are as follows: a *fracture board* to place under the mattress unless a commercial fracture bed is available; blocks if necessary to elevate the foot of the bed; two pieces of moleskin (about 4 in. wide and long enough to extend from the side of the foot to above the knee) with suspender-buckles attached; a spreader consisting of a piece of wood 5 in. long by 3 in. wide, to which is attached a strip of webbing about 1 in. wide and long enough to extend about 6 in. on either side, so that they may be fastened to the suspender-buckles; a piece of rope that is passed through a hole in the spreader and securely knotted, a pulley (with screws to attach it to the bed) over which the rope is passed, and weights suspended on the rope by means of which traction is made. Matches and an alcohol lamp are necessary to heat the moleskin to make it adhere. Gauze bandage may be needed to secure the moleskin. A splint, such as the Thomas splint, is used to support the leg if this is the injured part, to prevent eversion of the foot (the characteristic deformity in a fractured femur), and to flex the ankle slightly. The latter is to prevent stretching of the tendons which results in foot drop and impaired function of the ankle. Muslin bandages are required to secure the splint, and nonabsorbent cotton for padding.

Cotton or woolen socks and gloves may be used to protect feet and hands when casts or splints are applied to the extremities. Special linen is available in some institutions for patients in traction. Sheets, blankets, and spreads can be made in sections or openings cut and bound so that the entire body may be covered and the bed made to present a neat appearance.

Braces and Other Supports. When supports of metal framework or plaster are made removable by the use of adjustable canvas straps or other devices, they are called *braces*. These are used for the same purposes as casts and splints; that is, support, correction of abnormal bony alignment, and for the maintenance of rest to promote healing. Braces are ordinarily employed in the treatment of orthopedic conditions that are of long duration. At best they are uncomfortable and unless made to fit the individual and properly adjusted, they may do more harm than good.

Braces should never be used unless prescribed by the physician who also supervises the care of the patient. Muscles that are supported, and hence have no work to do, lose their tone. This may be prevented in most cases by removing the braces at regular intervals for massage and exercise. Such treatment must also be prescribed by the physician.

The metal framework and leather straps of braces are usually padded with felt. Soiled felt should be changed; canvas straps may be scrubbed with ordinary soap and water, and leather straps cleaned with saddle soap.

Crutches. During recovery from skeletal injuries and, in some cases, as compensation for useless or partially useless legs a patient must use crutches as an aid in walking. Many types are available, several of which are shown in Figures 257 and 258. Tripod crutches are sometimes used when the maintenance of balance is especially difficult. Springs have been introduced, rockers and wheels tried, and a variety of hand grips used. Adjustable crutches are especially desirable when they are rented or to be sold after short usage. Tips should be fitted with rubber caps. Sponge-rubber covers or pads are also available for axillary bars and hand bars. While the axillary bar should escape the axilla when the crutch is in use, many patients prefer to have it padded or made of a soft leather sling. White pads bandaged on are soon soiled and unsightly, and a heavy pad is likely to extend the crutch too much. The sponge-rubber cover is probably the most satisfactory type.

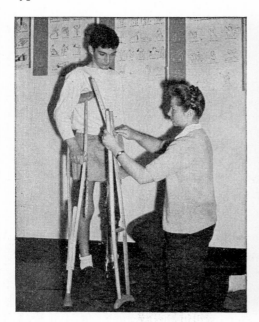 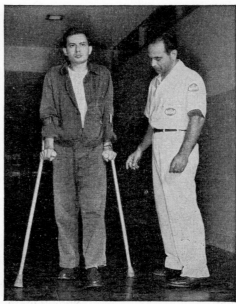

Figure 257 (*left*). Therapist adjusting crutches to correct length. (Courtesy of National Foundation for Infantile Paralysis, New York City.)

Figure 258 (*right*). When a patient can walk unassisted, greater attention is paid to the development of a proper gait. (Courtesy of Veterans Administration, Washington, D.C.)

It is essential that crutches be exactly the right length. Crutches that are too long cause pressure in the armpit and elevation of the shoulder girdle. Pressure on the radial nerve as it passes through the armpit may injure it and impair the function of the hands. When crutches are too short the user has to crouch and cannot get adequate leverage. The following directions for *measuring for crutches* are summarized from material in the book by Knocke and Knocke:[6]

1. Patient assumes an extended supine position with shoulder girdle relaxed (neither elevated nor lowered). If possible, patient should wear shoes (heels are low—about 1 to 1½ in.). The patient places the heels firmly against a footboard.

2. Measurement is made from the anterior axillary fold straight down to the footboard. (This permits space of at least 2 in. between the axilla and the axillary bar of the crutch.)

3. When crutches are obtained from the source of supply, the over-all measurement is made from the crutch pad to the rubber tip.

4. The patient assumes the position as stated in point 1 above. Then he grasps the crutches and holds them in position, crutch tips resting firmly against the footboard. At this time the position of the hand bar is checked and adjusted, as well as a final check of the over-all length of the crutches.

Patients should be thoroughly prepared for the use of crutches. In some instances they may be given practice before orthopedic surgery that will necessitate their use later. In all cases exercises should be taught that will strengthen the hands and

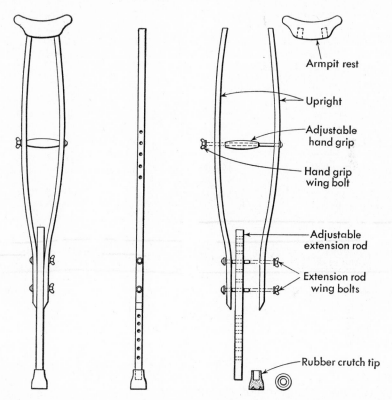

Armpit rest

Upright

Adjustable
hand grip

Hand grip
wing bolt

Adjustable
extension rod

Extension rod
wing bolts

Rubber crutch tip

Figure 259.   Wooden adjustable crutch. (Redrawn from *Let's Walk*. Air Forces Manual No. 49, 1944.)

arms and shoulder girdle (see Fig. 146). Bed patients can strengthen these muscles by the use of the trapeze and by pushing themselves up with their hands.

Unless the patient has had an opportunity to learn the proper use of crutches, considerable instruction is necessary. He must be taught to bear his weight on the hand bar rather than on the top of the crutch that fits under the arm. If the weight of the body is borne on the top of the crutch over any length of time, the arms may be seriously injured. Some of the gaits used include: "the four point," "three point," "two point," "swing to," "swing through," "rocking chair," and "tripod." The medical team should help the patient to adopt the gait, or several gaits, best suited to his needs. In cases where the injured leg is not to be used at all in walking, the weight is borne on the normal foot while both crutches are brought forward at once; then the normal foot is drawn in line with the crutches while the body is supported on the hand bars of the crutches. If the physician wishes the person to make some use of the injured leg, the crutches, like the feet, are put forward alternately, the sequence being (1) the left crutch, (2) the

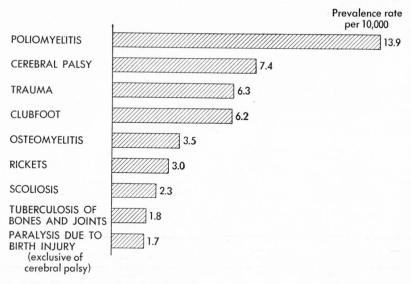

Figure 260. Leading causes of orthopedic impairments among children under age 21, United States, January 1, 1945. (Dublin, Louis I: *The Facts of Life from Birth to Death.* The Macmillan Company, New York, 1951.)

right foot, (3) the right crutch, (4) the left foot, and so on. Orthopedic and rehabilitation texts should be consulted for further details on crutch walking.

When crutches are used for a child over any appreciable length of time, they must be replaced frequently as the child grows taller; otherwise, he will develop postural defects that may be difficult to correct.

Mechanical devices that support the patient more completely than crutches are available for use in teaching patients to walk with an artificial leg or in other conditions that interfere with normal locomotion. These so-called *"walkers"* are a framework on large casters or wheels, which have an adjustable seat, crutches, hand rests, and foot supports. This type of apparatus gives the patient a feeling of greater security, because he knows that he can stop and rest at any time.

REFERENCES

1. Gold, Harry (ed.): *Cornell Conferences on Therapy,* Vol. IV. The Macmillan Company, New York, 1951, pp. 253-79.
2. Gold, Harry (ed.): *Cornell Conferences on Therapy,* Vol. V. The Macmillan Company, New York, 1952, pp. 164-85.
3. Howell, Trevor: *Our Advancing Years.* The Macmillan Company, New York, 1953, p. 52.
4. Christopher, Frederick (ed.): *Textbook of Surgery,* 5th ed. W. B. Saunders Co., Philadelphia, 1949, p. 216.
5. Knocke, Frederick J., and Knocke, Lazelle S.: *Orthopaedic Nursing.* F. A. Davis Co., Philadelphia, 1952, p. 160.
6. Knocke, Frederick J., and Knocke, Lazelle S.: *op. cit.,* pp. 465-67.

Additional Suggested Reading

Bick, Edgar M.: *Source Book of Orthopedics,* 2nd ed. W. B. Saunders Co., Philadelphia, 1948.

Buchwald, Edith, et al.: *Physical Rehabilitation for Daily Living.* McGraw-Hill Book Co., New York, 1952.

Funsten, Robert V., and Calderwood, Melita: *Orthopedic Nursing,* 2nd ed. C. V. Mosby Co., St. Louis, 1949.

Kessler, Henry H., et al.: *Principles and Practice of Rehabilitation.* Lea & Febiger, Philadelphia, 1950.

Lewin, Philip: *Orthopedic Surgery for Nurses Including Nursing Care,* 4th ed. W. B. Saunders Co., Philadelphia, 1947.

Magnuson, Paul B., and Stack, James K.: *Fractures,* 5th ed. J. B. Lippincott Co., Philadelphia, 1949.

Miller, Bernice L.: "Well-Leg and Well-Hip Splints," *Am. J. Nursing,* **48**:572, (Sept.) 1948.

Morrissey, Alice B.: *Rehabilitation Nursing.* G. P. Putnam's Sons, New York, 1951.

Rusk, Howard A., et al.: *Living with a Disability.* Doubleday and Company, New York, 1953.

Skinner, Geraldine: "Nursing Care of a Patient on a Stryker Frame," *Am. J. Nursing,* **46**:288, (May) 1946.

Watson-Jones, Sir Reginald: *Fractures and Joint Injuries,* 4th ed. Williams & Wilkins Co., Baltimore, 1952.

West, John P.; Keller, Manelva W.; and Harmon, Elizabeth: *Nursing Care of the Surgical Patient,* 6th ed. The Macmillan Company, New York, 1957, pp. 334-75.

CHAPTER 43. ACCIDENTS AND EMERGENCIES

1. INCIDENCE AND GENERAL PREVENTIVE MEASURES

Incidence.   Louis I. Dublin,[1] writing in 1951, gives an excellent summary of the known data on accidents. This is the major source of the following statistics on incidence: Annually 100,000 persons are killed and around 10,000,000 seriously injured. It is estimated that the cost per year is more than seven billion dollars.[2] In spite of these staggering figures it is encouraging to learn that the accident rate is declining.

Of the total deaths in this country 7 per cent are due to accidents; for the population as a whole accidents rank fourth among the leading causes of death. The rate is lowest at age 11 and continues to be relatively low up to 35 years; after this the rate increases until 75, when it is at least a thousand times greater than it is at 11 years. Infants under one year have a high rate, and indeed under 4 years the rate is relatively high. This might be expected, for the young child is venturesome and his safety depends upon the watchfulness of others.

The types of accidents commonest among infants are suffocation and mechanical injury from swallowed objects; in early childhood motor vehicles take the largest toll and they continue to be the major form of accident through youth, maturity, and middle age, although burning, drowning, and deaths from railroad accidents account for many fatalities in these periods. In old age (65+), falls are the chief cause of accidental death and injury.

Over half of the accidents reported occur in homes, it is estimated. This is considered such a serious health problem that the US Public Health Service has promoted and assisted with a number of state-wide studies of home accidents and, with state and local agencies, is fostering preventive programs. Some common home accidents are mechanical suffocation (in infancy), burns, scalds, conflagrations, drownings, and poisoning; falls are the commonest type of home accident among mature and elderly persons and they are most likely to occur on stairs. Accidental

Type	Crude death rate per 100,000		Mortality ratio: males to females	
	White males	White females		
FIREARMS	3.1	0.5	6.2	
DROWNING	6.5	1.1	5.9	
MOTOR VEHICLE	38.0	10.7	3.6	
ACCIDENTS (all forms)	97.7	42.8	2.3	
POISONOUS GAS	1.9	0.9	2.1	
CONFLAGRATION	2.2	1.4	1.6	
BURNS (except conflagration)	3.5	2.7	1.3	
ACUTE POISONING	1.2	0.9	1.3	
FALLS	15.9	18.6	0.9	

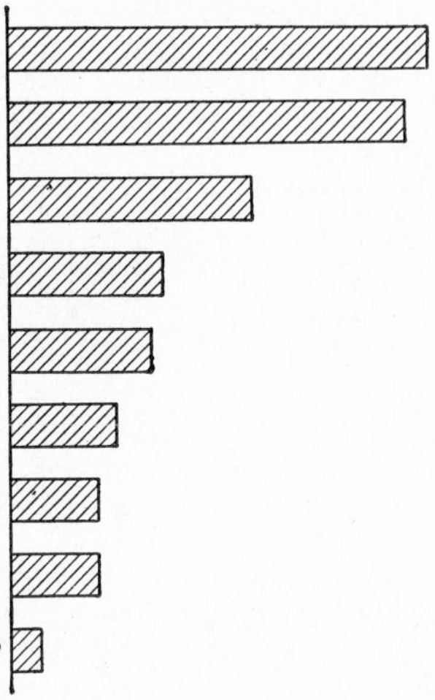

Figure 261. Sex ratio of mortality from specified types of accidents, white persons, United States, 1946. (Dublin, Louis I.: *The Facts of Life from Birth to Death.* The Macmillan Company, New York, 1951.)

death from firearms should be mentioned as a cause of death in homes. Although the death toll of 35,000 persons from motor vehicles in 1950 represents a declining figure, streets and highways are still among the major locations for accidents. About half as many persons in industry were killed "on the job," or off the job in 1950. It seems likely that accidental death rates from traffic and occupational hazards will continue to fall with the present intensive programs that are so obviously successful. If the same effort is put into the prevention of accidents in homes as has been exerted in industry, this rate will almost as certainly show a marked decline.

Table 18 summarizes the data available in 1951.

Prevention. Experts now stress public education as the single most effective measure in reducing the accident rate. It is urged in the reports of state-wide studies that accident prevention be stressed in educational programs for children, youths, and adults. Safety legislation and its enforcement constitute another aspect of the program. There are regulations to control traffic, construction of building and appli-

Table 18. Accidental Deaths by Age, Sex, and Type, 1951*

AGE AND SEX	ALL TYPES	MOTOR-VEHICLE	FALLS	FIRE BURNS†	DROWN-ING‡	RAIL-ROAD	FIRE-ARMS	POISON GASES	POISONS (EXCEPT GAS)
ALL AGES	95,871	36,996	21,376	6,788	6,489	3,631	2,247	1,627	1,497
Under 5	8,769	1,875	367	1,345	736	88	95	58	411
5 to 14	5,892	2,300	230	651	1,330	138	425	40	20
15 to 24	12,366	7,713	314	385	1,280	520	578	218	79
25 to 34	11,644	6,336	473	656	753	622	356	225	147
35 to 44	10,719	4,917	940	774	742	599	313	218	304
45 to 54	9,809	4,260	1,292	674	661	564	217	233	263
55 to 64	9,801	4,016	2,087	644	478	539	166	244	147
65 to 74	10,218	3,444	3,853	722	300	346	76	228	87
75 and over	16,465	2,082	11,805	925	167	196	18	162	35
Age unknown	188	53	15	12	42	19	3	1	4
SEX									
Male	66,873	28,075	10,295	3,945	5,640	3,024	1,964	1,177	917
Female	28,998	8,921	11,081	2,843	849	607	283	450	580
Per cent female	30%	24%	52%	42%	13%	17%	13%	28%	39%

* National Safety Council: *Accident Facts*, 1954 ed. The Council, Chicago.
† Includes deaths resulting from conflagration, regardless of injury.
‡ Includes drownings in water transport accidents.

1142

ances, light, temperature, injurious dusts, noxious gases, fire hazards, exposure to disease-producing organisms, radioactive substances, bathing where there is no protection from drowning, and to protect the public from many other hazards. An entirely safe, foolproof environment can, theoretically, be provided but this is no substitute for the individual's own awareness of danger. The role of the nurse in home safety and industrial health programs is an especially important one for she is the health worker who spends the greatest amount of time with the mother in the home and the employee in industry. The staff of the US Public Health Service have prepared, and are preparing, highly suggestive materials along these lines.[3, 4, 5] Consultant service from public and private health agencies is steadily raising the standards of safety education throughout the nation.*

Almost any contemporary discussion of the incidence of accidents includes some reference to the individual's physical and emotional state as a contributing factor. Physical fatigue as a contributing cause has been demonstrated by studies showing the higher frequency of accidents in the latter part of working periods. That physically handicapped persons *can* overcome the physical factor, however, is shown in a study cited by Dublin.

A person who has a series of injuries that can be attributed to carelessness is said to be "accident prone." It is generally believed that the emotional dissatisfaction, of which the person may be relatively unaware, underlies his carelessness. He may be indifferent to what happens to him or he may be seeking a temporary or permanent escape from an unhappy situation. Industrial health and personnel programs that recognize the psychological, as well as the physical, needs of workers have strikingly reduced the incidence of accidents. A modern industrial health plan provides the worker with satisfying employment and the legitimate rewards of accomplishment.

The Role of the Nurse.   If for no other reason than that nurses outnumber all other health workers, they have the greatest opportunity for teaching accident prevention. With health educators, physicians, and other workers of the health team they share the responsibility for teaching and practicing effective first aid. Since they are so constantly with the sick they should be especially well prepared to recognize early signs of emergency states during illness. If treated early, such states may be averted or their effects minimized. All nurses should have special instruction in safety education and in first-aid measures.

Chapter 36 is devoted to the immediate and later treatment of wounds. The reader is referred to page 948 for discussion of first aid in accidental mechanical injury.

2. EMERGENCIES INVOLVING LOSS OF CONSCIOUSNESS

Definitions.   The dictionary defines unconsciousness as "the state of being without sensibility and with reflexes abolished." Anyone with the most limited medical knowledge will realize that many persons are to all intents and purposes "un-

* A list of emergency first-aid items for homes appears in Appendix V.

conscious," but are not totally "insensible and without reflexes." Actually, unconsciousness is a relative term. The state varies in duration and depth; it may be self-limited and fleeting, or irreversible and leading to death. In some cases the subject is easily aroused, and in others he is unresponsive to all stimuli.

The conditions defined in the following paragraphs are characterized by loss of consciousness, brief or otherwise, complete or incomplete; all present common nursing problems although in each there may be additional, or peculiar, ones. Definitions of the conditions listed may be helpful as a preliminary to the discussion of the nursing care of the unconscious patient.

Fainting or syncope comes from the Greek *synkope,* a cutting short, a sudden loss of strength. Swooning or fainting is defined as a temporary suspension of consciousness from cerebral anemia. If consciousness is not rapidly regained the term syncope is not applicable.

Coma comes from the Greek *kōma,* deep sleep. It is defined as unconsciousness from which the patient cannot be aroused; *coma vigil* is a condition in which the patient lies with the eyes open but is unconscious.

Shock is derived from the French *choquer,* to shock; it may or may not be associated with unconsciousness, but normal awareness is always absent. "Collapse" is really another name for shock. The term collapse was formerly used to differentiate the prostration seen in cardiac crises, or other conditions found on medical services, from "shock" seen in surgery as the result of an accident or an operation. (Chapter 40 is devoted to the treatment and nursing care of the person in shock, or collapse.)

Convulsion comes from the Latin *couvulsio,* which is derived from *convellere,* to shake. William G. Lennox, writing in Russell L. Cecil and Robert F. Loeb's text,[6] says that all animals with an integrated neuromuscular system will have a convulsion if the stimulus is sufficiently powerful. Within each species individuals may differ widely in the strength of the stimulus required to induce convulsions. All conditions are said to result from a constitutional tendency toward the reaction in the presence of "an appropriate stimulus." Lennox suggests that in persons subject to convulsions, or seizures, both these conditions probably exist. They classify seizures into *genetic,* or idiopathic, in which the factor of heredity is believed by some to be dominant; and *acquired,* or symptomatic, those in which "some post-conceptual environmental conditions" seem to be the dominant factor. The latter include Jacksonian, traumatic, and organic epilepsy, tetanic convulsions, eclampsia, and syncope. Of these, they say epilepsy is the most dreaded. It is defined as a "symptomatic paroxysmal cerebral dysrhythmia."

Children are far more susceptible to convulsions than adults. They have not acquired as stable a neuromuscular system as they will later on. With infants a very moderate fever may be the only discoverable cause. Convulsions occur in abnormal pregnancies, and it is not known whether the irritation is chemical or mechanical. Such convulsions are called *eclamptic.*

When convulsive movements affect only a few muscles or a segment of the body, as, for example, the diaphragm, the face, or an arm, the condition is described as a *spasm*. A convulsion usually implies movements of the entire body.

Differentiation of Unconscious States. It is not the function of the person giving first aid, unless he is a physician, to diagnose the unconscious patient. However, the more nearly any one can distinguish between a relatively mild and fleeting state and a serious condition the more effective first aid he can give.

Syncope or fainting is the most common type of unconsciouness. It is fleeting, and the person recovers spontaneously—almost as soon as he assumes the horizontal position. It is most frequent in adolescence and occurs more often in females than in males. The direct cause is a diminished blood supply to the brain. Some common exciting causes are standing immobile, fatigue, hunger, and powerful emotion. It is not unusual for persons to faint at the sight of a bleeding wound or from fear during vaccination. The emotion that induces fainting, however, may be one of relief or joy as experienced on hearing that a beloved person is alive who was reported dead.

A premonition usually precedes fainting. There is a feeling of weakness and dizziness, often nausea, before the person falls to the ground. The face and lips blanch; the skin gets cold and clammy; there is complete relaxation with closure of the eyelids, although the pupils will react to light if the eye is opened. The pulse rate is increased, the respirations are shallow, and the blood pressure falls. All of these symptoms are of brief duration in typical syncope.

Lennox says that when syncope occurs frequently and is accompanied by cyanosis and spasms of the features and extremities it suggests epilepsy. An abnormal encephalogram may confirm this suspicion. A few persons with hypotension have a tendency to faint. (Such persons are urged to develop a strong physique, which may raise the blood pressure, and to avoid vasodilating drugs.)

Since recovery occurs spontaneously—as soon as gravity increases the brain's blood supply—treatment is unnecessary, although the patient should rest until the circulation is re-established and other symptoms disappear. Repeated syncope, or fainting associated with other alarming symptoms, should be reported to a physician. When fainting occurs during an illness, or a convalescence, the physician should be informed at once.

Coma is the prolonged state of unconsciousness which the nurse sees in the patient who is brought to the hospital in a critical state or in the seriously ill hospital patient. Russell Meyers and Mary E. Meyers[7] say the organism in coma has progressed to a "relatively advanced degree of suppressed activity."

The symptoms exhibited by patients in coma differ considerably since coma varies in depth and it may be associated with diabetes, meningitis, nephritis, toxemia of pregnancy, cerebral hemorrhage, brain injury, narcolepsy (a rare neurosis), hysteria, or drug poisoning, or any one of a long list of diseases. Meyers and Meyers list the causative factors in categories as, for example: (1) cerebral, (2) drug, (3) metabolic, (4) anemic, (5) psychogenic, (6) infectious, and (7) cardiovascular. They list over fifty diseases or conditions distributed among these seven categories that might cause coma.

Because effective treatment and nursing care are usually so dependent upon the etiology, the nurse's observation and report of the patient's symptoms are of utmost importance. The physician, unless he is thoroughly familiar with the case, makes a complete examination, including neurological tests, as described in Chapters 18 and 19. When the physician has not seen the patient before he is comatose the diagnosis is, of course, very much more difficult. Meyers and Meyers say that the patient whose empiric therapy happens to be effective may recover before a diagnosis has been made, but that this is unusual and, from the physician's stand-point, unsatisfactory. They speak of coma as a condition calling for "wide knowl-edge, quick thinking, sound judgment and prompt action." They say "there may be no second chance."

The physician's task of discovering the cause of coma is a difficult one; the nurse's task is equally, if not more, difficult in the writer's opinion. Because the patient cannot communicate with the doctor, the nurse, who watches over him, must do this for him and report his symptoms as she interprets them. What is more, she must supply the consciousness, the physical energy, and the will that the patient lacks in providing for his daily physical needs. Coma may be of short duration and of a critical nature; on the other hand, it may last for weeks, months, or years. In such cases those who nurse the comatose may feel that the patient's life is more theirs than his. He is as dependent upon a nurse as the newborn is upon his mother.

A problem sometimes faces the responsive person who comes across a comatose person sitting in a car or lying in the street. The problem is one of distinguishing between alcoholic stupor and other forms of coma. This is not easy. A few clues are that (1) the alcoholic can usually be aroused, (2) there is no irregularity in the pupils, and they will respond to light, and (3) paralysis of one side of the body, with a distortion of the face, is not present as it is likely to be in "a stroke," "apoplexy," *brain hemorrhage,* or "cerebral accident" as the condition is variously termed. Regardless of the cause, all comatose persons should be observed medi-cally; needless deaths have occurred because passers-by have assumed the un-conscious or confused person to be "drunk." The odor of alcohol on the breath, or its absence, is a relatively unimportant sign since the person with a cerebral hemorrhage may very well have had a drink just before the accident occurred; nor is it always possible to recognize the odor of alcohol on the breath of the in-ebriated. The comatose person should be taken to a hospital or to his home where medical attention is available.

Shock, unlike coma, is *always* a critical short-term physical state characterized by a circulatory insufficiency. Unconsciousness is not necessarily a prominent feature although complete unconsciousness and death follow irreversible shock, or severe shock that does not respond to treatment. Chapter 40 is devoted to a dis-cussion of shock; hemorrhage is discussed in Chapter 37. Whenever a person is injured he is examined for signs of hemorrhage and shock. The only conditions that take priority over them for first-aid treatment is asphyxia, or interference with respiration. The discussion of hemorrhage was placed earlier in the text because it was impossible to separate it from the discussion of the care of the wounded. A chapter was devoted to shock because of its importance in all medical and surgical services. It is impossible to describe postoperative care adequately without mention of the prevention and treatment of shock.

Convulsive seizures, as a cause of unconsciousness, can be differentiated from the other conditions mentioned *if* the nurse is present while the convulsive movements last. Sometimes the patient is not discovered until the convulsion has ceased, leaving him comatose. The fact that no spasmodic movements are observed should not rule out the possibility that a period of heightened tension and incoordinated movement preceded the passive stage.

Catalepsy, or a sustained muscular tension, accompanies some states of relative unconsciousness. In severe mental illness the patient stays in one position, sometimes a standing position, for hours or days, and appears to be unaware of his surroundings. In the coma of hysteria and other neuropsychiatric disorders the patient may exhibit no spasm or convulsion but a sustained muscular tension.

Observing and reporting the character of spasms, convulsions, fixed positions, or tension is an important nursing function. What the nurse should note and record are discussed later.

It is frightening to see a person in a convulsion; the observer may be so afraid that the patient is going to hurt himself that efforts to prevent mechanical injury may distract him, or her, from making the observations discussed on page 1154. The nurse should realize that the patient is rarely injured during a convulsion and that it is common for the physician to lack information about the seizure that would be most helpful in determining the cause.

Treatment and Nursing Care of the Person Who Is Unconscious, Including Those in a Convulsive State. Regardless of the cause, the fact that an individual is unconscious calls for a well-defined course of action. The following steps are based on the recommendations of Meyers and Meyers:

(1) Make a preliminary examination; (2) give first aid, including treatment of shock, if present; (3) transport to a place where facilities for treatment are adequate; (4) institute differential diagnostic procedures, including physical examination, x-ray, and laboratory tests; (5) provide for body needs, including oxygen, nutrition, fluid and electrolyte balance, elimination of waste, maintenance of body temperature within physiological limits, maintenance of physiological posture, movement, relaxation, and cleanliness, including protection from irritants and injurious objects; (6) re-examine at frequent intervals; (7) institute surgery if indicated; (8) continue to provide for body needs and continue to re-examine the patient until a cause has been established.

If the patient does not seem to be suffering from asphyxia, hemorrhage, or shock he is transported (unless he is in such a place at the time) to a place where he can be given adequate medical and nursing care. If there is any reason to suspect injury to the cervical vertebrae he should be moved in the supine position with the head extended; otherwise the prone position is advised to facilitate mouth drainage. Good alignment of body segments is important. The patient should be rolled "log-fashion," not lifted, onto the stretcher. Figure 262 shows a stretcher designed to reduce handling to a minimum.

In making a diagnosis the physician is urged by Meyers and Meyers not to accept what appears to be the obvious cause without justifying it with a thorough evaluation; this goes far beyond the usual physical examination. They discuss the variety of procedures that should be used in ruling out each of the causative factors (listed on p. 1147). There may be many contributory factors in coma; therefore, the physician is likely to x-ray the brain, to test the spinal fluid, the blood, and the urine; he may include liver-function tests and estimates of the basal metabolic rate; if there is fever or any sign of infection he will have suitable cultures made; he may order an electrocardiogram; and he always assesses the reflexes. If there is

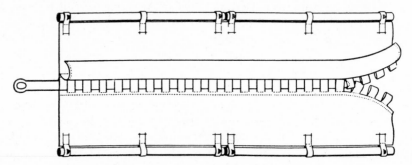

Figure 262. Separating stretcher to reduce movement of seriously injured patients to a minimum. Strong canvas construction, size 28 in. by 74 in. Halves interlock easily and are held together by a long metal strip. Used for ambulance patients and for operative eye, ear, and nose as well as other types of general cases, since the stretcher halves may be easily slid from under the patient. There are four rigid wood poles. (Courtesy of Melrose Hospital Uniform Co., Inc., Brooklyn, N. Y.)

reason to suspect poisoning he may suction and lavage the stomach. In children, and sometimes in adults, the stool may be studied for the presence of intestinal parasites. (Convulsions are a fairly common symptom of serious infestation, particularly in the young.)

In the examinations and tests, nurses play an important role, as described in Chapters 18 and 19; in providing for the patient's hourly and daily physical needs she plays the star role, and few persons survive prolonged coma without good nursing.

Maintaining a normal state of *nutrition* is perhaps the most difficult problem. Unless the swallowing reflex is present and the patient in, at least partial, contact with reality, it is impossible to feed him by mouth. He may not suck on a drinking tube and food placed in his mouth will stay there, or, worse, be drawn into the respiratory passage. There are two main choices in feeding the person in deep coma: intravenous feeding or intubation. Each has its disadvantages.

There are commercially prepared intravenous fluids that contain all the nutritional requirements except fat. (The intravenous administration of fat is in the experimental stage.) Fluids to be given by nasal tube can be prepared so that they provide a complete diet. They can be bought ready for use or made in the hospital or home. Intravenous feeding will ultimately traumatize the veins, just as the passage of the nasal tube will traumatize the nose, pharynx, and esophagus. Intubation must be skillfully managed to avoid insufflation of food and mucus when the tube is withdrawn. Donald Munro[8] favors feeding by nasal tube and advocates a high-caloric, high-vitamin, high-protein diet. He says that in spinal cord injuries the protein requirement is 150 gm of protein daily. Depending upon the adult's size, the feeding should provide from 2000 to 3000 calories. The feeding of children is calculated proportionately. While some physicians have advocated a continuous flow of nutrients through the nasal tube, it is more usual to give 200 to 300 cc every two or three hours. C. G. de Gutiérrez-Mahoney and Esta Carini[9] think that overfilling the stomach predisposes the patient to nausea and vomiting. This is dangerous because the vomitus can be insufflated so easily. They recommend oral feeding in small amounts as soon as the swallowing reflex is re-established. The quantity fed by mouth is increased as rapidly as the patient tolerates it until tube feeding can be dispensed with. (Nasal gavage is described in detail in Chapter 13.)

The maintenance of fluid and electrolyte balance depends upon the nature of the feeding, the amount taken, and the functioning of the organs of elimination. Excessive sweating, vomiting, and diarrhea can seriously upset the balance. The nurse must be aware of these dangers and assume her share of the responsibility for seeing that fluid and electrolyte balance is maintained either by intubation, or intravenous infusions, or oral feeding. She should realize that any other method than oral feeding is a poor substitute for normal eating. As soon as it is safe to do so she should start feeding the patient; first liquids and then solids, gradually increasing the amounts until intubation or intravenous feeding can be discontinued.

Elimination is a serious problem during comatose states. Sphincter control of the urinary bladder and rectum is often lost. The care of the incontinent patient is described in Chapter 14. Little can be added here to that discussion. An indwelling catheter will protect the skin from repeated contacts with urine which predisposes the patient to pressure sores; it will reduce the amount of linen and the quantity of cellucotton, etc., needed; on the other hand, a catheter is a foreign body in the bladder and its presence almost inevitably results in the development of a low-grade cystitis. Again, it is a question of a choice of two imperfect practices. Most physicians and nurses prefer to use a catheter of the Foley type, with tidal drainage, and thereby reduce the hazard of pressure sores. Normal elimination should be re-established as soon as possible, however.

Daily bowel elimination should be encouraged by including laxative foods in the tube feeding. Prune juice, for example, is very effective. If indicated, mild laxatives may be added to the feedings, and, if necessary, a colonic lavage given daily until the bowel resumes its tone and normal functionings. The bowel movement should be induced at the patient's regular hour for defecation, if this is known.

Feces can easily accumulate in the rectum until it is impacted, if the nurse does not make sure that there is adequate daily elimination. When there is stasis of the intestinal contents, as may happen if the ileus is paralyzed, it may be necessary to drain the contents of the alimentary canal by nasal intubation (see Chapter 29). This is indicated only in extreme cases.

Because the patient cannot say that he is hot or cold, he is dependent upon the nurse for this aspect of his physical comfort or protection. The body temperature is measured by rectum during coma, as one might suppose. This is some guide in clothing and covering the patient adequately and in regulation of the room temperature. Feeling the feet, as one would a baby's, tells the nurse whether the patient is overheated, comfortable, or cold. External heat should be applied with particular caution since the patient cannot protect himself from burns.

It is not unusual to find the unconscious patient in a gloomy environment, those taking care of him assuming that he is unable to enjoy his surroundings. The writer believes that this is an unwise position to take. In the first place, there is no exact measure of the patient's awareness, and, in the second place, the environment reacts on the patient's family and friends and on those in attendance upon him. The room should be kept at a comfortable temperature. It should not only be free from unpleasant odors and sights, but made attractive to the senses. The more normal and cheerful the environment, the less confusing it is to the person as consciousness returns, and the more normal the outlook of those who care for him. Positive factors such as change of furnishings, music, and perfumes might be studied for their effect upon the comatose, particularly if the state is believed to have a psychogenic origin and is prolonged.

Except for convulsive movements the deeply unconscious patient is motionless, but many comatose patients are also restless. They may vary from hour to hour or day to day in their awareness or depth of unconsciousness, and for this reason it is rarely safe to assume that the stuporous, irrational, and disoriented may not be in danger of falling from bed or otherwise subjecting themselves to injury if left alone. *Protection of the unconscious* from injury is an essential part of the nursing program. Bedsides, or homemade substitutes for them, should be used when it is necessary to leave the patient unattended. Munro points out that the patient's effort to free himself from tight restraints may be dangerous to a person with heightened intercranial pressure. The intuitive nurse who can discover the cause of the restlessness and relieve it often reduces the need for restraint to a minimum. She should explain to the patient what is going to happen and what is happening and hope that he understands enough to relieve some of his anxiety. She should, of course, remove causes of physical discomfort that lead to restlessness, if this is possible.

When the patient is deeply unconscious and motionless, the nurse must move the patient every hour. *Body movement* is essential for normal maintenance of many functions, but the nurse's most immediate concern is the prevention of pressure sores which can develop very rapidly. Change of position, adequate nutrition, and cleanliness are the chief means of reducing this hazard.

Contractures must be prevented during unconscious states by change of posture, placing the patient in physiological positions, rather than contracted ones, and occasionally by splinting joints when there is a tendency to flexion. The patient is kept in side-lying positions chiefly (see Chapter 15). Turning sheets reduce the effort involved and help to keep the body segments in good alignment. Pillows at the back are said to be contraindicated by one authority.[10] If the patient is well balanced and supported in the lateral position there is no tendency to fall over on the back. While the patient is side-lying, supports should be placed at each foot to prevent foot drop. The head should rest on a pillow of sufficient thickness to preserve the alignment of the cervical vertebrae.

The unconscious patient should not be left on his back because the relaxed tongue may fall over the glottis, and mucus cannot drain from the mouth while he is in this position. As he recovers he is turned on his back for certain periods, if he prefers this position.

Exercise of the arms and legs by the nurse will greatly reduce the harmful effects of immobility. Daily massage is also desirable. With returning consciousness the patient should be encouraged to participate in, and finally take responsibility for, exercising unless he is completely paralyzed. The patient should not remain bedfast any longer than is necessary. Even if he must be lifted, it is desirable to get him into a chair or move him by stretcher. He needs both the activity and the change of scene as his condition improves.

A firm bed is desirable. Sponge-rubber mattresses reduce the difficulty of preventing pressure sores, and sponge-rubber pads can be used in a variety of ways for support.

Nursing the unconscious may be complicated by the critical nature of the injury or its surgical treatment. In such cases the surgeon gives specific directions about the position of the patient and how he should be turned. Figures 255 A-D show the use of a lifting sheet in turning the patient with a spinal injury.

Cleanliness for the unconscious is not easily achieved. As in infancy, he is dependent upon the nurse. A daily bath is important for the stimulation of the circulation and to prevent skin lesions. Soap should be avoided and neutral cleansing agents substituted. Skin lubricants, such as the commercial preparation "Lubriderm," vegetable oils, or lanolin should be applied. Alcohol is drying, and therefore contraindicated in most cases. Incontinence should be managed, if possible, so that the bed is not soiled repeatedly, but if this occurs the patient should be sponged, dried, and the bed linen changed at once. "Keradex," a protective coating for the skin, might be helpful in such cases.

It is important to clean the mouth of the unconscious even more carefully than that of most patients. (Removable dentures should not be worn until consciousness returns.) During mouth cleansing the patient should be lying on his side with the head tilted so that water put into the mouth runs out into a basin, rather than down the throat. If this occurs there is little danger in rinsing the mouth with fluid introduced with the syringe. Motorized mouth suction is so helpful in caring for the unconscious that the apparatus should be rented when it is not otherwise available. Figures 61 A-C show the nurse using a toothbrush to clean the mouth of a comatose woman. A soft rubber catheter, size #20 or #22 French, is used in suctioning. The teeth should be brushed two or three times daily, and the mouth rinsed every few hours with water or a mouthwash. The lips should be kept lubricated with cold cream or a substitute.

Since the patient cannot blow his nose the passages may be occluded by encrusted mucus. Unless there is bleeding from the nose, or a head injury that contraindicates the procedure, the nurse should clean the nostrils as described in Chapter 12. Following a head injury, spinal fluid may drain from the nose. Any sign of this should be reported at once.

With deep unconsciousness the winking reflex may be absent; this takes away the patient's involuntary means of protecting the cornea and conjunctiva from injury. In such cases the eye can be protected by closing the lids with a dressing such as that shown in Figure 220. The dressing should be removed and the eye examined every few days. Untreated irritation may lead to permanent injury. The physician will order medication and possibly irrigation, if conjunctivitis develops.

Ears should be examined for bleeding if there has been a brain injury. Sterile cotton may be kept in them and any cleaning done, with the surgeon's knowledge, very gently, and with aseptic precautions. Evidence of bleeding or meningeal fluid draining from the ears should be reported at once.

For the family's sake, if not for the patient's, the hair should be brushed and combed becomingly. In cases of brain surgery it may be necessary to cut the hair or even shave the head. A head covering can be devised that is quite attractive. Shampoos cause minimum disturbance if given skillfully by several workers who, in helping each other, can shorten the time required for the procedure.

The *psychological aspects* of nursing the unconscious are more often neglected than the physical aspects. Medical workers, friends, and families make the serious mistake of talking in the patient's presence as if he could not hear.* They often speak discouragingly about his condition or perhaps complainingly of the care he requires. Even if they do not commit one of these gross blunders they increase the confusion in his mind by saying things he cannot understand. It is wise to assume at all times that the patient may be able to hear and, therefore, to refrain from saying anything in his presence that should not be said to him. As he seems to recover, but still cannot speak, a conversation between his intimates who are sitting with him may be encouraging, interesting, or entertaining, if they try to make it so.

A program of rehabilitation should be planned and initiated at once if there is a chance that the patient will survive the condition underlying the unconscious state. This optimism will communicate itself to the patient, and he will be encouraged to fight for a return to health, if he sees that others expect it.

---

* Various methods of communication with asphasic patients have been devised. In one method the alphabet has been divided into quarters, and then the individual letters identified by numbers. The patient is asked, "First, second, third, or fourth." Then, when the correct portion of the alphabet has been identified by the patient's nodding his head, he is asked, "First, second, etc., letter." This method is laborious, but in short-term illnesses has proved useful. Another method is based on the sign language; however, instead of using signs for individual letters, the various gestures represent phrases such as "I am thirsty."

Periods of unconsciousness are usually crises, but to those who have an untreated, or an uncontrollable, tendency to seizures, it may be a recurring state. Of such seizures, epilepsy is by all odds the commonest cause, although the term is used to cover a wide range of conditions. For an adequate discussion of epilepsy the nurse should consult the more detailed texts that are cited in this chapter. The following is a brief description of nursing care during any seizure, but with some specific reference to an epileptiform seizure as a common type.

During a convulsion the movements should not be restricted, but all objects that might injure the patient should be put out of reach. If the person is on a hard surface a pillow or other soft object should be placed under the head. Restricting clothing should be loosened, and since bladder incontinence accompanies a severe seizure, the bed and clothing should be protected from soiling, if possible.

To keep the patient from biting his tongue during involuntary movements of the jaw, a rubber wedge or padded stick should be placed between the upper and lower molars. If the mouth gag is not inserted early and the teeth are clenched, it must be omitted. Prying the jaws apart is likely to knock out a tooth, which is a more serious injury than a bitten tongue.

It is terrifying to most persons to watch a convulsion; therefore, other patients should be shielded from this sight. The victim also should be shielded and his privacy respected. Those who are subject to seizures can usually recognize early signs, or the aura, that precedes the convulsion. They will lie on a low bed or on the floor to avoid injury, and will seek out a person in whom they have confidence, if time allows.

Ignorance of its cause and the true nature of epilepsy has ostracized the epileptic until recent years. National and local programs to educate the public and improve the treatment of epilepsy is bearing fruit. With the insistence by experts that it has not been proven hereditary, that it does not necessarily result in mental deterioration, and that it can be greatly modified by treatment, there is a change in the attitude of the patient and the public.[11]

Louis S. Goodman and Alfred Gilman say that: "Considering the many important advances made in the field of convulsive disorders in the last few years and the active research currently in progress, epilepsy is now correctly termed the 'hopeful disorder.' "[*] They point out that drug therapy must be on an individual basis and sometimes combined with nutritional therapy, or even surgery. The anticonvulsant drugs, such as diphenylhydantoin, mesantoin, phenobarbital, trimethadione, are chosen and the dosage prescribed according to whether the seizure is classified as (1) grand mal, (2) petit mal triad, or (3) psychical or psychomotor epilepsy, or (4) a mixed type. Each is said to respond to different drugs.

A grand mal attack is one in which the patient gets cyanotic, has tonic spasms alternating with clonic movements, loses control of the bladder, and remains unconscious for a few minutes or longer. In a minor seizure there may be no convulsive movements or even noticeable loss of consciousness. The attack consists of transitory periods in which the person looks "vacant" and performs acts automatically

* Goodman, Louis S., and Gilman, Alfred: *The Pharmacological Basis of Therapeutics.* 2nd ed The Macmillan Company. New York. 1955. p. 179.

that he cannot later remember. Lennox[12] describes a variety of psychical and psychomotor states that often follow a history of convulsions and that are difficult to distinguish from hysteria or malingering. He calls this the psychical type of seizure. In any type, the object of treatment is to prevent seizures altogether or to make the patient's life as normal as possible, if they cannot be completely controlled. It is estimated that one person out of every 200 in this country has some form of so-called epilepsy. It is no longer believed justifiable to treat these potentially useful and happy elements of society as outcasts.

When convulsions occur and the nurse is present she should note the following and report her observations to the physician:

1. Was the patient warned? (Did he tell someone that he was going to have a seizure or did he prepare for it, or tell the nurse after the attack that he knew he was going to have a seizure?) Did he cry out or make a noise that attracted attention?

2. How did his appearance change? What position did the different segments of the body assume; were the eyes closed or shut, did they turn upward, downward, or sideways; was there a change in the size of the pupils, would they respond to light during and after the seizure? Did the skin and mucous membrane change color? Was there "foaming at the mouth"? Were the teeth clenched; was there any blood in the froth around the mouth?

3. What was the effect on the vital signs? How was the pulse rate affected? What was the respiratory rate?

4. What was the nature of the convulsion? When did it begin and how long did it last? What parts of the body were involved, and if it spread, how did it progress? Were the spasms tonic or clonic, or mixed, and did they change in character as the seizure progressed?

5. How was consciousness affected? Was the patient unconscious and how long did it last? Could he be roused to answer questions or follow directions? Was there urinary incontinence?

6. What was the aftereffect? Did the patient complain of pain or discomfort in any part of the body? Was there any change in speech following the attack? Was there elevation of body temperature?

No matter what the nature of the seizure, the nurse should maintain at least an outward calm since this is reassuring to all. Confidence is contagious just as is panic.

3. ASPHYXIA

Asphyxia comes from the Greek prefix, *a,* absence of, and *sphyxis,* pulse. It is a condition of unconsciousness, due to suffocation or interference of any kind with the oxygenation of the blood.

Causes.   The most usual causes include the following:

1. Mechanical interference with the entrance of air to the lungs which may be inflammation and swelling of the throat and larynx or the formation of a membrane, as in dipththeria; edema of the glottis in diphtheria, tuberculous laryngitis, cardiac and renal diseases; foreign bodies in the respiratory tract; pressure on the trachea or

bronchi from goiter, tumor, or aneurysm; water and mucus in the respiratory tract, as in drowning.

2. The inhalation of smoke, or poisonous gases, such as coal gas or illuminating gas, or the fumes of ammonia, or nitric acid, or the inhalation of ether in anesthesia.

3. Interference with the interchange of gases between the blood and air in the lungs, as in diseases of the heart or lungs, and in poisoning from carbon monoxide. In such cases the hemoglobin is saturated with carbon monoxide and is not free to combine with oxygen.

4. Weakness of the respiratory muscles, or convulsive spasms, as in croup or whooping cough; or paralysis, as in diseases or injuries involving the upper part of the spinal cord.

5. Paralysis of the respiratory center in the medulla. Normal function of this center depends upon the amount and character of the blood flowing through it. Respiration is stimulated by the carbon dioxide in venous blood. When this is markedly reduced a condition of alkalosis exists which, if severe, may paralyze the respiratory center.

6. Failure of the lungs to expand in the newborn.

Symptoms. The symptoms of asphyxia develop in three stages: In the *first stage* the venous blood flowing through the medulla stimulates the respiratory center, making the breathing more rapid (hyperpnea), labored (dyspnea), and distinctly audible. Respiratory muscles not used in quiet breathing are forced into action. The appearance of the patient is alarming—the lips are blue, the face congested, the eyes prominent and bloodshot, and the expression anxious. The venous blood also stimulates peripheral vasoconstriction and raises blood pressure. This stage lasts about one minute.

In the *second stage* convulsions occur as a result of further stimulation of the centers in the medulla, soon followed by coma.

The *third stage* is characterized by exhaustion. The patient's muscles are flaccid and the pupils widely dilated; blood pressure falls and the pulse is almost imperceptible, as the heart fails. The inspirations are prolonged and sighing, and the intervals between increase until breathing finally ceases. Death results from gradual exhaustion and paralysis of the centers in the medulla. Death from asphyxia may follow in 5 to 10 minutes after the onset of these grave symptoms.

Treatment. In all such cases of asphyxia the treatment consists in removing anything that might interfere with breathing, in establishing natural respiration with the least possible delay, and in treating the patient for shock. The first step is to remove any obstruction to the free passage of air, if possible. Foreign bodies, such as false teeth or a partial plate, should be removed from the mouth or throat. Mucus should be wiped out or removed with suction. The patient's position must be such as to keep the air passages wide open and to allow for free expansion of the lungs.

When fluid obstructs the lungs and bronchi, as in drowning, clothing should be loosened about the neck, chest, and waist and the patient then turned on his face, and his body raised at the waistline by means of a folded blanket or clothing. Pressure should then be applied, with both hands outspread over the lower ribs. Fluid from the stomach and lungs will run out by gravity from the esophagus and the trachea through the mouth and nose. The nose, mouth, and throat should be cleaned of mucus.

In asphyxia caused by closure of the larynx it may be necessary to introduce an airway. This can be achieved by introducing a rubber, plastic, or metal tube to keep the normal respiratory channel sufficiently open to allow the patient to breathe until the obstruction can be removed. Tracheal intubation is indicated whenever an obstruction to breathing is causing, or is in danger of causing, marked dyspnea, cyanosis, or exhaustion of the patient.

The articles required are a mouth gag, an intubator or introducer, an extubator for the removal of the tube, and a set of hard-rubber tubes graded to correspond to the size of the larynx of patients at various ages. Each tube is threaded with silk thread and attached to an obturator.

Successful treatment depends largely upon having the patient in a position that will enable the doctor to insert the tube. An adult is placed horizontally on the bed or table, with the head perfectly straight and firmly held. A child is wrapped and confined closely in a sheet, and is held upright by the nurse, with the back of his head resting on her shoulder and his feet securely held between her knees. Another assistant should hold the child's head up and backward as far as possible with the chin in a straight line with the trachea; this assistant also holds the mouth gag in place. The doctor sits directly opposite the patient.

A good light is essential. The doctor may wear a head mirror from which the light is reflected into the child's throat; otherwise, the child is held so that the artificial light or light from a window will shine directly into the throat.

Inserting the tube stimulates the secretion of mucus or it may have already collected. The head should be held to one side to allow this to escape. If the tube is properly inserted in the larynx, one or two coughs will be followed soon by quiet breathing, the color will improve, and the subject, worn out with struggling, usually falls asleep. If the tube is passed into the esophagus by mistake coughing will not occur, the color and breathing will not improve, and the string (attached to the tube and left hanging from the mouth) will gradually recede as the peristaltic action carries it down the esophagus. The string or silk thread should be left hanging from the mouth and observed for about 10 minutes; it is then either removed or passed around the ear and fastened to the cheek with Scotch tape. One objection to leaving the silk attached is that it is possible for a child, if not carefully guarded, to reach it and pull the tube out. Removal of the silk thread does not increase the danger from the tube passing into the trachea, because the whole tendency is to cough the tube up and out; however, the silk thread may be useful in removing the tube should it go into the esophagus.

The insertion of the tube should take only about two or three seconds. It should not last more than 15 seconds, because the breathing is obstructed during the introduction of the tube. Speedy and successful insertion depends to a great extent upon the assistance, judgment, and presence of mind of the nurse, as well as upon the skill of the surgeon.

In some cases of asphyxia a tracheotomy is performed. This is described on page 1041.

The *aftercare* in asphyxia is very important, and is the particular responsibility of the nurse. The intubation tube is usually left in two to seven days, according to the cause of the asphyxia and the condition of the patient. During this time he should be constantly watched and given the best nursing care, with particular attention to nutrition. The usual method of feeding is by nasal gavage. Special precautions must be taken to see that the catheter is in the esophagus, and also to prevent any liquid from accidentally entering the tube. When nasal feeding is not used, the patient's head is sometimes held much lower than the body, and liquids are given by mouth with a spoon. If there is difficulty in feeding without having liquid enter the tube, intravenous feeding must be used.

For the removal of the tube, the position of the patient is the same as for its introduction. After its removal, the patient must be very closely and continuously watched for any swelling of the throat, or for renewed difficulty in breathing; the physician usually waits, or is within immediate call, for a period of at least one hour.

The administration of oxygen may be indicated in the treatment of asphyxia. Opiates are contraindicated as are all drugs that depress the respiratory center.

In cases of asphyxia in which the larynx and trachea are open and there is no interference with the passage of air to and from the lungs, *artificial respiration* is indicated as treatment. If it is to be used, it should be started immediately. There are several methods of giving artificial respiration—that is, starting up respiration in a person in whom it has ceased. The Sylvester, Schäfer, Laborde, Howard, and Marshall Hall methods are generally known.

Other recommended methods developed within the last two decades are: the hip-lift method by Emerson, the hip-lift back-pressure method, the hip roll-back pressure, the Eve rocking method, and the arm lift-back pressure method (Holger Nielsen).

A nurse should become familiar with one or more methods and should practice them. Speed in action and perseverance are essential. The Schäfer and the Sylvester methods are commonly used, and lately the Holger Nielsen is said to be the method of choice because it is less exhausting to the resuscitator and there is little possibility of injuring the patient.

The *Schäfer* or the *prone-pressure method* saves labor and is said to be simple and not likely to injure the patient. It is described in the words of the writer more or less as follows:

It consists in laying the subject in the prone posture, preferably on the ground, with a thick folded garment underneath the chest and epigastrium. The operator puts himself athwart or at the side of the subject, facing his head, and places his hands on each side over the lower part of the back (lowest ribs). He then slowly throws the weight of his body forward to bear upon his own arms, and thus presses upon the thorax of the subject and forces air out of the lungs. This being effected, he gradually relaxes the pressure by bringing his own body up again to a more erect position, but without moving the hands.

The movements are repeated regularly at a rate of 12 to 15 times a minute until normal breathing begins or until the possibility of its restoration is abandoned. Efforts to revive the patient should be continued for an hour or more.

The *Sylvester push-pull method* consists in loosening the clothing, removing mucus or foreign bodies from the mouth or throat, and placing the patient flat on his back with a pillow or folded blanket between the shoulders, so as to raise the chest, extend the trachea, throw the head back, and keep the air passages open. The tongue is then grasped and held well forward by an assistant. Covering the fingers with a (clean) cloth makes it easier to maintain a grip on the tongue. The operator kneels at the head facing the feet of the patient and, grasping both elbows, moves the arms slowly outward from the body and upward above the head as far as they will go; this expands the chest and causes inspiration. The arms are held in this position for a few seconds, then brought toward each other, then downward to their original position against the last ribs, making pressure upon them so as to cause expiration. These movements are repeated at normal respiratory rate. Efforts to revive the patient should be continued for an hour or more.

"The *Holger Nielsen push-pull method* has been used for almost 20 years in the Scandinavian countries. The victim is placed in the prone position with one hand on top of the other and his head resting upon them. The operator kneels near the victim's head and grasps his arms above the elbows. He rocks backward drawing the arms upward and toward himself. After replacing the arms on the ground he rocks forward, places his hands on the midback—at the lower edge of the shoulder blades—and exerts pressure almost vertically downward. Twelve complete cycles are executed each minute. The arm lift produces active inspiration and the back-pressure results in active expiration."*

Hip-lift (Emerson) is a very effective method. The patient is prone. As the hips are lifted 8 to 10 in., the abdomen sags, the diaphragm is drawn downward, and the patient *inhales*. Returned to the initial position the patient *exhales* because the diaphragm rises, the floor presses on the abdomen, and the elastic lungs recoil. Study Figures 263 A-E; note that pressure in lifting is exerted on the hips, *not* the abdomen. (The use of a lifting sling reduces the resuscitator's fatigue.)

Laborde's method consists in applying rhythmic and forcible traction to the tongue, but this method is omitted from current texts and is apparently obsolete.

Archer S. Gordon et al., discussing the various methods of artificial respiration, come to the conclusion that Schäfer's method should be replaced by one of the more efficient push-pull methods. The Emerson method seems to the writer to be at once the most effective and practical of the methods that have been described. It is illustrated in Figures 263 A-F.

Any patient requiring artificial respiration is in a serious condition and is suffering more or less from shock for which treatment will be required. In cases of

* Gordon, Archer S.: "Newer Methods of Artificial Respiration," *Am. J. Nursing,* **52:**295, (Mar.) 1952.

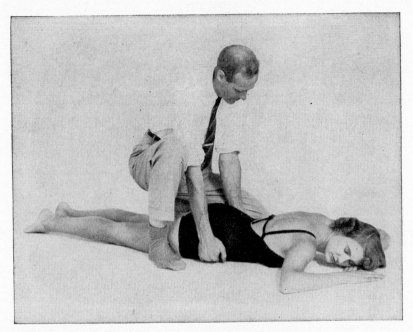

Figure 263A. Artificial respiration, using the Emerson method: Position for ease of lifting: The operator grips the hipbones with his hands. One knee is well *forward* of the victim's hip (and close in against the forearm). The victim's position, prone as for Schäfer artificial respiration, favors drainage of fluids from the mouth and maintenance of a clear airway. (Courtesy of Mr. J. H. Emerson.)

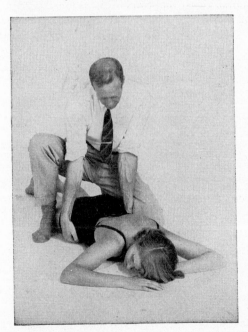 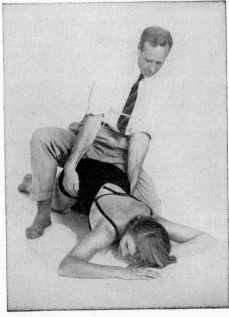

Figures 263 B and C. The rescuer sways, pivoting on one knee. Both arms remain straight, and very little effort is required. (Courtesy of Mr. J. H. Emerson.)

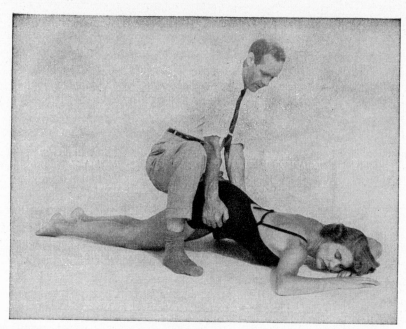

Figure 263D. Note that *both* hips are lifted off the ground. An 8- or 10-in. lift gets more air in than a very slight lift. As the abdomen sags, the diaphragm is drawn downward and produces *in*halation. (Courtesy of Mr. J. H. Emerson.)

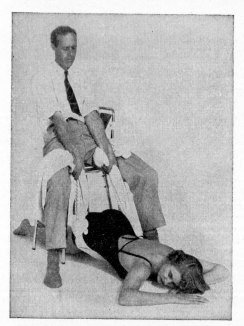 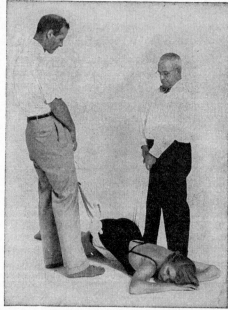

Figures 263 E and F. To make intermittent lifting during the process of artificial respiration over a long period easier, a towel, piece of clothing, etc., can be slid under the patient; these items must be placed well down where the patient bends and *not* across the abdomen. (Courtesy of Mr. J. H. Emerson.)

drowning, particularly, the patient will be suffering from shock due to cold, prolonged exposure, exhaustion, and fear of death. As soon as breathing has been established, the wet clothing should be removed and the patient wrapped in dry, warm blankets. "A brief return of natural respiration is not a certain indication for stopping the resuscitation. The patient must be watched and if natural breathing stops, artificial respiration should be resumed at once."* Heat should be applied to the extremities and friction using a warm towel to stimulate the circulation. Stimulants may be given by hypodermic. As soon as the patient is able to swallow, hot coffee, whisky, or brandy may be given by mouth. He should be kept quiet and in bed until fully recovered.

The *pulmotor* and *lungmotor* are mechanical devices used in giving artificial respiration. They are used by a doctor or operated by technicians in lifesaving stations, etc. It is not likely that a nurse will be expected to operate one. While waiting for the arrival of such apparatus the nurse or first-aid assistant should start artificial respiration at once, as any delay may result in death.

Oxygen may be administered in the treatment of asphyxia. The procedure is discussed in Chapter 27.

4. PULMONARY EDEMA

Pulmonary edema needs no definition for it is what the name implies—excessive fluid in the tissue spaces of the lungs. It is sometimes called pulmonary congestion, but the latter term is also used by the public for any inflammatory condition of the lungs while "pulmonary edema" is reserved for an alarming outpouring of plasma from the pulmonary capillaries into the tissue spaces and then into the air spaces, or alveoli, when the pulmonary lymphatics can no longer drain off the edema fluid. Unless the process is arrested by nature or therapy, the patient literally drowns in his own body fluids and dies of asphyxia. Death from pulmonary edema is really death from asphyxia since the fluid fills the spaces normally filled by air; death results from oxygen want.

Cause. Alveolar spaces can be filled with blood serum, or excess mucus following a chest wound, or the inhalation of irritating gases and substances to which the patient is allergic. Cecil K. Drinker's text,[13] or a comparable source, should be consulted for the full treatment of pulmonary congestion—its "active" forms, such as those just listed, and the passive form, generally referred to as "pulmonary edema," which is under discussion here and whose etiology is still obscure.

The direct cause of the outpouring of fluid from the capillaries is an increased permeability of their walls. What makes this, often sudden, change in the capacity of the capillaries to contain their contents is not thoroughly understood. Goodman and Gilman in discussing pulmonary edema say the mechanism is the same in the lungs and elsewhere in the circulation. "An increase in pulmonary hydrostatic pressure, a decrease in colloidal osmotic pressure, or an increase in pulmonary capillary permeability can lead to transudation of fluid into the alveoli."† They go

---

* American Red Cross: *First Aid Textbook,* rev. ed. Blakiston Co., Philadelphia, 1945, p. 93.
† Goodman, Louis S., and Gilman, Alfred: *op. cit.,* p. 94.

on to say that failure of the left heart is a common cause. Dickinson W. Richards, writing in Cecil and Loeb's text, says there are many causes, but the commonest is "hypertension in the pulmonary capillary bed secondary to left heart failure."[13a] He thinks a combination of factors brings about the condition, but he considers the cause essentially unknown. Margene O. Faddis and Joseph M. Hayman, Jr.,[14] in a very helpful presentation, point out that parts of the lungs that move least have been shown to be most susceptible to passive congestion. This ties in with Goodman and Gilman's suggestion that oxygen lack may increase capillary permeability. If this is true it is easy to see why the condition progresses so rapidly and often so fatally, and it suggests the importance of body movement in preventing pulmonary edema. Another etiological theory is that the increased capillary permeability is a response to vasomotor reflexes. This angioneurotic edema is seen in shock and epilepsy. Both of these conditions develop rapidly and have a good deal in common with pulmonary edema.

Symptoms.   The onset is usually sudden and is said to be, in some cases, unheralded by warning signs. The feeling of oppression in the chest may, however, develop gradually with mounting anxiety, whereas with a sudden onset and outpouring of fluid into the tissues the pain may be so great that the patient cries out in stark fear. A conspicuous symptom is an incessant cough producing a frothy, sometimes blood-tinged, sputum. The sputum gets increasingly copious until, if the condition is not controlled, the fluid gushes from the nose and mouth. Rales can be felt and heard all over the chest, and the breathing is increasingly moist, or crackly, as in the "death rattle." Breathlessness and cyanosis progress until the patient is gasping for air. The face is covered with cold sweat, the pulse gets steadily weaker, and the blood pressure falls. Attacks are said to be more common at night or in the early morning, and may be confused with asthma. It has been said that pulmonary edema may be fatal in a few hours or that symptoms may persist for 12 to 24 hours and then disappear. When fatal, pulmonary edema usually develops slowly and is accompanied by coma; the prognosis is always grave. It is one of the most deaded emergency states.

Treatment.   Fortunately, with the improvement of oxygen therapy, the lives of many persons with pulmonary edema are saved. If the cause is not removed there is a tendency to recurrence, however. Treatment, as in most cases, has two aspects: the preventive and the immediate ameliorative treatment.

The immediate treatment is that with which we are most concerned in this chapter. It has two main objectives: (1) to supply the oxygen needed and increase the gas pressure in the alveoli, and (2) to reduce the hydrostatic pressure in the pulmonary capillaries.

Oxygen is given immediately, no matter what the cause of the edema. If a positive pressure mask is available, this is the preferred method. (See p. 778 for description of this procedure.) Goodman and Gilman advocate the administration of not less than 50 per cent oxygen under 4 cm of water pressure. The positive-pressure mask offers a slight obstruction to expiration, which builds up gas pressure against the walls of the alveoli. This favors absorption of oxygen. (There are several varieties of positive pressure masks.) As the condition improves the pressure is gradually lowered at the rate of 1 cm of water every one to four hours. If a positive-pressure mask is not available, 100 per cent oxygen should be given at atmospheric pressure and the concentration gradually reduced after the first half hour, since pure oxygen should not be administered over a long period of time. Richards warns against the use of positive pressure in oxygen administration when pulmonary edema accompanies shock. He believes it reduces the amount of blood returned to the right atrium. If there is no drop in the systolic blood pressure, he says it is safe to assume that it is not having this untoward effect.

As soon as oxygen therapy is instituted, steps should be taken to reduce hydrostatic pressure in the lungs by decreasing the blood volume. Venesection, with the removal of 500 to 700 cc of blood, is advocated for hypertensive patients. A more universally employed procedure is to hold an abnormal supply of blood in the extremities by placing tourniquets around them near the axilla and the groin. Three tourniquets are applied. At the end of 15 minutes one is removed and applied to the free extremity; at the end of 30 minutes another tourniquet is removed and applied to the extremity that has had a 15-minute rest, and so on. With this rotation scheme, the maximum time any tourniquet stays in place is 45 minutes. Barbara C. Rothwell[15] suggests the use of a diagram and a system of recording to provide for accuracy when carrying out this procedure.

Richards advocates maintaining airways and suctioning the tracheobronchial tree or even bronchoscopic suction when patients are "choked with exudate."

Tourniquets must be adjusted tightly enough to be effective, but obliteration of the pulse means that they are too tight. As the condition is controlled the tourniquets are removed singly, in the same order of rotation and at 15-minute intervals. (The physician may prescribe slightly longer intervals in some cases.) It is believed dangerous to remove all tourniquets at once, for this would release a large volume of blood that might overtax the heart.

Drugs that may be ordered are atropine sulfate to "dry up" the secretions and a sedative to relieve the anxiety and pain. Atropine is said to be of doubtful value because the fluid is a transudate, not an exudate, and is therefore unaffected by the drug. Atropine may actually do harm by increasing the heart rate. Morphine sulfate may also make matters worse by depressing the respiration and by deadening the cough reflex that must be maintained. Meperidine may be more satisfactory. Rapid digitalization is recommended by Richards in "frank heart failure." Aminophylline given slowly, by vein, is beneficial in some cases.

When the critical stage is over the cause of pulmonary edema should be determined and treated, if possible. If an attack is anticipated, preventive measures should be instituted: Fluid intake reduced temporarily and 100 per cent oxygen administered for 30 minutes at 30-minute intervals. Bed rest and warmth are also advocated.

5. FOREIGN BODIES IN THE EYE, EAR, NOSE, OR THROAT

Removal of Foreign Bodies from the Eye.   Foreign bodies, such as dust, iron, coal, or ashes, may be carried into the conjunctival sac or may adhere to or be-become embedded in the cornea. Sharp particles may penetrate the chambers of the eye. When in the conjunctival sac, they often adhere to the inner surface of the upper lid. The patient can often tell the examiner where the particle is by indicating the point where he feels greatest discomfort. A good light should be focused on the eye, and both eyes should be kept open while they are moved from side to side and then up. If the particle is floating, E. Wolstein[16] says that after these movements it will often be found in the sac of the lower lid. The foreign body can then be removed with a moistened sterile cotton applicator. If the particle is not found, evert the upper lid as shown in Figure 211 (p. 910). In this maneuver the patient is asked to look down, the lashes are grasped and the lid is everted over a match or pencil, held horizontally against the eyelid. The mucous lining of the cartilaginous lid is examined, and the mois-tened applicator drawn over its surface (Fig. 264). If these operations are ineffective a sterile irrigation of the conjunctival sac may dislodge the mote. When all of these efforts are unsuccessful it is wise to put a drop of castor oil in the eye and fix a pad over the lid to keep it closed and inactive until a doctor can treat the condition. If the eye is very irritated a drop of mild silver protein (Argyrol)

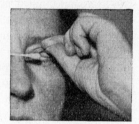

Figure 264. Subject about to remove a for-eign body on everted upper lid with a sterile moistened applicator. (See Fig. 211, Chapter 33, that illustrates steps in eversion of upper lid, prior to removal of a foreign body.) (Courtesy of Clay-Adams Co., New York City.)

or penicillin suspension may retard infection. Strict asepsis should be maintained.

When a corneal injury or an intraocular foreign body is suspected, the eye should be put at rest with a pad until a doctor can treat it. Corneal abrasions will show up as bright green patches after the instillation of 2 per cent fluorescein. E. Terry Coppin[17] describes a special metal cone to be used in detecting minute foreign bodies not easily found with ordinary x-ray techniques. Magnets are used to remove metal fragments from the eye.

If an eye has been injured by chemicals, Wolstein says it should be irrigated at once with large amounts of water, normal saline, or boric acid solution for a 5-minute period. After several minutes repeat the process.

Removal of Foreign Bodies from the Auditory Canal.   Foreign bodies found in the ear vary in size, shape, and substance, in their position in the canal, in their effect, and therefore in the symptoms to which they give rise. For instance, they may be small, hard, and smooth (like beads, stones, or buttons), easily inserted by a child, and pushed into the canal; they may, like peas and seeds, swell with moisture and block the meatus. They may be present for years, give rise to no symptoms, and be forgotten by the individual; or they may injure, inflame, and infect the canal and may cause deafness, dizziness, tinnitus, a reflex cough, and vomiting. Live insects especially produce acute pain and anxiety.

Foreign bodies rarely cause serious trouble unless they injure the tympanic membrane, while rupture of the tympanic membrane, removal of ossicles, purulent infection of the middle ear, inner ear, and meninges have resulted from *ill-directed attempts at removal.* Death has followed clumsy and misguided first aid when no foreign body was present.

Before attempting removal of foreign bodies, therefore, the surgeon will first note the symptoms and history, and will inspect the ear to determine the presence, nature, and position of a foreign body, and the condition of the canal. The nurse often prepares the equipment for this examination and may give some of the treatments that follow.

Removal by irrigation, or persistent syringing with warm water, is a method commonly used. This is the best and safest method, and is the only one that should be attempted by a nurse, or by anyone who is not an expert. Even syringing may do harm, and may be contraindicated if, for instance, there is danger of forcing the object in farther. Sometimes a preliminary treatment must be given: it may be necessary to relieve inflammation and swelling of the tissues before syringing, by applying an alcoholic solution of boric acid; or, when water will cause the object to swell (as in the case of a pea or seed), it is advisable first to syringe the canal with alcohol, which will absorb the water, prevent swelling, and may possibly shrink the foreign body. The instillation of oil or glycerin also helps to remove seeds. If the foreign body is an insect, it should first be killed by the introduction of a few drops of absolute alcohol, oil, or chloroform.* When dead, it usually floats out. Syringing with water will make a living insect move which causes great discomfort, even agony, to the patient.

When syringing the ear, incline the patient's head toward the affected side, as the force of gravity is to some extent helpful. (In the case of children, because the aural canal is straight, rotation in front of the ear with the finger sometimes helps to cause a round, smooth body to work its way outward.) The auricle should be held in the proper position for irrigating and the stream directed between the foreign body and the wall of the canal where the space is widest. Syringing should be continued gently until the body is removed, unless it gives rise to pain, vomiting, or other unfavorable symptoms; then it should be discontinued until further examination is made. To prevent chilling and earache, the ear should be carefully dried and absorbent cotton left in the meatus following the treatment. Any abrasion caused by the foreign body should be treated, and every precaution taken to prevent infection.

Removal by instruments is sometimes necessary, but this should be done only by a skilled otologist unless the body projects and can be easily grasped. As a rule,

---

* The writer was told by a person who lives in a region where medical services are unavailable that holding a light to the ear was a common practice when an insect was believed to have crawled or flown into the ear because most insects will be attracted by the light and come out of the meatus.

instruments are used only when syringing has failed or is contraindicated by the severity of the symptoms. In the hands of an unskilled person, an instrument may push the foreign body farther into the canal, may injure the tympanic membrane or the bony wall of the canal, and may cause such severe irritation, swelling, and inflammation as to necessitate a major operation (incision behind the ear into the canal).

Removal of Foreign Bodies from the Nose.   Flying insects and debris of various kinds are often drawn into the nose during inspiration. Children frequently push peanuts, safety pins, and other small objects into the nose. Should these objects lodge in the anterior nares, they may often be blown out before harm results. If they are visible in the nasal orifice, they may be removed with forceps, but great care must be taken not to force them in farther. When simple measures fail or when the object has dropped into the posterior nares, the patient should be taken to a physician who will light the cavity, discover the position of the foreign body, and remove it with special instruments.

Removal of Foreign Bodies from the Throat.   The experience of having food drawn into the respiratory tract instead of being directed into the esophagus is common to everyone. The presence of a foreign body in the larynx stimulates the cough reflex, which is nature's method of getting rid of the offending object. In most cases the foreign body will be coughed up into the mouth. Lowering the head brings gravity into play and helps throw the object out of the larynx. Many a mother has saved the life of a strangling child by picking it up by its feet and shaking a bead, a marble, or a crust of bread out of the respiratory passage.

If the foreign body passes the larynx, it will lodge in the trachea or bronchi, and in case it does not occlude the air passage, it may stay in this position without causing any serious damage for a few hours or possibly a day or two; however, if it is not removed by a surgeon within a short time infection results. In most large communities there are surgeons who specialize in removing foreign bodies from the bronchi (bronchoscopists). With highly developed skill and instruments designed for this purpose it is now possible to extract open safety pins, fishbones, and other objects equally difficult to manipulate, from almost any part of the bronchi.[18]

6. MOTION SICKNESS

Motion sickness is an individual reaction to constant or violent agitation of the fluid in the semicircular canals. Some persons are very much more susceptible than others. Those affected by the motion in a boat do not necessarily get carsick, and persons who suffer in plane travel may be comfortable in other vehicles. Most persons may be inexplicably free from it under conditions that usually cause them marked distress. It is thought that the emotional state, therefore, may help to induce the characteristic dizziness and nausea. When vomiting is added to these symptoms the subject may become very ill unless the resulting dehydration is corrected.

Because aviators are susceptible to motion sickness, military and commercial flying has stimulated the development of preventive measures. Leslie N. Gay and Paul E. Carliner say that dimenhydrinate (Dramamine) in oral doses of 50 to 100 mg every 4 hours for a period of 6 to 10 days "provides an ample margin of safety."* It is effective also in treating the condition. Herman I. Chinn[19] reports equally successful results with diphenhydramine (Benadryl)-scopolamine mixtures.

7. POISONING (ACUTE)

Ingestion of poison by mistake and with suicidal intention is, unfortunately, a fairly common emergency.† First aid is often given at home because time is of the essence. It would be a good thing if everyone understood the underlying principles of emergency treatment. The nurse may be called on to teach these and to put them into practice. In many cases there is no way of determining the nature of the toxic agent, and, as some authorities point out, time spent in trying to discover this before starting treatment in acute poisoning may cost the patient's life.

Nurses should be students of drug action so that they will recognize toxic symptoms in their patients. The signs of chronic drug poisoning should be part of the study of each potent drug. It is not within the scope of this volume to discuss the toxicology of even the commonest drugs. All that is attempted is an outline of the principles underlying the treatment of acute poisoning where an emergency situation exists.

In acute poisoning the person giving first aid may be seeing the patient for the first time. Immediate action is demanded. Information should be solicited, but first-aid measures can be initiated while the family, the friends, or the patient himself is explaining what happened. Needless to say, the services of a physician should be solicited at once.

First Aid or Immediate Treatment of Acute Poisoning. Goodman and Gilman[20] list the following steps in treatment: (1) remove the poison from the body, (2) administer antidotes, and (3) give supportive or symptomatic treatment.

Poison is removed from the stomach most effectively by gastric lavage. (See p. 838 for a discussion of this procedure.) This may be contraindicated when the poison is highly corrosive for the lavage might, in such cases, perforate the injured esophagus or stomach. Lavage should not be used when the poison is a convulsant drug, such as strychnine, for the procedure will induce or exaggerate convulsions. Goodman and Gilman point out that lavage not only removes the

---

* Gay, Leslie N., and Carliner, Paul E.: "The Prevention and Treatment of Motion Sickness," *Bull. Johns Hopkins Hosp.* **84**:470, (Mar.) 1949.

† A physician reports that in 1939 1 per cent of the children admitted to a large city hospital were brought there for treatment of poisoning. About a fourth of them were accidentally poisoned; about one-half were poisoned from the use of substances used therapeutically. (Gold, Harry [ed.]: *Cornell Conference on Therapy*, Vol. 4. The Macmillan Company, New York, 1951, p. 1.)

toxic agent from the stomach, but offers a means of introducing a saline cathartic into the stomach after the stomach is washed out.

Emetics are advocated in some first-aid texts. Goodman and Gilman state that "only in rare cases are such drugs of value." They suggest that of all the emetics apomorphine given hypodermically is most rapidly effective. Mustard water (in the proportion of one teaspoonful to a glass of tepid water) taken until vomiting occurs may be tried when a stomach tube and apomorphine are not available. Vomiting should not be induced in the comatose patient for he will almost inevitably insufflate the vomitus and, with it, the poison. The danger is obvious.

If the poison has not been ingested but is in contact with the skin, repeated bathing with running water is effective unless the irritant is insoluble in water. In such cases a bland substance that will dissolve the poison should be used as, for example, vegetable oil or alcohol, according to the nature of the toxic agent.

When contact with poisonous plants is suspected, a thorough scrubbing with yellow laundry soap is advocated. (Inoculations of susceptible persons are effective in some cases as a preventive but cannot be relied upon for control of poison ivy dermatitis.)

Because many ingested poisons are eliminated by the kidneys, the patient should be encouraged to drink as much water as he will take. This dilutes the toxic substance and thereby minimizes its harmful effect upon the kidneys.

Volatile substances that are eliminated by the lungs can be gotten rid of more rapidly if respiration is stimulated. Carbon dioxide should be administered only by specially trained personnel.

In Volume 4 of the *Cornell Conferences on Therapy*[21] there are two interesting chapters on household poisoning. A number of physicians reported cases in which the antidote used in treating the victim did more harm than good and was even a more dangerous substance than the so-called poison. One physician urged those who are unsure, or limited in the knowledge of antidotes, to resist the temptation to use them.

Goodman and Gilman point out that antidotes are of two kinds: chemical and physiological. Chemical antidotes are those that inactivate the poison by chemical reaction; physiological antidotes are substances that combat the harmful physiologic effect of the poison. An acid is, for example, a chemical antidote for an alkali; a drug that stimulates respiration is a physiological antidote for a respiratory depressant.

Even if the person giving first aid knows the specific antidote for the ingested poison, it is rarely available. Goodman and Gilman suggest the following household agents as antidotes one might expect to find and that are safe to use.

POISON	ANTIDOTE
For poisoning by heavy metals	Milk and egg white
For poisoning by any irritant (starch is especially effective against iodine)	Flour and starch water
For poisoning by alkaloids	Strong tea and diluted tincture of iodine

The following is a list of antidotes for common poisons as compiled from the discussion in Volume 4 of *Cornell Conferences on Therapy:*

POISON	ANTIDOTE
For nicotine poisoning	Potassium permanganate for lavage
For arsenic poisoning (including thera- peutic arsenicals such as oxophenarsine [Mapharsen] or Fowler's solution)	BAL (2, 3 dimercaptopropanol)
For poisoning by mercuric compounds	BAL (2, 3 dimercaptopropanol)
For effects of lead poisoning	Calcium (large amounts)
For cyanide poisoning	Sodium nitrite and sodium thiosulfate (in- travenously)
For most alkaloids	Potassium permanganate for lavage
For barbiturate poisoning	Picrotoxin and amphetamine sulfate (Ben- zedrine sulfate)

It should be understood that antidotes are often and most effectively used as a lavage in water solutions.

Pharmacology texts include the treatment of toxic doses in the discussion of every poisonous drug. Frank poisons usually give the antidote on the label of the bottle. Poisoning of children often results from ingestion of a cleaning fluid, a poison put down for insects or animals, or some other household chemical whose container may not be available or which may fail unfortunately to provide the needed information on its label.

Supportive, or symptomatic, treatment probably needs no explanation, but the authorities emphasize that it is as important as other aspects of therapy. There may be oxygen want or excessive loss of fluids; the patient may be in shock, or, if suicidal, in a critical emotional state. These and many other symptoms, or groups of related symptoms, demand either immediate attention or consideration after neutralizing and/or removing as much of the drug as possible from contact with the body. A person who has taken poison with suicidal intention is in need of psychiatric care.

8. POISONED WOUNDS CAUSED BY ANIMAL AND INSECT BITES

Hydrophobia or Rabies. This condition is *caused* by the bite of a rabid animal, usually a dog, although rabid cats and foxes are to be feared. The US Public Health Service reports that the disease of rabies is "widespread" in these and other animals in the United States and, in recent years, has been on the increase.[22] It is urged that the signs of rabies in animals be made known more generally. Rabid animals may be "furious" or "dumb." In the first case they are increasingly restless and irritable. They snarl and bark, cry or growl. They are inclined to wander, biting as they go.

The dumb type of rabies occurs in 20 per cent of the cases and is difficult to recognize. The progress is more rapid, and paralysis occurs within 2 or 3 days. The paralysis is noticed in the lower jaw. The animal's mouth should not be handled for fear of getting some of the infectious saliva into a skin abrasion on the human hand. Signs of excitement or irritability in the animal with dumb rabies are so slight as to be almost unnoticeable.

The *symptoms,* in man, develop in 14 days to 7 months after inoculation. The time depends upon the amount of virus introduced, the point of inoculation, and the susceptibility of the individual. When the bite occurs in tissues richly supplied with nerves, as in the face, the symptoms develop rapidly. These are headache, pain in the wound extending along the nerves, irritability, restlessness, sleeplessness, difficult breathing and swallowing due to spasmodic contractions of these muscles, and a marked increase in the flow of saliva. Convulsions usually follow. Death generally occurs on the third or fourth day after the symptoms appear.

The importance of *early treatment and prevention* cannot be exaggerated. The best method of prevention is the control of the disease in dogs through vaccination. This will be effected when the general public sees the urgency of this measure and proves it by widespread cooperation with health officers. This is of great importance as there has been an alarming increase in this country of rabies in animals, primarily dogs, during the past 16 years. When the symptoms have developed, this disease is invariably fatal. The only hope therefore lies in early treatment.

When an animal bites a person and there is any reason to believe it might be rabid, a tourniquet should be applied above the wound, if on an extremity, to keep the virus from entering the general circulation. The wound should be incised, and bleeding encouraged. It should then be cleaned with antiseptics, and a hot antiseptic dressing applied.

If the animal is known to be rabid, the Pasteur treatment should be given immediately. This consists in the injection of an especially prepared, standardized dose of an emulsion of the spinal cords of rabbits that have been treated with the virus. The emulsion is given subcutaneously in a series of 25 inoculations. It stimulates the body to produce specific antibodies and thus makes harmless the virus introduced through the animal's saliva. Although this treatment is very costly, it is the only positive remedy known for hydrophobia, and there should be no delay in using it, since, after the symptoms have developed, even this treatment is of no avail.

Paul W. Clough states that the Pasteur Institute reported that no case of rabies had occurred in vaccinated people who had been observed for 23 consecutive years. But he goes on to say that there is indirect evidence that in cases where the incubation period is less than 30 days, antirabies vaccine has little or no effect. This severe form of rabies mostly occurs in small children and in those severely bitten about the face and head. He says that investigations of the last ten years make it now possible to measure exactly the antigenicity of antirabies vaccine and to provide vaccines of uniformly high potency. He goes on to say: "They promise to yield methods for eliminating the antigenic substances which cause the paralytic accidents. They may also provide immune sera which should supplement the effect of vaccine and in part compensate for the deficiencies of the Pasteur treatment, which are probably greater than is now generally appreciated."*

In the event that it is not known whether the animal is rabid, if possible it should be kept alive and under expert observation in order to determine this. In hot weather animals may appear rabid when suffering from heatstroke. If the animal has been killed, the body should be sent to a laboratory where the brain may be examined. The presence of certain round or angular bodies, called *Nigri bodies,* found within the nerve cells or their processes is accepted as diagnostic of the disease.

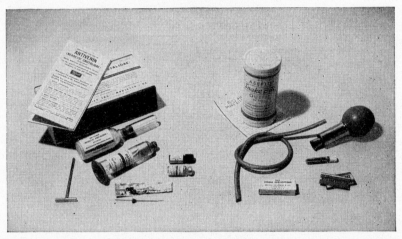

Figure 265. Commercially prepared and assembled snakebite outfits. (*Left*) Kit and instructions; ampoule with antivenim powder; vial-syringe of distilled water and metal plunger for preparation and injection of antivenin; needle with two points (foil container for needle in background); vial of iodine solution; vial of normal horse serum (for sensitivity testing and desensitizing). (*Right*) Kit and instructions; tourniquet; box that contains two ampoules of iodine solution and cotton-tipped applicators; suction cup with rubber bulb; ampoule containing iodine solution and applicator; razor blade. (Courtesy of Clay-Adams Co., New York City.)

Snakebite. If the bite is poisonous, pain, swelling, and discoloration appear within a few minutes; septicemia, prostration, and collapse may follow very quickly. The victim must have first-aid treatment at once and antivenin as soon as possible.

The purpose of the treatment is to prevent the poison's entrance into the general circulation and to relieve shock. Several tourniquets are applied at different levels above the fang marks, and the wound is freely incised lengthwise of the arm or leg; sometimes suction is applied to the incision, and bleeding is encouraged. The wound may be swabbed with pure carbolic acid or cauterized. Potassium permanganate has been used with some success. As the snake venom is not dangerous unless it enters the blood stream, the practice of sucking the wound has been advocated when other

* Clough, Paul W.: "Rabies; Some Current Problems and Recent Improvements in Measures for Its Control," *Ann. Int. Med., 34*:517, (Feb.) 1951.

means of suction are not at hand. There is slight danger to the person who sucks the wound if there is an abrasion on the lips or mouth. Complete rest, external heat, and stimulants are necessary to counteract shock. The tourniquets are removed one at a time (the one nearest the body first) if no symptoms of general poisoning appear.

Anyone exposed to the danger of snakebite is advised to provide himself with a protective serum or antivenom for the species he is likely to encounter. Unfortunately, this protective serum is not available for all types of poisonous snakes nor is it easily procured in every community in every country.

There is, however, a single antivenin (Nearctic-Crotalidae) which can be used for the bite of any and every North American poisonous snake, except the Gulf region coral snake (there is a special treatment for a coral snake bite).

Insect Bites and Stings.   Bites from poisonous spiders are treated in the same manner as snakebite. Bees, wasps, and other insects inject formic acid with their stings, and they are therefore treated with neutralizing alkaline solutions, such as ammonia water, bicarbonate of soda, soap and water, or a paste of baking soda. The sting, if visible in the tissue as a fine bristle, should be removed. This can be done by pressing firmly on the tissues around the wound with a round, hollow object, such as a key. Compresses moistened with an alkaline solution should be applied—hot applications are frequently more soothing. Shock is often marked when there are multiple stings. Bromides and morphine are given to relieve nervousness and pain.

If the bites result in severe itching, a weak solution of carbolic acid, which is a mild local anesthetic, relieves it.

9. INJURIES CAUSED BY EXTREMES OF TEMPERATURE (INCLUDING BURNS)

Types of Injuries from High Temperatures.   Heat exhaustion, heat cramps, heatstroke or sunstroke, and burns, including sunburn, are types of physiological response to high temperatures. They differ in symptoms and treatment. All but burns are most likely to occur under exertion since exercise increases temperature, the pulse and respiratory rates, and the loss of body fluids and sodium chloride.

Heat Exhaustion, Heat Collapse, or Heat Prostration.   This condition is said by Anna M. Baetjer,[23] in Kenneth F. Maxcy's text, to be the comomnest clinical condition resulting from exposure to heat. She describes it as circulatory collapse resulting from the failure of the body to compensate for the peripheral vasodilation and dehydration that occur in high temperatures not necessarily associated with exposure to the sun's rays. The symptoms of heat exhaustion range from very mild ones, such as dizziness, fatigue, and headache, to complete collapse and unconsciousness. Body temperature varies from subnormal to a slight fever. The blood pressure is low at the time of collapse.

The ingestion of sodium chloride and ample fluids will usually prevent this condition, and it is relieved by saline and glucose solutions. If the subject is conscious, fluids may be given orally; if not, they are administered intravenously. Drugs, such as cardiac stimulants, may be indicated in severe collapse, but re-establishment of blood volume is usually adequate treatment.

Heat Cramps. High temperatures associated with profuse sweating that accompanies physical labor in hot environments sometimes cause cramps in the chief

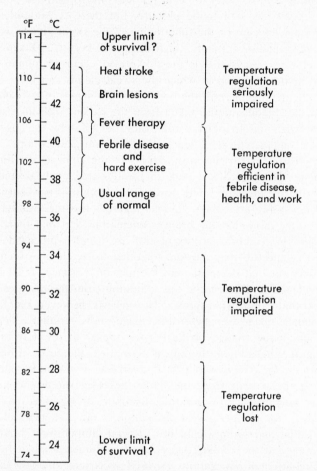

Figure 266. Extremes of human body temperature with an attempt to define the zones of temperature regulation. (DuBois, Eugene F.: *Fever and the Regulation of Body Temperature*. Charles C Thomas, Publisher, Springfield, Ill., 1948.)

muscles used. Baetjer says the onset is usually sudden and may occur during or at the end of the work shift. Studies have shown that heat cramps are the result of a fall in the sodium chloride content in the blood, caused by the loss of this salt in excessive sweating. The blood may be so concentrated that it is difficult to get a sample from a vein.

Cramps are said to be relieved at once by drinking water with salt or by intravenous injection of saline in severe cases. Glucose and drugs are said to have no effect on the painful muscles.

Heatstroke or Sunstroke.   According to Baetjer, there is no evidence that heatstroke and sunstroke differ. Both are due to the effect of the radiant heat of the sun. The condition is most likely to occur outdoors in tropical heat, but it may occur indoors. The etiology is said to be obscure, but there is evidently a breakdown in the sweating mechanism, or the functioning of the sweat glands, which results in alarmingly, and sometimes fatally, high fever. Robert C. Darling,[24] writing in Cecil and Loeb's text, says this is most likely to occur in climates where there is no relief at night; no period in which the sweat glands can rest. A hot dry skin is evidence of the derangement of the body's normal means of reducing its temperature. It is said that blood samples taken from the patient with heat stroke show no evidence of dehydration. In other words, they fail to show the loss of water and sodium chloride that is typical in heat exhaustion and heat cramps.

Baetjer says this is by far the most serious of the clinical conditions caused by hot environments. Darling calls it "one of the few true medical emergencies" and says it calls for heroic measures. The death rate is about 40 per cent if the temperature does not reach 43.3° C (110° F); if it exceeds this the fatality is 80 per cent or more. Autopsies show that the brain is edematous and that there is destruction of the cells of the cerebral cortex. Death is usually preceded by secondary vasomotor shock, and this may account for other tissue changes seen port-mortem.

Darling points out that diagnosis and the aim of treatment is clear cut, if there is sufficient evidence to differentiate this condition from the diseases of the central nervous system that cause hyperpyrexia. He suggests, however, that steps to reduce the fever should be taken even before the diagnosis is certain.

Since the fatal tissue changes in heatstroke appear to result from the excessive body temperature, the aim of therapy is to reduce the fever. Immersion of the body in ice water, or as cold water as is available, is the most effective method. After removing the patient from the bath, the body should be kept moist and fans played on it to produce evaporation. Rubbing, or vigorous massage, increases the cooling effect, for the peripheral circulation is often stagnant. Icecaps applied to the head, axilla, and groin are helpful. Rectal temperature should be taken at frequent intervals and the cooling measures discontinued when it falls to 38.9° C (102° F). (If cold colonic irrigations are used, as is sometimes the case, the mouth temperature may be a more reliable index. The delirium that accompanies hyperpyrexia prohibits the taking of mouth temperature in most cases.) A drop in temperature does not mean that the temperature may not soar again, calling for a repetition of the measures just described.

Intravenous fluids are usually contraindicated. Darling says they increase the danger of pulmonary edema and should be used with caution and only when there are definite indications. Blood analysis furnishes such indications.

Prognosis is said to depend upon the promptness and effectiveness of relief measures. According to Darling, all untreated cases die, and all would probably live if the symptoms were recognized and treated early. He believes that irregularity of temperature should be expected for several days in those who will recover. Persistence of coma and shock after cooling are grave signs. If brain damage is not apparent early, there is likely to be no evidence of it later.

Burns. Burns are *caused* by the exposure of the body to a very high temperature of either dry or moist heat, electricity, x-ray, radium, or corrosive poisons.

Burns may be *classified* according to the depth of the injury: (1) first-degree burns, simple reddening of the skin; (2) second-degree burns, dermatitis with the formation of blisters; and (3) third-degree burns, actual charring and destruction of both superficial and true skin, or the skin, subcutaneous tissues, and muscle.

Sunburn is usually a first-degree burn but it may well progress to the second degree, for blisters are not uncommon. Scalds are nearly always second-degree burns. Conflagrations usually result in charring with destruction of the skin and subcutaneous tissues, and burns from x-rays, radium, and radioactivity are especially feared because they are so penetrating in their effects.

The local *symptoms of burns* are known to many persons. The inflammatory process associated with all injury has been described in Chapter 36 and need not be repeated here.

Those who have not seen serious burns are horrified by the sight. In burns from moist heat the skin may be white and thrown into folds or rugae and some of the upper layer may be detached. Burns from conflagrations blacken and char the area. Because they destroy the nerve endings these burns may be, at first, less painful than more superficial ones which leave nerve endings exposed. The following are the most dreaded effects of burns: (1) immediate shock; (2) dehydration from seepage of fluid from the injured capillaries; (3) infection of the burned area with resulting toxemia; (4) contractions, with impaired function, and disfigurement; and (5) permanent ulcerative lesions from x-ray, radium, and radioactive substances. A less common result of burns is an anemia that is sometimes resistant to treatment. W. B. Castle, writing in Cecil and Loeb's text, says that local heating of the blood produces changes in red cells that makes them more fragile.[25] Shock, dehydration, and infection may be fatal, but in some cases the disfigurement and loss of function may be almost worse than death.

With the refinement of blood transfusion and intravenous therapy and with the discovery of the antibiotics, mortality from burns has been greatly reduced in recent years. Disfigurement and impairment of function are also far less serious than they were since plastic surgery and physical therapy have been greatly improved, and there is far more appreciation of the importance of rehabilitation.

Prognosis depends upon the extent of the burn, more than on its depth; it also depends upon the patient's age and condition, and most particularly on the knowledge and skill of the medical team.

Treatment of burns varies with their nature and extent. Sunburn, for example, may be such a mild dermatitis that it requires no treatment or, at most, a soothing, lubricating lotion or ointment; on the other hand, it can blister the skin and subject the patient to dangers of infection that must be avoided by aseptic dressings and even antibiotic therapy. Actually, it is far wiser to prevent sunburn with preparations that make a barrier between the skin and the sun's rays and by limiting exposure to sunlight. (For a discussion of this subject see Chapter 5.) Burns of small areas, such as one often suffers through carelessness when working around the kitchen, may be treated by an application of petroleum jelly, tannic acid jelly, or vitamin ointment. If the burn is deep a dressing should be applied. Large,

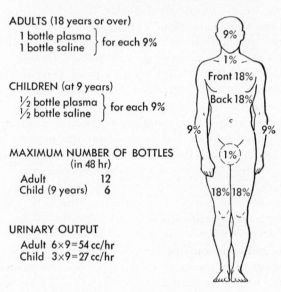

"THE RULES OF NINE"

Estimations of surface area, fluid replacement
and urinary excretion

I.V. fluid replacement for burns of 18% or over

ADULTS (18 years or over)

1 bottle plasma
1 bottle saline } for each 9%

CHILDREN (at 9 years)

½ bottle plasma
½ bottle saline } for each 9%

MAXIMUM NUMBER OF BOTTLES
(in 48 hr)

Adult   12
Child (9 years)   6

URINARY OUTPUT

Adult 6×9=54 cc/hr
Child 3×9=27 cc/hr

9%
1%
Front 18%
Back 18%
9%   9%
1%
18% 18%

1 bottle of plasma=500 cc (1 pt)

Figure 267. Burns are classified by extent and by depth. During emergency treatment, "the rules of nine" are useful in estimating the area burned. The head and each of the upper extremities are 9 per cent of the total body surface; the front of the trunk, the back of the trunk, and each of the lower extremities are 18 per cent. (Wallace, A. B. "Treatment of Burns," *M. Press,* **225**:191, [Feb.] 1951.)

but still not extensive, burns should be treated by a physician, especially if they might be disfiguring or might alter the function of joints. He will find it easier to apply the dressing of his choice if first aid is limited to the application of a thick pad of sterile wet gauze covered by clean waxed paper held on by a clean towel. If sterile gauze is not available, a clean and freshly ironed cloth is a fairly safe substitute.

Constitutional, or systemic, symptoms are negligible with such burns unless, as in the case of sunburn, there is extensive blistering with seepage. When this occurs the danger of dehydration must be guarded against. (In sunburn there is sometimes the possibility that the patient is suffering from sunstroke as well as the skin condition.)

Treatment of extensive, serious, thermal burns has been outlined in a number of excellent articles and monographs. The US Public Health Service has published a booklet on the treatment of burns as an aspect of the national defense program. The following steps are based on the recommendations of James M. Walker,[26] but they are paralleled in those of a number of authorities:

1. *Treat shock first.* Give whole blood if it is available; approximately 100 cc for every 1 per cent of the body area burned. Plasma is the best substitute for whole blood, if the latter is not available. (See Fig. 267.)

2. Give morphine (intravenously) if the patient is conscious and in pain. Avoid the use of morphine when patients are in profound shock, in which case they are probably unaware of pain, and when it is likely to cause nausea and vomiting.

3. If the patient is conscious and cooperative give electrolyte fluids by mouth in amounts equal to the blood infused. Use one-third sodium lactate (or citrate or bicarbonate) and two-thirds sodium chloride. These must be given intravenously, or by intubation, when the victim is unconscious, nauseated, or vomiting. The administration of blood and electrolytes should be repeated as the need is indicated by gross estimates of fluid balance (concentration of urine, record of intake and output, and estimated seepage from burned area) and by laboratory analysis of blood.

4. After shock treatment is instigated, remove clothing from over and/or around the burned area. Walker recommends minimal debridement, or removal of charred particles, in this first dressing, although most authorities stress a thorough cleaning. Petroleum jelly and pressure dressings are then applied to reduce to a minimum the loss of body fluids through seepage from the burned area. Figures 268 A-C show the application of such dressings. Note that they are made so that they can be adjusted quickly.

5. Give antibiotics (usually penicillin) and tetanus antitoxin parenterally. If the person has been previously immunized against tetanus, substitute toxoid for the antitoxin. Use such additional antibiotics subsequently as are indicated by cultures from the burned area.

6. Give a high-caloric, high-protein, high-vitamin diet, either intravenously, by intubation, or by mouth, as indicated by the patient's condition.

The local treatment of the burned area in deep and extensive wounds is primarily surgical, and it is a challenge to the best surgeon. The trend is probably toward early excision of the injured tissue with immediate grafting and closure of the wound. Frank R. Denham[27] urges immediate steps to avoid contractures. He recommends dressing the burned patient on an orthopedic table that exposes a large skin area and enables the surgeon to put the part under slight traction. After the dressing, traction and casts and exercise are all used to prevent contractures.

A difficulty in early skin grafting of extensively burned persons is that of finding sufficiently large areas of sound tissue to use for grafts. A waiting period may be necessary for this reason and to give the person in profound shock a chance to recover. The techniques of skin grafting and the types of dressing used vary with the surgeon and are undergoing constant refinement.

Changing the dressings of an extensively burned patient is a long-drawn-out, tedious, and painful procedure. It should be done in the operating room under strict asepsis. The patient is often anesthetized or kept under the influence of narcotics.

When the open-air method of treating a burned area is adopted, sterile bed linen is used under the area and a cradle (heated with electric lights) kept over the exposed part. Mattresses and pillows should be completely covered with waterproof fabric under the cotton covering. (It is necessary to protect them from the drainage of burns and from the odor of necrotic tissue.)

Control of odors is one of the most difficult problems in nursing the burned patient. It is ideal to treat him in a private air-conditioned room. When this is not possible a motorized air conditioner under the bed may help to control the odor. (The search for chemical deodorants will go on indefinitely until a satisfactory one is found. The writer has been told by workers in hospitals that "Atax-o"* is reasonably effective if sprayed around the room. It is said to be nonirritating, even if applied to the top layer of dressings or bedding.) Control of odor is extremely important. The patient may become immune to it, but he is usually aware that others notice it, are even actively nauseated by it. This adds to his mental distress, which is already acute.

Burned patients face disfigurement and possible limitation of function. Medical personnel should not expect them to be less than profoundly depressed. Doctors and nurses should encourage an expression of the patient's anxieties and should not dismiss them with trite remarks and false promises. The program of rehabilitation should have its emotional as well as its physical aspects. Diversion should be provided as soon as the patient can respond; occupation and self-help should be encouraged. Physical therapy is often started early in the form of massage, exercise, and, later, hydrotherapy.

Because pain is an unavoidable accompaniment of extensive burns, there is a tendency to overdo the use of narcotics, and so drug addiction may be added to the patient's troubles. The emotionally depressing effect of pain-killing drugs should be more generally recognized and their use carefully guarded.

The preceding discussion of the treatment and nursing care of burns should be augmented by the study of specialized texts and articles. The following suggestions on the treatment of special types of burns may be helpful:

In *burns caused by corrosive poisons,* the chemical substances may be *acids* or *alkalies.* Burns caused by acids should be irrigated freely with alkaline solutions to neutralize the acid. Limewater, weak ammonia, or a solution of bicarbonate of soda may be used. Carbolic acid or creosote should be neutralized by alcohol or whisky, after which a dressing of alcohol or a soothing ointment may be applied. Oil should not be used, as it hastens the absorption of carbolic acid. Burns caused by alkalies (caustic soda, caustic potash, or ammonia, etc.) should be treated with

* Glenbrook Co., New Haven, Conn.

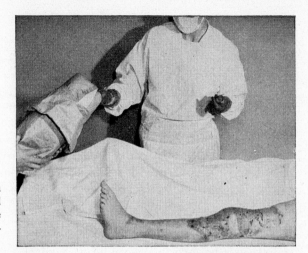

Figure 268A. Compression dressing of a burned leg: Burned extremity rests on sterile field. The physician is being handed a Surgipad.

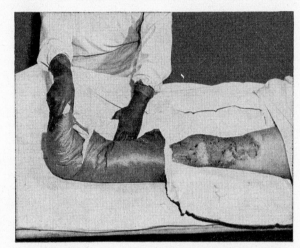

Figure 268B. The physician has partially wrapped the extensive burn with the large sterile dressing.

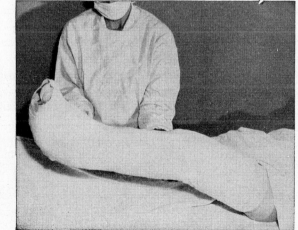

Figure 268C. The large dressing is held in place with a compression bandage. The bulk of the dressing is sufficient to make possible a resiliant compression bandage. (If immobilization is needed, there is sufficient bulk to the dressing to protect the extremity should a cast be applied.)

(Figs. 286 A-C, courtesy of Johnson & Johnson, New Brunswick, N. J.)

acid—boric, vinegar and water, or lemon juice and water. The amount of the solvent is more important than the neutralizing agent in it.

Burns of the eye are especially dangerous. Thermal burns of the lids are treated by irrigating with saline solution, then drying and applying a bland substance, such as castor oil—unless the patient can be taken to the doctor at once. When pain is severe, a wet dressing lessens the pain.

Burns of the conjuntiva and cornea are sometimes caused by boiling water, steam, lime, mortar, acids, powder, or molten metal. They occur most frequently among industrial workers. Treatment consists in the complete removal of the irritating substance as soon as possible. The conjunctival sac is irrigated with a solution that neutralizes the substance or renders it insoluble. A very weak tannic acid solution is used to remove lime, mortar, and other caustic alkalies. Copious washing is more important, however, than the neutralizing agent. A weak solution of bicarbonate of soda may be used to remove acids. Solids are removed as are foreign bodies, after which the sac is irrigated and precautions are taken to prevent infection. Cold compresses are usually ordered to relieve inflammation and prevent swelling and pain. Atropine is used as a sedative, and also to dilute the pupil and prevent adhesions. A bandage is occasionally applied in order to protect the eyes.

Frostbite.   This condition is *caused* by prolonged exposure to extreme cold. The parts of the body that are most commonly affected are the extremities because they are most distant from the blood-warming viscera and the ears, nose, and cheeks because they are unprotected by hair and clothing.

Pathology is described by William G. MacCallum as follows: "The noxious effect of the freezing is explained either as due to mechanical tearing of the cell as the ice crystals are formed, or to the concentration of salt around the crystals; or to the withdrawal of water from the cells to form the ice." The result is a serious inflamma tory reaction or gangrene. It is further explained "that the gangrene of the extremities which follows such chilling is by no means always directly due to the cold. On the contrary, it is the result of protracted ischemia from extreme contraction of the blood vessels or their obstruction by thrombi."[*]

The *symptoms* of frostbite are the following: the part tingles, aches, and feels cold at first but is soon numb and painless; for this reason the subject is often unaware of the danger, for when all sensation is lost the tissues have been seriously injured. Because vasodilation is the initial response to cold the area looks red at first, but vasoconstriction follows rapidly and then the area looks dead white. At this point it is "frostbitten."

Treatment of frostbite is aimed at re-establishing the circulation. Cold baths or compresses are used at first with the temperature increased to neutral and then to warm. Sudden vasodilation is undesirable because it may rupture the toneless vessels. The extremities are elevated, and glucose infusions containing procaine are given to supply nourishment and relieve pain in the affected parts. To prevent coagulation heparin is injected daily, and various circulatory stimulants are given.

---

[*] MacCallum, William G.: *A Textbook of Pathology,* 7th ed. W. B. Saunders Co., Philadelphia, 1940, p. 371.

If the skin blisters, dressings are applied and asepsis maintained. In severe cases gangrene develops in frostbitten fingers and toes, and amputation may be necessary. Smoking is prohibited because it induces vasoconstriction. Exercises are used to promote circulation, and after all threats of gangrene have disappeared, whirlpool baths are given for the effect of gentle massage. The temperature of the water advocated is about 37.8° C (100° F). First-aid texts formerly advocated rubbing the frostbitten area with snow when signs of frostbite are noticed. Some current texts say that any rough handling of the frozen area may cause further injury.

Chilblains are a chronic condition resulting from repeated exposure to cold that is not severe enough to cause the marked reaction just described. Maurice Newman suggests that the person who develops chilblains responds in an unusual if not abnormal way to cold and damp; others suggest that it is the effect of an irreversible change occurring during a former and severe frostbite. The following is taken from Newman's recent article on the subject:

Gourlay (1948) considers that the vasoconstriction of the subcutaneous arteries, as the result of exposure to cold, gives rise to interference with cellular metabolism with the formation of irritable metabolites. In normal subjects when the part is warmed the arterial spasm relaxes and the metabolites are removed and no lesion results. In chilblain subjects the arterial spasm does not relax on warming and more metabolites are formed at the site owing to increase of cellular metabolism due to warming the part. This causes irritation, oedema of the corium and interference with venous drainage, setting up a vicious circle and producing a chilblain. The patient complains of discomfort and itching. Symptoms, particularly itching, become more marked on warming. . . . The lesions may clear in a few weeks but relapses are common throughout the winter months. The redness is gradually replaced by a cyanotic tinge and pain may occur.*

Treatment may relieve chilblains but as they are likely to recur, Newman mentions sedative ointments, x-ray, and paravertebral sympathetic block. The latter would be used in extreme cases only.

REFERENCES

1. Dublin, Louis I.: *The Facts of Life from Birth to Death.* The Macmillan Company, New York, 1951, p. 242.
2. Leavell, Hugh R., and Clark, E. Gurney: *Textbook of Preventive Medicine.* McGraw-Hill Book Co., New York, 1953, p. 201.
3. Klem, Margaret C., et al.: *Industrial Health and Medical Programs.* US Public Health Service Publication No. 15, US Government Printing Office, Washington, D.C., 1950.
4. Kent, Frederick S., and Pershing, Madeline: "Home Accident Prevention Activities," *Pub. Health Rep.,* **67:**541, (June) 1952.
5. Collins, Selwyn D., et al.: *Accident Frequency, Place of Occurrence and Relation to Chronic Disease.* US Public Health Service Monograph No. 14, US Government Printing Office, Washington, D.C., 1953.
6. Cecil, Russell L., and Loeb, Robert F. (eds.): *A Textbook of Medicine,* 9th ed. W. B. Saunders Co., Philadelphia, 1955, p. 1486.

* Newman, Maurice: "Chilblains, a Review of a Common Winter Problem," *Med. Illus.,* **4:**591, (Dec.) 1950.

7. Meyers, Russell, and Meyers, Mary E.: "Management of the Comatose Patient," *Am. Pract. & Digest Treat.,* **1:**1031, (Oct.) 1950.
8. Munro, Donald: *The Treatment of Injuries to the Nervous System.* W. B. Saunders Co., Philadelphia, 1952, p. 5.
9. de Gutiérrez-Mahoney, C. G., and Carini, Esta: *Neurological and Neurosurgical Nursing.* C. V. Mosby Co., St. Louis, 1949, p. 135.
10. de Gutiérrez-Mahoney, C. G., and Carini, Esta: *op. cit.,* p. 137.
11. de Gutiérrez-Mahoney, C. G., and Carini, Esta: *op. cit.,* p. 196.
12. Cecil, Russell L., and Loeb, Robert F. (eds.): *op. cit.,* p. 1490.
13. Drinker, Cecil K.: *Pulmonary Edema and Inflammation.* Harvard University Press, Cambridge, 1945.
13a. Cecil, Russell L., and Loeb, Robert F. (eds.): *op. cit.,* p. 1016.
14. Faddis, Margene O., and Hayman, Joseph M., Jr.: *Care of the Medical Patient.* McGraw-Hill Book Co., New York, 1952, p. 301.
15. Rothwell, Barbara C.: "Nursing Care in Pulmonary Edema," *Am. J. Nursing,* **48:**700, (Nov.) 1948.
16. Wolstein, E.: "Eye Emergencies," *Canad. Nurse,* **43:**870, (Nov.) 1950.
17. Coppin, E. Terry: "Technique for Foreign Bodies in the Eyes," *Radiography,* **16:**239, (Oct.) 1950.
18. Gorham, A. P. (ed.): *Warwick and Tunstall's First Aid to the Injured and Sick,* 19th ed. Williams & Wilkins Co., Baltimore, 1952, p. 226.
19. Chinn, Herman I.: "Prevention of Air Sickness by Benadryl-scopolamine Mixtures," *U.S. Armed Forces J.,* **2:**401, (Mar.) 1951.
20. Goodman, Louis S., and Gilman, Alfred: *The Pharmacological Basis of Therapeutics,* 2nd ed. The Macmillan Company, New York, 1955, p. 1778.
21. Gold, Harry (ed.): *Cornell Conferences on Therapy,* Vol. 4. The Macmillan Company, New York, 1951, p. 1.
22. Federal Security Agency (Now Department of Health, Education, and Welfare), Public Health Service: *Rabies.* Health Information Series No. 30, US Government Printing Office, Washington, D.C., 1952.
23. Maxcy, Kenneth F. (ed.): *Rosenau's Preventive Medicine and Hygiene,* 7th ed. Appleton-Century-Crofts, Inc., New York, 1951, p. 940.
24. Cecil, Russell L., and Loeb, Robert F. (eds.): *op. cit.,* p. 518.
25. Cecil, Russell L., and Loeb, Robert F. (eds.): *op. cit.,* p. 1179.
26. Walker, James M.: "The Problem of the Extensive Cutaneous Burn," *Am. J. M. Sc.* **22:**233, (Feb.) 1951.
27. Denham, Frank R.: "A Simplified Method of Dressing and Skin Grafting Extensive Burns," *Surgery,* **27:**740, (May) 1950.

Additional Suggested Reading

American Red Cross: *First Aid Textbook,* 3rd ed. Blakiston Co., Philadelphia, 1945.
———: *First Aid Textbook for Juniors.* Blakiston Co., Philadelphia, 1949.
———: *Home Nursing Textbook,* 6th ed. Blakiston Co., Philadelphia, 1950.
Beecher, Henry K.: *Early Care of the Seriously Wounded Man.* Charles C Thomas, Publisher, Springfield, Ill., 1952.
Christian, Henry A. (ed.): *Osler and McCrae's Principles and Practice of Medicine,* 16th ed. Appleton-Century-Crofts, Inc., New York, 1947.
Cole, Warren H., and Puestow, Charles B.: *First Aid, Surgical and Medical,* 4th ed. Appleton-Century-Crofts, Inc., New York, 1951.
Federal Civil Defense Administration: *Emergency Medical Treatment.* US Government Printing Office, Washington, D.C., 1953.
———: *The Nurse in Civil Defense.* US Government Printing Office, Washington, D.C., 1952.

————: *Organization and Operation of Civil Defense Casualty Services; Part I, The First-Aid System.* US Government Printing Office, Washington, D.C., 1953.

————: *Organization and Operation of Civil Defense Casualty Services; Part III, Medical Records for Casualties.* US Government Printing Office, Washington, D.C., 1952.

Meek, Raymond E.: *Eye Hazards and Eye Injuries.* Commission for the Blind, State Department of Social Welfare, New York, 1949.

Olson, Lyla M.: *Improvised Equipment in the Home Care of the Sick,* 4th ed. W. B. Saunders Co., Philadelphia, 1947.

Perera, Charles A. (ed.): *May's Manual of Diseases of the Eye,* 21st ed. Williams & Wilkins Co., Baltimore, 1953.

APPENDIX I. SPECIAL ENEMAS

Anthelmintic Enema.   An injection of a solution containing a drug capable of destroying or expelling worms from the intestines. Pin-, thread-, or seat worms may be destroyed and expelled by repeated injections of an infusion of quassia, using ½ oz of chips to 20 oz of water. About ½ pt is the amount usually used, and the treatment is given daily until the worms are destroyed. Before giving the treatment, the bowel should be cleaned by a soap solution, so that the drug may come in direct contact with the worms and the lining of the intestines. Quassia is an astringent. It contracts the tissues and blood vessels, checks bleeding and inflammation, lessens the amount of mucus in which the worms may lodge, shrivels and destroys the worms. The patient should be encouraged to retain the solution for from 15 to 30 minutes.

Astringent Enema.   Alum, 2 oz, dissolved in 2 pt of hot water. The enema is not to be retained.

Other *astringents,* such as tannic acid (30 gr in 1 pt of water), are sometimes used to destroy worms, or germs in dysentery or cholera, and to relieve inflammation. They are usually given in the form of rectal or colon irrigations, the solution being allowed to run in very slowly and gently and to return immediately in order to avoid distention, pain, and irritation of the inflamed wall.

Carminative Enemas.   Given to prevent or relieve distention, a carminative enema is an injection into the rectum of a solution containing drugs which have a carminative action. Such drugs by their antiseptic action prevent the formation of gases and by their irritant action on nerve endings in the lining of the intestines cause the contraction of their muscular walls (reflex action) and expulsion of the gas causing the distention. Turpentine, asafetida, and alum are the drugs commonly used as in the following: (1) *Turpentine.* From 2 to 4 drams of turpentine may be added to 2 pt of soap solution. The turpentine must be very thoroughly mixed and dissolved. This enema is not to be retained.

Milk and Molasses. To prepare the enema, according to the amount ordered, heat from 3 to 8 oz of milk. To this add slowly an equal amount of molasses, stirring it in well and heating to 71.1° C (160° F) to mix thoroughly. The temperature of the solution when given should be from 38° to 40° C (100.4° to 104° F). The carminative action is due to the fact that the sugar in molasses is irritating to the lining of the intestines and the sugar and milk together produce gas that distends the intestines and causes pressure, peristalsis, and evacuation.

Rectal injections for a carminative effect are usually given as hot as the patient can stand (43° C or 109.4° F), the heat being a powerful stimulus to peristalsis and expulsion of gas. The injections should be given slowly, and when small amounts are used, the patient should be encouraged to retain it for from 10 to 30 minutes, or as long as possible. As the treatment is given for the relief of distention, note and chart particularly the amount of flatus expelled in the return.

Emollient Enema. This is an injection of some bland solution for the purpose of checking diarrhea or soothing and relieving irritation of an inflamed mucous membrane. Starch is commonly used. To prepare the solution, dissolve 1 tsp of starch in a little cold water, making a smooth paste. Then add slowly 6 oz of boiling water, stirring constantly. Allow the solution to cool to 40° C (104° F) and give with a catheter. The enema is to be retained. Laudanum (tincture of opium) is sometimes added to a starch enema to check secretions and peristalsis and to relieve pain and local irritation in diarrhea. When ordered, laudanum should be added just before the enema is given. Be sure that the full amount ordered is given. To ensure this, sometimes the drug is added to a small portion of the starch solution. After this is injected, the remaining solution is given.

Oil Enema. Before giving a soapsuds enema, an injection of oil is sometimes necessary in constipation to soften hard masses of feces. Oil enemas are, also, frequently given before the first bowel movement after operations on the rectum or perineum, such as for hemorrhoids or a perineorrhaphy, in order to avoid straining and injury to the sutures and wound. The enema may consist of 6 oz of olive oil, or to this may be added 2 oz each of castor oil and glycerin, to aid in the softening effect. The oil is prepared by warming it to a temperature of 38° C (100.4° F). An oil enema should be retained. It may be followed in 1 hour by a soapsuds enema or it may be retained from 2 to 6 hours before the cleansing enema is given.

Purgative Enemas. In obstinate constipation restal injections of various cathartics may be necessary to hasten or to cause free evacuation. The cathartics commonly used are glycerin, *fel bovis* or ox gall, Rochelle and Epsom salts (magnesium sulfate). Glycerin and ox gall both act as softening agents on hard fecal masses and by their irritating effect on the mucous lining tend to cause peristalsis and evacuation. The amount ordered (usually from 2 to 4 drams of glycerin or ox gall) may be added to a soapsuds enema or may be given in a small amount of warm water or normal saline solution and followed in 1 hour by a soapsuds enema. A small enema consisting of 3 oz each of glycerin and soapsuds thoroughly mixed is sometimes used; this is to be expelled.

Compound Medicated. Turpentine 4 drams, asafetida 2 drams, ox gall 4 drams, glycerin 4 oz with 2 pt of soapsuds. To prepare the enema, first mix the ox gall, if in crystals, with the turpentine, otherwise it will not dissolve. Also see that the utensils used are dry. Add the other ingredients and thoroughly mix with the soapsuds. The temperature of the solution when given should be 43° C (109.4° F).

Saline Enemas. Rochelle and Epsom salts may be given in a dilute or concentrated form. From 4 to 6 oz of Rochelle salts or from ½ to 4 oz of magnesium sulfate are the usual amounts prescribed for rectal injections. To prepare the solution, the amount ordered is added to sufficient hot water to dissolve the salts thoroughly. An enema (commonly called a 1.2.3 enema), consisting of magnesium sulfate 1 oz, glycerin 2 oz, and hot water 3 oz, is frequently used. When given in this concentrated form the concentration of salts in the intestines is greater than that in the blood and tissues. Fluid is therefore drawn from the blood and tissues by osmosis in order to dilute the salts in the intestines and render the concentration equal. The resulting accumulation of fluid in the intestines causes pressure that induces peristalsis and free evacuations.

The saline cathartics are sometimes given in dilute form by adding the amount ordered, first thoroughly dissolved in hot water, to a tap-water enema. When given in this dilute form, the concentration of salts in the intestines is less than that in the blood and tissues, the salts are not absorbed but they prevent the absorption of the water so that the intestines become distended with fluid, causing pressure, peristalsis and evacuation.

Rectal injections of the saline cathartics are particularly valuable in nephritis and some cardiac conditions when there is an accumulation of fluid in the tissues (edema).

APPENDIX II.   WEIGHTS AND MEASURES

DRY MEASURE

Metric		Apothecaries'		Household
16.0	gm	4	ʒ	1 tablespoonful
8.0	″	2	ʒ	1 dessertspoonful
4.0	″	1	ʒ	1 teaspoonful
2.0	″	½	ʒ	½ teaspoonful
1.0	″	15	gr	
0.6	″	10	″	
0.3	″	5	″	
0.2	″	3	″	
0.1	″	1½	″	
0.06	″	1	″	
0.03	″	1/2	″	
0.015	″	1/4	″	
0.008	″	1/8	″	
0.004	″	1/16	″	
0.0032	″	1/20	″	
0.0027	″	1/25	″	
0.0022	″	1/30	″	
0.0016	″	1/40	″	
0.0013	″	1/50	″	
0.0011	″	1/60	″	
0.001	″	1/64	″	
0.0006	″	1/100	″	
0.0005	″	1/120	″	
0.0004	″	1/150	″	
0.0003	″	1/200	″	

FLUID MEASURE

Metric	Apothecaries'	Household
1.0 cc	15 minims	¼ teaspoonful
4.0 cc	1 fluid dram	1 teaspoonful
32 cc	1 fluid ounce	2 tablespoonfuls
500 cc	1 pint	2 tumblerfuls
1000 cc	1 quart	

TABLE FOR SOLUTIONS

Prescribed strength	Amount of crude drug	Fluid to be added
1:1000	1 teaspoonful	to 1 gallon
1:1000	15 drops	to 1 quart
1/10 of 1%	15 "	to 1 "
1:500	2 teaspoonfuls	to 1 gallon
1:500	30 drops	to 1 quart
1/5 of 1%	30 "	to 1 "
1:200	5 teaspoonfuls	to 1 gallon
1:200	1¼ "	to 1 quart
½ of 1%	1¼ "	to 1 "
1:100 (1%)	2½ "	to 1 "
1:50 (2%)	5 "	to 1 "
1:25 (4%)	2½ tablespoonfuls	to 1 "
1:20 (5%)	3 "	to 1 "

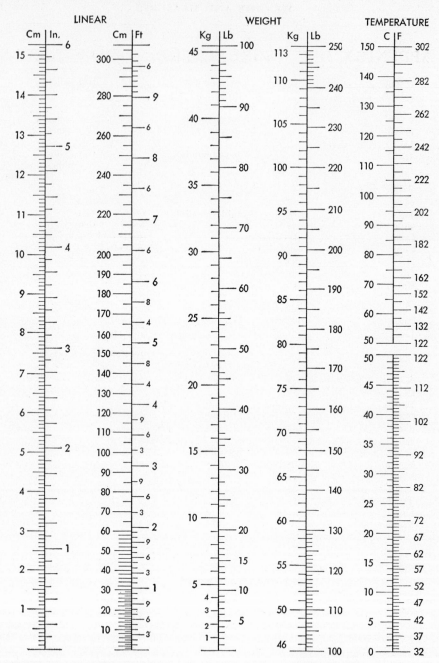

Figure 269. Comparative scales of measures, weights, and temperatures.

2.5 cm=1 in. 1 kg = 2.2 lb

To convert centigrade to Fahrenheit, multiply by 9/5 and add 32

To convert Fahrenheit to centigrade, subtract 32 and multiply by 5/9

APPENDIX III.   ABBREVIATIONS AND SYMBOLS

PREPARATIONS OF DRUGS

Abbreviation	Derivation	Meaning
Aq.	aqua	water
aq. dest.	aqua destillata	distilled water
Comp.	compositum	compound
Conf.	confectio	confection
D.	detur	give
Dil.	dilutus	dilute
Empl.	emplastrum	plaster
et	et	and
Fl.	fluidum	fluid
Inf.	infusum	infusion
Lin.	linimentum	liniment
Liq.	liquor	liquid
Lot.	lotio	lotion
Mist.	mistura	mixture
N.N.R.		new and nonofficial remedy
Ol.	oleum	oil
Pil.	pilula	pill
Pulv.	pulvis	a powder
S. fr.	spiritus frumenti	whisky
Sp.	spiritus	spirit
S. v. r.	spiritus vini rectificatus	alcohol
S. v. g.	spiritus vini gallici	brandy
Syr.	syrupus	syrup
Tinct.	tinctura	tincture
Troch.	trochiscum	lozenge
Ung.	unguentum	ointment
Vin.	vinum	wine

DOSAGE AND APPLICATION

Abbreviation	Derivation	Meaning
a̅a̅	ana	of each
Add.	adde	add to
Add. part. dol.	adde partem dolente	to the painful part
ad. lib.	ad libitum	as much as desired
C.	congius	gallon
C		centigrade
c̄	cum	with
cc		cubic centimeter
Cap.	capiat	let him take
Contin.	continuatur	let it be continued
Dim.	dimidius	one half
D. in p. aeq.	dividatur in partes aequales	divide in equal parts
Div.	dividatus	divide
Dur. dolor.	durante dolore	while the pain lasts
Ft.	fiat	let it or them be made
gm	gram	gram, grams
gr	granum, grana	grain, grains
gtt	gutta	a drop, drops
Garg.	gargarisma	a gargle
kg	kilogram	a thousand grams
L.	liter	a liter
lb	libra	pound
M.	misce	mix
m.	minimus	minim
ml	milliliter	a thousandth of a liter
N.b.	nota bene	note well
No.	numero	number
O	octarius	a pint
Part. vic.	partibus vicibus	in divided doses
Q.s.	quantum sufficit	as much as is sufficient
℞	recipe	take
s̄	sine	without
S. or Sig.	signa	give the following directions
S.o.s.	si opus sit	if necessary
Ss	semi	one half
Tsp	teaspoon	teaspoonful
Tbsp	tablespoon	tablespoonful
ℨ	drachma	dram
℥	uncia	ounce
℈	scrupulum	a scruple

TIME OF ADMINISTRATION

Abbreviation	Derivation	Meaning
A.c.	ante cibum	before meals
Alt. die.	alternis diebus	alternate days
Alt. hor	alternis horis	alternate hours
Alt. noct.	alternis noctes	alternate nights
A.M.		morning
B.i.d.	bis in die	twice a day
H.	hora	hour
H.d.	hora decubitus	at bedtime
H.s.	hora somni	at sleeping time
M. et N.	mane et nocte	morning and night
O.d.	omni die	daily
O.m.	omni mane	each morning
O.n.	omni nocte	each night
P.c.	post cibum	after meals
P.M.		afternoon
P.r.n.	pro re nata	when required
Q.h.	quaque hora	every hour
Q.2 h., Q.3 h. Q.4 h.		every two, three, or four hours
Q.i.d. or 4 i.d.	quater in die	four times a day
Stat.	statim	at once
T.i.d.	ter in die	three times a day

HOURS OF ADMINISTRATION

4 i.d.	8 A.M., 12 N., 4 P.M., 8 P.M.
Q.2 h.	6, 8, 10, 12, etc.
Q.3 h.	9, 12, 3, 6, etc.
Q.4 h.	8, 12, 4, etc.
Q.6 h.	6, 12, etc.
B.i.d.	10 A.M., 4 P.M.
T.i.d.	10 A.M., 3 P.M., and 6 P.M.
A.c.	½ hour before meals—6:30 A.M., 12:30 P.M., 4:30 P.M.
P.c.	8 A.M., 2 P.M., 6 P.M.
O.d.	10 A.M.
O.m.	6 A.M.
O.n.	8 P.M.

APPENDIX IV. NORMAL VALUES FOR BLOOD, STOOL, URINE, AND SPINAL FLUID*

NORMAL VALUES FOR TESTS OF KIDNEY FUNCTION

Phenosulfonphthalein	1 ml, intravenously	Urine	Total output	25 per cent or more in first 15 min; 40 per cent or more in 30 min; 55 per cent or more in 2 hr
Urea clearance	0	Blood and urine	Blood, 1 ml; urine, two 1-hr samples	75 to 125 per cent or normal

NORMAL VALUES FOR CLOTTING, BLEEDING, AND FORMED ELEMENTS OF BLOOD

Determination	Minimum quantity required (ml)	Normal value
Bleeding time	—	below $4\frac{1}{2}$ min
Coagulation time	5	4–12 min at 37° C
Sedimentation	4	Less than 0.35 mm/min
rate (two methods)	4	Less than .10 mm/hr
Hemoglobin	0.05	14–18 gm/100 ml, males; 12–16 gm/100 ml, females

* Reprinted by permission of the publishers from Thomas Hale Ham, editor, *A Syllabus of Laboratory Examinations in Clinical Diagnosis*. Cambridge, Mass.: Harvard University Press, Coypright, 1950, by The President and Fellows of Harvard College.

NORMAL VALUES FOR BLOOD, PLASMA, AND SERUM

Determination	Material analyzed	Minimum quantity required (ml)	Normal value
Amino acids (manometric ninhydrin method)	Plasma	2	3.4–5.5 mg/100 ml
Amylase	Serum	2	15–35 units/100 ml
Ascorbic acid (vitamin C)	Plasma	0.5	0.4–1.0 mg/100 ml (fasting)
Calcium	Serum	2	9.0–10.5 mg/100 ml*
Carbon dioxide (content)	Serum	0.5	26–28 meq/L†
Chloride	Serum	0.5	100–106 meq/L
Cholesterol	Serum	0.5	150–270 mg/100 ml
Cholesterol esters	Serum	0.5	60% of total cholesterol
Glucose	Blood	0.1	70–100 mg/100 ml (fasting)
Hemoglobin	Blood	0.05	12–18 gm/100 ml
Iodine, protein bound (thyroid hormone)	Serum	4	4–8 µg/100 ml
Magnesium	Serum	2	1–2 meq/L
Nonprotein nitrogen	Serum	0.5	15–35 mg/100 ml
Oxygen:			
capacity	Blood	3	19–22 vol. per cent
arterial content	Blood	3	18–21 vol. per cent
arterial percentage saturation	Blood	3	94–96 per cent
venous content	Blood	3	10–16 vol. per cent
pH (reaction)	Serum	0.2	7.35–7.45
Phosphatase, acid	Serum	1	0.5–2.0 units/100 ml
Phosphatase, alkaline	Serum	0.5	2.0–4.5 units/100 ml‡
Phosphorus, inorganic	Serum	0.2	3.0–4.5 mg/100 ml§
Potassium	Serum	3–4	3.5–5.0 meq/L
Protein			
total (macro)	Serum	0.5	6.5–8.0 gm/100 ml
(micro)	Serum	0.05	6.5–8.0 gm/100 ml
albumin	Serum	0.5	4.5–5.5 gm/100 ml
globulin	Serum	0.5	1.5–3.0 gm/100 ml
Prothrombin, clotting time	Plasma	0.3	By control plasmas
Pyruvic acid	Blood	2	0.7–1.2 mg/100 ml
Sodium	Serum	0.5	136–145 meq/L
Urea nitrogen	Serum	1	10–28 mg/100 ml
Uric acid	Serum	1	3–5 mg/100 ml

* Since the total serum calcium concentration is dependent on the serum protein concentration, evaluation of the significance of a serum calcium value requires a serum protein determination.

† Values in infants and children may be from 20–26 meq/L. Milliequivalents per liter equal volumes per cent divided by 2.2. The milliequivalent total CO_2 minus 1.3 is usually about equal to the HCO_3 expressed as milliequivalents per liter.

‡ The value parallels the rate of growth, diminishing from approximately 14 units/100 ml in infancy to 5 units/100 ml in adolescence and thereafter being maintained at approximately 3.5 units/100 ml.

§ In newborn infants values may be as high as 6 mg/100 ml, diminishing during the first year; in childhood they approach the normal adult value of 3.5 mg/100 ml.

NORMAL VALUES FOR STOOL

Determination	Minimum quantity required (ml)	Normal value
Stool fat	Representative sample	Less than 30 per cent dry weight

NORMAL VALUES FOR URINE

Determination	Minimum quantity required (ml)	Normal value
Albumin (quantitative)	10	0
Creatine	24-hr sample	Less than 100 mg/24*
Creatinine	24-hr sample	15–25 mg/Kg†
Diastase	2	Dilution of 1:4 to 1:16
Follicle-stimulating hormone	24-hr sample	Before puberty, less than 6.5 mouse units/24 hr; after menopause 104–600 mouse units/24 hr
Sugar		
total (quantitative)	5	0
total (roughly quantitative)	0.5	0
fermentable	1	0
fructose	1	0
galactose or lactose	6	0
osazone, differentiation of	5	0

* Per kilogram of body weight, the excretion is higher in women and children than in men, and still higher in infants.

† The value depends on the ratio of muscle to fat in the body mass of the patient. The higher the ratio the greater the creatinine excretion per kilogram of total body weight. Below this ratio [which] is low in infants, the excretion per kilogram is low.

NORMAL VALUES FOR SPINAL FLUID

Determination	Minimum quantity required (ml)	Normal value
Initial pressure	—	70–180 mm/water
Cell count	0.2	0–5 mononuclear cells (lymphocytes/mm)
Chloride	2	120–130 meq/L
Protein	0.6	15–45 mg/100 ml
Glucose	1	50–75 mg/100 ml
Colloidal gold	0.1	0000000000

APPENDIX V. EMERGENCY FIRST-AID ITEMS FOR A FAMILY OF FOUR PERSONS OR LESS*†

FIRST AID ITEM	QUANTITY	SUBSTITUTE	USE
1. *Antiseptic Solution* Benzalkonium Chloride Solution. 1 to 1000 parts of water.	3 to 6 oz. bottle	Organic mercurial compounds in water. Drug stores have them under several trade names.	*For open wounds, scratches and cuts. Not for burns.*
2. *Aromatic Spirits of Ammonia*	1 to 2 oz. bottle	None	*For faintness,* adult dose ½ teaspoonful in cup of water; children 5 to 10 drops in ½ glass of water. As smelling salts hold bottle under nose.
3. *Table Salt*	1 box	Sodium chloride tablet, 10 grains.	*For shock*—dissolve 1 teaspoonful salt and ½ teaspoonful baking soda in 1 qt. water. Have patient drink as much as he will. Don't give to unconscious person or semiconscious person. If using substitutes dissolve six 10-gr. sodium chloride tablets and six 5-gr. sodium bicarbonate (or sodium citrate) tablets in 1 qt. water.
4. *Baking Soda*	8 to 10 oz. box	Sodium bicarbonate or sodium citrate tablets, 5 grains	*For some slight protection against nerve gas*—dissolve 4 teaspoonfuls of baking soda in 1 qt. water. Wash parts of body exposed to nerve gas with it or saturate cloth and place over face as gas mask.
5. *Triangular Bandage* compressed, 37 x 37 x 52 in., folded, with 2 safety pins.	4 bandages	Muslin or other strong material. Fold to exact dimensions. Wrap each bandage and 2 safety pins separately in paper.	*For a sling; as a covering; for a dressing.*

* Federal Civil Defense Administration: *Emergency Action to Save Lives,* Publication PA–5. US Government Printing Office, Washington, D.C., 1951.
† These emergency first-aid items are assembled and then wrapped in a moistureproof covering that is placed in an easily carried box. A copy of the chart should be pasted inside the box cover; the box is then placed in the shelter area prepared.

1197

APPENDIX V. EMERGENCY FIRST-AID ITEMS FOR A FAMILY OF FOUR PERSONS OR LESS (Cont.)

FIRST AID ITEM	QUANTITY	SUBSTITUTE	USE
6. Large Bath Towels	2	None	For bandages or dressings: Old soft towels and sheets are best. Use as bandages or dressings. Cut in sizes necessary to cover wounds. Towels are burn dressings. Place over burns and fasten with triangular bandage or strips of sheet. Towels and sheets should be laundered, ironed, and packaged in heavy paper. Relaunder every 3 months.
7. Small Bath Towels	2	None	
8. Bed Sheet	1	None	
9. Medium First Aid Dressing 8 in. by 7½ in., folded, sterile with gauze enclosed cotton pads. Packaged with muslin bandage and 4 safety pins.	2	Must be bought	For open wounds or for dry dressings for burns. These are packaged sterile. Don't try to make your own.
10. Small First Aid Dressing 4 in. by 7 in., folded, sterile with gauze enclosed cotton pads and gauze bandage.	2	Must be bought	
11. Paper Drinking Cups	25 to 50	Envelope or cardboard type.	For administering stimulants and liquids.
12. Eye Drops, Castor Oil	½ to 1 oz. bottle with dropper	Bland eye drops sold by druggists under various trade names.	For eyes irritated by dust, smoke or fumes. Use 2 drops in each eye. Apply cold compresses every 20 minutes if possible.
13. Flashlight	1	Must be bought	Electric lights may go out. Wrap batteries in moisture proof covering. Don't keep in flashlight.
14. Safety Pins, 1½ in. long	15	None	For holding bandages in place.

Item	Quantity	Description	Use
15. *Razor Blades, Single Edge*	3	Sharp knife or scissors	*For cutting bandages and dressings, or for removing clothing from injured part.*
16. *Toilet Soap*	1 bar	Any mild soap	*For cleansing skin.*
17. *Splints, Plastic, Wooden,* ⅛ to ¼ in. thick, 3½ in. wide by 12 to 15 in. long.	12	A 40-page newspaper folded to dimensions, pieces of orange crate sidings, or shingles cut to size.	*For splinting broken arms or legs.*
18. *Tongue Blades, Wooden*	12	Shingles, pieces of orange crate, or other light wood cut to approximately 1½" x 6".	*For splinting broken fingers or other small bones and for stirring solutions.*
19. *Water Purification Tablets*	Bottle of 100	Iodine tablets; Chlorine tablets; Chlorine capsules sold under various trade names	*For purifying water when it can't be boiled, but tap water officially declared radioactive must not be used for any purpose.*
20. *Measuring Spoons*	1 set	Cheap plastic or metal	*For measuring or stirring solutions.*

1199

APPENDIX VI. THE LIQUID THERAPEUTIC DIET

Evaluation Chart (Speas-Newland)*

(Amounts given are for a sedentary male.)

FOOD†	AMOUNT	CALORIES	PROTEIN GM.	CARBOHY-DRATE, GM.	FAT GM.	CALCIUM MG.	PHOSPHORUS MG.	IRON MG.	VIT. A I.U.	THIAMIN MG.	RIBOFLAVIN MG.	NIACIN MG.	VIT. C MG.	VIT. D I.U.
Orange Juice	12 oz.	150	2.7	33.2	0.6	99	69	1.20	570	.24	.09	.60	147	
Eggs	3 T.	213	17.4	0.6	15.6	72	282	3.60	1,539	.15	.45	.45		
Karo, dark‡	2 T.	118		29.6		24	4	1.20				.08		
Sugar	2 T.	104		26.0										
Milk	20 oz.	423	21.5	30.0	24.0	723	570	.43	980	.25	1.05	.50	5	
Cream 20%	14 oz.	874	12.1	16.8	84.0	408	324	.25	3,484	.13	.60	.35	4	
Veg. (baby)‡	4¾ oz.	81	6.7	11.9	0.7	14	114	2.38	1,758	.18	.16		14	
Meat (baby)§	3½ oz.	103	15.2		4.1	9	115	2.10		.02	.22	3.12		
Tomato Juice	8 oz.	46	2.0	8.6	0.4	14	30	.80	2,100	.10	.06	1.40	32	
Rolled Oats	1 T.	24	0.9	4.1	0.4	3	22	.32		.03	.01	0.06		
S. Milk (dry)	4 T.	128	12.8	18.8	0.4	468	372	.20	16	.12	.72	0.4	4	
Homocebrin	5 cc.								3,000	1.00	1.2	7.37	60	1,000
Total		2,264	91.3	179.6	130.2	1,834	1,902	12.48	13,447	2.22	4.56	13.88	266	1,000
Recommended daily allowance NRC '48		2,400	70			1,000	1,500	12	5,000	1.2	1.8	12	75	400–800

* Speas, C. J.: "The Liquid Therapeutic Diet," *J. Tennessee M. J.*, 43:321, (Sept.) 1950.

† Food values from: Federal Security Agency, US Public Health Service: *Food Value Tables for Calculation of Diet Records* except ‡ items from Bowes and Church: *Food Values of Portions Commonly Used*, and § Swift and Co.

1200

Speas-Newland Liquid Diet*

Feeding Time	Feeding
6 A.M.	Beat together 6 ounces orange juice, 1 egg, 1 tablespoon Karo syrup.
8 A.M.	6 ounces milk, 4 ounces light cream, 1 tablespoon dried skim milk, mixed.
10 A.M.	Cereal gruel, made with 1 cup milk, 1 tablespoon of oatmeal, Pablum or enriched cream of wheat, 1 tablespoon dried skim milk, thoroughly cooked and strained with 1 tablespoon of sugar added.
12 NOON	Creamed soup, made with 5 ounces of light cream, 1 tablespoon dried skim milk, 3 ounces of strained vegetables (the 3 to 4 ounce prepared cans or jars of strained baby vegetables or meats may be used), 1 can or jar to a serving.
2 P.M.	Beat together 6 ounces orange juice, 1 egg, 1 tablesoon Karo syrup.
4 P.M.	Creamed soup, made with 5 ounces of light cream, 1 tablespoon dried skim milk, 3 ounces of strained vegetables (the 3 to 4 ounce prepared cans or jars of strained baby vegetables or meats may be used), 1 can or jar to a serving.
6 P.M.	8 ounces of tomato or orange juice.
8 P.M.	Beat together 6 ounces milk, 1 egg, remainder of the 4 ounces of dried skim milk, 1 tablespoon sugar. (Take vitamin preparation with this feeding.)

NOTE: The 6 A.M. and 8 A.M. feedings may both be taken at 8 A.M. for convenience if desired. It is necessary to be fed more often on a liquid diet. Three feedings a day are not enough. The patient feels overfed or hungry unless fed every two hours. If the patient is working, several feedings may be mixed together and placed in thermos bottles and taken to work. Salt feedings to taste. Malt, vanilla and other flavors may be used. It is not necessary to add the dried skim milk as recommended above; it may be added in greater amounts to any feeding as long as 4 ounces a day are consumed. The amount of dried skim milk may be increased or decreased as the doctor sees fit.

* Speas, C. J.: "The Liquid Therapeutic Diet," *J. Tennessee M. J.*, **43**:321, (Sept.) 1950.

GLOSSARY

MEDICAL TRADE-MARKED NAME*	NONPROPRIETARY NAME	USE(S)
Adrenalin(e)	epinephrine	Control of hemorrhage; relief of congestion of nasal mucosa; limitation of absorption of local anesthetics (thus prolonging duration, decreasing amount of anesthetic needed, and lessening danger of systemic toxicity); cardiac stimulation; control of bronchial spasm; control of nitritoid crisis
Amigen	an amino acid for intravenous use	Parenteral alimentation for maintenance of nitrogen balance
Amphojel	suspension of aluminum hydroxide	Gastric antacid, particularly indicated in treatment of hyperchlorhydria and peptic ulcer; treatment of intestinal toxemia because of adsorbent and demulcent properties; treatment of nephrolithiasis (when stones are composed of phosphate salt)
Amytal sodium	amobarbital	Hypnotic of intermediate duration; sedative
Argyrol	mild silver protein	Antiseptic applied to mucous membrane (upper respiratory infections, conjunctivitis, cystitis)
Atabrine	quinacrine	Antimalarial; control of some other parasitic infections
Aureomycin	chlortetracycline	Antibiotic for rickettsial, viral, and bacterial diseases
Avertin	tribrom(o)ethanol	Basal anesthetic; given by rectum
Basaljel	suspension of aluminum carbonate	Gastric antacid, particularly indicated for binding phosphate
Benadryl	diphenhydramine	Antihistaminic drug, particularly indicated for allergy diseases, the common cold, motion sickness, and Parkinson's disease
Benzedrine sulfate	amphetamine sulfate	Central nervous system stimulant; vasoconstrictor of mucosa of upper respiratory tract; mydriatic

* All such trade-marked names are indicated by an initial capital letter.

MEDICAL TRADE-MARKED NAME	NONPROPRIETARY NAME	USE(S)
Bromsulphalein	sulfobromophthalein	Dye for determination of liver function
Butesin	butamben	Local anesthetic with antiseptic action
Ceepryn	cetyl pyridinium chloride	Bactericide; nonirritating detergent
Decholin	sodium dehydrocholate	Rapid intravenous administration has been employed to measure circulation time; test usually follows that which determines venous pressure
Demerol	meperidine	Narcotic, particularly indicated for relief of pain, preanesthetic medication, relief of spasm, and during labor
Diaparene	methylbenzethonium	Bactericide, particularly indicated against *Bacillus ammoniagenes*
Dicumarol	bishydroxycoumarin	Anticoagulant used in prophylaxis and therapy of thromboembolic diseases
Divinyl ether	**vinyl ether**	General anesthetic, particularly indicated for minor operations of short duration when rapid induction and recovery are desired
Divinyl oxide	vinyl ether	*See* Divinyl ether (vinyl ether)
Doryl	carbachol	Parasympathomimetic agent, particularly indicated for peripheral vascular disease and urinary retention
Dramamine	dimenhydrinate	Treatment of motion sickness
Ethylene oxide	vinyl ether	*See* Divinyl ether (vinyl ether)
Evipal	hexobarbital	Ultrashort-acting hypnotic; sedative
Flaxedil	gallamine	Adjuvant agent in anesthesia for obtaining adequate skeletal muscle relaxation; prevention of fractures during electroshock seizure therapy; control of convulsions in tetanus
Holocaine	phenacaine	Local anesthetic limited to topical application—especially to the eye
Iso-Iodeikon	iodophthalein	Dye for x-ray examination of gallbladder
Lipiodol	iodized oil (such as poppy seed)	Contrast medium for x-ray examination of the lungs
Mapharsen	oxophenarsine	Treponemicide and spirocheticide, particularly indicated for treatment of syphilis, yaws, relapsing fever, trypanosomiasis, amebiasis
Mercuhydrin	meralluride	Mercurial diuretic, particularly indicated for treatment of cardiac edema

MEDICAL TRADE-MARKED NAME	NONPROPRIETARY NAME	USE(S)
Mercurochrome	merbromin	Bacteriostatic agent for "disinfection" of skin, mucous membranes, and wounds
Merthiolate	sodium ethyl mercurithio-salicylate	All-purpose antiseptic
Metaphen	nitromersol	Antiseptic for cutaneous and mucosal surfaces; disinfectant for instruments
Metycaine	piperocaine	Local anesthetic
Myanesin	mephenesin	Sketetal muscle relaxant, particularly indicated as adjuvant for general anesthesia
Nembutal	pentobarbital	Short-acting hypnotic; sedative
Neo-synephrine	phenylephrine	Sympathomimetic agent; vasoconstrictor agent; mydriatic
Novocain(e)	procaine	Local anesthetic
Nupercaine hydrochloride	dibucaine hydrochloride	Local anesthetic (with high toxicity)
Paludrine (British name)	chlor(o)guanide	Antimalarial
Pantopaque	ethyl iodophenylundecylate	Radiopaque material designed especially for myelography
Parenamine	an amino acid for intravenous use	Parenteral alimentation for maintenance of nitrogen balance
Pentothal	thiopental	Ultrashort-acting hypnotic; sedative
Phemerol	benzethonium	Germicide for metallic instruments and rubber articles; antiseptic for skin, tissues, and mucous membranes
Pitocin	oxytocin	Inducement of labor at term; control of post-partum hemorrhage; inducement of normal involution of uterus during puerperium; inducement of uterine contraction after Cesarean section
Pitressin	vasopressin	Antidiuretic, particularly indicated for relief of intestinal paresis and distention, diabetes insipidus of pituitary origin, determination of concentrating capacity of kidney, and intravenous urography
Pontocaine	tetracaine	All-purpose local anesthetic
Prostigmin	neostigmine	Parasympathomimetic agent, particularly indicated for relief of abdominal distention, prevention and treatment of atony of detrusor muscle of urinary bladder, and restoration of muscle power in myasthenia gravis

MEDICAL TRADE-MARKED NAME	NONPROPRIETARY NAME	USE(S)
Protargol	protein silver	Antiseptic for application to mucous membranes, particularly indicated for treatment of gonococcal conjunctivitis and gonorrhea
Resochin (German name)	chloroquine	Antimalarial
Seconal	secobarbital	Short-acting hypnotic; sedative
Spinocain	10 per cent solution of procaine	Local anesthetic
surgical Pitressin	surgical vasopressin	Relief of postoperative abdominal distention
Surital	thiamylal	Hypnotic; sedative
Terramycin	oxytetracycline	Antibiotic for rickettsial, viral, and bacterial diseases
Thioethamyl	amobarbital	Hypnotic; sedative
Urecholine	bethanechol	Relief of post-partum and neurogenic urinary retention, gastric retention after vagotomy, and postoperative abdominal distention
Urotropin	methenamine	Urinary antiseptic
Veronal	barbital	Long-acting hypnotic; sedative
Vinethene	vinyl ether	*See* Divinyl ether (vinyl ether)
Zephiran	benzalkonium	All-purpose bactericide; detergent

INDEX

1207